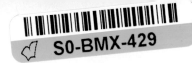

MANUAL OF

Clinical Behavioral Medicine
for Dogs and Cats

About the Author

Dr. Karen L. Overall holds BA, MA, and VMD degrees from the University of Pennsylvania and a PhD degree from the University of Wisconsin-Madison. She did her residency training in veterinary behavioral medicine at the University of Pennsylvania, and is a Diplomate of the American College of Veterinary Behaviorists (DACVB). Dr. Overall is also certified by the Animal Behavior Society as an Applied Animal Behaviorist (CAAB). She has served for more than 20 years on the faculties of both the veterinary and medical schools at the University of Pennsylvania where she has taught undergraduates, graduate students, and professional students with great joy and to rave reviews, and she ran the Behavior Clinic at Penn Vet for more than a dozen years.

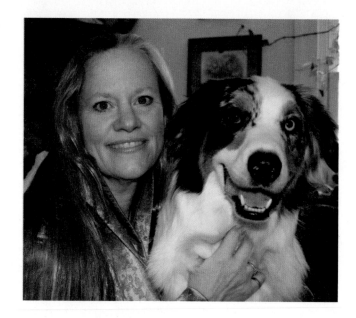

Dr. Overall has given hundreds of national and international presentations and short courses and is the author of over 100 scholarly publications, dozens of textbook chapters, and the text *Clinical Behavioral Medicine for Small Animals* (1997). She is the editor-in-chief for *Journal of Veterinary Behavior: Clinical Applications and Research* (Elsevier). Dr. Overall has been named the North American Veterinary Conference (NAVC) Small Animal Speaker of the Year, has been awarded the Cat Writer's Association Certificate of Excellence for "The Social Cat" column in *Cat Fancy* magazine, and in 2010 was named one of the *Bark's* 100 Best and Brightest—*Bark* magazine's list of the 100 most influential people in the dog world over the past 25 years.

Dr. Overall serves and has served on numerous governmental committees focused on canine health and behavior, including the Commonwealth of Pennsylvania's Canine Health Board, to which she was appointed by former PA Governor Rendell, and the U.S. Department of Defense's Blue Ribbon panel on canine–post-traumatic stress disorder (C-PTSD). She frequently consults with governments locally, nationally, and internationally about scientific, legal and welfare issues of pet dogs and behavioral assessment, welfare, and performance issues pertaining to working dogs, in which capacity she co-chaired the U.S. government's FBI Scientific Working Group on Dogs and Orthogonal Detection Methods (SWGDOG) for 7 years.

Dr. Overall's research focuses on neurobehavioral genetics of dogs, the development of normal and abnormal behaviors and how we assess behavior, especially as concerns working dogs. Her favorite collaborator is still her husband, Dr. Art Dunham, who understands how important it is to her to have a life of the mind and who shares her interests in political activism, art, classical music, and the value of travel for learning about languages, cultures, food, wine, and friendship. Having decided that the carrying capacity of their canine household was four dogs, they continue to live with four much loved, rescue Australian shepherds in a shifting array necessitated by the unfortunate disparities between human and canine demographics.

MANUAL OF
Clinical Behavioral
Medicine
for Dogs and Cats

Karen L. Overall, MA, VMD, PhD, DACVB, CAAB

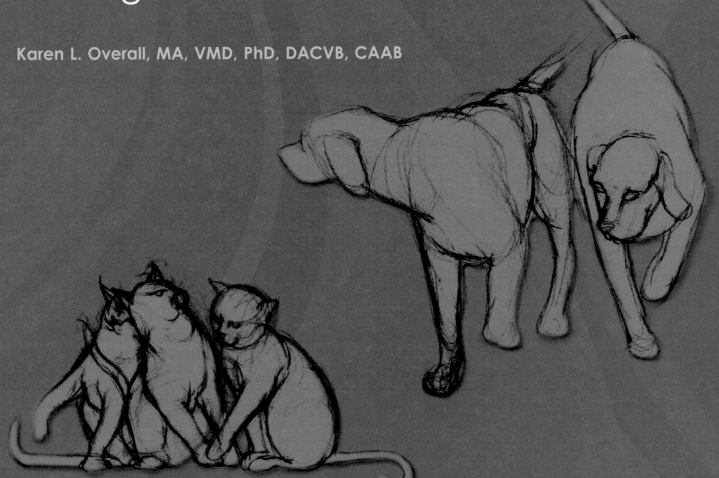

ELSEVIER
MOSBY

Elsevier
3251 Riverport Lane
St. Louis, MO 63043

MANUAL OF CLINICAL BEHAVIORAL MEDICINE FOR
DOGS AND CATS

ISBN: 978-0-323-00890-7

Copyright © 2013 by Mosby, an imprint of Elsevier Inc.

Notices

ISBN: 978-0-323-00890-7

Vice President and Publisher: Linda Duncan
Content Strategy Director: Penny Rudolph
Content Development Specialist: Brandi Graham
Publishing Services Manager: Catherine Jackson
Senior Project Manager: Carol O'Connell
Designer: Margaret Reid
Cover Photo: A.E. Dunham

Printed in Canada

Last digit is the print number: 9 8 7 6 5 4 3 2 1

 Working together
to grow libraries in
developing countries

www.elsevier.com • www.bookaid.org

Dedication

This text is dedicated to my dogs—all Australian shepherds, save one, who are always constrained by their circumstances to be both teacher and student—and to my husband. I love them all so much.

◇◇◇◇

- *For Maggie, smart, astute, and generous. Maggie possessed selfless courage. Everyone who met Maggie loved her, and she never met a human or another animal with whom she would not share. She was Tess's eyes and my constant companion. Maggie taught me to love unconditionally.*

◇◇◇◇

- *For troubled Tess, blind by 5 weeks and taken home at 8.5 weeks, who taught me about struggle, recovery, and forgiveness. Tessie had toughness but infinite sweetness, too, and far from being a throw-away at 5 weeks, she died in her sleep 1 month short of 15 years.*

◇◇◇◇

- *For feisty Little Bit, the only non-Aussie in the group, who showed me that sometimes pure orneriness has a place and that perseverance can make all the difference. Adopted at 13 years into a home of Aussies, she held her own among the big dogs, often barking back-up for them. She was cared for in her final illness at 22 years by the new dog, Flash. She captured all of our hearts.*

◇◇◇◇

- *For sweet Emma, who taught me that you can couple true devotion with rugged independence. We were inseparable, and when I could not be safely left alone she and Flash ensured that I never was.*

◇◇◇◇

- *For the indomitable Flash, my best and most critical teacher, who taught me how to heal, and how to help dogs to heal. Flash's lessons are on every page of this text, and it is from him I truly learned about mental suffering in animals and its redress. Flash convinced me of the power of redemption. Surely the most remarkable dog I have ever known, and who, with Emma, when I could not trust myself, ensured that I need not carry that burden. I miss him every second of every day, but his lessons endure and continue to inform the care of suffering animals and their distressed people.*

- *For Toby, who has taught me that interdependence can be more than okay but fun, and who remembers to wake up every day happy and full of wonder. Beauty and brilliance are seldom so well matched. He is the Rover to my Red, the Snowy to my Tintin, the Gromit to my Wallace, the Polo to my Marco, and he is sitting next to me as I write this. Watching him joyously learn and teach is to daily trace the footprints and heartbeats of Emma and Flash.*

◇◇◇◇

- *For Linus, the puppy mill rescue, who taught me the importance of not limiting one's expectations, and why we should never, ever give up. The last dog Flash helped raise, and the first dog for whom Toby apprenticed, Linus daily insists that life and dogs can and should be very, very funny, and always worthy of extended vocal commentary. Little Leaky Loopy Linus became Linus, Prince Ling, chorus master of the group howl.*

◇◇◇◇

- *For my handsome boy, Picasso, the boy who was "too much dog for a family with kids," and who came into a household awash in the deep sadness left by Flash's death. Pic pushed past despair to grow into and master Flash's jobs. He reminds me daily of the value of freedom and exploration, and that to touch is to live and love.*

◇◇◇◇

- *For Miss Buns/Bunny, who came to us at an advanced age, arthritic, painful, ill-kept, voiceless, thin, and fearful, who taught me that we can leave the pain behind to run on the beach while regaining our voices. Bunny was pure sweetness and adored by the boys. Cared for at the end by Pic and Linus, the death of this very quiet, little, old dog sucked all the oxygen from the atmosphere.*

◇◇◇◇

- *For the young, lovely, and quite fragile Missy Rose, a true West Texas cow dog and our newest family member, who continues to recover from earlier abuse and neglect to become a razzmatazz queen. She teaches me daily to remember to jump for joy.*

◇◇◇◇

- *And, finally, for my husband, Art Dunham, who taught me the true meaning of the words: for better, for worse, for richer, for poorer, in sickness, and in health.*

Preface

WHY AND HOW TO USE THIS BOOK

I want nothing less than to completely change how we practice veterinary medicine so that veterinarians and their staff are the driving force advocating for and enhancing patient welfare and for meeting the patient's cognitive and mental health needs. We must address the single most important aspect of our patients' well-being—their behavioral needs—using the same rigor and scientific approach that we use to vaccinate patients or treat them for diabetes.

Behavior is the core around which all other aspects of and specialties in veterinary medicine revolve, and it is the determining factor for which kind and how much veterinary care clients seek and patients receive. *Behavioral change* is how clients recognize that their dog or cat is physically ill and needs veterinary care, and yet most veterinarians are not sufficiently comfortable with their knowledge base in veterinary behavioral medicine to deliver any kind of behavioral care.

One of the reasons for this text is to help ensure every member of the veterinary team gains some comfort level with veterinary behavioral medicine, and that they do so using scientifically based findings as part of evidence-based medicine. By putting the behavioral needs of our patients first, we will also meet our own intellectual, physical, and emotional needs in a way that the modern routine practice of veterinary medicine may not currently permit.

At some point in their lives most people who became veterinarians realized that they liked to watch animals. I fear that we have forgotten how interesting watching cats and dogs can be and, as a result, in a sincere effort to deliver the most modern veterinary medical care, we have left from our business, teaching, and research models *the concept of the well-being of our patients*. I firmly believe that if we completely change our emphasis—and first focus on understanding our patients' behaviors and meeting their needs—we shall find ourselves practicing more advanced, state-of-the-art care, we will experience fewer injuries and less burn-out, and we will make a humane difference in our communities, in the lives of our patients, and in the lives of the humans who love the animals with whose care we are charged and entrusted.

This manual will help the practitioner to develop a hands-on, practical approach for meeting the goal of practicing veterinary medicine in a behavior-centered manner. I believe that veterinarians can be a force for good and can consciously participate in effecting cultural change that can address recycled, abandoned, and throw-away pets, and the abuse, neglect, entrapment, and fear that is the burden of far too many dogs and cats. To do this, we must make an effort to understand the dog or cat from the evolutionary/ethological perspective of a dog or cat in a way that addresses their cognitive, social, and mental health needs. If we do this, we will engage in a partnership with our patients based on shared and clear communication.

For such an approach to succeed, we must understand that all of our interactions with animals are based on the animal's ability to translate what we are signaling to them into a language or application that is meaningful to them. The animal then has to translate the resultant response back into signals that we, as humans, can understand. This is the rule for our interactions with our patients, and it is the rule for studies of the ability to "learn language" in primates and dogs (Aust et al., 2008; Conway and Christiansen, 2001; Hauser et al., 2001; Herman et al., 1984; Kaminski et al., 2004; Taglialatela et al., 2008; Petkov and Taglialatela, 2010; Pilley and Reid, 2011).

Understanding members of our own species can be difficult. Given the translations needed, understanding another species can mean that a lot goes wrong or is missed. *This Manual is intended to: (1) decrease the number of interactions that go wrong with your patients, (2) humanely address the needs of dogs and cats whose behaviors are contributing to damaging their relationships with humans and other animals, and (3) help veterinarians to treat patients who are experiencing painful mental distress, and the behavioral, social, and emotional fallout from such mental distress.*

Unfortunately, as was true when I wrote my first text 15 years before this one, veterinary schools have yet to make the commitment needed to encourage research in and teaching of veterinary behavioral medicine. Fewer than a dozen schools world-wide have dedicated, combined clinical, didactic, *and* active research programs in the field. I include research here because so few veterinary schools invest in those who can do rigorous research in this field, so progress using data-driven findings is slow. Yet the most common problems faced by veterinarians in general, community, and shelter medicine practice remain those associated with behavioral issues.

- The mildly annoying behaviors of the sweet but goofy dog who jumps on people become a lethal issue for this dog when his people hit hard economic times and have to move from a house to an apartment.
- The cat who is hit by a car is killed, not by the injury, but because the cost of fixing the injury is viewed through the lens of the annoyance his people feel at his lack of litterbox use.

Whether they are primary—the dog destroys the house when left alone—or secondary—the cat needs expensive care *and* shreds the furniture—behavioral problems affecting our patients and problematic behaviors for clients result in the death or relinquishment of more dogs and cats than do neoplasia, cardiac, and endocrine disease combined (Marston et al., 2004, 2005; Miller et al., 1996; Patronek et al., 1996; Salman et al., 1998; Scarlett et al., 1999; Salman et al., 2000; Shore et al., 2003; Shore, 2005). A quick review of reasons for relinquishment in Melbourne shelters (Marston et al., 2005) (Table 1) shows that even the "owner-related" reasons are influenced by aspects of canine behavior.

Dead dogs and cats do not eat pet food, do not need annual vaccinations, and never have to worry about fleas and ticks and the diseases they carry. Given that most behavioral problems develop or become fully pronounced during social maturity (~1-4 years of age if we consider both cats and dogs), it's a safe guess that dogs and cats euthanized or relinquished for behavioral reasons never use any complex veterinary services: they don't live long enough to need treatment for neoplasia or endocrine disease, to warrant a consult with a cardiologist, or to benefit from physical rehabilitation or specialized nutritional care. *The biggest untapped fiscal and intellectual "growth market" in veterinary medicine is in the pets lost from the veterinary population because of behavioral concerns.*

At some point in their lives, most pets display behaviors that would result in their death or relinquishment, were they in some other household (see Figure 1). Puppies have been known to be killed or seriously injured because of the way they were "disciplined" during housetraining. As veterinarians we view such stories as extreme examples of abuse, but we relentlessly tolerate "corrective" and often coercive training regimens administered by untrained "professionals" (AVSAB Dominance Position Statement: www.avsabonline.org/avsabonline/images/stories/Position_Statements/dominance%20statement.pdf and the Dog Welfare Campaign position statement: www.dogwelfarecampaign.org/why-not-dominance.php). Rather than collaborating with well-schooled and educated, humane trainers, we often simply abdicate any veterinary role in our patients' behaviors because we lack the expertise to intervene (Brammeier et al., 2006; www.

TABLE 1

Reasons Provided for Relinquishment of Dogs in Three Melbourne, Australia, Shelters (in Rank Order)

Owner-Related Reasons	Dog Behavioral Reasons
Accommodation/moving	Escapes
Owner health/personal reasons*	Hyperactive/too boisterous
Too much work/effort/ time*	Other (mouthing, housetraining, dog too demanding)
Abandoned	
Owner commitment*	
Financial	Barking
Did not choose dog*	Predatory behavior
Welfare issues*	Uncontrollable
Mismatch *	Destructive
Issues with children*	Digs
Wrong decision*	Separation anxiety
Not fitting in with family*	
Unrealistic expectations*	

Every issue with an asterisk (*) in the owner-related column has a direct link to dog behavior; the remainder could have a link. (Data from Marston et al., 2005.)

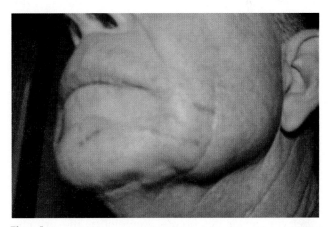

Fig. 1 The damage done by the paw of an 11-month-old Australian shepherd on his first night in his new home. He was originally relinquished to a rescue center because he was "too much dog for a family with kids."

avsabonline.org/avsabonline/images/stories/Position_Statements/how%20to%20choose%20a%20trainer.pdf).

Fortunately, we can change. If we wish to deliver the best and most modern care possible to our patients, *we must stop feeding into a cycle where pets are disposable.* We can and must lay the groundwork for an ongoing relationship that revolves around understanding and meeting the patient's cognitive, behavioral and social needs. We can most effectively establish this basis during our first few visits with the patient. These first few visits are the times when we will most profit by learning what the clients actually know about their dog or cat, and where more or better information can help.

In some practices, this need can be met by making licensed veterinary technicians responsible for behavioral assessment using standardized questionnaires on which they can then base humane and behavioral education (www.svbt.org). In other practices, extended appointment times with the veterinarians may be more appropriate. Some practices work with schooled, certified, and tested trainers to provide weekly question and answer sessions for owners of new or young animals (www.petprofessionalguild.com).

However we do it, we can and must work with our clients to ensure that we are their source for data-based information and advice about behavioral concerns, their pet's well-being, and how those two issues can affect the development of and our ability to treat medical conditions. *The time to address the importance of being able to handle a cat safely to get a blood sample is not when that cat is fractious and ill; it's when the cat is young and fun and happy to learn how to offer body parts for needle sticks.*

We need to be honest about the unwanted animal epidemic. Good data exist for the number of animals euthanized in many (but not most) shelters because of their behaviors; *no* equivalent data exist for private practices. This divide has allowed the veterinary community to view dogs and cats in the shelter system as divorced from the population of pets seen in primary practice. In fact, we may be worsening behavioral problems by this divide and by our inability to address problems in our patient population in a timely manner and as they develop. *If the veterinary staff does not ask about behavioral problems or can offer no tangible, on-the-spot advice for understanding, managing, or treating behavioral issues, we drive behavioral concerns underground* (Roshier and McBride, 2012a, 2012b).

We should let go of the myth that pets with behavior problems are best euthanized because there are plenty of "nice" pets in shelters who are problem-free and will otherwise never get homes. Remember, the primary reason pets are relinquished to shelters usually has something to do with their behavior, even if, as suggested by Marston (2005), the pets' behaviors may simply be a mismatch to those of the human household. Relinquishment of pets is behaviorally traumatic for them. *We need to change the illusion that well-behaved pets are something you simply get, into the reality that well-behaved and happy pets are something that we can all help create.*

All veterinary team members need to work with shelters and rescue groups to ensure that dogs and cats from our practices do not end up in the shelter population, *and* that the dogs and cats who *are* adopted from shelters can find humane and helpful care at veterinary practices who understand the often special behavioral needs of these dogs and cats. Clients whose dogs and cats need special handling and care are currently underserved (Anseeuw et al., 2006). If the focus from which all other services are delivered is seen as the behavioral

assessment, we can intervene early in the development of any condition that may cause the client to euthanize or relinquish a pet.

The severity of the behavioral condition is *not* the major determinant of whether a dog or cat will survive a behavioral condition (see Chapter 3: Changing Behavior: Roles for Learning, Negotiated Settlements, and Individualized Treatment Plans). Instead, the client's attitude about the pet is the single most predictive factor of whether the dog or cat will remain in the household and how much improvement the patient will experience. If the client: (1) understands the condition, (2) can minimize any perceived risk, and (3) can meet the animal's needs with a focus on the *pet's behavioral well-being,* that dog or cat will improve, regardless of how severe the behavioral concern. This finding suggests a clear role for centering a veterinary practice around veterinary behavioral medicine.

There are two tools that veterinarians must have to help clients understand their pets' normal behaviors and to address behaviors that are abnormal or that the client dislikes:

1. access to and an understanding of data-driven findings in the field, and
2. excellent communication skills in situations in which the client may feel uncomfortable.

Most veterinary schools teach neither of these. The people who will do best with the most difficult pet and clients are those who are best at listening to and communicating with both animals and humans.

Behavioral illnesses scare us and reveal our ignorance, weaknesses, and fears in a way that medical illnesses do not. With behavioral concerns, both clients and veterinarians feel personally responsible. Clients are often afraid to even ask their vet for advice about behavioral issues because they fear that they are responsible for the issues or will be thought to be responsible for them. Clients, like the rest of us, are afraid of appearing stupid, misinformed, careless, or irresponsible. Behavioral concerns provide the opportunity to encourage and teach compassion and empathy.

Although we all behave, we actually know less about behavior than we do about other veterinary or human medical specialties. We cannot encourage reliance on modern data until we understand that clients usually make the best decisions that they can with the tools they have available, *and they often have inadequate tools.* Neither clients nor veterinarians are helped by marketing and media efforts that focus more on drama and telegenicity than on providing clear, behaviorally relevant, accurate, helpful, and humane information.

Accurate information about veterinary behavioral medicine is something that veterinarians should and can own. In this text I have tried to meet the wishes of vets who want high-quality information, in easy to use formats, in language that they can share with the client, and in a manner that provides only the most essential, helpful references. Additionally, knowing that we do not teach client communication in veterinary school, I have attempted to explain the problems in ways that have proven useful to clients and veterinarians alike.

This text is divided into two primary sections: the explanatory, detailed text for veterinarians and the handouts for the clients. The handouts are also on the accompanying DVD, and they cover virtually all of the common diagnostic conditions and some of the common questions that clients have about management-related issues and normal behavior. There is a companion video that explains the foundation protocols for all behavior modification. The handouts mirror the material covered in the text, in language that should be accessible to most clients. The handouts are longer than most of us would probably like because populations of clients vary and veterinary knowledge varies. If the client knew nothing and the veterinarian knew nothing about the condition, the handout on the topic could be a stand-alone lesson and aid.

That said, these handouts are *best used* with the guidance of the consulting veterinarian and his or her staff. The handouts will be of most value when they are reviewed with the clients and the points most relevant to that particular patient highlighted for emphasis. In fact, this is how I use them for my clients.

Good veterinary behavioral care is individualized, and these handouts are best used as the framework for individualized treatment plans. The information in the handouts includes answers to questions that clients have had about the condition discussed, and relevant factors that the literature has shown to be involved in these conditions. Every point will *not* be relevant to every client or patient, but a joint review of the materials in the handouts is likely to produce extremely informative outcomes that will greatly help with the patient's care.

The text chapters use a topical approach. A narrative approach highlighting a review of the issues is used in the chapters that do not focus on specific diagnoses. For chapters focusing on common and specific behavioral complaints, the overview section discusses issues that unite the problems discussed within the topic and concerns that may exist for any of the issues discussed. For example, Chapter 6, Abnormal Canine Behaviors and Behavioral Pathologies Involving Aggression, contains a discussion on dog bites, breeds, and breed-specific legislation (BSL) because these issues are germane to any diagnosis involving canine aggression.

The text for each topic discusses the reasons for each of the complaints in a way that will allow the practitioner to evaluate whether the condition deviates from normal behavior, and if so, how best to determine the diagnosis.

1. Each diagnostic entity is discussed in an easy-to-review format that first lists the diagnostic criteria. These criteria are basically the definition of the diagnosis. There is no uniform, agreed-upon terminology in this field, which is a problem (Overall and Burghardt, 2006). In this text I have further developed a context-based, phenomenological terminology that is clear and becoming increasingly more widely used, while also discussing where other terminologies differ. These diagnostic criteria provide the context in which to evaluate the behaviors that concern you or client. Most behaviors that are of concern are non-specific in nature and can be shared by a number of normal and problematic conditions. Criteria for or a definition of the diagnosis provide the veterinarian with 2 things: the ability to interpret rare signs in a useful context, and the ability to not base the diagnosis on non-specific signs, which can be misleading and confusing. Instead, this approach encourages using changes in non-specific signs to evaluate improvements or decrements in the cat's or dog's behavioral condition.

2. The common non-specific signs seen for the condition are listed. The relevant signs and the contexts in which the client sees them should be noted in the record so that treatment targeted at the underlying reason for these behaviors can be monitored by using changes in signs and/or contexts in which they appear.

3. Rule-outs, including those that are medical, are briefly discussed.

4. A basic discussion of what is known about the neurochemistry or etiology of the condition is included. Included in this is whether any one group of animals is more at risk for developing the condition than any other.

5. Any common myths are reviewed.

6. Commonly asked client questions are listed and answered.

7. Treatment is discussed in terms of three core treatment foci:

   a. Management aspects of treatment: This core focus discusses behaviors and environments that can benefit from management and how that management is best addressed.

   • For example, the clients have a dog who is very protective of them, and whose behavior meets the diagnostic criteria for protective aggression. Whenever anyone comes to visit, the dog barks as soon as he hears an approach, and he barks and growls at the door when the bell is rung. The dog positions himself between the clients and the door, and the clients have to grab him and drag him away, growling, before they can let anyone in. This may seem like an incredibly simple circumstance on which to provide advice, but if you tone this down a notch . . . this is how most dogs behave at doors—most dogs are in the way, vocalize when visitors come, and have to be dragged from the door (which, incidentally, makes the behavior more intense).

- Management of this behavior will include the following, based on the outcome of a risk assessment:
  - The dog is placed behind a locked door (closed door, hook and eye or sliding bolt at the very top of the outside of the door) or a secure gate (one the dog is incapable of reaching through or jumping over) before anyone arrives. It's best to do this 15 to 30 minutes before an expected arrival so that the dog and humans have a chance to calm.
  - The dog can have a food toy, treat ball, chew toy, et cetera, to indicate that he is not being penalized and to keep him occupied.
  - No one is to visit these people without advance notice. If someone is coming to visit they must always call first, and should call a minimum of 15 minutes before they expect to arrive.
  - The dog is *not* permitted to visit with the guests if any human is afraid of dogs or of this dog, in particular.
  - If the dog is permitted to visit with the guests, he must be engaged in *and* progressing with a behavior modification program designed to make him less reactive and less concerned when people come to visit.
  - The dog can only visit with the guests if he is unable to do anyone damage. This means he is on a lead and head collar or harness and someone is responsible for monitoring him.
  - If the dog lunges at or threatens anyone, *or* if anyone feels that they have been threatened, the dog must return to his secure area.
  - If the dog is anxious, worried, or miserable, he should be allowed to return to his secure area.
  - If the humans are going to worry every second the dog is present, even if he is wearing a head collar, they are not ready to have him visit guests, and he should be in his secure area. This is better for everyone and has the advantage of ensuring that no tragedies occur.
  - If the guests and hosts are happy to have the dog visit under the above circumstances, the dog can be present if no one approaches the dog without asking permission of and guidance from the person holding the lead. Everyone must follow instructions. No one should stare at, reach for, or otherwise engage the dog until the dog is sufficiently calm to follow instructions, including those to sit and take a deep breath before being offered praise or a treat.

b. Behavior modification: As noted, most of the behavioral conditions that affect cats and dogs have a specific handout for the condition. The relevant behavior modification protocols and the specific handouts that may be helpful are listed here. The vast majority of patients will do well to start with the "Protocol for Deference," the "Protocol for Teaching Your Dog to Take a Deep Breath and Use Other Biofeedback Methods as Part of Relaxation," and the "Protocol for Relaxation: Behavior Modification Tier 1" which can be adapted for cats or dogs. No reactive patient should engage in a situations—physical or social—that could potentially make that patient more reactive until these programs can be performed flawlessly without the situation that sparks the reactivity.

c. Medication/dietary/supplement intervention: Specific medications and/or diets that may help are listed and discussed here. The medication dosages appear once, in the pharmacology section. The pharmacology chapter discusses the mechanism of each medication, patterns of effect, and dosing and half-lives so that individualized decisions about which medications to try first can be readily made.

d. Miscellaneous interventions: Miscellaneous interventions may include specific toys, harnesses, head collars, dog sitters, buggies, et cetera. Any further potentially beneficial hints are included in this section.

e. If there are any "pearls of wisdom" or "tips the pros use," they are found in the section on "Last words."

This text has benefitted from over a decade of comments by veterinarians, trainers, and clients on lectures, course notes, and on my earlier and broader text, and so it is hoped that this format will help even the busiest practitioner to move toward more humane and scientific behavioral care for their patients.

Acknowledgments

Textbooks are never completed without enormous amounts of help. For me, much of that help comes from clients and those attending lectures who make a comment or ask a question and from those who ask me about something I have written. Each experience makes me think more creatively and, I hope, more clearly. This is a field where much less is known than is unknown, so such questions/comments heighten the need for data and the premium on delivering scientific information fairly and in an accessible manner. This text would be poorer without such input . . . we are all students.

To everyone who expected this book much earlier, I apologize. After September 11th, 2001, there were a number of civic efforts in which I felt I must engage. I also was involved in writing dozens of grants and in writing (and rejecting) no fewer than four earlier versions of this book. And I needed time to address and recover from a number of professional and debilitating health issues.

For the 14 years I was on the staff of Penn Vet, the behavior program I oversaw faced challenges. By supplementing clinic fees with grants and a clinical research fund generated by memorial donations and long-distance consultations fees, I eventually built a program that paid for all of its clinical research, helped to pay student and assistant salaries, and provided all of its own supplies and equipment including desk chairs, lights, book cases, file cabinets, dog toys, printers, cartridges, clinic fax machines, video cameras and tapes, and wine, cheese, and snacks for the students at journal rounds, the first office computer, and many other needs. I was stunned when I finally found the detailed accounting—we'd really had nothing. But thanks to the clients and vets who supported the clinic, the vet students who took the behavior rotations and the vet students who worked in the office, we steadily gained ground and legitimacy. Finally, Hill's Pet Nutrition agreed to fully fund a 3-year residency, plus attendant research. I remain grateful to Hill's for their belief and investment and to Dr. Steven Zicker who shepherded the funding concept into reality.

Just when a full-time faculty position was finally created, my staff and I witnessed an IACUC violation that plunged me into a horrendous cycle of outcomes common to duty to report situations. I was devastated. My attempts to manage this situation gently and confidentially failed. Recovering from the aftermath and successfully refuting a litany of ensuing unsupported allegations, which at one point I was sure was not possible, took years.

At the same time my rheumatoid arthritis was becoming more debilitating, leaving me emotionally and physically bereft and incapacitated. I would not have made it through this period without the help of those acknowledged here. My husband somehow worked together with our dogs, Flash and Emma, to arrange that I was never alone during the months I could barely move from our bed. Emma and Flash so carefully collaborated and tag-teamed my care that I was always accompanied—even in the shower.

When my rheumatoid arthritis progressed to the point where I needed Flash simply to ambulate, we adopted Toby, a puppy born into Australian shepherd rescue, to be my service dog. Toby, who is very, very clever, learned to open doors, pull me from bed, support me on stairs, and turn keys. The extent to which I had any quality of life at all during this awful period was due primarily to the emotional and physical efforts of my husband and dogs, who provided company, a sounding board, encouragement, and respite from the self-loathing that I could have found myself in a position where I was dependent of someone else's competence, professionalism, and honor.

I have since learned that if you can focus on being grateful for the wonderful things in your life, you do not grieve so over what's lost. And so it is with very much gratitude that I have a number of people to whom I owe truly heart-felt thanks.

When I felt the most hopeless, Drs. Bonnie Beaver, RK Anderson, and Kersti Seksel called frequently. RK once told me he called because if he could hear me breathe, I was still alive. Dr. Sharon Crowell-Davis provided a real "steel magnolia" viewpoint and has only ever been helpful. Drs. Adelaide Delluva, Helen Davies, Ruben Gur, Christina Barr, Bill Bush, my aunt Giovanna Moore, Carol Murphy, and Chris Sandorello all provided unconditional support. I am extremely grateful to Dr. Urs Giger for his advice to focus on research. I'm equally grateful to colleagues everywhere who let me know that I had their support.

In 2001 I was solicited as a Faculty Excellence Scholar by Dr. Ted Valli, at the University of Illinois. Ted and Dr. Warwick Arden were wonderful to me. I have no words to express how difficult it was for me to decline a tenured position because Illinois could not also manage a position for my husband (and I hope that universities will ultimately truly value academic couples).

When I thought I should leave veterinary medicine, the enlightened dog training and veterinary communities (and their clients) voiced a different view. I am particularly grateful to Leslie McDevitt, Pat Miller, Angelica Steinker, and Paul Owens. The veterinarians in the greater Philadelphia referral area have always been just wonderful to me. I have been so fortunate with my clients, who are the best of the best. One client, Landon Pollack, ensured that he looked out for my interests, even when the result upset me. Landon has so grown into the role of guardianship in dogs that he has pushed frontiers of care in ways most of us cannot.

Carol Erickson of the local CBS TV station is responsible for the video that accompanies this text. She identified Andrea Korff as the producer, and the camera, sound, and make-up crew were all "borrowed" professionals. I am grateful to everyone involved for the lush final product, and am thankful that such a wonderful outcome was the by-product of a good friendship.

I am indebted to Dr. Colin Burrows who knew I needed stimulation, money, and community and so ensured that I returned to the ranks of speakers at the North American Veterinary Conference (NAVC). I cannot sufficiently sing the praises of the staff at NAVC. They are a model group.

Being able to travel internationally and lecture widely and frequently allowed me to encounter the most remarkable charity, *Dogs Trust* in the United Kingdom. *Dogs Trust* has 19 residential rehoming facilities for dogs. Their principals, Drs. Paul DeVile, Chris Laurence, Philip Daubeny, and, earlier, Andrew Higgins, other board members, and the absolutely marvelous Clarissa Baldwin, OBE, have been nothing but inspiring (and very helpful when I needed letters supporting some proposed legislation pertaining to dogs in the United States).

Tough times inform you about who your friends are and who they are not. After a particularly appalling interaction at a 2005 meeting, Dr. Walt Burghardt validated my impression of the exchange and—better yet—made me laugh with a comment about our divergent Second Amendment views. Despite our vastly differing politics, Walt has always been a good friend and a "big bro," a relationship we both credit to two attributes: tolerance and respect. Walt dragged me into the working dog field, a passion that solidified after September 11, 2001. When I had had a headache for 42 days and was hospitalized with a very scary diagnosis, Walt organized prayers for his atheist friend, and it was his and his wife Charlene's cell phone numbers that were taped to my hospital bed so that when I awoke at 3 A.M. I had someone to whom I could talk. During this time, my research assistant, Donna Dyer, also lovingly organized a prayer circle. I have learned we should be smart enough to cherish such gifts, even if we were not clever enough to think of them for ourselves.

I am indebted to Dr. Nancy Brown and her staff, and to Dr. Rafe Knox, who took such superb care of Tess, Emma, Flash, and Bunny. Flash's death from hemangiosarcoma was devastating for all of us, but no one ever gave up on him . . . no one. And because one can never know when one is wrong, I asked Fr. Al Murphy to pray for Flash when he was so ill, and it was a great comfort to me that he did so. Fr. Murphy has a keen understanding of the gifts of animals and his advocacy for dogs is well known and wide-spread.

I have become continually more appreciative of acts of kindness and generosity, so I need to thank at the vets at meetings at which I speak for offering to take me to dinner or direct me to activities and places they know I will love. I am particularly grateful to the vet at the California Veterinary Medical Association meeting who, when I asked for the location of a good book store, handed me her recently finished copy of Barbara Kingsolver's beautiful *Prodigal Summer*. It's a book I have now bought for others.

Drs. Kersti Seksel and Diane Frank provided the best year that that I ever had at Penn Vet. They volunteered to come and oversee clinics for a pittance so that I could have a research leave. Things did not quite work out as I had planned, but the experience reinforced to me the importance of community, especially in small or emergent fields. Simply, no specialty should be restricted to just one faculty member. All of the best knowledge is community based.

Along these lines I owe someone an apology. I have always taken great care to reference the ideas of those whom I cite and who stimulate me to think differently, but I missed an original reference. In my first text, I gave Dr. Victoria Voith sole credit for the *Nothing-in-life-is-free* and *Sit-stay programs*. I received the most generous letter and phone call from Bill Campbell, correcting my error, and I would like to acknowledge that I should have referenced his early writings, which contain these concepts and early foundations for these programs. Any revision of my first text will include the corrected references.

Meanwhile, although I sought and created a different, less authoritarian and more cognitive- and evolutionarily-based approach than that taken in the *Nothing-in-life-is-free* and *Sit-stay programs*, I am very grateful to Dr. Voith for sending me a laudatory note after my first text's publication. I have kept that note with the many others I have received, in part as a reminder to myself to tell people when I like something that they have done.

When I was trying to gain legitimacy and advancement for the behavior program at Penn Vet, I never stopped working. After too many 90-hour weeks, I realized that what I had neglected most was *life*. When I took advantage of my freedom, I was able to understand two essential things. The first was that I had always wanted a life of the mind, and now had a chance to have it. The second was that I had many, many friends all over the world.

Tony Trioli of Elsevier, was adamant in his support of a journal for this field and in his choice of me as Editor-in-Chief. Bringing the *Journal of Veterinary Behavior: Clinical Applications and Research* from concept to reality has been a true adventure. Watching it grow into a vibrant, well respected, oft cited academic journal is a real thrill, for which I thank those who have authored the papers we publish. I am thankful to Dr. Steve Arnold, who took me into his lab at Penn Med and taught me about molecular neuropathology. I had a great 8 years, but when I realized I was spending all my time writing grants and not enough actually doing the research and writing, I decided I needed to reverse those priorities. Dr. Freda Scott-Park, her husband David, and kids Ginny and Chris have often taken me in from my travels. David now insists I am an honorary Scott-Park, and I often see their views of Loch Lomond in my dreams. Mark Derr thinks more deeply about dogs than do most people I know. He has been a constant source of inspiration, support, laughter, and also a very good friend. Dr. Tiny de Keuster is a true sister in arms. Her efforts, along with those of Dr. Ray Butcher and the Blue Dog Trust, have made the Blue Dog bite prevention program the best and most accessible interactive learning program of its kind. Tiny is a model of what can be accomplished when you are determined, and how important it is to pursue and do the right thing. Her passion and friendship are beyond price. Tiny is also responsible for the wonderful photos of felines in this text because she introduced me to the photographer, Anne Marie Dossche, who has the most special and clear understanding of how cats see each other. Anne Marie's photographs made anything I wrote possible, and her generosity was overwhelming and extreme. I have had the great pleasure of wonderful intellectual and methodological discussions with Drs. Joanne van der Borg, Sófia Virányi, Adam Miklósi, Marta Gácsi, Barbara Schöning, and Kendall Shepherd. Drs. Kersti Seksel and Norm Blackman endeavored to keep me moving forward during a lovely if challenging month in Australia. When in tough economic times I adopted the rescue puppy who was to become my service dog, Dr. Jacqui Neilson made sure I had a video camera to record his every breath. When Flash died, Steve Dale, who has always championed behavioral causes in the popular press, had a brick laid at the American Humane Association that said "Flash—a dog who changed the world." He did, and I am so grateful that Steve and his wife, Robin, understood this. Dr. Paul McGreevy has always been steadfast in his support of my differing vision of thought, and I am indebted to him for all aspects of what that statement implies. Dr. Frode Lingaas has somehow always been there when most needed and has always made sure that my trips to Norway are full of Technicolor memories. Enduring closeness is not to be under-valued. Dr. Soraya Juarbe-Diaz has always been willing to help when the data and the journal threatened to overwhelm. Dr. Rhonda Schulman was an undergraduate when she first organized the student cadre of those running the behavior clinic. She was never surpassed, although Drs. Emily Elliot, Laurie Sponza and Tracy Barlup were in her league. Now a specialist, Rhonda and her husband, Dr. John Angus, have never paused in their support. Drs. Margie Scherk and Ilona Rodan embraced me and surrounded me with the world of cats. And Margie and I continue to have the most scintillating set of restaurant, travel, and meeting experiences wherever we are in the world. Sisterhood, indeed! When I was completing this text Dr. Karin Sorenmo harangued me to try one of the newer biological treatments for my rheumatoid arthritis, and I have not felt so well in 20 years (Toby isn't nearly as thrilled). She has my endless thanks. I have been so lucky to be shown people's home countries by the people who love them. Profound thanks are due to Drs. Helen Zulch, Quixi Sontag, Christine Halsberghe, Rudy de Meester, Seong Chan Yeon, Jaume Fatjo, Paty and Francisco Rosaldo, Moises and Rosa Heiblum, Chiara Mariti, Alessandro Cossi, and many, many others who have hosted and cared for me or directed me to cultural events they knew I'd love. Chris Osella and Angelo Gazzano have made me feel that I always have an intellectual and cultural home in Italy. All of these people have all shared their worlds with me and indulged and abetted my interests in food, culture, and great art. How could one not be better for such experiences and friends?

My post-September 11, 2001, grief and horror caused me to change course and focus on what could be done to aid working dogs, so I agreed to co-chair the Scientific Working Group on Dogs and Orthogonal Detection Methods (SWGDOG). One could argue (and I have) that I could have better used the 7 years I spent co-chairing this committee to publish books and papers, but one must start somewhere, and the introduction of scientific approaches can be rocky. This effort made me think more deeply canine behavior and introduced me to some wonderful people and dogs. Dr. Adee Schoon continues to impress me with her enthusiasm for science for the sake of the working dog. Jan Zoodsma and his wife Yteke have ensured that the enduring beauty of Friesland is etched on my soul. Jan has been an invaluable resource for my research and an excellent teacher about, and critic of, working dog skills and demands. Richard Davey taught me, generously and with humor, more about how governments work than I thought I needed to know (I was wrong). John Vandeloo (Australian Customs), Patrick Macisaac (RCMP), and Lee Titus (U.S. Customs) opened their hearts and facilities to me so that I could learn more about working dogs, and I am grateful for both. Many people gave me tours of government programs and taught me about explosives and other contraband about which I wish I did not need to know. Without a doubt I know that Rolf Krogh (Norwegian Customs) will always have my back, and that he will act only honestly and ethically on my behalf. Most importantly, Rolf and his dogs have confirmed my suspicion that the best working dog programs have first-class welfare and very happy dogs. These relationships remind me that none of us are islands of self-determination.

I have always thought that science was a way of discovering the truth, so I am thankful to David Kim, Yannick Nézet-Séguin, Valantin Radu, Anne d'Haroncourt, and Bruce Munro, among many, many others who have shown me that art can do the same. This book would not have been finished without the help of Hilary Hahn and Yo-Yo Ma, whom I have never met. It is to their recordings of the Bach Six Suites for Unaccompanied Cello (Ma; CBS Masterworks)[1] and Partitas and Sonatas (Hahn; Sony Classical)[2] that I listen while writing.

If this text has information that is accessible, it's because I benefitted from interactions with wonderful vet students. When I inherited the behavior program at Penn Vet, the clinic saw few cases and instructed few students. Within a short time, 99% of the senior class took the elective rotation and >90% of them elected to take it for the maximum three rotations possible. Primarily because of some very clever students, we were able to integrate behavioral medicine into other clinics and specialty fields. I am indebted to the Penn Vet classes of 1988-2001, for showing me what could be done by a motivated student body, and to all the students at vet schools around the world whom I have had the honor of lecturing. Students make you better thinkers and communicators and they seldom get credit for either. In the entire time I taught students, I never doubted I was doing exactly the right thing with my life.

Since 2002, the NAVC Institute (NAVC I) has offered a veterinary behavioral medicine course, thanks to Drs. Colin Burrows and Rick DeBowes. This course is the single best teaching experience I have had, and course participants say it is the best learning experience they have had. The form of this book is a direct result of the NAVC I course. Instructors have included Drs. Kersti Seksel, Jacqui Neilson, Lynne Seibert, Terry Curtis, Vint Virga, Soraya Juarbe-Diaz, and Martin Godbout. Working with them has been and is awesome.

The graduates of these courses are remarkable themselves, and they continue to help each other and the field after the course has ended. We have become an extended family of passionate advocates of better mental health care for the animals in our care and I am thankful to NAVC and the participants for creating an intellectual environment where this could occur.

I am grateful to the many people who read and re-read early parts of the text, suggested additional topics, and encouraged me to believe that it would be helpful, imperfections and all. Dr. Deb Bryant made the text much more clear by lecturing me that practitioners need easily accessible, focused information, and that the best path to this requires limiting the endless citations and digressions of which I am so fond. We compromised and I—mostly—managed to stick to a purely clinical focus in this text.

Elsevier has always been supportive of this field. Carol O'Connell was amazingly patient and a great help with the proofs. Jeanne Robertson provided the wonderful illustrations. Linda Duncan and Penny Rudolph provided much appreciated encouragement.

My husband, Arthur Dunham, is my best critic, and he has believed in me when I was positive that there was nothing meriting belief. Art also remains one of the rare, completely ethical academicians whom I know: he has overseen 22 successfully completed PhDs and all of those former students have academic jobs at universities or in government. Art is also a feminist.

My dogs—those gone and those still with us—are a constant source of inspiration, insight, and laughter. They are my window into dogs' minds and are always teaching, whether or not I am grasping the lessons. Flash, the dog whom I brought home thinking that the only intervention I could offer him was protection, became the best teacher I have ever had. He taught me about how troubled dogs view their world, and about compassion, which he had in abundance. He also taught me that if we allow them to do so, our pets and our patients will change us and make us better people.

I have tried to distill everyone's help, advice and enthusiasm into this text in a way that makes the practice of veterinary behavioral medicine informative, seductive, essential and humane, and firmly based in science. Any errors, omissions, mistakes, and misapprehensions, or fogginess of thought, however, are mine, alone.

[1]www.yo-yoma.com/music/bach-unaccompanied-cello-suites
[2]www.naxos.com/catalogue/item.asp?item_code=8.557563-64

Contents

PART I: UNDERSTANDING BEHAVIOR: MODERN PARADIGMS

1 Embracing Behavior as a Core Discipline: Creating the Behavior-Centered Practice, 2

2 The Science and Theory Underlying Behavioral Medicine: Terminology, Diagnosis, Mechanism, and the Importance of Understanding Reactivity, 45

3 Changing Behavior: Roles for Learning, Negotiated Settlements, and Individualized Treatment Plans, 56

PART II: CANINE BEHAVIOR

4 Normal Canine Behavior and Ontogeny: Neurological and Social Development, Signaling, and Normal Canine Behaviors, 122

5 Problematic Canine Behaviors: Roles for Undesirable, Odd, and Management-Related Concerns, 162

6 Abnormal Canine Behaviors and Behavioral Pathologies Involving Aggression, 172

7 Abnormal Canine Behaviors and Behavioral Pathologies *Not* Primarily Involving Pathological Aggression, 231

PART III: FELINE BEHAVIOR

8 Normal Feline Behavior and Ontogeny: Neurological and Social Development, Signaling, and Normal Feline Behaviors, 312

9 Undesirable, Problematic, and Abnormal Feline Behavior and Behavioral Pathologies, 360

PART IV: BEHAVIORAL SUPPLEMENTS AND MEDICATIONS

10 Pharmacological Approaches to Changing Behavior and Neurochemistry: Roles for Diet, Supplements, Nutraceuticals, and Medication, 458

PART V: SUPPLEMENTAL MATERIALS

References, 514

Questionnaires

Permission to evaluate and treat, 539
Short survey questionnaires to be used at all visits to monitor behavioral changes in cats, 540
Short survey questionnaires to be used at all visits to monitor behavioral changes in dogs, 544
Basic history questionnaire—cats, 547
Basic history questionnaire—dogs, 558

Client handouts

Foundation protocols for use in cats and dogs
Protocol for deference, 574
Protocol for teaching your dog to take a deep breath and use other biofeedback methods as part of relaxation, 580
Protocol for relaxation: behavior modification tier 1, 585

Discharge instructions specifically for dogs
Protocol for generalized discharge instructions for dogs with behavioral concerns, 599
Protocol for handling and surviving aggressive events, 605

Second tier of behavior modification protocols for cats and dogs
Tier 2: Protocol for teaching your dog to uncouple cues about your departures from the departure, 612
Tier 2: Protocol for desensitizing and counter-conditioning a dog or cat from approaches from unfamiliar animals, including humans, 614
Tier 2: Protocol for desensitization and counter-conditioning using gradual departures, 618
Tier 2: Protocol for desensitization and counter-conditioning to noises and activities that occur by the door, 620
Tier 2: Protocol for desensitizing and counter-conditioning dogs to relinquish objects, 622
Tier 2: Protocol for desensitizing dogs affected with impulse control aggression, 625

Protocols for understanding and treating specific conditions in cats

Protocol for understanding and treating cats with elimination disorders and elimination behaviors that concern clients, 628

Protocol for understanding and treating play aggression in cats, 635

Protocol for understanding and treating feline aggressions with an emphasis on intercat aggression, 637

Protocol for understanding, managing, and treating impulse control/status-related aggression in cats, 644

Protocols for understanding and treating specific conditions in dogs

Protocol for understanding and treating canine panic disorder, 647

Protocol for understanding and treating dogs with noise and storm phobias, 650

Protocol for understanding and treating generalized anxiety disorder, 655

Protocol for understanding, managing, and treating dogs with impulse control aggression, 657

Protocol for understanding and treating dogs with fear/fearful aggression, 663

Protocol for understanding and managing dogs with aggression involving and food, rawhide, biscuits, and bones, 666

Protocol for understanding and treating dogs with interdog aggression, 670

Protocol for understanding and treating dogs with protective and/or territorial aggression, 677

Protocol for understanding and treating dogs with separation anxiety, 681

Protocols for treating specific conditions that affect both dogs and cats

Protocol for understanding and treating redirected aggression in cats and dogs, 686

Protocol for understanding and treating obsessive-compulsive disorder, 688

Protocol for understanding and helping geriatric animals, 690

Protocol for preventing and treating attention-seeking behavior, 698

Protocol for treating fearful behavior in cats and dogs, 701

Protocols for using medication for both dogs and cats

Protocol for using behavioral medication successfully, 704

Generalized guidelines for using alprazolam for noise and storm phobias, panic, and severe distress, 714

Informed consent statements for the most commonly used medications, 716

Protocols for understanding miscellaneous behaviors in dogs and cats

Protocol for understanding and managing odd, curious, and annoying canine behaviors, 728

Protocol for understanding odd, curious, and annoying feline behaviors, 735

Protocols for preventing problems for dogs

Protocol for choosing collars, head collars, harnesses, and leads, 740

Protocol for handling "special-needs pets" during holidays and other special occasions, 750

Protocol for basic manners training and housetraining for new dogs and puppies, 753

Protocol for assessing pain and stress in dogs, 760

Protocol for preventing problems for cats

Protocol for assessing pain and stress in cats, 764

Protocols for preventing problems for both dogs and cats

Protocol for introducing a new baby and a pet, 767

Protocol for the introduction of a new pet to other household pets, 771

Protocol for teaching cats and dogs to "sit," "stay," and "come," 775

Protocol for teaching kids—and adults—to play with dogs and cats, 779

Protocol for choosing toys for your pet, 785

Protocol for activities for clients to practice with puppies and kittens, 791

Resources

Resources for information, tools, books, products, and other help, 794

Index, 797

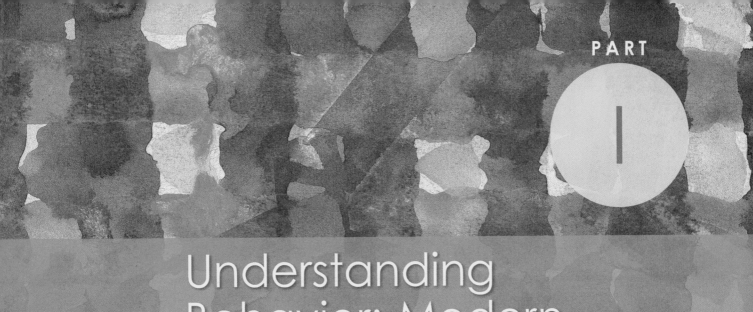

Understanding Behavior: Modern Paradigms

CHAPTER

1

Embracing Behavior as a Core Discipline: Creating the Behavior-Centered Practice

WHY CARE ABOUT BEHAVIOR?

Behavioral problems are still the primary reason why cats and dogs are abandoned, relinquished, or euthanized, and most of these cats and dogs are less than 3 years of age. This means that the average practice loses $2200 per relinquished cat and $3300 per relinquished dog, on average, in the most simple, basic services that are not delivered over an average 15-year lifetime. These estimates are based on the 2011 American Society for the Prevention of Cruelty to Animals (ASPCA) estimated costs for *minimum, basic, routine* veterinary care.* These estimates do not include grooming, boarding, products of any kind including food, any surgery including neutering, first-year care, or any emergency care. Even at this minimal estimate, you don't have to lose many patients to behavioral issues to realize lost income that could equate to the cost of equipment, a technician, a retirement plan, or an associate. More information about the role that behavior plays in pet loss and debility can be found in the Preface.

Clients recognize that their animals are ill based on their behavioral changes. If we use any aspect of behavioral change to inform us about somatic illness, *we should also be using such changes to inform us about behavioral illness.* Unfortunately, clients may not know enough about behavior to identify the concerns of their cats and dogs. As noted in Figure 1-1, clients may not notice all of the behaviors exhibited by their dogs or cats and may report to the vet only behaviors they do not like, whether or not these are "abnormal." For veterinarians to deliver the best holistic care possible, where they treat the whole dog and whole cat, they must understand when behaviors deviate from normal and how to help clients identify behaviors they like or dislike in a context that is meaningful for the dog or cat.

EVALUATING THE PATIENT: HOW OFTEN SHOULD YOU SEE CLIENTS AND THEIR PETS?

If we are to help clients raise and live with behaviorally healthy animals, we must be able to evaluate the normal behaviors of the dog or cat and any deviations from these. Ill animals are not behaving "normally." In fact, clients recognize that the dog or cat is physically compromised *because* of some change in his or her behavior. Behavior is at the core of the practice of veterinary medicine (Martin and Taunton, 2006) and specialty practices that include behavior encourage the use of other specialties (Herron et al., 2012). The same is true for general practices.

The opportunity to evaluate each patient in his or her "normal" baseline state occurs at new puppy/dog and kitten/cat visit and at wellness exams. Wellness exams should occur every few months through the first year of life; twice a year during the second year; and once a year until the dog or cat is segueing into later middle age or beginning older age, when evaluations should occur at least every 6 months (Table 1-1). This is more visits than is routinely recommended during the first 2 years of a dog's or cat's life, but this period of time is when the patient and his or her behavior is changing most profoundly. We need to observe cats and dogs during this time; teach clients how to observe them; and evaluate any behaviors or changes in behaviors that scare, worry, or concern clients or any member of the veterinary team.

APPOINTMENT LENGTH AND BEHAVIOR-CENTERED PRACTICES

Veterinarians have often made the mistake of charging for products and not charging for their knowledge, skills, and time. Behavioral medicine provides the veterinary team with an opportunity to change this unfortunate practice. There are numerous ways to structure fees for preventive appointments and consultations for behavioral concerns, but none of these fit well into a

*www.aspca.org/adoption/pet-care-costs.aspx; last accessed October 28, 2011.

What do clients notice and understand?*

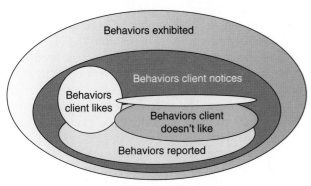

*One of the clinician's main jobs is casting this type of information within a context meaningful to the *dog or cat*. Can we create a tool that allows this type of assay for each patient?

Fig. 1-1 Conceptual diagram of how clients view cat or dog behavior. In this diagram, the set of behaviors exhibited includes ultra-normal behaviors (light color, left) through seriously pathological behaviors (dark color, right). Clients notice only a subset of behaviors, whether they are normal or abnormal. *Clients are most likely to notice and report behaviors that they do not like, without regard for whether these behaviors are problems for the cat or dog.* The role of veterinarians is to take this view of what clients notice and help them to interpret it *in a context that is meaningful to the cat or dog.* This is one of the goals of a behavior-centered practice.

15- to 20-minute appointment plan because you are doing more than evaluating the patient: you are educating the client, establishing a working partnership, and investing in the client's future willingness to invest in the health and care of their dog or cat.

For initial puppy and kitten wellness appointments, 40 minutes is sufficient time to:

- Accustom the puppy/kitten to the exam room and exam process
- *Listen* to the client when you ask if he or she has specific concerns or questions
- Review husbandry and care patterns in which the client is currently engaged
- Make recommendations about how to amend these patterns, if needed
- Provide some targeted education information; keep in mind that you will have at least two or, ideally, three puppy or kitten visits of this length and customize this information for each patient—if housetraining is the issue, your focus will be housetraining at this appointment; if chewing is the issue you will focus more on toys, supervision, and humane containment of damage at this appointment
- Examine and vaccinate the puppy/kitten

TABLE 1-1

Suggested Visit Frequency with Age for "Wellness" Appointments

Age	Frequency of Veterinary Checks	Behavior Landmarks of Interest
Through 16 weeks	Every 2-3 weeks or *more frequently if concerned*; consider weekly appointments if client is inexperienced in any manner (i.e., novice pet person, new species, new breed)	Housetraining/use of litterbox, development of appropriate inter-specific play behaviors; leash/car manners (cats, too); social exposure to novel humans and physical exposure to new environments and stimuli
>16 weeks to 1 year	Every 2-4 months	Sexual maturity from ~6-9 months of age; marking behaviors; onset of social maturity can be 9-10 months of age for some dogs
1-2 years	Every 6 months, *minimum*	Period of social maturity for most cats and dogs; end of social maturity for some dogs can be 18 months; cats may not be fully socially mature until 3-4 years; onset of most behavioral conditions
2-~8 years (depending on breed and size)	*At least* annually	Behavioral maturity; by 2 years of age, most behavioral conditions are becoming fully developed and will worsen without redress; at about 6 years, evaluate cognition and decide whether to initiate supplements or behavioral diets
≥8 years	*At least* every 6 months	Behavioral conditions associated with chronic illness or aging; consider supplements, diets, nutraceuticals; rehabilitative and cognitive therapy to keep the patient's body and mind flexible
≥12 years	*At least* every 3-4 months; more often if chronic condition identified	Possible cognitive changes associated with aging; may be painful because of degenerative changes; consider household, diet nutraceuticals, supplements, conditioning, accommodations for changes in elimination behaviors/mobility, conveyances (steps into car, slings for stairs, buggies, special bedding or flooring)

- Play with the puppy/kitten before and after examination; this is very important because the vaccine must come at a time when the patient is having a good time with enough time afterward to continue to have a good time

Subsequent puppy and kitten wellness appointments may take 30 or 40 minutes depending on whether the patient is attending a kitten or a puppy class and how well the integration into the household is going. If the patient is attending a class and everything is going well, you *may* be able to have a shorter appointment, but *do not forget that part of the appointment's purpose is to accustom the patient to the people, to the practice, and to new experiences in general.* Let these young animals explore the reception area, bathing area, treatment rooms, and exam rooms. If you are offering puppy or kitten classes, the exploration of all areas of the hospital can be a class exercise. For the puppy/kitten, having as much information as possible is a great buffer against fear.

Initial examinations for *newly adopted adult dogs and cats* take about 30 to 40 minutes. This is sufficient time to observe the patient, learn how he or she walks on a lead or moves around with unfamiliar people, review information about behavioral changes in new households, and discuss the common behavioral reasons that render adult animals available for adoption. You will also need to observe the patient and listen to how clients offer information and respond to questions you ask. Clients need to understand that "recycled" pets may have been relinquished at least in part because of a behavioral concern and that the entire range of the animal's behaviors may become clear only over the course of months. The veterinary team should make clear to the client that one of their goals is to help facilitate the transition.

Follow-up examinations may be successfully done in 20 minutes for adult animals, but this estimate assumes a healthy animal and a completely non-inquisitive client who truly needs very little information. Practices can best partition their time if they use a standardized questionnaire (see the end of this chapter) to survey the patient's behaviors at all appointments, if some members of the staff receive special training in choosing and fitting head collars and harnesses, and if early intervention and management-related advice is provided. Depending on the problem, support staff can take the patient and client into a less busy area and help them on the spot. Otherwise, the support staff can schedule a 15- to 30-minute appointment for a harness fitting or to review a housetraining handout (Table 1-2).

TABLE 1-2

Technicians as Consultants: Types and Tasks

Type of Consultant for Which Technician Can Develop Expertise	Tasks	Amount of Time Required per Client/Dog
Canine chew toy consultant	• Demonstration of types of chew toys • Discussion of potential risks and benefits of each type of chew toy • Evaluation of dog's style of chewing and appropriateness of choice for style	15 minutes
Canine food puzzle consultant	• Demonstration of types of food puzzles and toys • Discussion of potential risks and benefits • Discussion of cleaning and maintenance of toys • Discussion of when to use food toys and how to integrate them with meal feeding	15-20 minutes, depending on complexity of toy
Feline litter environment and hygiene consultant	• Discussion of normal feline elimination behaviors • Demonstration of types of litters and boxes • Discussion of cleanliness techniques • Recommendations for number of boxes needed and recommended locations based on discussion with client of housing arrangement and maps of various rooms • Discussion of types of cleaners/odor eliminators and how to clean	10 minutes if this is a new cat without problems; up to 30 minutes if there are multiple cats or any cat is having a problem
Feline kitten toy consultant	• Discussion/demonstration of the type of toys available • Discussion of the cat's playing style • Discussion of risks/benefits of different types of toys	15 minutes

TABLE 1-2

Technicians as Consultants: Types and Tasks—cont'd

Type of Consultant for Which Technician Can Develop Expertise	Tasks	Amount of Time Required per Client/Dog
Feline scratching consultant	• Nail trim mechanics and frequencies • Demonstration of scratching posts • Discussion of feline signaling using scratching • Discussion of how to build sandpaper or jute scratching posts/inclines • Discussion of nail caps	30 minutes if the client is concerned about inappropriate scratching; 15 minutes if the cat is new to the household or has no problems
Canine collar, harness, head collar, and lead consultant	• Discussion of mechanics of different types of collars, harnesses, et cetera • Discussion of different materials and their maintenance • Discussion and demonstration of fitting and use • Practice with client for fitting and use • Discussion of any potential risks and reminder for clients that nothing that can catch on anything should be left on unsupervised dogs	30 minutes for non-problematic dogs; for dogs who may be fearful, reactive or aggressive, multiple short sessions may be better than one long session, especially if coupled with instructions to have the client practice accustoming the dog to the harness or collar multiple times per day in short increments
Feline harness and carrier consultant	• Demonstration of harnesses, baskets, and carrier types • Fitting of harness/collar • Discussion of use situations	15-30 minutes depending on whether the client is having problems
Canine wrap consultant	• Discussion of the use of wraps and disclosure of what we do not know (e.g., the lack of controlled studies) • Demonstration of wrap • Fitting of wrap • Cautions about risks of wraps and need for supervision	15-30 minutes depending on whether the client wishes to have a wrap fitted
Canine eye shade/ear muff consultant	• Discussion of the use of eye shades, Doggles, ear muffs, ear plugs, et cetera • Fitting and demonstration of use	10-30 minutes depending on whether a demonstration or fitting is involved
Puppy and kitten preventive care consultant	• Discussion of the importance of handling puppies' and kittens' mouths and paws • Display and demonstration of types of nail clippers, inclined planes covered with sand paper for the dog's or cat's "self-use," and products for dental hygiene • Demonstration of toothbrushing and nail trimming • Coaching clients for nail trimming—this is important: clients must leave the practice feeling that they can trim nails	10-30 minutes depending on ease of execution
Canine housetraining consultant	• Explanation of normal elimination behaviors in dogs • Explanation of age-related elimination behaviors • Explanation and demonstration of techniques • Discussion of cleaning • Discussion of how best to integrate training for that specific dog's needs into the client's schedule • Review of how to train a dog to a litter box, if relevant • Review of handouts	≥30 minutes. This is one area on which no one should scrimp for time and instruction because dogs who exhibit elimination or marking behaviors in the house are often rehomed, euthanized, relinquished, or abandoned

Note: Technicians can be trained to act as consultants for specific types of labor-intensive tasks. Appointments with the specific consultant ensure that the client is receiving accurate information and manages time, costs, and expertise.

- It is optimal if someone on the staff, who is knowledgeable about and trained to play this role, is always available during normal working hours. Asking people to come back when their lives are already over-booked poses a risk.
- If practices are going to bill for the time of the staff, all fees should be disclosed and posted and based on time. There is no mandate that posted fees are charged, but charges *must* be transparent in advance. *Posting the cost for expertise in providing behavioral advice legitimizes the value of the service, but the fees must be commensurate with job description, talent and training, and information provided.*
- Some practices prefer to bundle all the fees for examinations, behavioral evaluation and coaching, and vaccinations for kittens and puppies into one package over some pre-agreed time period. If you are going to do this, make sure you post exactly what is included in the package. Are unlimited question-and-answer (Q & A) visits with the staff included for the first 3 months? Can clients see the veterinarian at no additional cost more often than for appointments scheduled with vaccines if they have concerns about physical health? What services will incur additional costs (laboratory evaluations, medications to treat illness, et cetera)? Package plans can be great practice builders and encourage terrific dialogue about behaviors.
- Some practices prefer to have staff or a trainer hired for the purpose of giving weekly evening classes for clients and charge on a per-class basis (e.g., maximum of six dogs and families per 2-hour session; weekly sessions for Q & A and fittings for and coaching for use of harnesses and head collars at $25 per session). See Brammeier et al. (2006) for advice on finding and utilizing trainers in veterinary practices.
- Some practices hire a trainer who will charge by the course. Courses can be divided by age and size but are best kept small (e.g., no more than six dogs or cats, with preferably two staff members). If the practice has the space to have a trainer offer basic manners courses for dogs and cats at the practice, these classes provide an income stream for toys, harnesses, and food and engage the practice staff in the commitment to behavior.
- Many practices hold group classes (e.g., two kitten classes, each separated by 2 weeks, and two to three weekly puppy classes of 1 to 1.5 hours' duration) as a "free bonus" for clients in the practice. The sole purpose of these classes is to answer questions and to allow the puppies and kittens to play and begin to learn about each other in a safe environment. The hidden advantage of this approach is that many clients have the same questions, and the group discussion of the answer is extremely informative. These clients may become their own support group while bonding to the practice.

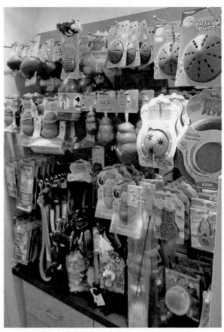

Fig. 1-2 An in-clinic display of behavioral tools (harnesses and head collars) on the lower left and toys above and to the right. (Photo courtesy of Dr. Steven Brammeier.)

- If the practice has a lot of first-time pet clients or a lot of clients with mild or management-based problems, it may be best to hold at least one session where the pets are not present so that the clients can focus on the information delivered and the veterinary staff running the session can listen to the clients. Choice of strategy is largely a manner of practice style, but whatever strategy is chosen, everyone will benefit.

Basic appointments should include a discussion of reasons some toys are preferred over others and the advantages and disadvantages of the various collars, harnesses, halters, leads, et cetera. If you have a display of these items, the display can serve to educate the client in appropriate choices and provide an income stream (Fig. 1-2), but you must also have samples available that show clients how the toys work and the harnesses fit. *This approach requires that a knowledgeable and helpful staff member is always available. (If you cannot fit the harness or show how the toy works or how to clean it, a client may wonder what else you don't know.)* See Table 1-2 for a list of tasks for which technicians can be trained to act as consultants, ensuring that clients get individualized attention and the most up-to-date, accurate information.

Having toys available in the exam room that encourage cognitive stimulation in cats and dogs can pique interest and engage both clients and pets. Whether the dog or cat shows interest in or plays with these toys may also tell you something about their level of distress.

For every harness, head collar, collar, halter, or wrap that is meant to help manage dog and cat behavior, laminate the illustrated fitting and use instructions and hang them on hooks in the exam rooms and waiting room. Even as we move to a paperless veterinary record, these materials provide tangible, pictorial information and give people a focus for the time spent waiting. Having these illustrated instructions instantly available also allows you to explain a tool that could help the client and patient as a segue to demonstrating the tool. This way there is no lapse in time between the suggestion and starting to implement helpful change.

LISTENING TO CLIENTS

Recent studies have shown that veterinarians, similar to physicians for humans, are not taught how to talk to clients in a manner that extracts important information while showing compassion and empathy. Clients cannot evaluate your medical skills; however, they *can* evaluate your ability to convey information, understand their concerns, and show empathy, and they do so on the basis, in part, of how well you listen. In one study, the median and mean lengths of time clients talked before being interrupted by the veterinarian were 11 seconds and 15.3 seconds (Dysart et al., 2011). Be conscious of this finding. Set a timer for a minute and see if you can allow the client to speak that long without interruption. If you are having trouble not interrupting, try sitting down. It's easier not to interrupt if you are not standing.

The main reason clients provide incomplete information to closed-ended questions is *interruption by the veterinarian*. Quite simply, clients are almost never provided with adequate time to talk about their concerns. As a result, the major concern or key piece of information is often delivered at the end of the appointment, when such concerns are least able to be competently handled.

Anyone who wishes to be good at behavioral medicine must be good at listening. One function of a standardized questionnaire is to start the discussion with the client. Questionnaires, especially if they allow for both open (e.g., "What concerns you about this behavior?") and closed (e.g., "How many times has the dog bitten?") responses, give clients some vocabulary for their concerns and some structure for thinking about related behaviors about which the veterinarian should know. Questionnaires also act as a form of note taking; rather than having to write everything down, the person interviewing the client can make notations to the client-provided report.

After reviewing the questionnaire, the veterinary staff can follow up with both specific questions (e.g., "Do you know if the cat uses the litterbox immediately after it is cleaned?") and more open-ended ones (e.g., "What outcome are you hoping for?"). If the client is provided the time at the beginning of the appointment to answer the questions fully, while the person taking the notes highlights points to which they need to return later, the client will provide much of the desired information. It's acceptable to interrupt if something is sufficiently unclear that it will be impossible to understand the next information, but the person taking the behavioral information must be able to guide the client back to his or her place in the discussion.

At the end of every appointment or visit, good listeners do one final thing: they ask if there is anything else that they should know and if there are any questions. As listening and communication skills improve, this last solicitation will tend to yield only small amounts of information. Regardless, it is essential to ask.

Questions to Ask of Clients with New Dogs or Cats That May Elicit Concerns or Gaps in Knowledge

New pets provide an opportunity to establish a dialogue with clients that will help ensure that the quality of that pet's life is the best it can be. Sample questions that may help you to learn where the client might need help follow:

- How did you get this cat/dog/puppy/kitten? Impulse buys or emotionally impulsive adoptions can work out, but it's important to assess whether the client has the knowledge base to care for the animal.
- Where did you get the pet? There are good public health reasons for asking this question. If the client has young children and a kitten is wormy and flea infested, both *Toxocara* and cat-scratch disease could be concerns.
- Why did you choose this specific animal (i.e., type of pet or breed)? Many people didn't make a choice, but if they did, chances are you will learn about something that is important to the client by asking.
- What are you feeding your new pet, and how do you think he or she is doing on that diet? This gives you a chance to combine behavioral advice (e.g., perhaps the kitten could have some or all of his dry food in a food ball) with nutritional advice.
- Have you noticed any problems with elimination? This question allows you to combine behavioral and medical advice and observations.
- Are there any behaviors about which you are concerned? Combined with the previous information, this question will help you to round out your understanding of the client's needs and knowledge base.
- Do you have any questions about anything pertaining to this new pet? Listen first. Probe and respond second.

PROVIDING QUALITY INFORMATION AT CLASSES AND APPOINTMENTS

Regardless of how you decide to handle your "new pet" appointments, consider putting together an *individually customized* packet/bag for *each* class/appointment. The packet/bag should include sample items and information in a folder with the pet's name. Creation of these packets/bags should be the responsibility of one or a few specifically chosen staff members.

- Samples of size- and style-appropriate toys can be included.
- Consider including the following handouts:
  - "Protocol for Teaching Kids—and Adults—How to Play with Dogs and Cats"
  - "Protocol for Choosing Toys for Your Pet"
- Treats and foods chosen for the breed and size of dog/cat can be provided in a small bag. Sources can be provided on an information sheet.
- Information on housetraining/litterboxes and choosing and using leads, harnesses, collars, et cetera, can be very helpful.
- Consider including the following handouts:
  - "Protocol for Choosing Collars, Head Collars, Harnesses, and Leads"
  - "Protocol for Basic Manners Training and Housetraining for New Dogs and Puppies"
  - "Protocol for Understanding and Treating Cats with Elimination Disorders and Elimination Behaviors That Concern Clients"
  - "Protocol for Understanding Odd, Curious, and Annoying Feline Behavior"
  - "Protocol for Understanding and Managing Odd, Curious, and Annoying Canine Behaviors"
  - "Protocol for Generalized Discharge Instructions for Dogs with Behavioral Concerns"
  - "Protocol for Handling and Surviving Aggressive Events"
- Include vaccination schedules, wellness schedules, and appointments already made in a calendar form that will encourage clients to add these to their calendar and/or stick them on the refrigerator.
- If the pet is of a type that might need a lot of grooming or special grooming, samples of dermatologically friendly shampoos can be included, along with a list of websites where good grooming products can be found.
- Suggestions for exercise should be tailored to the individual pet, but locations of dog parks or websites with information on hobby sports (yes, agility is a sport for cats, too) can be prepared by your practice staff and included for each new patient.
- Microchipping can help keep pets safer. Include information early in the sequence of visits and remind clients that shelters scan for microchips and will hold identified patients.

If these bags/packets are well tailored to the individual patient, you will have provided the client with an excellent foundation that should decrease the probability of a recycled or abandoned pet, while increasing the probability that if the pet displays problem behaviors, you will learn of them early on, not

later or too late. Note that the emphasis here is not on random, free samples. You may choose to provide some samples, but what you are delivering is thoughtful information targeted and personalized for each cat or dog. This practice encourages clients to understand that they are paying you for your knowledge—not as middlemen for products. For this reason, any product sample you provide should be coupled to the pet's needs.

APPOINTMENTS FOR OLDER PETS

A word on appointments for older pets is warranted. *People who have aging or geriatric pets often fear their loss.* These clients are already committed to quality and quantity of life for their pets and have a high probability of cooperating with recommendations.

We have more tools than ever before to help mitigate the effects of aging. *As pets age, they and their humans will benefit from the same types of in-depth care and creative suggestions provided at puppy/kitten and new dog/cat appointments.*

Appointment times and displays of helpful tools and toys should reflect the needs and commitment of these clients and the needs of cats and dogs in this life stage. The appointments should have the focus of keeping the aged dog/cat as healthy as possible and ensuring that the quality of life is as good as it can be. This may mean finding creative ways to exercise your patient's mind and body. Traditionally, the focus has been on mobility. We need to add to this an emphasis on encouraging the older dog/cat to use his or her brain. Games and cognitive exercise tailored to older pets (e.g., softer toys that are easier to manipulate and carry; food puzzles that are easier to manipulate, swimming/wading using an underwater treadmill) will enhance the interaction between clients and their pets, improving everyone's quality of life.

EVALUATING "NORMAL"

The biggest problem that veterinary practices have with evaluating and discussing normal behaviors with clients is that no one in the practice sees the patient exhibiting either globally normal behaviors or behaviors typical for the pet. *Most dogs and cats fear veterinary visits, so veterinary staff see these patients only when they are fearful.*

One study examined the behavior of dogs at veterinary hospitals and found that 106 of 135 (78.5%) dogs were fearful on the examination table (Döring et al., 2009). Of the dogs, 18 (13.3%) had to be dragged or carried into the practice; fewer than half of the dogs entered the practice calmly. Dogs who had had only positive experiences were less fearful than others, and dogs less than 2 years of age—who see vets often—were more fearful than older dogs—who see vets infrequently, suggesting that repeated exposure to veterinary practices may enhance fear to a certain age.

We need to question the extent to which these fearful behaviors interfere with our ability to assess patients and provide the state-of-the-art care they deserve and to what extent we cause or contribute to the fears of dogs and cats.

Visits to veterinary practices can be scary for our patients: the floor is slick, there are strange sounds and smells, there is not enough inter-personal approach space, the table is cold and provides poor footing, their people are tense, et cetera. Any dog or cat who is not physically ill should be able to walk happily in the door of the hospital. *If the patient is shaking, trembling, drooling, hiding, staying flat on the floor, scanning the environment, urinating, defecating, vomiting, or trying to leave, he or she is not happy.* We need to change this response for three important reasons:

1. We need to distinguish patients for whom early fear is a true pathological diagnosis from patients who are just afraid of what we are doing to them and where we are doing it. If most of our patients are afraid, we cannot adequately evaluate their early behaviors.
2. Although we can man-handle puppies/kittens and—usually falsely—dismiss fear as "normal," to do so sends the wrong message to the patient and to the client. We must realize that:
   a. We should not man-handle anyone.
   b. We will not be able to man-handle many of these patients as they age and grow without the greatly increased costs incurred by staff time, the effects of stress, and job-related injuries.
   c. Modern zoos have abandoned forceful handling. Children's hospitals are now open, engaging places where kids participate in the delivery of their care. Why are we still struggling with our veterinary patients?
3. The delivery of veterinary care may teach cats and dogs that humans can be threatening. This realization will contribute to the development or worsening of any behavioral problem.

These three factors suggest that, unwittingly and without malicious intent, the delivery of veterinary care can be a causal factor in the worsening of patients' behaviors.

Nothing in the experience of any puppy or kitten will have prepared it for the sensory overload that will occur at the first and subsequent veterinary visits.

- These babies will never have encountered the noise range and frequency that defines a busy veterinary practice.
- The general lighting is different and often invasive, and it's unlikely anyone has looked in the patient's eyes with a penlight.
- The global odor must be complex. Even if these puppies/kittens were born in a home with lots of

animals, they have never faced so many and such diverse smells at once.
- Most puppies/kittens will never have had the social experience of encountering so many humans and animals at once and in such close quarters.
- Many puppies/kittens may be walking for the first time on flooring that will steal their balance and traction.
- Finally, if the client is clutching at the patient or at his or her "restraints" (e.g., leads, harnesses, carriers, collars), the patient can only take this as a signal to react.

Is it any wonder that most animals never show their true behaviors at most veterinary visits?

Arousal levels are key to understanding why patients are at risk for learning fear at veterinary offices (see Chapter 2).

- Learning of adaptive fear at the neurochemical level in the amygdala and the hippocampus is modulated by cortisol levels (see Chapters 4 and 6 and the "Protocol for Teaching Your Dog to Take a Deep Breath and Use Other Biofeedback Methods as Part of Relaxation").
- As cortisol levels increase, brain-derived neurotrophic factor (BDNF) increases, which allows molecular memory to be made through the creation of new proteins (Peters et al., 2004) (see Fig. 3-5, *A* and *B*, in Chapter 3).
- This same process is involved in learning how to cope with arousal.
- Fear can be almost instantly encoded because the amygdala is "pre-adapted" to respond to perceived threats. However, behaviors associated with learning to cope with arousal cannot be encoded at the molecular level if the cortisol level is too high.
- An optimal range of cortisol produces an optimal range of BDNF and cytosolic response element binding protein (CREB).
- True complex, associative, and adaptive learning will occur at the molecular level only when CREB and BDNF are within this range.
- This is why in situations scary to the patient we see an almost invariant version of avoidance and withdrawal behaviors associated with arousal.

Fortunately, we can intervene. Our mitigation should focus on decreasing arousal and on increasing affiliative behaviors. We accomplish these goals by using calm environments, teaching patients that going to the veterinarian need not be scary, and avoiding situations that are perceived by the dog or cat as punishing or scary and instead ensuring that these experiences are seen as fun and rewarding. Cats and dogs who live at practices or who regularly come to the hospital with the veterinary staff are not afraid of the hospital environment. Why is this? For these patients, good experiences are the rule, not the exception.

WHAT CAN WE CHANGE?

Door Entryway

Doorways should provide sufficient space that no dog or cat is constrained to come within its personal approach distance of another animal (Fig. 1-3). This distance is 1 to 1.5 body lengths and varies individually with the patient. Large doors with porches or entryways can accomplish such avoidance easily (see Fig. 1-3). Windows, glass doors, and large panels of glass in doors also help. In urban environments, a double set of doors with large panels of glass can help accomplish the goal of avoiding abrupt introductions. Staff can be schooled to help orchestrate safe and non-stressful movement through doors.

Figure 1-3 shows a panoramic view of an entryway that was well designed with the patients' behavioral concerns in mind. Figure 1-3, *A*, shows that there are two double doors on each side of the reception area. This design allows dogs to go in one door and out another to avoid meeting each other, if needed.

Regardless, everyone can see who is coming and going, so avoidance and orchestration of movement of animals by staff are possible. Figure 1-3, *B*, shows that the reception staff has a clear and global view of both doors and the waiting area. The high ceilings give the illusion of even more space than the already large floor plan provides, which helps clients who may worry about their dog's reactions to other dogs. Figure 1-3, *C*, shows the wide open waiting area on one side of the reception area (note the large number of windows). There is a mirror image of this waiting area on the other side of the reception area, allowing dogs and cats or fractious animals to be separated. Figure 1-3, *B* and *C*, also shows that well-placed benches outside increase the amount of waiting area space and may allow many pets and clients to be calmer than they would be inside the hospital. Some exams and procedures may be best done outdoors where the patients can focus on other activities and not feel so entrapped.

Anyone who watches patients and clients in a waiting room is aware that few dogs, cats, or humans are comfortable. One study (Hernander, 2008) that

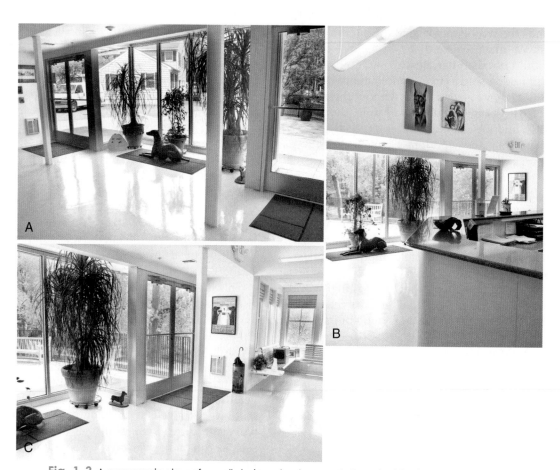

Fig. 1-3 A panoramic view of a well-designed entryway. **A,** Two double doors on each side of the reception area. **B,** A clear and global view of both doors and the waiting area. **C,** Wide open waiting area on one side of the reception area with plenty of windows. (Thanks to Hickory Veterinary Hospital, Plymouth Meeting, PA, for allowing photography.)

examined the role of waiting rooms in creating stress in the waiting room reported a number of conclusions that are important to consider if we are to be successful in creating behavior-centered practices.

- Although there was no difference between male and female dogs in the level of stress displayed, dogs accompanied by both a male and a female client were more stressed than dogs accompanied by only one client.
- Dogs who had recently been to the clinic had higher stress values than dogs who had not visited recently. This finding has profound implications for the invasive nature of some of the care provided by veterinary staff as perceived by the dogs.
- Dogs who stayed in waiting rooms that were not chaotic and had sufficient time to calm were less stressed than dogs who were moved quickly.
- Weighing dogs on the scale is much more stressful than sitting in the waiting room. This finding supports the idea that we should teach dogs how to be weighed and design scales and placement of them so that the dogs have some control over their participation in the process.

The busier the practice, the more crowded the waiting room can become. Urban veterinary practices may have limited space and should use schedules, exam rooms, and treatment areas sanely so that no patient has to sit in the waiting room with their human hanging onto them for dear life. If the client looks or sounds worried, so is the patient. Action must be taken to decrease patients' arousal levels immediately. Distressed patients often are calmer waiting in the car than they are in a busy and noisy waiting room. As an alternative, patients who are good with humans but might be afraid of other animals may be accommodated in the reception area through the creative use of barriers. Figure 1-4 shows a reception area with pass-through gates that can be closed, basically changing an open floor plan to one with concentric circles and visual barriers. Having such flexibility can be priceless.

We may do well to evaluate the stress level of each animal (and client), note these in the records, and use these to inform our handling procedures that day and to create a plan for reducing stress for handling and veterinary care in the future. The evaluation system used by Hernander (2008) is easy for any practice to implement and is presented in Table 1-3.

We can expand this scale to address many aspects of veterinary care and intervention. See Box 1-1 for the specific scales found in the separate questionnaire, "Scales to Evaluate Stress Level of Dogs at Veterinary Hospitals." A version of these scales for client use at the hospital or at home is available as a client handout ("Protocol for Assessing Pain and Stress in Dogs"). Similar questionnaires are available for cats and are discussed in Chapter 5.

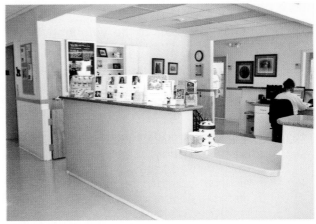

Fig. 1-4 Notice the gates on each side of the reception island. These can both be closed to create visual barriers for fearful animals. Also note the lower levels of the desk so that no one has to lean over a patient. Finally, notice that a visual inspection of the exam rooms is possible through the windows in doors. There is little chance of startling any animal if some common sense is used. In busy practices with fractious patients, windows and well-placed mirrors are safety measures. (Thanks to Hickory Veterinary Hospital, Plymouth Meeting, PA, for allowing photography.)

TABLE 1-3

Rating System for Assigning a "Stress Value" to Dogs in Veterinary Waiting Rooms

Stress Value	Dog's Behavior and Appearance
1	Calm, relaxed, seemingly unmoved
2	Alert, but calm and cooperative
3	Tensed, but cooperative, panting slowly, not very relaxed, easily led on lead
4	Obviously very tensed, anxious, shaking, whining, will not sit/lie down, panting intensely, difficult to maneuver on lead
5	Extremely stressed, barking/howling, tries to hide, needs to be lifted up or to be firmly forced when pulled by the lead (please do not do this)

Adapted from Hernander, 2008.

Flooring

The entryway may be perfect, but if dogs (cats are usually in carriers) slip on the floor on entry or cannot get purchase as they move across the room, you have lost the patient for that appointment. The patient knows that he or she has to go across that same floor to leave and will experience anticipatory anxiety throughout the appointment.

We install floors that we think are easy to clean and that will look clean. Most of these are too slick for animals with pads and claws, many of whom are already physically stiff with concern before entering the practice and who become more fearful when they

BOX 1-1

Scales to Evaluate Stress at the Veterinary Hospital (Based on Hernander, 2009; Döring et al., 2009)

Clinic Dog Stress Scale 1: Entry to the Clinic

Dog's behavior on entering the veterinary practice and in the waiting room (this section can be completed by a member of the reception staff). A total of 5 points is possible. Dogs with a score of 5 are distressed and need help. Dogs with zero scores are calm.

Stress Level	Dog's Behavior/Demeanor
0	Extremely friendly, outgoing, solicitous of attention
1	Calm, relaxed, seemingly unmoved
2	Alert, but calm and cooperative
3	Tense but cooperative, panting slowly, not very relaxed, but can still be easily led on lead
4	Very tense, anxious, may be shaking or whining, will not sit or lie down if exposed (may do so behind owner's legs), panting, difficult to maneuver on lead
5	Extremely stressed, barking/howling, tries to hide, needs to be lifted up or forced to move

Clinic Dog Stress Scale 2: Weighing the Dog

Dog's behavior on being weighed (this section can be completed by the veterinary nurse or technician who weighs the dog). A total of 5 points is possible. Dogs with a score of 5 are distressed and need help. Dogs with zero scores are calm.

Stress Level	Dog's Behavior/Demeanor
0	Extremely friendly, outgoing, solicitous of attention, eagerly gets onto scale
1	Calm, relaxed, seemingly unmoved, and walks easily onto scale and sits
2	Alert, but calm and cooperative, can get onto scale but not sit on it
3	Tense but cooperative, panting slowly, not very relaxed, but can still be easily led on lead, gets onto scale only with encouragement
4	Very tense, anxious, may be shaking or whining, will not sit or lie down if exposed (may do so behind owner's legs), panting, difficult to maneuver on lead, must be helped/encouraged to get on or stay on scale for 10 seconds to get reading
5	Extremely stressed, barking/howling, tries to hide, needs to be lifted up or forced to get onto or stay on scale for 10 seconds to get reading

Clinic Dog Stress Scale 3: Entering the Exam Room

Dog's behavior on being brought into the exam room (this can be completed by whomever guides the client and dog to the room). A total of 5 points is possible. Dogs with a score of 5 are distressed and need help. Dogs with zero scores are calm.

Stress Level	Dog's Behavior/Demeanor
0	Extremely friendly, outgoing, solicitous of attention
1	Calm, relaxed, seemingly unmoved
2	Alert, but calm and cooperative
3	Tense but cooperative, panting slowly, not very relaxed, but can still be easily led on lead
4	Very tense, anxious, may be shaking or whining, will not sit or lie down if exposed (may do so behind owner's legs), panting, difficult to maneuver on lead, avoids room
5	Extremely stressed, barking/howling, tries to hide, needs to be lifted up or forced to move into room

Clinic Dog Stress Scale 4: Examining the Dog

Dog's behavior on examination (this chart can be completed by the veterinary nurse or technician, in consultation with the veterinarian, if needed). This chart evaluates body regions that are involved in the stress response. Having as much information as possible will allow the veterinary staff to suggest interventions and to use the behaviors noted to assess improvement or debility. Rather than trying to remember if the dog is "worse" or "better" than at previous visits, this tick sheet allows the veterinary team to collect actual data and to use it to improve the quality of the dog's and client's experience. A total of 36 points is possible. Dogs with high scores are showing signs of stress and may be distressed. Dogs with low scores may be less distressed. Dogs with zero scores are calm.

BOX 1-1

Scales to Evaluate Stress at the Veterinary Hospital (Based on Hernander, 2009; Döring et al., 2009)—cont'd

Stress Level	Body Posture	Tail Posture	Ear Posture	Gaze	Pupils	Respirations	Lips	Activity*	Vocalization
0	Relaxed and moves on own	At rest for that breed or high	High and softly forward	Will look steadily at vet	Normal response to light	Normal–jaw relaxed	Relaxed	Flexible	None
1	Tense–can manipulate	Lower than at rest but not down	Moving back a bit	Looks only intermittently at vet	Normal to slight dilated	Normal–jaw tense	Firm	Inactive	Whine, cry
2	Rigid–hard to manipulate and a bit lower	Completely down	Fully back	Will not look at vet but scans room	Dilated, large amount of iris	Panting–dry	Licking lips	Paws flexed, may tremble	Whimper
3	Hunched–hard to see or examine belly and low posture	Tucked between legs	Ears back and down	Not scanning, looking steadily at distance or owner	Dilated, small amount of iris	Panting–dripping	Yawning and licking	Periodic trembling	Snarl, snap
4	Curled–completely withdrawn and belly maximally tucked	Clamped hard up to belly	As low and back as is possible	Staring fixedly and steadily at immediate fore-distance	Completely dilated–no iris	Profound panting, salivating, gasping	—	Uncontrollable trembling	Bite

Clinic Dog Stress Scale 5: Taking Blood from the Dog

This scale will be used only if blood is taken. The circumstance under which blood was taken should be noted below.

1. Laboratory evaluation: routine or because dog is ill (circle 1)
2. Tourniquet used? Y/N (circle 1)
3. Vein from which blood was taken:_____
4. Restraint level: (circle 1)
   a. None–dog sat still and butterfly catheter with digital pressure used
   b. Mild–vein held off manually
   c. Moderate–dog gently and minimally restrained physically while vein held off
   d. Severe–dog held down and restraint great

Stress Level	Body Posture	Respirations	Lips	Body Activity*	Forearm	Vocalization
0	Relaxed and moves on own	Normal–jaw relaxed	Relaxed	Flexible	Allows vet to pick up feet and forearm; forearm not stiff	None
1	Tense–can manipulate	Normal–jaw tense	Firm	Inactive	Allows vet to pick up feet and forearm; forearm stiff	Whine, cry
2	Rigid–hard to manipulate and a bit lower	Panting–dry	Licking lips	Paws flexed, may tremble	Allows touch but tries to withdraw forearm or body	Whimper
3	Hunched–hard to see or examine belly and low posture	Panting–dripping	Yawning and licking	Periodic trembling	Avoids all touch and needs leg held still	Snarl, snap
4	Curled–completely withdrawn and belly maximally tucked	Profound panting, salivating, gasping	—	Uncontrollable trembling	Avoids all touch and needs leg and body held still	Bite

BOX 1-1

Scales to Evaluate Stress at the Veterinary Hospital (Based on Hernander, 2009; Döring et al., 2009)—cont'd

Clinic Dog Stress Scale 6: Radiograph or Ultrasound of the Dog

Stress Level	Body Posture	Respirations	Lips	Body Activity*	Body	Vocalization
0	Relaxed and moves on own	Normal–jaw relaxed	Relaxed	Flexible	Allows vet to place as needed and remains loose and pliant	None
1	Tense–can manipulate	Normal–jaw tense	Firm	Inactive	Allows vet to place as needed but is stiff	Whine, cry
2	Rigid–hard to manipulate and a bit lower	Panting–dry	Licking lips	Paws flexed, may tremble	Allows vet to place by stretching out or manipulating areas and is rigid	Whimper
3	Hunched–hard to see or examine belly and low posture	Panting–dripping	Yawning and licking	Periodic trembling	Avoids manipulations by moving and stiffening, needs some restraint	Snarl, snap
4	Curled–completely withdrawn and belly maximally tucked	Profound panting, salivating, gasping	—	Uncontrollable trembling	Not possible to do without stretching and controlling head and legs	Bite

Clinic Dog Stress Scale 7: Trimming the Dog's Nails

Restraint level: (circle 1)

a. None–dog sat still and butterfly catheter with digital pressure used
b. Mild–vein held off manually
c. Moderate–dog gently and minimally restrained physically while vein held off
d. Severe–dog held down and restraint great

Stress Level	Body Posture	Respirations	Lips	Body Activity*	Feet/Legs	Vocalization
0	Relaxed and moves on own	Normal–jaw relaxed	Relaxed	Flexible	Allows vet to pick up feet and manipulate without resistance	None
1	Tense–can manipulate	Normal–jaw tense	Firm	Inactive	Allows vet to pick up feet, but stiff	Whine, cry
2	Rigid–hard to manipulate and a bit lower	Panting–dry	Licking lips	Paws flexed, may tremble	Allows touch to feet, but tries to withdraw them	Whimper
3	Hunched–hard to see or examine belly and low posture	Panting–dripping	Yawning and licking	Periodic trembling	Avoids all touch and needs foot/leg held	Snarl, snap
4	Curled–completely withdrawn and belly maximally tucked	Profound panting, salivating, gasping	—	Uncontrollable trembling	Avoids all touch and will not permit any access to feet without extreme restraint of body and feet	Bite

A discussion of the outcome of any assessment that is done should occur at the end of the appointment. This discussion provides an introduction to emphasizing quality of life and welfare issues and should flag extant problems that need redress. Done routinely, such screens lead to early intervention for most patients.

*Note if urinates, defecates, or releases anal sacs at any point since these behaviors can be associated with acute fear.

encounter a slick floor (Hydbring-Sandberg et al., 2004). Dogs and cats *can* learn to walk on such flooring, but they cannot do so if they are scared. We need to consider whether they *must* walk on such flooring and what decisions we can make to lessen their fear.

A better choice for humans and patients is rubberized flooring, which is widely available, attractive, and easily cleaned and maintained. The flooring in Figure 1-3 (and see Fig. 1-6 later) is Johnsonite ComforTech Cushioned Rubber Flooring (www.johnsonite.com). If renovation is not an option, rubberized mats that provide good traction can be used to create a trail from the door to check in to and through the exam room. If you do not know where you expect animals to walk in your practice, coat your shoes (or your pet's feet) in flour and go through your routine to determine where to put the mats. If pets or humans are going to stand in one place for any length of time, consider cushioning mats (www.gelpro.com).

Flooring in cages and runs also needs to be considered. Most high-quality cages are made of stainless steel and are loud, reflective, and slick. Yoga or other rubberized mats will make all the difference in how much control the patient has over movement and will help insulate the patient from concussive sounds and decrease the reflectivity of the cage environment. For older animals, cushioned gel mats provide much needed protection from hard surfaces and can be easily cleaned. All of these factors will contribute to making the patient calmer.

Runs are often made of cement, epoxy flooring, tile, or some version of a commercially slatted floor. Epoxy flooring can be designed to have excellent traction and still be easily cleaned. Epoxy flooring is still hard, and some padded bedding or flooring will be preferred by most patients.

Tile flooring is extremely hard on feet and joints when dry and is slick when wet. If the patient is already unstable or worried, the slickness of tile will increase his or her anxiety.

No dogs bear weight well on commercially available slatted floors because they force an unnatural weight distribution on various and shifting parts of the feet. Depending on the size of the slats or holes, smaller dogs can catch claws, toes, feet, or legs in this flooring. As shown in Figure 1-5, dogs are reluctant to bear weight fully on such surfaces if they have other choices. If the dog is a puppy mill dog or a rescue dog that has

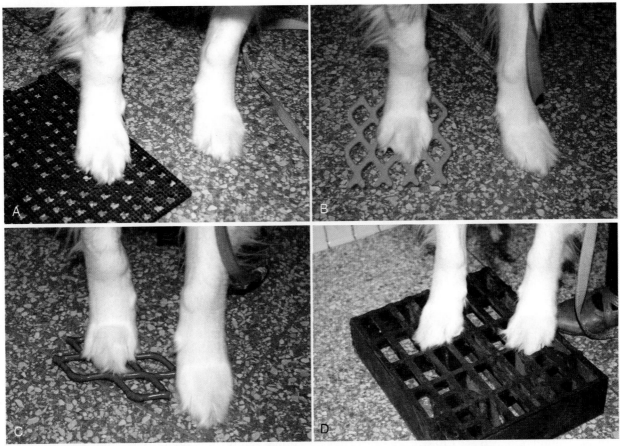

Fig. 1-5 A-D, Non-solid floors affect stability and hence anxiety and the ability to have control over normal behaviors in dogs. The dog used in these photos is young, athletic, agile, extremely compliant, healthy, and pain-free, and he still doesn't bear weight well on any of these non-solid floors. Such findings should inform decisions about cage and run flooring.

spent a lot of time in shelters that uses such flooring, the flooring may bring back extremely scary memories, and the dog will be distressed the entire time he or she is constrained to be on such flooring. Rubber/yoga/gel mats are a far better choice for cage flooring. All of these can be easily washed, and if patients dig in or chew on the lighter yoga mats, there are industrial grade rubber mats that resist wear.

All runs should be *dried and aired* before returning patients to them. Please understand the following:

- *Dogs and cats ask questions and work for information. Their most powerful currency is accurate and clear information.*
- Bleach and other disinfectants aerosolize and can *kill olfactory neurons.*
- Anxiety is associated with incomplete or uncertain information.
- Dogs get much of their information about the physical and social environments through olfaction. Regeneration of olfactory neurons takes days.
- If the dog is compromised in his or her information-gathering ability because of a stay at the vet's, he or she will learn that such stays are risky and should be avoided.

Scale

Even if we manage to get the patient in the door and to the reception area without anxiety, weighing the patient can be an anxiety-producing event. Scales are often placed in corners so that they are away from heavily trafficked areas. This makes sense only from the human viewpoint: from the dog's or cat's viewpoint, that scale is a nightmare. *Patients can feel trapped in a corner on a device that makes them feel insecure and without control.*

A better choice is a walk-through scale (the patient gets on at one end and leaves at the other) that is flush with the floor. In fact, in a renovation or new construction, these scales can be built with the non-slip rubber flooring over them (Fig. 1-6). The scale will still have some movement, but now patients have flooring that makes them stable and they are not trapped in a corner.

If the scale is always associated with some signal (a bell or a word) and the patient's entry onto the scale is followed by loads of praise and a tiny, high-value treat (e.g., a sliver of dried chicken, beef, fish, or shrimp), dogs can easily be taught to walk onto the scale and stand still without experiencing anxiety. To make this an even easier and more valuable experience, teach the patient to take a deep breath, which both relaxes the patient and keeps him or her still (see the foundation protocol, "Protocol for Teaching Your Dog to Take a Deep Breath and Use Other Biofeedback Methods as Part of Relaxation"). If you start to teach patients this protocol *the first time you see them*, regardless of age, you will have a tool that will help calm your patients for the rest of their lives.

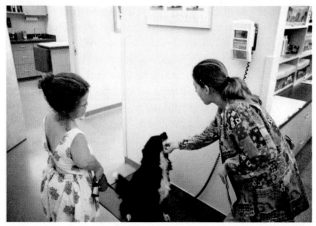

Fig. 1-6 This is an example of a digital walk-through scale that is flush with the floor and fitted with a non-slip surface. The flooring in this practice is all rubberized so that dogs and cats have a decreased chance of slipping. Dogs and cats still must learn how to use this scale because it moves a bit, but this learning is faster because they are calmer and more confident in their actions. (Photo courtesy of Dr. Steven Brammeier.)

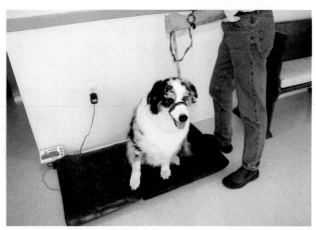

Fig. 1-7 A full-sized yoga mat was folded and simply placed over the scale so that the dog would not slip. This dog is extremely calm and willingly offered to sit. He is accustomed to being asked to go to a mat, and here he translated that to mean sit on the mat on the scale. The color choice was intentional because dogs can see blue. (Thanks to Hickory Veterinary Hospital, Plymouth Meeting, PA, for allowing photography.)

If you are using a digital scale—and you should be because it is quicker and less stressful for the patient—and you have to spend more than a few seconds "guessing" the patient's weight, your patient is not sitting or standing still, probably because of uncertainty or distress. If you have a walk-through digital scale, but it is not built into the floor, consider using a rubberized or yoga mat to cover it. Make the mat greenish yellow or blue, colors dogs can see, and teach your patients to "go to the mat" (many dogs will know this if they have done agility or worked with humane and forward-thinking trainers) and to associate the secure feeling of standing on an absolutely non-slip surface with praise and a reward the dog values (Fig. 1-7).

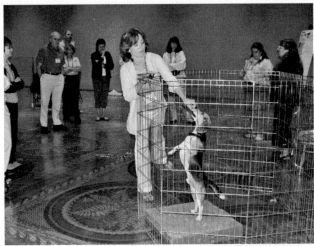

Fig. 1-8 As part of a laboratory for veterinarians on teaching patients to offer body parts, dogs were placed in X-pens to discourage the vets from forcing them to do anything (and the vets were to pretend that the beagles were exotic zoo animals who could mangle them if scared or hurt), and each group was assigned a task to accomplish. In this task, the blue box is a scale that has been covered with a non-slip pad. Because this dog never stops moving, the veterinarian realized that she could take advantage of his behaviors to have him stand on his back legs on the scale for treats. Someone else has to read the scale, but the weighing process was not traumatic for the dog (or the veterinarian).

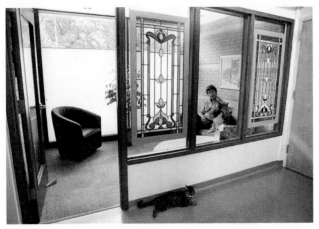

Fig. 1-9 This separate room can be used for many purposes. It has a comfortable and homey atmosphere, which may help some distressed patients and clients to be calm. (Photo courtesy of Dr. Steven Brammeier.)

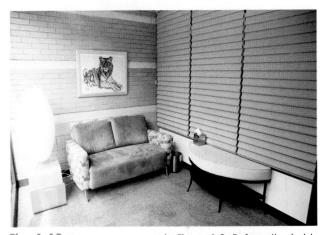

Fig. 1-10 The same room as in Figure 1-3, *B*, from the inside with the blinds drawn for privacy or for calming a fractious patient. (Photo courtesy of Dr. Steven Brammeier.)

For some dogs, sitting on a scale calmly is just not in their nature. This does not mean that they cannot learn to offer a behavior that allows you to weigh them (Fig. 1-8).

Finally, there are data supporting the idea that predictable and congruent sequences can minimize stress. If the dog is weighed after registration, but before sitting down to wait to be seen, the dog is less stressed than if he or she is taken to the waiting area and then recalled to be weighed (Hernander, 2008).

Waiting Area

With digitization, computerization of practices, and hand-held devices, there is no longer a real need for people to remain in a formal waiting area to check in or provide registration information if doing so is stressful for them or their pet. Paperless registration and history entry requires the time of a staff member up-front but also means you can ask for more information when the client is standing in front of you and prevent errors or incomplete information from entering your system. This saves the veterinarian time by ensuring that he or she does not have to sort through a paper record. It also ensures that everyone has access to the same and correctable information.

The smart use of a highly trained front desk staff and well-trained licensed/certified/registered veterinary technicians/nurses can be priceless. If you use paperless registration and history taking, the front desk staff can take and check all demographic and contact information, and the technician/nurse can review and enter history. The latter is best done in an exam room without distractions, even if the former is done in a waiting area.

Waiting areas are best if they are spacious and flexible. Judicious use of wheeled dividers (which may also be house plants) can separate fractious or scared animals from animals that are over-enthusiastic. Good designs will provide waiting areas with protected areas that do not make animals feel trapped.

Separate waiting rooms for cats may be beneficial for cats who live indoors without dogs. These areas can have glass and blinds so that everyone can monitor social activity from a distance (Figs. 1-9 and 1-10).

Giving the clients some control over where they sit and whom their pets might meet immediately lessens their anxiety. Dogs should be able to sit without being

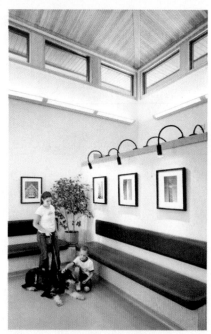

Fig. 1-11 This lobby is sufficiently large and airy that even large dogs can be 1 to 1.5 body lengths from other patients. This entire hospital uses rubberized, non-slip flooring. (Photo courtesy of Dr. Steven Brammeier.)

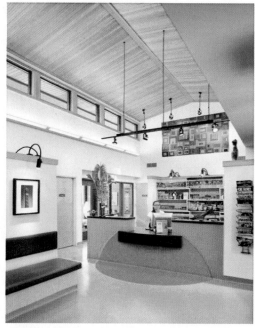

Fig. 1-12 This reception desk is not curved, but the practice has created space and the illusion of even more space in different ways. The desk is lowered so that no one hangs over the edge to see patients. The entire back side is open, providing another option for moving with a fractious pet. The open section of the reception area overlooks the separate room shown above, which also has windows and blinds, all of which can help manage fractious animals. This practice has skylights to provide natural light whenever possible. (Photo courtesy of Dr. Steven Brammeier.)

molested or vocally threatened by other dogs. This means that the minimum distance between patients should be 1 to 1.5 body lengths of the larger patient (Fig. 1-11).

If the waiting area does not have this amount of space, more attention can be paid to scheduling appointments so that wait times are minimized. Exam and conference rooms can be used to house fractious or concerned patients, or such patients can wait in the car.

If you know that you are going to see patients who can make everyone's life more complex—even if it is because they are just petrified—please consider asking the client to schedule a visit for the first or last appointment of the day. If your clients are local and can choose the last appointment, offer to call them as soon as the hospital/waiting area/exam area is quiet and when you know that you are within 5 minutes of being able to see them.

Waiting is painful for scared dogs and cats. Use of medication (e.g., benzodiazepines such as alprazolam) and behavior modification to teach dogs and cats to go to the vet is covered in Chapters 3 and 10.

A curved or circular reception desk that also has relatively low walls and multiple entryways can prevent the staff from leaning out and over the desk to look at the patient, which can be threatening to the patient, and can allow the staff to come around the divider quickly to greet clients and patients (Fig. 1-12). The curvature of the desk can prevent dogs who are closer together than desired from seeing each other.

The staff members in the reception area are primarily responsible for managing traffic flow and keeping everyone safe while they wait. *They should not answer phones.* In fact, phones and phone conversations are so disruptive and potentially upsetting for the patients that they should occur elsewhere, in a dedicated room that meets staff member needs, behind a closed door.

A rounded or circular waiting area also can facilitate flow-through traffic for an appointment so that you do not have clients and patients who have just completed their appointment mingling with those who are waiting for appointments. Having clients come in the front door and leave through a side or back door can also facilitate flow-through traffic. These practices make interactions between clients and patients safer (especially if contagious diseases are concerns), prevent congestion, keep noise and confusion levels lower, and respect patient privacy.

Discussion and payment of bills should be done in private. Anything that stresses the client will stress the patient as well as other clients and patients within earshot. If it is not possible to have such private discussions and meet the behavioral needs of the patients, the patients should wait in the car or the exam room. A paperless system would let the person responsible for processing payments come to the exam room, if needed, ensuring efficient use of time and space, privacy, and the least distressed situation possible for the patient and client.

Exam Room

Space Concerns

Exam rooms, similar to waiting areas, should be large. You will want to be able to fit any sized dog, at least two adults and two children (the average client family), and at least one veterinarian and one technician, plus any equipment you might need, into the room in a way that everyone still has their own personal space. Remember, the goal is to reduce stress, anxiety, and uncertainty for the patient. If the humans are crowded and socially uncomfortable, the dog or cat will be worried.

Everyone should be able to sit down. Dogs and cats are less reactive when sitting and so are humans. We tend to be physically more comfortable and feel less rushed if sitting. If one wishes to have an exam table in the room, it should be one that folds to provide extra floor space when needed, is movable, or is able to serve another function (e.g., acting as a desk for records and medications) (Fig. 1-13).

Issues Pertaining to Exam Tables

A patient should not be tied to an exam table unless the patient is fully anesthetized and this is for everyone's safety and/or surgical access. Such entrapment is traumatic to the patient and the client.

If patients are expected to be placed on an exam table that moves, they should be taught to sit calmly on it in a manner over which they have some control (Fig. 1-14). The use of a mat to which the patient is positively conditioned for an appointment can be a boon. Most cats and dogs can be taught to go to a mat, sit, and take a deep breath for a reward. Any good, certified/credentialed positive trainer who participates in modern continuing education can teach staff members and clients how to teach, condition, and reward this behavioral sequence.

Most exams of cats are best conducted in the client's or veterinarian's lap, for calm cats, and in the cat carrier for concerned cats (Anseeuw et al., 2006) (Fig. 1-15). Use of the exam table should be reserved for cats that have been conditioned to find this surface non-scary and comforting. If we condition cats from the time they are kittens to offer body parts for examination, including offering limbs and their neck for venipuncture (Fig. 1-16) (Seksel, 2001), we will ensure that these kittens grow into cats who will receive excellent veterinary care—and more accurate laboratory assessments—throughout their lives. When cats and dogs are fractious, scared, or embarrassing and difficult for the clients, veterinary care is delayed or avoided. This means that the patients are seen only when they are sicker and the situation is potentially tragic. Situations that delay care for cats are completely preventable.

The tendency is to place dogs automatically on exam tables, but unless the dog is routinely accustomed to

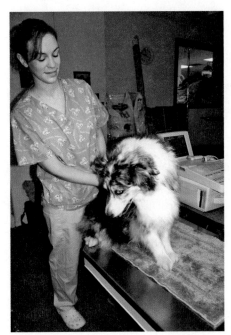

Fig. 1-14 This dog must undergo ultrasound thyroidal evaluation every 3 months. She has been taught to get onto her blue mat on the table, after which her collars and lead are removed and the table raised. The veterinary technician is standing behind the dog to ensure that she doesn't slip as the table moves. Notice that the dog is calm, rather than rigid and stressed. The technician is also calm. This dog has control over her own behavior. In fact, she is not being restrained. (Thanks to Veterinary Specialty Center of Delaware, New Castle, DE, for permitting photography.)

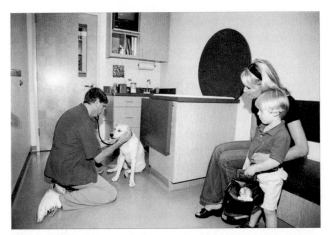

Fig. 1-13 An example of an exam room with flexible space. Note that the table is collapsed here to provide more floor space and to allow a large dog to be examined where he is comfortable. (Photo courtesy of Dr. Steven Brammeier.)

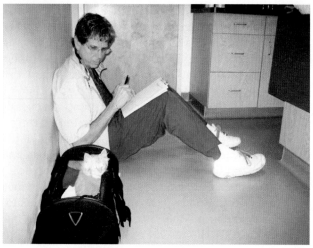

Fig. 1-15 Much of an exam can be done on a cat who is in his cat carrier. Note that this carrier has a zip top that provides easy access for humans but still allows the cat to "hide." (Photo courtesy of Dr. Steven Brammeier.)

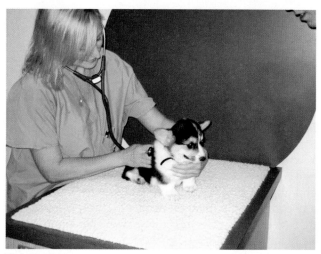

Fig. 1-17 This corgi pup is being examined without any serious restraint on a mat that provides him with traction. As he learns to undergo exams he will be calmer, and this is important because corgis are often carried or placed on tables for exams. (Photo courtesy of Dr. Steven Brammeier.)

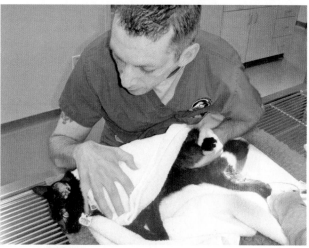

Fig. 1-16 Cats who must undergo treatment or examination on a table may be better off if there is a pad that provides warmth and traction (the red mat here) and when covered in a thick towel that allows gentle support of the cat while examining one body part at a time. The towel can also be used to cover the cat's head if this calms the cat. Here, a cat who has become accustomed to the mat/towel relaxed approach is having a blood sample taken using a butterfly catheter. Notice the lack of restraint and how calm the cat is. (Photo courtesy of Dr. Steven Brammeier.)

this (e.g., for grooming or showing), just the act of placing the dog on the table can be provocative. Some outmoded ideas for why dogs should be placed on tables include the false and dangerous idea that you do so to "dominate" the dog. We work best with dogs when we show them that we are humane partners. "Domination" and "dominance" have no role in our care of patients (American Veterinary Society of Animal Behavior [AVSAB] Dominance Position Statement: www.avsabonline.org/avsabonline/images/stories/

Position_Statements/dominance%20statement.pdf; Dog Welfare Campaign position statement: www.dogwelfarecampaign.org/why-not-dominance.php). There are few things more dangerous than having an unruly, large, inappropriately behaved dog on a table, in a position where he is unstable and can slip and where his face is level with yours.

There are modern, sane alternatives. As is true with cats, if you teach dogs, beginning when they are puppies, to offer body parts for examination and venipuncture, you will have less stressful exams, with more accurate laboratory assessments (Fig. 1-17). The stress for the patients, clients, and staff will be less, and you will see that dog at the first sign of any illness or concern.

If you think you may wish to put a dog on a table, help the client teach the dog to cooperate. Small dogs who are often picked up and carried may be accustomed to tables. If a blanket or mat is put down for them, they can learn to offer their teeth, belly, head, hind end, and forelegs (Fig. 1-18). For large dogs, consider teaching them to get up on the table on their own. A mat can be placed on the table, a chair or a set of steps brought to the table, and the dog can be taught to climb onto the table and sit on the mat for a single request (e.g., "table"). These are behaviors that can and should be practiced at home by the client.

Alternatively, and more preferably, large dogs can be examined while everyone is sitting. Fractious dogs often allow examination of one part of their body at a time if no one restrains them. Restraint is terrifying for most dogs with behavioral problems and can panic a problematic dog, rendering him or her problematic in veterinary contexts. Lack of control, especially in a context for which no understanding is possible, is a

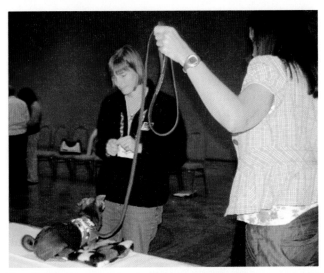

Fig. 1-18 This small dog has been conditioned to use a small mat for on-table exams. Here he is participating in a laboratory for veterinarians and is sitting on his mat so that he can be examined. Notice that the client is just keeping the lead out of the way. The lead is loose, and the dog is unrestrained.

profound stressor and is viewed as entrapment by many individuals.

Regardless of whether the dog is being examined on the floor or on a table, sitting on benches, chairs, the table, or stools relaxes everyone and ratchets down the dog's reactivity. For this strategy to work, sufficient space is needed so that the dog is not crowded and anyone who needs to do so can move. The practice of veterinary medicine is physically challenging. Newer, humane techniques recommended to promote behavioral well-being for our patients are also kinder to our bodies.

If the floor in the practice is not rubberized, consider the use of rubber or non-skid mats in the exam room, on the floor or on a table. Such mats may be especially helpful during venipuncture.

Clients can and should be encouraged to bring their own mats to use for their pet's exam.

- For lightweight cats, mats can be made of almost anything.
- For heavy cats who might slip and almost all dogs, mats should be rubber, have a rubberized backing, or be yoga mats.
- If clients bring their own mats, they can take them home and be responsible for washing them.
- Clients can also practice having the dog sit and offer body parts while he or she is sitting on the mat, making the next visit easier.
- If the records are flagged to indicate that a client has a mat, when the appointment is confirmed the client can be reminded to bring the mat and practice a bit before the appointment.
- Veterinarians can profit by taking advantage of clearance sales for out-of-style colors of rubber-backed

bath mats and yoga mats. The mats can be placed in bins in the waiting room and each exam room with a sign that informs clients about the benefits to teaching pets to use mats in veterinary care. An accompanying photo will sell the mat and the concept.

Once veterinarians stop struggling with patients, they often find that their staff has more time and less stress. *There are many hidden costs of behavioral struggles; only some of them are financial.*

Layout

Rooms should be designed for flexibility and movement. All of the tools the veterinarian will need—sinks, otoscopes, clippers, refrigerators, cupboards with syringes, swabs, et cetera—should be on one side of the room to decrease the number of times anyone has to step over or around the patients.

Lighting, Noise, and Busy-ness

Patients become aroused by overly bright, overly noisy, and overly busy exam rooms. Lighting should be as natural as possible. Large, preferably floor-to-ceiling, windows should be in each room. Patients are calmer and can have another focus when they can see the outside world. Fluorescent light is exhausting for humans who are constrained to work in it. Full-spectrum lighting can be easier on the eyes of the staff and patients, and flexible, variable intensity lighting should be available as needed. Such a plan allows patients to operate within more normal ambient light levels. For some cats, lowering the room lights may help them to be calmer. A small, targeted light can be used to examine their body parts as needed.

Rubberized floors provide traction, and they make the floor quieter. Hospital environments are noisy—sinks are metallic, tables are metallic, equipment is noisy, and cement walls reflect sound. Good materials to insulate walls and ceiling acoustically are available and can be designed into any new construction or retrofitted into older construction. Quiet environments allow the staff to lower their voices. This allows the patient to focus on the calm delivery of care without monitoring the auditory environment for sounds that signal threats and risk.

Planning for the design of the exam room and the procedures to be done should include the constraint of minimizing the numbers of entries and exits once the patient is in the room. For all patients, but especially for patients with behavioral concerns, busy-ness and movement signal potential risk and alert the patient to be watchful for threats. Quieter, calm appointments promote responses associated with decreased risk and need to assess it.

Finally, exam rooms should have windows and blinds in them. Being able to see into what one is walking minimizes risk. Blinds provide privacy and signals.

WITH WHAT CAN WE REPLACE RESTRAINT?

Most head collars can be better than muzzles for a veterinary exam. When used appropriately and by someone who is trained to monitor canine behaviors, head collars can prevent bites and control the dog's activity and direction (Fig. 1-19).

A combination of a good head collar and a good harness—using two leads—can position most dogs so that they are relatively unstressed, and not restrained or crowded by humans (Figs. 1-20 and 1-21) (see the "Tools That May Help or Hurt" section in Chapter 3).

Calm and Behavior-Centered Approaches to Vaccinations and Blood Samples

Calm and behavior-centered approaches can also be used to vaccinate a fractious animal. *Vaccinations are not emergencies,* so consider the vaccination an opportunity to work with the client to teach the patient how to prepare and receive veterinary care by offering calm behaviors and needed body parts. If the clients know the region on the dog or cat where the vaccine will be given (there are now protocols for this), they can teach the dog or cat to offer that area and expect pressure there. If the patient learns to tolerate the needed posture and pressure while at home receiving a treat, teaching the patient to do so at the veterinary hospital is not difficult. A good certified trainer who has had her or his knowledge assessed in a practical setting (www.ccpdt.org) can show clients how to condition dogs to the touching involved in vaccinations. A ball-point pen that retracts can be a good stand-in for a needle (Fig. 1-22).

The larger the gauge needle, the greater the probability of hitting a sensory nerve. The smaller the patient, the larger any gauge needle appears and feels. This is

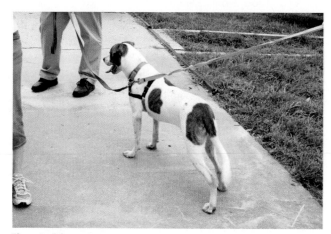

Fig. 1-20 This dog has exhibited some aggression to some approaching humans. For his exam, he was fitted with a front-control harness, which is clipped to his collar, and two leads, also clipped to the front. One person holds each lead, which allows a safer approach and exam, and no one has to restrain the dog physically, especially if he is being offered treats, as part of a learned behavioral sequence of "look at me" and "breathe" (see also Fig. 1-21).

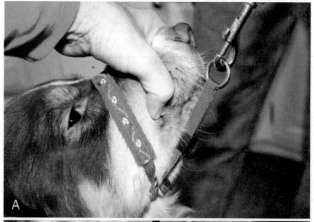

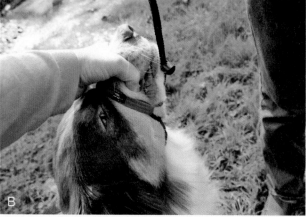

Fig. 1-19 Use of a head collar (**A**, a Gentle leader; **B**, a Black-dog Training Halter) to close a dog's mouth sufficiently tightly that he cannot open his mouth and bite. If someone who knows what they are doing and is humane is controlling the lead, head collars can help make veterinary exams calmer and safer and do both of these things while not engendering fear and anxiety in dogs.

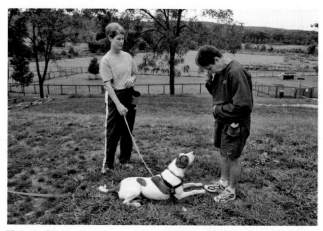

Fig. 1-21 This dog has been taught to lie down, take a deep breath, and look at the person giving the instructions for treats. Note the two leads, which will prevent lunging.

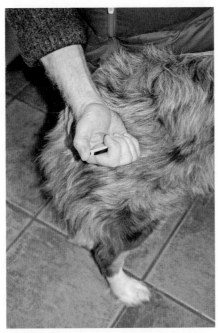

Fig. 1-22 Linus, a young Australian shepherd with some brain damage from his puppy mill past, is being "vaccinated" with a retractable ballpoint pen. Clients are happy to learn how to desensitize their dogs to needle-sticks. Here, someone could have been giving Linus treats as a reward for calm behavior, but he has done this so often, he was nonplussed.

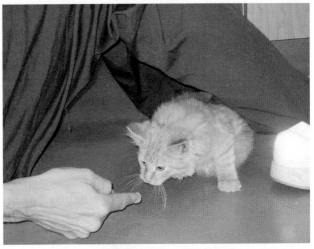

Fig. 1-23 Giving a kitten a treat (Vegemite on a finger) after an exam. (Photo courtesy of Dr. Steven Brammeier.)

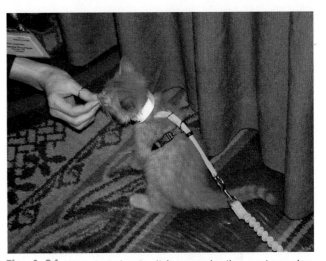

Fig. 1-24 Kitten learning to sit for examination and vaccination for a treat.

the logic behind using the smallest gauge needle possible to vaccinate patients. Some puppies/kittens do best with a 27-gauge needle. No animal should be vaccinated with larger than a 22-gauge or 23-gauge needle if trauma (and its effect on future time spent in procedures) matters. Sharpness matters: do not use the same needle to draw up the vaccine that is used to vaccinate the cat or dog; put a new needle on the syringe. The cost of this is less than a penny.

All patients being vaccinated should be otherwise engaged (e.g., playing with a tug toy, licking peanut butter, Marmite, or Vegemite off a finger, spoon, or exam table), calm, and happy and already should have had the repeated experience of having their skin gently manipulated and pinched until there is no longer even a startle from which to recover. In 20 to 30 minutes, you can teach most patients who have not had a bad experience to be calm during and quickly recover from vaccinations and needle-sticks. As soon as the vaccine is deposited, the area should be massaged while the patient is having a delicious treat, a good massage, a game of tug—anything that rewards him or her for allowing vaccination (Figs. 1-23 and 1-24).

Although this approach to vaccination is overly conservative, patients who cringe or cry at vaccinations are suffering more behaviorally than physically and are at risk of being damaged by veterinary manipulations. If we want patients to be partners in their care, we want their experiences to be as positive as possible. We

should err on the side of minimizing any potential distress because it is cheap and easy to do and may have a huge benefit for us (and our patients).

Consider that clients who think that their veterinary team is compassionate and empathic will trust them more and allow diagnostic and therapeutic intervention as recommended. Veterinarians who are resistant to changing any protocol that is potentially beneficial to the client and patient should query their resistance because it may flag a more global lack of flexibility in suggesting other behavioral solutions.

There are two reasons that most dogs are subjected to some kind of restraint for venipuncture:
1. We are taught to do this.
2. If you pick up one leg and the surface is not rubberized, the dog slips.

Instead, if we are using a head collar or have taught the dog to offer body parts, we can ask the dog to sit on a

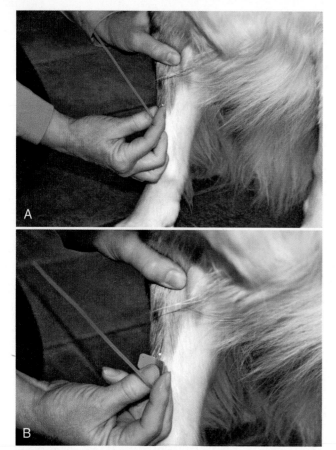

Fig. 1-25 A and **B,** A completely unrestrained dog has been taught to sit, stay, and take a deep breath, and the technique of using one finger to raise a vein and then using a butterfly catheter for venipuncture (the syringe to which the catheter is attached is being held out of the way for the photo) is shown. The leg is moistened first. These are impressive photos because this is a dog who has learned to panic when restrained—no restraint, no panic. The dog was rewarded with a treat after the procedure but not during it. When he was learning to do this, he was rewarded throughout the procedure.

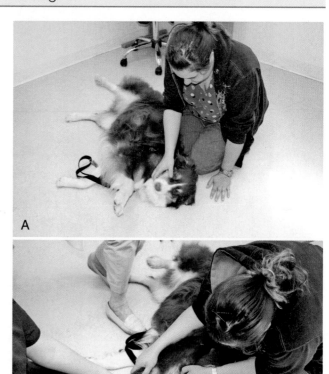

Fig. 1-26 A, A dog who has been trained to lie down and offer body parts for examination. The veterinary technician is petting him, not restraining him. The harness that this dog can be seen wearing is a Wiggles Wags and Whiskers New Freedom Harness. **B,** The same dog after venipuncture using a 21-gauge butterfly catheter. Notice how relaxed the staff and dog are. The veterinary technician is just holding off the vein after venipuncture. In the video taken at the same time the still photos were taken, one of the veterinary technicians noted that she wanted to show the video to her dog so that he'd get the idea!

mat and use a butterfly catheter and a cephalic vein *without* picking up the dog's front leg. A 21-gauge needle and catheter are adequate to get a good sample from a dog or a cat (Gilor and Gilor, 2011). The dog's blood pressure will help us obtain the sample quickly, he will not slip, he will not be off balance because one leg has been grasped, and he will be calm enough to take a treat offered while he is being stuck (Figs. 1-25 and 1-26).

If it is important to get a blood sample before a dog has been conditioned to offer his leg, consider getting the sample from the hind leg as the dog is moving through a door toward something (the outdoors) or someone (his person) that makes him calmer. By using a butterfly catheter and digital pressure, blood samples are extremely easy to obtain on standing, unrestrained or minimally restrained dogs, and the samples are excellent quality (Fig. 1-27). Samples can be drawn directly into the tube (Fig. 1-28). As practices move

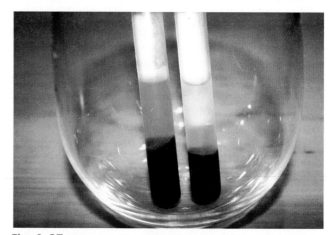

Fig. 1-27 These two blood samples were taking using different techniques. The sample on the left was taken with a 22-gauge needle and syringe with some restraint and the leg held off. The sample on the right was taken with a 23-gauge butterfly catheter from an unrestrained dog who was standing with hand-only digital pressure applied to her cephalic vein.

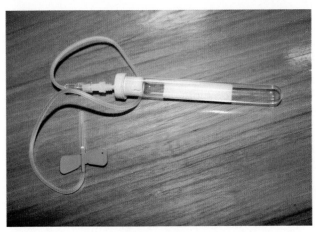

Fig. 1-28 Butterfly catheter with adapter for direct transfer of blood to the tube.

from restraint to a paradigm involving more cooperative patient care, staff may benefit from examples of lower stress handling (Yin, 2009).

Using little to no restraint requires that someone trustworthy is holding the lead and that everything possible has been done to minimize risk and quiet the environment. Samples that are easily obtained will be better quality. Hemolyzed samples adversely affect assays of bile acids, complete blood counts (CBCs) (including hemoglobin determinations), biochemistry, and coagulation tests. Coagulation test results can be profoundly affected by venipuncture technique (Gilor and Gilor, 2011).

Venous stasis is an important and confounding issue for coagulation testing that is highly sensitive to handling of the patient and the sample (Lippi et al., 2006). Although we lack complete validation for all sample values across all species for this technique in veterinary medicine, of 43 hematological/clinical chemistry parameters measured in humans, where samples obtained from needles and butterfly catheters were compared, only serum sodium and white cell and platelet count differed slightly, but significantly (Lippi et al., 2005).

Finally, behavioral stress plays a role in the results of laboratory evaluations. Stress has a significant effect on CBC results (the "stress leukogram": neutrophilia, monocytosis, lymphopenia, eosinopenia) and on glucose concentrations, including glucose concentrations in feline urine (Gilor and Gilor, 2011). If we wish to provide the best care for our patients, these are not trivial concerns.

What About Patients Who Previously Have Been Painful for Routine Care?

Some patients have learned that vaccinations, venipuncture, routine anal sac care, et cetera, hurt. Learned pain can lead to fear and anxiety (see Chapter 10). Once

the patient learns to be fearful, we must manage both the pain and the patient's perception of it, and the anticipatory anxiety that precedes the procedure and renders the patient more sensitive to pain. For some patients, clonidine or small amounts of benzodiazepines (e.g., alprazolam, lorazepam) given 1 to 2 times starting an hour or two before the visit may relieve the anticipatory anxiety (see Chapter 10). More fearful patients who respond to benzodiazepines or to clonidine may do best to start the medication 2 to 3 days before the visit, every 12 hours, possibly with an additional dose an hour before the appointment. For some patients, some amount of sedation may be desirable for which trazodone or dexdormitor may be helpful. Preventative pharmacological intervention seeks to address the anxiety caused by the appointment. If a benzodiazepine is used, some patients may experience less pain associated with the actual procedure. Topical lidocaine (5%) remains an underused strategy to help address and prevent pain directly. Clients can practice rubbing a thick ointment or cream onto the area of the body where the painful stimulus occurs (e.g., the leg used for venipuncture, the muscle where the vaccination is given, and the anal and perianal area manipulation for anal sac expression). By practicing manipulation, addressing the local pain associated with the stimulus and preventing and/or redressing associated anxiety, all patients can learn that there is nothing to fear at a veterinary hospital, and so can become easier to treat and more willing to display their true physical and behavioral signs.

The Wait

As noted earlier, if the appointment process is well planned, any wait for care will be short. That said, bathrooms should be big enough to include the patient comfortably. They should be situated in a manner that indicates whether a dog or cat is in the bathroom with the client and in an area where the door can swing widely and outward so as not to trap a dog. Signs can be wonderful: "Bathroom occupied by a human and a worried pet—please wait away from the door." If you do not think that your clients can adequately interpret the word "away," put a giant yellow spot on the floor at the distance you'd advise them to retreat. The sign would then read, "Bathroom occupied by a human and a worried pet—please wait no closer than the yellow dot."

No situation is always perfect. Waiting will happen. By providing a beverage area (tea, coffee, water) that is away from where animals are sitting, clients can calmly get a drink before returning to their pet. Any pet who has to wait for any amount of time or who will have a longer appointment (such as a behavior appointment) should be given a filled water dish. These are small things but make a huge difference in the quality of the veterinary experience for the patient and client. If clients and pets want to come to your practice, it's good for business, but it's even better for the welfare of the pets and the quality of medicine you are able to practice.

OVERALL HOSPITAL SENSORY EXPERIENCE—LIGHTING, NOISE, AND SMELLS

Dogs and cats see the world in different shades and spectra, hear a wider frequency range of sounds, and have more acute olfactory capabilities than humans. Unless we consider these attributes, the places where we care for canine and feline patients may not be meeting their needs.

Lighting

Natural light is as important to the people working at and visiting veterinary hospitals as it is to the patients. Veterinary staff work long hours, and high reflective light conditions can be stressful for staff and patients.

Cats have a minimum threshold for light detection that is 6 times lower than that for humans; dogs may do even better in dim light (Gunter, 1951; Miller and Murphy, 1995). In bright light, however, dogs have less acute vision than humans. Rhodopsin in dogs has a peak sensitivity to wavelengths of 506 to 510 nm and requires more than 1 hour to regenerate completely following exposure to bright light. Think about how compromised our patients may be with respect to information gathering if they are exposed to the glare of the lights of most veterinary practices!

Canine vision is exquisitely sensitive to movement, and dogs can recognize an object that is moving almost twice as well as when the same object is still. This could be one reason why dogs especially are more concerned when humans stand still and look at them than when some identifying movements are made.

The extent to which dogs experience binocular vision is less than for humans and depends on dog breed and head shape. Distribution of retinal neurons is not independent of nose length (McGreevy et al., 2004), factors we seldom consider when working with and around dogs.

Skylights, windows with vertical blinds, softer or full-spectrum light, and rheostats that can dim regional areas of any room will calm humans and animals. Bright overhead fluorescent lighting does not provide adequate lighting for tasks requiring close examination, so everyone is better served by flexible lighting that is as natural as possible, combined with ergonomically designed desk, table, exam, and work lights that provide brightness without creating eyestrain.

Blue-hued dimmer lights (dogs can see blue/violet and yellow/green), floor-level lighting, recessed lighting, or movement-triggered ambient lighting can save money and provide calm lighting conditions for patients who are kenneled, hospitalized, or recovering from surgery. Animals that are caged or kenneled for more than a few hours should have a window so that they can focus on more than their current condition. In the rare case of a dog or cat who is distressed by a window, it can be covered.

Noise

The extent to which noise is a concern for cats and dogs is seldom addressed. In addition, all of our interventions to render hospitals cleaner and more efficient enhance the noise level we and our patients experience. All one need do is observe the number of noise reflective surfaces to understand that noise—especially for species with enhanced acuity—is potentially damaging to patient care.

Dogs can detect frequencies of sound from 40 Hz to 50 kHz, whereas 20 kHz is the upper frequency range for humans. Dogs are most sensitive to sounds with frequencies in the 0.5- to 16-kHz range. Within this range, their sensitivity threshold can be *24 dB less than that for humans* (see Fay, 1988, for a more detailed discussion).

If the phones are behind closed doors, a major source of disruptive noise is removed. Rubberized floors and sound-absorbing walls and ceilings can further muffle sounds that might alert or distress patients. Surgery suites, treatment rooms, and recovery suites can be noisy places because of the number of metal surfaces. Calm human conversation occurs best at levels that do not exceed 75 dB, and most human conversations occur at 60 dB. Battery-operated, hand-held decibel meters are inexpensive (Extech Instruments Sound Level Meter; www.extech.com) and should be used to determine when environmental noise is interfering with patient well-being, an issue that likely should receive considerably more attention than it has in the past given the increasing recognition of the role noise reactivity plays for herding dogs and as a co-morbid factor for anxiety-related conditions in all dogs.

Laboratory rats experience increased urinary epinephrine and norepinephrine excretion at 100 dB, suggesting that they are showing hypothalamic-pituitary-adrenocortical (HPA) axis signs of stress (Ogle and Lockett, 1968). Humans experience the same effect at 90 dB (Falk and Woods, 1973). Human patients may experience increased sensitivity to pain—something we do not routinely evaluate well in canine and feline patients—associated with noisy recovery rooms (Minckley, 1968). The HPA axis has a low threshold for stimulation by noise (68 dB), a level exceeded by noise in the recovery room, acute care unit, and incubators in one human hospital study (Falk and Woods, 1973).

Exposure to loud and prolonged high-decibel noises by humans and patients is even more likely in veterinary hospitals. Daily peak values in kennels of all kinds routinely exceed 100 dB, and often reach 125 dB (Sales et al., 1997; Scheifele et al., 2012). In the United States, the Occupational Health and Safety Administration (OSHA) requires hearing protection for people working for 8 hours in environments above 90 dBA (A-weighted dB).* The two major contributions to kennel and veterinary hospital noise levels are vocalizations of dogs and human behavior related to husbandry (e.g., cleaning, feeding, moving animals). These sound levels—commonly experienced in any kennel or kennel-related situation such as veterinary hospitals—are sufficient to cause damage and stress in species whose hearing is less acute than hearing in dogs (Gamble, 1982). In one study of 14 dogs exposed to noise at one of two kennels, all dogs experienced measurable decrements in hearing ability with time (Scheifele et al., 2012).

Any mitigation of noise—whether through the use of noise-canceling headphones or by installing noise-absorbing panels—should be encouraged.

Smells

Careful, naturalistic tests of olfaction in two dogs indicated that they could detect odor at 1.14 to 1.9 ppt, lower, by 20,000-fold to 30,000-fold, than previously believed or reported based on laboratory data (52 to 32,600 ppt) (Walker et al., 2006). These sensory capabilities should inform how we handle patients and how we design the environment in which we treat them.

Bleach kills olfactory neurons, removing one modality for gaining information for our canine and feline patients. If the smell of bleach is obvious, any dog sniffing the surface will compromise his or her olfactory ability. Clients appreciate hospitals that smell "clean" or have no smell. Veterinarians primarily focus on meeting the client's needs for cleanliness. We need to give more thought to our patients' needs. Well-aired, clean, and dry environments are best for patients and humans. Air flow systems are now sufficiently sophisticated that 99% of particles larger than 5 µm can be trapped by filters.

Dogs and cats get information from all odors, and it may not always be the information that you intend. Many patients who have come from a shelter environment may walk happily through the door of a veterinary practice and then lower their bodies and cringe at the smell of disinfectants. To these patients, the disinfectant odor—coupled with cage sounds—means a shelter, and they may worry that they are to be relinquished again. *Patients with a relinquishment history will need and benefit from extra help to make "institutional" environments non-intimidating.*

Patients are often distressed during hospital visits or stays, and such information can be communicated through odorant molecules. Equally important to competent cleaning that involves drying surfaces and ensuring good air exchange may be the provision of olfactory information that indicates that pets can be safe and protected while at the veterinary hospital.

Calmer, happier patients, residents, and visitors will contribute to and promote an olfactory environment that conveys information about the lack of risk and threats to the patients in that environment. We should never underestimate olfactory effects on our patients. Unfortunately, pheromonal analog products are unlikely to accomplish the goal of providing calm information to patients. There is little to no evidence that such products are efficacious in any situations examined (Frank et al., 2010). Regardless, the chemical signaling of the patients would likely overwhelm any product and provide more timely, consistent, and verifiable information—especially in combination with redundant visual and auditory signals—than that provided by any analog product.

Other Animals

Dogs and cats are extremely good at reading the body language and auditory and olfactory cues of other dogs and cats. We do not use this to our advantage often enough. If clients have a particularly calm dog or cat in their household or one who actually likes to visit the vet, this dog/cat should accompany any other pets to visits. The day's patient may be too stressed to accept food treats, but the accompanying pet will not be, and the patient can learn from observing that pet get praise and treats.

In-house animals and calm pets may help nervous patients learn to handle veterinary visits better, but the in-house animal given this task must be suitable for it, and the patients must be observed to respond in a favorable manner for this to work. In small practices, if any of the staff have extremely calm, well-mannered, and tolerant dogs or cats, those animals may patrol the waiting room (Fig. 1-29; see also Fig. 1-9). Not only can the presence of normal, non-reactive animals calm visiting clients who are nervous, but also any cat or dog will recognize that a dog sleeping in the middle of a hospital floor does not feel threatened. The extent to which such interventions are successful depends on the realization that they are not passive, and responses of all animals involved must be monitored.

The second advantage to encouraging clients to allow their calm pets to accompany the distressed ones and to using resident or in-house animals who are able

*CDC National Institute for Occupational Safety and Health. Noise and hearing loss prevention. Available at: www.cdc.gov/niosh/topics/noise. Accessed June 20, 2012.

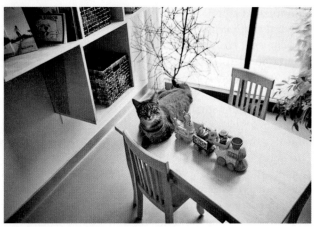

Fig. 1-29 A confident, happy resident cat—or dog—who visits most of the public spaces in a hospital—when other animals are not there—can communicate via olfaction that the hospital is a safe place to be (see also Fig. 1-9). (Photo courtesy of Dr. Steven Brammeier.)

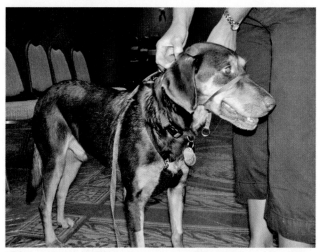

Fig. 1-30 A very tolerant and model "demo" dog who helped in a laboratory for veterinarians. This dog is wearing his collar, a head collar, and a no-pull harness and is happy to allow those participating in the lab to learn to fit and use these on him. He is frequently rewarded with praise and small treats.

to calm patients is in the ability to demonstrate successful calming exam and management techniques on a cooperative dog or cat. Clients may cognitively understand that their fearful dogs would benefit from a harness or head collar, but they do not understand at the gut level how to make this work until they have had a success with it.

Being able to fit and practice with devices on their calm pets or animals belonging to the staff or hospital is the best tutorial clients could have. We neglect the role that learning and first-hand successful experience can play in encouraging clients to buy and use products that promote their pet's well-being.

Any veterinary practice that does any amount of behavioral counseling, even if this is restricted to choosing devices used to walk the dog, should have an unflappable demonstration dog on the premises. Such dogs will allow clients to make mistakes successfully and allow themselves to be manipulated in ways that the patient may not (Fig. 1-30). Engaging with these "demo" dogs and cats also allows the veterinary staff to have a level of dialogue that would otherwise not occur. This dialogue and the trust such interactions engender will be personally and financially beneficial.

Staff Behavior

Few factors are more important—or more ignored—in terms of patient behavior than the behavior of the staff. Individuals working in the reception area can and should be trained to understand basic, normal behavior. This is almost never done, but these are the people who actually talk to the clients in a freely flowing format. Minimally, the reception staff should be able to recognize fearful, fractious, or overtly hostile patients and make recommendations about how to negotiate

safely their time in the waiting area and their passage to the exam room. The reception staff should also be sufficiently skilled at watching the patients to provide any potentially useful information directly to the veterinary staff. Electronic records can provide for real-time notes of their observations.

How to greet patients appropriately is the most important behavior for staff to learn. No staff member should make high-pitched noises when they see a patient unless they know how the patient will react. Most patients will become aroused by high-pitched noises (McConnell, 1990), and patients with behavioral concerns may become anxious, fearful, agitated, and antagonistic. If you have no relationship with a dog or cat, such greetings are considered scary and overly invasive.

Unless the staff member knows the dog or cat, he or she should calmly approach to no closer than the patient's inter-personal approach space and talk to the client. All staff should be able to allow the dog or cat to approach and sniff them. No one should stare at the patient or make sudden moves. Wooden behavior is not helpful, either, but soft, fluid, non-jerky behaviors that are contextual with the staff member's voice and the signals that the client is giving will tell the dog or cat that the approaching person is not a threat. If the client can greet the veterinary staff without fear and anxiety, the patient will recognize this. Client fear will render the patient more reactive.

When allowing a cat or dog to smell them, most people offer a closed fist. Everyone is taught this very inappropriate, closed finger greeting, yet dogs that have had bad experiences may view this gesture as a threat. Instead, a person wishing to greet an unknown dog should hold his or her arms loose and relaxed and gently and slightly extend an open hand. If the dog or cat wishes to explore, he or she will sniff the hand. If the cat explores further, a finger can be extended: cats engage in nose-to-nose sniffing, so this gesture mimics their normal behaviors.

Staff members should take the next cues about their behaviors from the cat or dog. If the patient backs away, no one should reach for him or her. The patient is supposed to be on a lead and so is in no danger of escape. Instead, the unfamiliar staff member can back up and continue to speak calmly with or guide the client and patient to a waiting area or exam room. This ongoing dialogue shows the patient that no one else was worried and nothing bad happened to them either for not approaching or for backing away.

No one should allow a client to discipline a patient for being worried or concerned. If these worried pets can get into a comfortable environment quickly, this will help them to relax. If treatment or testing does not contraindicate treats, the staff can spread tiny, high-quality treats around where everyone will sit and calmly talk to the client, explaining what will happen and taking a history while the patient learns that the veterinary clinic is not so scary.

Do not encourage anyone on the staff to bring their face into the face of an animal they do not know or to get down on the floor and try to engage a frightened animal in play. Such non-contextual behaviors tell frightened patients that the humans are clueless and a risk.

ROUTINE CARE—ROUTINE FOR WHOM?

Veterinary professionals have a set of tasks that they all view as "routine" care. For the patient, there is nothing "routine" about strange smells and sounds, slick surfaces, invasive prodding, having a stick or finger shoved up their rectum, having body parts grabbed, and then being stuck with a sharp object. By the time the cat or dog gets to the part of the appointment where they get their "routine" nail care, any pinch is going to render all memories of the experience as traumatic ones. The next nail trim will be neither quick nor routine. Clients can play a major role in preparing animals for veterinary visits, and if done well, this preparation may protect animals from thoughtless members of veterinary teams.

All puppies and kittens should be conditioned to be handled in ways that foster preventive veterinary care and facilitate veterinary examination. People love to pet puppies and kittens. Take advantage of this and provide your clients with a list of activities and the frequencies with which you want for them to practice these with their pets. If your clients cooperate, a number of things will happen:

1. The dog/cat will become used to veterinary manipulations and not fear them.
2. The client will come to understand what is involved in a good physical examination and will be a help, not a hindrance.

3. The client will become more attentive to their dog/cat and, if encouraged, report any concerning signs of behavioral change to you as soon as they are noticed. Realistically, the biggest benefit of having clients brush their pet's teeth daily may not be healthier gums and breath: it may be that the first time they have to struggle with the dog or cat or the dog growls, they will have flagged the onset of a behavioral condition and sought help when the condition is easiest to treat.

Demonstrate the activities in Table 1-4 to your clients and explain that if they participate in teaching their pet to be handled by them and the vet, the pet will be healthier and happier. If you think that a patient is going to need a certain kind of routine care (e.g., regional hair trims, injections, vision checks, medication, blood draws, ultrasounds), show the client how to practice these at home so that the manipulations are not unfamiliar to the pets. Encourage clients to link certain words ("settle," "puppy/kitty belly") to specific responses so that these can be used in a veterinary exam. Remind clients that because dogs and cats do not use the same type of verbal speech that we do, the clients will have to repeat the word frequently and praise and reward all appropriate responses.

All of the activities in Table 1-4 can also be practiced on animals out of puppyhood and kittenhood, but someone will have to teach the client how to work with their dog/cat based on the behavior which that individual animal displays. The beauty of doing all of this with babies is that they learn that it is routine and they never have any fear (Figs. 1-31 through 1-34). Older animals have learned that the world is an uncertain place or that they will be hurt. The place where the

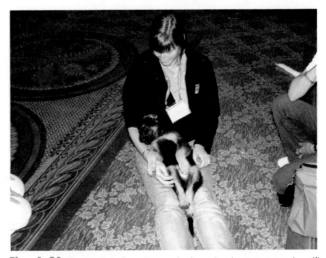

Fig. 1-31 Example of a puppy being slowly massaged until he stretches out onto his back. Clients can learn to do this and become familiar with normal physical appearances and behavioral responses. If you encourage them to do so the clients will call you when the dog deviates from these. Laps are great places for dogs and cats to learn physical examination skills.

TABLE 1-4

Activities for Clients to Practice with Puppies and Kittens*

Activity	How Frequently to Do It	When to Call the Vet
Firmly but gently stroke the kitten or puppy starting at the top of the head to the tail, and continue more gently to the tip of the tail 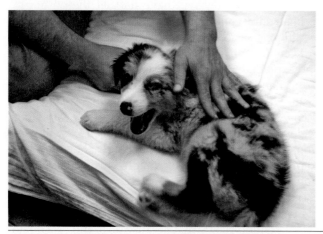	Multiple times daily	Become familiar with how your pet feels and report any lumps, bumps, scabs, changes in coat texture or behavior
With the puppy or kitten supported in your lap or gently supported on the floor, pick up the tail and look at the rectal area. Put the tail down and gently touch around this area (wash your hands, afterward)	Once a day as a kitten or puppy, at least weekly as an adult	If you see any swelling, or the dog or cat suddenly doesn't want you to touch around the tail base, or the tail is being held oddly, or if there is feces caked to the pet's bottom
Run your hands gently over the pet's face, and gently pick up each ear and look in it 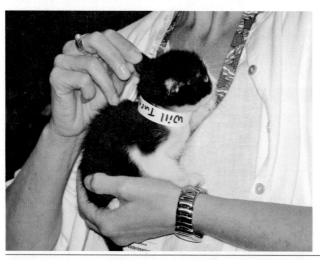	Once a day as a kitten or puppy, once a week as an adult	If the pet shies away before you get to the ear, yelps, cries, hisses, et cetera, or if there is swelling, discharge, or an odor. Normal ears are clean and pink and without odor
Run your hands gently over the pet's face, and gently wipe the corners of the pet's eyes while looking at the eyes	Once a day as a kitten or puppy, once a week as an adult	If the pet doesn't let you touch his or her face, moves away from you as you clean the corners of his or her eyes, vocalizes, or if there is a bad smell, something oozing from the eye, or the eye is swollen or red

TABLE 1-4

Activities for Clients to Practice with Puppies and Kittens—cont'd

Activity	How Frequently to Do It	When to Call the Vet
Stroke the pet slowly from head to tail until the dog or cat lies down ("settle"), then slowly stroke the sides until the pet is relaxed, and finally, move the legs gently and stroke the belly, gently rolling the pet onto his or her back ("puppy/kitty belly"). Gently run your hands over all of the nipples	Once a day as a kitten or puppy, once a week as an adult	If the cat or dog cries when any pressure is exerted, if you feel lumps, bumps, changes in texture, see wounds, see a rash, feel a swelling or hard area under a nipple, or smell anything foul

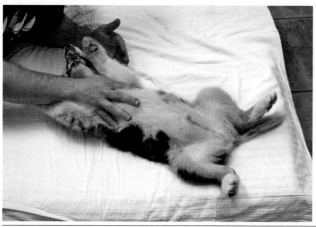

Activity	How Frequently to Do It	When to Call the Vet
When the kitten or puppy is relaxed in your lap ("settle"), gently move your hands from his or her side or belly and down each leg. Gently spread and flex all toes and claws	Once a day as a kitten or puppy, once a week as an adult	If the cat or dog won't let you touch the leg or paw, the pads are swollen or cut, nails are broken, if there is any discharge, the pads are cracked, or there is any odor or blood

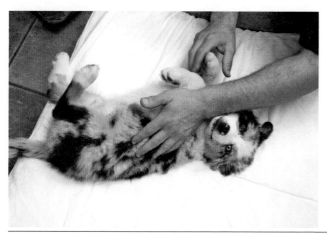

Activity	How Frequently to Do It	When to Call the Vet
Learn to file or trim the nails with the appropriate nail clipper and do this frequently, taking off the tiniest amount of nail when the pet is young so that they learn nail trimming isn't scary; putting treats on the towel your pet is sitting on can help	Multiple times a week as a kitten or puppy, once a week as an adult	If you could previously trim the dog's or cat's nails and now you cannot; this change could be due to a behavioral or physical problem

Continued

TABLE 1-4

Activities for Clients to Practice with Puppies and Kittens—cont'd

Activity	How Frequently to Do It	When to Call the Vet
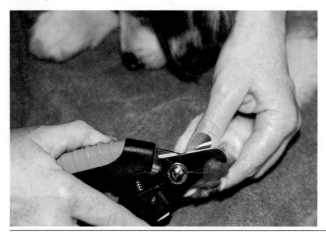		
Using pet toothpaste and a soft pet toothbrush, finger brush, or cloth, rub all the teeth and the nearby gums	At least weekly, but daily is better	If the gums bleed, if the cat or dog will not let you touch or open the mouth, if the dog or cat bites, growls, or hisses, if there is any foul smell or discharge
Give the puppy or kitten a "pill": Accustoming the pet to taking medication is essential for minimally stressful care. Normal, healthy animals can be given a "blank" daily. A "blank" is a small amount of cream cheese, peanut butter, sausage, hot dog, sardine, Marmite/Vegemite, cheese, a pill pocket—that is soft enough to be molded around a pill	Daily	By encouraging the dog or cat to take a "pill"/"blank" made of something they really love as a treat daily, when they need real medication, you will have a way to get them to swallow it without being overly suspicious. The ideal "blanks" are wolfed down without chewing

*This table is available as a client handout: "Protocol for Activities for Clients to Practice with Puppies and Kittens."

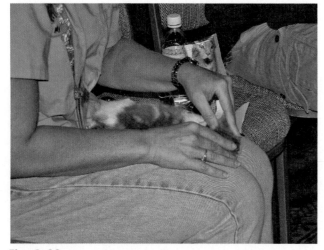

Fig. 1-32 The same massage technique being used on a kitten's head and back (the head is to the right). Note that the person is sitting with the cat in her lap and slowly working her way down the cat's sleeping body.

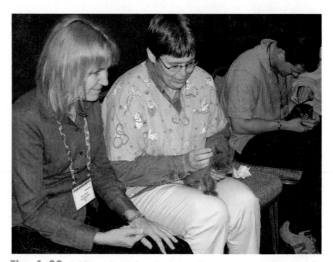

Fig. 1-33 A kitten learning to have her ears examined while sitting still on someone's lap. Notice the very gentle support and the fact that the person on the left is holding treats for the kitten.

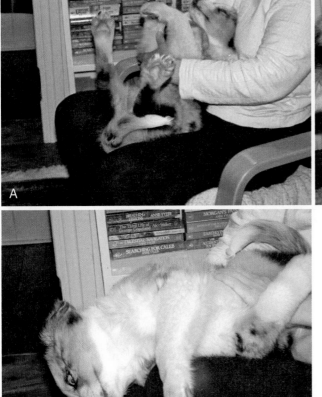

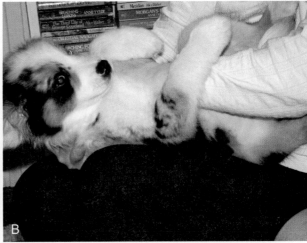

Fig. 1-34 **A-C,** These photos show the steps in teaching a puppy to learn to relax and be calm or "settle" and offer "puppy belly." If we just try to place a squirming puppy on his back (see also Fig. 1-31) he squirms more. If we start to rub and relax him, we can begin to guide him to his back (see also Fig. 1-32), If we rub very slowly but firmly the puppy will stretch out and go limp, allowing his neck and entire ventral area to be examined. The puppy in this photo, Toby, was 9.5 weeks when these photos were taken.

most caution is urged is in nail trims. Nail trims that go wrong are exquisitely painful and not forgotten. For this reason, clients delay nail/claw maintenance, worsening the situation.

Teaching young dogs and cats to offer nails for a trim, without restraint, and to stand in a way that their nails can be trimmed while they get treats are some of the most important behaviors that can be taught (Figs. 1-35 and 1-36) The dog in Figure 1-37 was scared and injured when someone tried to restrain him for a nail trim. He has been taught that if he will sit on the edge of a staircase, a stair, or a bench, as is shown in Figure 1-37, *A,* he will not be restrained. In Figure 1-37, *B,* the hair is moved off his nail and his foot steadied with one finger while the nails are trimmed. Someone out of the range of the camera is offering him a treat every time the person doing their trimming cuts a nail. As the nail is cut, the person says "treat" to cue the assistant. Because this nail trim is being done outdoors, the dog has less chance of feeling entrapped and is more likely to have other things on which to focus. Regardless, he was asked to get up and sit quietly on the bench before any nails were trimmed. Because the risks of causing a problem are so great, all dogs should be as calm and still as possible before a nail trim.

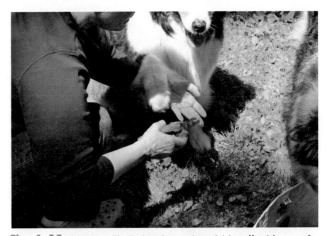

Fig. 1-35 This dog, Flash, has been taught to offer his paw for blood draw or nail trims in response to an outstretched human hand and the verbal request for "paw." By placing the paw on the hand, it is easy and quick to trim his nails, and no restraint is needed. The process is even quicker if another person offers the occasional tiny treat.

Because dogs so often have been hurt during nail trims, people may be reluctant to learn to trim their nails or become afraid of the dog. For people who really do not want to handle their dogs' feet and for the dogs who hate it, the smart thing to do may be to make the

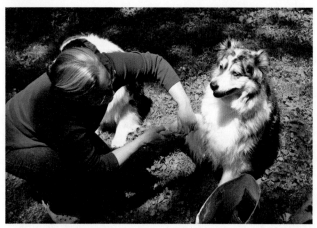

Fig. 1-36 This dog, Emma, is more reticent than the dog in Figure 1-35 but has been taught to have her paw held with the hair pulled back from the nails for the verbal request for "paw." Notice that neither this dog nor the one in Figure 1-35 is restrained, but they are on a non-skid surface (grass) and have been asked to sit before they were asked for their paws. Both dogs were offered treats throughout the trim but only if they sat quietly.

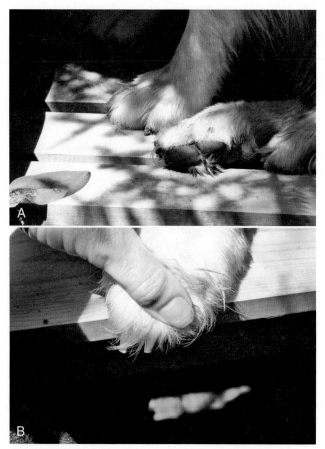

Fig. 1-37 A dog who was scared and injured when someone tried to restrain him for a nail trim. **A,** He was taught that if he will sit on the edge of a staircase, stair, or bench, he will not be restrained. **B,** The hair is moved off his nail and his foot steadied with one finger while the nails are trimmed.

dog his or her own giant emery board. A large, stable, angled piece of wood covered with sandpaper can be used by the dog to do his or her own nails. The client merely has to teach the dog to scratch (down with front feet, up with back feet (Fig. 1-38) by pairing the word "scratch" to the behavior and giving the dog a reward. Any competent and humane dog trainer should be able to teach this type of conditioned response.

EXTENDED OUTPATIENT WORK-UPS

Concerns for liability have often convinced the veterinary team to remove the client from the assessment and treatment phases. We should consider each client individually and ask whether they can help the patient to have a better experience. This may require some education of the client, and concerned practices can have the clients sign a liability waiver, but if the client is calm, his or her presence may be reassuring to the patient.

If the client is willing to stay with the patient during various steps of a work-up, the patient need not be tied or sequestered in a cage or run or unduly shifted around by people he or she does not know. If clients have been actively involved in teaching their pet to go to the vet, they may already have a mat that will make the patient calmer and have a sequence of signals that allow examination.

In Figures 1-39 and 1-40, veterinarians are participating in a laboratory designed to teach patients to offer body parts for examination. Here, the group was tasked

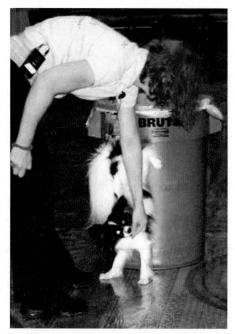

Fig. 1-38 A dog being taught to move her back feet up a surface, as a precursor for teaching her to file her own back toe nails on a sandpaper board. Angelica Steinker is the trainer demonstrating this technique in a laboratory for veterinarians.

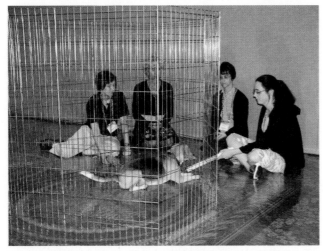

Fig. 1-39 Teaching a dog to lie quietly for targeting a stick that signals food treats. Here the target stick is a rolled set of papers.

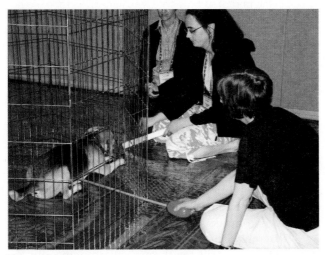

Fig. 1-40 Later in the sequence, the dog now targets the stick for the word "touch" and gets a treat for doing this and staying still while an "ultrasound probe" is moved over his side.

with teaching the dog to offer his abdomen for ultrasound examination. Figure 1-39 shows the early stages of teaching the dog to tolerate a probe, and Figure 1-40 shows the later stage. Because this laboratory was meant to stimulate everyone's creative thought process, participants had to make their own probes. Here, it's a Kong on a pointer.

HOSPITALIZATION AND IN-HOUSE PATIENT WORK-UPS

Hospitalized patients will not have their people present when scary things are happening to them. Regardless, if they have been taught to participate in any parts of their health care process, capitalizing on those learned rules will help them.

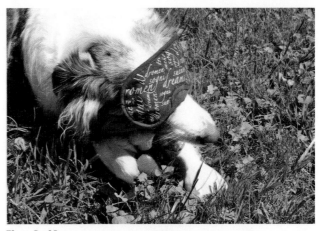

Fig. 1-41 This simple airplane eye mask is well tolerated by this young Australian shepherd who is photosensitive. It does not interfere with his ability to enjoy his toy.

Remembering that responses to unfamiliar, provocative, and distressing noises, smells, and lights can provoke an HPA-mediated stress response, our diagnostic and treatment ministrations could work against themselves. For these patients, a quiet, low-light room, with white noise and excellent filtration may help. If the lights cannot be lowered, consider Doggles (www.doggles.com) or a Calming Cap (www.premier.com) for amenable patients. In fact, if you know that your patients react to light and will have to be hospitalized, you can ask the client to teach the patient to become comfortable wearing one of these or a simple eye mask (Fig. 1-41). Not every patient can calmly wear these, but for those who can, there may be a benefit. For patients who cannot or will not wear anything over their eyes, and when low light levels are not possible, consider well-padded cages or runs and translucent curtains that dim the ambient light for the patient but allow some level of monitoring.

Patients should have familiar bedding from home, whenever possible, and any toys with which they comfort themselves. If the patient is going to be hospitalized for more than a day, ask the client to sleep in a tee shirt and bring it to you unlaundered to use in the patient's cage. The client must understand that the shirt will become stained. We know so little about olfaction; however, smells of home and familiar people may help modulate stress responses because we are providing some olfactory information that is meaningful to the patient.

PRE- AND POST-SURGICAL ENVIRONMENTS

Pre- and post-surgical environments never get the attention they need in terms of behavioral care. Many pre-anesthetic and anesthetic agents can affect cognition, perception of stimuli, anxiety levels, and overall reactivity, especially to noise. Acepromazine

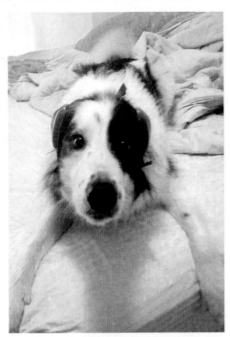

Fig. 1-42 A noise-sensitive border collie is wearing Mutt Muffs to block out ambient noise. (Photo courtesy of Angelica Steinker.)

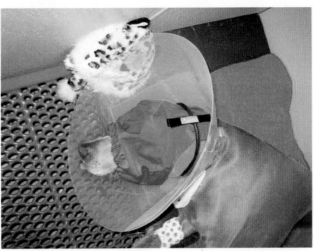

Fig. 1-43 This photo shows a Calming Cap on a patient recovering from anesthesia. These caps can protect dogs from the stimulation of bright lights and may calm them behaviorally. This dog has access to other objects that may help him recover more sanely and humanely: There is a pad on the kennel flooring (green in this photo) so he is on a firm, non-slip surface, he has an additional blanket, and he has one of his toys that smells like him and home. Other options include tee shirts that have been worn by the clients and towels that have been used to wipe down this dog and any of his housemates. If dogs have their own blankets or bedding that can fit in a cage or run, their use may help calm the dog. Clients will understand that the shirts, blankets, and bedding will have to be washed when returned home with the dog or cat. Note how reflective this cage is, making a calming cap or Doggles wise choices. Lining the cage with noise damping pads and adjusting the lighting would be even better. (Photo courtesy of Dr. Steven Brammeier.)

may render animals more noise reactive, a situation that is magnified for animals that are already noise sensitive. Because of this, all animals should be screened for noise reactivity before sedative treatment with dissociative agents such as acepromazine. We now have many more chemical agents available for restraint, anesthesia, and sedation, and we should make an effort to avoid medications that can cause or worsen behavioral pathologies. Although acepromazine at truly sedative levels and in combination with other medications can be excellent for physical pain control, we should ensure we are not inducing behavioral pain. Noise-sensitive animals may benefit from ear phones, ear plugs or Mutt Muffs (www.muttmuffs.com) if acepromazine is required in their premedication cocktail (Fig. 1-42).

Some anxious animals may require more preanesthetic medication, more of an induction agent, or higher flows of inhalant anesthesia than calmer animals. As noted, humans have a poor sense of smell compared with dogs and cats, and so we are unable to know whether smells are associated with calm for our patients. However, most humans have quite clear memories of the odor of something that is associated with a very good (e.g., cookies baking during the holidays) or bad (e.g., food poisoning) memory. Olfaction is one of the clearest sensory memories humans possess, and remembering the smell can induce the sensation of the remembered experience. We should at least entertain the thought that this can happen for animals, and if it does, we may also benefit from using worn client tee shirts in other places, such as supporting the patient's neck or anesthesia hose during induction and anesthesia.

The same lighting that allows us to monitor patients during recovery may adversely affect them. For these patients, eye masks (see Fig. 1-41) and Calming Caps (www.premier.com) (Fig. 1-43) may be extremely beneficial. Dogs can still see through these items, but the caps provide filtered, shaded light and may help some dogs calm because they can be fitted snugly. Some dogs panic when anything is put over their heads, and some dogs are too aggressive to fit with a Calming Cap when awake. Veterinary teams should remember that although the caps can be put on while dogs are sleeping, they must be removed from some patients before they are fully awake.

We should remember that we should be using cages to protect the dog while awakening and not simply as containment devices. If we put protection and meeting the animal's behavioral and mental health needs first, perhaps a cage is not the best choice.

Veterinary hospitals often prohibit clients from bringing their pet's beds, shirts, blankets, toys, dishes, crates, and sometimes even leads when the pet is hospitalized. The concern is that these items will be lost. In this age of computerized records that provide endless labels and hospital tags and that can create an inventory of the items that accompanied the pet and cell phones that can take photos, there is no reason to lose anything. We should make the effort to accommodate the patient's needs, even if they are not ours. When we make this effort, we will find ourselves trying to accommodate the dog's and cat's sensory needs.

BOARDING AND DAYCARE

If veterinarians have the physical space, boarding and daycare facilities, when done well, can sustain a practice in difficult fiscal times and can provide the staff with patient interactions that can boost morale. The key is in doing these well. Boarding and daycare situations require that animals partaking of the services get lots of social interaction and lots of cognitive stimulation and exercise. No one should just lock a dog in a run with two 10-minute walks per day and consider this an acceptable way to provide boarding or daycare.

Having dedicated staff, or a roster of support staff who share the duties and perhaps the income generated, can make all the difference. The dogs and cats who spend time at the hospital when well will develop good relationships with the staff with whom they routinely interact and will learn not to fear the practice if they have a good time. Private cages, runs, cubbies, small nooks, crates, et cetera, should be available for dogs/cats who need them and who need respite, but social or well-behaved dogs may benefit from supervised play and interactions indoors and outdoors.

Dogs need to be matched by size and behavioral style, and areas dedicated to these services should have flexible space that can be reshaped by dividers, crates, gates, or movable walls and screens. Training options with kind, humane, well-schooled trainers may produce additional income and some much needed skills in the dogs. Any pools or underwater treadmills used for rehabilitation can also be used for exercise that will help decrease anxiety: water pressing in on an animal, especially if it is warm, will relax the animal.

Surfaces should be non-slip, easily cleaned, and muffle noise. Any training/agility facility or shelter that offers training or classes will have such areas; a tour of the facilities in your area may give practitioners ideas about what will work for them.

Whenever dogs are loose, at least one and preferably two people must be available to monitor them and intervene, if needed. If you have arranged the facility correctly, such occurrences will be rare. Closed-circuit TV can also help monitor activities if the practice is large.

When housing cats, it is important to remember that cats experience increased serum and urinary cortisol levels when we *thwart* their ability to hide. This is one reason why examining a cat in a carrier or under a towel can be so helpful. Hiding is a coping skill in cats, and a behavior that is adaptive for small felines who can be both sit and wait predators and prey. The same types of creative changes that have been recommended for managing hospitalized or boarded dogs can be used for cats.

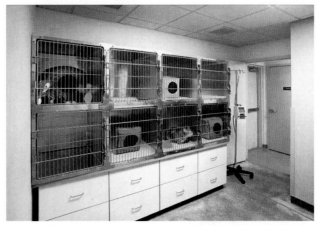

Fig. 1-44 A ward for boarding cats and cats needing relatively non-invasive care. Note that each occupied cage has a fleece cage pad to provide traction and to buffer noise and light reflection. The cage in the upper left contains the cat's nest from home and some of the cat's favorite toys. Both of these smell like home. A scratching post is provided in one duplex cage. There are no cages directly opposite these so there is no chance that cats can be scared or threatened by bully cats who face them. Cages are a form of entrapment. If animals are scared or distressed in a cage, that entrapment becomes behavioral and mental as well as physical. (Photo courtesy of Dr. Steven Brammeier.)

All cats who are caged or put in runs should have a place where they can hide; this can be a cardboard box turned sideways. Figure 1-44 shows some upscale, fabric cubbies for cats who wish to retreat. Some cages are expandable vertically or horizontally so that a climbing tree and litter box can be in one side, and bedding, feeding areas, and hidey-holes can be in another. For extended stays with cats who know each other, are social, and can get along or for cats who live at the clinic as blood donors, a more open and complex habitat can be created (Figs. 1-45 and 1-46). A screened-in porch and sitting area can be terrific for boarded cats as well as humans and should help by lowering stress and disease transmission risks (Fig. 1-47).

Wards, boarding, exercise, exam, and treatment areas that separate dogs and cats are best for cats. Separation allows individual needs to be met and allows the cats' areas to be separately soundproofed.

DEAD AND DYING HUMANS AND ANIMALS

Dogs and cats understand death—they may not understand "gone/absent," especially if they themselves were rescued. It is optimal for the client, patient, and canine and feline family if everyone can support dying animals. Pets should be allowed to visit with and explore dead human and animal companions, if they wish. Some nursing homes allow pets, but when it is impossible for the pet to visit a dying human or to learn firsthand that the human is dead, allowing the pet to sniff clothing and belongings may help.

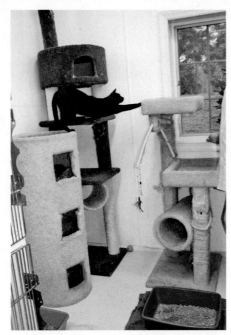

Fig. 1-45 A more complex habitat and housing choice for cats who get along and/or are boarded long-term. The key to making cats happy is clever use of complex three-dimensional environments with hiding areas. This room, which is smaller than one would think, accomplishes these goals.

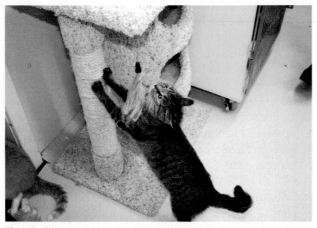

Fig. 1-46 Even if cats have to spend some time in a cage, if they can get out into an environment that has been enriched by smells, textures, and available activities, they will recover faster or be happier to be boarded and less stressed and distressed. Climbing trees and scratching posts like this one can be shared by sharing the central area between the cages in timed intervals throughout the day. Notice that these cages are on wheels. This means that a cat never has to sit facing someone who scares or threatens him and that cats can use a window as a time-share.

Death can be traumatic to pets unaccustomed to it, and no matter how well cleaned a room is, if an animal has died in it, expect the behavior of other animals—especially if they did not know the dead animal—to change. Some dogs or cats can become sufficiently distressed that they do not wish to enter the room. Respect those wishes.

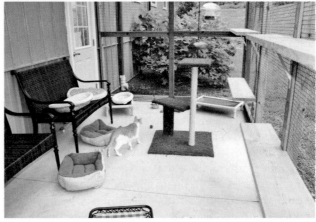

Fig. 1-47 A three-sided, screened-in porch designed for cats and humans. The bird feeders are a safe distance from the screening, and no perches face the birds directly. The perches allow the cats to associate or not and to look out over the horizon. The beds and climbing posts allow multiple cats to use the same area, interacting or not, by choice.

STAFF TOOLS AND EDUCATIONAL RESOURCES

Most continuing education (CE) in veterinary behavioral medicine focuses on diagnostics and therapeutics. Very little CE addresses the needs of the rest of the veterinary team or the information addressed in this chapter. There are some places to go for help:

The American Veterinary Society of Animal Behavior (AVSAB) has public and member sites and published position statements on topics such as punishment, socialization, dominance, et cetera (www.avsabonline.org).

Society of Veterinary Behavior Technicians (SVBT) (www.SVBT.org) provides ongoing CE through an annual seminar for veterinary technicians and provides helpful information to members online.

The Animal Behavior Resource Institute (ABRI) (www.abrionline.org) is now part of the American Humane Association (AHA) and provides videos and handouts helpful for all members of the veterinary team, including trainers.

The Association of Pet Dog Trainers (APDT) (www.apdt.com) provides CE for dog trainers and information for people interested in finding a trainer on its website. The Certification Council for Professional Dog Trainers (CCPDT) certifies Knowledge Assessed (KA) dog trainers who have participated in verified and approved CE and who have passed a rigorous exam on instruction skills, animal husbandry, ethology, learning theory, and equipment (www.ccpdt.org). Both the APDT and the CCPDT maintain lists of trainers.

The Pet Dog Trainers of Europe (PDTE) (www.pdte.org) sponsors CE in humane dog training and has an active website with humane position statements.

Most major CE meetings in the United States now include some veterinary behavioral medicine, and all staff would benefit from attendance because they can meet the experts in the field and ask questions of those involved in veterinary behavioral medicine. The American College of Veterinary Behaviorists (ACVB) (www.dacvb.org) and AVSAB hold a joint research meeting annually that is open to the entire community. The ACVB also has a public website with a membership directory and position statements.

WHAT ELSE CAN YOU DO TO ENSURE THAT YOUR PRACTICE IS BEHAVIOR-CENTERED?

At every visit, all veterinarians ask about physical health; *almost no veterinarians ask about behavioral health.* That *must* change. If the role the veterinarian can play in preventing behavioral problems is indeed large, veterinarians must also have a large role to play in intervention as behavioral problems develop.

Intervention is best done by surveying every animal at every visit using the same set of questions. In this way you follow specific behaviors through time and can learn whether a deviation is real or incidental. Canine and feline short questionnaires are attached and included in the handout section of this text and the accompanying DVD. These questionnaires have the advantage of not asking about clients' opinions. If you pursue a behavioral evaluation, you will get enough of those. Here, we need to know what happened.

If no one in the practice knows anything about veterinary behavioral medicine, these short questionnaire forms will allow the staff to elicit informative data from the client about specific behaviors that will suggest basic interventions. Please think of this assessment as an essential component to the "behavioral wellness exam" with which this chapter started. As behavioral history taking skills improve, you may be able to reduce the number of questions you ask to a few (Fig. 1-48). For this minimalist approach to work for you, you need to know what to say after the client expresses concern. The remainder of this textbook should help you to sound and be knowledgeable.

As you query clients about the behaviors, you may find that there is more going on than you realized, and you may wish to have the clients complete the full behavioral history questionnaire. This longer and more detailed form is found in the handout section of this text and on the DVD. The remainder of this text is devoted to making clear why certain patterns of behavior occur, whether one should worry, and how best to intervene. If your veterinary team takes these lessons to heart, you will have very few patients to refer to a specialist, and those who do require referral should be evaluated earlier in the progression of their condition—a boon for everyone.

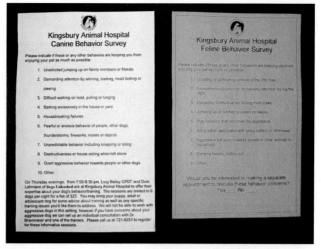

Fig. 1-48 One version of a very short questionnaire to review with clients at every visit. This questionnaire is from a practice where the veterinarians have had extensive training in veterinary behavior, attending numerous CE talks and the Institute courses offered by the North American Veterinary Conference (NAVC) (www.navc.com). These questions are found with the longer and short questionnaires at the end of the text and on the DVD labeled "Very Short Survey Questionnaire for Cats/Dogs." Note that this practice has hired a certified pet dog trainer to work with the clients in the practice. (Photo courtesy of Dr. Steven Brammeier.)

Short Survey Questionnaire to Be Used at All Visits to Monitor Behavioral Change in Cats

This short survey questionnaire can be used at any and all visits to check if the clients have any questions or complaints about their cat. Remember that clients might not even know that they have questions or complaints because they do not know what "normal" is. Also, myths about breeds, behavior, nature, and nurture are far more insidious in the client community than in the veterinary community. These questionnaires, when used at each visit together with the other, more detailed and specific tools provided, will tell you if further information is necessary and hint at some of the underlying factors contributing to the problems.

Clients may be uncomfortable with a behavior but not know how to ask if it is abnormal. These questionnaires will give clients the vocabulary and opportunity to discuss their pet's behaviors with their veterinarian in an efficient, consistent, and meaningful way.

If you know nothing about veterinary behavioral medicine, these short questionnaires will walk you through most of what you will need to ask. If you are experienced in asking about behavioral issues, you can shorten these questionnaires considerably. The complete and detailed version is attached here because authors have no way of knowing what readers know.

Survey questionnaire about general cat behaviors—to be used at all visits:

1. Client(s):	2a. Today's date: ____ /____ /____ 2b. Cat's date of birth: ____ /____ /____ ☐ Estimated ☐ Known
3. Patient's name:	4a. Breed: 4b. Weight: _____ lb/_____ kg 4c. Sex: ☐ M ☐ MC ☐ F ☐ FS 4d: If your cat is castrated or spayed [neutered], at what age was this done? _____ weeks/months (circle)
5a. Age in weeks at which your cat was adopted? 5b. How many owners has your cat had? 5c. How long have you had this cat?	a. _____ weeks/months (circle) b. ☐ 0 ☐ 1 ☐ 2 ☐ 3 ☐ 4 ☐ 5+ ☐ Unknown c. _____ months

6a. Is your cat (please circle):
     a. Indoor, only
     b. Outdoor, only
     c. Indoor/outdoor
	6b. How many litterboxes does your cat have:
	 ☐ 0 ☐ 1 ☐ 2 ☐ 3 ☐ 4 ☐ 5+
	 6c. What types of litter do you use?
	
	 6d. How often do you change the litterbox completely?
	 _____ times weekly/monthly (circle)
	 6e. How often do you scoop the box?
	 _____ times daily/weekly (circle)

7a. Does your cat leave urine or feces outside the litterbox?	☐ Yes ☐ No ☐ Don't know If you answered yes, a. Urine—Where specifically? b. Feces—Where specifically? c. Both—Where specifically?
7b. Does your cat "spray"?	☐ Yes ☐ No ☐ Don't know If you answered yes, where specifically?
8. Do you have any concerns, complaints, or problems with urination in the house now?	☐ Yes ☐ No If you answered yes, (a) Where is the cat urinating that you find undesirable (list all areas)? (b) How many times per week is the cat urinating in places you find undesirable? (c) At what time of day is the urination occurring? (d) Is the pattern different on days when you are home and days you are not home? (e) Are you at work during the hours when the cat urinates? (f) How many times per day does your cat usually urinate when he or she is not urinating in places you find undesirable?
9. Do you have any concerns, complaints, or problems with defecation in the house now?	☐ Yes ☐ No If you answered yes, (a) Where is the cat defecating that you find undesirable (list all areas)? (b) How many times per week is the cat defecating in places you find undesirable? (c) At what time of day is the defecation occurring?

For this and other questionnaires, see Section V, page 535, and the accompanying DVD.

	(d) Is the pattern different on days when you are home and days you are not home? (e) Are you at work during the hours when the cat defecates? (f) How many times per day does your cat usually defecate when he or she is not defecating in places you find undesirable?
10. Does your cat destroy any objects or anything else by chewing, sucking, or eliminating on them (e.g., furniture, rugs, clothes, et cetera) now?	☐ Yes ☐ No If you answered yes, what objects specifically does the cat destroy? Please list all of them and note which are destroyed when you are home or not home—please note if they destroy at both times—tick both columns: <table><tr><th>Object</th><th>When home</th><th>When gone</th></tr><tr><td></td><td>☐</td><td>☐</td></tr><tr><td></td><td>☐</td><td>☐</td></tr><tr><td></td><td>☐</td><td>☐</td></tr><tr><td></td><td>☐</td><td>☐</td></tr></table>
11. Does your cat mouth, bite, suck, or nip anything or anyone?	a. ☐ Yes ☐ No If you answered yes, to whom is this behavior directed? b. Is this a problem for you? ☐ Yes ☐ No
12. Does your cat exhibit any vocalization about which you are concerned?	☐ Yes ☐ No If you answered yes, what is/are the vocalization(s) and when do they occur: <table><tr><th>Vocalization</th><th>Situation in which it occurs</th></tr><tr><td>a. Yowling</td><td></td></tr><tr><td>b. Growling</td><td></td></tr><tr><td>c. Meowing</td><td></td></tr><tr><td>d. Hissing</td><td></td></tr></table>
13. Does your cat show any signs of hissing, growling, or biting?	☐ Yes ☐ No If you answered yes, what does the cat do and when does he or she do it? <table><tr><th>Sign</th><th>Situation in which it occurs</th></tr><tr><td>a. Hissing</td><td></td></tr><tr><td>b. Growling</td><td></td></tr><tr><td>c. Biting</td><td></td></tr></table>
14. Have you ever been concerned that your cat is "aggressive" *to people*?	☐ Yes ☐ No If you answered yes, why?
15. Have you ever been concerned that your cat is "aggressive" *to cats*?	☐ Yes ☐ No If you answered yes, why?
16. Have you ever been concerned that your cat is "aggressive" *to animals other than cats*? Does your cat hunt or prey on other animals?	☐ Yes ☐ No If you answered yes, why? ☐ Yes ☐ No If you answered yes, which animals and where?

17. Has your cat ever bitten or clawed anyone, regardless of the circumstances?	☐ Yes ☐ No If yes, what happened?
18. Has your cat had any changes in sleep habits?	☐ Yes ☐ No If you answered yes, what are these changes?
19. Has your cat had any changes in eating habits?	☐ Yes ☐ No If you answered yes, what changes have occurred?
20. Has your cat had any changes in locomotor behaviors or the ability to get around or jump on the bed, et cetera?	☐ Yes ☐ No If you answered yes, what changes have occurred?
21. Has anyone ever told you that they were afraid of your cat?	☐ Yes ☐ No If you answered yes, what did they say?
22. Has anyone every told you that your cat was ill-mannered?	☐ Yes ☐ No If you answered yes, why—what did the cat do that made them say this?
23. Do you have any concerns about your cat's grooming behaviors?	☐ Yes ☐ No If you answered yes, a. Little to no grooming b. Sucking c. Chewing d. Licking e. Self-mutilation/sores f. Barbering/trimming g. Plucking out clumps of hair
24. Is the cat exhibiting any behaviors about which you are concerned, worried, or would like more information?	☐ Yes ☐ No If you answered yes, please list these behaviors below:

Short Survey Questionnaire to Be Used at All Visits to Monitor Behavioral Change in Dogs

This short survey questionnaire can be used at all visits to check if the clients have any questions or complaints about their dog. Again, remember that clients might not even know that they have questions or complaints because they do not know what "normal" is. Also, myths about breeds, behavior, nature, and nurture again are far more insidious in the client community than in the veterinary community. These questionnaires, when used at each visit together with the other, more detailed and specific tools provided, will tell you if further information is necessary and hint at some of the underlying factors contributing to the problems.

Clients may be uncomfortable with a behavior, but not know how to ask if it is abnormal. These questionnaires will give clients the vocabulary and opportunity to discuss their pet's behaviors with their veterinarian in an efficient, consistent, and meaningful way.

If you know nothing about veterinary behavioral medicine, these short questionnaires will walk you through most of what you will need to ask. If you are experienced in asking about behavioral issues, you can shorten these questionnaires considerably. The complete and detailed version is attached here.

Survey questionnaire about general dog behaviors—to be used at all visits:

1. Client(s):	2. Date:
3. Patient:	4a. Breed: _____ 4b. Weight: _____ lb/_____ kg 4c. Sex: ☐ M ☐ MC ☐ F ☐ FS 4d: If your dog is castrated or spayed [neutered] at what age was this done? _____ weeks/months (circle)
5. Age in weeks at which your dog was definitively house-trained (e.g., no accidents in the house). If you adopted your dog as an adult and the dog was house-trained, just put in the adoption age.	_____ weeks ☐ My dog is not really house-trained

6. Does your dog "mark" with urine or feces?	☐ Yes ☐ No
	☐ I don't know
	☐ Not sure—I don't know what marking is
	If you answered yes,
	    a. Urine—where specifically?
	    b. Feces—where specifically?
	    c. Both—where specifically?

7. Do you have any concerns, complaints, or problems with urination in the house now?	☐ Yes ☐ No

8a. Do you have any concerns, complaints, or problems with defecation in the house now?	☐ Yes ☐ No
	If you answered yes,
	    (a) Where is the dog defecating that you find undesirable (list all areas)?
	    (b) How many times per week is the dog defecating in places you find undesirable?
	    (c) At what time of day is the defecation occurring?
	    (d) Is the pattern different on days when you are home and days you are not home?
	    (e) Are you at work during the hours when the dog defecates?
	    (f) How many times per day does your dog usually defecate when he or she is not defecating in places you find undesirable?

8b. Does your dog experience periodic bouts of diarrhea?	☐ Yes ☐ No
9. Did your dog destroy any objects that were not toys while teething?	☐ Yes ☐ No ☐ Unknown If you answered yes, what objects specifically did the dog destroy?
10. Does your dog destroy any objects or anything else (doors, windows, et cetera) *now*?	☐ Yes ☐ No If you answered yes, what objects specifically does the dog destroy? Please list all of them and note which are destroyed when you are home or not home—please note if they destroy at both times—tick both columns:

Object	When home	When gone
	☐	☐
	☐	☐
	☐	☐

For this and other questionnaires, see Section V, page 535, and the accompanying DVD.

11. Does your dog mouth anything or anyone?	☐ Yes ☐ No If you answered yes, what or whom does the dog mouth? Is this a problem for you? ☐ Yes ☐ No		
12. Does your dog exhibit any vocalization about which you are concerned?	☐ Yes ☐ No If you answered yes, what is/are the vocalization(s) and when do they occur?		
	Vocalization	**Situation in which it occurs**	
	a. Barking		
	b. Growling		
	c. Howling		
	d. Whining		
13. Does your dog show any signs of growling, barking, snarling, or biting?	☐ Yes ☐ No If you answered yes, what is/are the sign(s) and when do they occur?		
	Sign	**Situation in which it occurs**	
	a. Barking		
	b. Growling		
	c. Snarling		
	d. Biting		
14. Have you ever been concerned that your dog is "aggressive" *to people*?	☐ Yes ☐ No If you answered yes, why?		
15. Have you ever been concerned that your dog is "aggressive" *to dogs*?	☐ Yes ☐ No If you answered yes, why?		
16. Have you ever been concerned that your dog is "aggressive" *to animals other than dogs*?	☐ Yes ☐ No If you answered yes, why?		
17. Has your dog ever bitten anyone, regardless of the circumstances?	☐ Yes ☐ No If you answered yes, what happened?		
18. Has your dog had any changes in sleep habits?	☐ Yes ☐ No If you answered yes, what are these specifically?		
19. Has your dog had any changes in eating habits?	☐ Yes ☐ No If you answered yes, what are these specifically?		
20. Has your dog had any changes in locomotor behaviors or its ability to get around or jump on the bed, et cetera?	☐ Yes ☐ No If you answered yes, what are these specifically?		
21. Has anyone ever told you that they were afraid of your dog?	☐ Yes ☐ No If you answered yes, what did they say?		
22. Has anyone every told you that your dog was ill-mannered?	☐ Yes ☐ No If you answered yes, why—what did the dog do that made them say this?		
23. Is the dog exhibiting any behaviors about which you are concerned, worried, or would like more information?	☐ Yes ☐ No If you answered yes, please list these behaviors below:		

The Science and Theory Underlying Behavioral Medicine: Terminology, Diagnosis, Mechanism, and the Importance of Understanding Reactivity

DIAGNOSTIC TERMINOLOGY

There is still no consistent terminology in veterinary behavioral medicine. This lack of consistency has hurt collaborations, impeded progress in the literature, and confused veterinarians and clients who struggle to understand the dogs in their care.

There has been an unfortunate trend to lump aggressive diagnoses based on the victim (people [owner vs. stranger] directed vs. animal directed) (Bamberger and Houpt, 2006; Luescher and Reisner, 2008) as a way to achieve agreement on terminology, but when people using this strategy look further, the utility of phenotypic diagnoses is clear because they allow us to understand useful variation and to recognized clusters of behaviors that may be of greater and lesser risk. More *contextually discrete diagnoses* also make it easy for clients and clinicians to agree on *which behaviors to avoid* and *which to alter* in a manner that will *help the dog.*

Accurate diagnosis is particularly critical if the best care is to be provided to the patient. Veterinarians should also realize that particularly when destruction is involved the complaint is a true veterinary emergency. More pets are killed because of behavioral complaints than any other set of complaints (Miller et al., 1996; Spencer, 1993). The most common reason people abandon pets is due to behavior. Specific behavioral complaints accounted for 24 of 71 reasons for relinquishment (Salman et al., 2000). Dogs with behavior problems are relinquished after about 3 months; cats with behavior problems are relinquished after 1 to 2 years. Pets develop problems at social maturity—hence data that most dogs are kept for about 1.5 years before relinquishment (Salman et al., 2000). The breeds noted (Salman et al., 2000; Shore and Girrens, 2001) are also the breeds that are most frequently relinquished to shelters because of problems.

A case is made here for the approach suggested and expanded by Overall (1997, 2005a) and that is becoming more widespread. This diagnostic classification approach is based in classic ethology and relies on a context-dependent pattern of identification and enumeration of behaviors to create a *phenotypic, phenomenological diagnosis.* Phenotypically or phenomenologically diagnosed conditions are labeled on the basis of what the dog/cat does within specific contexts. As noted by Moyer (1968), phenotypic or phenomenological categories of diagnosis can be especially useful when aggression is a concern because (1) they allow us to identify specific behaviors or events that could provoke the aggression and permit avoidance of behaviors that would otherwise reinforce problematic and/or dangerous conditions, (2) they allow us to identify behaviors that can be modified *in a contextually meaningful way,* and (3) they presume nothing about the underlying neurophysiological and genetic basis of the behavior. *This last point is important because it acknowledges that numerous underlying mechanisms, whether genetic or cellular, can produce a similar, and possibly indistinguishable, constellation of signs. For example, we cannot begin to examine clusters of behaviors that may form phenotypes that are expressions of specific suites of genes until we have sufficiently large populations of patients who have been evaluated using objective and validated techniques.* Finally, the use of diagnostic criteria within a phenotypic/phenomenological diagnosis allows the clinician to interpret rare non-specific signs within a context in which the dog can be helped. For example, most dogs with separation anxiety do not mutilate their penis, but if you wish to stop the mutilation, understanding why the dog is so engaged may help guide your interventions (Ghaffari et al., 2007).

Archer (1988) criticized Moyer's classification because it distinguishes categories of aggression in a manner inconsistent with their neural basis. However, as is true for genetic associations, neuroanatomical aspects of any behavioral condition are complex and polymorphic. Gene by environment (G × E) effects are notoriously difficult to evaluate for heterogeneous, multifactorial behaviors that are quantitative and polygenic.

For our purposes, a modification of a *phenotypic/ phenomenological terminology can provide enough information to work at a level where we can intervene—the actual behaviors—while also permitting epidemiological data to be collected to test putative underlying mechanisms.* The definition of or criteria for a phenotypic diagnosis identify the pattern of contextual behaviors that commonly occur with the condition, allowing *patients with the condition to be grouped together in a consistent way on the basis of ethology and context that distinguishes these patients from unaffected dogs/cats or from dogs/cats with another, possibly related condition.* In other words, individuals more similar to each other than to those with other conditions are grouped together, which may permit recognition of underlying factors driving or contributing to the condition. There is no implication that all individuals with any diagnosis are equally affected, which is why it is so important to cluster patients on the basis of behavior and context.

It's interesting to note that specialists are often very willing to agree on these patterns but not on what the diagnosis itself should be labeled. What we call something can be less important than the criteria used to label it, *but what we call something can also be critically important if it affects the way we think.* If by the way we call or name something affects how we think about it, we should be extremely cautious and use labels only when we can provide criteria to assess them. How we group and label diagnoses is a function of knowledge, which we should hope evolves. By basing diagnoses on clearly identified and defined contextual behaviors, we can avoid both the unfortunate recent trend toward overly broad, non-informative diagnostic labels (e.g., human-directed aggression) and labels that confuse or bias the issue and may say more about our anthropocentrism than they do about our understanding of the condition (e.g., sibling rivalry). Collaborative efforts could reflect these truisms and allow the field of veterinary behavioral medicine to grow while heading toward a shared terminology. The approach used here can lead to that outcome. This approach has been used successfully to identify risk factors for pathological behaviors in chimpanzees, identify the severity of the condition, and follow responses to therapeutic intervention (Ferdowsian et al., 2012).

MECHANISTIC DIAGNOSES

It is essential to understand that *any phenotypic diagnosis could have multiple underlying mechanisms driving it.* In other words, not only are there a variety of diagnoses that may involve some aspects of anxiety (see Box 2-1 for a list of the non-specific signs of anxiety), but also within each diagnosis there is considerable phenotypic and mechanistic variation. These different mechanisms could be due to differences in regions of arousal in the brain that are aroused, differences in underlying neurochemistry, differences in molecular responses, and differences in genetic bases that facilitate the condition across the affected patient population (Fig. 2-1). For our

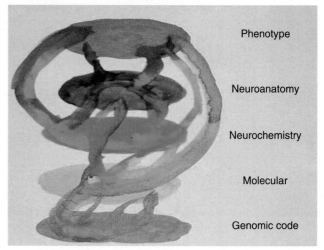

Fig. 2-1 Schematic illustrates the relative role that various mechanistic levels of diagnosis play in determining "response surfaces." Note that phenotype can be affected directly or indirectly. The extent to which the different levels interact directly or indirectly could be a function of intensity, duration, or type of stimulus. There is no way to know these effects in the absence of specific data collection. Here, the genomic code provides the set of choices that could effect—*but not necessarily will effect*—molecular and neurochemical expression of behavioral phenotypes. In essence, the genomic response surface acts to define "boundary conditions"—it tells you *what is possible, not what will happen.* (From Overall, 2005.)

purposes, this means that we should not expect all dogs who exhibit noise phobia, or all dogs who exhibit impulse control aggression, or all dogs who exhibit obsessive-compulsive disorder, or all cats who spray to be the same in terms of presentation, underlying brain regions involved, underlying neurochemistry, or underlying molecular basis (Overall, 2005a, 2005b). Certainly, these conditions need not be the same at the genetic level because one's genetic code informs what *could* happen, not what *will* happen.

Accordingly, different individuals with the same diagnosis could have very different "response surfaces" where they exhibit different behaviors, behavioral intensities, or frequencies; have different thresholds for reacting; and may have different physiological responses and different therapeutic responses than other individuals who meet the criteria for the diagnosis they share (Box 2-2 and Table 2-1). Clear use of terminology can help make apparent the parts that are consistent and that we can understand and separate them from the parts that are more complex. If we were able to characterize all of the response surfaces of the affected patients, we'd have an excellent description of the patterns of behaviors and reactivity within an affected population (Fig. 2-2). Such population-wide characterization is difficult but would be extremely useful because it allows you to *assess and assign relative risk.*

This type of approach is taken in genetic studies that are case-control studies, including those that underlie

BOX 2-1

Non-specific Signs of Anxiety

- Urination+
- Defecation+
- Anal sac expression
- **Panting***
- Increased respiration and heart rates
- **Trembling/shaking***
- Muscle rigidity (usually with tremors)
- Lip licking
- Nose licking+
- Grimace (retraction of lips)
- Head shaking+
- Smacking or popping lips/jaws together
- Salivation/hyper-salivation+
- Vocalization (excessive and/or out of context)
  - Frequently repetitive sounds, including high-pitched whines,* similar to those associated with isolation (see Yin and McCowan, 2004)
- **Barking***
- Yawning+
- **Immobility/freezing or profoundly decreased activity***
- **Pacing and profoundly increased activity***
- Hiding or hiding attempts
- Escaping or escape attempts
- Body language of social disengagement (turning head or body away from signaler)+
- Lowering of head and neck

- Inability to meet a direct gaze
- Staring at some middle distance
- Body posture lower (in fear, the body is extremely lowered and tail tucked)
- Ears lowered and possibly droopy because of changes in facial muscle tone
- Mydriasis
- Scanning
- Hyper-vigilance/hyper-alertness (may be noticed only when touching or interrupting dog or cat— may hyper-react to stimuli that otherwise would not elicit this reaction)
- Shifting legs
- Lifting paw in an intention movement+
- Increased closeness to preferred associates
- Decreased closeness to preferred associates
- Profound alterations in eating and drinking (acute stress is usually associated with decreases in appetite and thirst; chronic stress is often associated with increases)+
- Increased grooming, possibly with self-mutilation+
- Decreased grooming
- Possible appearance of ritualized or repetitive activities+
- **Changes in other behaviors including increased reactivity and increased aggressiveness (may be non-specific)***

The **most commonly** recognized signs* and least commonly recognized signs+ of anxiety identified via questionnaire by clients (Mariti et al., 2012).
Sources: Beerda et al., 1997, 1998; Overall, 1997; Overall et al., 2001; Rooney et al., 2007, 2009; Schilder and van der Borg, 2004; Tod et al., 2005.

TABLE 2-1

Example for Consideration of Interaction of Phenotypic Level of Mechanism with Others

Phenotype	A	B	C	D
	Abnormal variant A	Abnormal variant B	Abnormal variant C	Normal
Neuroanatomical variant	I	I	I	I
Neurochemistry	a	b	a	b
Molecular products	I'	II'	II'	II'
Genotype	b'	b'	b'	b'

In this example, the variants in the condition are due to some difference in environmental response. This could be a purely phenotypic effect where the behavior changes or is plastic without inducing changes in any underlying mechanistic level (abnormal variant B). Alternatively, the environmental response could affect learning and long-term potentiation, in which case the molecular level is affected and it, in turn, also affects neurochemistry (abnormal variant A), but may not alter neuroanatomical region activated. The environmental response could affect only neurochemistry, without affecting the molecular or neuroanatomical levels (abnormal variant C). Because the effects discussed here are ones within an individual across circumstances or time, no effects are seen on genotype. Over time, if abnormal behaviors are desired or convey some additional value, the genotype producing these may be favored. In this example we assume no change in genotype because of selection or epigenetic effects.

BOX 2-2

Understanding Patterns of Behavior within Levels of a Mechanistic Approach

I. Phenomenological, Phenotypic, Functional Diagnoses: Must Meet Necessary and Sufficient Terminological Criteria

A. Demographic patterns
 1. Global patterns of behavioral change with age and neutering (must follow individuals through time)
B. Suites of behavioral patterns
 1. Specific behaviors that occur
  a. Numbers of behaviors that occur (range, mean, predictive value)
  b. Co-variation in behaviors to define subtypes or subpopulations (Venn diagrams, *r* values)—must avoid spurious correlations
  c. Ontogenetic development of specific behavioral suites (ethograms) (must follow individuals)
 2. Elemental behaviors that are shared across diagnoses (may hint at underlying reductionist mechanism—i.e., the neurochemistry of stress)

II. Neuroanatomical Diagnoses

A. Region activated during normal versus abnormal behavior
 1. Level of activity
 2. Variants in patterns of activity
B. Neuron behavior
 1. Types
 2. Densities
 3. Overall activity

III. Neurochemical/Neurophysiological Diagnoses

A. Types of neurochemicals
 1. Activities
 2. Receptor types associated with these
  a. Activity of receptor gates
  b. "Metabolism" of receptors
  c. Conformation of receptors
B. Interactions of neurochemicals
 1. Neuron recruitment
  a. Regional activity
  b. Responses to behavioral changes

IV. Molecular Diagnoses

A. Molecular/conformational chemistry of receptors and neurotransmission
B. Gene product regulators of expression
C. Gene product regulators of function

V. Genetic Diagnoses

A. At the level of gene/locus
 1. Overall heritability (Mendelian pattern)
  a. Codon shifts
  b. Errors (loss or addition of part of chromosome—e.g., Marshall's disease, Down syndrome)
  c. Coding for different proteins
 2. Multi-factorial effects
B. At the level of genome
 1. Gene products
 2. Regulator genes
 3. Local environmental receptor effects

Note: Tests of mechanistic hypotheses must occur at the level of focus.

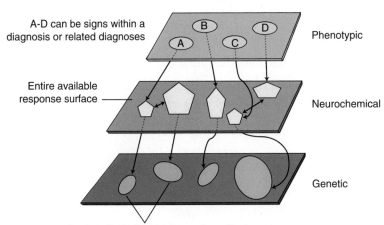

A-D can be signs within a diagnosis or related diagnoses

Entire available response surface

Dog's individual response surface. Each oval may also represent individual breeds or populations.

Phenotypic

Neurochemical

Genetic

Fig. 2-2 A model of various "response surface" interactions. In this schematic, only three of five discussed mechanistic levels—phenotypic, neurochemical, and genetic—are represented as three different response surfaces. Situation *B* is the one everyone hopes to find: one gene is responsible for one neurochemical change, and that change maps uniquely onto the problem behavior. The real world is more complex than this. In example *D*, one set of genes gives rise to one set of neurochemical responses, which then changes into another neurochemical response set. Each set of neurochemical responses gives rise to two separate phenotypes (*C* and *D*). In this case, the same genetic background can produce two diagnostic groups acting through two neurochemical mechanisms. For phenotype *A*, two neurochemical mechanisms are also involved, but they are each the result of two separate genes, which then produce two neurochemical responses that interact.

genome-wide associational studies (GWAS) (Diskin et al., 2009; Glessner et al., 2009; Wang et al., 2009). In these studies, numerous levels and types of assessment were used to decide who was affected versus who was unaffected with the phenotypic diagnosis of neuroblastoma and autism. Genomic patterns (single nucleotide polymorphisms [SNPs]) were compared for these two groups. Underlying genetic associations for subjects affected and those unaffected were tested statistically to ensure that patterns of association are not random. Done correctly, this approach suggests genes that *may* be involved in pathology.

We seldom have such an expansive level of knowledge in veterinary behavioral medicine, partly because of lack of standardization that would permit comparative studies of large populations. Newer methods of assessment (e.g., imaging, biochemical assays) have begun to contribute to our understanding of some mechanisms driving diagnoses of canine aggression, and these are discussed for the relevant diagnosis. It is now accepted that most canine and feline aggressions that are problematic or abnormal are rooted in anxiety (Luescher and Reisner, 2008; Overall, 1997, 2000), but specific information about differences in physiology, neurochemistry, et cetera, is largely lacking. Responses to newer behavioral medications that affect serotonin, noradrenaline, and other neurochemicals may allow us to imply mechanistic differences when, within the same diagnosis, not everyone responds to the same treatment.

ROLE OF REACTIVITY IN MANY BEHAVIORAL DIAGNOSES

Patterns of Reactive Responses for "Normal" and "Reactive" Dogs

The most problematic aspect of most behavioral pathologies is the underlying "reactivity" of the dogs. Regardless of the specific concern, the more reactive the dog, the more difficult it is to intervene in the developing behaviors to stop or redirect a problem behavior, and the easier it is to trigger the problem behavior. These patterns are illustrated in Figures 2-4 and 2-5 later in this section, but it may help to review the key role for arousal in reactive responses.

Roles for Arousal in All Forms of Anxiety

At the core of all anxiety conditions is the arousal level of the patient. Heightened arousal beyond a certain adaptive level prohibits accurate observation and assimilation of the information presented, interferes with processing of the information, and can adversely affect actions taken based on these earlier steps. The physical and behavioral environments are often factors in the level of arousal of the dog or cat. Although these environments may be completely within the normal range of encounters of dogs and cats, for some individuals they will be sufficient to trigger a problematic response. Given this, understanding the role the environment may play in the response provides help for treatment.

Manipulating the physical environment is often overlooked, yet environmental change can often be the first and easiest step in decreasing the patient's arousal levels. If our goal is to raise the threshold at which the cat or dog displays the signs associated with the diagnosis or the behaviors associated with the client complaint—and these behaviors could be normal—environmental manipulation may be simple and helpful (Fig. 2-3).

Figure 2-3, *A*, shows the effect of repeated stimuli, baseline levels of reactivity, and thresholds on the exhibition of behaviors. If the patient is already aroused, a stimulus that would be below the level at which he or she would react may cause reaction. If multiple stimuli are presented to the patient before he or she has returned to baseline levels, they may act additively, causing the patient to react more profoundly or in more situations than that patient would have otherwise reacted. This graph shows how important controlling the stimulus environment can be. Note that if you allow the patient to return to baseline between provocative events, you do not trigger the response. If you continue to force the patient to be exposed to provocative events, he or she reacts to ever higher levels. Because the reaction is profound and the duration of the decay of the response is lengthy, you cannot teach appropriate behaviors because the cortisol and epinephrine levels interfere with genetic transcription of information. You can only reinforce fear and avoidance, and over time will lower the threshold of reactivity. This application should resonate with veterinarians who have experienced treatment of patients using high levels of restraint (Overall, 2011).

Note that Figure 2-3, *A*, was developed using only patient A's response, and patient A is the most normal of the patients. The basal response level—the response surface of the patient—interacts across time with the intensity and frequency of the stimulus to produce the overall behavioral response.

Understanding Time Budgets and Reactivity in Practical Ways Useful to Clients and Patients

Figure 2-4 shows a static model for how reactive dogs differ from "normal," non-reactive dogs and how these differences can change with successful treatment. Note that the "normal" dog (Fig. 2-4, *A*) spends most of his time in calm, non-vigilant, non-reactive behaviors where he exhibits normal attentiveness. The next largest block of his time is spent in vigilant behaviors where

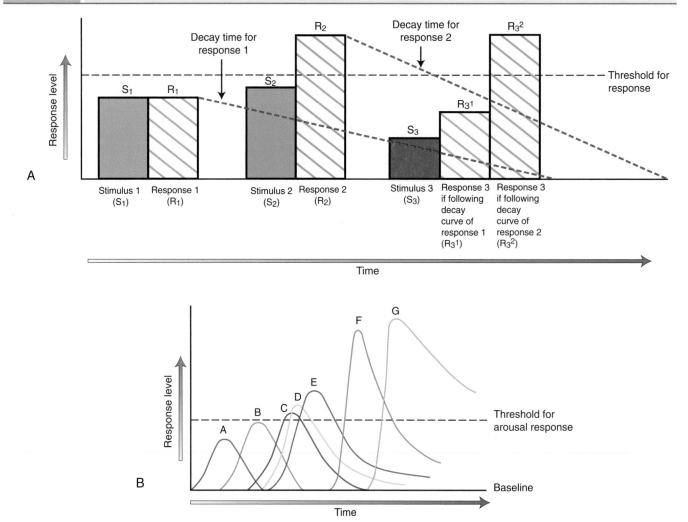

Fig. 2-3 A, The x axis represents time, and the y axis represents response level. R1 shows a response that is proportional to the stimulus—there is no overall behavioral reaction to this stimulus 1 because R1 does not reach the threshold level for the behavioral reaction *(horizontal dashed line).* The decay time—the time to return to baseline—is shown by the *colored dashed curves.* At stimulus 2, the summed proportional responses exceed the threshold, and the dog reacts (R2). At stimulus 3, even a small stimulus now causes a worsening in the response (R3) if the patient is still experiencing the R2 decay/recovery response because the responses are additive and the arousal level is still high. However, if the patient experiences stimulus 3 after R1 has sufficiently delayed or recovered, the additive level is not sufficient to trigger a response. This graph illustrates how important multiple stressors and the time over which they are experienced can be for the behavior of the dog or cat. **B,** This graph shows how patients with different types of reactivities may respond to the same stimulus and how reactivities can change with time. For simplicity, this graph assumes that the stimulus is the same for each patient, and that the threshold level does not change. In truth, with repeated exposure to distressing situations reactivity thresholds lower, allowing the dog or cat to react more quickly.

- Patient A reacts to the stimulus but not at a sufficient level to trigger the problematic response. Patient A's behavior decays to the baseline quickly.
- Patient B reacts to the stimulus at a level that just triggers the behavior but recovers, and his behavior decays to the baseline quickly.
- Patient C reacts to the stimulus in a way that exceeds the threshold for exhibiting the behavior, and because he had a worse reaction than patient B, he takes longer to return to baseline, but he does recover and return to baseline.
- Patient D reacts to the stimulus in a way that exceeds the threshold for exhibiting the behavior, and this changes his future behaviors and lowers his threshold for reactivity. Notice that beginning with patient D the slope of the curve increases—the patient is reacting more quickly. Patient D does not return to baseline. His recovery is incomplete, which increases the ease with which he will become distressed in the future.
- Patient E reacts to the stimulus in way that far exceeds the threshold for exhibiting the behavior, he remains reactive for longer than does patient E, he has a longer decay period for his response (during which he is easily stimulated to react inappropriately). Patient E reacts very quickly and does not return to baseline. His recovery is incomplete and he will view all future stimuli from the perspective of always being somewhat aroused and distressed. This is one model for patients with panic disorder.
- Patient F shows a very rapid response (see the slope of the curve) with a slow decay that never approaches baseline or the threshold below which he will react. Many small events trigger his response and speed the rate at which he reacts. He is always reactive to some degree, very much like a dog with generalized anxiety disorder.
- Patient G may or may not be at baseline, but he reacts almost instantly and to a quite high level. Once he reacts, he is very slow to calm. Patient G panics.

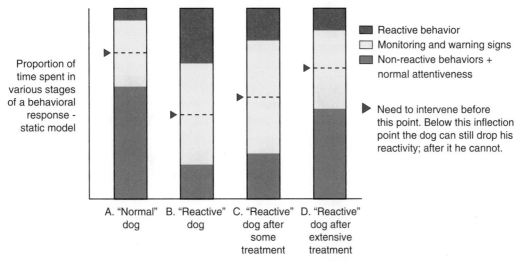

Fig. 2-4 Static model for how reactive animals differ from animals who are "normal" and how these differences can change with successful treatment. Here dogs are used as the model species, but this approach applies equally to cats. Green represents calm, non-reactive, and normally attentive behaviors; yellow represents monitoring behaviors with warning signs; red represents reactive behaviors. **A,** Dog A is a normal dog. **B,** Dog B is a reactive dog. **C,** Dog C is the reactive dog after some treatment. **D,** Dog D is the reactive dog after extensive treatment. The *triangle* and *dotted line* represent the point after which all intervention can be focused only on keeping everyone safe and on getting the dog out of the situation as quickly as possible.

he monitors the environment and may exhibit warning signs to learn if there are relevant threats or stimuli about which he should be concerned. The smallest proportion of the "normal" dog's time is spent in reactive behavior.

The reactive dog (Fig. 2-4, *B*) spends the least amount of his time in non-vigilant, non-reactive behaviors; most of his time in vigilant, monitoring, and warning behaviors; and more time in reactive behaviors than he spends in calm, non-vigilant behaviors. Note that the thresholds for reaction differ between non-reactive and reactive dogs, and that they change to become higher (more difficult to trigger) with improvement in the reactive dog.

The dotted line with the inflection point represents the midway point where vigilance could segue into reactivity. Any attempts to redirect the dog or to calm him so that he doesn't exhibit the reactive behaviors must occur before this point.

As the reactive dog begins to improve (Fig. 2-4, *C*), the proportion of his time spent in calm, non-reactive behavior increases, the proportion of his time spent in reactive behavior decreases, and the amount of time spent in vigilant, monitoring behaviors is either unchanged or increases. As dogs start to improve, they are uncertain, and although they may not have as many explosions of the problematic behavior, they may be more wary, uncertain, and vigilant.

Further into successful treatment, the reactive dog (Fig. 2-4, *D*) spends the most time engaged in non-reactive and calm behaviors; the least time in

problematic reactive behaviors; and an intermediate amount of time in vigilant, monitoring, and warning behaviors. The reactive dog's threshold for reactivity has also changed. This pattern mirrors the relative proportions of time allocation for the "normal," non-reactive dog (see Fig. 2-4, *A*), but the improved, reactive dog (see Fig. 2-4, *D*) still spends more time in vigilant, monitoring, and warning behaviors and in truly reactive behaviors than the normal dog. In other words, he is improved, may seldom react, and may look "normal," but he is not completely "normal." Without wise management, this dog could reach a level of reactivity where he would still react inappropriately. We do not know whether with continued treatment these dogs can both look like and be "normal" dogs, but if their needs are met and they are well managed by observant clients, *it will not matter because they will not exhibit problematic behaviors:* the clients will strive to keep the reactive tendencies of these dogs at a level below which the dog reacts, regardless of the social, environmental, or intrinsic/internal stimuli that trigger the reactions.

Figure 2-4 shows that one of the reasons reactive dogs are so problematic is that they spend the greater proportion of their time thinking about being reactive or doing so, and they have a relatively smaller window in which intervention is possible. *As unfair as it seems, people with reactive dogs get less time to intervene and must make that intervention go further than people with normal dogs under the same conditions.*

Figure 2-5 provides a more real-world example of the problem that reactivity poses for intervention.

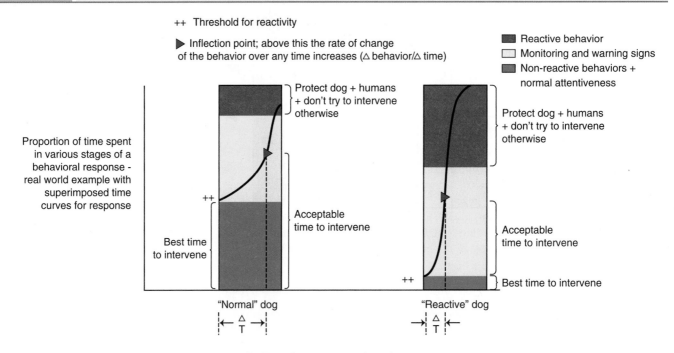

++ Threshold for reactivity

▶ Inflection point; above this the rate of change of the behavior over any time increases (△ behavior/△ time)

■ Reactive behavior
□ Monitoring and warning signs
■ Non-reactive behaviors + normal attentiveness

Proportion of time spent in various stages of a behavioral response - real world example with superimposed time curves for response

Protect dog + humans + don't try to intervene otherwise

Acceptable time to intervene

Best time to intervene

++

"Normal" dog

←— △T —→

Protect dog + humans + don't try to intervene otherwise

Acceptable time to intervene

Best time to intervene

++

"Reactive" dog

→ △T ←

△ T Time client has to convince dog not to react

Fig. 2-5 A more real-world example of the problem that reactivity poses for intervention. Green represents calm, non-reactive, and normally attentive behaviors; yellow represents monitoring behaviors with warning signs; red represents reactive behaviors. The superimposed curves show how normal and reactive dogs or cats change in response to a reactive stimulus. The reactive dog or cat has a lower threshold for any response, reacts more quickly to a level where he must simply be protected and moved out of the situation, and ends his behavior at a higher level of reactivity. The *triangle* represents the inflection point after which all intervention can be focused only on keeping everyone safe and on getting the dog or cat out of the situation as quickly as possible.

Normal, calm, non-reactive behaviors do not suddenly shift to reactive behaviors. There are transitions between behaviors and successful clients need to be able to recognize these transitions if they wish for their dogs to improve to the extent possible.

Note that in Figure 2-5 the non-reactive behaviors grade into the monitoring and warning behaviors, which then grade into the truly reactive behaviors. As soon as the gradation intensifies, behaviors change. The superimposed time curve for the response (the S-shaped lines) indicates how behaviors change with time for the "normal" dog and the "reactive" dog. The inflection point *(triangle)* marks the point beyond which rate of change of the behavior over time (△behavior/△time) alters quickly. In other words, beyond this point, any interventions are going to be difficult for the reactive dog. Once the vigilant and monitoring behaviors begin to contain elements of the reactive behaviors (overlap of red and yellow zones), it's best just to protect the dog and humans and not otherwise intervene. Just get the dog out of the situation as quickly as possible and don't try to "correct" or "fix" anything because it's not possible at this time. The *best time* to intervene is from the green zone through the overlap of green and yellow zones, and it is *acceptable* to intervene up to the

inflection point. Note that these rules hold whether the dog is "normal"/non-reactive or "reactive." The differences between the reactive and normal dogs are what matters.

- Normal/non-reactive dogs have a longer window of time in which they can be convinced to engage in another behavior than reactive dogs.
- Normal/non-reactive dogs have a higher threshold level (the beginning of the curve) for reactivity than reactive dogs.
- Normal/non-reactive dogs reach a lower point of reactivity than reactive dogs.
- Normal/non-reactive dogs take longer to reach their maximum reactivity and do so more slowly than reactive dogs.

For a client to be successful in treating a reactive dog—whether that reactivity involves a fearful response or an aggressive one—the client must understand these patterns and be able to indicate which of the dog's behaviors occur in *his* non-reactive zone, *his* vigilant zone, and *his* reactive zone. Only when clients can use and monitor these behaviors to inform how they will work with and intervene on behalf of the dog can any form of passive or active behavior modification become effective. Veterinarians may wish to engage with their clients in the exercise of listing "green," "yellow," and "red" behaviors for reactive patients so that plans are made, practiced, and modified as needed based on responses observed for each anxious and troubled dog.

What Contributes to a Dog Becoming "Reactive"?

The etiology behind the development of reactivity is unknown. The response surface interactions discussed earlier are likely important. In mice, cats, and dogs, there appear to be genetic lines or strains that are "more reactive" than others. Individuals from these groups have different response surfaces than "less reactive" lines and strains. There may also be in utero and epigenetic effects that contribute to overall reactivity of dogs in the same way that we know affect rodents and humans. Research comparable to rodent and human research is largely unavailable for dogs, but some early data suggest that these periods and effects should be more fully examined.

Pierantoni et al. (2011) showed that for 70 adult dogs who as puppies had been separated from their dam and litter at 30 to 40 days with 70 adult dogs who as puppies were not separated until after 8 weeks, early age of separation was a significant predictor for excessive barking, fearfulness on walks, reactivity to noises, toy possessiveness, food passiveness, and attention-seeking behavior. Dogs adopted early away from their litter were also more at risk for destructive behavior than dogs who had been permitted to stay with their litter through 8 weeks (Pierantoni et al., 2011).

There are few data on effects of anxiety on learning in dogs, but we know from studies on rodents and human children that chronic glucocorticoid excess—at any time, including pre- and peri-natally—interferes with learning at the cellular level (Yau et al., 2002). Chronic glucocorticoid exposure also appears to affect the structural development of the hippocampus—the brain region responsible for associational learning and its further integration into cortical function—and the amygdala—the region responsible for developing and modulating fear (Carter et al., 2002; Davis, 1997; Gogolla et al., 2009; LeDoux et al., 1990; Schafe et al., 2001; Wittenberg and Tsien, 2002).

Within the hippocampus, corticosteroids affect neuronal survival and excitability, cell proliferation, and gene expression and directly and indirectly affect the signaling mechanisms underlying learning and memory (Gould and Tanapat, 1999; Kim and Diamond, 2002; McEwen and Magarinos, 2001; Sapolsky, 2011). Chronic cortisol elevation appears to act as a translational gene regulator—a hormonal response element—that interferes with acquisition and consolidation of task learning in regions of the hippocampus (Lubin et al., 2008). Pre-natal stress and chronic ongoing stress in rats leads

to lower levels of extinction of cue-conditioned fear (Green et al., 2011), causes shrinkage of the hippocampus leading to memory impairment, and facilitates fear conditioning in the amygdala, especially for consolidation of auditory fear conditioning (Bisaz and Sandi, 2010); see Figure 2-6 for a schematic of how these factors are inter-connected. These effects may be more pronounced in some genetic backgrounds (Carola and Gross, 2010).

With respect to the levels of functional diagnoses and pathological integration described in Figure 2-6, pink lettering flags relevant neuroanatomical regions, and green lettering codes for associated neurochemistry. Purple shapes indicate subsequently affected neurochemistry, shades of turquoise shapes mark various molecular contributions to behavioral outcomes, and rust shapes indicate functional neuroanatomical and behavioral outcomes of all interactions. The most detrimental outcomes are indicated by darker colors. It's clear that the various underlying levels of any phenotype of behavioral pathology interacts across time in complex ways with that phenotype.

Stress that leads to the hypothalamic-pituitary-adrenocortical (HPA) cascade increases cortisol (left side of diagram). Cortisol adversely affects neuromolecular and neurochemical aspects of learning leading to apoptosis (cellular death) and decreased neurogenesis, synaptogenesis, et cetera, in the hippocampus (middle of diagram). Treatment with common medications augments learning in the hippocampus by enhancing receptor function and various growth factors that lead to hippocampal neurogenesis, synaptogenesis, et cetera (right side of diagram). Recovery from behavioral illness requires plump, healthy neurons that can communicate with other neurons through receptor stimulation of second messenger systems, leading to increases in protein kinases and neurotrophic factors that result in post-translational protein production resulting in new receptors, transcription factors, synaptic connections, et cetera.

Numerous studies, including those cited here, suggest potential mechanisms for the findings by Pierantoni et al. that puppies separated early experienced more fearfulness on walks, reactivity to noises, and overall enhanced reactivity as adults than puppies allowed to stay with their dams and littermates. One has to wonder whether humans willing to rush pups out the door act on any concept of providing the best environment for the bitch, and hence the pups, during pregnancy. If early adoption co-occurs with less-than-optimal breeding and pregnancy practices, pups can have real problems.

Prenatal exposure to maternal stress causes epigenetic methylation of glucocorticoid receptor promoter regions, which causes hyper-reactivity in rodents and humans (Radtke et al., 2011). In rodents, hippocampal expression of the glucocorticoid receptor gene and

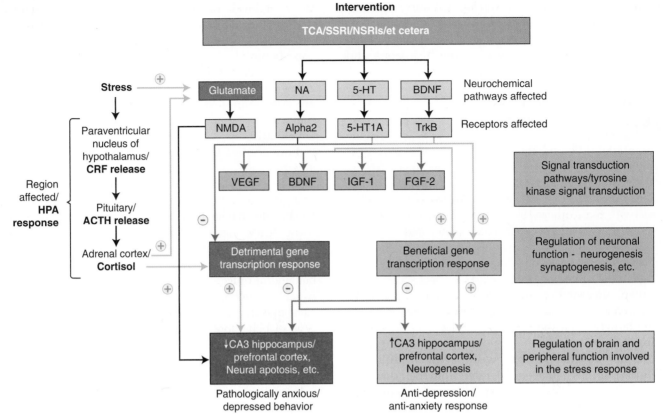

Fig. 2-6 Effects of stress and common pharmacological treatments (TCAs, SSRIs, NSRIs) for resultant behavioral distress/pathology on neurochemistry and related outcomes. Growth factor effects of treatment with psychotropic medications are likely critically important for clinical improvement and may require long-term treatment. *TCAs,* Tricyclic antidepressants; *SSRIs,* selective serotonin reuptake inhibitors; *NSRIs,* noradrenaline/serotonin reuptake inhibitors; *HPA,* hypothalamic-pituitary-adrenocortical response (this response occurs at the neuroanatomical level shown in Figure 2-1); *CRF,* corticosteroid releasing factor; *ACTH,* adrenocorticotropic hormone; *NA,* noradrenaline; *5-HT,* serotonin; *BDNF,* brain-derived neurotrophic factor; *NMDA,* N-methyl-D-aspartate; *TrkB,* protein kinase B; *VEGF,* vascular endothelial growth factor; *IGF-1,* insulin-like growth factor 1; *FGF,* fibroblast growth factor; *CA3,* region of the hippocampus especially involved in long-term potentiation and learning and used as a standard for functional morphological measures. (After Duman and Monteggia [2006], Rang et al. [2012], and others.)

behavioral responses to stress are modulated by the amount of care mothers give young in the first few days of life (Weaver et al., 2004), a process that likely also occurs in dogs. These studies show that task learning can be enhanced when stress and distress are mitigated. Raising puppies with their siblings and dam through 70 days, a time when most brain myelination is complete but when neuronal remodeling should be rapidly ongoing, provides such mitigation.

These emergent, complex neurobiological findings can be distilled to a few simple guidelines for breeding and raising pups, and all veterinarians should consider the implications with their clients.

- Considering the enhanced risk of relinquishment, abandonment, and euthanasia for dogs with any behavioral concerns, puppies should remain with their litters in the home of and with access to the dam through 8 weeks of age.

- Dams should have excellent pre-, peri-, and post-partum nutrition.
- Puppies, bitches, and dams should be exposed to humane conditions that minimize the risks of excess stress and fear.

This is a standard no puppy mill or farm can meet and with which some private breeders may struggle. Regardless, considering the overall contribution of "reactivity" to behavioral problems, true prevention is going to occur only when we meet the needs of the dogs and put their welfare concerns and quality of life first.

WHAT ABOUT CATS?

The same concerns pertain to reactivity in cats and to the diagnostic terminology governing feline behavioral diagnoses. For both cats and dogs, we fail to emphasize that far more important than choosing a label is:

- getting an exhaustive list of the behaviors the constitute the non-specific signs,
- attaching these signs to specific contexts,
- enumerating the patterns of the behaviors and responses with respect to any relevant provocative stimuli, and
- the value of using any response to perturbation in the social or physical environment (behavior modification, environmental change, social manipulation, pharmacological treatment) as a way to solicit data that can help inform classification of problems and aid in their resolution.

Given the large number of feral cats who are born and raised under less-than-optimal situations worldwide, the type of reactivity that affects puppies with poor beginnings should also affect cats. Unfortunately, there are few comparable data, but such studies could be done. The evaluation of the effects of early environments and stressors on later feline behavior may be complicated in cats because of their unique patterns of neurophysiological response and recruitment of neurons in the amygdala and hypothalamus. Cats have an atypical response to arousal in general when their hypothalamus is stimulated (Adamec, 1975a; Adamec et al., 1980a, 1980b, 1980c; Bernston et al., 1976a, 1976b; Bernston and Leibowitz, 1973; Bernston and Micco, 1976).

- Cats isolated from other cats for most of the first year of life exhibit a response characterized by galvanic skin responses and disruption of regular sleep rhythms.
- Excitation of the ventromedial hypothalamus and amygdala leads to a defensive response in cats.
- Stimulation of the lateral amygdala facilitates predatory attack and defensiveness in cats, but stimulation of the lateral amygdala using high intensity also recruits the ventral hippocampus in these behaviors, providing a partial explanation for why repetition is so problematic. The hippocampus plays a major role in associational learning.

These neural-stimulatory patterns affect how cats manifest pathological aggression and other anxiety disorders that may have explosive components (e.g., obsessive-compulsive disorder). These issues are addressed in Chapter 5.

Changing Behavior: Roles for Learning, Negotiated Settlements, and Individualized Treatment Plans

OVERVIEW

Thinking About Goals of Treatment

The goal of treatment for canine and feline behavioral concerns is a *negotiated settlement*. Everyone may not get what they want, but everyone *can* get what they need. This is true whether the behaviors of concern are normal behaviors that the clients dislike or will not tolerate or true behavioral pathologies that put the patient and others at risk. This negotiated settlement is obtained by identifying factors that can be changed through intervention, factors that can be avoided, and factors that require risk mitigation (Box 3-1).

Negotiated settlements can be created only in the context of honest discussion, the first step of which is to learn what the clients want as an outcome. Clients may not be able to have exactly what they want, but to negotiate a settlement that works for them successfully. Full disclosure of needs, concerns, fears, and annoyances/frustrations is essential. As clients discuss their concerns, fears, and distress, the "available space" for a negotiated outcome becomes apparent. With more information and a better understanding of the behavior and how it can be changed, this "available space" can only increase, and options that clients did not think were possible often become so.

The easiest way to learn what clients want is to ask them. Some clients do not have an appreciation of how much the dog or cat is suffering or how much risk may be present until they work through an extensive, exhaustive history questionnaire. The process of completing a history questionnaire informs the client's opinion of what they want and what a negotiated settlement can look like. Further discussion during the consultation allows clients to understand where and how their pet is troubled as they begin to understand normal behaviors/responses and the extent to which their pet deviates from these. If clients appreciate the level of distress that their pets are experiencing *and* understand that such distress can be alleviated humanely, they are more willing to meet the pet's needs

and become less focused on their fears and their desire for a "cure." We "cure" almost no conditions in this field, but—as with so many physical conditions—we can do a stellar job of controlling them, providing an excellent quality of life (QoL) for the pet and the client.

Good, standardized history questionnaires—*when followed by an informed review to establish agreement on terminology and validity of assessment*—do two things:
- They provide clients with an objective way to see their pets and their concerns.
- They form the first step in having someone listen to clients in a non-judgmental, helpful, and empathetic manner.

There are two sets of standardized history questionnaires included within this text and on the companion website: long questionnaires for cats and dogs with known behavioral concerns and short questionnaires for cats and dogs to use as routine screening tools at every appointment.

The concept of the outcome of a negotiated settlement helps clients to understand that although the cat or dog *may* never behave perfectly, *improvement, happiness, safety, and less stress for everyone all are attainable outcomes.* This concept also helps clients to understand that the processes of improving and negotiating relationships is lifelong and that they will continuously build on actions that have come before. As such, these settlements give clients permission to make temporary choices that may make their lives easier and increase their tolerance for handling the dog or cat. For example, boarding the dog during a family visit may be easier for the clients than having the dog present, especially if they worry (*regardless of whether the worry is justified*).

Negotiated settlements allow clients to understand that setbacks are likely, the route will not be linear, mistakes will be made, but improvement is still attainable, and recovery can be one of the ultimate goals. If everyone can focus on creating the best possible relationship with the pet, while meeting the dog's or cat's needs, treatment decisions can become much more clear and straightforward.

BOX 3-1

Factors to Be Identified in a Negotiated Settlement for Behavioral Concerns

1. Which aspects of the concern can be changed through avoidance?
2. Which aspects of the concern can be changed through intervention?
3. Which aspects of the concern require risk mitigation, and what plans does this mitigation require?

KEYS TO SUCCESSFUL INTERVENTION AND TREATMENT IN A NEGOTIATED SETTLEMENT

There are four required aspects of intervention to facilitate successful treatment as part of a negotiated settlement (Box 3-2).

1. Avoid the circumstances that provoke the behavior from the dog or cat or that are known to be a factor in the pet exhibiting the behavior.
2. Do not punish the dog or cat. Punishment merely tells the pet what *not* to do *and* will further raise levels of anxiety and reactivity.
3. Design and implement an appropriate behavior modification plan for *that* pet in *that* household using the techniques and strategies discussed later. Essential components of behavior modification include:
   a. Strategies designed to teach the dog or cat that they are happier and safer if they are calmer and less reactive
   b. Teaching the pet that he or she can take the cues about the appropriateness of their behavior from you and any normal pets in the household
   c. Teaching the pet that he or she does not have to react and can instead either avoid provoking situations or respond differently to those situations
4. Praise and reward the dog or cat for *any* behaviors considered acceptable or good, even if they are normal behaviors and occur when the pet is not interacting with anyone. *This is the most important part of treatment, and almost everyone ignores it.*
5. Approaches involving clear signaling, positive rewards, and predictable human behavior have been shown experimentally to be superior for training dogs.
   a. Client reports of their dog's obedience performance are higher when positive rewards are used (Hiby et al., 2004) and when the methods the clients use are consistent, clear, and reliable (Arhant et al., 2010).
   b. The ability to learn new tasks—and this is what behavior modification is for most clients and pets—is positively associated with the total rewards (praise, play, treats) that the dog receives and the patience that the client displays while teaching the dog the new behaviors (Rooney and Cowan, 2011).

BOX 3-2

Main Foci for Intervention as Part of Any Behavioral Treatment Plan

1. Avoid situations and triggers associated with the behaviors
2. No punishment
3. Behavior modification to teach dogs and cats to be calm and less reactive
4. Praise and reward all good behaviors all the time even if they are accidental or normal (e.g., sleeping)

All of these strategies are explained and demonstrated in the accompanying video, *Humane Behavioral Care for Dogs: Problem Prevention and Treatment.*

Do We Have to Wait until the Dog or Cat Has a Problem to Create a Set of Rules for Negotiated Settlements?

No! In fact, if everyone in the veterinary practice begins to model their puppy/kitten, new dog/cat, and wellness visits in the manner suggested in Chapter 1, everything that was just discussed can be implemented as a plan to *prevent a problem or intervene early* in problem development. This is called *anticipatory guidance.* Anticipatory guidance is used a lot in some human medical specialties, such as pediatrics, but it is underused in veterinary medicine. For a discussion of using this approach with children and dogs, see the "Protocol for Introducing a New Baby and a Pet" and the "Protocol for Handling and Surviving Aggressive Events."

Any method that can be used to treat a behavioral problem will work as well or better to prevent one. All of the protocols for treating specific behavioral concerns can be used to prevent full-blown problems and as early interventions. If veterinary staff use interventional protocols and behavior modification plans in this manner, we will save lives, have more fun, have more profitable businesses, and have better relationships with our clients and patients.

Prognoses and Predictors of Outcomes

Treatment of infectious or neoplastic conditions is largely dependent on the disease process and available interventions. The social and physical environment and daily behaviors of the family members of the ill dog or cat matter little for such treatment outcomes compared with the medications and other interventions used to treat the condition. *This situation is completely reversed for behavioral conditions.*

- Every single behavioral condition has a management component as part of the treatment.
- Every single behavioral condition can be made worse or better by the manner in which humans

interact with the dog or cat and by environmental alterations.

Because of this, prognosis is *not* well linked to diagnosis in veterinary behavioral medicine. Five main factors are generally thought to contribute to the success of treatment:

- client compliance,
- age of onset,
- predictability of outbursts,
- duration of the condition, and
- pattern of the behavioral changes in response to environmental, behavioral, and pharmacological intervention.

Of these factors, client compliance may be the most critical. This finding should not be interpreted to "blame" the clients for the pet's problems. With the exception of abusive or neglectful situations, most canine or feline behavioral problems are not created by people. It is true that people make mistakes, that they do not understand other species, and that it is possible to make any situation worse by inappropriate interventions. However, no study has been successful in showing that pets' problem behaviors/pathologies are attributable to similar problems in their people (Clark & Boyer, 1993; Jagoe and Serpell, 1996; Parthasarathay and Crowell-Davis, 2006; Voith et al., 1992). Interestingly, studies have shown that people who read their pets'

signals best, best meet their pets' needs, and find their pets charming and brilliant (Bradshaw and Nott, 1992; Rooney et al., 2001), suggesting a strong and profitable role for the veterinary profession in education of clients.

Boxes 3-3 through 3-6 outline good and poor prognosticators for behavioral conditions. Prognosis is best understood if client-driven and patient-driven factors are considered separately. A review of these lists suggests that the rate-limiting step for how well dogs and cats can become is the domain of their humans.

Are There Any Generalized Instructions That Can Be Quickly Given to Clients When They Express a Concern About Pet Behaviors?

Yes. If clients engage in the following behaviors, their pets either will never exhibit behavioral concerns or will start to improve. Depending on the problem, the type of improvement that the clients desire will require more specific and detailed help, but these are *three no-fail steps* (Box 3-7) that will help in any problem and that will form the basis of all the treatment interventions discussed in this chapter.

- Cease all punishment: no yelling, screaming, throwing things or pets, hitting, kicking, smacking, hanging or otherwise "disciplining" of the pet.

BOX 3-3

Client-Driven Factors Associated with Poor Outcomes

- Clients who cannot or will not comply with instructions meant to minimize risk, stress, and distress
- Clients who have a lack of understanding or acceptance of the dog's or cat's needs
- Clients who want or need to blame the dog or cat
- Clients who have an idealized world view of how their cat or dog "should" act and look
- Clients who are caught in a cycle of anger and fighting within the family that always seems to revolve around the dog and the dog's behavior
- Clients with lots of other stressors in their life: dogs and cats with behavioral concerns can be, but don't have to be, strains on marriages and family relationships
- Clients who have ill-behaved or unsupervised or unsupervisable young children
- Clients who live in very reactive, unpredictable households and environments
- Clients who do not like the cat or dog
- Clients who "need" a "quick fix"
- Clients who have and wish to adhere to a rigid timetable for improvement
- Clients with overly busy households, especially if they contain young children
- Clients who believe that children should be able to do anything they want with pets

- Clients with any perception or belief that the dog or cat is unpredictable and so inherently dangerous
- Clients with a continuing belief that the dog or cat is "unpredictable," even after a consultation with a specialist
- Clients who fear the patient
- Clients who are angry with the patient
- Clients who need to control all aspects of the patient's behavior
- Clients with dissention within the household over how treatment should be enacted, especially if one household member wants the pet dead or out of the house
- Clients who feel embarrassed or that a behavioral problem reflects poorly on them
- Clients who are unable or unwilling to avoid provocative situations
- Clients who are feeling especially financially compromised
- Clients who have used remote shock to "control" real or perceived aggressive behaviors
- Clients who experience adverse changes in financial or housing circumstances
- Clients who have seriously considered putting down the dog or cat and entertain this thought in most or all discussions involving the pet

BOX 3-4

Client-Driven Factors Associated with Good Outcomes

- Clients with a desire to understand the problem
- Clients with a desire to meet the needs of the dog or cat
- Clients with a willingness and ability to protect the patient
- Clients with an interest in quality-of-life (QoL) issues
- Clients who can recognize and identify patterns of behaviors when taught what to look for
- Clients who can recognize triggers and manipulate their environment and responses
- Clients who are flexible and willing and able to compromise
- Clients who do not feel embarrassed by the patient's behavior or who can disregard their embarrassment for the good of the dog or cat
- Clients who understand that some normal childhood behaviors are scary for pets
- Clients who help children to understand kindness and respect for animals
- Clients who like the dog or cat
- Clients who feel a special bond with their dog or cat
- Clients who have friends and/or family members who have struggled with and/or been helped by some form cognitive therapy and/or psychotropic medication
- Clients who live in less stimulating or more predictable environments
- Clients who can accept imperfection
- Clients who are willing and able to avoid as many problematic situations as possible
- Clients who understand that the behavior is not "normal" and that it is problematic for the dog or cat
- Clients who have never considered euthanasia

BOX 3-5

Patient-Driven Factors Associated with Poor Outcomes

- Concomitant severe organic disease, in the presence of any of the human factors associated with poor outcomes
- Exhibition of behaviors that require people to do a lot of physical, expensive, and time-consuming work (e.g., cleaning rugs, repairing doors)
- Bites/injuries to humans or other animals *whether or not these were accidental, serious, or warranted*
- Inattentive behavior to humans
- Early-onset, long-standing behaviors

BOX 3-6

Patient-Driven Factors Associated with Good Outcomes

- Recent behavioral change without long-standing history
- Behavioral changes that develop with time (the clients enjoyed puppyhood/kittenhood)
- Otherwise healthy
- Attentiveness to humans
- Exhibition of any behaviors that clients find funny, fun, interesting, endearing, or loving

BOX 3-7

Three No-Fail Steps to Avoid, Prevent, and Begin to Fix Any Behavioral Problem

1. Cease all punishment
2. Identify and avoid situations in which the undesirable behavior occurs
3. Watch for and reward behaviors that are acceptable and considered "good"

- Identify situations in which the behavior occurs and avoid those: for example, if the cat uses the carpet only when the litter hasn't been changed for 2 days, change the litter before 2 days.
- Watch for and reward the behaviors that you like and find acceptable: this often means telling the dog or cat that he is wonderful when he is asleep.

These three no-fail steps succeed because they encourage clients to meet the pet's needs, and they provide information about the pets with respect to what the clients want, not what they don't want. All of us work for information about which of our behaviors are acceptable or exceptional. Nowhere is this more true than for troubled cats and dogs, whose most valuable currency is accurate information.

UNDERSTANDING BEHAVIORAL INTERVENTIONS

What Can We Change or Manipulate?

In any situation involving problematic behaviors, there are three groups of environments that we can potentially manipulate and modify:
- physical environment,
- social and related behavioral environments, and
- pharmacological/neurochemical environment.

These environments are not independent. The extent to which psychotropic/behavioral medication may be warranted depends on the severity of the condition (how abnormal or problematic the neurochemical and behavioral responses are) and the ability to manipulate physical and social environments. Newer behavioral medications allow faster and more effective manipulation of the endogenous neurochemical environment, which helps to shape more appropriate neurochemical and behavioral responses to stimuli in the physical and social environments.

Roles for Arousal and Environmental Manipulation

Arousal

At the core of virtually all behavioral conditions, especially conditions related to anxiety, is the arousal level of the patient. Heightened arousal, *beyond a certain adaptive level*:

- prohibits accurate observation and assimilation of the information presented,
- interferes with processing of that information, and
- can adversely affect actions taken based on these earlier steps.

Non-adaptive arousal usually manifests as *fear*, which can have as a component *defensive aggression, or anxiety*, which can have as a component *offensive aggression*. Fear and anxiety are closely related but may not be identical at the neurophysiological level.

One should remember that when one diagnoses a problem related to fear or anxiety, one is doing so at the level of the phenotypic or functional diagnosis. Although much treatment and subsequent assessment focuses on changing the non-specific signs apparent at the phenotypic level, if psychotropic medication is used, we are intervening at the molecular and neurophysiological levels (which we then hope will help change the phenotypic level). New evidence about epigenetic effects suggests that effects at the molecular and neurophysiological levels may be governing the signs expressed by which we recognize the condition and the manner in which neurophysiological and molecular effects act (Krishnan and Nestler, 2008; Lubin et al., 2008; McGowan et al., 2009).

Anxiety is broadly defined as the apprehensive anticipation of future danger or misfortune accompanied by a feeling of dysphoria (in humans) and/or somatic symptoms of tension (vigilance and scanning, autonomic hyperactivity, increased motor activity and tension) (Overall, 1997, 2005a, 2005b). The focus of the anxiety can be internal or external. For an anxiety or fear to be pathological, it must be exhibited out-of-context or in a degree or form that would be sufficient to accomplish an ostensible goal (Ohl et al., 2008; Overall, 1997, 2000, 2005a, 2005b). The focus on context for the response and degree and form of behaviors informs all of our definitions of canine and feline behavior problems as discussed here.

We are quite good about recognizing situational anxiety in dogs where the stimulus is external (e.g., someone leaves the house, the client is out of sight), but we are not good at recognizing anxiety that is internally generated or found to be distressing by the dog (e.g., as in panic disorder, canine post-traumatic stress disorder, or generalized anxiety disorder (GAD); see Chapter 7 for a discussion of these conditions). Given what we now know about canine cognition, we must believe that true endogenous canine anxiety, such as that exhibited by dogs with GAD, occurs and can be recognized on the basis of the behaviors exhibited, across the contexts in which the behavior appears. The conditions specified in the general definition of anxiety should help us frame our criteria for diagnoses of pathological conditions involving anxiety and their assessments.

Accordingly, we should use as gauges of anxiety both behavioral and neurophysiological signs of anxiety. Behavioral signs of anxiety can include:

- increased vigilance,
- increased scanning,
- increased attentiveness,
- increased monitoring of the actions of others,
- increased or decreased motor activity, with an extreme of freezing,
- signs of autonomic hyperactivity (urination, defecation, trembling, shaking, panting), and
- offensive aggression.

Neurophysiological signs of anxiety can include (Beerda et al., 1997, 1998, 2000):

- tachycardic or bradycardic changes in heart rate (affected by norepinephrine [NE]),
- alterations in blood pressure (affected by NE),
- mydriasis (affected by NE),
- vasodilation/constriction (affected by NE),
- alterations in gastrointestinal function (which can result in subsequent diarrhea),
- changes in hypothalamic-pituitary-adrenocortical (HPA) axis function including effects of peripheral blood counts (note that chronic anxiety experienced secondary to chronic stress can blunt HPA axis function, which is why "changes" in function are emphasized),
- salivation,
- muscle tension and concomitant CK/CPK release (this muscle tension is the cause of dander release and damp fur/paws), and
- alterations in sleep and sleep-wake cycles (if the anxiety is long-term).

Fear is usually defined as a feeling of apprehension associated with the presence or proximity of an object, individual, social situation, or class of the above (Overall, 1997, 2005a, 2005b). Fear is part of normal behavior and can be an adaptive response. The determination of whether the fear or fearful response is abnormal or inappropriate must be determined by context. For example, fire is a useful tool, but fear of being consumed by it, if the house is on fire, is an adaptive response. If the house is not on fire, such fear would be irrational and, if it was constant or recurrent, probably maladaptive. Normal and abnormal fears are usually manifested as graded responses, with the intensity of the response proportional to the proximity (or the perception of the proximity) of the stimulus in the case of the "normal" fear and disproportionate or out-of-context with respect to the "abnormal" fear. A sudden, all-or-nothing, profound, abnormal response that results in extremely fearful behaviors (catatonia, panic) is usually called a phobia.

There are two conditions involving fear that affect many animals and that, when defined, will help in this discussion of treatment (also see the discussion in Chapters 7 and 9).

- *Fear/fearful behavior*
  - *Criteria:* Responses to stimuli (social or physical) that are characterized by withdrawal; passive and active avoidance behaviors associated with the sympathetic branch of the autonomic nervous system and in the absence of any aggressive behavior. Specific behavioral responses include tucking of neck, head, tail and all limbs, hunched backs, trembling, salivating, licking lips, turning away, hiding (even if the only hiding possible is by curling into oneself), averted eyes, et cetera. In extreme cases, urination and defecation are possible. Release of anal sacs may occur. Dander may become apparent, and fur may feel damp.
  - *Notes:* Fear and anxiety have signs that overlap. Some non-specific signs such as avoidance (which is different from withdrawal), shaking, and trembling can be characteristic of both. The physiological signs probably differ at some refined level, and the neurochemistry of each are probably very different. It is hoped that refinements in qualification and quantification of the observable behaviors will parallel these differences.
- *Fear aggression*
  - *Criteria:* Aggression (threat, challenge, or contest) that consistently occurs concomitant with behavioral and physiological signs of fear as identified by withdrawal, passive, and avoidance behaviors associated with the actions of the sympathetic branch of the autonomic nervous system. When these signs are accompanied by urination or defecation or when the aggression is active/interactive (i.e., defensive aggression)—even if the recipient of the aggression has disengaged from or did not deliberately provoke the interaction—the diagnosis of fear aggression is confirmed.
  - *Notes:* The actual behaviors associated with fear, fear aggression, and any aggression primarily driven by anxiety (see discussion on impulse control and interdog aggression, for example) are poorly qualified and quantified. In extreme cases, the conditions specified will be clear. If the aggression appears mild, it could be due to uncertainty

on the patient's part. Caution is urged in ruling out all other aggressions. The diagnosis that is most consistent and concordant with signs and criteria should be the one prescribed to the patient.

- Fear aggression does not have to occur consistently, although identification of the fearful stimuli will permit assessment of the extent to which the behaviors are consistent and pose a predictable risk.
- All of the behaviors associated with fear can occur with fear aggression, but when fear aggression is the consideration, aggressive behaviors usually occur before behaviors associated with extreme distress (urination/defecation/anal sac release, et cetera) occur or as they are happening.
- Finally, if the patient is affected by fear aggression, aggressive acts are most likely to occur if the patient is trapped or reached toward or as the provocative stimulus moves away while the patient is moving away and/or attempting to conclude the interaction.

Although anxiety and arousal may be the underlying stimuli that give rise to a fearful response, outright anxiety and fear differ because of neocortical processing and signaling that may be, but do not need to be, affected by the behaviors of other individuals involved in the interaction. Fear is characterized by physical withdrawal, decreased social interaction, and clear signaling that interaction will be truncated and that the subject/signaler wishes to disengage and is not an overt threat. Purely anxious behaviors can range from more overt, provocative ones to full withdrawal. *If clients understand this, they have a better chance of managing the dog humanely and avoiding injury.*

A lot has been written about the role for "appeasement" in fear and anxiety. We should have two concerns when this term is used in the context of fear or fear aggression:

1. "Appeasement" is seldom defined, given the context. A full understanding of risks, costs, and threats would need to be available to define "appeasement."
2. There may be more parsimonious explanations for the animal's behaviors that do not require extrapolation of some "emotional" or "motivational" state that is difficult to measure. Message and meaning analysis (Smith, 1977) provides a more discrete, judgment-free, and value-free way of interpreting complex social interactions by allowing us to know, for example, when one participant is signaling their withdrawal. This approach has an advantage over the motivational approach because it is based on behaviors without any assumptions about how these are interpreted by the dog. No one doubts that dogs and cats experience a complete range of emotions, but our attributions about them may be inaccurate, and what we assume to be a "motivation" may not

be as important to the dog or cat as it appears to us. If we are really to move into an era of research that maximizes welfare and QoL issues for our patients, we must be cautious about simplistic approaches that make our lives easier but that may not accurately reflect the dog's or cat's behaviors and their interpretation of them.

Environmental Manipulation

The physical and behavioral environments are often factors affecting the dog's level of arousal. Although these environments may be completely within the normal range of those dogs routinely encounter, for individual dogs certain environments will be sufficient to trigger a problematic response. Given this, understanding the role the environment may play in the response provides help for treatment.

Manipulating the physical environment is often overlooked, yet environmental change can often be the first and easiest step in decreasing the patient's arousal levels. If our goal is to raise the threshold at which the cat or dog displays the signs associated with the diagnosis or the behaviors associated with the client complaint—and these behaviors could be normal—environmental manipulation may be simple and helpful (Fig. 3-1; this figure also appears in Chapter 2).

Figure 3-1, *A*, shows the effect of repeated stimuli, baseline levels of reactivity, and thresholds on the exhibition of behaviors. If the patient is already aroused, a stimulus that would be below the level at which he or she would react may cause reaction. If multiple stimuli are presented to the patient before he or she has returned to baseline levels, they may act additively, causing the patient to react more profoundly or in more situations than that patient would have otherwise reacted. This graph shows how important controlling the stimulus environment can be. If you allow the patient to return to baseline between provocative events, you do not trigger the response. If you continue to force the patient to be exposed to provocative events, the patient reacts to ever higher levels. Because the reaction is profound and the duration of the decay of the response is lengthy (Pitman et al., 1988), you cannot teach appropriate behaviors because the cortisol and epinephrine levels interfere with genetic transcription of information. You can only reinforce fear and avoidance. This application should resonate with veterinarians who have experienced treatment of patients using high levels of restraint.

Note that Figure 3-1, *A*, was developed using only patient A's response, and patient A is the most normal of the patients. The basal response level or response surface of the patient interacts across time with the intensity and frequency of the stimulus to produce the overall behavioral response.

Because of these patterns of reactivity and arousal, the most unexploited of the possible manipulations involve the physical and social environments. Protecting dogs and cats from situations that they may find distressing or stressful promotes two changes essential for improvement:
1. Avoidance allows the dog or cat *not to react* to something. By not reacting, the patient does not learn with practice how to react more quickly, more frequently, and more intensely. Avoidance means patients do not experience generalization of an undesired response or lowering of the reaction threshold, both of which often occur with practice.
2. Avoidance promotes a *level of calm* that allows animals to *learn new behaviors and responses* and to take their cues better as to the appropriateness of their behavior from the context. This type of learning is not possible if the patient is aroused, stressed, or reacting.

Physical Environments
The physical environment includes:
• actual space considerations and the patient's perception of them,
• any visual, olfactory, or auditory stimuli,
• any other animals who share the environment,
• objects such as litterboxes, beds, and food toys, and
• objects that might change the dog's or cat's perception, such as curtains or the presence of background music.

Other animals are part of the physical environment—they take up physical space and use the same resources. They are usually, but not always, also part of the behavioral environment: a dog that can be seen through a window may be sufficient to trigger a reaction from a dog or cat indoors, although the outside dog was not part of any direct social interaction.

Because "perception" is so critical in the evaluation of the physical environment, clients' schedules and use of space must also be considered. Some problems, such as separation anxiety in dogs, may become apparent when the only environment that changes is the temporal one: day length shortens or the clients' schedules change. Part of the treatment must address this environmental change.

The physical environment may need to be modified because it is a direct part of the problem (e.g., insufficient space for exercise) or because changing the physical environment can help solve the problem.
• *Example 1:* In a shared, roofed kennel, comfortable, personal/individual doghouses with good visibility can divide the physical space in a way that allows the dogs in the kennel to choose not to interact. The doghouses all provide individual shelter so the dogs are not all crowded in the kennel in one place. As long as no bullies are present, this design can relieve social stresses imposed by group housing.
• *Example 2:* The dog becomes aroused and destroys the mail every day when it is put through the slot in

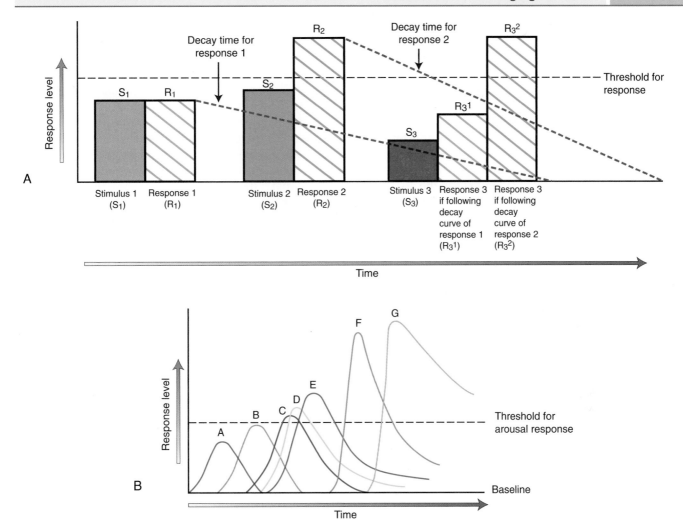

Fig. 3-1 A, The x axis represents time, and the y axis represents response level. R1 shows a response that is proportional to the stimulus—there is no overall behavioral reaction to this stimulus 1 because R1 does not reach the threshold level for the behavioral reaction *(horizontal dashed line)*. The decay time—the time to return to baseline—is shown by the *colored dashed curves*. At stimulus 2, the summed proportional responses exceed the threshold, and the dog reacts (R2). At stimulus 3, even a small stimulus now causes a worsening in the response (R3) if the patient is still experiencing the R2 decay/recovery response because the responses are additive and the arousal level is still high. However, if the patient experiences stimulus 3 after R1 has sufficiently delayed or recovered, the additive level is not sufficient to trigger a response. This graph illustrates how important multiple stressors and the time over which they are experienced can be for the behavior of the dog or cat. These graphs assume that the threshold level stays the same across time, but *with repeated distressing exposures threshold levels for reactivity lower.* **B,** This graph shows how patients with different types of reactivities may respond to the same stimulus and how reactivities can change with time. For simplicity, this graph assumes that the stimulus is the same for each patient, as is the threshold; however, *with repeated distressing exposures threshold levels for reactivity lower.*

- Patient A reacts to the stimulus but not at a sufficient level to trigger the problematic response. Patient A's behavior decays to the baseline quickly.
- Patient B reacts to the stimulus at a level that just triggers the behavior but recovers, and his behavior decays to the baseline quickly.
- Patient C reacts to the stimulus in a way that exceeds the threshold for exhibiting the behavior, and because he had a worse reaction than patient B, he takes longer to return to baseline, but he does recover and return to baseline.
- Patient D reacts to the stimulus in a way that exceeds the threshold for exhibiting the behavior, and this changes his future behaviors and lowers his threshold for reactivity. Notice that beginning with patient D the slope of the curve increases—the patient is reacting more quickly. Patient D does not return to baseline. His recovery is incomplete, which increases the ease with which he will become distressed in the future.
- Patient E reacts to the stimulus in way that far exceeds the threshold for exhibiting the behavior, he remains reactive for longer than does patient E, he has a longer decay period for his response (during which he is easily stimulated to react inappropriately). Patient E reacts very quickly and does not return to baseline. His recovery is incomplete and he will view all future stimuli from the perspective of always being somewhat aroused and distressed. This is one model for patients with panic disorder.
- Patient F shows a very rapid response (see the slope of the curve) with a slow decay that never approaches baseline or the threshold below which he will react. Many small events trigger his response and speed the rate at which he reacts. He is always reactive to some degree, very much like a dog with generalized anxiety disorder (GAD).
- Patient G may or may not be at baseline, but he reacts almost instantly and to a quite high level. Once he reacts, he is very slow to calm. Patient G panics.

the door. If a mailbox is installed at the fence, the mail carrier does not have to come to the door, and the dog does not become aroused. Also, the dog can no longer destroy the mail.

- *Example 3:* The dog meets the criteria for a diagnosis of territorial aggression and constantly monitors approaches to the house. When a person passes on the sidewalk, the dog begins to snarl and lunge at the window as soon as the person comes into view and continues to react until the person passes from view. A gate could be installed to keep the dog in the back of the house. Opaque film, curtains, or blinds could be installed on the window so the dog could not see the people passing.

- *Example 4:* The client's cat sits in the window. Whenever she sees the neighbor's cat come out the cat door and sit in the sun in her own yard, the client's cat becomes distressed and sprays the window. Closing the door to the room where the window is will not "fix" the cat's behavioral response, but it will stop it from being triggered. This may be enough of a change for the client. If the cat is otherwise distressed, this is *not* enough of a change *for the cat,* regardless of whether the client is content. However, closing the door may help lessen the frequency with which the behavior is triggered, which, when combined with medication, may be sufficient to raise that cat's reaction threshold. Closing the door also allows the client to avoid having to clean up sprayed urine, which helps the client to understand the cat's needs separate from her own anger and disgust.

- *Example 5:* The dog meets the diagnostic criteria for and has been diagnosed with inter-dog aggression secondary to GAD and noise phobia. Any loud, echoing noises make the dog more reactive and worsen the GAD. When this happens, the dog threatens his housemates. By having the dog wear Mutt Muffs (www.muttmuffs.com), the overall arousal level is kept low, the GAD triggers are minimized, and the probability of a dog fight is lessened.

In each of these examples, the overall threshold for reactivity was changed by some environmental manipulation. In some cases, the manipulation itself did not allow the behavior to rise to the threshold needed to react; in other cases, the manipulation altered the time frame over which multiple stressors could have acted. Alone, these types of manipulations will not "fix" the patient, but can prevent or decrease the occurrence of behaviors that are most distressing to the clients. Avoidance can also benefit the dog or cat. With time and the molecular changes associated with learning, the actual individual thresholds for each animal's reactivity may change because these dogs and cats may learn that they do not have to react.

When we are manipulating the environment to help negotiate a better or more acceptable behavior, we have to remember that *it is the dog's or cat's perception of the environment that matters*, not ours. If the clients do not know how the dog or cat will react to environmental change, they can collect the data by watching the response. In essence, clients can create their own situation-dependent response curves, as in Figure 3-1, for their own dog or cat and then craft their management tactics around these.

Because perception matters, clients will find that many of the behaviors exhibited by the cat or dog do not "make sense." One response to this is to tell the client that if the behaviors made sense, there would not be a behavioral concern. By definition, behavioral concerns or pathologies involve behaviors that don't "make sense" given the context. This logic can greatly inform environmental and social modification and avoidance.

In behavior cases, *the most successful clients are those who become partners in their dog's or cat's care.* For example, if the dog charges the door when visitors come, the client may try using a baby gate to keep the dog in the kitchen until visitors are settled. The goals are to stop the dog from lunging at the door and jumping up on people and to have the dog calmly greet the humans. However, if the dog perceives confinement as a punishment or if it makes him feel entrapped, this environmental change will not accomplish the ostensible goal because the dog may be more distressed or aroused. He will learn to associate the visitors or impending visitors with considerable anxiety that may make him more reactive.

The advantages of environmental manipulations are that they are relatively easy, they are usually reversible, and clients are readily able to identify changes in the dog's or cat's behavior. All of this presupposes that the clients are paying attention and not allowing their dogs or cats to continue to be exposed to a situation that makes them more distressed.

Social and Related Behavioral Environments

The behavioral environment includes the following:

- the humans with whom the cat or dog may interact,
- the conspecifics with whom the dog or cat may interact, and
- other household pets of a different species with whom the dog or cat may interact.

Interactions do not have to involve the patient to affect the patient: a group of five cats may play in a way that causes a reaction in the dog, but the dog and cats do not interact directly. In this example, if the dog barks or becomes fearful every time the cats roughhouse, part of the treatment may be to ensure that the cats play elsewhere until the dog can be calm when only two of the cats have social interactions.

When we alter the social and related behavioral environment, we focus on *behavior modification as way to construct new rule structures for interactions.* We also may decide to *manage some situations by altering the social environment so that the behaviors do not occur*, rather than engaging in behavior modification that would change interaction rules. Such changes may be temporary while the patient acquires the skills needed to be less reactive, or they may be part of the routine used to manage the problem. If the clients maintain their focus on meeting the animal's needs while obtaining the most humane and manageable outcome for all, they will generally make good decisions about changes in the social environment.

Pharmacological and Neurochemical Environments

The pharmacological and neurochemical environments include:

- the endogenous neurochemical environment of the patient's own, changing neurochemical state,
- the hormonal environment in which the neurochemical environment is found (intact vs. neutered dogs and cats),
- any disease that may affect the patient's neurochemistry or interaction with the physical and social environments (e.g., endocrine imbalances, sensory or physical limitations), and
- exogenous medications, diets, supplements and nutraceuticals that can affect the patient's neurochemistry (see Chapter 10).

None of the above-mentioned environments is independent: they all interact, and perturbation in one can cause a shift in another (Fig. 3-2). The behavior/phenotype of the dog's or cat's behavior is the result of the effects that the social and physical environments have on his neurochemistry, the effects of the dog's or cat's neurochemistry on various regions of the brain, and the effects that stimulated regions of the brain have on both the neurochemistry and the molecular changes in the brain; in turn, these all affect the resulting behavior. The genetic background (the genomic code) of the patient tells us only what *could* happen and not what *will* happen. Even when diseases are heritable in a simple manner, their phenotypes and presentations can be altered by interaction with the environment.

What Happens When Environments Change?

Clients often wish to know what to expect when one or more of the aforementioned environments is changed. Discussions should involve desired or expected change, but clients benefit from understanding that all cats or dogs with the same problem as their cat or dog are not the same. If clients learn to think about the interacting levels of response as shown in Figure 3-2, this should make sense: there are many paths to get to any behavioral presentation or phenotype.

We cannot know to what extent any pet's response is due to the pet's genetic background or to the interaction of that background with the various environments. The concept of a response surface was developed to help understand how patterns of behavior can individually vary with exposure to different environments depending on genetic background.

The response surface in Figure 3-3 theoretically represents the space created by the behavioral traits in question, the environments in which they are displayed, and the genetic environments that contribute to them.

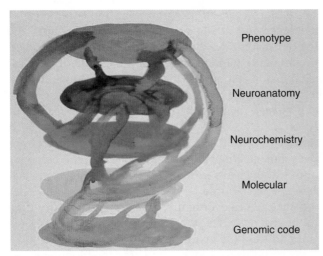

Fig. 3-2 Levels of response that are affected by the external environment to form a behavioral response. Interactions can be direct (e.g., between the behavioral and neurochemical levels) or indirect (e.g., affecting the behavioral level through molecular changes stimulated because certain areas of the brain were activated, which stimulated neurochemical-based molecular shifts that altered response choices—learning). (From Overall, 2005.)

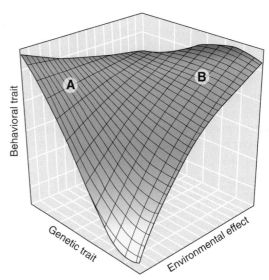

Fig. 3-3 A response surface for a series of expressions of a behavioral trait across different genetic and physical environments. *A* and *B* represent individuals who look the same (same color), but for whom the genetic and environmental contributions to their behaviors are vastly different. (From Overall, 2005.)

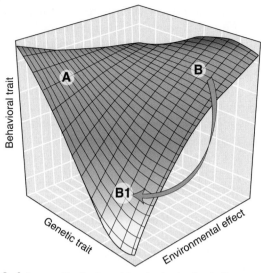

Fig. 3-4 Two patients, A and B, who look alike in the presentation of their behavior. The underlying contribution of their genes to their behavior differs here, and when exposed to a series of environments, one of them alters his behavioral response surface considerably (patient B1) compared with the other (patient A). This difference in response suggests that the underlying mechanisms for their response are not identical. This means that patients A and B, although they have the same diagnosis and appear similar in the presentation of their complaint, may require different types of treatment. (From Overall, 2005.)

In Figure 3-3, patients represented by *A* and *B* appear to have the same condition, as indicated by their representation by the same color. Their responses to different environmental manipulations will expose how they are different. As patient A is exposed to a range of environments from the right to the left of the environmental axis, she remains unchanged; however, when patient B is exposed to the same range of environmental changes, her behaviors alter dramatically and shift to location B1 in Figure 3-4.

Treatment interventions often identify patients with different response surfaces. If veterinarians begin to treat enough behavior cases, the most common styles of response surface within their population of patients become apparent, allowing patterns of successful intervention to become clear.

WHAT BEHAVIOR MODIFICATION IS AND IS NOT

Behavior modification *is not:*
- correction,
- training,
- a "sit-stay" program,
- learning by compulsion,
- "earn to learn,"
- a "leadership program,"
- "nothing in life is free,"

- adversarial,
- painful,
- tedious, and
- scary for the dog or human.
  Instead, true behavior modification involves:
- shaping behaviors in a non-threatening context,
- possible implementation of classic desensitization (DS) (e.g., the patient learns not to react to stimuli that increase in intensity) and counter-conditioning (CC) (e.g., the patient is rewarded for exhibiting a preferred behavior that is incompatible with the undesirable one)—*these techniques do not have to be used at first and can come as part of more intensive secondary treatment*, and
- replacing a set of rules that encourage reaction, regardless of context, with a new set of rules that allows the animal to relax and take his or her cues from the contextual environment; for this to happen, there must be clear signaling and learned trust from both parties and reliability from the humans.

This approach to behavior modification is more complex than traditional approaches, which primarily emphasize only the second point: DS and CC. DS and CC are discussed later, but they are mentioned here to show that true behavior modification is about more than classical and operant conditioning. It is about understanding that pathologies are sets of rules that govern neurochemical, physiological, and behavioral responses. By concentrating on those aspects of responses, we can change the rules that the patient is using to ones that produce calmer, happier, and safer responses.

The approach discussed here is *not* the same as engaging in basic "training" or obedience exercises. It is *not* the same as using much publicized "sit-stay"/"earn-to-learn" programs. In simple training and obedience and in sit-stay/earn-to-learn programs, the dog or cat complies with the instruction (usually called a "command") and exhibits a specific suite of physical behaviors in response to that command. These physical behaviors are exhibited *whether or not the cat or dog is calm and able to learn from the exercises and whether or not the cat or dog wishes to engage in such behaviors.* Such exercises are not true behavior modification and are likely not meeting the patient's needs. True behavior modification seeks to change rule structures, and such change is not simple.

If the cat's rule structure is that he hisses every time the boyfriend visits, there are a number of ways we could address the problem.
- We could use avoidance and stop the hissing almost instantly by not exposing the cat to the boyfriend. This may not meet everyone's needs.
- We could also use a seriously aversive stimulus (e.g., a shock), but hissing does not occur in isolation. By teaching the cat that he will experience pain and fear when he hisses, he may avoid all interactions with

humans or he may stop hissing and move directly to a full frontal attack of the boyfriend.

- One concern with aversive techniques is that the association is made with the stimulus and the behavior, neurochemical/neurophysiological state, and cognitive state at the moment the aversive stimulus is delivered.
  - This may not be the moment that the individual controlling the timing is trying to choose.
  - As a result, the behavior affected is not the one that was anticipated to be affected.
  - The result is an animal who has now learned to respond in ways that were unanticipated and that are damaging to the patient and may be damaging to others.
- The most humane and lasting way to stop the hissing focuses on altering the reaction and cognitive process that is driving the hissing.
  - This means that we must change the cat's neurochemical response (the green zone in Fig. 3-2).
  - Changing the neurochemical response will allow the cat to learn a new rule (using the blue and yellow zones in Fig. 3-2) that enables him not to be afraid (blue zone in Fig. 3-2) and to remain calm and respond appropriately when approached by the boyfriend (red zone in Fig. 3-2).
  - When the cat learns that such approaches are possible, within his control, and perhaps even pleasant, he makes changes at the molecular level (green zone in Fig. 3-2) that will govern future responses (red zone in Fig. 3-2).
  - The extent to which any responses are possible is defined by the genomic response surface, which includes the broad, underlying heritability of any factors involved in the behavior and the inducible genes or gene products that can be activated.

We want to alter the behavior as early in its sequence as possible, so that series of behaviors do not become part of the problematic response. If we can teach each dog or cat that:

- he or she does not have to react,
- a reward is given for not reacting, and
- he or she will feel better for not reacting.

We make available to these dogs and cats an array of choices that were not previously available to them. This is helpful because of the following patterns of behaviors.

- Problematic behaviors are more "stereotypic" than non-problematic ones.
- Normal dogs and cats are characterized by a large array of very *flexible responses*.
- Problematic and troubled dogs and cats are characterized by a *narrow array of characteristic responses given certain sets of contexts.*
- One role of treatment is to *increase the patient's range and flexibility in choice of responses.*

Attention to and use of natural canine and feline postures matters.

- Dogs and cats are less reactive when sitting than when standing because they must go through more movements to lunge or leave.
- Dogs and cats are less reactive when lying down compared with sitting for the same reasons.
- To effect behavioral change, we must use this type of information about body posture and understand how it affects reactivity, vulnerability, and overall ability to react to change the dog's or cat's attitude about relaxation and assumption of deferential or anxiety-reducing behaviors.
- Animals may use "obedience-type" postures such as sitting and lying down as part of a behavior modification program, but *the context in which they are used is different.* That difference is the crux.
- Quite simply, we are encouraging certain body postures only when and *because they correlate with underlying physiological responses.*
- *When behavior modification is done correctly, we are rewarding the physical signs of the underlying physiological state.*
- If we focus on rewarding ever more relaxed, nonreactive postures and physiologies, we actually *enhance the patient's ability to learn cognitively that they do not have to react and that they will feel better for not reacting.*

There is a lesson here for the veterinary staff: we are also more attentive and less reactive if we are sitting down, a strategy that would help many of our patients.

WHERE DO REWARD STRUCTURES FIT HERE?

The conventional wisdom of operant conditioning is that rewarded behaviors are repeated and all animals will work for rewards (see Box 3-8 for a list of types of rewards). Although this is true, we should also understand that *evolution has guaranteed that the most valuable reward of all is good information.* Dogs and cats (and humans) work for information, especially as it pertains to risk. If animals are always worried about risk—which is a component of behavioral

BOX 3-8

Type of Rewards

- Information, especially about risk
- Food
- Touch
- Praise
- Play
- Attention
- Social access
- Chewing or access to special chew toy
- Avoidance of discomfort

pathologies—providing information that helps manage and mitigate those risks and the behavioral and physiological changes such concern induces will help alter behaviors for the better.

UNDERSTANDING LEARNING

There are two aspects of learning that are essential for the veterinary staff and clients to have some comfort level with: (1) the neuroanatomical, neurochemical, and molecular changes involved in learning and (2) learning theory. Learning theory tells us how best to deliver the information in the way that best informs the needed molecular changes.

Learning Basics

Learning is generally defined as the acquisition of information or behavior through exposure and repetition. Reinforcement is key for learning. Reinforcement can be either positive, encouraging repetition of the behavior, or negative, discouraging repetition of the behavior. *Positive reinforcement* encourages desired behaviors because it marks and identifies the preferred behavior to the patient by coupling it with a reward (e.g., praise, food, toys, love). *Negative reinforcement* discourages the behavior because the animal is rewarded with a more favorable experience not just when they cease the undesirable behavior, but also *as a result of ceasing it.*

It is important to realize that negative reinforcement is completely different from punishment, where no reward structure is in place (see later discussion).

Learning at the Neuroanatomical, Neurochemical, and Molecular Levels and Factors That Affect Learning

Regional Roles for Brain Structures

Regions of the brain differentially affect the types of behavioral responses exhibited. Imprinting is a learning process that pertains only to very young animals where they develop recognition of and attraction for animals of their own kind and/or individuals who are exposed to them during the relevant time. The neurophysiology of imprinting is both similar to and different from standard memory. Imprinting correlates with increased ribonucleic acid (RNA) synthesis in the intermediate medial hyperstriatum ventrale (IMHV) in the dorsal forebrain. Electron microscopy has demonstrated increases in the synaptic area of the IMHV after imprinting, and the rate of neuronal firing in the IMHV is subsequently altered. Lesions of the IMHV quickly alter the ability to imprint but leave associative learning unimpaired. The type of learning in which we are most interested for altering behavior is associative learning.

At the broadest level, the primary structures of importance for associative learning are the cerebral cortex, hippocampus, and amygdala. Other mesocorticolimbic circuits using the nucleus accumbens and ventral pallidum are essential in stimulating different types of reward structures that affect learning. Although these regions of the brain are identifiable in terms of types and distributions of neurons and receptors, it's important to remember that each part of the brain connects with other parts of the brain. These interactions are complex and incompletely understood but are likely affected in some behavioral pathologies. In the broadest terms, the hippocampus is the main region where associational learning occurs.

Associational learning is among the simplest kinds of "signal/stimulus-response"–type patterning. Associational learning is characterized by changes induced by repeated, high-frequency stimulation.
- The basic associations we teach are often of this type.
- Any simple request/response falls into this grouping: "Sit, Ariel. Good girl! Here's a treat!"
- In this example, we have a signal—the request/cue/stimulus ("sit") and the reward (the treat).
- The praise ("Good girl!") can act as a reward itself or as a signal to reinforce that the treat is coming.
- If the praise acts as a signal that the treat is coming, it can act as a marker of when the desired behavior is first exhibited, which can help to reinforce a quick and clear associated response. This is the basic principle underlying the use of a clicker.

Associational learning also can occur in the cortex, which is particularly relevant for dogs and cats because this is the way olfactory learning works, but there is ongoing signaling between the hippocampus and cortex.
- Whenever associational learning occurs in the hippocampus, connections with the cortex facilitate decisions about action as part of the cortex's role in integrating information and forming reactions as part of "executive function."
- Executive function includes understanding and acting on rule structures that allow action in some situations and inhibition of action in others in a contextually flexible and measured manner that depends on using selective sensory information. In short, the cortex is where choices are made that drive actions and behaviors.

The amygdala, which is involved in fearful responses, is located at the ventral end of the hippocampus. The following associations are established (Davis, 1997; Ehrlich et al., 2009; Le Doux, 2000; LeDoux et al., 1990) and relevant for fearful cats and dogs.
- An intact amygdala is required to learn fear.
- Fear can be and is adaptive in context, and some of the earliest learning that is done in any species is avoidance learning, which usually involves some level of contextually relevant fear.

- Fear can also be learned in pathologies, and heightened reactivity in the amygdala has been postulated to underlie some behavioral and cognitive conditions and pathologies.
- The respective locations and activity levels of the paired amygdala and hippocampal structures are not independent, and the locations within them that are stimulated may affect the phenotype of behavioral conditions.
- Different patterns of behavioral response associated with different fear responses (e.g., salivating, shaking, increased respiratory rates) can be obtained by stimulating different regions of the amygdala (Davis, 1997).

Although fear must involve the amygdala, various "reward" systems involve parts of the cortex, substantia nigra, and miscellaneous parts of the "limbic system" (Davis, 1997). More recently, attention has been directed toward the circuitry for reward structures, an essential part of much associational learning. This research may greatly inform the way we consider the concept of "motivation," which is often considered—but seldom defined and measured—as an important component for changing behavior through learning.

- There appear to be at least three separate neuronal representations for the *"wanting"* (often referred to as the motivational/incentive salience component), *"liking"* (often referred to as the hedonistic component), and *"prediction"* components of the same reward within the nucleus accumbens to ventral pallidum segment of mesocorticolimbic circuitry (Smith et al., 2011).
- This finding supports the concept that *new rules* that provide accurate information about *risk* and *predictability* will help troubled dogs and cats.
- As discussed subsequently, these findings also highlight the importance of ensuring that the right physiology is rewarded to ensure that we maximize the "liking" and "wanting" parts of the reward system.
- Recognition memory has two components: recollection (remembering the episode in which an item was learned) and familiarity (knowing that an item was encountered without remembering the learning episode). The hippocampus primarily supports "recollection" (Song et al., 2011), but lesions of the hippocampus impair both familiarity and recollection.
- The reason that this is important for veterinary patients is that recognition memory is one form of declarative memory, which is so often assessed only verbally. Because recognition memory focuses on the ability to judge whether an item was previously encountered, it can be assessed in well-designed spatial tests that use specific exploratory behaviors to assess cognition both in young animals who are learning and in aging animals who may become cognitively impaired.

Regardless of the type, learning at the neuroanatomical level involves multiple regions of the brain in a complex, dynamic, but structured manner.

Cellular and Molecular Aspects of Learning

At the cellular and molecular level, learning is defined as cellular and receptor changes that are the result of stimulation of neurons and the manufacture of new proteins. These new proteins/receptors then change the way the cell responds when next stimulated.

- It's important to remember that no cell/neuron acts on its own: region of the brain, neurochemical tract, and interactions with other cells are critical for determining response.
- For animals to learn at the molecular level, they must make new proteins.
- These proteins can form new neurochemicals, new receptors, new ion channels, new cell membranes, or new cell structures—any component of the neuronal signaling pathway.

Cellular learning—long-term potentiation (LTP)—can take place in different regions of the brain, including the amygdala, parts of the cortex, the substantia nigra, and miscellaneous parts of the "limbic system" (Davis, 1997). The tools of learning theory and operant conditioning—positive reinforcement, negative reinforcement, and punishment—primarily use different neurochemical tracts or way stations (Table 3-1).

- Positive reinforcement uses opiate and dopaminergic systems.

TABLE 3-1

Neurochemical Systems Thought to Be Involved in Basic Reinforcement Paradigms

Neurochemical System Involved	Positive Reinforcement	Negative Reinforcement	Punishment
Dopamine	X	X	
Opioid	X	X	
Norepinephrine/noradrenaline		X	X*
Serotonin		X	

*With subsequent effects on corticotropin-releasing hormone.

- Punishment involves the flight, freeze, or fight pathways of the norepinephrinergic sympathetic systems.
- Negative reinforcement likely involves some complex association of both of these plus the serotoninergic system.

These neuroanatomical and neurochemical associations are poorly understood at best, but ongoing research will be informative.

- Research in mice on reward circuitry for the three components of rewards ("liking," "wanting," and "prediction") (Smith et al., 2011) has shown that dopamine-stimulating drugs enhance only the motivation/incentive salience component of rewards, leaving the learned prediction signals and the "liking" or hedonistic components untouched in the mice.
- Opioid-stimulating drugs increase hedonic liking and firing of neurons in ventral pallidum but do not alter signals about earned predictive values of a reward cue.
- Finally, prediction signals do not change during dopamine or opioid stimulation of the nucleus accumbens (Table 3-2).

Given these very broad patterns of effects of dopaminergic, norepinephrinergic/noradrenergic, serotoninergic, and opioid systems, we can begin to see that neurochemical patterns are intimately connected with learning and ability to learn. This association is discussed in Chapter 6 in the context of *using anti-anxiety medications to speed the rate at which newly learned responses can be acquired.*

Reward Structures

How Rewards Work to Influence Molecular Processes

It is critical to understand reward structures and what these mean at the cellular and molecular level for behavior modification. Behaviors are reinforced or learned best if every time they occur they are rewarded. At the cellular level, repeated reinforcement insures better, more numerous, and more efficient connections between neurons (Carter et al., 2002; Duman, 2004; Duman et al., 1997; Wittenburg and Tsien, 2002).

- Stimulation is induced when a neurochemical in a synapse triggers a receptor to engage it.

- This stimulation of the receptor engages second messenger systems in the post-synaptic cell, usually those involving cyclic adenosine monophosphate (cAMP). The end result is LTP.
- By itself, this initial process represents "early phase LTP" (E-LTP) and short-term memory (STM).
- STM/E-LTP is short-lasting and RNA-dependent and protein synthesis–*in*dependent, and the result does not persist or become self-potentiating unless the stimulus is consolidated into "late phase LTP" (L-LTP).
- E-LTP can be induced by a single train of stimuli in either the hippocampus or the lateral amygdala.
- L-LTP is a more permanent form (Schafe et al., 2001).
- L-LTP/long-term memory (LTM) requires repeated stimulation of cAMP, requires induction of cAMP response element binding protein (CREB) (a nuclear transcription factor), and is long-lasting, protein synthesis–dependent, and RNA transcription–dependent.
- When stimulation continues, brain-derived neurotrophic factor (BDNF) enhances neurotransmission by stimulating CREB and potentiates what is called "activity-dependent plasticity" at synapses (e.g., learning), particularly in the region of the brain most involved in learning, the hippocampus.
- This effect can also occur in the lateral amygdala and is one modality postulated to be involved in learned or conditioned contextual fear.

This neurobiology is important to consider in the context of reward systems. It explains why *continuous reward works best in acquiring a behavior* (E-LTP and STM) and why *intermittent reward acts best to maintain a learned behavior* (L-LTP and LTM). This neurobiology explains why a really excellent reward can help you learn or reinforce a behavior quickly and why a really horrible experience can quickly stimulate the amygdala to encode learned panic or phobia at the molecular level.

Because so many behavioral problems of cats and dogs are based in anxiety and fear, the neuromolecular biology of scary events and the role for the amygdala should be further considered.

- Events that induce panic or phobia all share the trait that those afflicted are unable to escape the stimulus.

TABLE 3-2

Model for Which Neurochemicals Affect Postulated Reward Paths

	"Liking" (Hedonistic Component for Reward Structures)	"Wanting" (Motivational/Incentive Salience Component for Reward Structures)	Prediction Component of Reward Structures
Dopamine	No effect	Enhances	No effect
Opioid	Enhances	No effect	No effect

Adapted from Smith et al., 2011.

- The amygdala itself is an incredibly complex structure (although measuring only a few cubic millimeters). The efferent tracts from the amygdala that control some higher forms of integration of behavior in the cerebral cortex, hypothalamus, brainstem, et cetera, are shaped by their regional origin in the amygdala.
- The lateral amygdala is likely the site where memories of conditioned (learned) fear are created through a process involving neuronal plasticity. If the lateral amygdala is lesioned or made inoperable, it is impossible either to acquire a fear or to express a previously acquired fear (LeDoux et al., 1990).

The *extracellular environment* of the amygdala is responsible for the maintenance of memories about fear (Pizzorusso, 2009). Perineuronal nets composed of chondroitin sulfate proteoglycans (CSPGs) render fears difficult or impossible to "erase" (Gogolla et al., 2009). This "resistance" is not present at birth, so fear is more difficult to learn early in development, and resistance to recovery from fear comes harder once the CSPG landmark is reached. Such findings complicate our understanding of learning but also suggest potential future interventions.

Differential Effects of Reward Type

When one considers rewards—or aversive stimuli—that best induce these quick learning experiences, it is important to consider them in terms of their evolutionary value. Evolutionarily tightly coupled rewards—ones that selection has shaped to be of particularly high value—are those directly coupled to survival: food, freedom, elimination, mating. Evolutionarily less tightly coupled rewards—ones on which survival should not hinge—will be of lesser value: praise, play. When one considers the molecular biology of learning within the evolutionary context of very pleasurable or very fearful stimuli, it should be clear how behaviors can best be modified.

Concerns for Aversive Stimuli and "Treatments" at the Molecular Level

Whether it is the result of an underlying behavioral pathology or of an aversive/punishment-based training plan, *chronic glucocorticoid excess interferes with learning at the cellular level* (Duman and Monteggia, 2006; Yau et al., 2002). Chronic exposure has also been proposed to affect hippocampal neuronal structure (Hajszan et al., 2009; Schmidt and Duman, 2007, 2010). Chronic cortisol elevation may act as a translational gene regulator—a hormonal response element (HRE)—in regions of the hippocampus. As noted, learning requires that new proteins are made. CREB is involved in transcribing the genetic code for proteins. HREs such as cortisol stop CREB from reading the genetic code and so stop transcription of new proteins.

Induction and maintenance of cellular and molecular learning—LTP—requires the induction of CREB proteins that are required to transcribe the genetic code of the proteins. The amount of CREB made depends on the amount of BDNF available to stimulate it. Furthermore, the level of any stress response and the subsequent level of cortisol affect the number of BDNF receptors—trkB receptors—that are recruited (Duman and Monteggia, 2006; Peters et al., 2004).

- If the stress/arousal level is too high or too low, a sub-optimal range of trkB receptors is recruited (Fig. 3-5, *A*).
- This is important because BDNF levels affect levels of CREB proteins that help decode the genome in a dose-effect relationship.
- If the BDNF levels are too high (high stress situations) or too low (low stimulation/arousal situations), insufficient CREB is available for the genomic decoding needed for transcription of proteins.
- Unless the range of BDNF is within the optimal zone for CREB production, learning at the cellular level does not occur (Fig. 3-5, *B*).

The LTP that is induced after a stressful event is maintained during slow wave sleep only if BDNF and cortisol lie within certain ranges. This indicates that the effects of BDNF act as an indicator for the scale of the stressor effect, whereas cortisol acts as an indicator for the scale of the stress reactions in an integrated manner (Peters et al., 2004). Clearly, if we wish our patients to consolidate what we are trying to teach them with behavior modification, we must ensure that their arousal and stress levels are sufficient for attentiveness but not high enough for the distress that will compromise their ability to learn and get well (De Quervain et al., 2009).

All of these findings are relevant for dogs who are learning to acquire true job skills (e.g., finding explosives, guiding a blind human) as well as dogs whom we hope will benefit from behavior modification.

- The factor that prohibits most dogs from completing working dog training programs is their fearful/anxious/uncertain response to novel or complex environments.
- Fear/anxiety will adversely affect successful implementation of behavior modification programs for troubled dogs and cats.
- Accordingly, the use of medications that can relieve anxiety is virtually always helpful.
- These data suggest that training environments should be as humane as possible and rely *neither on aversives nor fear.*
- Task learning—including learning associated with replacing one set of problematic behavioral rules with another that is more adaptive and humane—is enhanced when stress and distress are mitigated.
- We can affect levels of stress and distress by modifying the physical environment, the social/behavioral

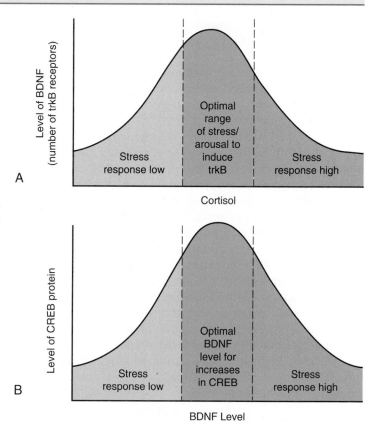

Fig. 3-5 Cortisol increases with the stress response (**A**, *bottom*, x axis). The number of BDNF receptors/trkB receptors made depends on an optimal level of cortisol in a bell-shaped, dose-effect relationship (**A**). The amount of BDNF that stimulates trkB receptors affects the amount of CREB protein available to help transcribe the genetic code in another bell-shaped, dose-effect relationship (**B**, *top*). CREB is most available in moderate stress/arousal situations. (Modified after Peters et al., 2004.)

environment, and the exogenous and endogenous neurochemical environments using medication, diets, and supplements (see Chapter 10).

HOW LEARNING THEORY CAN INFORM US

Leaning theory offers six main tactics for *stopping* unwanted and undesirable behaviors, regardless of whether the behaviors are normal:

- habituation,
- extinction,
- desensitization,
- counter-conditioning,
- flooding, and
- avoidance/aversive conditioning.

Some knowledge of the terms and techniques used in learning theory is essential for veterinarians wishing to help behaviorally troubled patients. With the development of certification programs for dog trainers, veterinarians would be well served by affiliating with well-educated certified dog trainers (see www.ccpdt.org for one example; see www.petprofessionalguild.com for an example of a group committed to force-free training) or developing that expertise within their practice.

Understanding the Main Processes

Habituation is an elementary form of learning. It involves *no rewards*. It is merely the cessation or decrease in a

response to a stimulus that is the result of repeated or prolonged exposure to the stimulus.

- The stimulus can be positive, neutral, or negative.
- Stimuli associated with potentially adverse consequences (negative stimuli) might be more difficult than other stimuli to extinguish with habituation, especially if such responses are adaptive. For example, sounds associated with predators (e.g., hawks) should be difficult to habituate in prey species (e.g., sparrows) because such attention has been selected for, and the response is adaptive. The predator (the stimulus) does not have to be present very often for the response to be rewarded.
- Prolonged exposure to a stimulus that provokes *an adaptively anxious response* does not induce habituation. Instead, it can induce hypervigilance, exhaustion, and increased anxiety, which may or may not become pathological, given other factors in the environment.
- Rewards will interfere with habituation. If responses that are to be diminished are *even occasionally rewarded*, the *habituation response will be inhibited*.
- When habituation is recommended for behavior modification, the goal is the attenuation of a response to something novel but *non-threatening*.
- The response to be habituated is associated with an increase in intensity or frequency of exposure to the stimulus in circumstances where nothing horrendous happens. For example, a doorbell may startle a

new puppy, but as the pup hears it more frequently in a benign context she can habituate to it. However, if the puppy is rewarded inappropriately for reacting in any way to the doorbell, she will overcome habituation.

- Three phenomena associated with habituation are helpful to understand.
  - *Stimulus generalization* is the quick habituation to a new stimulus when the new stimulus is only slightly different from the old one. Doorbells differ in tonal qualities. With a very short exposure to the new doorbell, it is treated as the old one was if nothing else changes.
  - *Spontaneous recovery* can occur if there is an extended time between last exposure to the stimulus to which habituation occurred and re-exposure to the stimulus. If a ringing doorbell becomes a rare occurrence, the puppy may react if it starts to ring again as a result of spontaneous recovery. *Spontaneous recovery* is usually easy to reverse if no overt fear is involved.
  - *Dishabituation* is the reinstatement of a habituated response as a result of exposure to a stimulus that provokes a response similar to the original. Classic examples involve mildly fearful responses: if habituation had just occurred to a certain hand gesture and another movement occurred that was also worrisome for the animal, the animal could *dishabituate* to the hand gesture. *Rehabituation* is the rule unless the event is compounded and made more fearful or the animal's reaction is extreme.

Extinction is the process by which normal or conditioned responses are decreased or attenuated by exposure to a stimulus that has in the past gained a reward but that no longer does. *Extinction is the cessation of a response that occurs when reinforcement is stopped.* The classic example of an extinction response in dogs involves dogs who jump on people for attention. If people continue to pet a jumping dog, the dog continues to jump (e.g., the dog is rewarded with petting for jumping). If people stop petting the dog when the dog jumps and ignore the dog until she is still, the dog will extinguish her response over time because the reward is no longer there.

- There is a pitfall for extinction: *resistance to extinction.* Any form of intermittent reinforcement—even occasional petting of the dog in response to her jumping—will encourage the repetition of the response. The more valuable or desired the original reinforcer/reward (e.g., petting) and the longer the reinforcement has been ongoing, the greater the resistance to extinction. Resistance to extinction can also occur without continued reinforcement, if the initial reward was good enough and if it is tightly coupled to the behavior (e.g., the dog jumped up and managed to grab and eat 250 g of butter).

- The intensity or frequency of the behavior that is the focus of extinction usually increases at the beginning of an extinction process. There may be an association between eliciting the reward and the intensity or rapidity of the performance of the behavior that gains the dog the reward: a dog may be petted only for jumping many times, not once. Regardless, the dog already has one learned response that has been rewarded in the past (e.g., jumping) and so the dog will continue to offer that response as a way to get information about whether some form of jumping will be rewarded.

- For extinction to work and for resistance to extinction to be overcome, *the absence of the rewarding response must be complete and consistent.* Caution is urged because resistance to extinction is a very common phenomenon and occurs with very little reinforcement.

- *It is also important to realize that extinction does not work well for behaviors that are self-rewarding (chewing/scratching), innate (urine marking), or truly pathological.*

- *The use of extinction for truly troubled/pathological behaviors should be avoided at all costs.* True extinction requires the ability to learn a new response. As discussed, distress and excessive stress interfere with learning. Anyone who attempts to treat a true behavioral pathology with extinction may inadvertently be using flooding, which almost always will worsen these patients.

Desensitization (DS) is a decrement in response to a certain stimulus that is obtained by gradually exposing the dog or cat at a sub-threshold level to the stimulus that elicits the concerning response. An external reward is not necessarily involved in desensitization, but it may help speed the process *if* the person giving the reward is correctly rewarding a calm response rather than just sitting and not reacting.

- If a puppy has become fearful of the doorbell, using a recording of the doorbell at a level below that to which she reacts may help her to become less fearful. For this to happen, the recording must be played very softly at first so that she does not react. The sound level is raised gradually at increments designed to elicit no response until the volume reaches the level of the real doorbell.

- Slowly increasing sub-threshold exposures are key to desensitization.

- Going too quickly, the patient's threshold for exposure can be exceeded. If this happens, it is possible to worsen the fear by further sensitizing the dog.

- This is one technique where the desired outcome is possible *only* when the physical behaviors (not reacting by showing fear) are mirrored by the underlying physiological state. *Dogs who merely sit still to comply with an order while remaining distressed are not being desensitized and are not having their needs met.* We must separate compliance from true treatment effects.

Counter-conditioning (CC) changes, controls, or stops an undesirable/problematic behavior by teaching the cat or dog to engage in another behavior—preferably one that is favorable and fun—that competitively interferes with the execution of the undesirable behavior.

- CC is usually coupled with DS. When done correctly, it results in *response substitution:* the development and exhibition of a positive/desired behavior or behavioral sequence that is *incompatible* with the expression of the unwanted behavioral sequence.

- The puppy who is fearful of the doorbell will alter her behavior faster if she is first taught to sit and to relax in exchange for a treat. One of the reasons that treats are so often used in CC involves the relationship with sympathetic arousal and food intake. If the puppy is aroused and distressed, she will not be able to eat because her physiological responses are governed by the sympathetic branch of the autonomic nervous system (ANS). This is the branch of the ANS associated with the classic flight/fight outcome that is the response to increased levels of norepinephrine/noradrenaline. To eat, the parasympathetic branch of the ANS must be governing the puppy's actions. She must be quiet and calm. All of her body language must be congruent and indicate that she is calm and attentive. Not only does this sequence allow the puppy to use a behavior rewarded with a food treat as a behavior that is competitive with her fearful response, but also this is the situation in which the puppy is able to learn at the molecular level that not being afraid is also self-rewarding.

- Once the puppy can reliably sit calmly and take a treat for doing so, this sequence can be added to the DS plan so that she is rewarded for not reacting by exhibiting behaviors that are incompatible with the fearful response (e.g., sitting quietly) and with learning and enhancing a fearful response (e.g., a calm, relaxed response that does not trigger cortisol spikes or increase in norepinephrine).

- If at any point in the joint DS/CC response the puppy starts to act anxious or inattentive, the tape recording should be lowered in volume until she can relax again. This is key—sitting and staying is merely a facilitator for the relaxation response, and we should not reward sitting and staying without that relaxed response unless we wish to teach the dog to be internally distressed while giving few outward cues. There is no sense to having the dog sit and stay if she is panting, salivating, her pupils are dilated, her ears are back, and she is clearly distressed. This is antithetical to a counter-conditioned response. This is why the first steps in changing any behavior focus on teaching the dog to relax (see the "Protocol for Teaching Your Dog to Take a Deep Breath and Use Other Biofeedback Methods as Part of Relaxation"). CC with DS can be time-consuming because the exercises must be repeated until the dog does not

respond inappropriately to the stimuli. Combined DS/CC is best done in frequent, short intervals so that we increase the probability that everyone is paying appropriate attention and so that it can fit in with real-world experiences in a number of contexts.

- Clients who are least successful with CC often rush the process and worsen the dog's response. Clients must be warned of this risk, especially if they are embarrassed by their dog or are determined that their dogs must be elite performers.

- Problem dogs have special needs. These needs do not reflect on the intelligence of the dog or on the abilities of the clients. Although the clients did not cause the dog's behavioral problems, they are constrained to accompany the dog on the path that will best alleviate the dog's suffering if the dog is to get better.

Flooding involves prolonged exposure to the worrisome stimulus at a level that provokes the response. The intent is that, with exposure, the patient will stop reacting to the stimulus.

- In contrast to desensitization, where the goal is to expose the dog or cat to a worrisome stimulus at a level *below* that which will trigger the response, flooding exposes the cat or dog to a worrisome stimulus *at* a level that triggers the response.

- Unfortunately, with distressed or troubled patients, flooding usually only sensitizes the patient to the stimulus and makes them worse. The molecular biology of learning explains why this is the case.

- Because flooding can be so injurious, it should be recommended only exceptionally for targeted, very specific, and very mild avoidance or fear situations in normal patients where the veterinarians and clients can monitor both the behavioral and the physiological signs of distress that flooding could provoke.

- Flooding can cause a complete shutdown and collapse of a patient. The classic situation in which flooding is often and incorrectly and cruelly advised is the introduction of unfamiliar cats.
  - Clients are often asked to put their new cat in one crate and their original cat in another and place the crates close to each other.
  - What is usually not mentioned is that the inability to escape, the entrapment—whether from a cage or a stimulus that the patient views as fearful—can cripple an animal behaviorally for life because they experience a condition called *learned helplessness*. In learned helplessness, the actions of the dog or cat do not affect the outcome of the manipulation, regardless of the actions taken. The patient learns that all behavioral responses are ineffective, and he or she stops offering any responses. In laboratory situations, rodents who are taught that no behavior results in escape from

a swimming pool cease to offer behaviors and drown.

- The client handout, "Protocol for the Introduction of a New Pet to Other Household Pets," provides informed, humane alternatives to flooding when introducing new pets.
- If the behavior is not readily altered using humane techniques, there is no reason to resort to risky and inhumane ones. Risk mitigation and avoidance should be the next option and provides respite for the patient while a new treatment program—generally involving medication—can be developed.
- Patients cannot have a good behavioral relationship with their people if they fear them and vice versa.

Avoidance/aversive conditioning/punishment involves the presentation of an aversive stimulus in response to an inappropriate or undesirable behavior. Punishment is now thought of as being of two kinds: positive punishment, where a punisher is applied, and negative punishment, where a reward is removed.

- Positive punishment occurs when the probability of a behavior occurring decreases because of something unpleasant happening after the behavior occurs.
- Negative punishment occurs when the probability of a behavior occurring decreases because something pleasant was removed after the behavior occurred. One of the best examples of this is the human who immediately walks away from the dog any time the dog jumps on the person but who stays and pets the dog anytime the dog sits calmly. Here the reward that is removed is the human's attention.

When most people discuss punishment, they are discussing positive punishment.

- The stimulus is intended to abort the behavior *and* to decrease the probability of its occurrence in the future. In most situations where the event is interrupted or aborted, the probability that the behavior will be exhibited in the future is *unaffected.*
- If the probability of the behavior occurring is unaffected but the behavior stops only whenever the stimulus is presented, the process that is ongoing is not punishment, but it can be abuse.
- For the requirements of punishment to be met, a probabilistic decrement in the occurrence of the behavior must occur.
- When punishment is used, for it to be most successful the stimulus designed to abort the behavior must be delivered as early as possible—certainly within the first 30 to 60 seconds of the onset of the behavioral sequence (including the cognitive part of the sequence, where the behavior is conceived) or within a second of the offending behavioral process—*and* the stimulus must be consistent and appropriate.
- The critical factors in punishment include:
  - timing, which requires that behavior is viewed as a process,
  - consistency, which involves vigilance and avoidance,
  - appropriate intensity, which requires that the dog's or cat's behavior is closely monitored and well understood, and
  - presence of a conditioned response. The presence of a conditioned response means that *when the undesirable behavior ceases, there must be some favorable stimulus or reward* for the dog or cat that signals that the dog or cat is now engaging in an acceptable behavior. *This is the most frequently ignored aspect of treatment.* Secondary cues can be used for distance situations.
- The value of using a stimulus that meets the above-listed criteria in a manner that can truly interrupt the behavior is based on the Rescorla-Wagner model of conditioning, where the startle or interrupter is an unconditioned stimulus (UCS) (Rescorla and Wagner, 1972). Learning does not automatically occur with any pairing of conditioned stimulus (CS) to UCS. Learning depends on the:
  - animal's previous experience,
  - presence of other stimuli, and
  - relevance to the animal of the pairing of the CS/UCS.

These are all factors in why punishment is usually a bad idea and why electric shock is problematic for addressing any behavioral concern. Following a startle, the pup can be taught a more appropriate behavior, such as sitting and staying, but *only* if he stops, is not scared, and can attend to his human and take the cues as to the appropriateness of his behavior from his human. Here, the discriminative value of punishment makes clear the difference between rewarded desirable behaviors and undesirable ones.

Behavioral change is reliant on the second phase, which requires no aversive stimulus. *If people do not ignore good behavior and instead always reward it, the punishment issue won't arise.*

- People resort to physical punishment when they do not understand alternatives or are afraid. Punishment levels may best reflect the human's stress level, especially with respect to shock of any kind, including invisible fences that deliver shock.
- If we truly wish to use punishment as the correction method of choice, it does not have to be physical. The best punishment is nonphysical: the withdrawal of interaction. In response to withdrawal of attention and interaction, dogs and cats will begin to offer behaviors. If clients understand this, they can pick the behaviors they prefer (e.g., sitting, sleeping) and reward those behaviors.
- If the withdrawal of interaction and attention is done correctly, this technique becomes one of negative reinforcement: the human withdraws attention based on very specific behaviors and immediately returns the attention once those behaviors cease.

Negative reinforcement is associated with true positive reinforcement because not only is attention returned when the problematic behavior stops, but also specific behaviors are identified by being rewarded (the presentation of positive reinforcement).

- Punishment is never an "easy out" and has a high probability of backfiring unless the client understands that its focus is to decrease the probability of future inappropriate events.
  - Pain of the type caused by pinching/scruffing/pinch collars, hitting, or electric/shock/e-collars increase anxiety and any associated aggression.
  - Species-specific responses are also important to consider. "Scruffing" a dog is likely to cause pain in puppies because flexor dominance does not persist in puppies, and this is not a common behavior seen in dogs after a certain age. In thousands of cases of noted naturally occurring aggression of various forms between dogs, scruff-shaking was noted to be rare and unusual (Schilder & Netto, 1991). In a study of mother-pup behaviors of litters from 190 breeders, 97.2% of breeders never witnessed scruff-shaking administered by the mother to pups (Hallgren, 1990). Accordingly, "scruffing" by humans is inappropriate to use in dogs. However, flexor dominance does persist in kittens, and one sees adults of the same species use this response to interrupt kitten behavior. However, we should be aware that when humans attempt to mimic the behaviors cats are exhibiting, we are likely to cause pain because we lack the ability to gauge the force of our intervention in terms of any assay meaningful to the cat. This concern is valid in the absence of any anger from the humans.
- Punishment may be best used early in the development of the course of undesirable behavior, but *we do a poor job of identifying the beginning of undesirable behaviors, so the application for this advice is severely limited.*
- Random punishment is abusive and usually leads to learned helplessness.
- Most people use both punishment and negative reinforcement poorly. They usually engage either in scary, abusive behaviors (e.g., "dominance downs," "alpha-rolls," "staring down") based in a profound misunderstanding of dog and cat behavior and principles of learning theory or in disengagement by ignoring all behaviors. Neither engagement in abusive behaviors not disengagement is really helpful for changing behavior and can often render behaviors worse (Blackwell et al., 2008; Herron et al., 2009). Rewarding good and desired behavior is easier for most people than engaging in punishment or negative reinforcement. Rewarding good and desired behavior also helps answer questions that

dogs and cats may be asking, and it aids in the acquisition and repeated use of behaviors humans prefer (Hiby et al., 2004; Rooney and Cowan, 2011).

CONDITIONING, TIMING, AND REINFORCERS

The above-described techniques all use operant/instrumental conditioning, which uses a reinforcement (reward or punishment) structure. These differ from classic/Pavlovian conditioning because of the reinforcement structure.

Classic/Pavlovian conditioning does not require an external reward structure for cementing associations because the response is paired to a stimulus that is an innate one. The classic example pairs the sound of a bell (conditioned stimulus [CS]) to the presentation of meat (unconditioned stimulus [UCS]) to a dog. The dog salivates (unconditioned response [UCR]) when he sees the meat. If the sound of the bell is paired with the presentation of the meat, later when the meat is removed, the dog will salivate (conditioned response [CR]) when the bell is rung (CS). Classic conditioning can occur and be useful in training situations (if you correctly train a puppy to eliminate on a cue, you may be taking advantage of this—see Box 3-9), but the vocabulary and techniques of instrumental conditioning are most relevant to helping troubled pets and their distressed humans.

More Terminology That Will Help You Talk to Trainers and Help Your Patients

- Using a *lure* refers to using a reward to increase the dog's or cat's attention and interest to *shape* the behavior to that desired. For example, to teach a cat or dog who does not know the word "sit" to sit, the treat is held in front of the nose and moved back over the cat's or dog's head until sitting (which is the easiest choice in this exercise) occurs. Once the dog or cat executes the behavior, the lure is given, and the dog or cat is rewarded. Lures are used only for behavioral requests that are not yet known to the dog or cat, as a way of helping him make the association between the request and the desired outcome or response. Once the dog or cat exhibits the desired response, he is rewarded with access to the item (e.g., tennis ball or rare steak) that was moved to encourage him to get into a certain posture or to provide a certain response. Lures should not be needed as the desired/appropriate response is learned, but you should still reward the dog or cat for any appropriate or desired response to any request.
- A *target* is an object of focus. The target can be an object, such as a stick with a large tip, or it can be a body part, such as a finger or knee. The dog is usually

BOX 3-9

Using Pavlovian Conditioning to Housetrain a Puppy

Here, the response that will serve as the focus and the UCR is not involuntary, like salivating, but reflexive—urination. When a bladder is full (UCS), emptying it (urinating, UCR) becomes self-rewarding. Food treats are unlikely to compete with the reward of actual micturition. The CS is the location in which elimination occurs or the cue that tells the dog to eliminate (or both).

CS = A Location

Puppies will urinate wherever they are in the house when they have to urinate. If the client can anticipate this need and continually take the dog to the appropriate spot (CS), the act of micturition (UCR) in that area will become a CR. If the client wishes to reinforce a specific elimination posture, substrate preference, or elimination on command, instrumental conditioning involving a reward (praise or food) can be used. This will not reinforce the elimination behavior, but when done correctly, it could help with other choices.

CS = A Verbal Cue

As soon as the puppy *begins* to squat (UCS) say "Go wee" (CS). It helps if the pup's bladder is full and you can correctly predict when she will squat. The act of micturition—still a UCR—will now become a CR with the CS now being the phrase "Go wee." Instrumental conditioning involving a reward can be used to hasten the acquisition of the associated cue and compliance with the cue, but urinating is self-rewarding. Here, accurately pairing the words to the squat that will release the urine is what's important.

asked to follow the movement of the target and/or to put a body part on it. The dog is most often asked to touch the target stick with his nose, but you could also ask him to touch it with his shoulder or hip if you don't want him to have his teeth or face near it. These behaviors are usually taught through *shaping* techniques. Teaching these patterns is called *target training.* Although not a true behavior modification technique itself, target training can help the dog accomplish the behavior modification program.

- *Conditioning* refers to associations between stimuli and responses.
- *Reinforcement* is the process that involves a stimulus or event that *increases the future probability that a certain behavior or class of behaviors will be performed.*
  - Positive reinforcement increases the probability that a behavior will occur because a reward was given after the behavior.
  - A positive reinforcer is a stimulus or an event that occurs after a response that leads to an increase in that response in the future.

- Negative reinforcement increases the probability that a behavior will occur because a negative stimulus was removed after the behavior occurred.
- A negative reinforcer is an aversive event or stimulus that increases the frequency of a behavior, usually through escape or avoidance
  - Negative reinforcement shouldn't be confused with punishment. As noted earlier, punishment uses the application of an aversive stimulus to decrease the probability that a response will occur again. *Negative reinforcement* is the withdrawal of a stimulus, which increases the probability of a behavior being repeated.
  - In negative reinforcement, the animal responds more quickly to avoid a stimulus.
  - The classic example of negative reinforcement is actually the "correct" use of choke collars: when the animal stops, the collar releases, and the animal is rewarded with release from pressure.
    - As long as the dog walks calmly and well, there is no pressure.
    - If the dog bolts, the collar tightens.
    - The tightness can be released only by the dog slowing and walking calmly.

This is the theory. Unfortunately, most people using these collars, "choke" the dog, as anyone who has walked through enough waiting rooms and dog parks well knows. It is for this reason—that these collars are so hard to use correctly and so simple to use incorrectly—that most people now recommend no-pull harnesses for tricky walkers.

- One of the principles that makes no-pull harness use successful is that of negative reinforcement: these tighten and stop the dog when the dog lunges forward. When the dog stops lunging, the harness loosens and stays loose if the dog walks at a pace that matches the human's pace.
- No-pull harnesses have the added advantage of providing some safe and humane leverage so that if a dog must be quickly removed or turned from a bad situation it is possible for the average human to do so without injuring the dog.

The reinforcement structure used in instrumental conditioning is commonly simply presented as the four choices of positive reinforcement, negative reinforcement, positive punishment, and negative punishment as shown in Table 3-3.

- Both negative reinforcement and punishment differ from *omission training,* in which animals are taught that they are *rewarded for not responding.* For example, a dog that does not bark gets a treat. The signal (or *secondary reinforcer*) "quiet" can indicate that the absence of sound will engender a reward. This technique is grossly misunderstood and under-exploited in veterinary medicine.

TABLE 3-3

Classic Set of Reinforcement Structures Used in Operant Conditioning

	Positive (Add Something)	Negative (Remove Something)
Reinforcer	Positive reinforcement (add something pleasant, rewarding)	Negative reinforcement (remove something unpleasant, aversive)
Punisher	Positive punishment (add something unpleasant, aversive)	Negative punishment (remove something pleasant, rewarding)

- *Stimulus and response generalization* occurs when an operantly or classically conditioned response is provoked not only by the object or event that originally provoked it but also by objects or events that are similar to the original stimulus.
  - The most common example of stimulus and response generalization in dogs is to people in uniforms: if a delivery man or meter reader initially scared the dog or provoked a protective response, this response may be generalized to others in uniform even though the circumstances might not be the same.
  - The more similar the original and subsequent stimuli, the more similar and intense the response.
  - Stimulus and response generalization may be associated with the development of profoundly anxious or fearful and phobic responses, and understanding this pattern may be tantamount to diminishing the worrisome behavior.

Bridging stimuli (recordings, signals) are stimuli that link the reward to an action when there is a time delay. When used correctly, such stimuli can be used to tell an animal to continue to relax because the reward is forthcoming.

- One example of the use of bridging stimuli involves dogs who become distressed when left alone. If we learn by videotaping the dog that the dog can be alone 30 minutes before beginning to be distressed but the client has to be gone 2 hours, we can teach the dog to associate a bridging stimulus—a light turning on—with the ultimate return of his person. If a light turns on every ½ hour and the dog is first conditioned to waiting for the signal of one light, then two lights, then three lights, the client will have developed a signal for the dog that tells the dog that his person will be home in 2 hours.

Overlearning is a phenomenon that is frequently used in training for specific events but may be underused in preventing fearful responses in dogs.

- Overlearning is the repeated evocation and expression of an already learned response. This accomplishes three things:
  - it delays forgetting,
  - it increases the resistance to extinction, and
  - it increases the probability that the response will become a "knee-jerk" one, or response of first choice, when the circumstances are similar. This last aspect can be useful in teaching any animal to overcome a fear or anxiety. This technique is also useful for performance dogs.

Overshadowing is the reduction in the influence of multiple stimuli by working on decreasing the response to one. Minimizing the effects of one stimulus decreases the effects of the others. This is a critical part of the paradigm for treating fears and anxieties, although it is seldom explicitly identified.

Shaping is a learning technique that works well for animals that do not know what a perfect response would look like.

- Shaping works through gradual approximations and allows the animal to be rewarded initially for any behavior that resembles any part of the behavior that is the desired outcome.
- For example, when teaching a puppy to sit, rewarding a slight squat will enhance the probability that squatting will be repeated. This squatting behavior is then rewarded only when it becomes more exaggerated and, finally, when it becomes a true sit.
- *Autoshaping* is classic conditioning that occurs simply because of repeated exposure (e.g., the cat comes when the can opener sounds).
  - One example of autoshaping that can be extremely useful involves teaching *"autosits."*
  - In this case, the dog is taught to sit whenever he or she encounters a certain stimulus, a certain cue, or both.
  - Example 1:
    - The dog is asked to sit at every curb and is rewarded when he complies until he is reliable (he always sits calmly at the curb when you ask).
    - Then he is taken to curb and not asked to sit and rewarded only when he sits. Waiting for the dog to offer the behavior is key.
    - If these periods of rewarding the dog for sitting at your request at the curb are interspersed with periods of decreasing frequency in which the dog is rewarded for sitting—at the curb—without a request, the dog learns that he is rewarded for the sitting at the curb in this context and that the cue does not have to be there.
    - This is an example of what trainers call *"fading the cue."*
  - Example 2:
    - The dog is asked to sit, as previously discussed, every time a car passes until she is reliable.

- The dog is now asked to move back from the curb or road on request using the cue/request "over."
- The request for "over" is first taught, as was "sit," in a benign, non-provocative situation, where the human takes a step to the side, and guides the dog using a voice signal and/or a movement of the lead/harness. As soon as the dog follows, the dog is rewarded.
- Once the dog can execute "over" in a variety of circumstances, she is taken to where she will encounter passing cars. As soon as the car approaches, the request for "over" is given. The dog is rewarded.
- Once the dog reliably moves "over" when cars pass, "sit" is added to the request "over." The scenario will look like this:
  - "Maya, 'over,' please. [Dog moves aside.] Good girl. Maya, 'sit,' please. [Dog sits.] Good girl!"
- Now the dog is ready to fade the cue for "sit" first so that "over" comes to mean "please move over and sit." This scenario will look like this:
  - "Maya, 'over,' please. [Dog moves aside and sits.] Good girl. [Dog is rewarded as she finishes her sit.]"
- Once the dog is reliable and moves over and sits each time a car passes for the cue "over," you can fade the cue for "over." You stop and wait as the car begins to pass: the dog is rewarded only when she moves over and sits. The cue for the dog to move over and sit consists of you stopping when a car is approaching to pass.
- If you execute the rewards correctly, you can now fade the cue given by stopping and instead allow the dog to use the approaching car as the cue to move over and sit.

If the dog appears confused at any point, the terrific thing about positive reward systems is that you can move back to the last place where the dog really understood the concept and rebuild from there breaking the task down into steps as small as needed. You cannot do this if you were shocking, yelling at, or hitting the dog.

Chaining and *back-chaining* are two concepts that are illustrated in the example of moving away from cars and that feature prominently in the language of trainers.

- A *behavior chain* is a series of responses linked together by a continuous sequence of cues.
  - The reward (the reinforcer) comes at the end of the chain for the desired response, but each cue becomes *not just a request but a marker* that the previous behavior was successfully completed.
  - The example of moving away from the car is a behavioral chain.

- The request to "sit" following the "over" request served as a marker that "over" was accomplished successfully.
- *Chaining* is the process by which multiple behaviors are linked together by a continuous sequence of cues where each cue acts as both the reward (reinforce) for the successful execution of the first behavior and the request for the next behavior.
- *Back-chaining* is the process where the last behavior in the chain is taught first, then the penultimate behavior is taught, et cetera. Stronger, more desired, more probable, more common, more familiar responses (e.g., "sit") reinforce weaker, less desired, less probable, less common, less familiar responses (e.g., "over"), a principle defined by Premack (1959).

Local enhancement is a form of trial-and-error learning that is combined with observation. Because of the observational component, learning occurs faster. For example, a puppy learning to go through a dog door will eventually figure it out, but the puppy will learn faster if she watches another dog go through the door.

Constructional aggression treatment (CAT) and *behavioral adjustment training (BAT)* are techniques recently in vogue that are borrowed from functional and behavioral analysis. These techniques are primarily used to treat dogs who are fearful of something (e.g., another dog, an approaching human) by teaching them that they have control over access to a stimulus that makes them fearful based on their behaviors. These techniques are most commonly used for autism spectrum disorders where traditional behavior modification has failed or is impossible to implement. In both BAT and CAT, the "reward" involves increased distance between the patient and the stimulus inducing the fear.

- In BAT, the dog is supposed to be kept under the threshold where he would react during exposure to the stimulus that scares him by using desensitization, and when he shows that he is able to decrease his attentiveness to the stimulus, he is rewarded by being allowed to move away from the individual who scares him. The offending stimulus need not disappear.
- In CAT, the constraints about sub-threshold responses from the patient are not as clear, but the idea is similar: the fearful dog is faced with the object of his fear—generally another dog or a human—until he shows some indication he is not responding as fearfully and that he is able to offer and voluntarily attend to other stimuli (e.g., he can flick his tail or turn and look at you). When the fearful dog shows signals of broader attention, he is rewarded by the departure of the object of his fear.
  - There are some concerns with CAT that need to be discussed.
    - In CAT, ensuring that the dog is "sub-threshold," as in BAT, is not usually discussed. Without this aspect, this technique is a

flooding technique. Without exception, flooding will render all but the mildest and most specific fearful/reactive associations worse.

- Even if flooding is not involved, both BAT and CAT are forms of negative reinforcement. Simply, the reward is the release from having to be in the presence of the upsetting stimulus. This is the same principle on which the use of choke collars is based, and these techniques carry the same risks of recidivism or worsening of behavior that choke collars carry.

- When these techniques are used to treat dogs who are afraid of other dogs, the dog serving as a "intruder" or model dog may be inadvertently subjected to huge numbers of threats and a large amount of stress/distress because of the behaviors of the fearful dog. The welfare of both dogs in these types of interactions is a concern. Unless there is a specific and detailed protocol for assaying welfare concerns of *both* dogs, these techniques should not be used.

- Unless the timing of the handler is exquisite and the understanding of dog signals is complete, it is very easy to reinforce an inappropriate response with both BAT and CAT.

- If the goal is to teach the dog that he can tolerate avoiding other dogs, there are ways to do this using positive reinforcement that are less risky than CAT or BAT.

- If dogs learn to have the expectation that if they just stand there the other dog will leave, we have provided them with some very seriously flawed real-world applications.

- One major concern is that there are many ways to avoid something and we cannot know which one of these is being truly "rewarded" in CAT and BAT. In contrast, rewards mark specific, suitable behaviors that are identifiable. Done correctly, rewards can help alter neurochemistry and can allow us to use physical cues about underlying physiological states to our and the patient's benefit in our treatment of worried dogs and cats. This is not the case for BAT and CAT. Proponents will argue that they can tell when dogs are distressed, which would affect cortisol levels and the ability to learn, but caution is urged. We are already placing the dog in a situation he would not choose, prohibiting escape or outright aggression and chase, and not giving him information about which specific behaviors or signals leading to a response are helpful. We are not rewarding offered small behaviors that could help him, and we are not recognizing that dogs can ask questions by offering small behaviors. Given this, it is likely that we may be teaching dogs to give us less, not more

information. Excellent trainers can teach dogs *not* to indicate distress. As a result, these dogs are not experiencing a neurochemistry conducive to relaxing and learning more suitable and more plastic responses, as *would* be the case were desensitization and counter-conditioning correctly used. These less trendy techniques are safer, easier, and more effective and carry with them very little risk. *CAT and BAT are not low-risk techniques* and are not recommended for most situations or people without extensive training in physiology and learning theory.

- Finally, we should acknowledge that since the techniques of CAT and BAT made their appearance there have been changes in interpretation and explanation that were not in early versions. Now it has sometimes been suggested that the patient's behaviors must include relaxation or exhibition of confident behaviors, not just non-reaction to the stimulus, for the stimulus to move or the patient to be allowed to move from the stimulus. If this is true, this is nothing more than routine desensitization and counter-conditioning as discussed here and historically.

Look at that (LAT) is a derivation from the "Protocol for Relaxation: Behavior Modification Tier I," as developed by McDevitt (2007). If we remember that dogs work for information and that risk assessment is an issue especially for worried, anxious, and fearful dogs, it makes sense that dogs should want to survey their environment to collect information. The intent of the "Protocol for Relaxation: Behavior Modification Tier I" is to teach the dogs to control adverse reactivity and instead learn that they need not react adversely, given situations that provoke them, and—ultimately—that they will feel better and can more accurately assess situations when they relax and stop reacting. When the dogs are doing any of the relaxation exercises, they are allowed to collect information if (1) they are not distressed to start, (2) viewing the focus of their information does not cause them to become more reactive, and (3) they can look calmly back at the person working with them. Distressed dogs cannot stop looking at the stimulus, hesitate in returning their focus to the person, or react when looking at the stimulus. These are all cues that people can use to decide where the individual dog's threshold lies. LAT puts the behavior of looking to collect information on cue so that the dog is rewarded for assessing the situation in a nonreactive manner and then returning his or her focus to the person. This technique allows the handler to take advantage of the dog's normal cognitive process and use it to show the dog that, yes, he *can* look at things that worry him, and if he looks right back and is calm, good things happen.

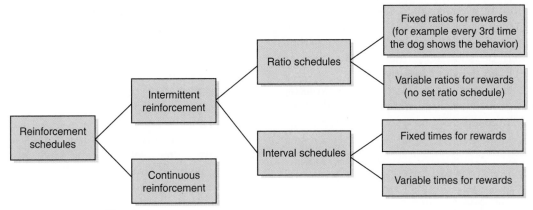

Fig. 3-6 Flow chart explaining types of reinforcement schedules.

REINFORCEMENT SCHEDULES AND TIMING OF REWARDS

A *schedule of reinforcement* is important for teaching or learning *a behavior and for maintaining it* (see Fig. 3-6 for a flow chart). There are two main types of reinforcement schedules: *continuous* and *intermittent*.

- In a *continuous reinforcement schedule,* every occurrence is rewarded. This type of schedule produces the *fastest acquisition of a response.*
- *Intermittent schedules* are best for *maintaining an acquired response.* Intermittent reinforcement schedules can be of two types: *ratio schedules* and *interval schedules.*
  - In ratio schedules, the animal is provided with a reward on either a *fixed* or a *variable basis* depending on the number of times the animal executes the behavior correctly.
    - *Fixed ratios* mean that the reward comes, for example, every third time the animal successfully executes the behavior.
    - *Variable ratios* are exactly that—sometimes the reward comes after two correct responses, sometimes after five, et cetera.
  - Interval rewards come after a set interval of time that also can be either fixed or variable.
- Most clients are actually using *variable interval rewards* because the time lapse between the correct performance of the desired behavior and the reward usually varies unless someone is attending to and measuring it.

Second-order or *secondary reinforcers* are signals that can be used at a distance that convey that the reinforcer is coming.

- Commonly used second-order reinforcers are words ("Good girl"), hand signals, and clickers or whistles.
- By carefully pairing these with the reward with which the desired response has already been paired, second-order reinforcers can elicit and maintain the same response as the reinforcer would.

- This rule also holds for negative reinforcement. In fact, the sound the collar makes as it pulls and then slips is supposed to act as a secondary reinforcer where the sound stops the behavior. Observation would seem to indicate that few people use this device as intended, suggesting that such tools are best abandoned, especially if there are other tools to replace them that are easier to use, more humane, and more effective.

Other Important Things to Know About Timing and Rewards

In operant conditioning, learning is fastest if the positive reinforcer/reward is presented immediately—within 0.5 second—of the desired behavior. Delayed and intermittent reinforcements slow the acquisition of the response but work well to reinforce its maintenance because they enhance resistance to extinction.

In addition to timing (quantity), value (quality) is also important. The more an animal values a reinforcer, the more quickly and reliably the animal will acquire the response. Food treats that the dog does not usually get (e.g., cheese) will be better than his standard kibble in teaching a new behavior. When working with a fearful dog on the street, he may require a different reward than he would when working with him in a quiet room. For some, but not all, dogs, the tougher the circumstances are for them to handle, the greater the value of the reward will need to be. Not all dogs value food above all else; some value play with a ball or Frisbee or massage. Designing behavior modification programs that have a high probability of success requires understanding what the dog values.

Finally, factors that affect arousal/attentiveness must be considered. According to the Yerkes-Dodson Law (Yerkes and Dodson, 1908), performance increases with cognitive and/or physiological arousal but only to a point. If any kind of arousal becomes too high, performance decreases (Mendl, 1999). The molecular basis of this finding was discussed earlier with respect to interacting levels of cortisol, BDNF, and CREB (Peters et al., 2004). For practical purposes, this means that rewards should be something that the dog or cat strongly desires but doesn't cause frenzy.

For a wonderful, quick, and easy source that explains training terms, go to www.clickertraining.com/glossary (last accessed August 31, 2011).

APPLYING ALL OF THIS SO THAT CLIENTS AND STAFF CAN IMPLEMENT HUMANE BEHAVIOR MODIFICATION USING TREATMENT PROTOCOLS

This text includes a complete series of client handouts included on the companion website. Every condition discussed includes a reference to a client handout that explains the condition and provides specific suggestions for intervention. For some of these, the *trio of foundation protocols* as discussed later will also be needed.

All handouts are written for a broad audience and anticipate that the reader may know nothing. It's understood that many in the veterinary and training professions—and that many clients—are more knowledgeable than is assumed here and may not need the degree of hand-holding that the handouts provide. However, it is wise to err on the side of providing more, rather than less, information. If the veterinary staff reviews the handouts with the clients and highlights the parts that they believe are essential for the clients to know, everyone will benefit.

ESSENTIAL STEPS IN BEHAVIOR MODIFICATION AND PROTOCOLS THAT MATCH THESE STEPS

The essential steps for the behavior modification discussed in this text are found in the accompanying video, *Humane Behavioral Care for Dogs: Problem Prevention and Treatment*. This video demonstrates the key parts of the *trio of foundation protocols* that are used for all behavior modification:

- "Protocol for Deference"
- "Protocol for Teaching Your Dog to Take a Deep Breath and Use Other Biofeedback Methods as Part of Relaxation"
- "Protocol for Relaxation: Behavior Modification Tier 1"

"Protocol for Deference"

The "Protocol for Deference" can be used for cats and dogs but will be most useful in dogs and young, rambunctious cats. If cats are started on this protocol when young, they are likely to become more interactive with their humans and stand a good chance of having their needs better understood and met by their humans. This protocol is a set of instructions that allows anyone's pet to:

1. begin to learn to be calm,
2. learn that they can ask questions of people, and
3. learn that they can get guidance about what is expected or whether they need worry if they just sit calmly.

Together, these three points teach dogs and cats that they learn better, feel safer, and have more control in creating favorable interaction if they are calm.

These three points make this program completely different from "leadership," "earn to learn," "nothing in life is free," and other similar programs that are often recommended for dogs. In contrast to these other programs, the "Protocol for Deference" is based on understanding and using innate social and cognition systems. For dogs, especially, this program capitalizes on the apparent ability dogs have to ask questions about their environment, risks, social interactions, et cetera, in a way that is obvious to their people. This basic program asks pets to do one thing: sit calmly and look at the human whenever anything is desired or needed. Sitting is an especially deferential behavior for dogs that signals that the dog is seeking and receptive to information. If the dog is quiet, calm and relaxed, and looking at the human, the dog can understand and use any information that the human can share with the dog.

"Protocol for Teaching Your Dog to Take a Deep Breath and Use Other Biofeedback Methods as Part of Relaxation"

Dogs and cats, similar to humans, cannot learn new behaviors if they are distressed. In fact, we all produce best the needed brain chemicals to make lasting memory if we are attentive enough to watch carefully but not so attentive that we are overly concerned. Most dogs and cats about whom clients are concerned and/or who have truly pathological behavior are not calm enough to learn and use new information, especially if part of that information is learning to be calm.

This protocol focuses on dogs because most people will actually implement it for dogs. A feline aficionado could easily also use it successfully for cats. The protocol teaches clients how to teach their dog to take a deep breath and how to use other biofeedback tools to prepare the dog to relax so that the dog can learn how to change his or her behavior in a way that makes everyone happier and calmer.

The three important signaling tools used here that involve biofeedback are:

- "look,"
- "breathe," and
- "smart-pet": petting a dog in a manner that avoids unhelpful arousal and encourages useful focus.

Smart-pet relies on teaching the clients to pet the dog using only long, slow strokes that provide some pressure and muscle massage. Clients are completely unaware that rapid petting and scratching causes arousal and inattention in dogs, but that appropriate petting can calm dogs and reinforce the physiological effects of being calm (Kostarczyk and Fonberg, 1982). In fact, clients do not know what "rapid petting" is—they just unconsciously touch, pet, and scratch dogs in ways that provide stimuli of which the human is unaware. Smart-pet slows clients down and calms the dog or cat. This way both parties can pay attention to each other and interact purposefully in an informed and relaxed manner that promotes learning. As soon as the client touches the dog or cat, she can start to apply gentle pressure while v-e-r-y s-l-o-w-l-y moving her hand down the dog's or cat's back and over muscle groups. If the client is doing this correctly, one stroke will take 10 to 20 seconds (that's a long time), and she should be able to feel the cat's or dog's structure. Clients will need to be coached in this, and it is worth the time it takes to do so because if they can learn how the dog or cat responds physiologically to different external cues of rhythms from them, they can understand how their arousal state and guidance can affect their pet. These three signaling tools are demonstrated in the video, *Humane Behavioral Care for Dogs: Problem Prevention and Treatment*.

"Protocol for Relaxation: Behavior Modification Tier 1"

This protocol contains the essential, basic behavior modification program on which all more complex programs using DS and CC will be built. This protocol can be used for both cats and dogs. The protocol comprises the following sections:

1. introduction,
2. starting out—roles for spontaneous reward and using the "shaping" technique,
3. description of the protocol for relaxation—tier 1,
4. a note about food treats,
5. understanding the reward process,
6. getting the dog's or cat's attention,
7. avoiding problems,
8. format for the protocol,
9. protocol task sheets and tips for implementing these, and
10. suggestions for future repetitions.

Underpinning this program is the successful use of the "Protocol for Teaching Your Dog to Take a Deep Breath and Use Other Biofeedback Methods as Part of Relaxation" and the "Protocol for Relaxation: Behavior Modification Tier 1." Fundamental and unique to the approach taken in these tiered approaches is the encouragement of specific behavioral responses in a manner

that alters brain neurochemistry to encourage relaxation and learning. Taken to the next level, this program is a form of cognitive therapy for dogs and cats. This program, as originally published in 1997 (Overall, 1997) and modified and expanded here, had as its roots and inspiration—not the "sit-stay" and other obedience-based programs so commonly in use—but the types of cognitive and biofeedback approaches developed and recommended by Wolpe (1969) and Beck (1975), combined with the molecular/neuropharmacological approaches being supported by the U.S. National Institute of Mental Health.

Clients should be encouraged to use these programs *only* in ways that help the dog. It is very easy for clients to assume that because the dog sits, the dog has learned something. The dog may have learned, but if the client did not reinforce the right behavior, *the dog may have learned to be more uncertain*. This is what is problematic about routine sit-stay and training types of programs: they focus on the tools that you can use to get behavioral, physiological, and cognitive improvement (e.g., sitting, which is a stop signal in dogs), not on the improvement itself. One sequela is that dogs may be rewarded for sitting even if they are anxious and scanning the horizon.

In contrast, we focus on the improvement itself, knowing that there are many ways to succeed. The key is to recognize and reward only calm, progressively calmer, more adaptive, less reactive, more flexible behaviors that will allow the dog to make choices about engaging in more contextually appropriate ways. The dog can get to the point where he realizes that he has some control over the way he responds and the way he feels. Once the dog acquires this level of skill and flexible behavior, improvement is extremely rapid.

For clients to help their dogs achieve such improvement, they need to be able to know whether, when, and how the dog is improving. For them to do this, we must encourage them to measure the outcomes that their work with the dog is producing. Measurements in veterinary behavioral medicine are rare, and we must make an effort to reverse that trend and create more objective standards and outcomes.

There are numerous ways to measure outcomes, and they are not equally easy for all people. Some suggestions follow. These suggestions can also be found in the "Protocol for Relaxation: Behavior Modification Tier 1."

1. Clients can video themselves and others working with the dog every day. They can compare the same exercise each day, noting all of the postures that worry them and all of the postures that they think are good. They can then discuss the video with the veterinary staff and/or any certified trainer who has the knowledge to help with this issue.
2. Clients can video the dog performing the behavior modification program once a week and compare specific behaviors by the week. Measures taken from

the video may include the number of times the dog scanned the room, the number of times the dog licked his lips, the dog's respiratory rate, and the number of repeats of an exercise before the dog was calm and perfect for it. There are many, many things that clients can measure if they are given some guidance.

3. Clients can count and record the seconds until the dog complies in a happy way. As the dog improves, these intervals should be shorter, but the client will need to ensure that as the dog's mastery of sitting for all the exercises improves, allowing progression through them to be faster, he remains calm.

4. The clients can have the dog repeat the exercise using some criteria they have established for how often the dog must be "perfect" in her position and calm before they move on to the next step. In these types of measures, common assessments may include:
   a. having the dog succeed 3 out of 4 times during four repeats of the exercises over 2 days,
   b. having the dog succeed 9 out of 10 times during one or two repeats of the exercises on 1 day, and
   c. having the dog succeed 8 out of 10 times during one or two repeats of the exercises over 2 days.

Note the pattern here: in these types of measures, you need a better success rate to advance over a short period of time than you do if you are going to advance more slowly over a period of days. These types of measures are common validity tools and are most useful when the dog is learning something that has a clear endpoint.

Regardless of how clients decide to measure their dog's progress, they should be encouraged to advance only when there is true progress and when the dog has learned something helpful. If the client complains that they are "stuck" and cannot advance, that's when they need your help and/or the help of a qualified trainer who truly understands both behavioral modification and conditioning strategies. If there is no one in your area who does this, consider subsidizing the training of a gifted technician so that he or she can learn these skills.

TOOLS THAT MAY HELP OR HURT

Most humans will rely on some tools to help them interact with their dogs and cats safely and in a manner that they find acceptable. For cats, such tools may be restricted to an identification collar or an implanted microchip, if the cat gets outside, or a cat carrier or lead/harness for visits to the vet. Yet cats can walk on leads and engage in sports like agility. Cats will benefit from these interventions as will dogs. If we wish to have a truly positive effect on feline behavior, we need to understand their evolutionary history and realize that as cognitive individuals they likely need more

stimulation than being left alone indoors and meal feeding affords. In this respect, cats may be the big growth market for the humane use of tools and gizmos.

Collars, Harnesses, Head Collars, and Leads

A client handout, "Protocol for Choosing Collars, Head Collars, Harnesses, and Leads," is available at the end of the text and on the DVD. The main points are highlighted here.

Collars

The main purpose of collars should be identification. Clients need to understand that (1) the tags must be up-to-date (and that they should keep a copy of their rabies vaccination certification in a safe place because it is the legal proof of rabies vaccination in countries that require this), and (2) they are on a collar that fits safely and comfortably. Collars should be breakaway collars through which one or two fingers can slip comfortably or be fitted sufficiently loosely that it remains on the animal when the dog or cat lowers her head, but should the collar become entangled, the collar will slip from the animal. If clients are not cautious about the fit of collars, animals can strangle, or collars can become imbedded in their skin resulting in injury or death. Breakaway collars are particularly important for cats, who are very good at forcing their bodies into small places where a collar could become entangled.

Microchipping has allowed large numbers of pets to be returned to their humans, and in the United States may buy a dog or cat extra time at a shelter if the chip is detected. All shelters in the United States are supposed to have microchip readers and scan every entering animal for them. A microchip tag on a collar acts as a failsafe.

Choker/Prong Collars

Dogs are often routinely fitted with something like a choker collar as part of a training program. Choker collars are usually made from chain, leather, or a rolled, braided nylon. When used correctly, choker collars are actually one of the best examples of true "negative reinforcement": when the dog pulls, the collar tightens, and either the sound or smallest amount of pressure indicates that the dog has engaged in an undesirable behavior; when the dog stops, the pressure is released (and in the case of a chain the sound of slippage occurs) *and* the dog is unimpeded. The release from the negative stimulus (the tightening of the collar) is the reward.

Unfortunately, virtually no one uses choke collars in the described manner. Instead, most dogs placed on chokers "choke." When they are allowed to pull on the collar and permitted to sustain the pull, these dogs learn to override the choker. In doing so, they are also at risk for laryngeal damage, esophageal damage, and ocular damage (Fig. 3-7) (Pauli et al., 2006). In a

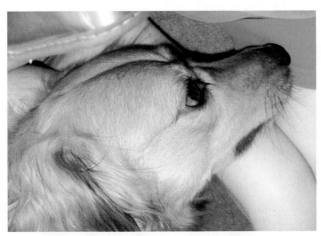

Fig. 3-7 Scleral hemorrhage that occurred when a flat buckle collar became constricted during play with another dog when the client was present and observing the dogs. Chokers are even more constricting in such situations. (Photo courtesy of Dr. Soraya Juarbe-Diaz.)

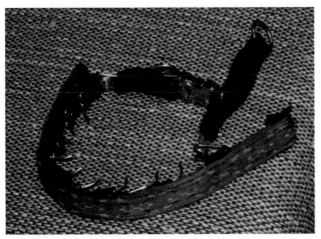

Fig. 3-8 A modern prong collar, with a covering that disguises the prongs and makes them less apparent for those passing by.

retrospective study on spinal pain, injury, or changes in dogs conducted in Sweden, Hallgren (1992) found that 91% of dogs with cervical anomalies experienced harsh jerks on the lead or had a long history of pulling on the lead. Use of chokers was also overrepresented in this group. This study strongly suggests that such corrections are potentially injurious. The dog who pulls harder has no choice: dogs will always push against pressure, which means they all pull harder.

Prong collars are actually a special case of a choker collar (Fig. 3-8). As the dog pulls, the bent, paired prongs of an adjustable sized collar tighten. If the dog slows or stops pulling, the prongs release. Because the prongs are not continuous, they are often thought to be less potentially injurious and damaging to dogs. There are no data to support this opinion. If the dog is very forceful, the prongs can become embedded in the skin, a pattern some humans choose when they sharpen the prongs. Particularly abusive humans routinely sharpen

the prongs. Remember, it's impossible to "sharpen" a harness or head collar.

Because of new developments in other collars, head collars, and harnesses that render these safer and easier to use and more humane for dogs, *traditional choke collars and prong collars are ideas whose time has passed.*

For people whose dogs don't bite who dislike the idea of harnesses and head collars, a modified neck collar with a baffle is now available. The Scruffy Guider has three neck straps that can be adjusted for a snug fit. The collar tightens down when the dog pulls in a manner similar to a fabric choke collar, but there is a baffle that prevents the collar from tightening beyond the point where it is just flush to the neck, plus two other baffles on the collar itself. The baffle on the part of the collar attached to the lead works better than a martingale to snug the collar without putting direct pressure on any one place on the neck. These baffles are well padded but solid and unbendable and so provide structure for the collar as it wraps around the neck—something not present in standard choke collars. This is not the solution for an out-of-control dog, but it is another tool that may work for some dogs.

Figure 3-9, *A,* shows an unattached Scruffy Guider, and Figure 3-9, *B,* shows Linus modeling a fitted Scruffy Guider. Figure 3-9, *C,* shows a young dog successfully and safely wearing a Scruffy Guider.

Head Collars

Head collars are similar to horse halters: they act as a basket that holds the dog's cheeks and jaws and stay on the dog by fastening high on the back of the neck. There is generally at least one strap that fits over the bridge of the dog's nose, and one that fits over the back of the neck. The lead is attached in the middle of the halter, to the nose strap but under the chin. This is just like how a lead is attached to a horse halter but is a major change for many people accustomed to attaching a lead directly to something around a dog's neck. A number of head collars are now widely available: the Halti, the Gentle Leader Canine Head Collar (formerly called the Promise System), the Canny Collar, Respond, the Control collar, the Infinity Lead, et cetera (Figs. 3-10 through 3-16).

The Halti is intended to be fitted with a second collar because it fits loosely. It also cannot be as easily tightened by pulling forward, but it fits some very jowly breeds well and snugly. The Gentle Leader gives most dogs a better fit, requires no second collar, and can be used with a lead to correct inappropriate behaviors and prohibit biting. Both of these collars have undergone many improvements in their first decades, including narrower nose straps and ergonomic buckles that resist breakage.

Because the company that manufactured the Gentle Leader, Premier Pet Products, was sold in 2010 to Radio Systems Corporation, the largest manufacturer of electronic and shock collars, many trainers, vets,

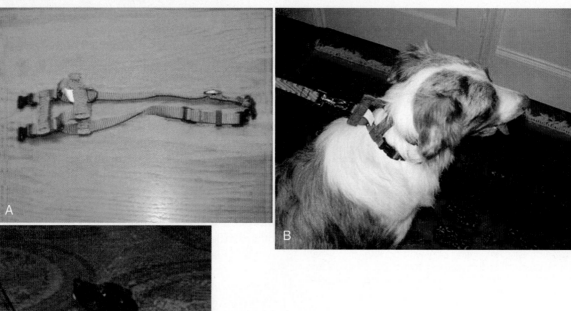

Fig. 3-9 A, Unattached Scruffy Guider. **B,** Fitted Scruffy Guider modeled by Linus. **C,** A young dog successfully and safely wearing a Scruffy Guider.

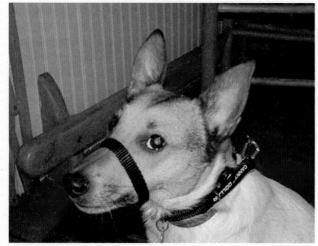

Fig. 3-10 Snap demonstrating a Canny Collar, a type of convertible collar where the nose loop can be incorporated into the collar so that the dog can quickly be wearing a type of flat buckle collar without having to disconnect or remove the head collar. This is a boon to people who have enthusiastic dogs who also may wish to go to a dog park. The lead attaches at the back of the neck with this head collar.

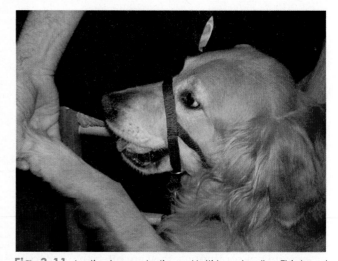

Fig. 3-11 Austin demonstrating a Halti head collar. This head collar has a jaw strap that many dogs find more comfortable, and it fits many fat-faced dogs, such as mastiff breeds, more comfortably than head collars with one nose strap. Unless it fits snugly, it may come off (there is now a martingale adaptation to prevent this risk), and you will not be able to close the dog's mouth tightly, if desired. The lead attaches under the throat with the Halti.

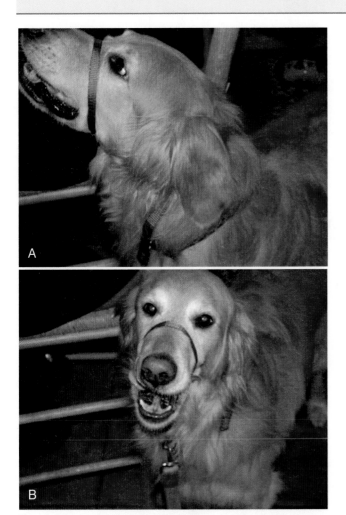

Fig. 3-12 Austin demonstrating two views of a Gentle Leader head collar. **A,** Austin showing the snug fit at the top and back of his neck and the correct placement of the nose loop so that it sits *behind* the corners of the mouth. In this case, the lead attaches under the throat. **B,** Front-on view of Austin showing an appropriate fit and that he can open his mouth, yawn, lick his lips, eat and drink, and even bite someone when no pressure is put on the lead. This snug fit allows the person with the lead to close the dog's mouth and stop or prevent a bite.

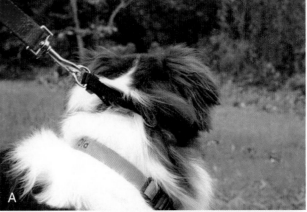

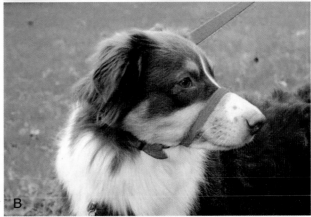

Fig. 3-13 **A,** The Black Dog Infin8 head collar uses a martingale type of attachment for the lead at the back of the neck. **B,** The nose loop of the Infin8 head collar wraps around the nose then clips to the side of the collar allowing the collar to adjust easily to the dog's movement and head shape. These head collars are made of cotton webbing and so are unlikely to slip.

behaviorists, and clients have been looking for other sources of head collars and harnesses from companies that do not use, endorse, or sell products that involve electric shock. The good news is that the number of alternative product choices is growing and will likely continue to grow.

At present, unless the dog is fat-faced, there are two collars that best close an aggressive dog's mouth when used appropriately: the Gentle Leader and the Black Dog Training Halter (www.blackdog.net.au) (see Figs. 3-12, *B*, and 3-14). If the client does not need to be able to close the dog's mouth tightly, there are many other head collars and harnesses that will meet the client's needs.

Head collars are wonderful for most dogs and people. They spare the dog's larynx and esophagus and so are one of the ideal choices—along with harnesses—for dogs with laryngeal damage, tracheal collapse, or cervical (neck) damage involving disks, bones, nerves, or muscles. Head collars also ride high on the back of the dog's neck so that when the lead is pulled forward or the dog pulls in the direction opposite to that of the lead, this part of the collar tightens a bit and puts a small amount of steady pressure on this area of the upper neck near the head. Not only is this generally very safe, but also this pressure is the exact kind of signal that dogs communicate to other dogs when they wish to control them or stop.

The Black Dog Training Halter does an excellent job of closing a dog's mouth and maintaining it closed (see Fig. 3-14). This head halter is among the easiest to fit, is well tolerated by dogs, and communicates well with the dogs. The webbing is cotton, which means that it doesn't slip once sized.

As with all equipment, check your leads, harnesses, collars, and head collars routinely for damage and replace anything that is questionable. Nothing lasts forever, defects occur, and wear is normal. The head

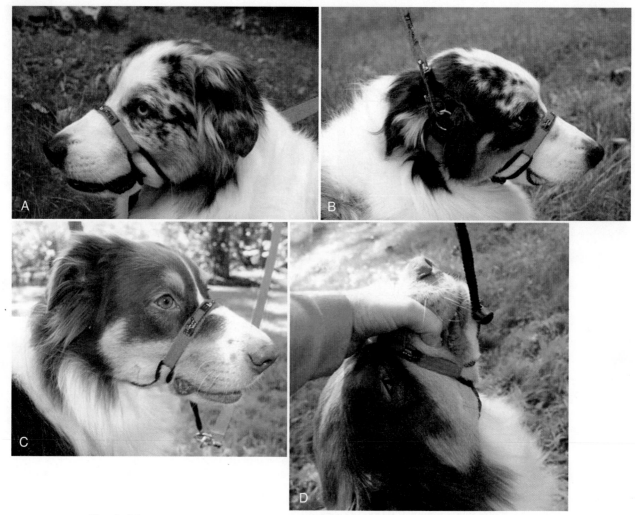

Fig. 3-14 A, The Black Dog Training Halter has a nose loop that is padded and held in place by easily adjustable mouth and neck pieces (control cords) that are secured under the neck. The lead attaches under the neck so that the dog's mouth can be gently closed, if needed. **B,** The Black Dog Training Collar fits snugly behind the neck, and the lead attaches under the throat to the adjustable control cords, which lock after adjustment to the dog's size and head shape. **C,** The Black Dog Training Halter used on a dog at rest. **D,** The Black Dog Training Halter used to hold the mouth shut. The toggle adjusts to fit the nose loop securely.

collar in Figure 3-16 suddenly tore across a stitched area, but no one was injured.

Bark Collars

There are two types of collars commonly recommended for stopping or reducing barking: shock/static electric/shock collars (e-collars) and citronella collars. Both of these are aversive devices and punishers. Before anyone considers the use of any device to stop barking or vocalizing, it is essential to understand that barking, whining, and howling provide information. If the dog is barking in an appropriate context, there are more humane ways to modulate the noise. For example, expressing interest in the focus of the bark, indicating that you know the bark contains information, and then thanking/rewarding the dog when she quiets because you are responding usually works.

If dogs are barking because they are pathologically distressed, aversive devices either will have no effect on them or will render them more anxious. The neurochemical and stress responses explained earlier in this chapter detail why this is so.

If one has a dog who exhibits "nuisance" barking, the adverse effects of shock/e-collars and citronella collars may be expected to be less, but the data support neither this assertion nor one of efficacy. An early study using citronella collars and shock collars for control of barking in the clients' home showed that the citronella collar decreased barking by 88.9%, and the shock collar decreased it by only 44% (Juarbe-Diaz and Houpt, 1996). This study suggests that an aversive/disruptive stimulus alone was not sufficient to account for the findings. Pain may have caused repeat vocalization,

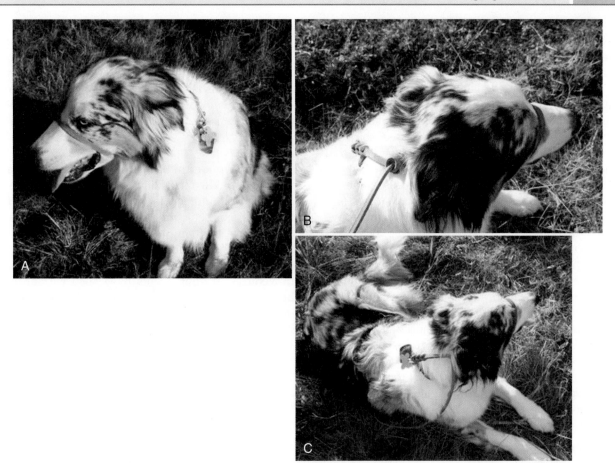

Fig. 3-15 An easy-to-use and easy-to-fit version of a leather figure 8 head collar, the Infinity Lead, is being made as a prototype by a company, Service Dog Designs, that makes custom equipment for service/assistant dogs and their partners. This simple head collar is designed so that the lead attaches at the top of the neck, behind the head. A lanyard attaches it to the dog's neck collar for additional security. Leather requires special care, and anyone using leather leads, harnesses, collars, or head collars should know and meet these care needs. This prototype has huge potential, given its simple on-off assembly, its ease of fitting, how readily dogs take to it, and how well it manages pulling. **A,** The nose loop is snugly fitted over Toby's nose by adjusting a leather connector under Toby's chin. **B,** The back part of the figure 8, the neck loop, is slipped over the head behind the ears and gently secured at the bottom of the skull/top of the neck using the leather ratchet. The lanyard attachment that can hook to a regular neck collar is shown in **A** and **B. C,** The entire lead and head collar as it would be used is shown, complete with lanyard attached to a regular neck collar.

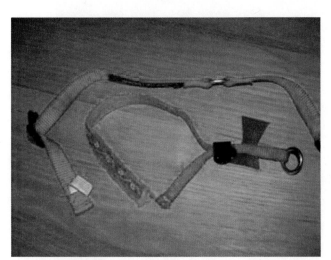

Fig. 3-16 Gentle Leader Canine Head Collar with a spontaneous tear not due to age or wear.

accounting for the differences in response. Regardless, clients thought that the citronella collars were "more humane." Is this so?

In one study that examined the use of shock versus citronella collars to stop barking in kenneled dogs, both collars significantly reduced barking compared with controls; however, the citronella collars did so more quickly (Steiss et al., 2007), a finding supported by other studies (Juarbe-Diaz and Houpt, 1996; Moffat et al., 2003). It is possible that such a quick response occurs because the citronella collar acts as a true, contextual, disruptive stimulus, without being painful; however, plasma cortisol levels were not different among the three groups (shock, citronella, and control) and there was no difference in the activity levels of the dogs among the treatment groups (Steiss et al., 2007). Fewer repetitions were required using the citronella collar than the static electric/shock collar, again indicating that pain may have interfered with learning or caused an opposite response to that desired. This finding suggests that stress levels are always high in kenneled dogs and that the dogs merely learned not to bark when wearing the collar, which is an avoidance behavior. Juarbe-Diaz and Houpt (1996) noted that barking returned to previous levels once collars were removed. None of these studies evaluated roles for context, pain, and stress/distress, but other studies that did so for applications of shock are discussed in the section on non-treatments, at the end of this chapter.

Because citronella collars can still cause fear and become phobic stimuli, and because some dogs have adverse reactions to the essential oils, spray collars without citronella have been studied (Moffat et al., 2003). Both spray collars without citronella and collars with citronella were associated with a reduction in barking that was statistically significant over control collars. These data all merit thoughtful consideration. If the finding by Moffat and Landsberg (2003) is true, this can only mean that timing and some form of intervention—acknowledging the dog—matter. Accordingly, expressing interest in the focus of the dog's bark and indicating that this vocal signal contains information, followed by some signal to the dog that acknowledges this transfer of information ("Good boy, Picasso, I've got it. Thanks!"), will interrupt the barking as well as any device.

If there are real emergencies (e.g., burglars/rapists) or if the dog is home alone, normal dogs will bark, if the individual dog is predisposed to do so, whether anyone listens.

Harnesses

There are wonderful harnesses available now that are intended to do more than simply contain the dog. Simple containment is acceptable only when the dog has no behavioral issues when leash-walked. This means that simple harnesses are acceptable *only* for dogs who do not pull or jump and who do not growl, lunge, or snarl at humans, dogs, other animals, or vehicles. If your clients have such extraordinarily behaved dogs, simple harnesses and collars are adequate for leash walks. For all other dogs, the no-pull harnesses discussed here are wonderful tools for dogs who do not need, do not wish to use, or cannot use head collars.

Cat harnesses need to hold the cat securely to prevent escape and not impede walking/climbing. With lovely harnesses available for kittens and cats (Fig. 3-17), there

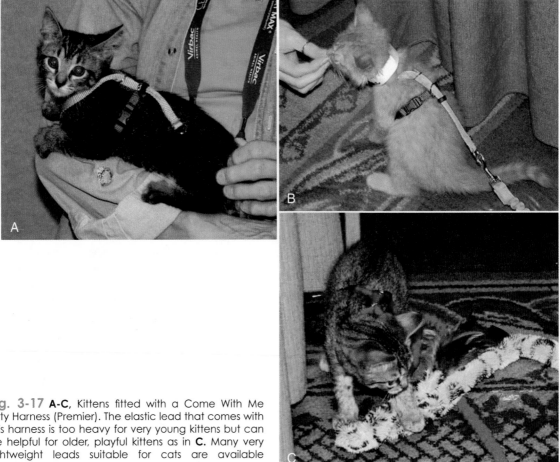

Fig. 3-17 A-C, Kittens fitted with a Come With Me Kitty Harness (Premier). The elastic lead that comes with this harness is too heavy for very young kittens but can be helpful for older, playful kittens as in C. Many very lightweight leads suitable for cats are available commercially.

is no excuse not to start leash-walking kittens and taking them for car rides as soon as they enter the household. Cats who are reared with the expectation that they will meet people, travel, and go for leash walks tend to be easier to handle, will be less fearful of such situations because of exposure, and will be less stressed at veterinary visits.

The new design of the Sporn No Pull harnesses has padding that goes under the forelegs and through which the straps—attached to the band under the neck and again at the back—freely glide. The lead is attached at the back over the shoulders so that if the dog pulls, the straps tighten. The intent is that the dog slows and then releases himself to move forward again. The dog shown in Figure 3-18 took part in a laboratory where he also quite tolerantly and correctly was fitted with a Gentle Leader Canine Head Collar.

No-pull harnesses fit under the dog's front legs and loop over the dog's shoulders so that when the dog pulls, his front legs are pulled back and he slows his pace. A number of these harnesses, including the SENSE-ation harness, the original no-pull harness, exist: the Lupi, the Sporn No Pull Harness (see Fig. 3-18), the DreamWalker Harness (Fig. 3-19), Easy Walk Harness (see Fig. 3-20), the Freedom No-Pull Harness from Wiggles, Wags & Whiskers (see Fig. 3-22). The Freedom No-Pull Harness has a special collar that is sewn with two different-sized metal tabs. The loose, lead-like part of the harness fits through one of the loops and goes under and around the legs and is attached to the other loops, under the neck, using a clasp. The lead is attached to the loose part of the harness over the dog's back. The back part of the harness can be tightened for a better, more responsive, fit.

The Lupi doesn't have any clasps or tabs, instead relying on a system of concentric loops that are fitted around the dog's front legs and over the back. The lead is affixed to the back portion, which slips to tighten if the dog pulls. The Lupi is a little easier to fit to very hairy dogs or for people whose hands are very arthritic. Both of these fitting patterns sound complex and like topological puzzles. They are not. Once the client has the device in his or her hands, the fit becomes self-explanatory.

The SENSE-ation Harness (see Fig. 3-21), the New Freedom Harness, and the DreamWalker Harness are "power-steering for dogs." Some of these are more complex than others to fit. The DreamWalker Harness can challenge anyone's spatial skills, but the instructions are so good and logical that with a small amount of practice, fitting these makes complete sense. The handle is a little bulky, and people accustomed to traditional leads may take a while to get used to this, but for anyone who needs instantaneous control over a dog's movement, this is a great solution. Unfortunately, although it is possible to purchase the DreamWalker Harness on many sites online, it is no longer being manufactured. This is a concept that needs to be re-developed and re-released in a simpler and easier to use form.

Linus models the Gentle Leader Easy Walk Harness in Figure 3-20. Note in Figure 3-20, B, that Linus' lead is attached to a ring in the center of the chest strap. Sizing can be tricky with these harnesses, and the amount of hardware in the front can cause the harness to sag on some dogs. For these dogs, the SENSE-ation harness or custom-fitted Freedom No-Pull Harness from Wiggles, Wags & Whiskers may be preferable. As mentioned earlier, because the manufacturer of the Gentle Leader, Premier Pet Products, is now owned by Radio Systems Corporation, the largest manufacturer of electronic and shock collars, a number of trainers, vets, behaviorists, and clients have been looking for other sources of head collars and harnesses from companies that do not use, endorse, or sell products that involve electric shock. A number of alternative products from the growing range of those available are listed here.

In Figure 3-21, A, Bunny is wearing a SENSE-ation Harness. The front attachment is clear. The hardware in this no-pull harness is not bulky and fits smoothly against the chest. Bunny is older, arthritic, and small, so this is helpful. In Figure 3-21, B, you can see that the SENSE-ation Harness is fitted so that the angles on the shoulders are as recommended in the instructions, which are just excellent. This fit allows fully unimpeded shoulder and foreleg girdle motion.

In Figure 3-22, Picasso is wearing the Freedom No-Pull Harness from Wiggles, Wags & Whiskers. This is a back and front fit harness that comes with a dual lead for more control or for very worried humans. A center strap fits between the dog's legs and attaches to a belly band that clips around the belly and chest. The

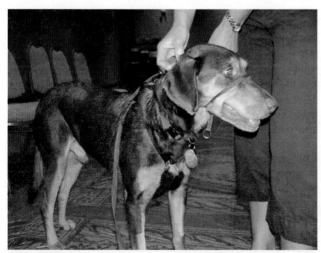

Fig. 3-18 A dog wearing a well-fitted Sporn No Pull Harness (and a head collar).

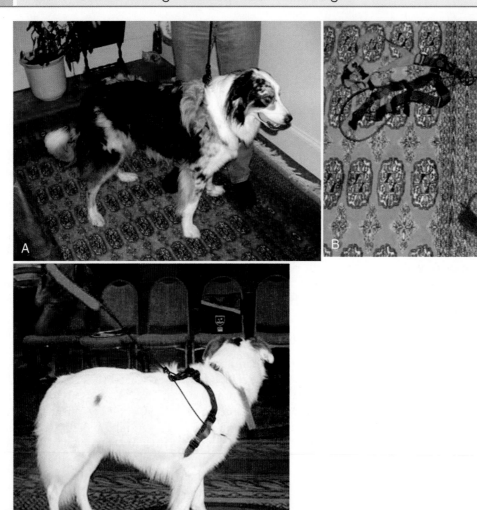

Fig. 3-19 **A,** Toby demonstrating the DreamWalker Harness. The instructions make this fit easy to understand, and if the harness is stored correctly, putting it on the dog each time is not a challenge. **B,** Toby's already fitted/sized DreamWalker Harness as it comes off the dog. You can see why reading the instructions and practice are so important for getting this on the dog correctly and quickly. **C,** DreamWalker Harness well fitted to a border collie showing the set of cords that help with steering.

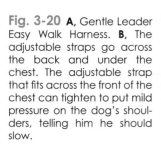

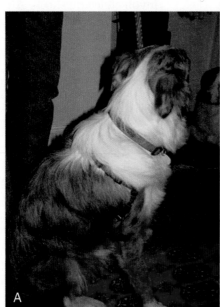

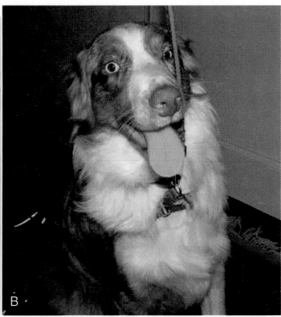

Fig. 3-20 **A,** Gentle Leader Easy Walk Harness. **B,** The adjustable straps go across the back and under the chest. The adjustable strap that fits across the front of the chest can tighten to put mild pressure on the dog's shoulders, telling him he should slow.

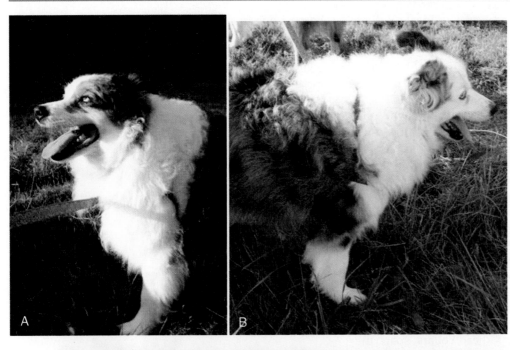

Fig. 3-21 **A**, Front attachment of the SENSE-ation Harness is clear. The hardware is not bulky and fits smoothly against the chest. **B**, The SENSE-ation Harness angles on the shoulders, as recommended in the instructions. This allows full shoulder and foreleg girdle motion.

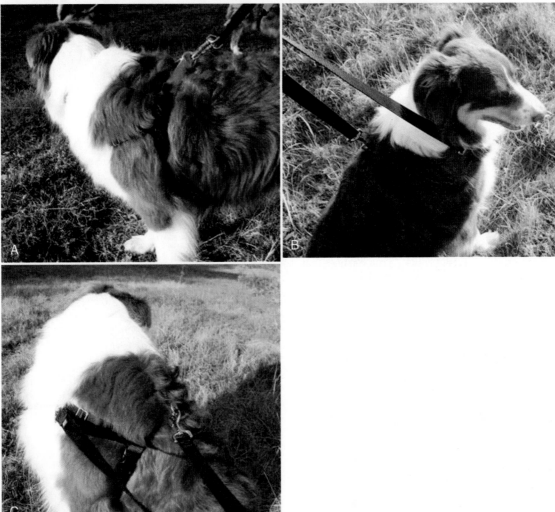

Fig. 3-22 Freedom No-Pull Harness from Wiggles, Wags & Whiskers. **A**, Back lead attachment with both leads attached to it. A single lead could also attach here. Note that the buckle is well away from the shoulder and front arm motion. **B** and **C**, Picasso with one of the leads attached to the back lead attachment and one to the front lead attachment for more control.

belly band is made from velvet and so is ideal for dogs who chafe if rubbed or who fuss at webbing. Each part of the harness is adjustable making a good fit easy, and all of the buckles are out of the way of the elbows. The instructions do an excellent job of explaining all fitting options and adjustments.

No-pull harnesses are wonderful for dogs who pull or lunge. These are *not* appropriate devices to fit to dogs whose biggest problem is biting, nipping, or grabbing because they do nothing to control the dog's mouth or head. Furthermore, reaching around the dog's head and neck to fit these harnesses could be dangerous if the dog is aggressive to people.

When fitted correctly, these harnesses will easily allow children and people with arthritis to walk their dogs pleasurably and calmly *if* the dogs are not huge and strong. Huge, strong dogs, especially dogs who are poorly mannered or unmannered can override these harnesses and end up dragging their person down the street while inflicting self-induced rope burns. These "no-pull" harnesses, similar to head collars, spare the dog's neck so that dogs with laryngeal, tracheal, esophageal, or spine problems can be more safely exercised. Caution is urged against fitting no-pull harnesses too tightly: too tight a fit could impede circulation in the dog's front legs.

Although not true harnesses, some vests developed for sporting and working dogs can fit snugly enough to act as harnesses for dogs who do best when hugged or squeezed. Figure 3-23 shows a Web Master Harness fitted snugly to a dog who has compromised vision and who worries about anything that suddenly appears in his visual field. The snugness of fit calms him, but the harness also provides the added security of a handle that allows anyone walking this 50-pound dog to lift him out of a potentially distressing or dangerous situation. The chest piece helps to encourage a pulling or lunging dog to move back (Fig. 3-24). This harness has reflective trim for nighttime walking. Because of the snug, 5-point fit and padding on the underside, this harness does not compromise any canine activity (Figs. 3-24 and 3-25).

A flyball harness can accomplish many of the same goals as the Web Master Harness (Fig. 3-26). By providing a solid y-front against the chest (Fig. 3-26, *A*), the Black Dog Flyball Racing Harness provides additional guidance for the dog and encourages the dog to pull less. This harness provides the safety of a handle (Fig. 3-26, *B*) so that the dog can be stopped, if needed.

Leads

High-quality fabric leads are now cheaply and widely available and should be most people's routine lead.

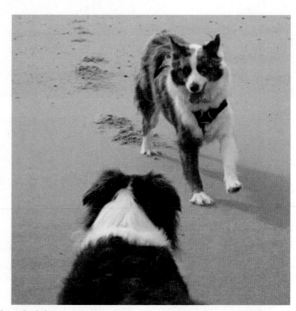

Fig. 3-24 The front of the Web Master Harness helps to pull the chest back and secure the dog if the dog pulls.

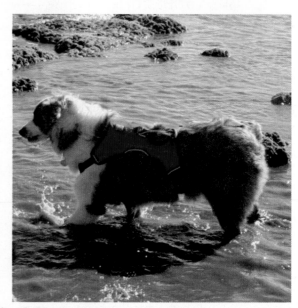

Fig. 3-25 The handle and reflective trim of the Web Master Harness provide safety in uncertain situations.

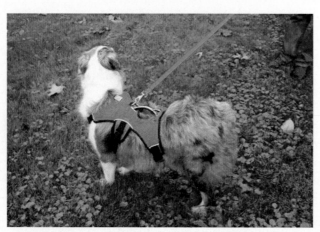

Fig. 3-23 Linus wearing a Ruffwear Web Master Harness.

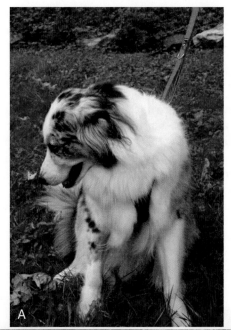

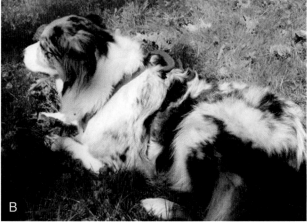

Fig. 3-26 A, Solid Y-front against the chest, which provides additional guidance for the dog and encourages the dog to pull less. **B,** Provides the safety of a handle to stop the dog, if needed.

They are flexible, hard to break, washable, and relatively maintenance-free. No one should be using metal chain link leads: they are hard on people's hands and do not lend themselves to humane guidance and control. Leather leads must be maintained, oiled, and frequently checked for failing stitching or leather. Regardless, no dog should be tied for more than a few minutes, and then they must be supervised to ensure that they are safe. Tying out dogs is a terrible idea; does not meet the dog's needs; and may put humans in the area at more risk of tripping, falling, being lunged at, or being injured by the dog. Tying dogs is inhumane to everyone. The client handout that expands on this information is "Protocol for Choosing Collars, Head Collars, Harnesses, and Leads."

Muzzles

In contrast to head collars, muzzles are not containment and control devices that work with the dog to alter or shape his behavior. Muzzles are intended to do exactly one thing: prevent the dog's teeth from contacting anything else. Although some dogs appear to behave more calmly when wearing a muzzle (possibly, in part, because their people are calmer), this is not a universal experience.

- No one should believe that a muzzled dog cannot injure someone.
- Muzzles can be weapons and can do serious harm to humans and other animals when they make forceful contact of the type common when the dog is trying to remove the muzzle or trying to escape and flinging his head around.
- Muzzles *do not* render dogs less aggressive and may reinforce a *heightened level of threat behavior* because there is no "cost" to the threats: the dog is not removed from the social interaction and does not engage in a true fight.
- Any dog who could injure a child without a muzzle may also injure that child while wearing a muzzle because more behaviors than just biting are involved in injury.
- Unless the muzzle is custom-fitted with respect to the dog's head size and shape, and unless it has a basket that rests comfortably around but does not touch the distal muzzle, the dog may still be able to bite.
- All dogs should be able to drink and take treats through muzzles.

If clients wish to use a muzzle as part of an informed program of behavior modification so that they worry less about their dog biting a human or another animal, a muzzle may work for them. For this to happen, three requirements must be met. *One requirement pertains to the human, another to the muzzle, and the third to how the clients use the muzzle.*

1. The clients understand that their anxiety and fear is contributing to heightening the reactivity of the environment for the dog, and so they are using the muzzle, in part, to mitigate concerns that make them less able to monitor and work sanely with the dog. Knowing this, they ensure that they work with the dog as recommended, and they seek competent behavioral help at the first sign of any worsening behavior.
2. The muzzle must be fitted and maintained by someone who knows what they are doing and should be padded and have multiple straps to ensure that it stays comfortably and safely in place.
3. No dog should be forced into a muzzle. Dogs should be taught to place their face willingly into the muzzle and stand to have it tightened. This can be done through a process of desensitization using food treats to accustom the dog gradually to placing her

head *voluntarily* into the muzzle and having the straps tightened. If the clients are good at teaching their dog to wear a muzzle happily, chances are that they will also be good at the behavior modification that could help address the problem for which the muzzle is being used.

If the clients cannot meet or do not understand these requirements, muzzles could be dangerous in their household, and muzzling the dog will do harm to him or her. Examples of well-fitted muzzles are shown in Figure 3-27. The dog in Figure 3-27, *A* and *B*, is wearing a front fit no-pull harness. Note that for the dog in Figure 3-27, *C* and *D*, the muzzle does not stop the dog from exhibiting aggressive behavior; however, it does allow the client to stand calmly back from the dog and

not jerk on the lead. The ability to engage in this type of helpful and non-reactive response is primarily a function of the client, not the tool.

Location Devices and GPS for Pets

Location devices are underused both in the monitoring of pets and in the teaching of basic manners training. These devices have been developed to monitor movements of individuals needing more care (e.g., young children, cognitively compromised older adults) and to monitor the location and/or potential theft of objects. There are two major classes of monitoring devices: devices that emit an auditory signal to let the human know when the cat or dog is moving beyond a pre-set

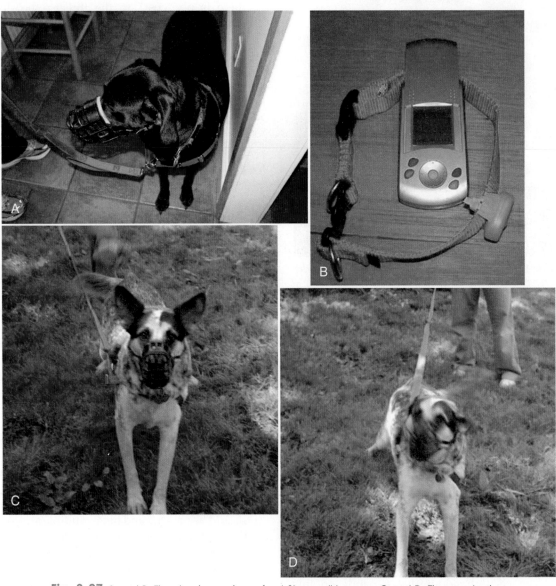

Fig. 3-27 A and **B**, The dog is wearing a front fit no-pull harness. **C** and **D**, The muzzle does not stop the dog from exhibiting aggressive behavior. However, it does allow the client to stand calmly back from the dog and not jerk on the lead.

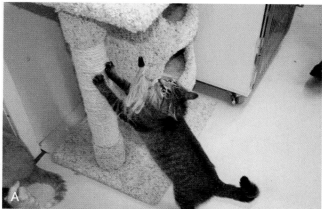

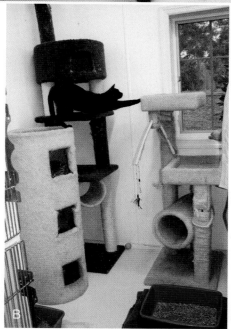

Fig. 3-36 **A** and **B**, Indoor and outdoor enclosures that meet all the needs for a group of shelter cats.

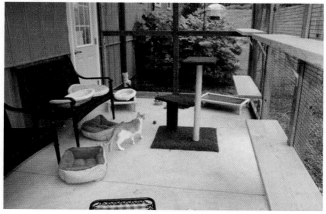

Fig. 3-37 This enclosure and many cat condos were built over the course of a weekend with volunteer labor from Eagle Scouts and less than a few hundred dollars of materials, including the fiberglass roofing. The concrete slab had been poured and cured before the Scouts got to work.

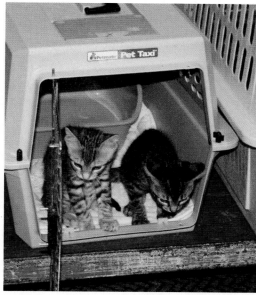

Fig. 3-38 Kittens partaking in a lab for veterinarians on the importance of early handling. They have a litterbox (with a tiny amount of litter not visible) and a blanket in their transport crate.

needs of the dogs can be met. Puppies need to eliminate every 30 to 60 minutes when awake and approximately 20 minutes after eating. Puppies who are sleeping will awaken every 1 or 2 hours and need to go out. For dogs of any age, crates are best used for housetraining when someone is available to notice that the dog is signaling a need to eliminate and can take the dog out, praising elimination in appropriate areas and rewarding it with play, freedom, and love (see the client handout "Protocol for Basic Manners Training and House Training for New Dogs and Puppies").

Crates can be useful in housetraining puppies and in protecting them from the dangerous world of electrical cords, outlets, glassware, et cetera, when no one is supervising them. Crates should be large enough for the dog to stand up and turn around in without having to hunch down; should be able to contain water, food/treats, toys, and bedding; and for pups or kittens left inside for an extended time, contain a box or area for elimination (Fig. 3-38).

Crates are not for everyone all the time and not for some animals ever. Figure 3-39, *A* and *B*, shows the teeth of a dog who was incarcerated in his crate 23 of 24 hours per day through 10 months of age when he was relinquished to a rescue. His chronic chewing on the crate damaged the lingual surfaces of all of his canines. Figure 3-39, *C*, shows a dog who is very distressed when left in a crate and has developed gum lesions as a result of his chewing.

Dogs who do not go willingly into their crates and seem happy to be there should not be contained in crates. What the human may perceive as secure, the dog

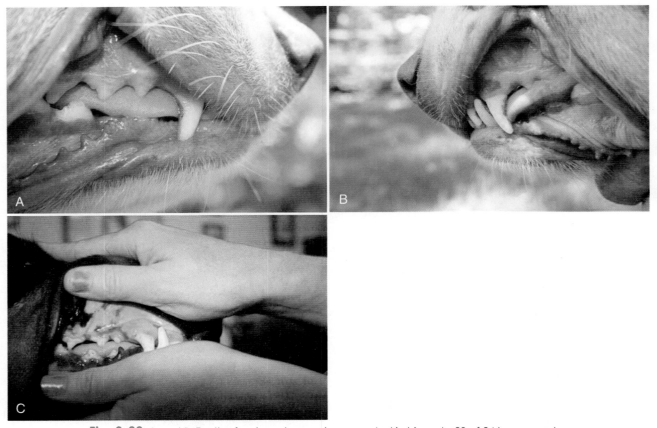

Fig. 3-39 **A** and **B**, Teeth of a dog who was incarcerated in his crate 23 of 24 hours per day for 10 months. Chronic chewing on the crate damaged the lingual surfaces of all of his canines. **C,** The lesion on the gum over the canine is the result of chewing on the crate in distress when left.

could perceive as entrapment. If the dog's crate is left open when everyone is home and the dog chooses to spend time in it with door open, chances are that dog will be content when the door is closed. Regardless, all dogs left in crates should periodically be videotaped. No dog who exhibits real or increasing signs of true distress should be forced to remain in a crate. Dogs have been known to break all of their teeth and nails in attempts to escape crates. Increasing the size of the crate or changing the style is generally not sufficient to render the dog content because the issue is that the dog feels entrapped and panics. Figure 3-39, *B* and *C*, shows damage to the lingual side of all canines associated with chewing on crate bars. The lower canine can be seen in Figure 3-39, *C*.

All dogs are different, and how they respond to crates should be frequently assessed before assuming a specific behavioral response. The dog in Figure 3-40 is actually locked out of her crate because she would otherwise choose to spend all of her time in it. The crate is in a large, airy kitchen; has water, a blanket, and toys; and, most importantly, spares this puppy the clumsy interactions with the older dog in the household who is blind and always knocking the pup down. Instead, emphasis was placed on having the older dog wear a

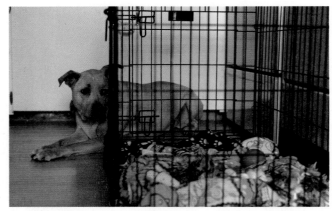

Fig. 3-40 This dog is locked out of her crate because she would otherwise choose to spend all her time in it. The pouch on the dog's collar is a Quiet Spot, designed to hold tags safely and without noise. (Photo courtesy Kristen Penkrot.)

bell so that the puppy had some control over avoiding clumsy and undesired attention.

Some dogs feel more secure in protected spaces. Figure 3-41, *A*, portrays a Saluki who panicked when placed in a large, open run with a window. She urinated and defecated, knocked over her food and water, and

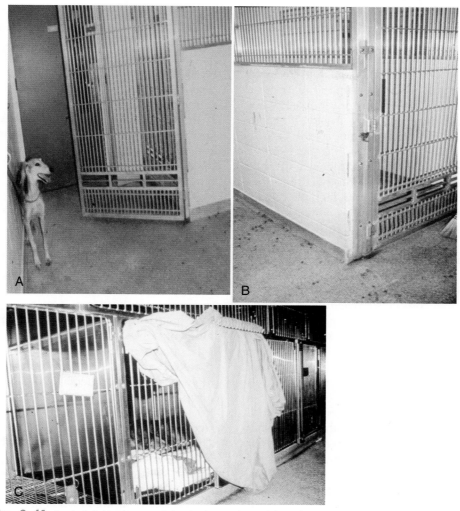

Fig. 3-41 **A,** A Saluki who panicked when placed in a large, open run with a window. **B,** The blood on the walls of the run is due to the escape behaviors that resulted in ripped toenails of the dog in **A. C,** The dog from **A** in a small, low cage covered with a sheet.

ripped out toenails (Fig. 3-41, *B*) trying to escape the run. Minutes later, when this dog was placed in small, floor-level cage with a sheet providing a darkened environment, she calmed. Open spaces are terrifying for this dog.

Finally, no one should believe that dogs who are crated will behave the same whether or not they are in the crate. Figure 3-42 shows a dog who is profoundly aggressive in a frenzied manner whenever anyone approaches the cage. When removed from his cage he was concerned, hiding behind his person. This fearfully aggressive dog had no choice but frank and profound aggression when he could not remove himself from the stimulus (us) that he found so distressing. This photo is an object lesson in how we are obligated not to render our patients worse and not to cause them to suffer by containment and other tools designed to "help" them.

Gates help separate dogs—and some cats—who live in the same household. Sometimes separation can

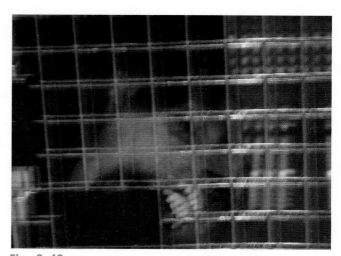

Fig. 3-42 A fearfully aggressive dog in a small crate. His only option when approached was to attack the door of the crate. He is so frenzied that the entire crate bounces around. Truly fearful dogs are trapped when they cannot escape, reducing their choices to attack or freeze.

prevent problems that may be developing. Dogs who fight over certain toys or treats (e.g., rawhides) may be able to enjoy them separately when separated by a gate. Dogs who eat at vastly different rates can be accommodated by a gate that allows the slow eater to remain part of the social system but at the same time protects her and her food from the dog who would force her out of the way and steal her food. No aggression needs to occur to engender a problem behavior that can be helped by gates.

Dogs who are aggressive to each other usually, but not always, continue to threaten each other through a gate because they can see each other. In fact, the threats usually escalate because they can: there is no physical "cost" to threatening the other dog. Figure 3-43 shows the exception to this rule. Here, the dog contained by the gate, who is blind, is aggressive to most other dogs. The gate works for her because she doesn't see the other dogs well enough to threaten them, but they see the gate and know that she cannot reach them, so they can live amenably together. In fact, the puppy, who has never been together with the incarcerated dog, is slowly managing to steal one of her favorite toys.

For many cats and dogs, the sane choice is a true barrier (e.g., a door) that is locked with a key (left hanging on a nearby peg in case of emergency), a sliding bolt, or a hook and eye. Bolts and hooks and eyes should be placed at the very top of the door so that no one who is casually thinking of opening the door can easily do so, and no small children can open the door. If the patient can threaten another pet or human through a gate or window, a solid door is needed to contain the patient. Dogs and cats can both time and space share. If the pet poses a risk to certain humans or animals, when those are present, the pet is behind a locked door. If two pets are equally fierce in depriving the other of his or her right to exist, they can share the rest of the family by having a rota where one is sequestered while the other is out. This type of plan works best if each pet has his or her "own" room. Scent is one of the currencies of communication for dogs and cats. If the animals are adversaries, they will not wish to sleep on bedding smelling of the other pet. Humans could be sharing these rooms, but the plan should be to contain one pet before releasing the other for group family time.

Visual and Auditory Barriers

For some animals, their overall arousal level will drop if their visual, auditory, or olfactory perception is changed. Dogs who worry about lightning storms may do well with an eye mask (Fig. 3-44), Doggles (Fig. 3-45) (www.doggles.com), or Calming Caps (Fig. 3-46). Dogs who have difficulty with sounds may benefit from ear plugs or noise-canceling headphones. Mutt Muffs (Fig. 3-47) (www.muttmuffs.com) are made especially to protect canine hearing and damp sensory exposure in high-noise environments. Dogs who can engage in normal, favored behaviors (see Fig. 3-44) are benefiting from the use of these devices. Although not tested in a rigorous scientific manner, some music for dogs (e.g., Through a Dog's Ear, www.throughadogsear.com; Pet Music, www.petmusic.com) may mask worrisome sounds and/or provide a calming environment for the dog with little risk of side effects.

Many people are curious about CDs that will help "desensitize" dogs to the sounds of storms. By the time dogs are truly phobic of storms, humane care involves medication and behavior modification. It is unlikely that any exposure to a CD will be helpful until their treatment has progressed, if then. CDs of storms may not be sufficiently realistic or target the specific triggers

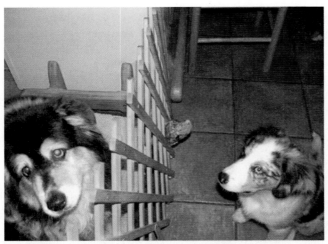

Fig. 3-43 A gate being used to contain a dog who is aggressive to other dogs in the household (Tess, the black dog on left). This works because she is blind and so does not threaten dogs on the other side of the gate. The other dogs know this and are calm. In fact, Toby, the puppy on the right side of the gate, is slowly stealing the blind dog's favorite toy: a chicken that is being squeezed through the gate.

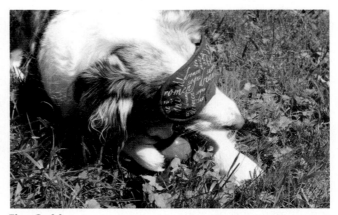

Fig. 3-44 A simple eye mask can be fitted well and comfortably. Linus' mask blocks some visual stimuli, but doesn't interfere with preferred activities.

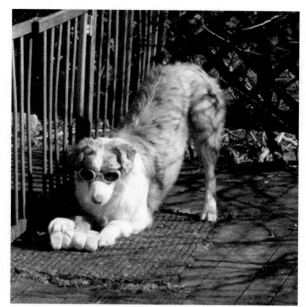

Fig. 3-45 Doggles that are fitted well do not interfere with the dog's preferred activities.

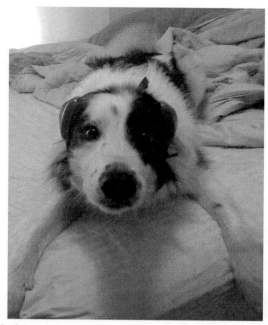

Fig. 3-47 Mutt Muffs on a noise and storm phobic dog. (Photo courtesy of Angelica Steinker.)

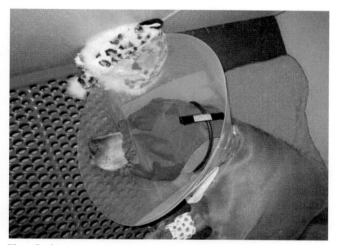

Fig. 3-46 A Calming Cap placed on a dog recovering from anesthesia to reduce the amount of ambient and reflective light to which the dog is exposed. Not all dogs are good candidates for these if they worry about anything being placed over their heads. The cap will be removed when the dog is awake, so it's essential that it can be removed without distress or risk.

that cause that individual dog to react. The best use of such CDs is likely as the dog is beginning to show signs of being concerned about noise. Such exposure must conform to the rules of learning theory, as discussed earlier.

Remote Devices—Mousetraps to Scat Mats

Most remote devices are considered remote punishers. All remote shock (collars, boundary devices, and Scat Mats) devices are aversive. Whether they actually meet the criteria for true "positive punishment" is debatable because the usual response to experiencing such stimuli is to avoid the stimulus but otherwise engage in the behavior. Cats whose sofas are covered with Scat Mats, which shock anyone touching them, instead choose to sleep in locations not covered by Scat Mats. To ensure the cat slept on no furniture, each piece would require its own device.

Even when well timed to interrupt the pet's behavior because the trigger stimulus is the pet's behavior, as is true for citronella collars to stop barking, whether the dog ceases to bark depends on *his or her reasons for doing so.* Distressed dogs just become more distressed when sprayed in the face because now they are being further stimulated and surprised. Very confident dogs learn to bark loudly and quickly to empty the citronella chamber because they can: any dog can learn to tell by weight how much liquid is left. Some dogs have adverse skin or respiratory reactions to scented sprays, and some dogs panic when their face is sprayed. The disruptive stimulus is actually the "psst" sound that the sprayer makes, but even this could cause fearful dogs to become more fearful (Moffat et al., 2003). When fitted with these types of remote bark collars, most dogs learn to bark below the level that triggers such collars, rendering their utility limited at best if the intent was to teach the dog to stop barking. Dogs bark for rational reasons. Understanding these reasons is far more important and a far superior approach to attempting to suppress the bark.

Remote Devices That Can Positively Reward Pets

True Operant Conditioning Machines

The remote devices about which there is too little discussion are the remote reward systems, such as the Manners Minder. Thanks to a series of programmable settings based in sound learning theory, auditory signals cue the dogs that if they move away from whatever is stimulating them (the door), rewards will be dispensed in a way that positively reinforces nonreactive behaviors (Fig. 3-48).

Feeding Puzzles and Toys (Including Kong Time)

Dogs and cats can now acquire huge numbers of calories quickly and for almost no effort. Most pets in the United States are overweight. Food puzzles and toys provide physical and mental exercise and are wonderful for most pets. Anything that helps animals to move around, aids them in eating more slowly, and encourages them to think about food is a good idea.

Figures 3-49 and 3-50 show examples of food toys that dispense kibble or dried treats. Both of these toys can be adjusted to make getting the food relatively easier or harder. Numerous companies are making such toys, so toys should be chosen with the pet's needs, durability, safety, and ease of cleaning in mind. Biscuits, which are usually calorically dense and quickly eaten, can be placed in toys specifically designed to slow their consumption while encouraging high effort manipulation. The Big Kahuna Biscuit Bouncer (Figs. 3-51 and 3-52) comes in two hardnesses (black is harder) and multiple sizes, and it can be washed in the dishwasher. Stuck biscuits can be removed with a bottle brush or chopstick.

As part of their evolutionary history, cats have always eaten many small meals a day. In contrast to dogs who can and will hunt cooperatively to kill and share larger prey, domesticated cats hunt primarily alone and so focus on smaller prey. Catching and handling enough food historically has taken more than the

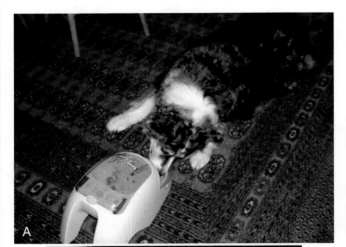

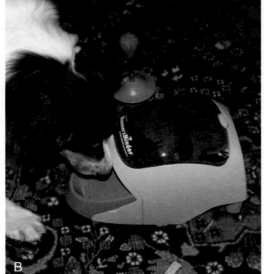

Fig. 3-48 A, A dog lying down to receive treats from a remote positive reinforcement device. The original version of this was called Treat and Train and needed a power outlet. **B,** The newer version is battery operated and renamed Manners Minder (modeled here by Picasso). Both devices have the same excellent learning programs developed by Dr. Sophia Yin.

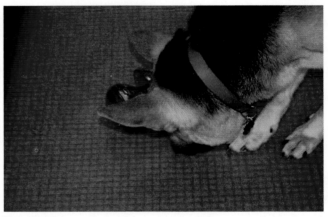

Fig. 3-49 A mushroom-shaped, wobbly food dispensing toy.

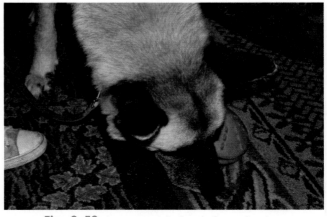

Fig. 3-50 A saucer-style food dispensing toy.

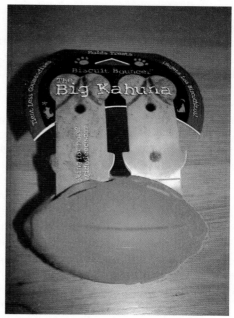

Fig. 3-51 The Big Kahuna toy specifically for biscuits.

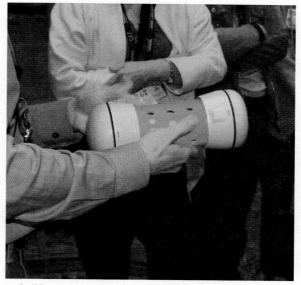

Fig. 3-53 The Pipolino cat food dispensing device has a center chamber whose holes can be adjusted for different sizes and shapes of kibble and for different ease of release. The design allows the device to roll and dispense dry food when batted.

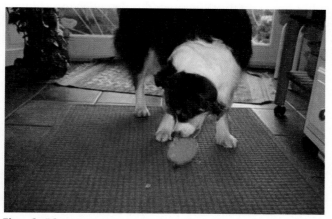

Fig. 3-52 A very energetic, always hungry Australian shepherd is seriously slowed in his biscuit consumption through use of the Big Kahuna. As a result, fewer biscuits last longer, and he gets considerable physical and mental exercise throughout at least part of the day.

5 minutes it takes them to eat a bowl of prepared food. As a result, the average pet cat is getting a full day's worth of calories in minutes and without any physical and mental stimulation. This is antithetical to what it means to be a cat. Toys like the Pipolino (www.pipolino.ca; www.pipolino.eu) (Fig. 3-53) have been developed to provide cats with mental and physical stimulation by mimicking actions that will trigger some of the hunting behaviors. For the Pipolino to dispense food, it must be batted and moved. Because the holes are adjustable, the task can be made harder for more forceful cats so that they have to work to get their food. While that sounds like an affront to all of "catdom," cats are happier,

healthier, and thinner when stimulated. Before cats are left to rely on such devices, clients need to ensure that the cats can physically use and behaviorally understand the device. Most learn how to use these toys quickly if no other food source is provided.

Food toys and puzzles, especially for cats, can be made for almost no cost. Small amounts of kibble can be left in paper muffin cups on three or four shelves of various book cases. Wine and beer often comes in segmented cartons. Dry kibble can be put in a few, but not all, of the partitioned holes. Wet food can be frozen and floated in a water dish. Small Kongs are perfect for freezing wet or a combined wet and dry food for cats. If the cat will eat only warm, moist food, this, too, can be placed in many of the food puzzle toys, the smallest size of which usually works for cats. If the cat goes outside in hot weather, she may enjoy a floating popsicle of cooked chicken or chicken liver frozen in its own broth. Dogs love such treats, and they cost almost nothing in time or money to make.

For dogs who may be home for extended periods alone, their meals can be provided by Kongs that are released at pre-determined times (Fig. 3-54). This type of delivery system is best for food that cannot spoil, but for some clients with long working hours, this type of device can be a great choice. Three cautions are warranted:

- These machines should not be placed on high tables because the filled Kongs are heavy and could hit and injure the dog who is waiting for them.
- Contrary to what the box says, *this is not and should not be viewed as "daycare in a box."* No one should

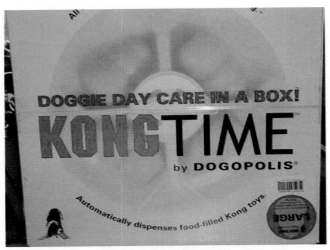

Fig. 3-54 An automated device that delivers filled Kongs at pre-determined times.

substitute food for true daycare, and if this is the intent in using this device, the clients need to find competent daycare.

- No one should assume that food toys will "ease the signs of separation anxiety/distress." In fact, truly distressed dogs cannot eat. Such toys can be used as *diagnostics for the condition* (they will be untouched when the client returns home) and may be used as *markers of when the dog begins to improve* when given competent treatment (the food will begin to be eaten when the client is gone). *No one should assume that treating any pathological anxiety is as simple as providing food.* To do so is to do the dog or cat a disservice.

Fences and Invisible Fences

Standard Fences

Dogs and cats with behavioral concerns should never be left alone outside, supervised. Unless there is a solid fence in place, most of these animals should never be left unrestrained by a lead and harness/head collar. This is for both their protection and the protection of others. Dogs and cats with behavioral concerns are at risk from people acting in ways that are unpredictable and that may seem unpredictable to them, and should something untoward occur, it is always the dog who will be "blamed." The first step in helping distressed animals is to avoid provocative situations.

Dogs who are aggressive for any reason should always be closely supervised. The only type of fence that can be used for them is one that is real and not flimsy.

- If the fence is post and rail, it must be lined with chicken wire or some type of grid.
- If it has spaces, they must be small enough to prevent the dog from reaching through it and grabbing someone.

- If the fence borders a busy area, the dog must be both supervised and leashed so that the dog's behaviors do not worsen because of the constant stimulation.
- If the fence borders a truly busy area, the clients should consider a second fence that provides a buffer zone between the fence for the dog and the fence for the property. Dogs who scare or injure people— whether or not the person was complicit—often do not get a second chance. Although breed-specific legislation (BSL) is unfair, unfounded, and unhelpful for preventing dog bites, dogs of certain breeds will be more harshly judged than others. The BSL debate has only served to make people more reactive about dogs.

The simplest way of keeping dogs safe and sane is to protect them. This may mean that dogs with problems do not get to chase balls unimpeded in their yard, but it does mean they will live long enough to remember chasing balls when they were young.

Dogs should not be left alone, outside, contained by fences for safety reasons. They should also not be left in these circumstances because these circumstances do not meet the dog's cognitive, social, and exercise needs. In one activity budget study of 55 Labrador retrievers living in Australia, videotaped data collection showed that during the daylight hours these dogs spent 74% of their time being inactive, whereas during the night hours they spent 95% of their time being inactive (Kobelt et al., 2007). The amount of time these dogs spent near the door or checking the door was also not trivial. Locking the dogs in the yard did not provide them with the exercise they needed. The dogs studied got almost no exercise, even if they had a canine companion. The bulk of their exercise occurred *only* when a human emerged from the house, and it was also only then that those dogs who had canine companions played with their companions. The human and canine interaction so needed by the dogs—their stimulation— was functionally impeded by containing them in the yard.

Live Wire Fences

Live wire fences for dogs and cats are terrible ideas because they will be well avoided by those they seek to contain but place all other neighboring cats, dogs, and humans at risk. Any dog who leaves the property to roam will learn to go around or over a live wire fence in a way that was not injurious to them. Whether they would work that hard to return is debatable because the association they would now make about the periphery of their home is that it is a risky place for them.

Invisible/Static Shock/Electric/Electronic/ Radio Fences

Invisible/electric/static shock fences are *not* substitutes for solid, visible, and functional fences. The only dogs for whom these are suitable are dogs who don't need a fence anyway.

Invisible/static shock fences are designed so that an auditory signal alerts the dog (or—and we should be appalled—the cat) that he is approaching the fence wire—which he cannot see—where he will be shocked. The intended response is targeted avoidance response. There are numerous problems with this situation.

- If the reward on the other side of the fence is sufficiently great or beneficial, the dogs will learn to run through the fence quickly to leave. They will learn not to cross it to return. If freedom, the chance to explore, horse manure, a neighbor's dog, et cetera, were the stimuli for leaving, they are obviously not present at home, and so returning is not a "reward" worth the "cost." There are numerous reported incidents where dogs leave home but wait just outside the boundary for the fence to be turned off before coming back onto the property.
- If people drag the dogs across the boundary where they will be shocked to bring them home, they will associate *that action* with the shock. There are cases of bites to humans that have occurred only in this circumstance. One could argue that such bites are justified because the human is hurting and scaring the dog. Certainly the dog now has reason not to trust the human.
- If the fence is sufficiently close to the road/sidewalk and a known human or dog is passing, the dog may cross the boundary to meet them. Because the person may be in the shock zone the dog remains in it and is repeatedly shocked. There are a number of reports where dogs with no history of aggression have bitten in this situation (Polsky, 2000).
- A real fence provides real protection against marauding humans and neighborhood dogs: an invisible fence provides no such protection. In fact, dogs left inside invisible fences are excellent victims for predators, unkind humans, and dangerous dogs.
- If the dog has any aggressive or protective tendencies, any fence makes the dog more reactive—not less reactive. Invisible fences are exactly that—invisible to humans and dogs. An innocent human could cross into the area that the dog is now patrolling simply because they did not know the fence was there. There are numerous reports of human injury under exactly these circumstances. The human would never behave in the same manner with a real fence, avoiding injury by the dog.
- For the neurochemical reasons discussed in the section on shock that follows, shock will change the dog's behavior for the worse and will stop more behaviors than just straying. It's a myth that invisible fences provide dogs with more freedom. In fact, these devices violate the principles of three of five freedoms that define adequate welfare for animals:
  - Freedom from pain, injury, and disease
  - Freedom to express normal behavior
  - Freedom from fear and distress

Tie-outs and Chains

Tie-outs and chains are now being increasingly prohibited by law. Dogs who are tied, regardless of modality, get less exercise than freely moving dogs, are more at risk from abuse from humans and interference from and attacks by other animals, and become more reactive than dogs who are not tied. Dogs who are tied/chained are over-represented in dog bite statistics, where co-variantes in the United States include lack of a dog license and lack of proof of rabies vaccination (Overall and Love, 2001), suggesting that tying a dog may be one sign of irresponsible ownership. The use of tie-outs and chains is antithetical to meeting the dog's welfare needs.

Containment Fences and Habitats for Cats

In an attempt to meet cats' needs for more intellectual and physical stimulation, while also meeting the concerns of wildlife and neighbors with gardens, a number of companies are now making "cat fences" or cat containment habitats (www.purrfectfence.com, www.catfencein.com, www.catterydesign.com). Some fencing merely stops cats from leaving the property; some fence designs protect gardens and prey from the cats. All of these enrich the cat's world humanely, by keeping them safe while allowing them to explore.

NON-TREATMENTS: TOOLS THAT DO NOT WORK AND TOOLS THAT HURT

Removal of Body Parts

Tooth Removal

Animals whose teeth have been removed can still do damage. Occasionally, they will stop biting (Houpt, 1991), but this appears to be the result of a less worried response by clients that alters the underlying cycle. Large dogs have powerful jaws. It would be a mistake to believe that because a dog is without teeth he has been rendered "safe" and can no longer cause injury. Many countries have outlawed this procedure, and it is moving toward restriction in the United States.

Limb or Tail Removals

If animals are mutilating a body part, removal of the "offending" part, unless it is severely necrotic, is unlikely to help in the treatment of the problem. The problem is not local; it is global, and unless the neurochemical ramifications of the problem (e.g., the anxiety) are treated, the problem will not resolve. The animal will just chew more proximal parts. Many countries (but not the United States) prohibit the removal of any body part unless it is necessary for the good and well-being of the animal, an approach that is sane, humane, and limiting.

"De-barking"

Cutting or crushing of the vocal cords ("de-barking") has often been used to decrease kennel noise and/or to decrease the noise made by certain breeds. This is a painful, injurious procedure that may compromise the dog behaviorally and medically. Anyone who has heard wolves, coyotes, or foxes in the wild or who has seen a single movie, video, or television show featuring any of these animals must be struck by how quiet they are compared with the domestic dog. Whether we selected for such enhanced canid vocal behaviors directly (e.g., as for hounds) or, similar to additional estrous cycles in Belayev's "domestic" foxes (Trut, 2001), these behaviors were the result of co-variant traits, no one should doubt that such enhanced vocal behaviors in dogs are the result of human choice. As such, breed-associated behavioral traits should inform potential adopters as to the behavioral profile needs of the dog, and breeders should ensure that this is the case. Surgical mutilation is not a solution for poorly informed humans. "De-barking" is increasingly frowned on and is moving toward illegality in the United States.

Immersion

Whether the patient is a cat or a dog, no matter how much clients wish for this to be the case, troubled animals don't just "get over it" or "grow out of it." Because clients sometimes believe these events could happen, they will continue to expose animals to situations that the cat or dog finds distressing without realizing that what they are doing is "flooding" the patient. As noted earlier in this chapter, *flooding almost without exception renders dogs and cats with problematic behaviors worse because they cannot escape the stimulus that they find the most provocative.* As a result, not only do their original problems worsen, but also the patients may become more reactive in different ways.

The most common way in which cats are flooded is one where the client assumes that cats are fussy and that they will not understand them, so the client leaves the cats to sort out their relationships on their own. Whether this scenario involves the introduction of a new cat or cats or ongoing household relationships, clients who think that the cats will work it out are not monitoring the cats' behaviors, largely because of this mistaken belief. Care should be taken by the veterinary team to learn how well clients watch cats, what they actually know about feline behaviors, how much they understand of *the cat's perspective of events* (crawling around at cat height can be informative), and how they would assay or recognize problems. This approach involves true anticipatory guidance for one of the most common pet species for whom behavioral and welfare needs are often not met: cats.

One underappreciated example of flooding is seen in "dog parks." Clients who have dogs who are fearful of or reactive to another dog often think that if they take the dog to the dog park the dog will learn to be less fearful or reactive either by watching the other dogs or by interacting with them. In fact, there is a growing body of data that suggests dogs at dog parks may be disproportionately reactive.

Even when those surveyed express satisfaction about dog parks, recommendations include separate play areas for large and small dogs, separate areas for different types of play, including free play, and recognition of the fact that safety issues exist and that dogs' behaviors should be monitored for appropriateness (Lee et al., 2009 [this reference also contains a number of creative plans of parks for those wishing to create them]; Shyan et al., 2003). That so many clients are unsure of what constitutes appropriate behavior is a concern.

If clients wish to make use of dog parks, which can be a fabulous addition to communities, they should ask why other dogs and people are there. If the answer hints at the dog having a behavior problem, caution is urged. People who decide to take their dog to a park to "expose" him to other dogs should realize that they will meet others with the same goals and will now have to contend with two problem dogs. This is not unlike the situation where people with aggressive dogs only walk their dogs at 5 AM and 1 AM. Unfortunately, they are likely to meet others who also have difficult dogs at these times.

Dog parks are not a treatment for behavior problems. However, the appropriate use of dog parks can contribute to the well-being of dogs and their people in well-managed situations. Some guidelines follow.

- Clients should attend the park without their dogs the first time. They should talk to the people, meet the other dogs, learn about schedules, and learn about how well people police their own dogs. If feces are left in the open without appropriate disposal, this may portend a group that either has few appropriate guidelines or is lacking or absent in their reinforcement.
- Clients should be open about their dog's needs and flexible in scheduling time. Some parks have fenced, lockable runs for dogs who are aggressive to other dogs and assigned times that ensure these dogs can run free but do so safely for everyone.
- Dogs with behavior problems can benefit from dog parks if their activities are restricted and carefully monitored. The views of the other users of the park must matter. Open dialogue is essential.
- Clients should feel comfortable videotaping the dogs interacting so that they can take that video to their veterinarians and other professionals for a discussion of which behaviors are appropriate and which worrisome.
- If clients are using parks to expose their dogs to either people or other dogs, they must be doing so

as part of a treatment plan overseen by a professional and with full disclosure. Many people with normal dogs will be willing to help people with worried dogs. Many people with worried dogs will have the same questions that the client has. Many visitors to dog parks may think their dog is "normal," and instead that dog is concerned. *However, immersion itself is not a treatment.*

- *Finally, clients should be encouraged at every opportunity to consider the source of information about their dog's behavior.* Dog parks can be ideal places for folklore and inappropriate/wrong information exchange. Clients must understand this, and having a veterinary team who can share actual data and scientific rationale increases the chances that valid information exchange will occur.

Many pet supply stores allow/encourage clients to bring their dogs to the store. Unfortunately, this is often an opportunity for another inappropriate immersion experience for dogs with behavior problems. Clients should be appropriately cautioned because pet supply stores pose risks that may not be present in most other environments.

- Food treats, such as rawhides, are often in open bins in pet supply stores and may provoke aggression in dogs who care very much about or protect some food items.
- Shelves are heavily stocked and high in most pet supply stores, impeding visual assessment of who is approaching. The risk of a person or a dog suddenly appearing in the dog's visual field or next to the dog is high.
- Pet supply stores often have relatively crowded aisles meaning that dogs are always within their inter-personal approach distance of 1 to 1.5 body lengths.
- Pet supply stores may be noisy, and if they include grooming or adoption facilities, they may also house animals who are distressed.
- Pet supply stores often hire people without training who will not recognize when an animal is distressed and so at risk. This means that they may interact inappropriately with a dog who is concerned.
- Other people with dogs may not recognize when a dog is distressed or at risk. This means that they may interact inappropriately with a dog who is concerned.
- Worried dogs cannot easily escape or back away from unwanted interactions in pet supply stores.

Some pet supply stores may have staff who are willing to help with exposure programs that are being conducted under the guidance of veterinary or other professionals, but for this to work, the person overseeing the program needs to be involved in the orchestration of exposures. When these needs are met, pet supply stores cease to be bastions of immersion and flooding and can be useful resources for the implementation of DS and CC.

Shock

To understand people's willingness to shock their dogs and cats (and sometimes horses), one important association needs to be acknowledged: *people reach for tools such as shock when they feel helpless to address their pet's behavioral concerns and when they feel that this is the only way that they can keep their pet safe and alive.*

Unfortunately, companies that make and market shock collars prey on these concerns, claiming that their products keep pets safe and save lives. There is *no* published evidence to support these claims, but there is now considerable evidence published in the peer-reviewed literature that refutes them.

Anyone considering the use of shock for behavioral problems—whether it is a remote/bark activated shock collar, a remote controlled collar, an invisible fence, or a device such as a Scat Mat that shocks anyone who touches it—should know:

1. The use of shock is not treatment for pets with behavioral concerns.
2. The use of shock is not a way forward.
3. The use of shock does not bring dogs back from the brink of euthanasia; instead, it may send them there.
4. Such adversarial techniques have negative consequences that are dismissed/ignored by those promoting these techniques.

We have known for decades that aversive stimuli such as shock work to teach avoidance and cessation of behavior. In the extreme form, this cessation of behavior is called "immobility." It is this criterion of "immobility" by which learned helplessness is accessed (Seligman, 1971).

Few people appear to understand that *cessation of behaviors may not be a hallmark of "improved behavior,"* especially when the welfare of the animal is considered (Mendl, 1999). When animals experience a shock and exhibit cessation of behavior, they cease *all* behaviors that they associate with the experience, including good, calm, and normal behavior. Exposure to uncontrollable shock has been shown to affect a range of factors including social interactions. Rodents exposed to shock that they cannot control or escape show lower social interaction and investigation, and exhibit alterations in interactive behaviors seen in social defeat situations (Amat et al., 2010). Such findings have important implications for dogs and cats subjected to shock.

This unfortunate and unpublicized sequela has been demonstrated by Schilder and van der Borg (2004) using guard dog–trained German shepherd dogs. Dogs who were shocked in training, but not when the evaluations were made (which may have been years later), showed a lower ear posture in free walking and more stress-related behaviors than dogs who had never been shocked in training. These differences were also found when the dogs participated in obedience training and manwork/protection training and work.

In addition to the noted behavioral responses associated with stress and distress found in dogs that had been trained with shock, the researchers found that the behavioral differences were most profound when the person associated with the shock (the owner or handler) was present. These data supported findings from a previous study (Beerda et al., 1997), which also documented alterations in the HPA axis in dogs that were shocked compared with dogs experiencing no shock. Schilder and van der Borg concluded that:

1. This type of training, in general, is stressful.
2. Receiving shocks is painful for the dogs.
3. The dogs learn a context-dependent concern—the presence of the handler and his or her commands announces the reception of shocks.

It is important to note that despite these differences, these dogs all continued to work, meaning that even superstar dogs are adversely affected by the use of electrical shock in training. Most of the dogs and cats subjected to such aversive techniques are not superstars and have not been selected to withstand the amounts of rough handling and tough situations for which police dogs are selected. If superstar working dogs suffer, pet dogs and cats will suffer worse.

Schalke et al. (2007) evaluated the use of remote shock when used to stop dogs from touching a rabbit dummy in a group of naïve laboratory dogs chosen for their shared derivative and husbandry history. Three partially randomized treatment groups were evaluated: dogs that responded to receipt of shock immediately and only when touching the dummy (treatment group—aversion and/or avoidance), dogs that did not respond to a recall command about "hunting" the dummy (treatment group—here), and dogs under conditions in which the shock was delivered unpredictably and out of context (treatment group—random). Dogs in all treatment groups experienced cortisol increases associated with shock compared with baseline values. In the context in which the timing was immediate (treatment group—aversion and/or avoidance), the stimulus clear (rabbit dummy), and the behavior discrete and unambiguous (touching the rabbit dummy), the increase was least in both relative and absolute terms. The increase in cortisol was the highest for dogs in the random group by more than an order of magnitude compared with the contextually clear aversion and/or avoidance group.

With respect to behavior, context is everything. When one considers the constraints of the controlled and measurable methodology under which trained scientists collected these data, one cannot be surprised at the discussion in the final paragraphs, which can leave no room for misinterpretation. The authors state: "The results of this study suggest that poor timing in the

application of high level electric pulses, such as those used in this study, means there is a high risk that dogs will show severe and persistent stress symptoms. We recommend that the use of these devices should be restricted with proof of theoretical and practical qualification required and then the use of these devices should only be allowed in strictly specified situations" (Schalke et al., 2007, page 379). These data and conclusions are borne out in Figures 3-55 through 3-57.

Simply, shock will not help the animals to exhibit behaviors that would be safer, happier, and preferred and could do them serious neurochemical and

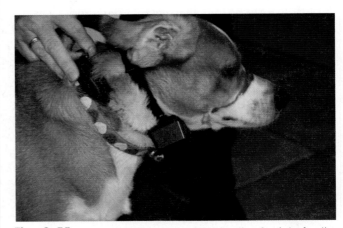

Fig. 3-55 A beagle who was seized by the Society for the Prevention of Cruelty to Animals (SPCA) as part of a successfully prosecuted abuse case, with the shock collar he was wearing when seized. There is scar tissue under the prongs of the shock collar. The scar tissue and lesions across the dog's nose and by the sides of his mouth are due to skin sloughs associated with the use of a Gentle Leader Canine Head Collar that was fitted too tightly so that he could not open his mouth (see also Fig. 3-56). The intent of both the shock collar and the head collar was to stop this dog from barking. The scar tissue at the side of the mouth (see also Fig. 3-56) appears to be due to self-trauma when the dog tried to remove the head collar. These photos were taken 2 months after the dog was seized, at which point his skin had healed to the extent possible, his hair had re-grown, and he had gained some much needed weight (and then some).

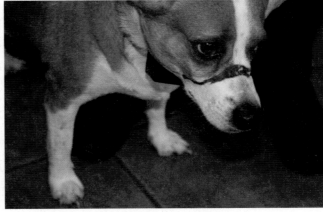

Fig. 3-56 Healed skin slough after inappropriate use of a head collar.

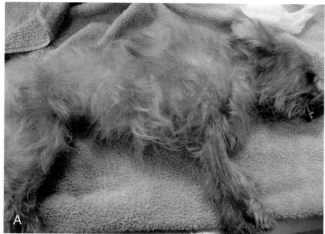

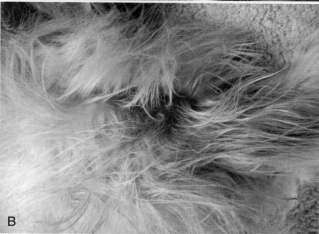

Fig. 3-57 A, A dog who died apparently after being electrocuted by a shock collar. The collar had been recently fitted to the dog to control the dog's barking. The clients arrived home to find that the dog had hemorrhaged, with blood pooling from the nose and throat. The dog was dead on arrival at the veterinarian's where these photos were taken. The dog has been washed to show the bruising of skin, which along with extreme muscle contraction and respiratory and cardiac paralysis, is characteristic of electrocution (Drobbie, 1973; Green et al., 1972). One area of cutaneous hemorrhage is shown in **B,** The clients declined a forensic necropsy because they were heartbroken and not interested in litigation.

behavioral harm. Companies that make devices that shock (the vast majority of them worldwide are now made by Radio Systems Corporation [RCS], the parent company of PetSafe products and Premier Pet Products) use wording that appears to underplay mechanism and risk when marketing and describing their products. The ScatMat "emits a mild, harmless static pulse when touched" (www.petsafe.net/products/pet-proofing; accessed June 21, 2011). "PetSafe ScatMat trains pets to stay away from areas where you don't want them by giving them a harmless little static shock. These Scat Mats have three levels of intensity that you can adjust for varying animal sizes or stubbornness" (www.safepetproducts.com/scat-mat-for-cats-and-dogs.html; accessed June 21, 2011).

Numerous videos are available on YouTube that show the adverse effects of these devices on dogs and cats (and humans) (regardless of the uninformed comments that may accompany the videos). These adverse effects are the reason that the use of electronic shock with dogs and cats is illegal in some states in Australia, all of Wales, and a growing number of other countries, regions, and municipalities.

In my patient population, dogs who have experienced the use of shock collars in an attempt to treat their aggressive behaviors before the consultation are at increased risk for euthanasia compared with dogs with similar conditions who have not been shocked. *The use of shock in the treatment of behavioral conditions is abusive, is doomed to fail, and will make situations less, not more, safe and reliable.*

For the time and money anyone would invest in any shock-producing product, their efforts and currency would be better spent hiring a competent, certified, humane dog trainer and/or a specialist in veterinary medicine. Members of the veterinary profession should be appalled that many online sites advertising products that use shock claim that they are "veterinarian approved." Were the pet food or pharmacological companies to produce and market a product like the family of devices that deliver shock and make the claims that these products make, the U.S. Food and Drug Administration would require data that detailed the range of responses of dogs or cats using the devices with respect to breed, circumstantial variation in response, epidemiology, and outcome. Companies making and marketing shock products appear to have managed to convince people who should know better to recommend as treatment interventions unproven solutions *that have been documented to cause harm.* No drug would be licensed if it produced the results that the peer-reviewed articles pertaining to shock have reported.

Although neither behavior nor welfare for companion animals is taught at most veterinary schools worldwide, veterinarians should value their reputations more than to allow any company to tarnish them for profit that comes at the expense of their patients.

Euthanasia

Euthanasia is not a *treatment* option. Euthanasia is the outcome of failed anticipatory guidance and failed, inadequate, or incomplete treatment interventions.

Pets are no longer considered disposable in most of the industrial world. If veterinary medicine and veterinarians wish to achieve their full potential, dogs and cats with behavior problems or about whom clients have concerns/complaints cannot be considered disposable. The best time for veterinarians to invest in ensuring that they euthanize their patients *only for humane relief* is the time when veterinarians spend the *least* amount of time with the patient: *before* the dog or cat exhibits any behavioral problems.

If veterinarians trained their staff in educating clients about normal behavior and common age-related behavioral concerns, vets would start a dialogue that would allow people to seek help at the first—not last—sign of any behavioral concern. For this to happen, veterinarians need to invest in education for all members of their staff, including the reception, kennel, and nursing staff. Suggestions can be found in Chapter 1. *If veterinarians make this investment, euthanasias and relinquishments because of behavioral concerns will become rare, and clients will be held to a greater standard of responsibility.* In a study of client and veterinary attitudes about whether behavior problems affected adoptability from a shelter, only serious behavioral problems were considered to render dogs and cats unadoptable (Murphy et al., 2013). *With behavioral concerns, worsening is a matter of time left untreated and repeated practice of problematic or pathological behaviors.* Only the truly exceptional behavioral concern appears suddenly and full blown. With early screening and intervention, behavior problems will not worsen and euthanasia and relinquishment rates should drop.

There are some cases where euthanasia may be the only acceptable outcome, but these are rare, and they all focus on safety. There are dogs and cats who pose such a danger to others in the environment—both humans and other animals—that it is impossible to keep them safely, unless one does so for a living. Sanctuaries for these animals exist, but they are rare and can protect only the exceptional animal. The key to addressing this heartbreaking situation, which also contributes to professional burnout, is to *address the behavioral concerns early* (Fig. 3-58). *None of these animals, even those with neurological reasons for aggression, showed that level of aggression consistently throughout their life or no one would have chosen to live with them.*

There are some profoundly abnormal and aggressive puppies. Because these pups may never have experienced "normal" behaviors, every intervention possible, including medication, must be used as early as possible in the hopes of remodeling their neurons in a direction that benefits their neurochemistry. These puppies will always have some "special needs" aspects, but even these puppies can improve to the point where few would ever witness evidence of their early pathology. If the extent to which these puppies improve depends on the client, the same is true for dogs and cats who may have been more "normal" as youngsters. Treatment and prevention require ongoing, thorough history taking and follow-up by the veterinary staff and honest assessment of the client's needs and expectations. Clients' needs and expectations can change as a function of their knowledge, and the veterinary team should serve as a major resource to gain such knowledge.

Most behavior cases can improve to a level that the dog or cat is not a burden or risk and has an excellent

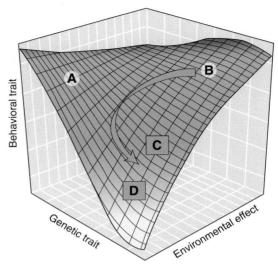

Fig. 3-58 The role for early intervention is clearly shown in a response surface diagram. Both *A* and *B* look "normal." Regardless of what happens environmentally, *A* copes, but *B* does not. *B* continues to worsen through *C* until reaching *D*. The drop to the worst behavior of *D* is precipitous, once it starts, but early on there is a lot of space to work between *B* and *C*. It is easier to return to *B* from *C* than from *D*, and it is harder to become worse if you are starting at *C* rather than *D*. If clients understand these downhill patterns, and if they believe that the veterinary team can provide helpful information, they will avail themselves of needed help. (From Overall, 2005.)

QoL. These dogs and cats can become truly happy. Because so much of this depends on environment, risk of euthanasia depends on environment. Veterinarians should always look for ways to minimize risk that can also benefit the dog or cat. *The only advocate for the patient's behavioral and physical needs is often the veterinarian.*

For dogs or cats who cannot stay in the home in which the problem is a concern, rehoming is possible *if the new home can meet the patient's needs.* The veterinarian is essential in helping the clients and any potential adopters understand what these needs are. *This means that veterinarians are the conduit to good, data-driven, evidence-based information about behavior and that they must be aware of their limitations.* There are now sufficient numbers of behavior specialists worldwide that veterinarians should always seek more input before deciding that euthanasia is the only choice. A list of international specialty groups is found in the handout, "Resources for Information, Tools, Books, Information, Products, and Other Help."

ROLES FOR MODELING GOOD AND NORMAL BEHAVIORS

Clients often ask if getting another dog or cat will "help." Studies on separation anxiety in dogs have shown no greater incidence of separation anxiety in households without another dog than in ones with one (King et al., 2000a). It is possible to have completely normal cats and dogs in households with cats and dogs who have true behavioral problems. Animals with behavioral problems will not spontaneously learn how not to have them by watching problem-free pets.

The situations in which another animal might help involve observational learning where having a normal animal from whom the patient is able to take their cues is helpful. Also, kittens and puppies learn appropriate behavior from older dogs and cats, and they may also learn how to learn.

The older dog in Figure 3-59 is teaching the puppy to play tug and letting the puppy set the pace. The puppy pictured exhibited the same behaviors to other puppies when he matured. There are no published data on any long-term benefits of learning to learn (but see Marshall-Pescini et al., 2008), but it may be more important than we know.

Humans can also take advantage of a dog who exhibits appropriate behaviors to encourage a puppy to learn these behaviors (Fig. 3-60). There are good experimental data suggesting that under some circumstances dogs are good at observational learning. In one well-designed, well-controlled study of working dogs, puppies who were offspring of working dog mothers and who were able to watch their mothers work had superior scores on later tests for training as a working dog than did puppies who did not watch their mothers or puppies who were born to non-working mothers, whether or not they could watch them (Slabbert and Rasa, 1997). Dogs can learn from watching humans exhibit successful problem-solving behaviors and from watching human cues (Miklósi et al., 2000; Pongrácz et al., 2001, 2003).

These findings should lead us to conclude that dogs may learn to display desired behaviors more quickly if they can watch another dog do so. However, in the case of a dog with behavioral problems, the patient needs to be sufficiently improved that they are ready and able to attend to the other dog and can benefit from observational learning. An example of this type of situation is shown in Figure 3-61 where a dog who has a history

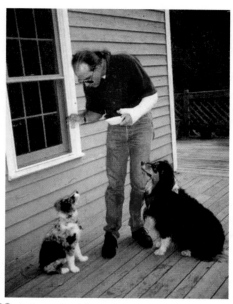

Fig. 3-60 A 9-week-old puppy, Emma, learning to sit for a food treat while an older dog, Tess, is present for her to use as a model. The older dog is also sitting in response to a request to do so and receiving treats.

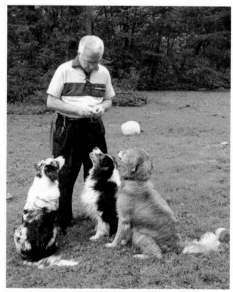

Fig. 3-61 The golden retriever in this photo, Austin, worries about other dogs and has never been able to play with them because he becomes too aggressive. The black Australian shepherd, Flash, is teaching him how to play with other dogs without becoming aggressive and is serving as a model for his behaviors. The golden retriever is rewarded when he mirrors the other dog's behaviors. The sub-adult, merle Aussie on the left, Toby, is also being rewarded for ignoring the golden retriever.

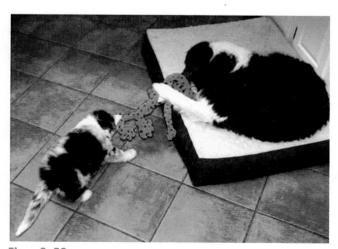

Fig. 3-59 An older dog, Flash, teaching a 9.5-week-old puppy, Toby, how to play tug. The puppy determined how hard he had to pull, and the older dog did not feel the need to acquire the toys. These are behaviors that are viewed, although they have not been tested, as hallmarks of normal play between mature adult dogs and puppies.

of aggression to other dogs (the golden retriever) is learning to model his behaviors on a dog who is completely contextually appropriate with other dogs (the black Australian shepherd). It is important to note that the model dog is not simply non-reactive: *he is completely appropriate*, which means he signals well to the golden retriever that he is no threat and he lets the golden retriever take toys from him without incident. The golden retriever is still not wholly comfortable, but whenever he growled or barked, the other dogs ignored him, later offering solicitous behaviors.

Dogs who read social situations well and fluently may also be excellent "mediator dogs," signaling clearly to clients when another dog is exhibiting behaviors that are a concern for social stability and that may put other dogs or humans at risk. Once clients know what to look for, they can often identify these "supra-normal" dogs who often interpose themselves between people or other dogs in ways that change interactions for the better. It's difficult to see these interactions in real time, but they are clear on video, again reinforcing that a video camera is an essential tool for people interested in behavior.

Dogs who have difficulty understanding and interpreting social situations may be able to take their cues from another, appropriate dog as is the case in Figure 3-62. The great Dane suffers from a number of anxiety-related conditions. The breeder noticed that he was less reactive and calmer whenever he was able to be with his sister. The client and breeder went together to a shelter to find a dog with behaviors similar to those of the sister, and the patient immediately began to take all of his cues from her, greatly improving his QoL.

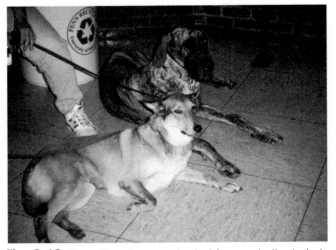

Fig. 3-62 The collie mix was adopted from a shelter to help the patient, the great Dane. The patient relies on his housemate to decide whether he needs to react to a social interaction. If she is calm, he is calm.

COGNITIVE THERAPY FOR ANIMALS

Roles for Fast Mapping, Strong Inference, and Data from Dogs

Research on the cognitive abilities of canines has begun to reach its stride (Hare and Tomasello, 1999; Hare et al., 1998, 2002; Miklósi et al., 2004). Kaminski et al. (2004) showed that dogs have the ability to "fast map." Fast mapping was originally defined as a cognitive process whereby a new concept is learned or a new hypothesis is formed based on a single exposure to some source of information. This concept of fast mapping has been most frequently applied to learning language.

Current thought tends toward a broader pattern for cognitive abilities and processes that allow animals (including humans) to use information in a probabilistic manner (e.g., if not this, then probably that), to include acquisition of a relation between a word and the object, activity, or thought process labeled by the word (the referent). The test for such a process is to learn whether the subject can infer a new word, or cognitive association for an activity, or a thought process, and retain this information in a format that allows recall and demonstration of function.

Kaminski et al. (2004) demonstrated that fast mapping of words occurred for a border collie named Rico. In both identification and retention trials, Rico was able to label and remember the label for a novel item in a manner significantly different than expected by chance, as demonstrated by repeatedly retrieving the one novel item in a group of eight items, for which the rest of the items were known. The process of fast mapping using referential thinking can be extended to specific classes of objects and activities, as demonstrated by Pilley and Reid (2011). Chaser, another border collie, has been shown to know the names of 1022 specific nouns and to identify items individually ("the big ball") and by class ("balls"), using specific referential sets of activities ("paw," "nose," and "take") (Pilley and Reid, 2011). The video can be found at http://dx.doi.org/10.1016/j.beproc.2010.11.007 (accessed February 25, 2013).

Such studies have been and continue to be replicated in other dogs and other animals. Type of previous exposure and experience (e.g., how and what one has learned and what the relationships are between those tested and testing) can affect outcomes. This is important to know if we are going to attain the level where "conditioned responses," "behavior modification," and "biofeedback for dogs" becomes "cognitive therapy."

- There is no doubt that dogs can learn that there are consequences. Conditioned responses and behavior modification are built on this premise.
- There is no doubt dogs can influence and attend to physiological correlates of their behaviors. This is

what allows biofeedback to work, and it is why being fearful facilitates learning associates of fear and increased fear at the molecular level.

- There is no doubt that dogs distinguish between events and experiences that make them feel good (chewing a bone, playing with a ball, being petted, swimming) and experiences that make them feel bad (avoiding a shock, leaving when someone starts to scream, hiding under a bed to escape being hit or bitten).

Accordingly, dogs should be able to link all of the above in a cognitive manner that allows them to decide to control their responses to certain circumstances, by choosing strategies that make them less reactive and calmer and happier. In this sense, if people work with their dogs as described here, there is no reason not to expect that couplings of dogs and humans who work best could not attain this level of "cognitive therapy."

A story will help illustrate this potential: Linus is a young male Australian shepherd. Linus' current family includes two adult humans and three other Aussies, one male 2.5 years older than he, one male 0.5 years older, and one female 8 years older. These dogs are all rescues. Linus was a puppy mill dog who was illegally sold by 6 weeks and relinquished to rescue by 7 weeks, from whence he came into his home.

Linus is undersized; when he was adopted he had no body fat, his ribs showed, and he was small. He did not respond to humans but interacted with other dogs fairly normally. The older male Aussie took responsibility for teaching Linus to play and about the environment and protecting him when needed. Linus did not respond to humans at all for the first 6 weeks he was in his new home. During this time, he was fed an enriched, high-protein puppy diet supplemented with large dosages of omega-3 fatty acids and other polyunsaturated fatty acids. Sometime during his seventh week in his new home (approximately >14 weeks of age), Linus began to respond to humans and progressed in his interactions with them rapidly.

Linus was worked with intensively using behavior modification and conditioning to teach him how to manage—without distress or reactivity—experiences and environments that scared him. By the time he was 4 years old, it would have been difficult for anyone to know he had had problems unless they watched him when he was in a stressful situation. As part of his conditioning to explore novel environments, he was taught to jump onto and run quickly back and forth on a segment of a very large trunk of a downed tree that was more than 20 meters in length. He was rewarded with food and praise, and using chaining he was taught to "jump on your log," "run the log," "turn," "up," "off," "over" (meaning to jump clearly over the log). When he became proficient, and anytime he did this thereafter, he was told he was "smart and brave."

Because of a series of storms and in the search for a wandering dog, Linus ended up off his property in a heavily wooded and treacherous preserve. To return to his property with the other dogs, it was necessary for him to walk across an angled thin tree that crossed a fast-moving stream and that had fallen on a fence over which he would then need to jump. The other dogs did this first in response to a verbal request to "go." When it came time for Linus to do this, he was scared and balked. He was asked to "jump on your log," as this was nothing more—conceptually—than his log trick—thinner, angled, over water, and with a jump at the end. He tried three times and each time did not move quickly enough not to fall. On his fourth try, as soon as he had traction he was told he was "smart and brave": he ran along the tree and cleared the fence. In this case, the phrase "smart and brave" marked a successful, happy outcome he could choose in response to the request to "jump on your log." This is cognitive therapy using fast mapping. See Figure 3-63 for the behavior that started the chain.

Dogs and cats are cognitive and social, and we have just begun to understand what that means for helping them recover from behavioral conditions. Good studies on how animals communicate about risk and learning with other animals are needed if we are to advance further.

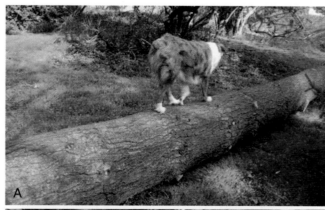

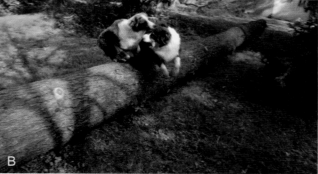

Fig. 3-63 A, Linus on his log, where he has been taught to walk and run back and forth for treats ("jump on your log"). **B,** Linus and Picasso responding to the request "over."

SUMMARY AND FINAL THOUGHTS ABOUT TREATMENT

Treatment of any behavioral problem is neither linear nor simple. All of the modalities used to treat behavioral concerns can also be used to prevent them, and we should emphasize this finding to our clients. Regardless, the following simple steps will work:

- avoid situations that distress the pet,
- avoid punishment,
- work with the dog or cat with some form of behavior modification (and possibly medication and/or diet change) to expand their choice of reactions, and
- renew the focus on rewarding these cats and dogs for every single behavior that is liked or favored.

No two animals with the same condition will be alike because they live in different environments and, in contrast to every other specialty in veterinary medicine, the social and physical environment can determine the extent to which a pet with any behavioral problem can improve. We now have more tools than ever to help these troubled pets and their distressed humans. The accompanying treatment protocols are designed to help the veterinary staff customize treatment plans, using clear and modern information, in a way that is meaningful, helpful, and humane to the clients and patients alike. A suggested pattern for developing discharge instructions and treatment plans for clients with troubled dogs and cats is presented in Box 3-10. This outline of topics to be covered and types of information that should be included can be adapted to any behavioral situation in a way that is helpful to the clients and will provide them clear information about treatment plans and outcome expectations.

BOX 3-10

Outline Approach for Structuring a Thought Process for Treatment of Dogs and Cats with Behavioral Concerns

1. Enumerate clients' chief complaints or concerns.
2. List observations by the veterinary team, and ask whether these observations match clients' concerns.
3. List any specific/special concerns of the veterinary team (e.g., the client has debilitating rheumatoid arthritis and the dog is large and ill-mannered).
4. List the differential or tentative diagnoses.
   A. Include in the list medical problems that are historical or noted at the time of the behavioral assessment.
5. List clients' goals, taking into consideration items 1-4 above. Note for discussion goals that are achievable, under which conditions they may be achievable, and which goals may face constraints (this can be done tentatively, at first, and then reviewed with specifics at the end of the consultation and assessment).
6. Provide a paragraph summary of the case that includes all notable events. This summary should be concise but sufficiently detailed that any staff member could read it, close their eyes, and adequately and accurately imagine the case.
7. Create a specific treatment plan that addresses all of the following:
   A. Helpful or appropriate environmental change or modification.
      (1) Within this category consider a risk assessment, where warranted, and discuss options that will protect both the dog/cat and anyone whom the dog/cat might injure.
         a. Emphasis on risk assessment is essential for any case in which aggression may be a likely occurrence or for which there is a realistic risk. All risk assessment requires anticipatory guidance. Such guidance may include direction to or providing the client with resources to help them better understand the dog/cat so that risk can be minimized (e.g., Blue Dog program: www.thebluedog.org).
      (2) Discuss any potential use of gates, crates, or locked doors that allow dogs and cats to time and space share.
      (3) Discuss any potential use of head collars, harnesses, collars, muzzles, leads, et cetera, and the circumstances under which they should or should not be used and where warnings apply (e.g., head collars should not be left on unsupervised dogs because they could catch on another object and strangle an entrapped dog; muzzled dogs can still do serious injury by knocking someone over or by hitting them repeatedly with the muzzle—all good basket muzzles can also be weapons).
   B. Specific behavior modification plans.
      (1) Provide clients with instructions and demonstrations of any specific behavior modification suggested.
      (2) List specific handouts or programs given to clients.
      (3) Provide resources for help for implementing programs (e.g., re-checks with one of the vets or technicians/nurses, scheduled sessions with a competent humane dog trainer (www.petprofessionalguild.com/).
      (4) Ask clients to provide you with updates and/or schedule re-checks at certain intervals.
         a. Most clients have questions within a few days of the consultation. Tell them to e-mail or call you within this time period with their list of questions.

BOX 3-10

Outline Approach for Structuring a Thought Process for Treatment of Dogs and Cats with Behavioral Concerns—cont'd

b. Checking in within a couple of weeks to see how the implementation of the plans is going is helpful.

c. In-person or e-mail/video re-checks should occur after 8 weeks—this is the time that clients need to treat dogs with some medications before they can determine that they are not helping.
  i. Medication strategies should be amended as needed.

d. Monthly rechecks are helpful.
  i. Encourage clients to use video to help them assess progress or problems.
    (a) Clients should have provided a pre-exam video. This video could act as their baseline video.
    (b) Otherwise, before treatment begins, clients should video dogs in four to five circumstances that can be replicated. Some of these should be non-reactive situations (e.g., sleeping, walking in the door from a walk, playing with their favorite toy), and some should be situations in which they react (e.g., being approached by another dog or human, eating when the other dog is present).
    (c) Every 7 to 10 days, clients should take another video of their dogs in at least these same four to five circumstances. Clients should be encouraged to video new or curious behaviors also, but the point is to monitor behavior over time.
    (d) Videos should be reviewed for changes that can be discussed. It is optimal if the veterinarian also has a copy of the video.

e. For dogs engaged in active behavior modification, re-checks every 4 to 6 weeks may help tweak strategies.

f. Re-checks—via video or in person—should occur if there is any backsliding or concern or as often as the client wishes because relieving clients' concerns aids treatment outcomes.

(5) Emphasize the basics of successful behavior modification and appropriate landmarks.

(6) Explain the difference between acquiring and reinforcing a behavior.

(7) Explain the role of avoiding inappropriate behaviors for learned behaviors.

(8) Emphasize humane techniques and avoidance of positive punishment.

(9) Demonstrate appropriate timing and reward.

(10) Discuss types, uses of, and differing reactions to rewards.

(11) Provide lists of specific behaviors to watch for that indicate concern and behaviors that indicate progress (see the "Protocol for Deference" and the "Protocol for Teaching Your Dog to Take a Deep Breath and Use Other Biofeedback Methods as Part of Relaxation," in addition to the discussions of normal signaling and behavior in Chapters 4 and 5).

(12) Emphasize the *appropriate* use of specific interventions, such as dog walkers, attending agility classes, and attending nose work classes. Be very specific in guidance for how these interventions should and should not be executed.

C. The potential use of medications, supplements, dietary, and nutraceutical interventions.

(1) Discuss with clients expected effects and when these can be seen.

(2) Discuss monitoring for undesirable effects, and list the most common of these for clients.

(3) Assess and discuss with clients how any behavioral medications, supplements, diets, nutraceuticals, et cetera, could interact with medications that the patient is taking for other conditions.
  a. Ensure that you list all medications, specialty diets, et cetera, taken for any reason at each re-exam, along with the patient's weight should dose alter.

8. Decide how you will track outcomes.

A. Although clients favor subjective evaluations, a combination of subjective and objective evaluations is preferred.

B. If clients can provide video, objective assessment may become possible.

C. Clients can count events. If you use their complaint list as a basis, most clients can help with planning objective ways to assess change.

9. Recognize and discuss why assigning a prognosis is complex in veterinary behavioral medicine. Prognosis depends on conditions both intrinsic and extrinsic for the patient. Review Boxes 2-3 through 2-6 with the clients.

10. Remind clients that outcomes depend on:

A. Their ability to meet the welfare needs of the patient.

B. Their ability to protect the patient from the world and the world from the patient, if needed.

C. Their ability to observe the patient accurately and act on those observations.

D. Their ability to comply with the recommended treatment plan and to engage in a dialogue with their treatment professionals about this.

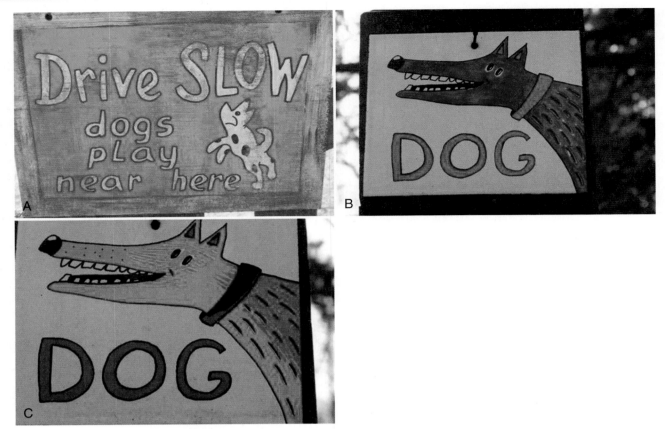

Fig. 3-64 **A-C,** Signs hung on a gate for a property with multiple dogs.

Is There Anything That We Have Missed?

Yes. Clients should always let people know they have pets, regardless of the kind of pet and regardless of whether the pet has problems. This is part of good citizenship and helps to incorporate pets into the community. There are two reasons for alerting people to the presence of pets.

- In an emergency, emergency personnel will look for animals whom they know are present, so an emergency sign is a good idea. Most cities in the United States now have emergency plans that include pets and stock. Clients can buy stick-on emergency signs and complete them, vets can give them as gifts, or clients can make their own. The sign needs to indicate how many pets of each kind exist and whether any have special needs. For example: *In case of emergency please rescue the three dogs and two cats. One dog is old and deaf and will be in the bedroom upstairs.* Such signs do not guarantee that pets will survive tragedy, but they can only help and ensure that the time that the emergency worker spends is well spent. Clients should post the sign on the door or a window near it.
- If people know that there are pets on the property and they are afraid of the pets, don't like them, or allergic to them, they have been put on notice and can make

their decisions accordingly. These types of signs are especially important if the resident cat or dog has any aggressive propensities. The signs do not have to assign blame to the dog or cat and should not do so but should clearly announce their presence and ask people to ring, knock, call, et cetera, first (Fig. 3-64). Signs attributing certain behavioral propensities (e.g., "Trespassers will be eaten") should be avoided.

Last Words

At the heart of the treatment and prevention of behavioral problems is an understanding that all species work for accurate information. Nowhere is this more obvious and applicable than in the co-evolved relationship between dogs and people. Dogs ask questions with their behaviors. The responses they receive determine their next behavior after being processed by a brain neurochemistry that may not be normal or helpful. If we can provide information that allows our patients to engage in accurate, helpful risk assessment that lowers anxiety and allows them to learn about more adaptive behaviors that help them to feel better and think more clearly, we will have achieved the goal of using advances in neurobehavioral genetics to promote humane care and the best possible mental health for those entrusted to our care.

Canine Behavior

CHAPTER 4

Normal Canine Behavior and Ontogeny: Neurological and Social Development, Signaling, and Normal Canine Behaviors

OVERVIEW OF NORMAL DOG BEHAVIOR

Why Domestic Dogs Are Special

Dogs have a relationship with humans unlike that of any other "domestic" animal. Dogs have been selected over time for true collaborative work with humans, and such selection has historically resulted in dog breeds and the attendant groupings, regardless of which organization defines the groupings (e.g., American Kennel Club [AKC], Federation Cynologique Internationale [FCI]).

Molecular data support that dogs separated from wolves 15,000 to 135,000 years ago (Cadieu et al., 2009; Leonard et al., 2002; Lindblad-Toh et al., 2008; Pang et al., 2009; Parker et al., 2004; Savolainen et al., 2002; Sutter et al., 2004; Vila et al., 1997; Vonholdt et al., 2010). Molecular and anthropological data support that dogs of different morphologies who were likely engaged in different tasks have lived together with humans for at least 15,000 years (Boyko et al., 2009; Castroviejo-Fisher et al., 2011; Morey, 1994; Pang et al., 2009). Stand-alone anthropological evidence supports that dogs have lived intimately with humans for at least 30,000 years (Bienvenido et al., 2009; Derr, 2012; Germonpré et al., 2009, 2012; Ovodov et al., 2011). For the past 3500 years or more (consider dogs portrayed in ancient Chinese and Egyptian art), there have been well-defined breed clusters or groups comprising dogs of different shapes and sizes who engaged in related tasks.

Regardless of the debate over timing, we should appreciate that one of the forces associated with speciation may have been a special, collaborative working relationship with humans that ultimately resulted in morphological variation in dogs as a relatively—perhaps profoundly—late development in the human × dog relationship. We accept that humans have changed dogs. We seldom consider the extent to which dogs may have changed humans. Our unique relationship with dogs may be due to convergent evolution of canid and human social systems that was *the result of like groups meeting and recognizing the power of collaborative efforts*, followed by *secondarily derived, homologous changes in brain function* (Saetre et al., 2004) that have allowed modern humans and dogs to rely on each other.

Dogs, as a species separate from wolves, likely co-evolved with humans over thousands or tens of thousands of years, during which time they may not have been fully "domesticated." "Domestication" may have occurred when we began to develop breed groups intended for specific tasks, which happened 3000 or more years ago. In contrast to wolves, who require handling by humans early in their ontogeny (beginning by at least 14 days of age) to minimize fear and reactivity to humans, *most dogs can adapt to delays in handling and exposure, and their normal, innate sensitive periods are greatly expanded from those of wolves*. When dogs cannot adapt or when they seem to have short sensitive periods, such patterns are indicative of pathology. In dogs, it is likely that this *sensitive period expansion* occurred concomitantly with changes in molecular and neurochemical function and gene expression (Saetre et al., 2004) that may represent some of the *true outcomes of active "domestication."* In contrast to dogs, but similar to other non-domesticated species, *cats have a relatively short and truncated sensitive period for exposure to humans, which may be associated with or evidence of lack of tampering associated with "domestication."*

Both humans and canids live in extended family groups, provide extensive parental care, share care of young with both related and non-related group members, give birth to altricial (completely dependent, immature) young that require large amounts of early care and sustained amounts of later social interaction, nurse for an extended period before weaning to semi-solid food (dogs do this by regurgitation; humans use baby food, but the concept is the same), have extensive vocal and non-vocal communication (it has been estimated that 80% of all human communication is nonverbal) (Smith, 1965, 1977), and have a sexual maturity that precedes social maturity. These shared characteristics may have allowed dogs and humans to recognize similarity in each other that allowed exchange of information and that led to later "domestication" and changes on the parts of both dogs and humans related to task management.

Behavioral Ontogeny in Dogs

Early Brain and Behavioral Development in Dogs

Myelination of cranial nerves V (trigeminal), VII (facial), and VIII (vestibulocochlear/auditory) is present at birth. These nerves are associated with essential functions of eating, balance, and body-righting. As is true for other animals, myelin is almost completely absent from the brains of newborn puppies but appears during the first 4 weeks, at the same time ribonucleic acid (RNA) synthesis is increasing at a rapid rate (Fox, 1971). In humans, myelin is first deposited in the peripheral nervous system (PNS), the central nervous system (CNS) in the brainstem and cerebellum, and in components of some major motor systems just before and after birth. Myelination of the human brain cortices occurs well after birth and progresses over decades (Volpe, 2008). Dogs undergo a gradual increase in myelination of the spinal cord, motor and sensory roots, and efferent pathways starting at birth and progressing through 3 weeks, which is reflected in the development of olfactory, thermal, and tactile capability and in increased mobility associated with development of vision. PNS and CNS development is reflected in development of motor responses and reflexes in young pups. This period of gradual myelination is followed by more rapid myelination of the somatosensory cortex at about 4 weeks and a more even distribution of myelination of the visual and auditory cortex by 6 weeks (Fox, 1971). As with humans, myelination is slowest in the frontal lobe. As brain development progresses, canine behavior becomes more complex, and the markers for onset of "socialization" or sensitive periods appear to be neurodevelopmental.

Much of what is known about early social development is the result of work done by Scott et al. in a laboratory on five breeds of similarly shaped dogs (wire-haired terriers, Shetland sheepdogs, cocker spaniels, beagles, and basenjis), using a relatively small number of litters over 2 decades and observing pups beginning at 3 weeks of age (Scott and Fuller, 1965). These studies remain landmarks. We still lack comparable data on most breeds, yet such data could be relatively easily collected across breeds, as demonstrated by Schoon and Goth Berntsen (2011), who provide excellent data on neurodevelopmental landmarks from birth for 10 litters of Belgian malinois raised under controlled conditions.

The following broad conclusions appear to hold for most dogs:
- The "neonatal period" covers the period from birth to 13 days of age when puppies are dependent on rudimentary locomotor skills and use tactile signals to locate and orient toward dams and littermates. During this period, puppies vocalize if separated from their dams. Olfactory ability is present but poorly characterized in dogs this age. Few data about tactile signaling exist, yet given its early importance it should help structure brain development.
- The mild stress of daily and early handling is beneficial for puppies and allows them to cope better with later stresses (Selye, 1952). Excessive stress should be avoided because chronic, excess secretion of adrenocorticotropic hormone (ACTH) has been correlated with a decreased ability to learn.
- From days 13 to 20, puppies become more coordinated, open their eyes, and begin to startle to sound. The change in motor abilities coincides with eruption of teeth at approximately day 20 and with improved vision. This period is traditionally called the "transition period."
- Tail-wagging behavior becomes apparent at the end of this 20-day period, and there is considerable variation across breeds in this development. No one has investigated the extent to which use of the tail in signaling may reflect an effect of neurodevelopment but this is an important question.
- If pups are exposed to passive observers beginning at 3 weeks of age, they will approach and explore the observer.
- If pups are not exposed to passive observers until 7 weeks of age, they must habituate to the observers before they approach and explore. This habituation took 2 days in the laboratory setting (Bacon and Stanley, 1963, 1970; Freedman et al., 1961; Love and Eisenberg, 1986; Scott and Fuller, 1965).
- Dogs isolated from humans through 20 weeks became fearful of humans (Agrawal et al., 1967) and had impaired learning ability (Melzack, 1968; Melzack and Scott, 1957; Thompson and Heron, 1954).
- Even if kept with their mothers, by 12 weeks of age, puppies chose to wander extensively, a finding that anyone who has raised puppies has witnessed.
- Pups that were kept in kennels beyond 14 weeks were very timid and demonstrated a lack of confidence in any circumstances other than the kennel. These dogs would not voluntarily leave the kennel and became truly phobic of anything novel (neophobia) (see Scott and Fuller, 1965, for summary data).
- Different breeds responded differently to various rewards and restraints and differently with respect to various social contexts (Plutchik, 1971), and these patterns were replicable.

Based on these data, the period from 3 to 12 weeks was called the "socialization period," from which a number of context-specific developmental periods were identified as "socialization periods." These periods became prescriptive with respect to types and extent of exposure that were thought to be required to produce "normal dogs." *Instead, such data are best viewed within the context of a "sensitive period" (Bateson, 1979), which implies risk assessment.* There are environmental and genetic aspects of all behaviors (see Figures 3-3 and 3-4 accompanying discussions in Chapter 3), and some individuals may benefit from earlier exposure than others. If the opportunities are available, non-pathological dogs will expose themselves when they are able.

A concept of a *sensitive period* takes such variation into account and *is best defined as period when animals can best benefit from exposure to certain stimuli, and if deprived of such exposure, there is an increased risk of developing problems attendant with the stimulus.* In other words, when animals are neurodevelopmentally able to respond to stimuli, they will benefit from exposure, and if they lack exposure, they could develop behavioral problems associated with the omission (Bateson, 1979; Cairns et al., 1985). This does not mean that all exposure is equal, that all dogs are ready for all exposures at the same time, that you stop exposing the dog when the dog is out of the sensitive period, or that if exposed, no dogs will have problems.

Given what we know about sensitive periods, exposure, and neurodevelopment, we may wish to replace the concept of a "socialization period" with one that uses the concept of a sensitive period as the time when we should ensure that dogs have access to the relevant stimuli. When dogs are neurodevelopmentally able to respond to the stimuli, they will do so unless they are impeded. This approach also includes exposure to new environments, something that a technical definition of "socialization period" does not include.

We also should remember the role for cortical development in how a puppy learns to respond to different stimuli and understand that the time/developmental period of imposed change matters to the dog. A study comparing 70 adult dogs who as puppies had been separated from their dams and litters 30 to 40 days with 70 adult dogs who as puppies were not separated until after 8 weeks showed that early age of separation was a significant predictor for excessive barking, fearfulness on walks, reactivity to noises, toy possessiveness, food passiveness, and attention-seeking behavior. These dogs were also more at risk for destructive behavior than dogs who had been permitted to stay with their litter through 8 weeks (Pierantoni et al., 2011). Clearly, there are potential roles for both the hormonal effects of stress/distress and the developmental phase in these findings. Considering the enhanced risk of relinquishment, abandonment, and euthanasia for dogs with behavioral concerns, welfare and behavioral standards should mandate that puppies remain with their litters in the home of and with access to the dam through 8 weeks of age (Box 4-1).

General guidelines for exposure based on the available data are found in Table 4-1.

Roles for Play

Play appears to be important in every species in which it has been studied. Although play has been thought to have numerous roles in behavioral development and maintenance from enhancing coordination and locomotor activity to encouraging problem-solving ability and enhancing cognition (Spinka et al., 2001), it may be especially effective in *teaching animals how to make mistakes successfully and in established baselines for well-honed, broad, basic communication skills.* This hypothesis is supported by data showing that dogs who received more playful interactions from their people were less fearful in new environments (Tóth et al., 2008).

TABLE 4-1

Sensitive Periods and Associated Neurodevelopmental and Behavioral Landmarks*

Age/Relevant Sensitive Periods	Neurodevelopmental Landmarks	Behavioral Patterns and Most Relevant Stimuli for Exposure	Problems That Might Occur if Exposure during Relevant Period Is Missed
0-13 days	Continued maturation of cranial nerves and myelinization of somatosensory and motor brain regions	Handling especially involving tactile and thermal stimuli	Hyper-reactivity Altered sensitivity to touch (consider the role for tactile stimuli and attendant neurodevelopment in dogs with docked/bobbed tails and docked ears)
13-20 days	Startle reflex Responsive to auditory stimuli Responsive to visual stimuli	Handling by humans and dogs Exposure to novel auditory and visual stimuli, without rational bounds	Concerns with visual and auditory acuity (based on laboratory animals)

TABLE 4-1

Sensitive Periods and Associated Neurodevelopmental and Behavioral Landmarks—cont'd

Age/Relevant Sensitive Periods	Neurodevelopmental Landmarks	Behavioral Patterns and Most Relevant Stimuli for Exposure	Problems That Might Occur if Exposure during Relevant Period Is Missed
3-8 weeks	Teeth begin to emerge at 3 weeks Tail wagging at 3 weeks; most dogs begin to wag their tails before 8 weeks (possibly not most basenjis) Increased locomotor capabilities beginning at about 3 weeks associated with beginning to approach novel people and more interactive motions with other dogs Puppies start following each other at about 3 weeks Rapid myelination of the somatosensory cortex begins at about 4 weeks More even distribution of myelination of the visual and auditory cortex occurs by 6 weeks	Pups begin to eat semi-solid food by about 3 weeks and solid food by about 5 weeks Pups will begin to explore and interact with other dogs As the period progresses and they become more coordinated they will engage in pouncing, rolling, rough and tumble play, mouthing, grabbing, and growling at other pups or older dogs who play with them Species identification may occur by 2.5-3 weeks of age. Pups raised only with cats from 2.5-13 weeks of age do not recognize dogs (consider the concern of raising dogs of one breed with only dogs of that breed—a common occurrence in very small breeds)	Heightened reactivity to dogs Heightened reactivity to other species including humans Lack of inhibition both in arousal levels and in behavioral responses to arousal Animals learn to be calm and settle or relax, and such learning has profound responses for how they later handle situations that are potentially anxiety-provoking (see Chapter 2)
5-7 weeks through 12 weeks	Myelination of cortex continues and by week 8 there is sufficient myelination with sufficient connectivity that the patterns seen in adult EEGs are first seen in EEGs of pups (this does not mean the individual is fully neurologically mature given what we now know about neuronal pruning and remodeling)	Beginning at about 5 weeks as frontal cortex myelination continues pups will begin to recognize "other" and interact with and seek out other species, including humans. This interaction is more complex than the approaching that they will begin to do at 3 weeks Maximum distress, as indicated only by vocalization, occurs at week 5 of development (Gurski et al., 1980) At 5 weeks dogs begin to hone their intra-specific skills First true pathological fear responses reliably reported for laboratory animals in genetically susceptible lines Interaction with humans intensifies beginning at ≥6 weeks Housetraining is most successfully begun at about 8.5 weeks when there is sufficient cortical development to (1) make an association with preferred substrate and (2) understand that inhibition of micturition may be desirable	Fear of humans and other species Fear of approaches of humans Lack of learned inhibition for elimination of feces and urine

Continued

TABLE 4-1

Sensitive Periods and Associated Neurodevelopmental and Behavioral Landmarks—cont'd

Age/Relevant Sensitive Periods	Neurodevelopmental Landmarks	Behavioral Patterns and Most Relevant Stimuli for Exposure	Problems That Might Occur if Exposure during Relevant Period Is Missed
		Mounting of littermates starts at about 5-6 weeks	
		Dogs begin to bark by 4-5 weeks and growl shortly thereafter. Amount of vocalization and age of onset is affected by breed	
		By 7 weeks of age the dams of the dogs Scott et al. studied had naturally weaned all of their pups, although they remained with them through 10 weeks	
		The earliest age at which a dog can/should be sold is 8.5 weeks. Most dogs would benefit from longer, not shorter, stays with their families (see Box 4-1)	
		Frequency of play behaviors in free-ranging dogs increases through week 8 and begins to decrease slowly starting at weeks 9-10 (Pal et al., 2010). It is likely that non–free-ranging dogs may have a longer period of frequent play, given the right stimuli	
10-12 through 16-20 weeks	Rapid period of myelination slows by 10 weeks	Intense period of learning how to explore and about novel environments	Neophobia Lack of plasticity in responses Inappropriate play and lack of play
		At about 8-10 weeks of age dogs have sufficient cortical development to associate experiences or stimuli with the sensation of fear and may become more hesitant and discriminating in their previously unfettered, exuberant responses (Fox and Bekoff, 1975)	
		This response is normal and adaptive, and involves learning about (1) risk and (2) how to make a mistake successfully	
		Play becomes rougher and appears to be about successfully making and learning from mistakes	

TABLE 4-1

Sensitive Periods and Associated Neurodevelopmental and Behavioral Landmarks—cont'd

Age/Relevant Sensitive Periods	Neurodevelopmental Landmarks	Behavioral Patterns and Most Relevant Stimuli for Exposure	Problems That Might Occur if Exposure during Relevant Period Is Missed
14-20 weeks	Major myelination is complete, and pruning and neurogenesis are ongoing	Dogs not allowed to explore new environments by 14 weeks will not voluntarily do so. If forced to do so, they freeze and become extremely distressed Normal marking behaviors may begin to appear as dogs approach sexual maturity	Neophobia Profound panic Plasticity of response is characteristic of normal behaviors. Lack of plasticity in response is characteristic of abnormal behaviors Ability to have a plastic and flexible response and to have neurons that facilitate it is learned at both the behavioral and neuromolecular levels

These periods indicate when dogs are first most receptive to the noted stimuli. There is no implication that dogs ever stop learning from their experience. Data support the concept of repeated, ongoing neurological and molecular remodeling with exposure, as occurs in humans.
EEG, Electroencephalogram.

BOX 4-1

Case Against Very Early Puppyhood Adoption

- By 3 to 4 weeks of age, pups start to follow each other (Scott and Fuller, 1965).
- By 5 weeks of age, they rush at an opening as a group. The more activity there is at the opening, the more frenzied the puppies will become (Scott and Fuller, 1965).
- In both kennel and field situations, the strongest attachment to location and companions occurs at 6 to 7 weeks. If separated from either family members or the location where raised, puppies become severely destabilized (Elliot and Scott, 1961). This response can be mitigated if all littermates are exposed to a variety of fairly benign circumstances, both as an intact litter and in smaller groups early in life. Separation from each other or a place at 6 weeks of age causes recidivistic changes in the puppies' behavioral development. *These findings constitute one of the strongest arguments in favor of the abolition of puppy mills.* They also provide insight into why so many puppies that are placed at a very young age develop or continue to have behavioral problems.
- Stress at 6 to 7 weeks affects the pups' ability to learn about housetraining (see section on stress and learning in Chapter 2). Puppies begin to form substrate and location preferences for elimination by 8.5 weeks. This is the period when they first have sufficient cortical development to learn about substrates and choose to act on them, while also having sufficient physical and behavioral abilities to inhibit elimination. Dams have stimulated pups to urinate and defecate until about 3 weeks of age. From 3 to 7 or 8 weeks, puppies eliminate whenever necessary, with little regard to location. Few people understand that young pups cannot inhibit elimination, and so they resort to punishment (see client handout, "Protocol for Basic Manners Training and Housetraining for New Dogs and Puppies").
- If breeders are willing to housetrain the puppy and encourage its independence by ensuring that the pups are exposed to novel people and environments, there may be no costs and sometimes some benefits to keeping the puppy longer than 8.5 weeks. The amount of time involved in exposure is often smaller than anticipated: Fuller (1967) noted that semi-isolated puppies avoided the pitfalls of restricted exposure in as little as two 20-minute periods a week.
- Puppies respond best to objects, such as leashes, between 5 and 9 weeks of age (Scott and Fuller, 1965). Breeders can help puppies by starting to fit them with head collars, harnesses, and leashes (see client handout, "Protocol for Choosing Collars, Head Collars, Harnesses, and Leads").
- Puppies separated from the dam and litter at the time of weaning display up to 100 vocalizations per minute (Elliott and Scott, 1961). This argues that one should not concomitantly wean and place dogs.
- Hand-reared puppies explore novel stimuli more than kennel-reared puppies when evaluated at 8.5 weeks of age because this is the major stimulation available to them.

Continued

BOX 4-1

Case Against Very Early Puppyhood Adoption—cont'd

- Separation of pups from their mothers at 6 weeks of age had a negative effect on the physical condition, health, and weight of pups (Slabbert and Rasa, 1993).
- Pettijohn et al. (1977) provide data that indicate that *toys have no effect on relieving separation distress, but that social stimuli do.* Humans may be preferred to dogs for relief of the social exposure stress that occurs at 7 to 8 weeks of age, the time when dogs are developmentally able to explore and learn from people.
- Some breeds that have been developed for work in groups (e.g., hounds) when reared alone until 16 weeks of age lose the capacity for spontaneous play. Play can be elicited, but these dogs play differently from dogs who were able to associate with other dogs (Adler and Adler, 1977).
- In dogs from 47 different breeds studied from birth to 9 months of age, "socially deprived" dogs

were antagonistic when greeted by humans and exhibited agonistic behavior in response to human approach, whereas dogs that had adequate "socialization" exhibited normal, friendly greetings and were well adapted in other social circumstances (Feddersen-Petersen, 1994).
- Adult dogs, who had been separated from their dam and litter from 30 to 40 days, experienced a greater incidence of excessive barking, fearfulness on walks, reactivity to noises, toy possessiveness, food passiveness, attention-seeking behavior, and destructive behavior than dogs who had been kept with their litter through 8 weeks (Pierantoni et al., 2011). This is some of the strongest evidence that dogs should neither be separated from their litters nor the influence of the dam nor adopted into a new home before 8 weeks of age.

In dyadic relationships of dogs participating in free play, sex of participants does not affect play, but age does: older dogs play more forcefully than younger dogs (Bauer and Smuts, 2007). Play and play signals also appear to modulate interactions between younger dogs and more forceful older dogs in dyadic play. Play signals given by younger dogs alter the course of more forceful interactions by older dogs (Bauer and Smuts, 2007), likely by making intentions more clear.

Dogs playing with other dogs play with toys differently than dogs playing with humans. When dogs play with humans, they are more interactive and less likely to continue to hold the toy (Rooney et al., 2001). Humans play with dogs using vocal, tactile, and visual/postural cues that can affect how dogs play. When humans display the lunge and bow aspects of the canine play bow, dogs increase play, and lunging increases play duration and frequency (Rooney et al., 2001). If the humans added vocal signals, play was enhanced. Effective human play with dogs enhances the relationship between the dog and the human, reduces the incidence of behavioral problems, and encourages humans to think that their dogs are very clever (Rooney and Bradshaw, 2002, 2003).

Play signals affect how dogs interpret the information provided by interactions between humans. In staged contests between humans, dogs whose humans give play signals approach more quickly than dogs whose humans provide no signaling information (Rooney and Bradshaw, 2002). Because play behavior involves a number of signaling modalities (vocal, visual, tactile, olfactory [licking, sniffing]), the redundant signals involved minimize the risk of mistakes in communication and help young animals learn about

managing mistakes and quick changes in interactive behavior.

Early Exposure, Puppy Classes, and Vaccination Programs

Dogs should be allowed sufficient safe access so that when they enter their individual sensitive periods, there is no impediment to them exploring the relevant environment or having the relevant social interactions. The earlier dogs can learn about the broad-scale social and physical environment in which they are to live, without inducing fear, the better. If dogs are protected from stimuli, they may react inappropriately when exposed later (Scott, 1963; Bacon and Stanley, 1970).

If the pups had healthy dams, are healthy themselves, and are engaged in a modern vaccination program, they can be exposed to as many situations as possible. Of 24,000 guide dog puppies who began vaccination at 6 weeks of age and were re-vaccinated every third week through weeks 12 to 16, fewer than 6 pups ($\frac{2}{100}$ of 1%) who were healthy during the vaccination series got sick (Appleby, 1993). If there are available puppy classes or puppy play groups, any pup physically and behaviorally able to participate should do so. If pups shy from these groups or classes and gentle continued exposure does not alleviate their response, they need help immediately.

Very early fear is a problem for pups. Historically, pups from lines of dogs genetically selected to show fearful behaviors show the behavioral and physiological effects of fear by 5 weeks (Murphree et al., 1967, 1969). Pups from lines of dogs commercially bred for research purposes show almost the same distribution of fearful behaviors at 5 weeks of age as do their dams and sires at 1.5 to 2 years (Overall et al., unpublished). Puppies who are shy, worried, or anxious throughout early veterinary visits are likely to exhibit the same behaviors as adults at 1.5 to 2 years of age (Godbout et al., 2007). Early intervention is essential for such dogs.

One study has suggested that there could be a beneficial effect of pheromonal analogue collars on one of a series of behaviors studied, early excitability in class, and hence on learning in puppy classes, based on owner surveys (Denenberg and Landsberg, 2008). Even if this effect were real—and the data, techniques, and analysis are problematic (Frank et al., 2010)—the magnitude of the effect appears mild, especially considering that it uses a tool (ranks of owner responses) that may exaggerate mild and/or rare outcomes. There are no data to suggest that pheromonal products are helpful for early fears, and so treatment with interventions whose mechanisms are known to work should not be delayed. Early intervention, often involving medication, is essential for these dogs so that they have a decent quality of life.

Claims have been made that some types of handling and stressors, including those discussed in early neural stimulation, protect dogs from effects of later stress (Battaglia, 2009). Only one study has evaluated early neural stimulation in a blinded, controlled, rigorous manner, and this study showed that it had no effect on the dogs chosen for the evaluation (Schoon and Goth Berntsen, 2011). However, as the authors note, the dogs tested were purpose-bred to become mine-detection dogs and already lived in an extremely enriched environment where they were intensely handled and interacted with daily as part of their routine protocol. This is exactly the environment in which you would expect not to see an effect because the control dogs are also highly, albeit slightly differently, stimulated. For dogs raised in homes, kennels, or commercial breeding facilities where dogs are behaviorally deprived, early stimulation of any kind is known to be beneficial.

Brain Changes and Social Maturity

The time between the end of myelination of the cortex and concomitant development of normal social and exploratory behavior (8 to 12 weeks) and the development of sexual maturity is considered to be the "juvenile" period (Scott and Fuller, 1965). Dogs are sexually mature by 6 to 9 months of age. If the dog is to be a breeding dog and does not show signs of sexual maturity by 6 to 9 months of age, further consultation is warranted. Sex hormones may interact with various neurodevelopmental systems, but no data exist on the effects of early versus later neutering on these systems in dogs, with the possible exception of correlates on long bone growth. Regardless, both neutered and intact animals are affected by behavioral concerns and pathologies.

We lack information on dogs that is now available for humans (and rodents), but it may be safe to assume that myelination and neuronal pruning occur rapidly for the first few months of life and then slow until social maturity, as is the pattern in humans. Social maturity is a period of renewed but progressive myelination and regressive pruning that is associated with changes in neurochemical profiles and shifts in behavior (Sowell et al., 1999). Behavioral changes attendant with canine social maturity begin at approximately 12 to 18 months. There is likely considerable variation attached to this estimate because of breed and size differences and because some dogs are still bred and selected for certain tasks. Such concerns are reduced for humans.

Social maturity is usually thought to end at about 24 to 36 months of age. The period of social maturity has never been well measured behaviorally, physiologically, or neurochemically through functional imaging in dogs, and so these are approximate ages around which much variation should occur, but if changes occur as they do for humans, these are reasonable landmarks. Given shared selection pressures on the development of behavior, we should expect dogs and humans to experience similar age-related developmental brain changes.

Humans are sexually mature at some point between 8 and 13 years of age, but are not socially mature—based on functional imaging and neurochemical evidence—until well into their 20s or 30s. As humans age from 6 to 17 years, cerebral gray matter volume decreases, and white matter and corpus callosum volumes increase, suggesting increased ability to integrate and act on information, when measured by magnetic resonance imaging (MRI) (De Bellis et al., 2001). Standard MRI assays reveal profound differences in size-by-age trajectories of brain development between males and females as they mature through age 27 years (De Bellis et al., 2001; Lenroot et al., 2007). Using diffusion tensor MRI, age-related (5 to 30 years) changes are seen in many areas of the human brain (i.e., deep gray matter, subcortical white matter, major white matter tracts) in a pattern that suggests that connections between the frontal and temporal lobes develop more slowly than other regions.

Patterns of change in maturation of the human frontal cortex appear to improve cognitive processing, a hypothesis supported by congruent data from electrophysiological, positron emission tomography, and neuropsychological studies on normal cognitive and neurological development (Sowell et al., 1999). Trajectories for regional brain maturation can be affected by trauma, indicating how important connecting tracts are in the development of adaptive behaviors. Children with post-traumatic stress disorder (PTSD) have larger prefrontal lobe cerebrospinal fluid volumes and smaller regional measurements of the corpus callosum than age-matched unaffected children; this finding is amplified for boys with PTSD (De Bellis and Kreshavan, 2003). We should hypothesize that the same pattern can occur with dogs.

These neurobehavioral developmental patterns that occur with social maturity have important implications for learning and acting on what is learned. The frontal cortex is especially involved in response inhibition, regulation of "emotion" and emotional outburst, organization of activities, and forethought involved in planning and problem solving in all species. It is unfortunate, especially given our evolved relationship with them, that we lack comparable data for dogs as they move from puppyhood through social maturity, but as imaging technologies become more accessible such data may emerge.

Why It Is Not about "Dominance"

The human social system is a fluid hierarchical one that is based on ability and/or age but that is grounded in the context of deference. Dogs also have fluid social structures where day-to-day interactions are largely based on deferential behaviors, especially where dogs are known to one another, and on behaviors designed to elicit information about risk in situations where they are not known to each other. Combat is the exceptional choice for resolution of conflict in both canids and humans. When combat is the first choice for conflict resolution, it is an abnormal, out-of-context behavior. Instead, agonistic behavior is generally accompanied by an elaborate display structure designed to minimize damage to the individual. Both canid and human social systems use signals and displays that minimize the probability of outright battle and the damage that could be incurred during fights.

Deferential relationships in neither dogs nor humans are structured as linear hierarchies. Most concepts involving "dominance" in dogs are outdated, something that the behavioral community has finally recognized (American Veterinary Society of Animal Behavior [AVSAB] Dominance Position Statement: www.avsabonline.org/avsabonline/images/stories/Position_Statements/dominance%20statement.pdf and the Dog Welfare Campaign position statement: www.dogwelfarecampaign.org/why-not-dominance.php). Many situations in which "dominance" is implicated in hierarchies may be artifacts. The study of relationships between fewer than six animals will automatically produce a numerical rank order hierarchy that is linear (Bernstein, 1981; Boyd and Silk, 1983; Rowell, 1974; Syme, 1974), but the ranks produced are unable to account for the social complexities that are noted. Instead, deferential behaviors are dependent on context and are based on knowledge, age, size, and the situation in which individuals are interacting. More information in language useful for clients can be found in the client handout, "Protocol for Generalized Discharge Instructions for Dogs with Behavioral Concerns." It is not surprising that humans were able to incorporate dogs into our social groups, as we were incorporated into theirs.

HOW DOGS COMMUNICATE

Understanding Non-vocal Signals

Because dogs and people do have such similar social systems and use so many of the same signals, it has been very easy for people to assume that when a dog gives a signal that resembles a human signal, the message is exactly the same and that it means exactly the same thing (Smith, 1965). We have shared signals, but we should also understand that animals who do not use verbal speech in the manner we do and who do not have opposable thumbs may have their own signals that we could benefit from learning, rather than always expecting us to learn their signals. When humans allowed dogs to teach them to play using canine signals (bow and lunge), the relationship between the human and the dog improved, and dogs who had not played now played enthusiastically (Rooney and Bradshaw, 2001).

Behavioral descriptions are usually made on the basis of either structure (e.g., descriptions of postures or sounds) or consequences (e.g., the effect of the behavior on the individual exhibiting the behavior, others in the behavioral environment, and the behavioral environment itself). A good description of these concepts can be found at the Animal Behavior Society website (www.animalbehavior.org/ABSEducation/laboratory-exercises-in-animal-behavior/laboratory-exercises-in-animal-behavior-ethograms). The difficulty in veterinary behavioral medicine often arises when descriptions of measures and consequences are confused or given an associational or causal link without actually testing whether that link is valid or true. For descriptors to have scientifically valid causal or associational links, we would have to measure or assess whether these terms characterize what they were intended to characterize, an effort that is seldom made.

Early Behaviors

Early canine behaviors can be divided into et-epimeletic (care-seeking), epimeletic (caregiving), and allelomimetic (group-activity) behaviors. Until about 4 weeks of age, the relationship between the mother and puppies is primarily epimeletic. Box 4-2 contains the traditional classification of these stage-associated behaviors. Many of these behaviors are also seen later in life and can be understood by referring to this ontogenic history.

BOX 4-2

Epimeletic, Et-epimeletic, and Allelomimetic Behaviors

Epimeletic behaviors include:
1. Licking the pup's anal and genital regions and eating urine and feces
2. Grooming and licking faces
3. Pushing pups with the nose to encourage them toward warmth and feeding opportunities and to stimulate postures associated with respiration and other physical and physiological functions
4. Carrying straying puppies
5. Guarding pups
6. Suckling
7. Regurgitation
8. Carrying food for puppies

As they age, puppies perform rutting and whining, *et-epimeletic behaviors*. These include:
1. Tail wagging, with their tail low in a deferential solicitation gesture
2. Yelping
3. Licking the mother's face, nose, and lips
4. Jumping up and pawing at the mother
5. Following the mother closely

Group or allelomimetic behaviors that puppies exhibit as they move into their more social periods include:
1. Sleeping together
2. Feeding
3. Walking, running, and sitting or lying together
4. Investigating things as a group
5. Barking or howling as a group
6. Grooming other group members
7. Sniffing and nosing other members of the group

SYSTEMATIC APPROACH TO UNDERSTANDING CANINE SIGNALS

Canine Visual Communication—What Can Dogs See?

Dogs are born with an immature and relatively non-myelinated visual system. Vision improves rapidly through 20 days of age.

With a 97-degree binocular field, dogs have relatively poor binocular vision compared with humans, but the extent to which they experience binocular vision depends on dog breed and head shape. Dogs have better lateral vision than humans, which may affect how they learn to understand the behaviors of other dogs. It should be noted that canine vision is exquisitely sensitive to movement—which is likely related to their excellent lateral vision—and *dogs can recognize an object that is moving almost twice as well as when the same object is still.* This finding has profound implications for dogs who are reactive to humans or other dogs.

Eye radius, a measure of size, positively correlates with the length and width dimensions of the skull but not with cephalic index, a measure of shape, rather than size (skull width/skull length × 100). Among breeds of domestic dogs, retinal ganglion cells range in distribution from a dense concentration in a strong area centralis, with virtually no visual streak, to a strong, horizontally distributed visual streak and almost no area centralis (McGreevy et al., 2004).

- Skull length was negatively correlated with peak area centralis density of ganglion cells but positively correlated with peak density of ganglion cells in the streak (e.g., long-nosed dogs have few ganglion cells in the area centralis but a lot of ganglion cells in the streak).
- The ratio of ganglion cell densities in the area centralis to cells in the streak was negatively correlated with skull length (i.e., the more cells in the area centralis compared with the streak, the shorter the skull).
- Dolichocephalic dogs have strong visual streaks and relatively low densities of ganglion cells in the area centralis, and brachycephalic dogs have concentrated ganglion cells in the area centralis and low to no concentrations in a visual streak.
- Red/green cones (medium to long wave) were denser in the temporal region than in the area centralis in brachycephalic dogs and less concentrated in the temporal retina in dolichocephalic dogs. Blue cones (short wave) were sparse compared with red/green cones in all dogs.
- The number of ganglion cells correlates positively with skull size. McGreevy et al. (2004) did not examine the extent to which skull shape and size may have affected distribution of olfactory neurons, but it may be prudent to expect an effect.

We seldom consider what selective breeding to produce dogs of different shapes, looks, and work attributes has done to the senses of dogs, but it now appears that there may be effects for some aspect of how dogs see. If this is true, some of the behaviors seen in long-nosed versus short-nosed dogs may be the result of how they perceive their world.

Dogs see in rudimentary color vision (dichromatic), and they are sensitive to short-wave (bluish) light. Dog color vision is sufficiently discriminating so that they can pick out an object based on color (Neitz et al., 1989). Dogs have two classes of photopigment in cones with spectral peaks at approximately 429 nm (blue) and 555 nm (green), the peak of sensitivity for light-adapted eyes. In bright light, however, dogs have less acute vision than humans. Rhodopsin in dogs has a peak sensitivity to wavelengths of 506 to 510 nm and requires more than an hour to regenerate completely after exposure to bright light. The extent to which rods and cones develop is dependent on early exposure to a full range of ambient light conditions and to critical nutrients docosahexaenoic acid (DHA).

Non-vocal Signaling—Visual Signals Using Body Language

Body posture in dogs is an easy factor to assess in the signaling repertoire, but we too often ignore it. A quick review of common postures will help in understanding what dogs are communicating and what their next movement might be. Numerous popular videos, posters, and books on canine signaling are available (e.g., Collins S. *Tail Talk: Understanding the Secret Language of Dogs.* Chronicle Books, San Francisco, 2007), but we still lack a good, detailed, extensive, and agreed-on ethogram. *Replicable, rigorous quantitative studies using sequence analysis within interactions is labor intensive but much needed.* Some general patterns can still emerge. Table 4-2 provides an outline of some of the common signals seen in dogs and what these signals can convey.

Text continued on p. 141

TABLE 4-2

Common Signals Given by Dogs and the Context and Circumstances in Which They Are Usually Seen*	
Signal	**Context/Circumstance**
Barking	Alerting—loud, single-syllable repeats Warning—often a more complex bark that is deep and with changing pitch Attention-seeking—bark is high-pitched and often repetitive
Growling	Warning—usually deep Play—multi-tonal and often ending with a higher pitched sound Distance increasing signal—in both play and warning growls separation usually results, although in play it has to do with chasing or the back-and-forth actions common in normal play
Crying	Et-epimeletic Attention-seeking Solicitation of social interaction May indicate some level of distress
Whimpering	Et-epimeletic Attention-seeking Solicitation of social interaction May indicate some level of distress or uncertainty More common in very young pups
Whining	Et-epimeletic Attention-seeking Solicitation of social interaction May indicate some level of anxiety or distress Isolation
Howling	Elicit social contact Group cohesion Long-distance communication signal Individual and group identification Statement of presence (indicating that you are there) May indicate some level of uncertainty/anxiety (social contact is reassuring)

TABLE 4-2

Common Signals Given by Dogs and the Context and Circumstances in Which They Are Usually Seen—cont'd

Signal	Context/Circumstance
Moans	Pleasure Contentment
Tail and ears up, one forefoot in front of the other 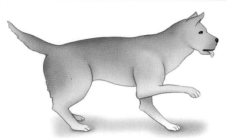	Ready to participate Alert
Direct gaze Note the direct gaze into the face of the human to the right and the erect ears. This dog is being taught to "look" 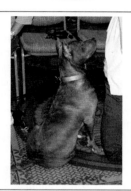	Seeking information Confidence—indicated by the dog waiting for the input of the other; it may be a signal that decreases distance and increases interaction Challenge—only if the sender/signaler is stiff and pupils dilated; it may be a signal that increases distance or decreases interaction Absence of threat and fear
Averted gaze Note: Much is often made about an association between fear and whether you can see the whites of the eyes, but much of the ability to see the whites and assess "meaning" depends on posture. In this photo, the gaze is averted only, and the whites are seen because the dogs are attending to something out of the postural range and they do not wish to turn their entire bodies to focus of the stimulus 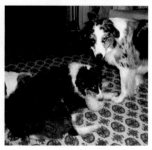 In the photo above, the dog is showing the white sclera of his left eye because he is monitoring the behavior of the person with the second long lead. Here he is avoiding an interaction. Notice the lowering of the head 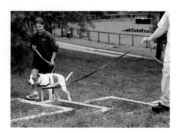	Fear—this assessment depends on the duration of the gaze and the rest of the body signals Avoidance Withdrawal Extreme deference Absence of a challenge—which may not be the same as deference in confident dogs Can be a distance decreasing signal, especially in play when it allows the other dog to make the next move Attentiveness to something out of postural view area

Continued

TABLE 4-2

Common Signals Given by Dogs and the Context and Circumstances in Which They Are Usually Seen—cont'd

Signal	Context/Circumstance

In the photo above, the red merle dog is growling while staring at the dog seated in the rear. All of the dogs are averting their gaze from the dog issuing the threat. They have also stopped their activity, recognizing the threat for what it is. Behaviors such as stopping may abort further aggression, as was the case here, but it would be incorrect and simplistic to interpret any of these behaviors as "appeasement" signals. No one is being "appeased" here. The three dogs who are redirecting their gaze are signaling that they are not threats, and they have stopped to ensure further accurate transmission of information. They are deferring the control of the situation—at this point—to the dog issuing the threat. In essence, they are waiting to see if the aggressive dog decreases his reactivity and threat postures in response to their signals (he did) or whether he becomes more reactive and threatening. The next step in the sequence that defines the outcome will be their response to his follow-up to the averted gazes of his housemates. In this case he walked to the dog at the back and licked at the corner of this dog's mouth. The dog at the back then offered a play bow and everyone moved on. *The frequency of the need to defer to another dog, conveying that you are not a risk, may be a good assay of the stress level in the household or that felt by the dog(s) exhibiting the deferential behavior*

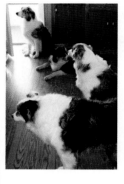

Belly presented
The puppy soliciting play with an open belly is the littermate of the dog standing

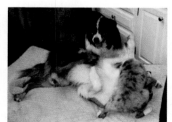

The dog on the bottom is in the process of presenting his belly as part of play with a new puppy, which is being overseen by the oldest dog in the household

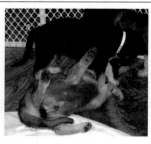

Deference
Relaxation
Solicitation of social sniffing— here this acts as a distance decreasing signal
Stretching—whether this is purely a physical action or also indicates size is not known
Note: The word "presented" here matters. Not all dogs who show their bellies "present" them. Instead, extremely fearful and withdrawn dogs who do not wish to interact and who may feel cornered will roll onto their backs and curl up with their limbs folded over their chests and bellies. These dogs are signaling that they do not wish to interact and that they are concerned. If that dog also is staring at the approacher with the head down so the neck is not visible, the dog may bite if approached

TABLE 4-2

Common Signals Given by Dogs and the Context and Circumstances in Which They Are Usually Seen—cont'd

Signal		Context/Circumstance
Tail tucked when belly exposed	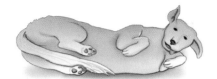	True fear Referred to as "submission" in old literature, but caution is urged because this behavior can occur without a contest. Relative social rankings are fluid and context-dependent in dogs, so such terminology is best avoided Withdrawal from interaction Concern
Tail tucked when belly exposed with urination		Profound fear
Jaw relaxed and open; tongue out	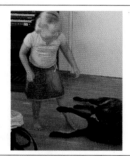	Deference Willing to interact Calm
Grin† Here the grin is given with an open mouth: the dog on the left is not a threat as conveyed by the rolled top lip, but the bark and the opening of the entire mouth convey that play/chase has been too exuberant. The Labrador retriever on the right gets the message	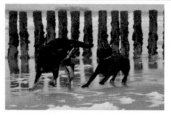	Deference—teeth show but lip is rolled back to reveal gum Lack of a threat Some level of comfort—if seen in one-on-one interactions Willingness to continue ongoing interaction without threat Distance decreasing signal
Piloerection The bimodal pattern of piloerection so commonly associated with fear aggression	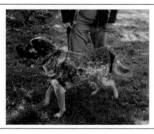	Arousal Uncertainty—generally if hair is raised only over rump Fear—generally if hair is raised in a bimodal pattern over rump and shoulders
Piloerection restricted to neck or along entire dorsum	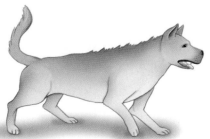	Very confident, aroused dog

Continued

TABLE 4-2

Common Signals Given by Dogs and the Context and Circumstances in Which They Are Usually Seen—cont'd

Signal	Context/Circumstance
Rigid stance, stiff torso 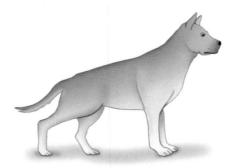	Arousal Assertiveness Possibly forceful Distance increasing signal that encourages avoidance of interaction, if extreme Confidence and potential to interact present, depending on approach, if less extreme Notes: (1) Attention to other signals must be paid, and all signals should—and will—be congruent in these dogs; (2) by itself, this signal says nothing about aggression
Tail above horizon or topline 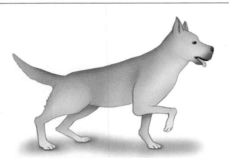	Confident dog Assertiveness Dog actively attending to social and physical circumstances
Tail below horizon or topline 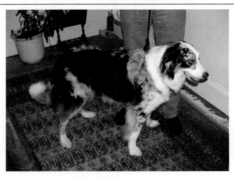	Less confident—this assessment depends on the patterns of the individual dog Less focused or attentive Relaxed—this assessment depends on the patterns of the individual dog Note: All interpretations of tail postures require knowing what is typical for the breed. Dogs without tails cannot be easily evaluated for such signs, and breed groups such as sighthounds always have lower, tucked tails
Tail wag This dog is wagging his tail while growling. Note the direct gaze and ears that are up and forward. This dog is fearfully aggressive, but the closer he is approached, the fewer choices he has. Here, the wagging tail likely indicates that an interaction that humans will view as negative will occur if they approach. 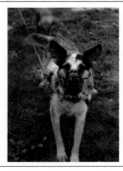	Willingness to interact—the interaction does not have to be good; type of interaction will depend on integration of all other signals

TABLE 4-2

Common Signals Given by Dogs and the Context and Circumstances in Which They Are Usually Seen—cont'd

Signal	Context/Circumstance
Tail tip wag, stiff	Confident Assertive Can be seen with frank aggression Potentially offensively interactive
Neck erect or arched	Confident Challenging Aroused Possibly forceful
Neck displayed—head deflected to the side 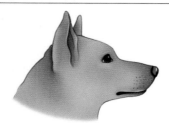	Deference Lack of any threat
Ears erect 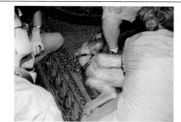	Attentiveness Gathering information Assertive Confident
Ears back Note that the ears are back, the dog's back is turned, he is closed to the interaction as indicated by the tucked tail, and forelegs and hind legs pulled to close off his chest and belly. Note the averted look that shows the sclera. He is avoiding another dog who is staring at him 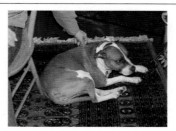	Concern Uncertainty, anxiety Fear—ears may move and not always move in the same direction Withdrawal Unwillingness to engage or comply
Ears vertically dropped 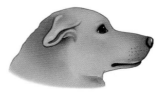	Deference Withdrawal from interaction True fear and concern Less assertive, lower "ranking" dog in group—caution is urged for assuming or imposing absolute ranks in dogs Inability to engage or comply

Continued

TABLE 4-2

Common Signals Given by Dogs and the Context and Circumstances in Which They Are Usually Seen—cont'd

Signal		Context/Circumstance
Snarl/growl only with incisors and canines apparent Notice that the square mouth threat is accompanied by erect ears and body stiffness	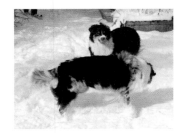	Assertion True, confident threat Activity halting signal Confidence Offensive aggression
The above close-up photo shows the square jawed snarl with full closed teeth. The upper lip is *not* rolled back over the gums	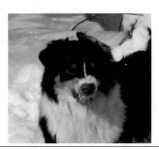	
Snarl/growl with all teeth and back of inside throat and ventrum of neck apparent	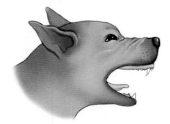	Defensive aggression Fear Distance increasing signal Avoidance preferred, aggression as a last resort Representation of individual as an accurate or true threat Classic redundant signal that clearly indicates intent
Body lowered	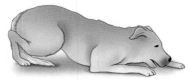	Deference Relaxed Defensive Withdrawn Lack of activity/interaction Distance increasing or decreasing depending on the context and congruence of the rest of the signals
Licking lips		Uncertainty Anxiety "Appeasement" Et-epimeletic Distance decreasing Solicitation of information

TABLE 4-2

Common Signals Given by Dogs and the Context and Circumstances in Which They Are Usually Seen—cont'd

Signal		Context/Circumstance
Flicking tongue		Uncertainty Anxiety "Appeasement" Et-epimeletic Distance decreasing Solicitation of information Fear Aerosolization of volatile compounds
Raising forepaw The dog in the foreground is showing a very clear intention signal to pursue the other dogs as part of a threat sequence. Notice that both other dogs are turning their necks away from each other and the dog in the foreground. The dog in the back also has his paw up signaling a change in movement away from the threat	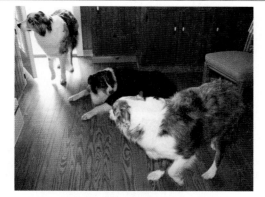	Intention signal—usually for movement or a change in behavior Distance decreasing signal Solicitation of interaction/ attention Deference—waiting and off-balance
Paws out, front and down, rump up, broadly wagging tail	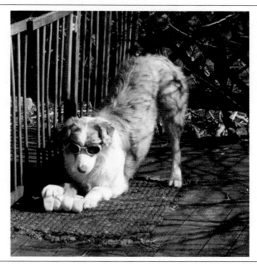	Play bow Body bow Classic play posture Distance decreasing signal Solicitation of attention Deferential signal—the dog is off-balance and vulnerable

Continued

TABLE 4-2

Common Signals Given by Dogs and the Context and Circumstances in Which They Are Usually Seen—cont'd

Signal		Context/Circumstance
Paw pressure/touch	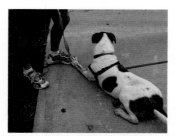	Uncertainty Passive monitoring of activity Early warning signal for movement
Perpendicular posture (T-posture)	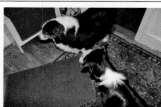	Threat Challenge Request for information about intent Confidence Assertiveness
Mounting or pressure on back or shoulders of another dog		Challenge Solicitation of information Assertiveness
Licking at the corners of another's mouth The young puppy is licking the corner of the mouth of the older dog as a deferential signal seeking information. Notice that the older dog's neck is showing and his head is turned signaling that he is no threat to the pup	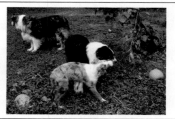	Et-epimeletic Information seeking Deference Solicitation of signals/information
Blowing out lips/cheeks		Anticipation—positive or negative Uncertainty Anxiety—if very fast
Popping or snapping of upper and lower jaw ("bill pop" sound)		Capitulation Intent to comply as a less desirable outcome Pushiness Assertiveness Note: If this is accompanied by licking of the lip on one side of the face and turning that side of the neck to the recipient, this is a true deferential gesture but one that has been negotiated. Such an outcome would not have been the signaler's first choice

*The photos in this table illustrate some more complex examples of the signals to illustrate why all aspects of the signaling system matter and why congruence between signaling systems is valuable.
†Photo courtesy of Dr. Tiny de Keuster.

These associations will be helpful in conducting the information assessment as discussed subsequently.

- When looking at any dog, the first thing that we should assess is how the dog is standing. What is the relationship of the tail, head, and neck to the back or topline?
- Is the head tucked?
- Is the hair up on the back or the neck, and if so, where? Where the hair is raised matters because not all piloerection is signaling the same thing.
- Is the neck stiff, in which case the head will appear pulled in and the shoulders bunched, or is the neck extended and relaxed, giving a long line?
- Is the head and neck fluid and firm but turned away from the other dog? Dogs who are showing that they are no threat expose their necks. This is one of a series of deferential behaviors.
- Can the teeth be seen? The amount of tooth and gum visible is important and dependent on context. Dogs who are no threat show all their teeth, the underside of their throat, and the inside of the back of the throat.
- What about the tail? Is the tail up, down, tucked, or curled? Is the tail in motion? If the tail is moving, is all of it moving, or is just the tip vibrating? Is it moving and high, or is it moving and low? We need to know because there are profoundly different implications for these postures. Tails affect how dogs balance (Wada et al., 1993), but they also affect how reliably the signaler is perceived to communicate by another dog. When exposed to a dog robot whose tail length and wag frequency could be varied, dogs of all sizes more readily approached the robot with the long, wagging tail versus the one with the short, still tail (Leaver and Reichem, 2008), suggesting that longer moving tails may provide more or more reliable information. Given the constraints of canine visual abilities, movement may render tail signals more visible. There may also be information in whether the tail moves from left to right or right to left. Quaranta et al. (2007) showed that dogs indicated specific differences and whether they recognized the approaching human by changes in tail wag direction and deviation, something likely to be readily observable to another dog but less so to an inattentive human. In one study (Bradshaw and Brown, 1990), most of the interactions associated with wagging tails were aggressive interactions, but tails that wagged loosely below the horizon correlated with a friendly approach. Regardless, the greater the frequency of wagging, the more aroused the dog. Tail movement may also involve olfactory and auditory cues because air is moved.
- Where are the feet, and how are the limbs held? Are the limbs stiff, in which case most dogs are angled a bit forward? Are the legs widely spaced, or are they simply in a relaxed position under the dog in a place driven by the anatomical constraints of that particular dog?

All of these behaviors must be interpreted within the bounds of the relevant context. A context is a set of events, conditions, and changeable recipient characteristics that modify the effect of a signal on a recipient's behavior. Context includes both immediate and historical factors. Sources of contextual information include the characteristics of the recipient and the sources external to the recipient (i.e., the signaler and the setting). If the signal itself does not provide enough information, the role of context is critical. One criterion by which abnormal behaviors are gauged is whether they are contextually appropriate. Some behaviors about which clients complain could be normal, appropriate, in-context behaviors, but still undesirable.

Figure 4-1 provides a good example of why these postures and relational body positions matter. If clients and the veterinary staff do not know what *normal* body postures are for the dog, they are incapable of understanding when these postures become *abnormal or worrisome*. If the staff and clients do not understand what signals and postures are routine for the dogs in certain circumstances, they cannot know that these have changed and may merit concern.

The best investment any client or clinic can make in behavior is a *video camera*. If clients take still photos or videos at least once a week while the puppy is becoming a dog and at least once a month once the dog is 1 year old, they will see problems or concerning behaviors as they develop, when it is easiest to intervene.

Veterinary practices should have charts and descriptions such as those in this chapter on the wall, laminated as teaching aids, or available as handouts so that the postures can be discussed at each visit as part of behavioral wellness exams and anticipatory guidance.

Basic Canine Signals

The dog in position 1 in Figure 4-1 is calmly attending to the environment. He is neither overly aroused nor disengaged. He is allowing the information in the surrounding physical and social environments to inform his behaviors. In these illustrations, the model dog is a German shepherd. *It is essential that a dog's individual behaviors are understood and interpreted in the context of the breed/morphology of the dog because you can interpret deviations from normal only within the context of "normal" for that individual.* You need to ensure that colloquial information about breed biases and assumptions is not driving the client's description or the veterinary staff's interpretation.

German shepherd mixes, as portrayed here, often have erect ears, strong heads, and sloping backs. Pay attention to the degree of slope in dogs who are at risk

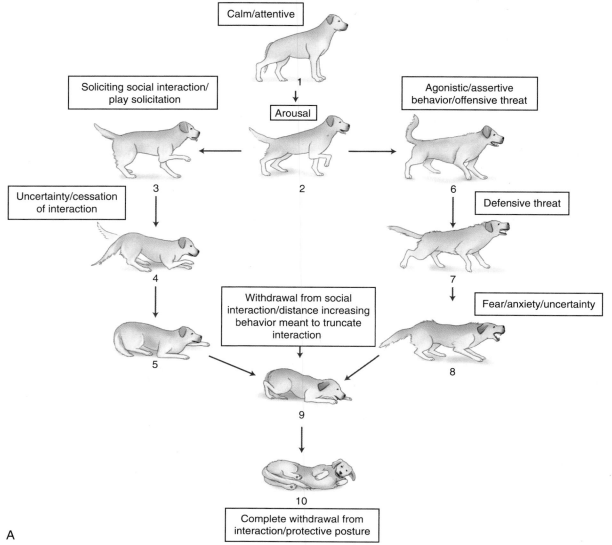

Fig. 4-1 A and **B,** Classic canine behavior postures using a shepherd mix type dog and soft-eared mixed-breed dog as models. Note that the terms as labeled are not those of the original authors. While these behaviors are portrayed as directional sequences, order is not deterministic. For each step portrayed, it is possible that the dog not only could go backward but also could move on through a series of behaviors not portrayed before displaying another of the hallmark behaviors illustrated. (Adapted from Overall, 1997, with permission from the Monks of New Skete, 1991).

for hip dysplasia. *Dysplastic dogs may be in pain and have orthopedic or neurologic impediments to signaling clearly.* This is a serious concern when meeting dogs and humans whom they do not know if their behaviors are to be clearly understood.

Under normal and healthy conditions, the tail, when at rest, hangs loosely in only a slight arc to the ground. For dogs of other morphologies, the posture associated with calm attendance to the environment will differ. *Encourage clients to photograph or videotape*

their dogs when they are calm so that they know what calm looks like.

The dog in position 2 is aroused. The head and neck have moved forward, the dog's ears have begun to rotate a bit more forward. The dog's hind legs are more widely spread, and the rear feet are now parallel to provide more stability. The hind end musculature is tenser than in position 1. The tail is raised above the topline and straight. One front foot is elevated in what has been called an "intention movement." Intention

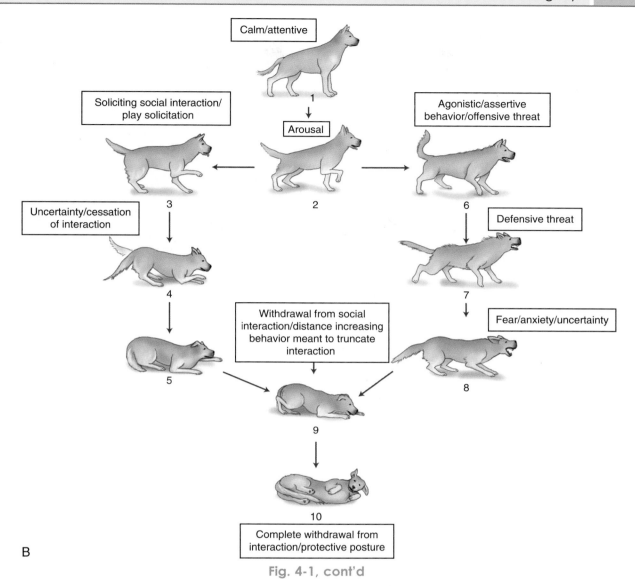

Calm/attentive

1

Arousal

2

Soliciting social interaction/
play solicitation

3

Agonistic/assertive
behavior/offensive threat

6

Uncertainty/cessation
of interaction

4

Defensive threat

7

Withdrawal from social
interaction/distance increasing
behavior meant to truncate
interaction

5

Fear/anxiety/uncertainty

8

9

10

Complete withdrawal from
interaction/protective posture

B

Fig. 4-1, cont'd

movements signal a willingness and likelihood of changing positions. Note that the intention movement itself does not tell you in which direction the dog will move or whether the arousal is friendly or agonistic.

The dog in position 3 has a topline that is close to horizontal to the ground. The raised tail is clearly moving, widely and loosely without tension. Compared with position 2, the head and neck are relaxed, and the dog's jaw and ears are loose and relaxed. The forepaw is raised, and this dog could easily put the ventral surface of his forelegs flush with the ground, while keeping his hind end up in the air. Were he to do so, this behavioral posture would be called a "play bow."

In position 4, the entire dog is sinking toward the ground. His forelegs are flush with the ground, but his entire back end is also sinking down. His tail is

becoming still. His head and neck are also lowering. His ears are going back. This dog is becoming increasingly uncertain and disengaged. Disengagement in the face of uncertainty is a normal and adaptive behavior in dogs and most other social animals. This dog is taking himself out of the interaction and becoming smaller and less apparent as he does so. He is becoming still, which attracts less attention, but he is watchful.

In position 5, the dog has committed to the withdrawal. He is using the ground to anchor himself. His neck is withdrawn as he sinks into himself. His tail is still and wrapping around his hind end, closing any activity and beginning a process of disengagement and withdrawal that is complete in position 10. Compare this posture with an intermediate posture seen in Figure 4-2, where some of the dog's movements are constrained by a wall.

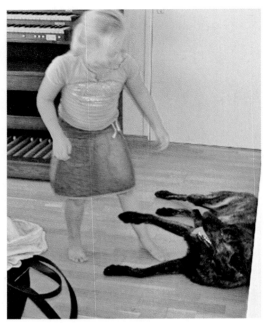

Fig. 4-2 A girl approaching a young Belgian malinois whom she knows. The dog is lying down and rolling over, but her back is against the wall, limiting her mobility and signaling options. This dog is happy to have the girl approach to pet her belly: her hind legs are bent and open; her front legs are open and relaxed, not held tightly together; she is rolling onto her back in a way that will expose her belly; she is looking at the girl with a loose, relaxed jaw; and her tongue is calmly lolling from her mouth.

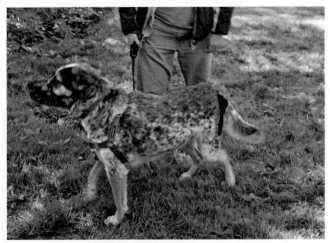

Fig. 4-3 A dog with true fear aggression shows the bimodal dorsal piloerection pattern classic for fearful, anxious, and uncertain dogs.

The dog in position 9 is even more withdrawn than the dog in position 5. He is flush with the ground; his tail is limp and tucked; his neck is withdrawn; his ears are soft, down, and back; and his head is close to the ground. This is a canine cringe. He is looking at the focus of his attention so that he can accurately assess risk, but he must look up, through his brow, because his head is lowered. Notice that the dog's back feet and toes are arched in case he has to move away.

The dog in position 10 is not "submissive," as is traditionally thought. He is not submitting. He is completely closed to outside interaction and withdrawn in a protective mode. He is not only as small as possible, but he also is rolled into a ball with his tail up across his belly, between his legs. His legs are pulled over his belly and chest. His neck is invisible because his snout is tucked. *This dog wants nothing more than to be left alone and to be thought invisible. These behaviors are protective behaviors associated with fear and entrapment and should not be the object of anyone's training method.* This dog will resist interaction, and if he truly feels a threat or is reactive, he may bite if someone reaches for him.

Position 6 represents what happens when, instead of play (position 3), the response and sequelae to arousal is agonistic. The dog in position 6 is stiff, he is leaning

further forward and has moved his center of mass and balance. His back legs are widespread, providing him with a stance from which he could pivot to a number of other postures. His tail is raised up, stiff, and wagging at the tip, a reminder that a wagging tail indicates only a willingness to interact—not the quality of that interaction. His neck is tensed, as are the muscles of his face and head. His ears are rotated forward and his jaw is tense and squared. Piloerection is uniform down the dorsum and, possibly, down part of the tail. The jaw is squared, and the ventrum of the neck is not obvious and is instead tucked up by the squared shoulders, head, and jaw. This is an assertive dog who would be confident in a fight or attack. This is the type of posture that is seen in learned or natural assertive, offensive threats.

The dog in position 7 has become more defensive. His body is still stiff, but it has lowered. The tail is no longer stiff and has also lowered. The ears are no longer forward and have begun to rotate in unconnected directions as the dog seeks to sense threats from all acoustic angles. The ventrum of the neck shows, and the dog's jaw is no longer square. The pattern of piloerection is changing and is no longer uniform but beginning to show the bimodal pattern that is fully developed in position 8. This dog is showing only a defensive threat. He could become more assertive and aggressive, more fearful and aggressive, or less reactive, depending on the response received to his threats.

The dog in position 8 is a fearfully aggressive dog who mixes the signals of these two painfully reactive states. He is low to the ground and crouched. His tail is low and arced toward his hind end. His ventral neck is fully exposed, and his dentition is fully exposed. His ears are floppy and rotating. The bimodal pattern of piloerection being most prominent over his shoulders and rump is now fully pronounced (Fig. 4-3). This pattern is seen only in fearful, anxious, or uncertain dogs. Confident dogs, such as the dog in position 5, may raise their hair over their entire dorsum or only over their shoulders and ruff but not over their rump. The dog who is showing position 8 is disclosing all of his vulnerabilities and weapons. He is displaying that he is not a threat. This is less an "appeasement" behavior than it is a set of signals to encourage increased distance and disengagement.

No one signal is completely clear in its meaning when alone. Congruent signals are important for clear understanding of behavior. This means that the tail posture and movement will match the overall body height and facial signals. *The more congruent all the signals are, the more certain the signaler is.* When information is important, redundant signals are the rule whether the focus is encoding genetic information or social information.

The same approach can be taken with facial expressions. In Figure 4-4, the *x* axis is labeled as "increasing fear" from left to right, and the *y* axis is labeled as "increasing aggression" from top to bottom. The *x* axis could also be called "increasing uncertainty/anxiety," and the *y* axis could be called increasing "assertiveness/agonistic behavior." The overall determination of the dog's signaling behavior *as made by the receiver of the signal* will depend on:

1. the extent to which all facial and body signals agree,
2. the order in which signals are shown or the direction in which they develop (e.g., is the dog becoming more or less reactive?), and
3. whether and how changes in signaling correlate with follow-up responses from the receiver of the original signal. It is important to realize that for distressed dogs this last point may be more a function of previous experiences and learning/memory pertaining to the distress than of the current context.

Interpretation of behaviors depends on context, and the social and signaling behaviors of others are a major contributor to context.

Aspects of faces to which attention should be paid are the height and position of the ears; the shape of the brow ridge, which can be changed by facial muscle contractions; the relative posture of the head to the top of the neck; the position and activity of the lips; and any movement of the nose. When considering face 1 in Figure 4-4, we see the face of a dog that corresponds well to body posture 1 in Figure 4-1. The ears are erect but not sharp and rigid. The ears are forward but not fixed. The eyes are attentive but not narrowly focused, and the brow ridge is not tense. The jaw and lips are taut without being loose and in motion or rigid. The nose is not dripping liquid, and the nostrils are likely changing shape as the dog senses the ambient environment. The dog's head is sitting high on the neck. This is the face of a dog who is surveying his environment in an attentive, relaxed manner.

As we move from face 1 to face 7, the dog's head sinks into the neck. The chin is slightly tucked, but the lips and cheeks are softer in face 7 than in face 1. The ears are no longer rigid: in face 4, the ears first lose their rigidity and then begin to fold back and down. By face 7, the ears are fully back and down and flaccid. The brow ridge is no longer firm in face 4 and is completely soft in face 7. The nose may be dripping liquid. The eyes in face 7 are softer and are in more motion than in faces 4 and 1.

As we move from face 1 to face 3, an already alert head becomes aroused and forceful. The dog's head does not lower, but because of contracture of neck muscles and raising of hair, the neck in face 4 is larger than the neck in faces 1 and 2. The ears move even more forward, becoming narrower and more rigid as we move from face 1 through face 2 to face 4. The brow ridge is pronounced in face 4 and frames tightly focused eyes. The muscles of nose and cheeks are contracted in face 4, rippling the nose and tensing the cheeks. The jaw is square and set. In face 4, the canines are the most readily visible teeth. Neither the inside of the throat nor the underside of the neck is easily seen.

By face 9, the underside of the neck and the back of the throat are apparent, indicating that the animal is posing no risk and disclosing the size of his weapons. The ears are neither flaccid nor rigid but instead are moving. They are partially erect and configured in different directions, indicating a large amount of muscle tone and the potential for quickly changing signals. The hair on the back of the neck is up but the overall neck is no longer thick and threatening. The brow ridge is not apparent, and the dog does not have a complete field of vision with the head and nose elevated. The nose may be dripping. While we cannot hear this dog, this set of facial signals correlates with variable, high-pitched barks, growls, and whines. Face 1 correlates with low growls and more continuous, sustained vocalizations.

The dog with face 7 is usually considered fearful, but he could be anxious or uncertain. The dog with face 1 is usually considered aggressive, but he could be assertive or displaying offensive aggression. Offensive aggression is a normal part of canine behavior, but it is also a behavior that is trained for some protection dogs. The dog with face 7 is usually considered fearfully aggressive, and it may be best to say that he is conveying mixed and changing signals because he is not wedded to one set of responses. Instead, this dog is trying to negotiate as little damage as possible and could flee without biting, as can be seen in body posture 8. Dogs with faces 4, 5, 7, 8, and 9 all will intensify their behaviors if abruptly approached and given no options. Only dogs with faces 4 and 7 are likely to freeze. Dogs with faces 5, 8, and 9 will be more likely to bite but only if given no escape or no signals that de-escalation is possible.

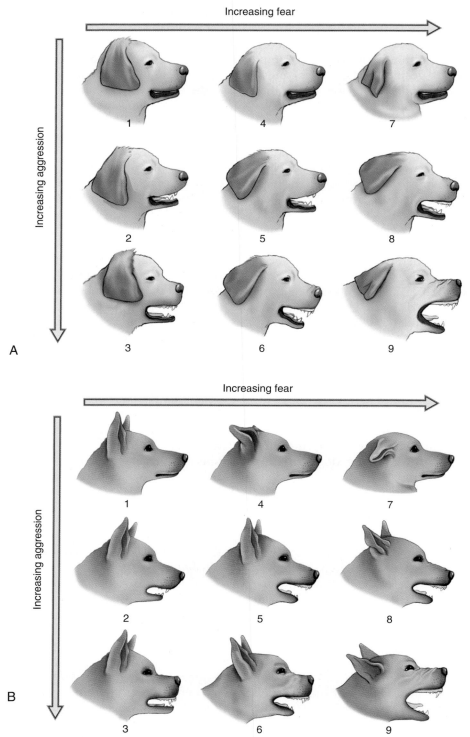

Fig. 4-4 A and **B,** Classic facial signals using a German shepherd mixed breed dog and a soft-eared mixed breed dogs as models.

It is important to remember that behavior is a dance, not a series of line drawings or snapshots. In Figure 4-5, the behavior of two wolves engaged in a complex sequence is captured in line drawings made from a few still shots from film. All wolf signaling behaviors are likely conserved in dogs. Artificial selection has favored more elaborate signaling in some groups of dogs. These drawings wonderfully illustrate how fluid canine behaviors are, *emphasizing the extent to which dogs ask questions to gain information and rely on redundant signaling to ensure that they are clear.*

In Figure 4-5, *A,* the individual on the left puts his paw below the neck on the shoulders of the individual on the right. Concomitantly, he is also gently but firmly grabbing the jaw of the individual on the right. The individual on the left has a loosely hanging tail, a normal stance, and ears that are back and shows no piloerection. The individual on the right has an elevated and stiff tail, cocked and forward facing ears, and a stiff back. *Note that the individual on the right has turned his neck so that it is visible by the individual on the left.* This posture is maintained in Figure 4-5, *B.*

Turning the neck away from another dog, especially if done with a fully open mouth, signals that there is no risk to the second dog. Full disclosure of the number, size, and health of teeth/weapons potentially involved is important because it minimizes the chance that the behavior is misunderstood or becomes more antagonistic (Figs. 4-6 and 4-7). Contrast these postures with

those of the dog in Figure 4-8, which shows face 4 from Figure 4-4.

In Figure 4-5, *B,* the individual on the left has backed up. He is no longer touching the individual on the right, and every aspect of his posture is the same except that his mouth is softly open. His mouth is neither slack nor stiff, but there can be no mistake that his jaw is a bit loose. This behavior has been called a "deferential grin or grimace." By backing away and waiting, the animal on the left is asking a question and providing time for the animal on the right to respond. In

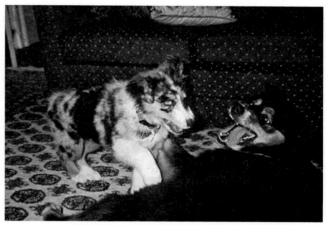

Fig. 4-6 A 2.5-year-old Australian shepherd *(right)* playing with a 9-week-old pup who is about to land on and grab her. *Notice that the older dog shows the side of her neck and all of her teeth.* She is ensuring that the interaction is interpreted as play and that the young dog understands that she is not a threat. This is interesting because the older dog has been almost completely blind from congenital cataracts since 5 weeks of age.

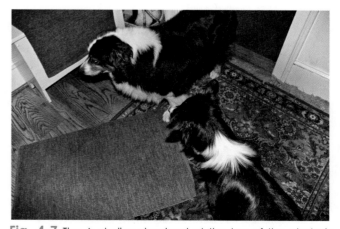

Fig. 4-7 The Australian shepherd at the top of the photo is being threatened by the border collie at the bottom. To show he is not a threat, thereby diffusing the situation, he turns his head and exposes the side of his neck, changing the orientation of the classic T-challenge in a small but meaningful way.

Fig. 4-5 **A-D,** The classic line drawing of a wolf interaction from Schenkel (1967). (Adapted from Schenkel, 1967, with permission.)

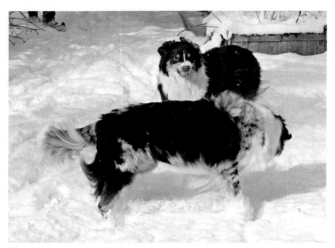

Fig. 4-8 The red Australian shepherd is showing the closed mouth and fairly serious threat shown in face 4 of Figure 4-4. These dogs are circling each other and having a serious disagreement. Note the hair up over the neck and shoulders of the merle dog in front.

Figure 4-5, *B*, the response of the animal on the right is to stiffen a bit (look at the back legs) but not do much else.

In Figure 4-5, *C*, the animal on the left intensifies his response and asks the question again. The animal on the left is now exhibiting the body posture of the other animal. This is a heightened state of arousal, and when behavior changes in this manner it can be viewed as a threat. The agonistic level of the interaction has changed because the animal on the left still cannot learn whether the animal on the right is a true threat to him. He can learn if this is so by provoking the situation by raising the level of threat given.

In Figure 4-5, *D*, we see the outcome of the question posed in Figure 4-5, *C*. The animal on the right is no threat. Instead, he lowers his body and tail, tucks his tail and limbs to indicate that he is not a threat, and is withdrawing from the interaction; also, he licks the mouth of the animal on the left. Licking the mouth is a behavior derived from et-epimeletic solicitation behavior. Dogs who lick the corners of the mouth or the lips of any species are asking for information. Sometimes this information is olfactory, and it is not unusual to see dogs who have been away from other dogs across a pasture or wood open their mouths in response to licking of their lips and teeth by the dogs who did not accompany them. *This type of behavior doubtless provides information about food and about behavioral state as respiratory samples likely carry much neurochemical information.*

The role for a deferential grin/grimace, with or without licking, has been underemphasized. Figure 4-9, *A*, shows a border collie exhibiting the grin, which exposes her upper gum, to her humans. Note that her

nose is wrinkled. This is a solicitous signal that is shown to ensure that the others in the interaction understand the lack of aggressive "intent" and will be shown only to someone whom the dog trusts. For an example of this behavior offered to another dog, see Figure 4-21, *E*, later. The Dalmatian in Figure 4-9, *B*, is exhibiting the deferential grin, but in this case it is part of a signal that is communicating the dog's anxiety as part of being needy. This Dalmatian was diagnosed with attention-seeking behavior and separation anxiety. The constant licking of the nose and lips (Fig. 4-9, *C*) that accompanied the grin is due to anxiety. Note that both of these dogs show their canines, and both wrinkle their noses, making these signals difficult for someone who does not watch dogs all the time to understand. These dogs are both sitting, and it is common, but not mandatory, for dogs exhibiting these signals to be sitting or lying down. Normal dogs have no difficulty understanding these signals.

Licking the lip/corner of the mouth of other dogs is normal behavior that initially solicits feeding (et-epimeletic) from an older dog and develops into a behavior that is both deferential and involves seeking information (Fig. 4-10). Clients need to understand this ontogenic history so that they interpret the signal correctly.

There are some general patterns of behaviors that, if they can be recognized, will help clients and veterinary staff to understand better and help their canine patients. The aggressive components of agonistic behavior can include:

- stalking, with the head and tail down but with the ears pricked, the back arched, or the hindquarters raised,
- chasing, pouncing, and spraying,
- the perpendicular posture, or T-posture, where one dog stands with his or her head or neck over another dog (see Fig. 4-5, *B*),
- a mobile or distant T-posture (Fig. 4-11; see also Figs. 4-7 and 4-8),
- walking around an adversary in a stiff-legged gait with neck arched and neck and tail raised with or without a stiffly wagging tail,
- overt attacking and biting,
- specific attacking of the face and shoulder with seizure and shaking,
- piloerection,
- baring of teeth with the vertical retraction already described, and
- turning the head away from an adversary.

Turning the head away has been characterized as an "appeasement" gesture; this is probably inaccurate. Only a very confident animal can afford to back down at the apex of a disagreement, so this signal is better understood as one that communicates to the receiver that if he or she will do the aggressor's bidding, the aggressor is willing not to let the aggressive act escalate

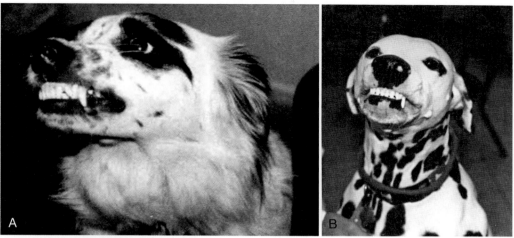

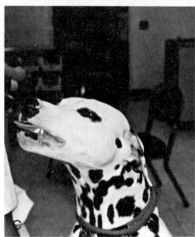

Fig. 4-9 **A,** A border collie with a grin that leaves her upper gum exposed and her nose wrinkled. This "grin" indicates an intent to show no aggression and is given only to humans she trusts. **B,** A Dalmatian showing a grin that communicates anxiety and neediness. **C,** The same Dalmatian licking his nose and lips, which is a symptom of his anxiety.

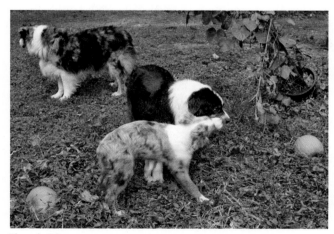

Fig. 4-10 A 7-week-old puppy licking the corner of the mouth of a 14.5-year-old dog as part of a deferential greeting behavior. The puppy had just entered the household as a rescue. The licking at the corner of the mouth is an et-epimeletic (care-seeking) behavior.

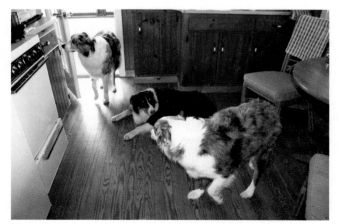

Fig. 4-11 This photo displays a mobile and more distant T-threat. The dog in front is staring at the dog in the back at the doorway and is assuming a nose-to-shoulder challenge, long distance. Both the red dog in the middle and the dog at the back are averting their gaze and turning their necks to show that they are not a threat.

further. Dogs who turn their heads and necks display that they are no threat (see Figs. 4-6 and 4-11).

Defensive and deferential behaviors usually involve a *greeting approach* designed to lower arousal levels:

- the forequarters of the body are lower than the hindquarters,
- the head and neck are usually extended and swung from side to side, and
- the side or the dorsum of the neck is bared.

If such defensive or deferential behaviors are successful, the behavioral sequence proceeds through flexing of the back, going down on one hip, and ultimately rolling over and presenting the neck and the inguinal region for sniffing or licking by the other animal.

Signaling behavior involved in *active defense* includes behaviors that show that the recipient of the initial aggressive display will respond should the challenge continue. Piloerection and snarling with visible teeth are common under these circumstances. These are exaggerated behaviors, and exaggeration may indicate that the signaler is not willing to aggress actively but will actively defend itself. These animals will also turn their heads away and, while baring their teeth and showing eyes, bare their neck. This is not a contradictory signal. The signaler is conveying a message to the aggressor that the signaler is willing not to engage, but if the aggressor pursues the attack, the signaler will retaliate rather than acquiesce.

Passive defensive behavior can involve:

- sitting,
- crouching,
- running away,
- licking of the lips and showing of teeth,
- the submissive "grin" with the lips retracted horizontally,
- the tail between the legs,
- the ears depressed and an indirect gaze,
- forepaw raising,
- rolling onto the back with the legs extended,
- lateral recumbency with an elevation of the topmost hind leg to give access to the inguinal region,
- recumbency and complete inhibition of movement in a tonic immobility,
- urination and/or defecation, and
- a silent, quiet stance while the aggressor places its feet on the animal's back.

The last signal listed is a signal by default—what the animal is really doing is not meeting a challenge. It is important to remember that when animals do not do something, they are still conveying information. Absence of a signal can function as a signal itself.

Aggressors who have already made the decision to attack usually do so with a stealthy approach. This approach may include crouching body posture and a lowered head and changes in ear postures. As aggression intensifies, ear postures change from erect to flattened. The first clue that an individual might become aggressive to another animal is the intense nature of the physical orientation demonstrated toward the potential victim.

In contrast, friendly approaches include bounding, a head position that is level with or above the body, decreased body tension (this is probably a correlate of not tensing muscles for attack), loose ears that possibly may be folded back and down, and a very loosely carried body (Fox and Bekoff, 1975).

Size also matters in understanding interactions between dogs and roles played for clarity of signal. When faced with a dog robot, larger dogs were more likely to approach the model, approach without stopping, return to approaching if they paused ($P < 0.08$), and touch the robot as part of their approach (all $P < 0.05$ except as noted) (Leaver and Reichem, 2008). Smaller dogs may be more hesitant because should they misinterpret the signal, it increases their own risk. Additionally, small dogs may not view some visual signals given by larger dogs with the clarity possible for dogs who are similarly sized or larger than the signaler. Uncertainty in visual signaling may be a concern for brachycephalic breeds whose eyes and brains are rotated compared with dolichocephalic breeds (Roberts et al., 2010), especially considering that the distribution of retinal neurons depends on whether the dog is brachycephalic or dolichocephalic (McGreevy et al., 2004).

Finally, as is true with the finding of puppies raised with cats, if dogs do not experience a variety of types of dogs and other animals when young, they will have difficulty reading and understanding their signaling behaviors. We assume that social decisions that are made are "informed," but this may not always be true. An informed decision is a response that is characteristic of the recipient of communicatory signals (Green and Marler, 1979; Hailman, 1977; Markl, 1985; Smith, 1977). In abnormal, out-of-context situations—the sphere of most behavioral problems—the recipient may not be able to be informed, and difficulty in understanding signaling is at the core of many anxiety-related conditions. In problematic social interactions, any number of steps could be affected.

- The receiver of the signal may be unable to read or interpret the signal correctly.
- The receiver of the signal may be able to read/ interpret the signal but may be unable to process the information they read or interpret appropriately.
- The receiver of the signal may be able to read/ interpret the signal and process the information it contains but may be unable to formulate an appropriate response.
- The receiver of the signal may be able to do all of the aforementioned correctly but may be unable to signal their responses well or clearly in a timely and contextually relevant matter.

Any or all of these steps could be affected in pathological or troubled social behaviors. It is essential that the veterinary staff, trainers, and clients understand signaling as part of their assessment of interactions between dogs and between humans and dogs. Dogs play better and more enthusiastically with people who understand and offer canine signals (Fig. 4-12) (Rooney and Bradshaw, 2001). Play postures can be assumed to be important because they appear to be innate and not learned: hand-reared puppies use play postures (Bekoff, 1972, 1974, 1977).

It is important to interpret canine behaviors from the dog's contextual viewpoint. Behaviors associated with the development of agonistic behavior are also those associated with play:

- stalking other pups with the head and tail down and the hindquarters up with ears erect,
- chasing, ambushing, and pouncing on littermates,
- standing over a littermate with the head and tail erect and the neck arched,
- circling a littermate while wagging the tail with an erect, assertive walk,
- attacking and biting, primarily around the littermate's neck and face,
- piloerection, primarily on the back of the neck,
- snarling and showing teeth, primarily the canines,
- a direct stare at littermates without dilation of the pupil,
- shoulder and hip slams,
- placing forepaws on a littermate's back,
- boxing,
- mounting with or without pelvic thrusts, and
- wagging only the tip of an erect tail.

The sets of associations discussed can provide information about any interaction. For individuals who will watch and examine the same dogs interacting over time, shifts in body postures can be indicative of social shifts in households. See Figures 4-13 and 4-14 for an example. The family photo album or video collection will contain clues for understanding problems among family pets that will illustrate any developing conflict.

Figures 4-13 and 4-14 show an adult dog who is 3 years of age in a classic and wholly normal play posture with a puppy who is 9 weeks of age. In Figure 4-13, the adult is giving the classic play bow, and the puppy is relaxed and stretched out with her upward paw ready to reach for the older dog.

In Figure 4-14, the adult and the pup are engaging in mutual cheek chewing. This behavior is often ritualized in older dogs and can be used to determine if the recipient is a threat. If this behavior is a threat, it is used to intensify a challenge. Because Figure 4-14 shows

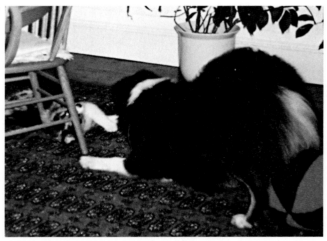

Fig. 4-13 A 2.5-year-old dog and a 9-week-old puppy playing.

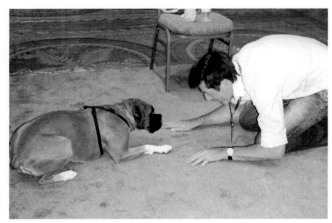

Fig. 4-12 This boxer was said to "not be able to play." When a human played with him the way dogs play, by assuming the same bow and lunge postures, the dog not only played, but he also was completely focused on the first person who had ever made sense to him.

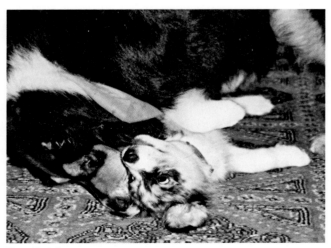

Fig. 4-14 The adult dog has taken the side of the puppy's head in her mouth in play. No one is injured here, and this is normal play behavior.

early play, this behavior is ritualized and mutual, demonstrating to both dogs that there is no threat and the actions are truly play. Other clues include the floppy nature of the puppy's limbs, the loose, relaxed ears exhibited by both dogs, and the exposed belly of the puppy. Dogs feeling threatened or closed to social interaction tuck all of their limbs over their chest and belly.

Figures 4-15 and 4-16 show a less joyous relationship. In Figure 4-15, the older dog has sequestered all the toys, and the younger dog has turned her head and neck away, while putting her ears stiffly back. This is not a relaxed dog, but one who is trying to avoid a confrontation. The older dog is staring at the youngster, her face stiff, her ears stiff and forward, and her countenance intense. In Figure 4-16, the older dog is being called away from the younger. Her entire posture, which is stiff, shows that she is not happy with the situation.

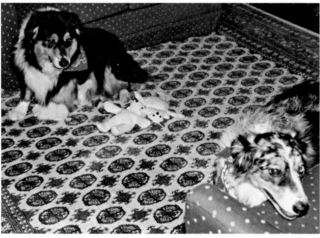

Fig. 4-15 The same dogs 4 months later when the puppy is 6 months old.

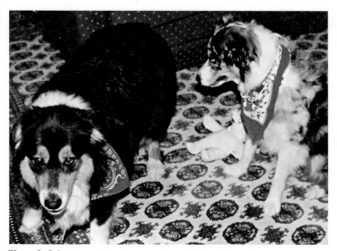

Fig. 4-16 The older dog on the left, being called away from the younger dog minutes after Figure 4-15 was taken.

When the younger dog is 18 months of age and in the midst of social maturity, the body language is clear (Fig. 4-17). The older dog is staring at and clearly threatening the younger dog. Notice that dog is occupying more of the couch. The younger dog is looking obliquely away, clearly signaling that she is not a threat. In fact, she is not even sitting down; she is merely perched, another true sign that she might need to flee quickly. Were this not the case, she could easily curl up in that area. She would have to go through many more behaviors to leave than she does by assuming this posture.

Figure 4-17 provides insight into the future. A few months later, the older dog attacked the younger, rupturing some ocular vessels. Over the next year, the aggression intensified to the point that the younger dog engaged in preemptive attacks whenever she saw the older one and became fearful of other dogs. Separating the dogs allowed them to remain in the household, become independently happy, and, for the younger dog, to have other dog friends free from fear (see the section on inter-dog aggression).

In the end, context matters. Figure 4-18 shows why not all piloerection signals are a concern but that they always signal information. The standing dog is a Rhodesian ridgeback who has limited choice about how he presents his pelage. Dogs can learn about other dogs and vagaries of breed, such as bobbed tails, but they also learn to interpret another dog's signaling because of congruent signals given by other body parts. In Figure 4-18, the ridgeback's ears are really loose, as are his lips, and the pups are clearly playing. The beagle is pushing back with all four feet and giving a deferential grin/grimace, reinforcing the idea that this is play, not a threat. Notice, too, that although these pups are mismatched in size, their play is equal, and the ridgeback is not over-running the smaller dog.

Figures 4-19 and 4-20 show the adult version of a big dog/little dog play. The little schnauzer is considerably

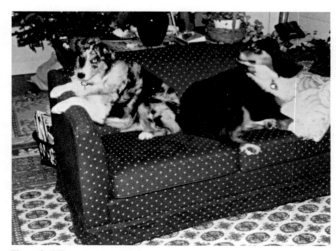

Fig. 4-17 The same dogs shown a full year after Figures 4-15 and 4-16. Note the relative body postures of the dogs.

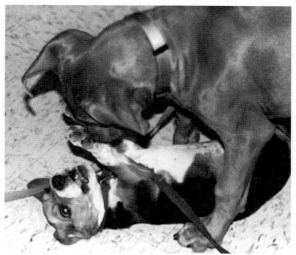

Fig. 4-18 A beagle playing with a Rhodesian ridgeback puppy.

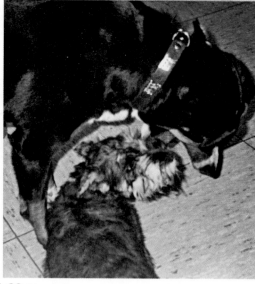

Fig. 4-20 Play between a miniature schnauzer and a Greater Swiss Mountain dog.

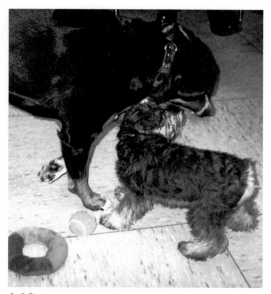

Fig. 4-19 Two household dogs of different breeds playing.

disadvantaged in size and with respect to signaling capabilities—he has no tail and is fluffy enough that even if he does piloerect, it will be tough to see. That said, his ears, which have not been docked, are floppy and relaxed. He has leaned into hind legs, and he has a broad stance with both forelegs and hind legs. If he were being serious, his legs would be stiff and long. If we look at the Greater Swiss Mountain dog, his stance is relaxed as can be ascertained by the fact that he is off-balance. His hind legs are broad and unevenly spaced; little weight is on his right hind leg, and his left forepaw is raised, signaling that he will change directions.

The neck of the Greater Swiss Mountain dog is out and down—a concession to the height difference—but it is not stiff, and his hair isn't raised. Additionally, his ears are loose and floppy because this interaction is all about play. Finally, the mouth of the big dog is open wide, even exposing his teeth. This is because he is no threat and is communicating that clearly by showing all his weapons.

An open-mouth response to rough play is shown in an intensified form in Figure 4-20. Notice that the schnauzer has completely turned its neck, also showing that he will relinquish the control of the play bout, at this point, to the larger dog. These two photos elegantly hint at the ballet that is dog play.

Figure 4-21, *A*, shows the young dog grabbing the black dog's ear and side of the neck in a play challenge. The black dog has turned and held his neck away, showing that he is not a threat, and the puppy is lying down and partially under the black dog. The puppy must reach up to grab the black dog.

In Figure 4-22, the puppy in Figure 4-21 is grown up and now raising a puppy himself. Note that the same play behaviors are recapitulated and that the older male who raised this dog is now supervising his play with the new pup.

We should remember that play is a behavior that has many roles. Play functions to (Fagen, 1981):
- stimulate communal behavior,
- facilitate social interaction,
- mold adult behavior, particularly through the role of the learning curve,
- establish early, strong social relationships,
- enhance physical and mental dexterity,
- improve coordination,

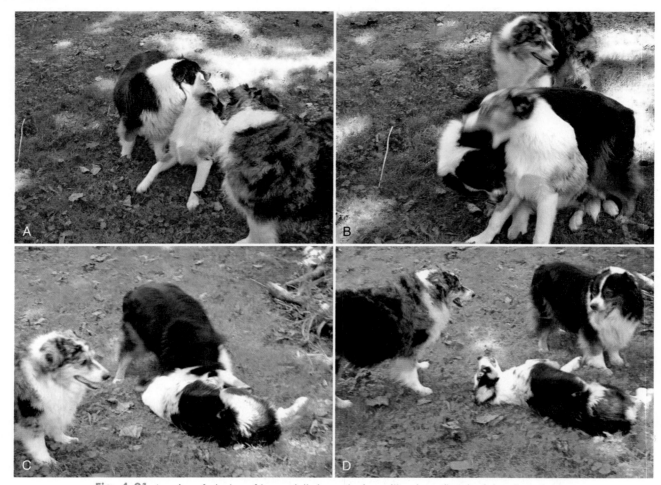

Fig. 4-21 A series of photos of two adult dogs playing with a juvenile who is less than 1 year of age. Dogs, similar to most social animals, engage in their most personal behavioral exchanges in dyads. Dogs will play in groups but they, like us, can focus on only one other dog at a time, although they can quickly shift their focus to another dog. **A,** The young dog is grabbing the black dog's ear and side of the neck in a play challenge. The black dog has turned and held his neck away, showing that he is not a threat, and the puppy is lying down and partially under the black dog and showing no signs of distress. **B,** The black dog is grabbing the puppy's leg as the puppy grabs his neck. Note that the black dog is standing over the puppy and that this entire posture is fundamental to how dogs wrestle. **C,** The black dog is grabbing the puppy as the puppy pulls him down using his mouth and forelegs. What is most interesting in this photo is the second adult, who is carefully monitoring this activity. **D,** The black dog has disengaged and handed off control to the merle adult dog on the left. That dog is carefully watching the puppy who is showing warning signs of rolling over to reach up and grab her. As the other adult assumes control of the interaction, she gives a sharp bark, which is a redundant signal ensuring that everyone is in agreement about relative roles.

- provide a venue for safe experimentation and the first, demonstration of ritual and ritualized behaviors,
- provide puppies with an outlet to learn about social rules and predictability through sequences of events,
- provide puppies with an outlet for exploration, and
- provide them with a safe outlet for increasingly complex problem solving.

In short, play teaches animals about social relationships and how to make mistakes successfully within them. Given this, we should encourage clients to understand normal play behavior and have their dogs participate in it, whether it is with dogs or humans.

Canine Vocal Communication—What Can Dogs Hear?

Dogs can detect frequencies of sound ranging from 40 Hz to 65 kHz, whereas 20 kHz is the upper frequency range for humans. Dogs (and cats) can discriminate one-eighth to one-tenth tones (Ewer, 1973; Neff and Diamond, 1958). Dogs are *most sensitive* to sounds

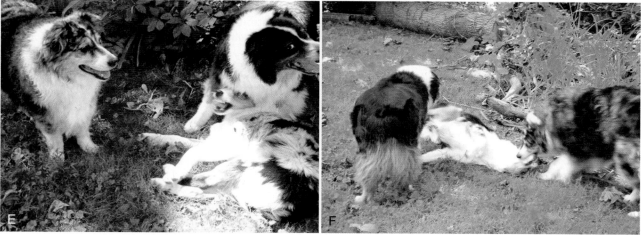

Fig. 4-21, cont'd E, The roles have switched again, and both adults have disengaged, although the puppy is still ready and willing to play. Notice that you can see all of the puppy's upper front teeth and the gums. The beagle in Figure 4-18 is doing the same thing, and the dog in Figure 4-9, A, is engaging in a similar behavior in a different but related context. He has rolled back his lip—a signal that is found only when two conditions are met: the dog is comfortable with and not threatened by whomever is receiving this signal, and the signaler wants to ensure that everyone understands that his behavior is play. This is an important distinction because many people who are unfamiliar with or misguided about dogs think that all showing of teeth is problematic and a threat. **F,** Both dogs are attending to the puppy; while the black dog noses the puppy's crotch while pushing against his legs, the merle adult grabs the puppy's mouth gently in her jaws in response to some of his grabbing behaviors. No one was injured at all in any part of this sequence, but the sequence emphasizes that wrestling in dogs involves their mouths and teeth because dogs don't have opposing thumbs (a primate trait). Dogs have thicker skin than humans, and some of these same wrestling behaviors could mildly injure humans. If the human became angry in response, this would be an out-of-context and problematic response for the dog.

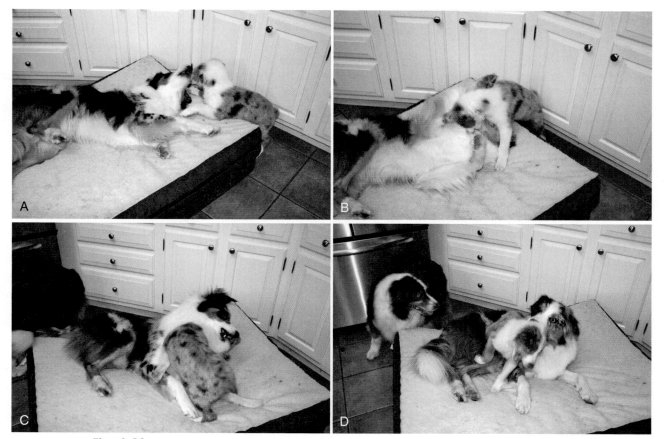

Fig. 4-22 A-D, The puppy from Figure 4-21 is grown up and now raising a puppy himself. The same play behaviors are shown.

with frequencies in the 0.5 to 16 kHz range. Within this range, their sensitivity threshold can be *24 dB less than that for humans* (see Fay, 1988, for a more detailed discussion). Bear in mind that the daily peak values in kennels of all kinds routinely exceed 100 dB and often reach 125 dB (Sales et al., 1997). These capabilities inform the vocal signals that dogs use.

Canine Auditory Signaling—Signals Using Sound

Canine vocal communication has been categorized into five basic sound groups based on overall function:
- infantile sounds, including crying, whimpering, and whining,
- warning sounds, including barking and growling,
- eliciting sounds, including howling,
- withdrawal sounds, including yelping, and
- pleasure sounds, including moans.

Wolves bark when strangers approach a pack and growl when challenged or when eating, but they whine when greeting each other. Howling acts as a social coordinator in wolves. The preservation of neotenic behaviors that has occurred in domestic dogs has exaggerated this role. Barking in domestic dogs announces the presence of someone and may identify the approacher. It has been said that stray dogs seldom bark (Beck, 1973), but few good data are available. If you do not wish to be located, not barking is smart.

Whining and howling behaviors are et-epimeletic behaviors. Whining is among the first sounds a puppy makes. Howls carry a long distance, and wolves are said to distinguish strange adult howls from strange pup howls and answer only the former (Harrington and Mech, 1982).

McConnell (1990) looked at two specific signals that are frequently used by trainers: (1) short, rapidly repeated, rising notes that are postulated to elicit a "come" response and (2) one long note that has been asserted to elicit a "stay" response. Short, rapidly repeated notes elicited a "come" response, but one long note did not elicit a "stay" response, as many handlers believe. The solitary long note was associated with decreased motor activity. Signals that inhibit behavior may have two main varieties (McConnell, 1990): signals that are designed to slow or soothe, such as the long continuous notes that have little frequency modulation, and signals that are designed to stop, which consist of one, short, rapidly descending note (McConnell and Baylis, 1985). In this context, it is interesting that canids use short, rapidly repeated whines to elicit an approach by conspecifics (Cohen and Fox, 1976).

Vocal sounds associated with agonistic behavior include growling, barking, snapping of the teeth, gaping (which is a noisy, yawning display), and pawing with or without growling. Much frank aggression is quiet.

Dogs do not continuously bark in response to every stimulus, and they do not use the same bark in all circumstances. We can measure aspects of vocalizations by using sonographs/spectrograms—voice spectrographs—of the vocalizations. Using recordings of dog barks, Molnar et al. (2006, 2008, 2009) demonstrated that, regardless of their experience with dogs, most humans would correctly identify a dog who was vocalizing in a fight and one who was vocalizing when a stranger approached. Less agreement was found for dogs who vocalized on walks, in play, when alone, or on being given a ball. This finding is important because it means that *people may be confident that they recognize a frank aggressive or alert response, but that they may not know that they do not accurately identify the information contained in barks or other vocal signals in other situations.* Yet, we can demonstrate that the information contained in vocalizations across such situations is different.

In a study that examined growls in three contexts (play, when guarding a bone, and when approached by a threatening stranger), Faragó et al. (2010) found that play growls differed from growls in the two agonistic contexts with respect to frequency and formant dispersal: play growls had higher frequencies and lower formant dispersal. Although lower frequency growls usually correlate with larger dogs, it's important to note that growl frequency has a functional component that can be altered by contracting the muscles of the throat. Formants—the amplitude peaks in the spectrum considered—can also be functionally altered: when a dog stretches his neck, he behaviorally lengthens his vocal tract and disperses formants, making him appear "larger" to someone who has made the general association between these vocal characteristics and dog size. Maros et al. (2008) demonstrated that such information content is recognized by and affects dogs. Dogs' heart rates were measured in response to a series of auditory cues and found to increase significantly after hearing a recording of a dog barking at a stranger.

Yin and McCowan (2004) demonstrated that classes of barks and other vocalizations are consistent among different dogs, given the specific context. They identified three contexts (play, isolation, and disturbance) where the 10 pet dogs tested vocalized in ways that were sufficiently similar that it was clear that the signature of the bark was associated with the context (Fig. 4-23). When this happens, we know that dogs are communicating useful, context-dependent information, and we can learn from it.

Another study of canine vocalization that compared barks from dogs with a diagnosis of separation anxiety with barks from dogs who were unaffected showed patterns similar to those reported by Yin and McCowan. The bark of the unaffected dog in Figure 4-24 is an alerting bark, similar to the high-frequency, solitary note shown by dogs in play, but the repetitive, atonal, complex barks of the dog with separation anxiety

	Disturbance	Isolation	Play
Farley			
Freid		None	
Keri			
Louie			
Luke			
Mac			
Roodie			
Rudy		None	
Siggy			
Zoe			

Fig. 4-23 Three contexts where 10 dogs vocalized in ways that were sufficiently similar that it was clear that the signature of the bark was associated with the context. (From Yin and McCowan, 2004.)

Fig. 4-24 The vocalization of a dog who is alerting to someone he can see passing by his window. This bark is similar to the high-frequency, solitary note shown by dogs in play.

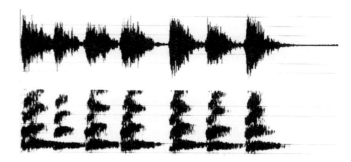

Fig. 4-25 The repetitive, atonal, complex barks of a dog with separation anxiety resembles the vocalization given in both the play and the isolation contexts.

(Fig. 4-25) resemble the vocalization given in both the play and the isolation contexts (Overall, unpublished). Dogs can clearly recognize the information provided in such signals, and for us to understand dog behavior, we must do so also.

Humans have been shown to classify the "emotionality" of canine vocalization with respect to tone, pitch, and inter-bark interval (Pongracz et al., 2005, 2006). Taylor et al. (2008, 2009, 2010) manipulated both formant dispersions and fundamental frequency and learned that lower formants and fundamental frequencies were rated as belonging to larger dogs, and participants gave more weight to formants, which more accurately reflect vocal tract length because they correlate with the weight of the dog.

Dogs are cognitive and complex, and their signaling behaviors are a reflection of these characteristics. Dogs use signals to convey information and to provoke the social situation to gain information. When we evaluate or classify canine behaviors, we need to be acutely aware of these patterns and how inadequate our labels can be for conveying such complexity.

Canine Olfactory Signaling—What Can Dogs Smell?

Dogs have the greatest olfactory acuity of any domestic species.

- We used to understand that dogs could detect concentrations of a substance at $\frac{1}{100}$ of the strength that humans can detect (Moulton et al., 1960)—at diluents of $\frac{1}{100}$ to $\frac{1}{10,000,000}$ (Becker et al., 1962). Careful, naturalistic tests of olfaction in two dogs indicated that they could detect odor at 1.14 to 1.9 ppt, *lower— by 20,000-fold to 30,000-fold—than previously believed or reported* based on laboratory data (52 to 32,600 ppt) (Walker et al., 2006).
- Dogs have 2.831^8 olfactory cells and 7000 mm^2 of surface area (humans have 2.31^7 olfactory cells and 500 mm^2 surface area).
- Dogs can detect fingerprints 6 weeks after they were placed on a pane of glass (King et al., 1964) and can individually identify twins based purely on odor (Kalmus, 1955, cited in Houpt, 1991).
- In a test to determine whether an individual can reliably discriminate between humans and identify an individual regardless of the origin of the body

odor, gauze pads soaked with secretions from exocrine, eccrine, and sebaceous glands were tested in a rigorous experimental design (Toner and Miller, 1993). The dogs investigated were experienced police dogs; they had a 93.3% success rate in correctly discriminating not only the scent of the individual but also the body part from which the scent came. If clothing was used, the accuracy increased to 100%, suggesting that a large scent pool helps.

Viral respiratory conditions affect dogs' ability to smell. Dogs apparently recover their sense of smell 6 weeks after infection with nasal respiratory viruses. The extent to which intra-nasal vaccination affects odor detection capabilities has not been reported, but the effect is likely non-trivial.

We should remember that illness, vaccines, cleansing agents (e.g., bleach kills olfactory neurons), et cetera, all may have an effect on olfactory ability, which could affect signaling. Because humans have a relatively poor sense of smell, they underplay any role for changes in olfactory ability in relationships between dogs and humans or other dogs. If we watch the dogs, they do not have this constraint.

Canine Olfactor Epithelium and Olfactory Receptors

Dogs have an exquisite sense of smell partly as a result of a large and complex olfactory epithelium. The area of the olfactory epithelium in some dogs has been cited to be 170 cm^2 (Bear et al., 2001), and the number of olfactory neurons has been estimated to be 1 billion.

ORs are found on ciliated membranes of olfactory sensory neurons in the olfactory mucosa. Efficient odor discrimination requires that ORs bind with odorants and that this process trigger a signal transduction pathway that allows information to be processed and acted on via connections in the olfactory bulb and brain cortex. Absence of, or blocked, ORs means that little information is available later for cortical processing. Naturalistic testing has shown that the threshold at which dogs can detect odor, 1.14 ppt and 1.9 ppt, is much lower—by 20,000-fold to 30,000-fold—than previously reported (Walker et al., 2006).

OR genes are members of the G protein–coupled receptor (GPCR) superfamily, which contains approximately 1300 genes in dogs (Olender et al., 2004) and is one of the largest gene families in mammals (Buck, 2000, 2004). All GPCRs have seven transmembrane domains, of which the intracellular and extracellular loops are polymorphic in all species studied, including dogs (Tacher et al., 2005), and are important for odor discrimination. Perception of odor relies on three stages of processing in the brain after OR binding: memory of odor quality, memory of odor intensity, and range of intensities and qualities over which the odor is generalized (Masek and Heisenberg, 2008).

The question arises whether specific dogs or breeds are particularly skilled at odorant detection. It is often asserted, but seldom tested, that genetic differences in olfactory abilities exist across individuals and breeds (Issel-Tarver and Rine, 1996; Rooney and Bradshaw, 2004). If dogs vary in ability to detect odors, are dogs who are more skilled more efficient in initiating the signal transduction cascade, or do they have different alleles encoding ORs with greater odorant affinity (Robin et al., 2009)? Studies suggest that attribution of "ability" is not going to be straightforward.

No studies couple true, measured, olfactory acuity to specific haplotypes/genotypes. Some small studies have begun to compare variability in genotypes with respect to dog breeds and/or performance of dogs in specific tasks. These studies suggest that there has been no strong selection for more variable OR genes or proteins. It is possible that there may have been stronger selection pressure to maintain the structure of the parts of the OR associated with odorant binding than to maintain the part of the protein involved in signal transduction. If this is true, it may mean that dogs with particularly acute olfactory detection capabilities may perform so well because they are particularly good at processing and acting on olfactory information, not detecting it. If so, aspects of communication between the dog and handler may be more important for the success of detection dogs than has previously been believed (Gazit and Terkel, 2003b; Goodwin et al., 1997; LeFebvre et al., 2007; Szetei et al., 2003).

Canine Olfactory Signals—Signals Using Smell

Little has been published on normal social aspects of marking in domestic dogs, including scent marking with feces and anal sac secretions. Scent marking has been more fully investigated for non-domestic species and is thought to play a profound role in intra-specific hierarchical organization (Gosling, 1982; Kleiman, 1966; Peters and Mech, 1975; Ralls, 1971; Rieger, 1979). Comparable data for domestic dogs are limited, but scent is likely to be important in subtle interactions.

Anal sac secretions are normally eliminated with feces and leave a unique odor (Bradshaw et al., 1990; Natynczuk et al., 1989). Anal sacs can be forcefully expressed by scooting. The extent to which this would leave a physical and olfactory cue has been under-investigated in the literature. Anal sac secretions can provide an individual identification for greetings between dogs that know each other (Fox and Bekoff, 1975). This may be the basis of part of the social role that ear sniffing can play in hierarchical interactions (Overall, 1995b). Anal sacs are often emptied when the dog is excited or distressed, suggesting a signaling capability that is often noted but seldom explored.

Scratching may disperse scent, but dogs seldom scratch the exact area where they urinated or defecated. It is impossible to rule out the role of the interdigital glands, merocrine sweat glands (pads), or sebaceous glands (found on hairy, interdigital skins) (Bradshaw and Brown, 1990) in the role of marking by scratching. Scratching, whether accompanied by urine or feces, provides a two-pronged visual display.

- First, the animal exhibits a species-specific posture during the scratching.
- Second, the animal leaves olfactory and visual marks (Bekoff, 1979a, 1979b).
  - Urine deposits of male dogs do not appear to repel conspecifics (Bekoff, 1979b; Scott and Fuller, 1965). This does not mean that urine deposits of dogs do not contain information. Other information may be provided by urine, including data about the specific individual involved, specific identification of the social group involved (implied by Scott and Fuller, 1965), sex, recency of visit, duration of visit, food eaten, and health status. All of these cues could allow dogs to make decisions about how to allocate their time and energy in that physical area.
  - Olfactory communication can act as passive social behavior and may act to decrease active agonistic interactions.

The extent to which olfaction plays a role in modulating social interactions can be affected by sexual dimorphism.

- Males are more likely to mark with feces than are females (Sprague and Anisko, 1973).
- Male dogs are more strongly attracted to the urine of an estrous bitch than they are to the vaginal or anal sac secretions of the bitch (Doty and Dunbar, 1974), but males need mating experience to respond to estrous versus anestrous females (Beach and Gilmore, 1949).
- Males without mating experience also appear to respond to these substances, but the other attendant changes in their behavior have not been well investigated.

Countermarking is marking with urine on another dog's urine (*overmarking*) or in the close vicinity of (*adjacent marking*) another dog's urine. Reproductive wolves to whom others defer countermark more than other wolves, and the presence of testosterone during the breeding season can increase urine marking in both sexes of wolves (Asa et al., 1990; Mertl-Millhollen et al., 1986).

In laboratory studies where urine was presented to dogs, males overmarked more than females (and usually over estrus females) (Dunbar, 1977, 1978). This pattern has been thought to indicate that the males were masking the presence of the female's urine from other males (Dunbar and Buehler, 1980), but, given the sensitivity of canine olfactory capability, the information received in response to an overmark may suggest how one should spend one's efforts, depending on demography of other dogs present. If this is true, how one overmarks is as important as what one overmarks.

- Lisberg and Snowden (2009, 2011) examined countermarking in dogs (Labrador retrievers) in parks. Both males and females investigated and marked at scentposts (locations, usually with a visual landmark, where dogs serially countermark).
- Tail position is important in signaling relationships between and behavioral intent in dogs (de Meester et al., 2008, 2011; Quaranta et al., 2007).
  - Tail base position may co-vary with any pattern of countermarking.
  - Males and females with high tail base position urinated, investigated urine, and countermarked more than same-sex dogs with a lower tail base position (Lisberg and Snowden, 2011).

Patterns of overmarking differ from patterns of adjacent marking. For overmarking:

- Males in general overmarked urine more frequently females, but they did so equally for known and unfamiliar dogs.
- Intact males overmarked urine of intact females more often than urine of intact males.
- As previously noted, males and females with higher tail positions countermarked more than same-sex dogs with lower tail positions.

For adjacent marking:

- No sex adjacent marked more than the other.
- Males and females adjacent marked only the urine of unfamiliar dogs.
- There was no effect of tail base height on any aspect of adjacent marking.

These data suggest that urine marking at a minimum provides information about identity, sex, potential sexual receptivity (and when relevant), and familiarity and social relationship among dogs. Urine marks are available over time, whereas the visual signal of the dog marking is available only at the moment. For dogs who exhibit indoor urine marking associated with anxiety, this finding may be important.

Both visual and olfactory signals—and the type of information contained in them—are important *to the dogs*. Urine marks are unique in that they can be revisited over time and compared with the urine of other dogs or the same dog over time. These types of information are important to dogs, and dogs make keen distinctions: the urine of spayed females is not as interesting as the urine of intact females regardless of estrus status to intact male dogs (Lisberg and Snowdon, 2009), suggesting that different types of information are used for different tasks. This same complex pattern of information gathering should apply to dogs who mark with feces or anal sac secretions, dogs who roll in feces, and dogs who mark using other parts of their body by rubbing against an object or person.

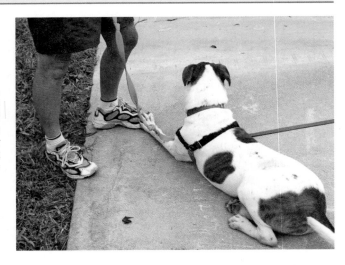

Fig. 4-26 A 10-month-old dog in a rescue center during a behavior modification session designed to help him to learn not to react to approaches of some strangers. His foot is resting on the shoe of the volunteer with whom he has been working and whom he trusts as others move around. This tactile gesture allows him to monitor the movements of the person helping him without having to look at the person. He is unable to take his attention from busy movements of people in the near distance.

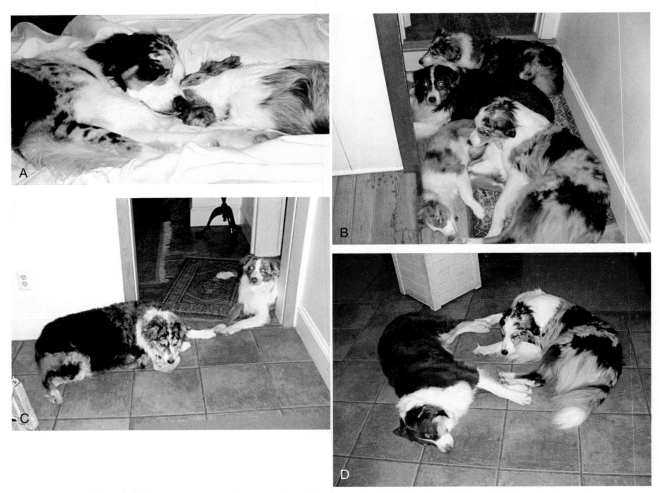

Fig. 4-27 Patterns of tactile behaviors with dogs who live together. **A,** An older dog on the left, sleeping with a young puppy on the right. The pup's head is under the face of the older dog. **B,** The black dog is days from dying of hemangiosarcoma. The other dogs, including the 5-month-old puppy, went everywhere with him as a group and stayed with him when he rested. **C,** The older dog *(left)* and the 5-month-old puppy *(right)* the day after the black dog, the oldest dog in the household, died. **D,** A new, 11-month-old rescued Australian shepherd was brought into the household 3 days after the black dog's death. This photo was taken after new dog's first dinner in the new home. The other dog is the now the oldest male. Look at the positioning of the feet.

Tactile Signaling

Tactile signaling in dogs gets almost no attention. This is a mistake. Tactile signaling is among the first signaling to develop in dogs, and tactile stimulation enhances neurodevelopment.

Clients do not realize that they can signal most clearly if their verbal signals match their tactile ones. The single place where this is most important is in petting dogs. People routinely arouse their dogs when petting them by petting in quick, short strokes all over the dog's head, face, and shoulders.

Instead, if we want a thoughtful, calm dog who looks to us for information that is helpful to him, conventional petting must be replaced with long, slow strokes, deep muscle pressure, and massage (see the client handout, "Protocol for Teaching Your Dog to Take a Deep Breath and Use Other Biofeedback Methods as Part of Relaxation," for "smart pet" instructions). Clients are often unaware of the role that their tactile signaling plays for animals. Rapid petting can reflect the client's own level of concern or anxiety or lack of attentiveness to the dog's responses and needs. By videotaping clients with their dogs, mismatches in communication can be identified. Dogs are so attentive to tactile signaling that they may respond to casual signaling from the client as if it were meaningful and so react in a context that the client did not know existed and may find problematic.

Dogs who are uncertain of, are fearful of, or need to control humans often rest a paw against the human (Fig. 4-26): as soon as the human moves, the dog has warning of a change in behavior and can become alert. Dogs who may be unable to interact actively with someone can still monitor their movements if the dog's back is turned to the human but resting to any extent against the human's foot. Tactile signaling has not enjoyed the attention from the research community that it deserves (Fig. 4-27).

Problematic Canine Behaviors: Roles for Undesirable, Odd, and Management-Related Concerns

Problematic behaviors can be loosely divided into two groups: (1) variants of normal behaviors that annoy clients but that respond well to understanding and management and (2) truly abnormal behaviors that are distressing to dogs and humans. Both of these sets of concerns can result in a dead, abandoned, relinquished, or euthanized dog. Where dogs fall on the continuum of "normal" to "abnormal" behaviors will determine the best types of interventions, as shown in Figure 5-1.

MANAGEMENT-RELATED BEHAVIOR PROBLEMS AND CONCERNS THAT DO NOT RISE TO THE LEVEL OF A DIAGNOSIS

Behavioral concerns that don't rise to the level of a diagnosis and management-related behavior problems are usually variants of normal behaviors that annoy clients but that respond well to understanding and management.

- Behavioral concerns that don't rise to the level of a diagnosis may be extreme variants of what could be normal canine behaviors or exhibition of normal canine behaviors but in contexts that may be undesirable or extreme.
- Management-related behavior problems are normal behaviors in most circumstances, but some of them can progress to become part of a behavioral pathology.

This chapter addresses the following common canine behaviors about which clients often have questions or complaints:

- digging,
- jumping, scratching, bolting, and barking at the door,
- grabbing people and/or other pets as they go through the door,
- barking and patrolling when outside,
- mounting/humping,
- rolling in feces,
- eating feces,

- mouthing/grabbing/biting, and
- dogs who never seem to stop moving.

The information and techniques in this section can be applied to any canine behavior that the client does not want or like and which is not due to underlying pathology. If dogs' behavioral, cognitive, and physical needs are met, dogs can learn to substitute different behaviors for those which the clients dislike, will not tolerate, or wish to stop. An expanded version of the information in this section is found in the client handout, "Protocol for Understanding and Managing Odd, Curious, and Annoying Canine Behaviors." *Remember, the keys to successful solutions always involve a humane human response that meets the pet's needs.*

All the behaviors discussed in this chapter are normal canine behaviors. As with all behavioral concerns, the extent to which we understand the behavior to be "normal" depends on:

- the context in which the dog exhibits the behavior,
- the intensity of the behavior,
- the ability of the dog to be interrupted, and
- the extent to which exhibition of the behavior affects other facets of the dog's life in an undesirable way.

All of the behaviors discussed here could become so extreme that they would meet the diagnostic criteria for obsessive-compulsive disorder (OCD). Because we do not understand the early stages of OCD and how it develops, it is important that any client whose dog is exhibiting any of these behaviors should be encouraged to discuss them with their vet, and any dog exhibiting these behaviors should be screened for more serious behavioral issues. Anticipatory guidance is important for management-related concerns.

DIGGING

Most dogs dig, although some do so zealously. Digging can involve raking or scratching a surface a few times before sniffing, eating, defecating, urinating, or turning in a few circles before sleeping.

Understanding behaviors from the dog's view

Normal   Less normal   Truly abnormal/pathological

Dog's behaviors: This is the universe of what is possible. The dog can vary, although the extent to which this is true depends on interactions between the learning and behavioral environments and any limitations posed by the genetic environment.

Intervention level

None/encourage   Client education: Client education, as noted*
                        Environmental change*   Direct redress of pathology*
                        Interaction change*
                        True behavior modification*

*These are not independent

Fig. 5-1 Conceptual diagram of the range of behaviors exhibited by dogs and which types of intervention will be needed or work best. The extent to which the dog's behaviors are less normal and more abnormal is represented as darkening color of the oval from left to right. The intervention level required is matched to the level of pathology.

Why Do Dogs Dig?

Dogs dig:
- to aerosolize existing scent,
- to leave a scent mark of their own,
- because the objects they find are interesting or "play" back with them (e.g., tree roots),
- to search for or find an animal that they hear or smell,
- to extricate something to eat or on which to chew (e.g., truffles, old bones),
- because they are curious and no one is paying attention to them, and
- because they are hot and are trying to cool down, or because they are cold and trying to create shelter.

Roles for Olfaction

- When dogs dig, they aerosolize scents that may have been hidden.
- Most of the information dogs obtain about their physical and social environments is likely done through olfactory means. This may be why dogs sometimes scratch before they eliminate: in addition to learning about who was there before them, they contribute to the olfactory environment when they eliminate, and they wish to gauge how to spend their "olfactory currency."
- Scratching before and after elimination may convey considerable olfactory information itself about a dog's seasonal behaviors, estrus states, social companions, and intruders.
- Dogs tend to scratch more when they are not on their own property or in areas where other dogs pass frequently.
- Scratching is another form of marking that has both visual and olfactory components. We know little about scents that are transferred from dogs' paws, but we do know that this is one body region where dogs can "sweat" and that there are sebaceous glands between the dog's foot pads. Sebaceous glands are the source of oily secretions that may be largely invisible but heavily informative to dogs because of the sensitive canine sense of smell.

Hidden Objects and Play

When dogs dig, hidden objects become found. It's possible that the dog buried a bone where he is digging, but while digging, dogs also discover roots of trees, rocks, old bulbs, et cetera. These are all objects that enrich the dog's intellectual and olfactory environment. In the case of roots and plants, many of these objects "play back." Humans tire pretty quickly when they play a game of tug with the dog—roots of oak trees "play" without tiring.

Roles for Auditory Cues

Dogs may also dig because they hear or smell another animal. Moles, voles, groundhogs, spiders, field mice, white-footed deer mice, et cetera, all burrow to some extent. If the dog sniffs, listens, and paws a bit and then moves on and repeats these behaviors, the dog is likely following cues about where another living animal has been. Some dogs may do this only in snow: some rodents have very elaborate burrow systems and trails under snow, which interest many dogs. When people report attentive behavior, punctuated by listening, scratching, and pouncing in snow, the dog is likely trailing a rodent.

Intellectual Curiosity

Dogs often dig just because they are curious. Attributing every behavior that annoys humans to "boredom" is simplistic and misses the point for the dogs. Dogs that are very social, curious, or active may just be exploring their environment whenever they dig. If their people were to play with them, these dogs might not dig. If they had a companion or went to an inter-active daycare center, they might not dig. If provisioned with appropriate areas for digging in a manner that stimulated their mind (e.g., sand or soil boxes with hidden toys; small pools with floating toys), they'd still dig, *but* their behavior would not be distressing to the clients.

Thermoregulation

Dogs may dig to thermoregulate. During hot weather, dogs dig because the earth is cool. Dogs cool by putting their belly on soil. Dogs can dig holes in the snow or dirt to create a cave-like environment where, if they curl up, they can stay warmer than they would if they were exposed.

How Can We Meet a Digger's Needs?

- Bury rawhides or other treats or toys in a bucket or tub of dirt/sand and let the dog find them.
- Fill small, sturdy plastic pools with water and float food toys (at least one model of Kong floats) and/or "food-sicles" (treats frozen in broth in yogurt containers). "Food-sicles" are mentally stimulating and helpful in the hot weather and can use the same skills involved in digging.
- For dogs who like to dig in really wet areas, fill a kiddie pool with water. Other objects that they find interesting can be added.
- Some newer food toys have expanded on the idea of the original Buster Cube, providing both easier (Roll-A-Treat Ball) and harder puzzles. The premise for all of these items is that when the toy is batted or moved, the treats fall out. The dog is rewarded for getting the exercise of chasing the toys and for the intellectual part of figuring out how best to get the treats.
- For dogs who dig to thermoregulate, provide other thermoregulation choices (e.g., pools, fans, digging pits created by filling kiddie pools with wet sand and placing them under shade trees, allow the dog in or provide a heated dog house in the winter, et cetera). Some vets have cooling/warming packs, if additional heating and cooling is needed.

Are Some Breeds Likely to Be Diggers?

Many dogs dig because they are of a breed that we asked to dig. Jack Russell terriers, Glen of Imaal terriers, fox or rat terriers, et cetera, all were developed to track, chase, and kill earth-dwelling animals. For these dogs, clients may consider earthdog trials (see www.akc.org/events/earthdog for information) where the dog's skill is directed to an appropriate venue for—digging.

JUMPING, SCRATCHING, BOLTING, AND BARKING AT THE DOOR

Jumping can be a normal behavior, and for some smaller or herding dogs we have encouraged that the dogs jump for work, and we have encouraged jumping in play. Sometimes we think it's cute that dogs will jump. Jumping, barking, lunging, and bolting are all behaviors that commonly occur at doors and annoy humans. Unfortunately, humans exhibit behaviors that accidentally encourage these patterns and teach the dogs to perform better the exact behaviors the humans find most annoying.

Following are common *situations created by humans* that turn into *problems for the dogs*.
- Problem A:
  - Dogs have been selected to bark to alert humans to visitors. When people open a door, they do not ask the dog to sit and be quiet before they actually open the door to whomever is on the other side. The dog is now aroused and made more aroused by barking, and standing, at the door in way that the new person is right in front of them when the door opens.
- Solution A:
  - Ask clients to acknowledge the bark, attend to what's going on, and ask the dog to sit and be quiet, then tell the dog that he is brilliant when he sits quietly. Wait until this happens. No one must open a door immediately, and by doing so clients may further stimulate a dog who is already overwhelmed.
  - Quiet can be maintained for many dogs by quickly offering the dogs a toy and telling them they can get up when they "take it." Dogs cannot bark annoyingly with their mouth full, they self-reward for being quiet, and dogs with toys are less likely to jump and instead greet everyone by carrying a toy around and wiggling. This solution is so simple that—of course—few people think of it.
- Problem B:
  - When dogs start to lunge at or through doors or jump on people who are entering, their humans tend to pull the dog back by the collar. Dog push against pressure: this means that when you grab a collar, it tightens under the dog's throat, and the dog lunges harder. Humans then tend to yell at the dog who, understandably, is now fairly confused.
- Solution B:
  - Ask the dog to sit quietly, as noted, or use a physical cue to stop the dog. The client can place a hand gently against the dog's chest so that the dog backs up.
  - Clients concerned about grabbing, biting, or fleeing have two other choices.
    - Isolate the dog behind a baby gate elsewhere before they expect guests. The dog can be let out to join the people when the door is closed, the greetings are completed, and people are calm and sitting down.
    - Put a head collar on the dog when home to supervise him and allow him to drag a light lead that slips through furniture. When someone comes to the door, clients can do the aforementioned plus:
      - Take the lead.

- Ask the dog to sit and ensure that he does so by gently pulling up on the lead.
  - Close the dog's mouth by *gently* pulling forward on the head collar. The dog can then have a toy. If he doesn't like toys, he can have a treat for being quiet. The dog must have a reward once he is calm and quiet; praise is not enough.
  - If clients believe that the dog might snap at or bite the person at the door, *they should not have the dog at the door.* The dog should be behind a baby gate, in a crate out of the way, or locked behind another door. Visitors need to know that the dog might snap or bite and not be able to interact with the dog. Some dogs are too reactive to humanely introduce to visitors, even when on leads and head collars. These dogs are best protected from people, which, in turn, protects the people, too.
- Problem C:
  - People tell dogs what *not* to do but never tell them what *to* do.
  - The dog who is barking at the door wants to ensure that his or her people pay appropriate attention.
  - While the people are telling the dog "no," the dog is saying "yes, yes, there is someone here." The result is some profound cross-communication, which results in the humans raising their voices.
  - There is no need to yell at the dog—the problem is not deafness; it is inadequate signaling.
  - There is an additional liability associated with yelling at the dog—the human becomes upset. This bodes poorly for the dog.
- Solution C:
  - The dog barks.
  - The bark is verbally acknowledged ("Good boy, Flash!").
  - The client goes to what the dog sees or hears ("You're right, Flash, FedEx is here.").
  - The client thanks the dog ("Thanks for letting me know, Flash.")
  - The clients asks the dog to sit and be quiet ("Can you sit and give me a smooch, boy?").
  - The second the dog sits, the client tells the dog she is brilliant and rewards the dog with praise, with a treat, or with a toy ("Oh, you are so wonderful, take your toy!").
- Problem D:
  - Dogs scratch at the door because:
    - There is someone on the other side of it.
    - They have to go out.
    - They get some attention for doing so.
- Solution D:
  - Use a Plexiglas shield on the door to decrease client distress and increase client patience if damage is a concern.

- If the dog is trained to "knock" to go out, or if she trains the client that this is what scratching means, the dog must be let out.
- Alternatively, hang a rope of bells so that the dog hits the bells before the door. Reward the dog for ringing the bell using praise and access to the outdoors. This solution can be combined with a plexiglass shield. Again, if the clients have asked the dog to tell the clients when the dog needs to go out, going out must be part of the reward.
- Make creative use of scratching by putting sandpaper over the part of the door where the scratching occurs. This will keep the dog's nails smooth while also stopping him from damaging the door.
- Encourage clients to go to the door immediately to see if anyone is there. Dogs will intensify their behavior until they get the person's attention.
- Clients can hasten the dog's understanding of his role in starting or stopping this type of "door alert" by using a reward for being quiet. It's a good idea to keep a treat jar or toy basket by the door for this purpose.

GRABBING PEOPLE AND/OR OTHER PETS AS THEY GO THROUGH THE DOOR

Many dogs who grab humans—and who are normal—are just excited. Some dogs who grab humans are not normal and may need to control humans in order to have some sense of security. *We are not discussing the latter group of dogs here.* They are discussed in Chapter 6 and in the "Protocol for Understanding, Managing, and Treating Dogs with Impulse Control Aggression."

Many dogs who grab humans or other dogs as they go through doors are dogs from herding breeds. Not everyone understands that the dog is "just herding you," and many other pets become frightened or injured.

The rule for these dogs is simple: there is a toy basket inside and outside every door and the dog must take a toy and sit quietly before any door is opened (Fig. 5-2). Clients should continue to request that the dog stays as the door opens, then quickly release the dog and let him take himself out of the way. This works if the clients are consistent.

BARKING AND PATROLLING ACTIVITIES THAT OCCUR ON THE STREET

Dogs watch what's happening in their world by looking through windows or doors. Dogs are cognitive and will monitor these activities. We have selected some breeds to be especially vigilant. If the client is not home, these behaviors become reinforced because they are self-reinforcing: your dog sees someone, he barks, he becomes stimulated by his own barking, and then whoever was in the street moves on and the situation

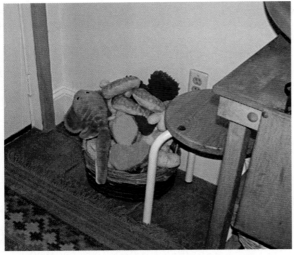

Fig. 5-2 Toys can be kept in a basket placed by the door so that dogs can be handed the toys before going through the door. This prevents the dogs from grabbing humans in their excitement to go outside.

changes. If the dog is inclined to be protective, the situation is even more self-rewarding: he alerted, he protected, and the person who threatened his home left! He succeeded!

Intervention must focus on encouraging the dog *not* to exhibit these behaviors when no one is home.

- Use of a shock in this situation is akin to chopping off a dog's leg to stop jumping.
- Blinds, curtains, barriers, gates, large and spacious crates, et cetera, provide an environment that protects the dog from the stimulus.
- Dogs should be provisioned with other stimulation (e.g., food puzzles, automatic treat delivery systems).
- When clients are home, they should follow the instructions for dogs who are rowdy at doors.
- Clients can also teach dogs to check with them frequently. Ask the dog to sit at the door, and then call him away. If the dog is given a treat every time he leaves the door, calling him from the door will become much easier. By doing this and providing stimulation that does not rely on those who pass by, clients render the dog's behavior easier to interrupt.

MOUNTING AND "HUMPING"

Mounting and humping are not about "dominance" and usually not about sex.

- Both intact and neutered/desexed dogs can mount.
- Both males and females can mount.
- Unless this behavior is part of a sequence in a dog fight or agonistic interaction—in which case the actual behaviors are very different (such behaviors are stiff, directed toward the shoulders and neck, and the dog is very focused and quiet)—most mounting is about affiliation or wanting to be with others or is used as an attempt to get attention.

- Dogs will hump people when they are happy and want the people to interact with them.
- Humping is involved as a part of the sequence involved in sex or masturbation. The form is very different from the affiliative form: sex and masturbation involve fast, repetitive motions, leaning with the face and neck on the object of desire, and facial signal changes. Both male and female, neutered and intact dogs can masturbate.
- It's a normal behavior.
- Because this behavior can be normal and we know that dogs will work for information and a salary, if clients do not wish to be humped or mounted, they can ask the dog to stop and sit and reward that behavior instantly. If the dog goes back to mounting them, they must leave and ignore the dog. They cannot laugh or think this is "cute" and expect to extinguish the behavior (see Chapter 3).
- Because humping can be an affiliative and "claiming" behavior, dogs will often hump dogs of the other sex (usually it's the male who humps the female). Sometimes these dogs will urine mark over the dog they hump and sniff their vulva or prepuce for residual urine. Changing the odor of the urine may change the behavior, but there are no studies to support this. Anecdotal recommendations include feeding herbal mint and chlorophyll.

ROLLING IN FECES

Many dogs roll in feces (Fig. 5-3). The feces chosen is usually that of other dogs or of other species and not the dog's own feces. Feces are often placed on clear signposts by other canids (Figs. 5-4 and 5-5).

Hypotheses about why dogs do this include:
- rolling to disperse and thus lessen the effect of the original scent,
- covering the original scent with the dog's own,
- making a visual statement about the other animal's mark,
- covering themselves in another animal's scent for camouflage,
- using the scent as an insect repellant,
- obtaining chemicals from the feces that help nervous system development and immune health, and
- gaining information from the scent about who the animal was, when the animal last passed through, to whom the individual is related, what the animal had recently eaten, et cetera.

Clients need to understand:
- dogs are washable,
- if unsupervised, dogs who like to do this will do it more often than less often,
- dogs share this information with other dogs and can introduce another dog to the joys of rolling, and

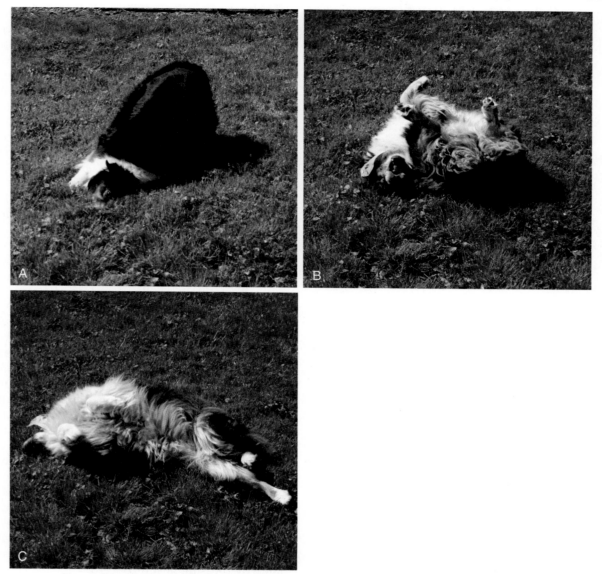

Fig. 5-3 A-C, Photos show how a roll in feces or other objects with the possibility for scent transfer occurs. The dog usually starts with smearing the side of the face and the neck, then moves so that the shoulders and back are also touching the area, and finally rolls back and forth in a stretched-out manner using the back and hips.

- if clients wish to stop the dog from doing this, they must interrupt them as early in the sequence as possible (e.g., as soon as the dog begins sniffing intensely, call the dog away and reward him for returning).

EATING FECES OF OTHER SPECIES

Ingestion of another animal's feces can be either a normal behavior or one of desperation. Starved animals will eat the feces of others. Puppies kept in pet stores and bred in puppy mills/farms may not be fed enough if the pet store or puppy dealer wishes to keep them small and so may be both hungry enough to eat their own feces and under-stimulated enough to use feces as toys. Virtually all pet store puppies and dogs come from puppy mills/farms and likely received inadequate food, care, exercise, et cetera.

Dogs who are *inappropriately punished* for elimination may become ultra-fastidious as a way to avoid the pain and anxiety that they have come to associate with elimination. Some of these dogs will ingest their urine or feces immediately after elimination or as they are eliminating.

Finally, some dogs ingest feces (coprophagia) as a manifestation of OCD. These dogs need more than just management-related help and would benefit from a visit to a specialist in veterinary behavioral medicine.

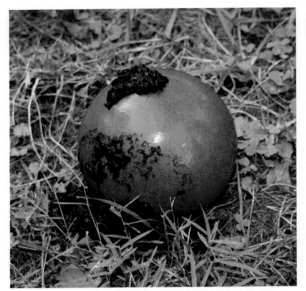

Fig. 5-4 A bocci ball with fox feces that was placed on top of it when it was left outside.

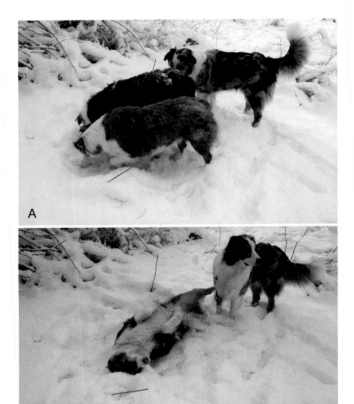

Fig. 5-5 A, Dogs who roll in feces can find feces, even under snow. **B,** One dog rolls in the feces, dispersing it, and leaves a large, visual snow signal that the feces were found by a dog who dispersed them.

Many dogs enjoy snacking on the feces of other individuals. They may enjoy cat feces because the feces are high in protein and animal muscle that is not fully digested. Dogs often love the feces of herbivores (e.g., deer, rabbits, cows, horses), and it has been suggested that this is because these species all use bacteria in their digestion and the bacteria form a source of protein themselves and may help immune function. Additionally, consuming the feces of herbivores can be a good way to get partially digested herbs and grains, such as oats.

Ingestion of feces is not a behavior that is easily amenable to change because it is *normal*. The keys to *controlling* eating of feces are simple but difficult to implement continuously:

- the dog must be prevented from ingesting the feces to begin with, and
- clients must monitor the environment so that they see the feces before the dog does and can call him away.

Any dog who ingests feces should be screened for parasites at least every 6 months, even if the dog is taking a heartworm preventive that also controls nematodes. Other parasites may be involved. Warn clients that some parasites may be transmissible to humans.

If the dog ingests only canine feces, the solution is easy: clean up all dog feces found, including those deposited by other dogs. It is harder to know where the feces of squirrels, rabbits, deer, foxes, raccoons, cats, et cetera, are, and so it is more difficult—and in some cases, impossible—to remove them.

Some dogs can eat feces through muzzles. Muzzles may send other messages to the neighbors about the dog. Some dogs become incredibly unhappy in a muzzle, and the quality of their life declines. Muzzles should be reserved for situations where they are mandated by pressing health concerns.

MOUTHING, GRABBING, AND BITING

Mouthing, grabbing, and biting are common complaints of people who have inadvertently played too roughly with their dog. Mouthing and biting can also be normal behaviors in young dogs. As such, they are almost always amenable to change, but prevention is key. *Veterinarians must be in charge of providing anticipatory guidance and risk assessment.* No puppy should be encouraged to mouth/grab/bite. If these are issues, veterinarians should assess risk to all those with whom the dog interacts and the dog himself or herself. The handouts "Protocol for Generalized Discharge Instructions for Dogs with Behavioral Concerns" and "Protocol for Handling and Surviving Aggressive Events" may help.

Puppies will "mouth" naturally because they use their teeth and mouths much as we use our hands. It is a simple matter to abort this behavior when it is first starting, but mouthing can be tremendously difficult to stop it if it has been ongoing for a long time.

- Clients should be encouraged to consider whether the behaviors that they see in pups are ones they wish to see in their adult dog when they are rushing at a crowded and busy time such as a holiday season.
- Help clients consider the worst-case scenario and take preventive action to avoid or abort mouthing and biting by understanding normal behavior and using that understanding to shape behaviors that they wish to see and that are possible to see in adult dogs.

If mouthing and biting behaviors have just started, they can be aborted easily. The more that these behaviors are reinforced, the tougher interruption, avoidance, and cessation will be.

- Mouthing and biting are self-rewarding behaviors and so can intensify easily if they are practiced with people who have not considered them thoughtfully.
- Clients can intervene in mouthing and biting if they learn about age-related normal behavior and how best to shape appropriate and desirable behaviors, given the breed and adult size of the dog.
- No dog, regardless of size, should feel that he has to mouth or bite someone to get anything that he needs, including attention.
- Steps to addressing these concerns are straightforward:
  - Clients must stop interacting with the puppy and freeze as soon as they are mouthed or grabbed. *This is the most difficult advice with which to get the clients to comply.* It is hard to be quiet and still when faced with a cute puppy, but this technique works.
  - If clients pull away from the puppy, they are encouraging the pup to pursue the "game."
  - Clients can use a gentle verbal cue to signal that the interaction is finished ("no," "stop," "uh-uh") and *gently* extricate or remove body parts while *gently* holding the body of the dog. If clients want to use a verbal signal to flag an activity that is ending, they must not yell. Otherwise, the signal is a punisher, not a flag.
  - Clients should be apprised of how fragile young animals can be and cautioned about the dangers of physical discipline.
- If clients quickly offer the puppy something on which she can chew (e.g., a stuffed toy, a ball, a chew toy) and praise her when she takes it, they will have successfully redirected the behavior (see "Protocol for Teaching Kids—and Adults—to Play with Dogs and Cats" and "Protocol for Choosing Toys for Your Pet" for helpful ideas).
- Because attention from the human is what the pup wants, appropriate play with toys is an essential step for avoiding injury and discouraging inappropriate

and potentially dangerous behaviors (see "Protocol for Teaching Kids—and Adults—to Play with Dogs and Cats" and "Protocol for Preventing and Treating Attention-Seeking Behavior" for specific suggestions and "Protocol for Understanding and Managing Odd, Curious, and Annoying Canine Behaviors" for specific stepwise advice).

If simple *redirection, which is a trading or substitution strategy* (e.g., your arm for a wonderful fuzzy squeak toy) does *not* work, people have often been taught to "startle" the dog to get him to stop the behavior. It's important to define "startle." The application of a novel or less familiar stimulus at a level *below* that which scares that dog but that is sufficient to get the dog to stop what he is doing and focus on the client can act as a *disruptive stimulus*. If the advice to "startle" the dog is used in this context, it's fine. No one should scare, injure, or confuse a dog. We tend to think of sharp sounds like whistles and shrieks as a way to "startle" a dog. This may work without frightening the dog, but disruptive stimuli can also suggest that positive things may follow. Once clients understand the concept, they will readily identify disruptive stimuli that work for their dog.

- In addition to being a conditioned stimulus, the noise the can opener makes can be a disruptive stimulus for cats fed tinned food.
- The characteristic sound a bag of cookies makes can be a disruptive stimulus. The smell of microwave popcorn can be a disruptive stimulus.
- If the dog treats are kept in tin or a mason jar, the sound it makes when opened is readily recognized and can be a disruptive stimulus.

Clients will always think of true punishment first, so we need to expand their thought process.

- Physical violence, physical struggles, physical discipline, and physical punishment will almost always make dogs who mouth, grab, or bite do so faster and more fiercely.
- Sometimes this worsening in behavior is a response to being hurt or scared.
- Sometimes the worsening in behavior is a contextual attempt to get information about potential threats. Regardless, it is not what is needed.
- Instead, we need to emphasize to clients that dogs ask for information and that they should not be punished when they do so. Rather, clients must respond with accurate information that provides a clear and humane rule structure and a safe expectation. In the most simple case, a default of quietly sitting (a natural deferential and "stop" signal in dogs) and looking at the client for cues can be used in almost all situations, and it saves dogs' mental health and lives.

Can We Truly "Teach" Bite Inhibition?

There are few data that show that we can teach bite inhibition. However, we can *enhance* biting and grabbing behaviors by rewarding the dog exhibiting them. This is exactly what happens in rough play or when we accept such behaviors from young puppies and continue to interact with them because they are small or we think that they "did not mean it."

For any behavior in which there is variable expression, whether in intent, content, frequency, or context, we can have an effect on that behavior through our responses. In other words, *where there is variation, there is the possibility of selecting and changing any behavior.* This means that we can encourage dogs to enhance an obnoxious or worrisome behavior *and* preferred behaviors, such as encouraging a dog to take objects or treats gently rather than grabbing and biting. It's unclear whether we truly teach dogs to "inhibit" a bite, grab, or mouthy behavior. It's far more likely that we teach them that these behaviors will not be rewarded, but other, more palatable behaviors will gain them rewards of some kind. The standard approaches for enhancing a preferred behavior are discussed in Chapter 3 and will work here.

- Dogs who did not have early experience in learning about variation and its sequela, modulation, may have more trouble than others. Dogs who were raised without other dogs, locked in a kennel, ignored, never given toys, et cetera, may have trouble learning any response other than the one they practiced the most. In the case of the toy, it may *not* be that they never learned to play, but that *they learned not to play.*
- Dogs who had early and/or extensive experience in protecting themselves or in adaptive survival strategies may have difficulty in relinquishing these strategies until they can understand that they are experiencing less risk than they thought or than they formerly experienced. Only when they can understand experiencing variation in risk can they learn to try varying responses to different risks.

Both of these groups of dogs may grab too hard or grab and mouth in circumstances that could appear atypical and could be worrying.

Under most normal circumstances, the general belief is that dogs learn bite inhibition from other family members because they make mistakes and are "corrected" for them. Other puppies and adult dogs often bark or shriek at the offender and, with time, may give open mouth threats or grab the offending pup. There are actually very few data on this subject, and fewer data that look at the effects of singleton or early orphaned pups or effects of breed on the development and type of mouthing behavior.

- The take-home message to clients *must* be that humans are unable to read dog behaviors in the context and the way in which canine family members do and cannot hope to mimic the relevant canine behaviors used in dog-typical "corrections."

Accordingly, we should redirect—*not punish*—inappropriate/undesirable mouthing/biting behaviors by rewarding behaviors that are better and desired. The first step in this process is to ignore the dog when she is mouthing or grabbing; however, if the dog's response is already fully developed, this is a difficult strategy to implement. Instead, if the mouthing can be anticipated, it can usually be stopped and/or redirected to a toy using the three foundation protocols—"Protocol for Deference," "Protocol for Teaching Your Dog to Take a Deep Breath and Use Other Biofeedback Methods as Part of Relaxation," and "Protocol for Relaxation: Behavior Modification Tier 1"—to teach dogs that not biting/grabbing is rewarded.

Some breeds or lines of dogs, such as herding dogs, may grab more readily than others because they have been selected to do so. *This does not mean that anyone should tolerate being grabbed simply because the breed is one selected for herding and guarding.* If people think that some breeds should grab, *inappropriate grabbing will be tolerated,* and the dog's behavior will become more risky with age and practice. Individuals who exhibit behaviors that are thought to be typical for breeds or lines *can and should be redirected* to appropriate targets for mouthing or grabbing (e.g., toys). Most herding and guarding behaviors do *not* involve mouthing, grabbing, and biting. Grabbing and biting in these contexts are last resorts, not first. Only for predatory *behavior,* which can be a normal, adaptive behavior, is routine biting part of a normal repertoire. Note that predatory behavior is *not the same as predatory aggression.* The latter is a diagnosis of a behavioral pathology.

If mouthing/grabbing/biting do not respond to early intervention, redirection, and access to outlets that dissipate energy and provide cognitive exercise, the contexts in which these behaviors occur should be explored further for anxiety-related behavioral pathologies. Bear in mind that most mouthing/grabbing behaviors and a lot of biting behaviors in dogs presented to routine veterinary practices are behaviors that have been inadvertently, mistakenly, or deliberately reinforced earlier in the dog's life. Prevention is key, but the same behavior modification principles used there and discussed in Chapter 3 can address these learned behaviors.

DOGS WHO NEVER SEEM TO STOP MOVING

Most dogs that people think are hyperactive because they never seem to stop moving are not hyperactive: they are high-energy dogs whose needs are unmet. Almost all dogs can benefit from increased *aerobic* exercise. Tired dogs are happy dogs, and they have ecstatic people! Activities that allow dogs to reach their aerobic scope (assuming that they have no physical contraindications) include:

- leash walks over trails and/or uphill,
- running with the dog (or riding a bicycle with the dog running alongside),
- play with flying disks or launched balls,
- agility,
- scent work over a long, complex course,
- lure coursing,
- earthdog trials, and
- swimming, especially if the dog will chase and retrieve a ball.

All of these activities are more calorically expensive and stimulating for the dog if other dogs are involved. Nothing wears out a dog like another dog. Obviously, the dogs must be companionable. Caution is urged for non-critical use of "dog parks"; this is addressed in discussions of general treatment strategies (see Chapter 3) and discussions of inter-dog aggression (see Chapter 6).

Clients who may not be able to have their dogs engage in these types of aerobic activities could still wear out their dogs by using *intellectual exercises,* including some scent work. For example, teaching the names of toys and asking for them by name multiple times per day will stimulate many dogs. Scent work is becoming increasingly popular and may be an activity advantageous for most dogs. Scent work encourages calm, non-reactive approaches to problem solving and rewards focus and follow-through (Thesen et al, 1993). In this sport, sequestering dogs who are not working is common. Other dogs are not in the immediate vicinity when one dog is working, and instructors are able to make accommodations for "reactive" dogs because of this. Finally, olfactory neuron stimulation may benefit cognition (see discussion in Overall and Arnold, 2007).

Assess the dog in terms of breed, age, and individual temperament or personality. Ask if the dog's behaviors seem extreme, given this. If the dog appears to be active because he is hyper-reactive or anxious, conduct a full behavioral history and assessment that will lead to a diagnosis.

Abnormal Canine Behaviors and Behavioral Pathologies Involving Aggression

The vast majority of problematic behaviors and true behavioral pathologies are rooted in anxiety and the neurochemical/neurophysiological response to that anxiety (see Box 2-1 in Chapter 2 for the non-specific signs of anxiety). For ease of use of this manual, behavioral conditions affecting dogs are divided into two groups: diagnoses involving aggression and diagnoses not involving aggression.

Diagnosis and treatment of canine aggression remain controversial, often volatile, issues; however, most dogs can improve with treatment. The roles for terminology, mechanism, and reactivity are discussed and graphically illustrated in Chapter 2 and are applicable when discussing canine pathologies. Early diagnosis and treatment can make the difference between life and death for dogs affected by these conditions and between living in a safe environment or one replete with risk.

EPIDEMIOLOGY AND OUTCOME OF DOG BITES, RISK, AND BREED-SPECIFIC LEGISLATION

Overview of Canine Aggression

Aggression is best defined within a given context as an appropriate or inappropriate threat or challenge that is ultimately resolved by combat or deference. This broad definition encompasses the standard definition of agonistic behavior and is consistent with definitions of terms involving types of hierarchies affected by limited resources (Immelmann and Beer, 1989).

Aggression from dogs can be an appropriate response, and a defensive bite or attack may be an appropriate form of aggression. Over history, dogs have been selected to exhibit responses protective of their humans. Remember, dogs do not have opposable thumbs or verbal speech and so use their mouths when engaged in protection and when trying to ascertain whether protective behaviors are necessary.

- A dog who attacks visiting friends as they hug their hosts is responding inappropriately and out of context.

- Dogs who defend their people from rape, theft, attack, or attempted murder are considered heroes regardless of whether they do so by merely being present, by inflicting an element of fear and surprise regardless of their behavior, by growling, by baring their teeth, or by biting. This form of aggression is usually considered to be appropriate, and in context. We prefer that the aggression is proportional to the threat posed, which is interesting because such a preference relies on the dog's ability to make fine, contextual decisions. Dogs are cognitive, but dogs who are anxious, by definition, may not be able to make these distinctions.

- When trying to decide whether an aggression was appropriate, given the context, or inappropriate and out of context, it helps to remember that normal behaviors are variable and flexible; pathological behaviors are inflexible and relatively stereotypic.

- The term "provocation" must be discussed in the context of a dog known to be aggressive in certain circumstances compared with a dog that has never reacted in those circumstances. If a dog is known to have a propensity to behave inappropriately in certain contexts (i.e., petting or reaching over its head), she may be "unintentionally provoked" (*sensu* Podberscek and Blackshaw, 1991a) by what would otherwise be considered a normal gesture. For abnormal animals, "normal" gestures will not be "normally" perceived. Dogs exhibiting inappropriate, out-of-context aggressions are not misbehaved or poorly behaved—*they are clinically abnormal and must be regarded as such.*

- For any dog exhibiting any potentially aggressive behavior or when clients complain about any aggressive or potentially aggressive behavior, the following must be determined.
  - In what context did the behavior occur?
  - Was the behavior contextually appropriate?
  - Did the behavior involve threats or combating/fighting?
  - How did the incident resolve?

Inherent in this assessment is an understanding of the extent to which the dog inhibited her own aggression in response to a changing context. Social situations are not static; they are a continuous interplay between signal and response. A dog with aggression associated with underlying anxiety will have more difficulty responding to changing situations than a dog without such anxiety.

- Dogs who bark or growl can be potentially as dangerous as dogs who bite, but some idea of the extent to which the dog has been able to inhibit itself can be obtained from the dog's reactions. A dog who never reacts in a given context—and who has been exposed to it—probably does not have a problem with that context. This is not a guarantee that no problem could develop in the future, but such information provides a reference point for when the dog was last problematic. *This is why screening each patient, at each visit, for behavioral problems and concerns is so important.*
- Reactivity of the dog can be determined from the dog's behaviors (Boxes 6-1 and 6-2). Barking can be an alerting behavior. Snarling or lip lifting (usually silent at first), growling, and snapping or biting represent increasing levels of aggression. Body posture usually parallels vocal behaviors: lying down is a less reactive posture than sitting, which is a less reactive posture than standing. This does not mean that a dog who is lying down cannot bite. It does mean that the dog who is lying down must proceed through more behavioral sequences before he or she is in the position to bite, giving another individual more time to react or to anticipate a problem.
  - No one should be misled by the myth of the "tail-wagging dog"; a wagging tail is only an indication of willingness to interact—not of the tone of the interaction. A dog that is standing rigid, hair up, ears back, barking, growling, baring its teeth, and wagging its tail will be very willing to interact in an extremely aggressive manner, given the appropriate cue or stimulus.
- By definition, a first bite means that the dog has never bitten before; it does not mean that there have been no aggressive events or that the dog cannot or will not bite in the future.
- Whether dogs bite may be a threshold issue: completely normal dogs can bite if the threshold is sufficiently lowered (e.g., abuse of or threats to them or their people).
- Aggressive dogs should not be described as "vicious." Viciousness connotes an underlying state involving retribution that cannot be evaluated in dogs. Aggressive dogs can be determined to be "dangerous," which is a more useful distinction.

Epidemiology of Dog Bites

An extensive review of the literature concerning dog bite injuries reveals that the only robust data are those supporting the following conclusions:

- There is a substantially greater injury and fatality rate for children compared with adults.
- Boys are injured and killed more often than girls, indicating that human behavior may be a major factor.
- There is a preponderance of owned family dogs involved in bites and fatalities.

The data on dog bites have been dominated by catastrophic bites as defined by those attended in an emergency setting. The vast majority of fatal dog bites are to older, debilitated adults and very young children. See Overall and Love (2001) and Patronek and Slavinski (2009) for detailed reviews of the data and the study statistics.

A careful reading of the literature supports three conclusions regarding breed:

- Breeds most represented in dog bite data vary over time (which may indicate changes in breed preference by owners rather than changes in breed-specific aggressive tendencies per se).
- Breeds most often represented in published data are popular ones, and no single breed may be represented in bite data in proportion to its actual population.

BOX 6-1

Canine Signals to Evaluate When Aggression Is a Concern

- Posture of head, back, and tail
- Position of ears
- Activity and height of tail
- State of piloerection
- Eye and mouth positions
- Vocal cues: barking, growling, snarling/lip lifting, snapping and biting*

This could be orderly progression of signals, but in profound cases it will not be and need not be progressive.

BOX 6-2

Considerations for Determining Intensity of Aggression

- Where is the dog on the continuum of barking, growling, snarling/lip lifting, snapping, and biting, and is this a change?
- Are physical signals congruent?
- Was warning given by the dog before the threat or bite?
- Can the behavior be interrupted?
- Can the behavior be inhibited?
- Can the behavior be redirected with activity?

- "Pit bull" is often applied, without biological basis, to a range of dog types, regardless of the underlying genetic stock (this problem may be magnified in communities that have experienced a previously publicized pit bull–type dog attack) (Lockwood and Rindy, 1987; Sacks et al., 1989).

We lack excellent data on dog bites that would be useful for most clients because we lack databases of registered dogs and owners and data on the relative population numbers of different breeds (Collier, 2006; Overall and Love, 2001; Patronek and Slavinski, 2009). Without these data, we cannot calculate a breed-by-breed bite-related index, which has been so useful in understanding Dutch dog bites (Cornelissen and Hopster, 2010), or the population attributable fraction percentage for each breed, which would provide a more accurate bite frequency assessment.

Cornelissen and Hopster (2010) examined all bites, not just catastrophic ones. Their findings parallel the generalities in the literature.

- First, and in keeping with other studies, male humans are more frequently bitten by dogs than females, and children are bitten more frequently than adults. However, in more recent studies (Shuler et al., 2008), boys were not bitten more often than girls, an odd victory for gender equality that may hint at how children's play styles have changed over the years.
- Second, children were bitten in non-public places more often than adults and were bitten intentionally more often than adults. These findings strongly suggest that the *risk to children from dog bites is a correlate of responsible adult oversight.*
- Third, although showing the global pattern of experiencing more bites to the head and face, children in this study had no or more minor injuries than adults, an uncommon finding in the literature. This pattern may suggest that some population-level (probably cultural) differences exist between these populations and those in the literature, which is heavily biased to studies on dogs in the United States.
- Fourth, *60% of people bitten could identify a trigger that resulted in the bite.* This means that we can educate people about triggers, what they mean to the dog, and how to respect the dog's perception of the situation and prevent accidents.
- Fifth, most people could readily identify the biting dog's breed using a chart of breeds and breed characteristics that the authors provided, but *no single breed was over-represented in the pool of dogs that did the biting. The breeds that were most common were the ones most likely to have bitten.* These findings support the data of a number of comparative (Overall and Love, 2001) and original (Drobatz and Smith, 2003; Shuler et al., 2008) studies. Simply put, controlling breeds is not sufficient to control dog bites.

Situations in which bites occur need to be thoroughly, rigorously, and consistently reviewed and documented by health care personnel, using validated assessment tools. The appropriateness of the situation, the extent to which a bite is provoked, the nature of the provocation, and the behavioral tendencies of the dog involved (including whether the dog has received a behavioral diagnosis involving aggression) must be evaluated (de Keuster et al., 2006). This aspect is particularly important given the association between dog abuse and child abuse and the extent to which violent behaviors are learned and practiced (Felthous and Kellert, 1987).

The specialist community has not been willing to engage in creating a consensus terminology in veterinary behavioral medicine, despite numerous attempts to encourage this (Overall, 2005; Overall and Burghardt, 2006). As a result, data on dog bites and associations with diagnoses involving aggression have not been collected in a manner that allows for comparative studies. Unfortunately, this situation has tacitly encouraged an approach of categorizing aggression by the victim such that we understand even less about underlying mechanisms than would be the case using the types of mechanistic diagnoses defined in this text (Duffy et al., 2008; Segurson et al., 2005; Takeuchi et al., 2001; van den Berg et al., 2010). Only when we can share accurate diagnostic information can specialists develop a cohesive approach to understanding and treating the mechanisms underlying pathology.

ROLE OF HUMAN SELECTION IN DOGS AND DOG BREEDS FOR BEHAVIORS SUCH AS AGGRESSION

All behavior has environmental and genetic components. The variation in the genetic component is sufficient to produce a wide array of individual behavioral phenotypes in the absence of any specific breed. The extent to which behavioral plasticity is a function of genetics is complex.

Humans, as the agents of selective breeding, may have removed some of the advantages of plasticity through domestication while selecting for traits that have little adaptive or survival value (e.g., coat colors, particularly those associated with defects: white boxers are usually deaf). One function of establishing and maintaining a breed is to canalize some of the overall genetic variation within the species (and within the breed). Although domestic canine breeds have a relative body size that spans two orders of magnitude, such variation in size is absent in wild canids. The process of domestication itself relieved many of the pressures for which wild canid body size was a response, allowing the underlying genetic variation to respond to artificial selection.

Selection, natural or artificial, cannot act if there is no underlying genetic variation. Some variation (termed "additive genetic variance" by quantitative geneticists) must be present for a trait to be developed. This is easy to understand with physical traits such as coat color but is harder to see with behavioral traits such as "protectiveness." "Protectiveness" is actually a constellation of behaviors: watching, following, guarding, and reacting to keep one group separate from another when needed. Breeding for traits that are this complex and variable produces a continuum of protective behaviors, some of which may not be desired or expected. Some of these behaviors will be inappropriate because they are not complete or forceful enough, and some will be unacceptable because they are too forceful and out of context (Figs. 6-1 through 6-3). If breeders of dogs prefer more forceful behavior and do not care whether it is appropriate or in context, it is very likely that within a few generations, the distribution of protective dog behaviors will look like that in Figure 6-2, in which case more dogs behave inappropriately.

The chance of someone encountering an inappropriately behaved member of this breed increases. However, if breeders act responsibly and choose to breed only dogs that have behaviors that are considered "optimal," the proportion of appropriately behaved dogs increases; over time, the genetic variation may decrease, which may help to reduce the probability of undesirable traits appearing.

Caution is urged regarding any generalizations about inappropriate breed-based behaviors. Breeds selected for one or a few particular and specific behaviors may be more at risk for developing undesirable variation for *those behaviors,* and when dogs of a certain breed develop a behavioral pathology, that pathology is informed by breed (Overall and Dunham, 2002). This *does not mean* that dogs selected for protective behaviors are more aggressive than dogs for which this selective pressure was absent. It *does mean* that that particular

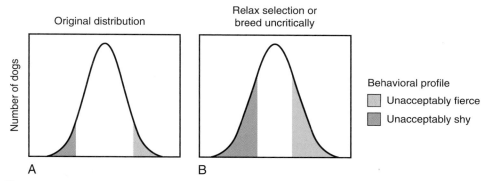

Fig. 6-1 Graph *A* represents the hypothetical distribution of behavioral phenotypes for a random breed. The individuals in the blue area of this curve are considered too shy to perform the task for which the breed was developed or are too shy to be desirous as pets. The individuals in the orange area of this curve are considered too fierce to perform the task for which the breed was developed or are too fierce to be desirous as pets. Selection has limited the spread of the less desirable population members by not breeding them, and in this example breeding of unaffected members maintains the represented distribution. Graph *B* shows what happens, all other forces being unchanged, if selection is relaxed or breeding is uncritical, and the undesirable members are included or encouraged in the breeding population. The relative proportion of dogs with both undesirable phenotypes of behaviors increases.

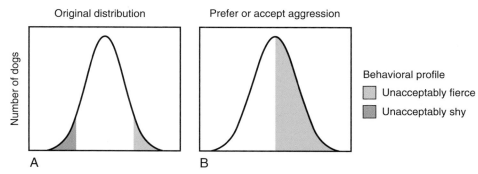

Fig. 6-2 Graph *A* is the same as graph *A* in Figure 6-1 and is originally maintained in the same way. Graph *B* represents what happens when the unacceptably fierce animals are preferred, and selection acts to reinforce this through preferential breeding and culling of unacceptably shy animals. The relative proportion of the unacceptably fierce phenotype of dog increases.

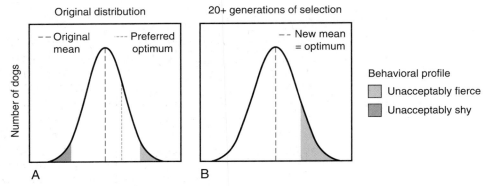

Fig. 6-3 Graph A shows a distribution similar to graph A in Figure 6-1 and is originally maintained in the same way. In this case, the original mean represents the mean phenotype of the selected behavior in the breeders' populations. The line marked *preferred optimum* represents the phenotype of the behaviors that breeders prefer and have selected for by breeding only dogs that have phenotypes close to it. Graph B indicates what happens after more than 20 generations of breeding for the preferred optimum. In this case, the mean of the behavioral phenotypes in the population has shifted to the preferred optimum, and as a result, the proportion of dogs with the undesirable behavioral phenotype of unacceptably shy has decreased to nil, whereas the proportion of dogs with the undesirable behavioral phenotype of unacceptably fierce has increased, along with an increase in the proportion of dogs with the highly desirable optimum phenotype.

breeds *may* be more at risk for developing a disproportionate number of dogs who exhibit inappropriate, out-of-context protective aggression given the selection/breeding conditions outlined previously.

Regardless, the following should be understood by anyone who interacts with dogs.

- Any dog, regardless of breed, can exhibit inappropriate behavior.
- *Any dog can bite, and the vast majority could likely be pushed to do so under some awful circumstance.*
- If there is a bite or collision, dogs who are large, muscular, tenacious, and who have powerful jaws will do more damage—even by accident—than dogs who do not have these attributes.
- The data on hormonal contributions to canine aggression are not strong, and all are correlational.
  - Un-neutered male dogs who bite tend also to be un-licensed and un-vaccinated, suggesting that the pattern may reflect human responsibility, not biology.
  - Castration has been reported to decrease aggression to other dogs in 62% of cases (Hopkins et al., 1976), but there are no data on true effects on problematic behaviors or specific diagnoses. In general, testosterone acts as a behavior modulator that allows dogs to react more quickly and intensely and for a prolonged period of time. Clients should be told this.
  - For females, there is evidence that for dogs younger than 6 months of age who are *already* exhibiting signs of "dominance"/impulse-control aggression, ovariohysterectomy renders them more aggressive (O'Farrell and Peachey, 1990; statistical analysis in Overall, 1995c). *In utero*

androgenization is a concern for many species but remains largely un-investigated in dogs (Compaan et al., 1993; Vandenbergh, 1971). One study (Kim et al., 2006) compared incidence of "aggression" in neutered female working dogs and dogs who were anesthetized but not neutered. The neutered dogs were more reactive/"aggressive" in some circumstances, but because no sham surgeries were used, as is the routine in rodent studies, the effect may have been attributable to surgery/recovery. This is not a trivial issue given roles for altered mental states associated with anesthesia, pain, learning, and inflammation.

- What should veterinarians recommend with respect to neutering for dogs showing some aggression?
  - If the patient is a young (<6 months) bitch puppy, she may benefit from one or two heat cycles, if the clients are responsible and she will not be bred. This means that any "protective" effect of early neutering on mammary neoplasia will be forfeit. The dog should also be engaged in active treatment for her behavioral concerns.
  - If the dog is male, neutering may diminish reactivity, but there is a huge learning component to any aggression. Clients should be realistic. The dog should also be engaged in active treatment for his behavioral concerns.
  - No aggressive animal should be bred because we cannot rule out genetic contributions.
  - If the dogs are shelter puppies or dogs and we do not know their propensities, our focus is preventing unwanted puppies, and this concern should trump hormonal concerns of risk. Neuter the dogs.

In short, the vast majority of dog bites can be prevented by responsible dog care and training, and by supervision of interactions of dogs with those who may be most at risk for injury (primarily children). No dog should be left alone with any child younger than age 2 because the child cannot get away from the dog and an accident could happen. Young children (3 to 6 years old) should always be supervised with dogs so that they can learn safe and humane interactions with dogs and so that they respect the dog and her needs.

For hands-on, gut-level learning for children (the group of people most likely to be victimized by inter-specific misunderstanding), it would be difficult to out-perform the lessons taught in the Blue Dog CD (de Keuster et al., 2005). In this clear interactive video, children (and their caregivers) are able to try out their behavioral responses on a virtual dog and learn about what could happen with a real one. Scientific validation of the beneficial effects of this program continues, with early studies showing that the Blue Dog video reduces errors made by children 3 to 6 years old with respect to

their responses to dogs' behaviors (Meints and de Keuster, 2009). That said, we should understand that until children are 8 to 12 years old, what they cognitively know and can recite may be somewhat divorced from what they do when the circumstance arises. Practicing behaviors can help teach responses but cannot override neurodevelopment. Until children's brains are sufficiently mature to act rationally on material that they have mastered, their caregivers need to show responsible oversight. Table 6-1 explains the neurodevelopmental stages of children and their effects on dogs.

Caregivers and other adult observers also need to be aware that not all children treat animals kindly or fairly. Table 6-2 lists canine behaviors that may indicate that the dog is distressed because of the child. Refer also to Table 6-3 for assessing damage done during aggressive events.

A growing number of resources are available that should help even the most clueless among us to understand canine signaling—if we read the signals. The best references address the point of view most often neglected—the dog's. Two short popular books should heighten the

TABLE 6-1

Developmental Stages for Children and Their Effects on Dogs

Age of Child	Developmental Milestone(s)	Typical Child Behaviors Affecting Dogs	Typical Normal Dog Behavior	Diagnoses in Abnormal Dogs That Could Put Children at Risk
0-6 months	Reflexive behaviors	New noises: crying, screaming, babbling	Sniffing	Predatory aggression
	Sitting up/creeping	New smells	Licking	Fear aggression
		Grabbing fur, body parts of dogs	Avoidance, at first	
6-24 months	Fine motor skills improve	Increased noise/chaos	Freezing or avoidance	Fear
	Crawling/cruising	Exploration of dog's body with hands, mouth, teeth	Waiting for food	Fear aggression
	Walking/running Curiosity/exploration			Pain aggression Food-related aggression Possessive aggression
2-5 years	Autonomy/tantrums	Interactions with dog:	More distant withdrawal	Fear aggression
	Gross/fine motor coordination improve	Interrupt sleep/rest	Avoidance	Pain aggression
	Egocentricity	Fondling	Offering of toy	Food-related aggression
	Magical thinking/ fantasizing	Chasing games	Soliciting food	Possessive aggression
	Animism/ anthropomorphism	Removal of toy/food		Protective/territorial aggression
	New friends enter household	Sharing human/dog food		Impulse-control aggression
		New friends enter household		Fear
				Inappropriate herding behavior
5-9 years	Intense curiosity Experimentation	Interactions with dog: Teasing	Curiosity Following	Inappropriate play Fear aggression

Continued

TABLE 6-1

Developmental Stages for Children and Their Effects on Dogs—cont'd

Age of Child	Developmental Milestone(s)	Typical Child Behaviors Affecting Dogs	Typical Normal Dog Behavior	Diagnoses in Abnormal Dogs That Could Put Children at Risk
	Independence/ decreased adult supervision	Reprimanding/punishing	Playing with toys	Pain aggression
	Poor deductive/ generalizing powers	Bossing	Playing roughly	Possessive aggression
	Desire for control	Roughhousing/tug of war	Sleeping in specific child's room	Territorial/protective aggression Play aggression Impulse-control aggression Fear Inappropriate herding behavior Inappropriate play Play aggression
9-12 years	Increased peer influence	Interactions with dog:	Accompanying specific child	Impulse-control aggression
	Increased sense of responsibility	May take responsibility for feeding, grooming, exercising	Aerobic play	Fear aggression
	Concrete operations	Increased teasing/ rough play	Sleeping in specific child's room	Play aggression
	Problem solving	Abusive interaction may begin		Protective/territorial aggression
	Increased deductive/ generalizing powers			

Note: This table is also found in the client handout "Protocol for Surviving and Handling Aggressive Events."
From Love and Overall, 2001.

TABLE 6-2

Warning Signs in Dogs That Can Indicate Distress Associated with Children

- Acute change in a dog's normal behavior (e.g., withdrawal or increased circling and patrol behavior; changes in amount or character of vocalization)
- Change in eating habits, particularly if dog will eat only when the child is absent or if the dog suddenly shows food-guarding
- Increased reactivity of pet (e.g., barking, growling, patrolling, lunging in new or lesser circumstances)
- Changes in sleeping/resting activity and locations
- Changes in behaviors associated with behavioral diagnosis and increase in or appearance of gastrointestinal signs (vomiting, regurgitation, diarrhea) associated with stress
- Signs of separation anxiety only when left with children (e.g., vocalization, destruction, elimination, salivation, increase or decrease in motor activity)
- Frank aggression—even without a specific diagnosis—in the presence of children

Note: This table is also found in the client handout "Protocol for Surviving and Handling Aggressive Events."
From Love and Overall, 2001.

interest of most veterinarians and dog lovers. *Tail Talk* (Collins, 2007) is a beautifully photographed, informative book that could have a home in the waiting rooms of all veterinary surgeries. The *Canine Commandments* (Shepherd, 2007) offers parents a translation of canine behavior and needs that will allow them to learn to meet their dog's needs humanely and to understand that by doing so they will keep their children safe.

When considering canine aggression, we must begin to ask what kind of people we wish to be. Cornelissen and Hopster (2010) hint at this in one laudatory statement: *"We found that all dogs can bite and therefore one*

TABLE 6-3

Assessing Damage Done during Aggressive Events

The following scale is an adaptation of one widely used to assess damage caused by dogs during an aggressive event (Dunbar, 2011; Wrubel et al., 2011); this table is also found in the client handout "Protocol for Surviving and Handling Aggressive Events."

Severity Level	Threat or Bite Characteristics
1	Posturing, growling, lunging, or snarling behavior occurred without teeth touching skin (i.e., mostly mild agonistic, intimidation behavior). *Note: These behaviors may be completely normal.*
2	Teeth touched skin, but no puncture wounds > $\frac{1}{10}$ inch were inflicted. Marks or minor scratches from paws and nails (minor surface abrasions) may have been incurred. Abrasions more likely to be horizontal than vertical. *Note: These may be normal behaviors, and no to minor injury may be normal. The extent of injury is often associated with the amount of movement of the individuals involved and their relative masses.*
3	Punctures were half the length of a canine tooth and resulted in 1-4 holes from a single bite. No tears or slashes were incurred, and the recipient was not shaken side to side. Lacerations are in a single direction. *Note: Movement and mass matter here because force = mass × acceleration. This consideration should factor into all interactions with dogs, including those involving play (dog-dog and human-dog).*
4	A single bite resulted in 1-4 holes, with ≥1 holes deeper than half the length of a canine tooth. Deep bruising from prolonged pressure and contact results. Contact and punctures were incurred from more than the canine teeth. Tears and/or slash wounds resulted, and shaking—as evidenced by lacerations in multiple directions—was involved. *Note: The extent of damage done in this circumstance not only may be affected by mass and movement but also by dog morphology. Jaw size and mass and distribution of jaw muscles matter and should be a consideration when evaluating to what extent any inhibition could have been involved.*
5	Multiple bites at severity level ≥4 incurred in a concerted, repeated attack. *Note: The context in which this type of bite can occur matters, and dogs who are defending people have been known to exhibit these behaviors. In the absence of any justified context, these dogs are extremely dangerous.*
6	Any bite that resulted in death of any individual (dog, human, cat, et cetera). *Note: It is important to realize that dogs will hunt if hungry and that accidental bites can have fatal consequences. This is the best justification for evaluating the appropriateness of the behavior given the context in which it occurs.*

Adapted from Association of Professional Dog Trainers website (www.apdt.com): Dr. Ian Dunbar's dog bite scale. An assessment of the severity of biting problems based on an objective evaluation of wound pathology. www.apdt.com/veterinary/assets/pdf/Ian Dunbar Dog Bite Scale.pdf. Accessed August 3, 2011; and Wrubel KM, Moon-Fanelli A, Maranda LS, Dodman NH. Interdog household aggression: 38 cases (2006-2007). J Am Vet Med Assoc 2011;238:731-740.

should always be careful when interacting with a dog, even a family dog and during play."

When we choose to share our lives with another species, particularly one with large canine teeth, no verbal speech, and no opposable thumbs, we assume some risk. We assume risk in all social interactions even when we share our lives with those whose teeth, speech, and thumbs are like ours, as evidenced by accident and divorce rates. *Yet the far greater risk is assumed by the dogs, who are expected to translate human language to "dog" and who can be relinquished and euthanized at will, even if it wasn't their "fault."* Humans have a stunning propensity to desire a "guarantee" of "safety" over an acceptance of responsibility that includes assessing and acting on risk. In fact, it is this propensity to need a guarantee of "safety" that has so misguidedly driven breed-specific legislation (BSL) and most of the inhumane training techniques based on outdated, inappropriately applied concepts of "dominance."

Scientific studies too numerous to list here have shown that the benefits to humans of interacting with pets range from the physical to the emotional. The defining relationship in a child's life that turns that child into a humane adult can be their relationship with a dog. We can understand, minimize, and wisely assume risk. What we gain from our relationships with dogs certainly outweighs the costs of such education.

CANINE BEHAVIORAL PATHOLOGIES

Behavioral Diagnoses Primarily Involving Pathological Aggression

Maternal Aggression
Diagnostic Criteria and Description
- Consistent aggression (threat/challenge/contest) directed toward people or other animals by a bitch

who has puppies, is about to have puppies, or is experiencing pseudocyesis (false pregnancy).

- Attacks are unprovoked by the approaching individual and may occur as a result of any near movement, not just that associated with an approach to the bitch or puppies.
- Injury of the pups is almost always accidental.

Common Non-Specific Signs

- Growling, snarling, lunging, and rarely biting in response to being approached by humans or other animals when "nesting."
- Most approaching individuals are able to avoid the bitch before she grabs them.
- Some bitches will "nest" with and defend toys or blankets
- Intensity of the threat is generally related to proximity of approacher: the closer the individual, the more intense the aggression.

Rule Outs

- This condition is likely a medical condition and related in part to reproductive hormones.

Etiology, Epidemiology, and Risk Groups

- This is a recurring condition for susceptible dogs and may appear at each heat or breeding.
- *If the dog is continually annoyed (from her perspective), she may injure, kill, or eat pups or destroy and consume blankets and toys.* Clients should watch for signs of increasing reactivity on the part of the bitch and avoid stimuli associated with such reactivity.

Common Myths That Can Get in the Way of Treatment or Diagnosis

- This is a normal behavior.
  - Although some inexperienced or worried dams may occasionally be uncertain, if the dog is reacting this way routinely, either she is overly/pathologically concerned or she is being continuously harassed by the focus of her aggression. *Abuse and inappropriate treatment should be on the rule-out list.*

Commonly Asked Client Questions

- Will this happen if the dog is bred again?
  - It often does. Some dogs become less reactive with mothering experience.
- Should the bitch be spayed?
  - If this aggression is associated with repeated pseudocyetic events, spaying the dog may be the most humane choice. *No dog should be bred before 2 years of age, more than once a year, or more than four times in their lifetime.* The health, welfare, and well-being of the bitch matter.
  - If the bitch is aggressive during more than one pregnancy, her quality of life (QoL) is suffering, and she should be spayed.

Treatment

- Management:
  - Provide a truly secure location for the bitch and her puppies. Nest boxes/whelping pens should protect the mother and pups and provide an unobstructed view of anyone who could approach.
  - Provide warning of an approach by talking to the dog. Anxiety worsens when dogs have incomplete information or must monitor the environment. Early warning can relieve related anxiety.
  - Quiet rooms or rooms with classical music or white noise and/or dimmed light may help some dogs, but there are no data.
  - Provocation of the dog can be avoided by cleaning bedding and providing food and fresh water when she is elsewhere. If the dog has learned to like walking on a leash, using the leash to take her for a walk without the pups may help her to re-evaluate her level of concern.
  - Restrict visitation to the dog. As the pups move in to week 3, they will begin to benefit from the ability to meet other dogs and other species. Encourage this. If the mother is still reactive by week 6, take her away to do something she can enjoy while the puppies learn to explore new social and physical environments. Her protective behaviors could restrict their interactions at a time when the pups can most benefit from exposure, and she could inadvertently injure the pups.
- Behavior modification:
  - All dogs can benefit from learning to relax. If there is a known risk that this condition could occur, relaxation and deferential behaviors taught before pregnancy and used throughout nursing should help.
- Medication/dietary intervention:
  - Although this condition likely has hormonal components, no interventions are recommended beyond spaying 2 months after the pseudocyetic event or after the pups are weaned.
  - Any medications used could pass into the mother's milk.
- Miscellaneous interventions:
  - Breeders should inform anyone who has a dog from this line about this concern.
  - An honest appraisal of any patterns in the pedigree will help determine whether the occurrence of this behavior in one pregnancy may be exceptional. Dogs from any pedigree with recurrences of maternal aggression would benefit from early genetic and behavioral counseling.

Helpful Handouts

- "Protocol for Generalized Discharge Instructions for Dogs with Behavioral Concerns"
- "Protocol for Handling and Surviving Aggressive Events"

Last Words

- See the following discussion of bitches who kill their puppies as a special case of predatory aggression.

Predatory Aggression Involving Dam and Pups
Diagnostic Criteria and Description
- Consistent aggression (threat/challenge/contest) directed toward puppies by the mother in the absence of threatening or injurious behavior by the puppies.
- Attacks are unprovoked and inappropriate, given the age of the pups.

Common Non-Specific Signs
- Growling, grabbing, shaking, biting, with or without mutilating, with or without killing the puppies.

Rule Outs
- Starvation of mother, acute pain, profound neurological disease.

Etiology, Epidemiology, and Risk Groups
- This appears to be a heritable condition that runs in family lines.

Common Myths That Can Get in the Way of Treatment or Diagnosis
- Management practices are often blamed, but there are no published data.

Commonly Asked Client Questions
- Will this happen if the dog is bred again?
  - Clients must understand that the risk for this to recur is great. The condition has been known to occur in surviving female offspring. Few data exist, but a fatal version of this condition has been noted to occur in at least three generations of laboratory dogs. If the clients are vigilant, they may prevent injury to the pups, but we do not know if these puppies are otherwise affected by their odd early development or any potential co-morbid risks *in utero*. If the clients breed a surviving female offspring, they should disclose that this condition is in their line.
- Should the bitch be spayed?
  - We do not understand this condition, but for the sake of everyone, spaying the bitch may be the most humane choice.
- Are other puppies not related to this bitch at risk?
  - The risk is unclear. There have been reports of dogs who killed their own puppies also attempting to kill or killing puppies of other bitches. These dogs may, but do not have to, behave normally with adult dogs. Caution and vigilance are urged.

Treatment
- Management:
  - Prevent pregnancies, and early wean and hand-raise pups with the help of another adult dog (male or female) who likes puppies.
- Behavior modification:
  - None.
- Medication/dietary intervention:
  - None recommended.
- Miscellaneous interventions:

- Breeders should query everyone who has a dog in this dog's line and inform all interested parties of the results of the queries.
- An honest appraisal of any patterns in the pedigree will help determine whether the occurrence of this behavior in one pregnancy may be exceptional.
- Once it is known that this condition has appeared, efforts should be made to ensure no affected dog is mated, and clients with related dogs should be cautioned.

Helpful Handouts
- "Protocol for Generalized Discharge Instructions for Dogs with Behavioral Concerns"
- "Protocol for Handling and Surviving Aggressive Events"

Last Words
- This condition is rare, but it is awful.
- If this condition appears in a breeding colony, especially of working dogs, or in a family line, careful records, especially of the female lines, should be kept with respect to nutrition, vaccination history, overall medical and behavioral health, and behavioral and developmental landmarks. The sooner excellent records are kept, the sooner correlated deviations may be spotted.

Play Aggression
Diagnostic Criteria and Description
- Consistent, out-of-context aggression (threat/challenge/contest) that occurs in contexts in which play behaviors (play bows, yips, shoulder blocks, et cetera) would normally occur or where these would be relevant.
- Play aggression is often most clearly seen in solicitation of play, but it involves actions that would actually discourage play (biting, pain).

Common Non-Specific Signs
- Barking, grabbing, growling, jumping, and biting to get people to play and with increased intensity as play progresses.
  - Some growls may change in pitch and volume as a result of increased stimulation or in response to increased rough play by people.
  - A play growl can be distinguished from a serious one, and clients should be taught to discriminate. Play growls are usually high-pitched, short, and repeated frequently. True aggressive growls are lower pitched and prolonged.
  - Change in the tone of the growl may not always be present.
  - Changes in the pitch of the growl can happen too abruptly to detect safely.
  - Some dogs give other signals that they are becoming aggressive during play: the hair on the neck may go up, the ears may flatten, and the pupils may dilate.

Rule Outs
- None.

Etiology, Epidemiology, and Risk Groups
- Puppies who have been hand-reared may play differently than puppies reared with their parents and siblings. These dogs do not experience the real-time feedback that they would have received were they to injure family members, and so they may not inhibit behaviors well.
- Some older puppies and young dogs exhibiting play aggression may never have learned to play appropriately. This condition may be the result of abandonment, lack of interaction in humane shelter or kennel/crate situations, or restricted access to other dogs in normal play situations.
- The dog may never have learned to play appropriately because the clients proactively encourage rough play. *No puppy or dog should ever be slapped about the face and head in the course of play or be offered a hand or arm to grab in play.*

Common Myths That Can Get in the Way of Treatment or Diagnosis
- Playing roughly with a puppy makes that puppy "tough."
- Smacking the dog so that he comes back at you will make the dog into a more protective dog for the family.

Commonly Asked Client Questions
- How do I get my husband/son/boyfriend/father/ et cetera to stop playing so roughly with the dog?
  - This diagnosis—and dog bites to children—are more common when human males are involved. Male humans play more roughly with dogs than females. The veterinary staff should acknowledge this and screen families for concern.
  - Most people who play roughly do not understand the risks to the dog. Clients need to understand the role for early learning and that dogs who bite are liability risks, could seriously injure someone, and could end up relinquished or euthanized.
  - Informed clients can accept that they must protect the dog and themselves and that they are responsible for helping the dog play in ways that are fun for everyone.

Treatment
- Management:
  - The normal, accepted, or contextual range of social play behaviors is well defined compared with abnormal, unacceptable, or out of context behaviors. The first step in managing interactions is to understand which ones are normal and which ones are not. Having the clients video themselves playing with the dog will indicate where the problem lies.
  - As a first step, instruct clients to play only with toys. Toys should be bigger than the dog's head so that the dog can make a mistake and still not bite the human.
  - Once the dog takes the toy, it is acceptable to play tug if—and only if—the following safety rules are adhered to:
    - The dog can mouth only the toy.
    - At the first instance of any part of the dog connecting with the client's arm, the game stops, and the client removes his or her attention from the dog.
    - The dog must sit and be calm to start the game again.
    - The dog can relinquish the toy in exchange for another or for the request to "drop it."
    - If the dog quits the game, that's fine.
    - If the client wishes to quit the game, the dog can be asked to sit and told he or she is brilliant. Whether the dog keeps the toy depends on whether she will destroy or ingest it.
- Behavior modification:
  - Modifying the behavior of the *human* will help modify the behavior of the dog.
  - People have little idea that puppies are fragile.
  - The vet staff should demonstrate appropriate toys and play techniques for all puppies and at any visits with young dogs who seem rough and/or whose people have scratches on their hands, forearms, legs, or face.
  - All play should take place only with toys.
  - Clients should be taught to play with the dog only in a manner that allows the client to control the intensity of the interaction. Done correctly, the dog is taught to take the cues as to the appropriateness of his or her behavior from the client.
  - Puppies need targets for full-on, rough and tumble play. The best targets are other puppies or adult dogs who like puppies and play and who are known to play appropriately. Play groups are wonderful ideas if the participants are well matched.
- Medication/dietary intervention:
  - Some diets and supplements address the role for polyunsaturated fatty acids (e.g., docosahexaenoic acid [DHA] and eicosapentaenoic acid [EPA]) in retinal and neurological development (see Chapter 10).
- Miscellaneous interventions:
  - Young dogs rescued from shelters may come to their new home with profound play aggression. Head collars and no-pull harnesses (e.g., Freedom Harness from Wiggles, Wags, and Whiskers; www.WigglesWagsWhiskers.com) can stop these dogs from jumping. Head collars (e.g., Blackdog Training Halter; www.blackdog.net.au) can stop these puppies from grabbing. Such tools must be used gently and humanely and in association with behavior modification that teaches the dog to sit, relax, and play appropriately with toys.

- If the dog still needs a head collar to relinquish a toy in a few weeks, the behavior modification is not being done.
- A humane, certified dog trainer, whom the veterinary staff have interviewed, seen work, and checked references and credentials, may be very helpful in teaching the clients play techniques suitable for their household.
- Some dogs with play aggression hide and charge people to incite play.
  - Some people (e.g., ill adults, older adults, young children) can be seriously injured if knocked over or grabbed by a dog.
  - If the dog wears a bell on a breakaway collar, warning will be given of his or her movement.
  - If the potential victims cannot use this warning, ensure that the dog is kept behind gates or doors when these people are present.
  - These dogs need aerobic exercise outlets.
    - Leash walks are important because studies have shown that dogs prefer the household member who walks them (Mariti et al., 2013), but these walks are not usually aerobic.
    - Running (e.g., running after a Frisbee, running after a flyball, or running through deep snow), swimming, running on an underwater treadmill, and chasing other dogs all can help dogs reach their aerobic scope. Such exercise will help these dogs.

Helpful Handouts
- "Protocol for Handling and Surviving Aggressive Events"
- "Protocol for Generalized Discharge Instructions for Dogs with Behavioral Concerns"
- "Protocol for Basic Manners Training and House-training for New Dogs and Puppies"
- "Protocol for Deference"
- "Protocol for Preventing and Treating Attention-Seeking Behavior"
- "Protocol for Choosing Collars, Head Collars, Harnesses, and Leads"
- "Protocol for Teaching Kids—and Adults—to Play with Dogs and Cats"
- "Protocol for Choosing Toys for Your Pet"

Last Words
- The difficulty lies in distinguishing rough play that the animals have learned in their interactions from other animals or people from truly abnormal behavior.
- It is extremely easy for humans to contribute to making this condition worse.

Fear Aggression
Diagnostic Criteria and Description
- Aggression (threat/challenge/contest) that consistently occurs in dogs exhibiting behavioral and physiological signs of fear.

- Behavioral signs of fear include withdrawal and passive (looking away) and active avoidance (attempting to leave or hiding) behaviors.
- Physiological signs of fear include signs associated with the sympathetic branch of the autonomic nervous system: increased heart rate, increased respiration, shaking, trembling, salivation, mydriasis, lack of appetite, uncontrolled urination, uncontrolled diarrhea/loose stool, anal sac expression.
- The more profound the signs and the more signs that are present, the more certain the diagnosis.
- Affected dogs would prefer to avoid frank aggression, but if cornered or given no choice, they will bite.
- Affected dogs tend to bite at last, not at first, and the bite follows vocal and physical warning by the dog.
- Affected dogs tend to be consistent in the triggers of their behavioral response (e.g., all new people, tall men on dark nights, dogs who approach from the back, et cetera), and they can generalize (e.g., all men, regardless of height and time of day) if their human confirms that their concern is valid.
- The focus of the aggression could be humans or members of other species.
- Because these dogs give clearly recognized warning, they are often reinforced by having the focus of their aggression leave. Learning that threats cause others to leave is swift and easy and needs to be considered in treatment.

Common Non-Specific Signs
- Body postures associated with fear aggression include a lowering of head and body, tucking of the tail, piloerection, ears moved back, wrinkled muzzles, horizontal and then vertical lip retraction, and snarling.
- Vocal threats, such as growling/snarling/barking, generally occur while the dog is backing up with the tail tucked and back arched.
- Affected dogs will often try to avoid the situation first, but they must monitor the actions of the individual of whom they are fearful.
- Affected dogs are often *hypervigilant* in contexts that may provoke the fear aggression and/or contexts in which aggression has been previously demonstrated.
- These dogs threaten while backing up and may lunge if the focus of the aggression turns their back. These dogs may lunge in part because they cannot monitor the threat. Lunging/biting provides them with some control, allows them to assess a response to their increased aggression, and encourages the focus of the threat to leave.
- Affected dogs can remain aroused for a considerable time after the event.
- In contrast to anxious dogs, who must provoke a situation, dogs with any component of fear to their response prefer to avoid an encounter, if possible.
- In a pairwise comparison of the behaviors of dogs with fear aggression or "dominance" aggression

(now usually called "impulse-control aggression" or "conflict aggression"), possessive aggression, and protective aggression (Borchelt, 1984), a re-analysis of the data (Overall, 1997) showed that of the six behaviors studied (barking, growling, baring teeth, snapping, biting, and staring), only barking was exhibited more frequently in fear aggression.

Rule Outs

- Any condition that impairs the dog's mobility or ability to monitor the environment may cause previously unaffected dogs to show signs of fear aggression.
  - As aging dogs begin to experience visual or auditory impairment they may become fearful and uncertain and react aggressively. If the client recognizes this pattern, intervention to announce approaches and rewarding a calm response will help.
  - Once the dog's condition has stabilized, if they had not previously exhibited fear aggression, it usually resolves if it was associated only with the debility.
- Fear aggression is a common sequela to pain.
  - The most common pain that dogs experience is that induced by veterinarians. Although we are doing a better job of addressing pre-, peri-, and post-surgical pain, we do a poor job of avoiding and controlling pain and anxiety from routine procedures (e.g., vaccination, nail clipping).
  - Pain may also be a factor in the development of fear aggression toward other dogs if age and size mismatches occur. Large, young, boisterous puppies may make poor companions for smaller, older, arthritic, and painful dogs.

Etiology Epidemiology and Risk Groups

- Because of the manner in which the amygdala and the hippocampus interact (see Chapter 2), fear is easily reinforced and learned. Fear is adaptive, in context. Even non-contextual fears and accompanying aggressive responses are learned if they spare the dog from further, longer, or repeated exposure to the fearful stimulus. We do not focus on teaching animals how to recover from fearful events as these events are occurring.
- It is likely that a genetic predisposition is responsible for animals who recover from fearful events well and quickly and animals who recover poorly. If the dog learns that the aggression is adaptive for him (the person whom he fears leaves him alone), he will hone his aggressive responses.
- We know that heritable fear in dogs has been confirmed in pups as young as 5 weeks. We lack similar information for fear aggression.
- Dogs who have been abused or ill-treated and learned to survive such treatment may be at enhanced risk for fear aggression.
- Dogs experiencing inappropriate punishment (e.g., hitting, shocking) may be at enhanced risk for fear aggression. Affected dogs may associate approach of the person with the punishment experience.
  - In situations in which punishment has been inappropriately or excessively used or when there is any suspicion that this may be the case, veterinarians should screen other pets and humans in the household for signs of abuse. Animal abuse is associated with spousal and child abuse, and most abusers hone their abuse skills on pets and captured animals.
- Dogs who have been kept in situations where they cannot escape those who threaten or scare them but who learn to control proximity by threat (many shelter dogs) may be at enhanced risk for fear aggression.
- Dogs who have been teased but limited in their response (e.g., because of a fence that allows someone to poke sticks at the dog but does not permit his escape) may be at enhanced risk for fear aggression.
- Cornered, cage/kenneled, entrapped dogs—even if the entrapment is in their mind—with this diagnosis are more at risk for frank aggression (Fig. 6-4). The vast majority of aggressive events with affected dogs do not involve biting.
- Fear aggression can be a common condition in part because its exhibition may have been adaptive for the dog (e.g., consider abandoned and feral dogs when they are not treated kindly).
- This condition can appear in young dogs but appears to worsen and become fully developed as dogs pass through social maturity, based on incidence data (Borchelt, 1984).
- The occasional dog may develop fear aggression idiopathically, but caution is urged for attributing an idiopathic basis for dogs whose histories are incomplete.

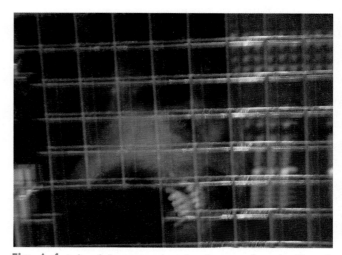

Fig. 6-4 A fearfully aggressive dog in a small crate. His only option when approached was to attack the door of the crate. He is so frenzied that the entire crate bounces around. Truly fearful dogs are trapped when they cannot escape, reducing their choices to attack or freeze.

Common Myths That Can Get in the Way of Treatment or Diagnosis

- "Flooding" has sometimes been recommended as a treatment for fearful dogs, including dogs that are fearfully aggressive. Flooding requires exposing the dog to the stimulus that provokes the response, at the level that provokes the response (see Chapter 2 for a comparison of this technique and desensitization), without recourse until the dog is no longer reactive.
  - The use of flooding is almost always inappropriate, and it is abusive in this situation.
  - Exposing a fearful or fearfully aggressive dog to a stimulus of which he is afraid but cannot escape will make the dog worse.

Commonly Asked Client Questions

- Should we take the dog to a pet supply store and/or a dog park to expose him to other dogs?
  - No. Please see the discussion of flooding. There is also a discussion in Chapter 3 on the use and abuse of dog parks and pet supply stores. Dog parks, shopping centers, and pet supply centers are potentially provocative places for dogs who are not normal. Most of the staff in any store situation will not have adequate training about dog behavior to recognize when a dog poses a risk.
  - The only "exposures" likely to help are those conducted under controlled circumstances by professionals. With guidance, controlled exposures designed to help the dog may be arranged at dog parks, shopping centers, or pet supply stores, but they must be carefully thought out, planned in advance, and orchestrated with full disclosure and the cooperation of others. See the discussions on management and behavior modification that follow.

Treatment

- Management:
  - All situations in which the dog exhibits fear aggression must be avoided until the dog can be desensitized to the stimuli that provoke him. This means that if the dog shies away, growling, whenever it meets another dog, dogs must be avoided until the behavior modification program is well under way.
  - Physical punishment/discipline has no role in the treatment of any aggressive dog, but it is particularly awful for dogs with fear aggression. Fearfully aggressive dogs become worse when punished/disciplined and may have no recourse except to bite.
  - Never corner a fearfully aggressive dog. Although the dog may have backed up while growling, once cornered, it will have no choice but to bite if further frightened.
  - Dogs with fear aggression should not be reassured that it is "all right." It is not all right, and

they know it. To tell them this reassuringly while petting them may reinforce the abnormal behavior, but it also is conflicting information for the dog.
  - Instead, extract the dog as calmly and safely from the situation as is possible.
  - Neither punish nor praise the dog, but calm the dog. Some dogs are calmer when exposed to steady pressure or to quiet rooms.
- Dogs with fear aggression must be protected as the first step in helping them to recover. Protection prevents further learning at the molecular level of problematic and abnormal behaviors.
- Dogs with fear aggression will do best when walked on head collars or harnesses that allow the clients to interrupt their behavior humanely if they react and to get them away from the provocative stimulus as soon as possible. The Web Master Harness by RuffWear can be snugly fitted, which some dogs find comforting, and has a handle. The Freedom No-Pull Harness from Wiggles, Wags, and Whiskers gives clients traction to redirect the dog physically, if needed.
- Behavior modification:
  - Behavior modification must focus on:
    - teaching the dog to look at the client when requested to do so,
    - teaching him to couple looking at the client to sitting and taking a deep breath as the first step in learning to relax, and
    - using these behaviors in a good and humane desensitization and counter-conditioning program.
- Medication/dietary intervention:
  - Treatment with behavioral medication is the humane choice for these dogs. The medication of choice depends on whether the dog panics when he encounters the stimulus and whether he engages in hypervigilance. We can divide medication use into two groups: fear aggression that is shown in a number of circumstances and fear aggression that is shown at the veterinary practice, whether or not it's a sequela to pain.

Fear Aggression Shown in a Number of Circumstances

- First-pass medications include selective serotonin reuptake inhibitors (SSRIs) such as fluoxetine with or without tricyclic antidepressants (TCAs) such as amitriptyline.
- If the dog is hypervigilant, gabapentin alone or in combination with TCAs/SSRIs may help.
- If the dog panics, the panicolytic benzodiazepine (BZD), alprazolam, can be given to interrupt the panic, as a preventive, or as an interventional medication for potential encounters (see handout, "Generalized Guidelines for Using Alprazolam for Noise and Storm Phobias, Panic, and Severe Distress"). The

dogma has been to avoid BZDs in dogs who have fear aggression because they may be "disinhibited." Pharmacological and rodent data suggest that this concern pertains only to truly "inhibited" behaviors (and these dogs are not inhibiting their aggression). The larger issue may be that the BZDs, which go through the *N*-desmethyl-diazepam metabolic pathway, are sufficiently sedative that the dog is more, rather than less, uncertain. Alprazolam does not use this metabolic pathway and so is anxiolytic and panicolytic without being sedating at therapeutic dosages (see Chapter 10).

- For dogs that are globally hyper-reactive and affected by fear aggression, the use of a centrally acting alpha agonist (clonidine) plus a SSRI and/or TCA may be helpful.
- Other classes of anti-anxiety medications may be useful for dogs who do not respond to the aforementioned agents. This diagnosis may be a candidate for treatment with nasal oxytocin.

Fear Aggression Shown at the Veterinary Practice

- If the dog becomes distressed during or as a result of a veterinary intervention and the dog is not undergoing a procedure/treatment that would prohibit treatment, give the dog a BZD (preferably alprazolam) as soon as possible to abort the profound distress and to help the dog not to learn to associate the distress with the circumstances. Although it is true that the clinician will not know whether the dog will experience an undesirable side effect, a veterinary practice is a good place to monitor for these, and dogs and clients can sit quietly in a calm area for 30 minutes to see if there is an effect and/or a side effect.
- If the dog is known to become distressed as soon as it is apparent that a veterinary trip will occur, the dog can be pre-medicated with alprazolam 2 hours and 30 minutes before the visit (see "Generalized Guidelines for Using Alprazolam for Noise and Storm Phobias, Panic, and Severe Distress"). Clonidine can also be used 1.5 hours and/or 30 minutes before the visit for dogs who do not respond to BZDs.
- If the dog is painful and/or ill and anxious, consider using both pain medication and anti-anxiety medication as needed (BZDs may be best unless respiratory compromise is acute; nasal oxytocin may have potential in this situation).
- Miscellaneous interventions:
  - As the dog begins to improve, use of a "safety signal" or another dog who is normal and after whom the patient can model his behaviors may help.
  - Toys that the dog associates with fun and that can hold his attention can act as safety signals. If clients are able to anticipate when they are going to encounter the provocative stimulus and they can

get the dog to concentrate on the safety signal before and during the encounter, the dog can learn that he can manage the event without distress.
- Dogs who are able to learn from other dogs can benefit from a normal dog who is not reactive to the stimulus as a model, once the affected dogs are calm enough to be able to learn new behaviors. The affected dog should be able to execute flawlessly tier 1 of the behavior modification programs ("Protocol for Relaxation: Behavior Modification Tier 1") before this technique will be useful. It's also helpful if the model dog has completed the behavior modification programs. Normal dogs learn these programs quite quickly.
- Dogs who react to very specific stimuli that can be anticipated can benefit from devices or behaviors that interrupt their normal response.
  - If the dog reacts only to dogs he can see approaching him, consider using eye shades or Doggles (www.doggles.com) to alter his visual impression of the approaching dog.
  - If the dog reacts only to dogs going away from him, try to position him so that all passing dogs are approaching him. This means that the client has to turn around a lot, but techniques like these allow the dog to have some control over his behaviors and to learn that he does not have to react and feel awful.
- All of these ancillary interventions are facilitated by appropriate and effective medication use.

Helpful Handouts

- "Protocol for Deference"
- "Protocol for Teaching Your Dog to Take a Deep Breath and Use Other Biofeedback Methods as Part of Relaxation"
- "Protocol for Relaxation: Behavior Modification Tier 1"
- "Tier 2: Protocol for Desensitizing and Counter-Conditioning a Dog or Cat from Approaches from Unfamiliar Animals, including Humans"
- "Protocol for Understanding and Treating Dogs with Fear/Fearful Aggression"
- "Protocol for Understanding and Treating Canine Panic Disorder (PD)"
- "Protocol for Using Behavioral Medication Successfully"
- "Generalized Guidelines for Using Alprazolam for Noise and Storm Phobias, Panic, and Severe Distress"

Last Words

- A lot has been written about the role for "appeasement" in fear and anxiety, and we should have two concerns when this term is used in the context of fear or fear aggression:
  - Is "appeasement" defined, given the context? (It virtually never is.) A full understanding of risks, costs, and threats would need to be available to define "appeasement."

- Are there more parsimonious explanations for the animals' behaviors that do not require extrapolation of some "emotional" or "motivational" state that cannot be measured? The answer here is almost always "yes." Message and meaning analysis provides a more discrete, judgment-free and value-free way of interpreting complex social interactions by allowing us to know, for example, when one participant is signaling their withdrawal. This approach has an advantage over the motivational approach because it is based on behaviors without any assumptions about how these are interpreted by the dog.
    - No one doubts that dogs and cats experience a complete range of emotions, but our attributions about them may not be accurate, and what we assume to be a "motivation" may not be as important to the dog or cat as it appears to us. If we are really to move into an era of research that maximizes welfare and QoL issues for our patients, we must be cautious about simplistic approaches that make our lives easier but that may not accurately reflect the dog's or cat's behaviors and their interpretation of them.
- Fear aggression is one of the common conditions to have co-morbid diagnoses. These dogs often panic or are reactive in other circumstances. It is important to screen all dogs thoroughly to ensure that all diagnoses are treated.
- If any family has more than one dog with fear aggression and they are not deliberately rescuing afflicted dogs who need help, take a close look at the family and ensure that no abuse is ongoing.
- No one should ever be bitten by a dog affected with fear aggression. These dogs give clear and extensive signals about their concerns and are honest about their behavioral patterns. This is the easiest of the aggressions to avoid.
- For veterinary visits, and because pain and anticipation of the visit may be involved in fear aggression, topical analgesics such as lidocaine gel may help with vaccinations, venipuncture, and anal sac expression and may facilitate desensitization to these manipulations as discussed in Chapters 1 and 3.

Pain-Related Aggression
Diagnostic Criteria and Description
- Aggression (threat/challenge/contest) exhibited in contexts associated with injury, illness, or treatment/intervention that could potentially cause adaptive (nociceptive and inflammatory) pain or exacerbate maladaptive (neuropathic, functional, and central) pain (*sensu* Hellyer et al., 2007; Reid et al., 2005).
- The aggression exhibited is greater than that required to indicate concern and to effect cessation of the offending stimulus.

- Because all aggressions have a learned component, if a dog has learned that he is made painful for a specific treatment/manipulation, he may exhibit signs of pain-related aggression *before* the actual treatment/manipulation. For example, the dog may splint and guard his abdomen while growling before he is actually touched or reached for.
- Evaluation of pain is difficult but increasingly possible.
    - Common signs of pain in dogs include guarding/protecting body parts, thrashing, restlessness, inability to rest normally, vocalization, and unusual attention to the painful area.
        - Dogs who have a history of another aggressive condition before the onset of the painful condition show fewer defensive behaviors before reacting than do dogs who have no history of other aggressive diagnoses (Camps et al., 2012).
    - Pain scales suggest that these behaviors may move from intermittent to more continuous behaviors as pain worsens (Firth and Haldane, 1999), and aggression may be part of a normal progression.
    - Whether the dog is in pain and experiencing pain aggression are ascertainments of degree and correlation. Conditions that are known to cause pain (i.e., fractured legs) could render the animal resistant to manipulation.
    - Domestic animals do not have opposable thumbs and so may use their mouths to grasp and restrain.
- For this diagnosis to be made, fear must not be primary (although anticipation of pain and the attendant anxiety may be involved), and the *behaviors must be in excess of those required to indicate the animal's concern and may precede manipulation.*
- Although this aggression occurs in the absence of behavioral and physiological signs of fear and avoidance behaviors, fear, fear aggression, and avoidance may become sequelae.

Common Non-Specific Signs
- Baring teeth, growling, snarling, lunging, and biting at the first perception of pain or behaviors that signal that a painful procedure/intervention may be about to occur.
- An aggressive response to the slightest touch is abnormal.
- Biting should be a last resort in canine communication, not the first resort.

Rule Outs
- Primary neurological disease including blindness and/or deafness. Inability to anticipate an approach can lead to fear.

Etiology, Epidemiology, and Risk Groups
- The experience and expression of pain are highly variable and individual.
- Clinicians must remember that the intensity of the pain experienced may be much greater than would be predicted on the basis of behavior alone.

- No one should assume that because animals are not complaining they are not hurting. Absence of patient complaints and dramatic behavioral displays can lead to under-treatment.
- In such cases, by treating the inapparent pain, the presence of pain may be confirmed by the display of more normal, happier behaviors and the abatement of pain aggression.
- Arthritis can also stimulate pain aggression.
  - A push on the shoulders or the rump or a small child's landing on a dog with arthritis or dysplasia may cause pain and could cause pain aggression.
  - Children in the 18- to 36-month-old age group are frequently implicated in this type of aggression because of their tendency to play roughly, coupled with their lack of coordination and judgment.
  - Children and dogs both can exhibit unpredictable behaviors; it is critical to teach young children appropriate ways to interact with dogs.
- It is important to remember that interactions with other dogs and cats can also cause pain aggression.
  - Dog fights result in painful wounds, and lacerations and punctures can teach the recipient to be fearful or fearfully aggressive to the aggressors.
  - In profound cases, the recipient of the aggression (the victim or defensively aggressive dog) may generalize her fear or fearful aggression to all dogs or to all large, dark dogs, for example.
  - Puppies, similar to small children, can inadvertently traumatize an older, arthritic dog, leading to avoidance, fear, or fearful aggression on the part of the older dog.

Common Myths That Can Get in the Way of Treatment or Diagnosis

- All of the following are wrong and inhumane:
  - Dogs don't feel pain the way we do.
  - Pain is a great immobilizer.
  - Pain is nature's way of telling you something is healing.
  - It will feel much better when the pain stops if the pain is allowed to occur.

Commonly Asked Client Questions

- Isn't it normal for a dog to bite when he is painful?
  - Not at first, and not for relatively minor interventions. We become concerned when a dog's first response is to bite and when dogs bite when experiencing any amount of painful stimulus but do not appear to be afraid. One concern here is a hypersensitivity to touch (e.g., allodynia, neuropathic pain, functional pain).
- Has my dog been abused? He never used to bite when given veterinary care.
  - If you know the dog's history and this behavior is a new development, the dog has likely not been abused. If the client is permitted to accompany the dog through as many treatment and intervention procedures as possible, this concern diminishes.
  - If you do not know the dog's history, abuse is always possible, but this type of behavioral concern can also develop in dogs who have had a flawless upbringing and no risk factors.
- Must we control the pain to control this response?
  - We should assess the primary pain and its perception and *treat both the pain and the anxiety*. Pain must be assessed in a consistent manner. One tool is the Glasgow pain scale (Table 6-4) (Holton et al., 2001).

Treatment

- Management:
  - Behavioral assessments of pain may be more helpful than pain assessment scores or physiological measures in terms of possible interventions (Hansen et al., 1997; Hardie et al., 1997; Holton et al., 1998a, 1998b, 2001).
  - Investing in a practice standard that encourages calm, humane, behavior-centered care may minimize the likelihood of this condition developing because of associations made.
  - Environments that are less noisy and where movement can be anticipated may have an effect on this condition. There are no data.
- Behavior modification:
  - If clients teach dogs to be manipulated and offer body parts for manipulations, they may decrease the probability of pain aggression developing.
    - The manipulations most important to learn include offering nails for trimming, having teeth brushed, offering ears for routine ear cleaning, offering limbs for venipuncture, and offering hind ends for temperatures and anal sac expression.
  - If clients teach dogs to wear head collars, these can help relax and control dogs during procedures.
  - Desensitization and counter-conditioning to the veterinary practice, the clinician, the treatment room or ward, or any aspects of the procedures may be needed once pain aggression develops. Such behavior modification will help with future veterinary care.
- Medication/dietary intervention:
  - We must treat the pain that precedes this condition. Behavioral assays conducted before and after treatment for pain using oxymorphone or fentanyl demonstrated return to normal behaviors with analgesia (Hansen, 2003).
  - Anxiety associated with the potential to experience pain can be treated with BZDs and/or other related compounds such as gabapentin.
    - Unless the dog is sedated by the BZD, the dog is unlikely to become more aggressive. This is especially true if he was not inhibiting any aggression before medicating him.

TABLE 6-4

Glasgow Pain Scale

This instrument requires that the clinician stand outside the kennel or cage and assess the dog. The authors recommend that street clothes are worn because of learned associations of lab coats and scrubs. The questionnaire consists of a number of questions, each of which have several possible answers. Clinicians are asked to select the best choice.

1. Look at the dog's posture, does it seem:
   a. Rigid
   b. Hunched or tense
   c. Neither of these
2. Does the dog seem to be:
   a. Restless
   b. Comfortable
3. If the dog is vocalizing, is it:
   a. Crying or whimpering
   b. Groaning
   c. Screaming
   d. Not vocalizing/none of these
4. If the dog is paying attention to its wound, is it:
   a. Chewing
   b. Licking or looking or rubbing
   c. Ignoring its wound
5. Now approach the kennel door and call the dog's name. Then open the door and encourage the dog to come to you. From the dog's reaction to you and its behavior when you were watching it, assess its character. Does the dog seem to be:
   a. Aggressive
   b. Depressed
   c. Disinterested
   d. Nervous or anxious or fearful
   e. Quiet or indifferent
   f. Happy and content
6. Now look at the dog's response to stimuli. If the mobility assessment is possible, then open the kennel and put a lead on the dog. If the animal is sitting down, encourage it to stand and come out of the kennel. Walk slowly up and down the area outside the kennel. If the dog was standing up in the kennel and has undergone a procedure that may be painful in the perianal area, ask the animal to sit down. During this procedure, did the dog seem to be:
   a. Stiff
   b. Slow or reluctant to rise or sit
   c. Lame
   d. None of these
   e. Assessment not carried out
7. The next procedure is to assess the dog's response to touch. If the animal has a wound, apply gentle pressure to the wound using 2 fingers in an area approximately 2 inches around it. If the wound is impossible to touch, apply the pressure to the closest point to the wound. If there is no wound, apply the same pressure to the stifle and surrounding area. When touched, did the dog:
   a. Cry
   b. Flinch
   c. Snap
   d. Growl or guard wound
   e. None of these

Definitions Needed to Complete Glasgow Pain Scale

Posture	Rigid: Animal lying in lateral recumbency, legs extended or partially extended in a fixed position
	Hunched: When animal is standing, its back forms a convex shape with abdomen tucked up or back in a concave shape with shoulders and front legs lower than hips

Continued

TABLE 6-4

Glasgow Pain Scale—cont'd

	Tense: Animal appears frightened or reluctant to move; overall impression of tight muscles; animal can be in any body position Normal body posture: Animal may be in any position; appears comfortable, muscles relaxed
Activity	Restless: Moving bodily position, circling, pacing, shifting body parts, unsettled Comfortable: Animal resting and relaxed, no avoidance or abnormal body position evident, or settled, remains in same body position, at ease
Vocalization	Whimpering: Often quiet, short, high-pitched sound, frequently closed mouth (whining) Crying: Extension of whimpering noise, louder and with open mouth Groaning: Low moaning or grunting, deep sound, intermittent Screaming: Animal making continual high-pitched noise, inconsolable, mouth wide open
Attention to wound area	Chewing: Using mouth and teeth on wound area, pulling stitches Licking: Using tongue to stroke area of wound Looking: Turning head in direction of area of wound Rubbing: Using paw or kennel floor, et cetera, to stroke wound area Ignoring: Paying no attention to wound area
Demeanor	Aggressive: Mouth open or lip curled showing teeth, snarling, growling and snapping or barking Depressed: Dull demeanor, not responsive, shows reluctance to interact Disinterested: Cannot be stimulated to wag tail or interact with observer Nervous: Eyes in continual movement, often head and body movement, jumpy Anxious: Worried expression, eyes wide with white showing, wrinkled forehead Fearful: Cowering away, guarding body and head Quiet: Sitting or lying still, no noise, will look when spoken to but not respond Indifferent: Not responsive to surroundings or observer Content: Interested in surroundings, has positive interaction with observer, responsive and alert Bouncy: Tail wagging and jumping in kennel, often vocalizing with a happy and excited noise
Mobility	Stiff: Stilted gait, slow to rise or sit, may be reluctant to move Slow to rise or sit: Slow to get up or sit down but not stilted in movement Reluctant to rise or sit: Needs encouragement to get up or sit down Lame: Irregular gait, uneven weight bearing when walking Normal mobility: Gets up and lies down with no alteration from normal
Response to touch	Cry: Short vocal response; looks at area and opens mouth, emits a brief sound Flinch: Painful area is quickly moved away from stimulus either before or in response to touch Snap: Tries to bite observer before or in response to touch Growl: Emits a low prolonged warning sound before or in response to touch Guard: Pulls painful area away from stimulus or tenses local muscles to protect from stimulus None: Accepts firm pressure on wound with no reaction

From Holton et al., 2001.

- Gabapentin was developed to treat neurogenic and myogenic pain and so may have widespread use in pain aggression.
- Alpha-2 agonists may be extremely useful for treating *both the pain and the anxiety* associated with it and are reversible (dexmedetomidine canine dose, 5 μg/kg intramuscularly or intravenously; reversed by atipamezole, 0.025 to 0.1 mg/kg intravenously or intramuscularly).
- N-methyl-D-aspartate receptor antagonistics such as amantadine (3 to 5 mg/kg orally every 24 hours) are extremely useful for *both the type of pain worsened by anxiety and the anxiety, itself.*
- TCAs and SSRIs are often used to treat *neuropathic and myogenic pain and the anxiety that may co-occur and/or augment the pain.* These agents will potentiate the effects of opioids, which may be helpful for painful dogs. For these to work as well as possible, treatment needs to be continuous and daily.
- Miscellaneous interventions:
  - Muzzles will stop bites, but muzzles can be potent weapons when the dog swings his head. Muzzle use can backfire by allowing the dog to exhibit and practice more aggression and a greater continuum of aggressive behaviors than would have otherwise been the case.
  - Head collars are often more helpful and appropriate for helping to provide safe control of dogs, and they are under-used during veterinary procedures.

Helpful Handouts
- "Protocol for Generalized Discharge Instructions for Dogs with Behavioral Concerns"
- "Protocol for Deference"
- "Protocol for Teaching Your Dog to Take a Deep Breath and Use Other Biofeedback Methods as Part of Relaxation"
- "Protocol for Teaching Cats and Dogs to 'Sit,' 'Stay,' and 'Come'"
- "Protocol for Relaxation: Behavior Modification Tier 1"
- "Generalized Guidelines for Using Alprazolam for Noise and Storm Phobias, Panic, and Severe Distress"
- "Protocol for Using Behavioral Medication Successfully"
- "Tier 2: Protocol for Desensitizing and Counter-Conditioning a Dog or Cat from Approaches from Unfamiliar Animals, including Humans"

Last Words
- Veterinary staff often think that pain aggression is normal when animals are badly injured or have undergone painful procedures. This need not be true, and the assumption that it is true subjects the patient to physical and behavioral suffering.
- Treating pain at each possibility is essential. For animals with pain aggression, any procedure may be cause for anxiety, which will heighten their already elevated response to pain. Use of topical analgesics such as lidocaine gel may help with vaccinations, venipuncture, and anal sac expression and may facilitate desensitization to these manipulations (see Chapters 1 and 3).

Territorial and Protective Aggression
Diagnostic Criteria and Description
- Protective aggression can be defined as aggression (threat/challenge/contest) that is consistently demonstrated when an individual/group of individuals is approached by another individual/group of individuals in the absence of a contextual threat from those approaching.
- Territorial aggression can be defined as aggression (threat/challenge/contest) that is consistently demonstrated in the vicinity of a mobile (e.g., car) or stationary (e.g., yard), circumscribed area when that area is approached by an individual/group of individuals in the absence of an actual, contextual threat from those approaching.
- For both conditions, the aggression intensifies with decreasing distance, regardless of attempts at intervention, correction, or the desire to interact on the part of the approaching individual(s).
- These diagnoses should be made only after the relevance of the context in which it occurs has been evaluated. Clients may not realize that the dog valued something about a location or that their relationship with another dog, cat, or person contributed to their response.

Common Non-Specific Signs
- Heightened attentiveness and vigilance as the object of the aggression approaches, barking, snarling, growling, and grabbing/biting.
- The form of aggression intensifies with proximity.
- Because these conditions are about protecting something/someone, grabbing without actually doing a lot of damage is common because the dog is attempting to stop and hold the approacher.

Rule Outs
- Any condition that could affect pain or mobility and that could make a dog feel trapped may result in a more reactive dog.
- Blindness and deafness can render dogs more reactive, especially as they are adjusting to their impaired sensory function.

Etiology, Epidemiology, and Risk Groups
- Territories can be floating/transient/seasonal or more permanent.
- Dogs can protect an inappropriate location as its territory (e.g., a park bench) or an appropriate location but in an inappropriate context (e.g., the gate of the house from the homeowner).
- Dogs may exhibit territorial aggression toward any species or combination of species.
- Some dogs become territorial about their crates and the surrounding area or the places they sleep.
- Some dogs have a specific individual approach distance that they protect. In this sense, they have a mobile territory—the space around them—and become aggressive toward anyone who invades that space.
- Confined spaces, such as cars, crates, fences, or restrictive chains, may intensify territorial aggression.
- The hallmark of territorial aggression is that the dog is *not* aggressive when he is *removed from the territory.*
  - A dog who protects the area around his food dish might not protect his personal space when he is lying in the living room.
  - Chained or enclosed animals may have a heightened sense of a territory to defend, and so affected dogs may be more reactive if chained or enclosed.
- Fences, including electric fences, remove any ambiguity about territorial boundaries and will render a dog more secure and confident in its inappropriate aggression.
- Territorial aggression is most obvious when the dog is in the yard and a person or a dog passes or when the dog is inside and a stranger knocks on the door or enters the room.
  - Most or all dogs will bark to warn or announce the visitor. This is a normal first step in the sequence of behavior characterizing protection.

- Dogs with territorial aggression do not respond to human requests/guidance and can become so aggressive that visitors cannot safely enter.
- In territorial aggression the dog persists in the behavior despite cues indicating a contradictory context.
- Dogs affected by protective aggression perceive that the client is threatened and there is no actual threat.
  - Triggers include the entry of visitors through doors or into the house, approaches on the street or approaches when the dog and client are in a vehicle.
  - These dogs are always vigilant, but some affected dogs use raised voices or swift movements as triggers. These are stimuli that may be unpredictable, and so they worsen this aggression, which is based in underlying anxiety.
  - Touching or hugging the client can trigger protective aggression.
  - These dogs must be distinguished from dogs who are watchful and make good decisions about when to react.
    - In each case, the dog often positions itself between the possible threat and its person.
    - True protective aggression occurs when there is no real threat and the dog reacts inappropriately and out of context.
    - Instead of maintaining distance, the dog lunges, nips, herds, growls, or bites.
    - Appropriately behaved dogs monitor the newcomer's activities quietly, with their back turned only to their person.
    - In situations involving movement, appropriately behaved dogs may preserve these relative postures by maintaining a separation between their person and the newcomer.
    - It is acceptable to be vigilant; it is unacceptable to respond in a manner that contradicts the contextual significance of any cues.
    - Regardless, vigilant dogs should be sensitive to client desires and requests.
  - In territorial and protective aggression, the dog persists in the behavior *despite cues* indicating a contradictory context.

Common Myths That Can Get in the Way of Treatment or Diagnosis

- Dogs are supposed to be "protective."
  - Although this is a true statement and it is clear that humans specifically selected for characteristics of exaggerated protective behavior in many breeds, the expectation is that the dog can distinguish between a real threat, in which case the dog is just protective, and the approach of someone who is not a threat. This is a condition where context is everything.
- If the dog doesn't threaten people who approach, he will not learn to protect you from a threat. You must encourage dogs to threaten people.

- Encouraging inappropriate and pathological behaviors only renders such behaviors more abnormal. It does not make anyone safe. In fact, dogs who are inappropriately protective and territorial are real risks. Normal, in-context protective behaviors require a dog who recognizes "normal," can distinguish between it and "abnormal," and can temper his response to the context.
- Protective and territorial aggression are about access to resources, and social animals are supposed to protect resources.
  - In terms of future ability to understand genetic and neurochemical bases of these behaviors, "resources" may be best defined to exclude people and space. When the prevailing belief was that everything was due to a struggle over "dominance," the term dominance aggression often included the diagnoses of food-related, protective, and territorial aggression, plus impulse control/"conflict" aggression. This is an inappropriate characterization. Protective and territorial aggression can occur independently of other aggressions or in concert with them as part of a control complex. Not all assertive behaviors are predictors of impulse-control aggression. By keeping phenotypic diagnoses crisp, we can best recognize and enumerate contexts in which the aggression is likely to occur and design effective treatment plans to address them.
- Herding dogs or dogs of herding breeds are always aggressive in these contexts.
  - Part of herding behavior is guarding. That guarding and the attendant "rounding up" behaviors should always be appropriate and contextual. Being a member of a herding breed does not justify or excuse pathological aggression, and most members of these breeds are not affected. However, when a member of one of these breeds is affected, the form the behavior takes is likely to be shaped by the types of behaviors that breed uses for herding.

Commonly Asked Client Questions

- My dog is very quiet and laid back. Can I rely on her to protect me if something happens?
  - Most dogs will protect most people if the threat is clear. This is true regardless of age, size, and breed of the dog.
- My dogs sleep right through package deliveries when we are home. Can they be relied on to protect the house?
  - Most dogs behave differently if their people are home compared with when their people are gone (assuming they wake up). If protection of property is important to clients, they should install an alarm system. Alarm systems will often result in decreased home insurance costs. Inappropriately

or pathologically behaved dogs result in increased home insurance costs.

Treatment

- Management:
  - Dogs with territorial aggression should never be left alone, outside, confined, or unsupervised because they may pose a risk to any individual (human or animal) unable to perceive where the dog believes its territory to be.
    - A fence allows the dog to know exactly where the boundary of his or her property is and to patrol and protect it. Instead of becoming less aggressive, territorially aggressive dogs are often *more* aggressive when fenced because there is no doubt about boundaries.
    - Solid fences prevent any cost to the aggression to accrue because the dogs can threaten but not bite.
    - Because there are no outward signs of an electronic fence, intruders do not recognize the boundary and may cross it.
    - Motivated dogs will endure a shock to cross an electronic fence in pursuit of something they want—even if what they want is freedom to run—and dogs who are territorially or protectively aggressive will endure a shock to pursue someone.
      - Dogs who are shocked become more reactive, not less reactive.
      - There are reports of non-aggressive dogs biting whomever is next to them when they cross an invisible electronic fence and are shocked.
  - Similarly, dogs with protective aggression must not be put in situations in which they believe that they have to protect.
    - Instead, the dog can be placed behind a locked door (closed door, hook and eye or sliding bolt at the very top of the outside of the door) or a secure gate (one the dog is incapable of reaching through or jumping over) before anyone arrives. It's best to do this 15 to 30 minutes before an expected arrival so that the dog and humans have a chance to calm.
    - The dog can have a food toy, treat ball, chew toy, et cetera, to indicate that he is not being penalized and to keep him occupied.
    - No one is to visit these people without advance notice. If someone is coming to visit, they must always call first and should call a minimum of 15 minutes before they expect to arrive.
    - The dog is *not* permitted to visit with the guests if any human is afraid of dogs or this dog in particular.
    - If the dog is permitted to visit with the guests he must be engaged in *and* progressing with a behavior modification program designed to make him less reactive and less concerned when people come visit.
    - The dog can visit with the guests only if he is unable to do anyone damage. *This means he is on a lead and head collar or harness and someone is responsible for monitoring him.*
    - If the dog lunges at or threatens anyone *or* if anyone feels that they have been threatened, the dog must return to his secure area.
    - If the dog is anxious, worried, or miserable, he should be allowed to return to his secure area.
    - If the humans are going to worry every second the dog is present, even if he is wearing a head collar, they are not ready to have him visit guests, and he should be in his secure area. This is better for everyone and has the advantage of ensuring that no tragedies occur.
    - If the guests and hosts are happy to have the dog visit under the discussed circumstances, the dog can be present if no one approaches the dog without asking permission of and guidance from the person holding the lead. Everyone must follow instructions. No one should stare at, reach for, or otherwise engage the dog until the dog is sufficiently calm to follow instructions, including to sit and take a deep breath before being offered praise or a treat.
- Behavior modification:
  - Behavior modification should focus on addressing the dog's heightened vigilance and arousal.
  - Dogs with these conditions will benefit from learning to sit and to take a deep breath on cue and on learning to relax in situations where there are no threats.
  - Once the dog has demonstrated that he can be calm and happy in non-stimulating environments, desensitization and counter-conditioning can be used to teach the dog gradually that he does not have to react unless a true threat exists.
  - Until the dog is absolutely reliable, the protective measures discussed should continue.
  - These dogs are at risk for breakthrough events when the social environment is stimulating. These conditions are based in anxiety, and we are focusing on ameliorating and containing that anxiety using a clear and humane rule structure (desensitization and counter-conditioning). If the rules change suddenly—the approach of very rowdy unpredictable kids or adults—the dog may not have a rule that helps him to cope with such change.
    - If these types of events are expected to be part of the dog's experience, the behavior modification programs must address them (e.g., you desensitize the dog to recess at school using audio and video and then staged recesses before exposing him to the real thing).

- Regardless of whether it is rational, if anyone is going to worry about the dog's behavior during a gathering, the dog should be protected in a room away from everyone. The risk of the dog reacting to inappropriate human behavior or being blamed for it is too great.
- Medication/dietary intervention:
  - Diets that are relatively lower in protein may render some dogs less reactive; the evidence for this is weak and complex. However, this is an inexpensive and easy intervention to try. Unless dogs have a medical condition or are serious working and performance dogs, most of them do not need ultra-high-protein foods.
  - There is anecdotal evidence, but little hard data, to suggest that some diets high in DHA/EPA or nutraceutical supplements (e.g., CALM by ROYAL CANIN) may render these dogs less reactive. DHA can be supplemented, separately, with an aim to provide the dog with 1200 to 1500 mg/day of DHA.
  - Nutraceuticals alone have been reported to lower activity levels, and heightened activity is one of the behaviors associated with these aggressions (e.g., Zylkene (alpha-casozepine), Anxitane (L-theanine), Harmonese, Calmex (L-theanine, L-tryptophan, and other ingredients). Most of the data for these compounds are weak, and the effects may be relatively minor, but side effects are rare.
  - Medications should be chosen on the basis of their expected effects on anxiety.
    - If the dog is fairly explosive, the SSRI fluoxetine may help. If the dog is constantly vigilant, gabapentin may help. If the dog is exceedingly worried, the BZD alprazolam may help.
    - Alprazolam can be given before planned gatherings to lower the dog's arousal levels.
    - Clonidine may be helpful before planned gatherings in hyper-reactive and hypervigilant dog's.
    - Combinations of medications may be beneficial.
    - Because these conditions affect social interactions, they may be suitable test situations for the effects, if any, of intranasal oxytocin.
- Miscellaneous interventions:
  - Head collars can be hugely helpful in these conditions. When fitted well, they can both guide the dog from a situation and close his mouth, preventing any injury.
    - When people know dogs are unlikely to injure them, they behave more normally, which can relieve the contextual anxiety involved with these conditions.
  - Muzzles will stop dogs from biting but do nothing to affect any other aspect of these conditions. Because the perceived threat is still present, a muzzle is most likely to increase the dog's reactivity and level of aggression.

Helpful Handouts
- "Protocol for Deference"
- "Protocol for Teaching Your Dog to Take a Deep Breath and Use Other Biofeedback Methods as Part of Relaxation"
- "Protocol for Relaxation: Behavior Modification Tier 1"
- "Protocol for Generalized Discharge Instructions for Dogs with Behavioral Concerns"
- "Protocol for Handling and Surviving Aggressive Events"
- "Tier 2: Protocol for Desensitizing and Counter-Conditioning a Dog or Cat from Approaches from Unfamiliar Animals, including Humans"
- "Tier 2: Protocol for Desensitization and Counter-Conditioning to Noises and Activities That Occur by the Door"
- "Protocol for Understanding and Treating Dogs with Protective and/or Territorial Aggression"
- "Protocol for Handling 'Special-Needs Pets' during Holidays and Other Special Occasions"
- "Protocol for Using Behavioral Medication Successfully"
- "Generalized Guidelines for Using Alprazolam for Noise and Storm Phobias, Panic, and Severe Distress"

Last Words
- The biggest problem with these conditions is that some degree of contextual, innate "territoriality" is desired in most pet dogs because people want their dogs to protect property. Clients need help with distinguishing when behaviors are neither normal nor desirable.

Inter-Dog Aggression
Diagnostic Criteria and Description
- Inter-dog aggression (threat/challenge/contest) may be described as consistent, volitional, "proactive" aggression that is not contextual given the social signals, threat circumstances, or response received from the focus of the aggression.
- Absence of any signal or interaction from the animal that is attacked before the attack/aggressive encounter is sufficient to rule out normal squabbles/bickering/disagreements that all social animals experience.
- As with other diagnoses for abnormal and pathological behaviors, at some level, the behaviors involved with aggression are normal behaviors, and it is this confounding of normal and abnormal behaviors that has so confused our understanding of this extremely problematic and pathological condition in dogs.
- This diagnosis is associated with social changes in relationships and interaction that occur as animals move through social maturity and their brain chemistry changes, but it is not defined by either hierarchy or social maturity. *This pathology depends on and*

is defined by the contextual response of the dogs involved. This is a subtle but important distinction that supports the contention that social shifts and occasional threats can be normal.

- A change in behavior of both parties is not necessary, although it may be usual with time, exposure, and repeated harassment by one dog.
- This condition is usually associated with changes in social relationships, behaviors, and possible perceived changes in relative social "hierarchy" that are often related to the development of social maturity in at least one of the involved parties. The individual who worries about the maturation-related changes can be the aggressor who demonstrates offensive aggression or the victim who usually comes to demonstrate defensive aggression.
- Less injurious/lethal inter-dog aggression has been reported (Bamberger and Houpt, 2006; Orihel and Fraser, 2008; Wrubel et al., 2011) and may be a variant of "normal" behavior.
  - Dogs in shelters may have had bad experiences with other dogs, especially if stray, and may be unable to control their inter-personal approach distance in shelters. Many of these dogs can learn to habituate well to broad groups of other dogs given targeted, controlled exposure over relatively short time periods (e.g., 11 days) (Orihel and Fraser, 2008). Although termed a variant of "inter-dog aggression," this very moderate form of "aggression" may have to do with reactivity and/or uncertainty rather than true pathology as discussed here.
  - Dogs with inter-dog aggression may also have territorial aggression and generalized anxiety disorder (Bamberger and Houpt, 2006), suggesting that a range of behavioral patterns may be included in a diagnosis of inter-dog aggression, *not all of which are as specific as the diagnosis discussed here.* This may be especially true for many classifications of inter-dog aggression involving male dogs (Beaver, 1993; Borchelt, 1983).
  - Triggers for some forms of inter-dog aggression include attention from clients, presence of food, excitement/noise in general, items with which the dogs were playing, movement through passageways, small spaces, and access to valued areas including beds or furniture (Wrubel et al., 2011). That 50% of the "fights" involved injuries requiring veterinary treatment and that half of the clients also had difficulty separating dogs during a fight and had to separate them physically support the suspicion that this diagnosis has been used for two phenotypic populations of dogs: (1) dogs who exhibit social squabbling associated with attention-seeking behaviors and (2) dogs who are quite serious about their aggression and would take advantage of situations where one dog could victimize the other (e.g., tight spaces,

passageways). There are no data indicating ultimate treatment outcomes where one group of patients is highly controlled and separated when unsupervised correlates with the behavioral patterns, but such a finding would make sense.

- It must be understood that the population heterogeneity for this condition ranges from "normal," boisterous behavior, to mild true aggression, to the full pathological aggression discussed here. We do not understand the behavioral trajectories for any of these patterns.
- It is likely that the more "normal," less pathological forms of inter-dog aggression involve dogs who can live companionably much of the time and are not aroused unless a stimulus is present. Clients should know this and know that dogs recognize inequities in resource allocation (Range et al., 2009).
- As for most behavioral conditions, the pathology is unknown, but at least one of the four skill sets that normal dogs should possess is impaired in the aggressors in inter-dog aggression:
  - reading signals correctly,
  - correctly processing/understanding the information in those signals,
  - making a plan to act appropriately on the signals by utilizing the information in them once they have been read and processed, and
  - successfully and clearly signal and act on that plan.
- This condition is most commonly manifest between known dogs, especially dogs who live together. There are cases of true inter-dog aggression between dogs who do not know each other, where the aggressor's pathology likely rests with these same impaired signaling pathways. Unfortunately, the dogs whom these pathological dogs encounter usually go away, so the pathology is rewarded.
- Affected dogs are sometimes seen as chronic bullies. Bullying may not escalate, but inter-dog aggression almost always does.

Common Non-Specific Signs

- Dogs with inter-dog aggression are characterized by subtle signs where one dog tries to control the other dog.
- These signs are often missed by humans. Humans most commonly notice that there is a problem between the dogs when there is an outright fight.
- The aggressor tried to control the victim through the use of subtle threats and challenges.
- Challenges from the aggressor usually fall into one of three categories—displacement of victim, control of victim, and threat of victim (Table 6-5)—and can include:
  - blocking access to a bed or crate,
  - lying on or in front of a couch or chair (blocking access),
  - lying or pushing them on the other dog,

TABLE 6-5

Hallmarks of Aggressor Behavior (Offensively Aggressive Dogs) and Victim Capabilities (Defensively Aggressive Dogs) That Can Be Useful to Distinguish Dogs Involved in Inter-Dog Aggression

Classes of Behaviors Exhibited by Aggressors to Victims	Factors in Most Victim Behaviors That Can Be Rewarded in Treatment
Displacement of victim from resting places	Behaviors are *appropriate* to the context
Control of activities, access, sites, resources used/favored by victim	Behaviors are *fluid or labile*
Threats (e.g., stares) to victim	Dogs *recover and learn from mistakes*

- stealing the other dog's biscuits, rawhides, or toys,
- blocking access to the other dog's food (standing in front of the food or standing in front of the entry to the room where the food is),
- shoving past the other dog to get out or in a door or car first,
- using halls, doorways, and steps as situations to control the other dog and its access to areas or escape from them,
- ritualized displays including an approach where the challenger approaches the other dog nose to shoulder,
- staring,
- vocalizing (aggressive barks, snarls, growls), and
- frank aggression.
- These behaviors can occur alone or in combination and may be self-limiting or can escalate within a few minutes to outright aggression with grabbing and biting.
- By themselves, these behaviors are designed to elicit information from the other dog in the interaction, but the information received from the victim has virtually no effect on the course of the behaviors of the aggressor.
- Early in the development of this condition, there may be a lot of exaggerated posturing and vocalizing. As the condition progresses, these clear signs diminish. Snarls become silent, and attacks may occur with little warning.
- Region of the body grabbed matters.
  - Victims who have learned that they will be injured may start to show defensive aggression, grabbing the ears, cheek, or side of the neck of the aggressor to abort the offensive aggressive attack as it is occurring (Fig. 6-5). This pre-emptive strike ensures that the victim's neck cannot be grabbed.
    - Defensive behaviors by victims may be the first sign of aggression clients recognize. They then think that the victim is the "problem" dog.
  - Early in the development of the pathology, the aggressor grabs the shoulders, dorsal neck, and legs.

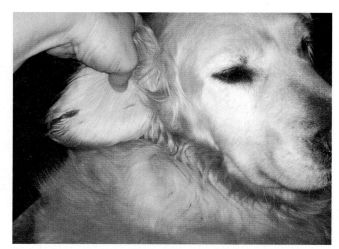

Fig. 6-5 A golden retriever who was thought to be the victim, or defensively aggressive dog, in an inter-dog aggression scenario. Note that the dog's ear is torn, and there are scratches or grooves made by teeth on his nose. In fact, this dog was the aggressor or the offensively aggressive dog in the pair. Clients often miss that the dog who has been repeatedly threatened will make an effort to protect herself as the aggression intensifies. If the dog who is being victimized can grab the aggressor's ear and/or side of the head first, she controls where the aggressor's jaws can go, and she directly prevents any bite to her throat, neck, or shoulders. (Photo courtesy of Cheryl Taylor.)

- Later in the development of the pathology, the aggressor grabs the sides, the underbelly, and the ventral neck and shakes and twists the skin and/or dog (Fig. 6-6).
- Later attacks share many commonalities with predatory attacks.
- As with most pathological conditions, the behaviors exhibited by the aggressor/offensively aggressive dog are most stereotypic and less fluid and flexible than the behaviors exhibited by the victim/defensively aggressive dog.

Rule Outs

- Endocrine (e.g., thyroidal) conditions and seizure disorders can become apparent as dogs move through social maturity (e.g., before 4 years of age) and so should be ruled out if any physical signs that could support them are present. The note

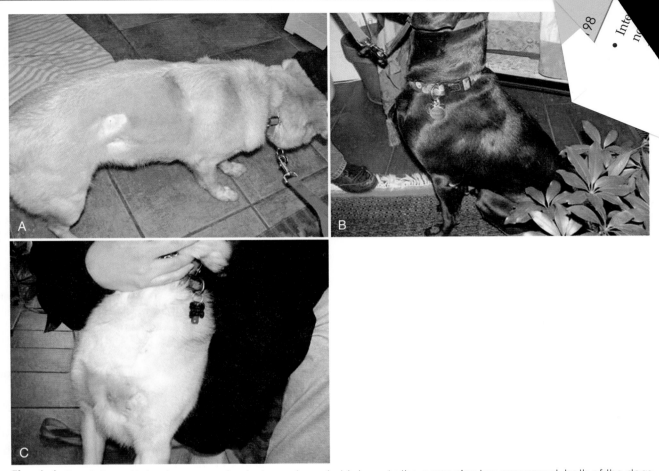

Fig. 6-6 The victims of inter-dog aggression between household dogs. As the aggression has progressed, both of the dogs in two separate cases have received offensive wounds to the flank. The victim in **A/C** also has throat wounds from the most recent fight.

about reactivity and thyroidal function found in the section on impulse control aggression has relevance here, also.

- Pain-related aggression can look like the early stages of inter-dog aggression because it can be induced when one dog bumps into another or when they have close contact.
- Any infectious or toxic agents that can affect behavior could alter the manner in which dogs interact with each other, but the pattern of change and the response from the other dog in the interaction differs. Dogs who are the recipient of aggressive behavior from an ill housemate know that the pattern is not associated with their own behavior but with something else, and they usually either avoid or try to help and care for the dog who is behaving inappropriately.
- Aging dogs can become intolerant of other dogs because they cannot see or hear them and/or because they are painful, arthritic, and slower and less able to react, but aging dogs do not seek out other dogs to victimize, and aggressive responses to

interference are most likely to be normal, contextual behaviors.

Etiology, Epidemiology, and Risk Groups

- Inter-dog aggression can be highly variable, but it generally appears at social maturity (approximately 18 to 24 months of age in dogs with a range of 12 to 36 months).
  - Various ages of onset have been reported by clients, but these may reflect when they noted the development of the condition. Wrubel et al. (2011) reported a mean age of onset of 36 months with a range of 15 to 48 months, in keeping with the association with social maturity.
- Changes in social relationships *also* occur in dogs *who are not affected by problem aggressions,* and these changes occur during this same developmental time period.
- During the period of social maturity, all social animals experience huge upheavals in neurochemistry, so it is not surprising that this is when we fully appreciate truly problematic social interactions.

r-dog aggression is more common between—but not restricted to—dogs of the same sex. Relatively minor, sporadic sparring seems common in households with young male dogs, but true, serious inter-dog aggression has been reported to be more common in households with young female dogs (Sherman et al., 1996; Bamberger and Houpt, 2006; Wrubel et al., 2011).

- Inter-dog aggression appears to be about social relationships between the dogs and how the affected or aggressor dog perceives his or her relative social status or role and his control over that status/role.
- Inter-dog aggression can occur between dogs that are unknown to each other and/or between dogs that are known to each other. When threats or fighting are seen in dogs who are *unknown* to each other, it is important to rule out two reasons for the fighting other than inter-dog aggression:
  - normal behavior, which may involve some posturing, especially as dogs get to know each other, and
  - problematic behavior involving fear or fear aggression. For fearful dogs, see the "Protocol for Understanding and Treating Dogs with Fear/Fearful Aggression."
- Some dogs who are aggressive to housemates are also aggressive to dogs with whom they do not live, whether they are known or unknown.

Common Myths That Can Get in the Way of Treatment or Diagnosis

- Fighting between dogs is "normal" if no dog is injured.
- The younger dog should "submit" to the older, "dominant" dog.
- There is a "dominant" dog, and all dogs should do whatever that dog wishes.
- The older dog is always right.
- The fighting is the result of "spoiling" one of the dogs.
- Dogs who live in the same household and fight will not kill each other.
- The "top dog" makes the rules and should be respected.
- If you leave the dogs alone, they will "settle it."
- This is just "sibling rivalry."
  - These are all erroneous perceptions and potentially injurious or fatal to household dogs. These myths are responsible for forcing dogs to suffer and assume that the aggression seen in this condition is "normal." It is not. These myths also absolve clients of all responsibility for interpretation and intervention. *These myths have no place in modern veterinary behavioral medicine.*

Commonly Asked Client Questions

- How do I know which dog is "alpha"/"dominant"?
  - There is no "alpha" or "dominant" dog in a home, which would imply one dog makes all decisions and sets the pace for all interactions and activities.

Relationships between dogs are not absolute. They change with age, health, and—most importantly—context. In a household where the dogs are normal, no one dog feels the need to control the other dogs all the time. Similar to people, sometimes control will not matter, and sometimes the dog who is less pushy may have a skill or interest that the rest of the group can use or follow.

- If there is no "dominant" dog, what is this about?
  - Inter-dog aggression is about the relationships between dogs, and how those relationships are viewed by the dogs involved. Even if dogs do not like each other, they should not feel that they "must" fight with each other. Needing to fight or feeling that you "must" control another dog's (or person's) behaviors is not normal behavior. In fact, an overriding need to control or dispatch another individual—regardless of how they behave—is pathological in any social species. There are four types of problems that could lead to such pathology, and they all involve signaling and communication.
    - One individual cannot read the signals of the other individual.
    - One individual can read the signals but not process the information in the signal.
    - One individual can read and process the signal but cannot make a plan to act on it appropriately, regardless of the information it contains.
    - One individual cannot successfully signal the plan and successfully act on it.
- If the dogs are fighting with each other because one of them doesn't understand signaling, why are we talking about giving them anti-anxiety medication?
  - Dogs who exhibit out-of-context or inappropriate responses to other dogs actually suffer from anxiety disorders: they cannot adequately assess the risk associated with the other dog and so provoke the situation in an attempt to get more information or to preempt any challenges. Think of this as a failed rule: every time they try to get information, they cannot use that information so they become more anxious and aggressive.
- If this has to do with one dog maturing, won't it just improve with time?
  - Unfortunately, no. The dog who is victimized learns that the dog threatening or attacking him is unreliable. *With repeated exposure to aggressive interactions, both dogs in the interaction become more anxious and reactive and often more aggressive.*
  - Uncontrolled, repeated exposure without escape or remediation is a form of flooding, which should be avoided because it does damage to dogs.
- Should we take the dog or dogs to dog parks where they can learn to play and get along with other dogs?
  - Dog parks are wonderful places for people to socialize while their normally friendly, appropriately behaved dogs play, run, exercise, and just visit. The

key words are *normally friendly, appropriately behaved dogs.* Too many people have thought that dogs who are aggressive to other dogs will improve if they are allowed to play with other dogs.

- Instead, such dogs may improve their skills at victimizing other dogs.
- Exposures of dogs who have been involved in episodes of inter-dog aggression should occur only under guidance from people helping to treat the dog. If the decision is made to use such exposures, full disclosure is needed, and encounters must be planned with everyone's approval. Someone should also video the event to ensure that no dog is placed in an untenable situation that may be apparent only on review.
- The issue of using pet supply stores and dog parks as part of a potential treatment program is discussed in depth in Chapter 3.

Treatment
- Management:
  - Management is the key part of treating this condition. Treatment of inter-dog aggression focuses on setting and maintaining a new set of social relationships that will *relieve everyone's uncertainty and—most importantly—keep everyone safe.*
  - Once clients understand which behaviors are normal and which are problematic, they should be able to identify the relative victims (defensively aggressive dogs) and the relative aggressors (offensively aggressive dogs).
  - Most of the behavior modification could be helpful without correct identification of victims versus aggressors, but everyone will be much more successful in preventing, anticipating, and fixing problem interactions if the relative role of each dog in the relationship is understood.
  - If there are more than two dogs in the household, the clients may have an advantage in learning about the relationships between the dogs. A third dog often acts as a "mediator" dog (Fig. 6-7).
    - A mediator will be watchful of the interactions of the other dogs, and the dog whom the mediator dog actively watches is usually the aggressor.
    - The mediator dog often chooses to accompany one dog; this tends to be the victim dog (the one who may be exhibiting defensive aggression).
    - The mediator dog often physically comes between the aggressor and the victim, turning the victim away from any active or passive threats from the aggressor.
    - The mediator dog often blocks the view of or access to the victim dog.
    - The mediator dog may intervene by physically blocking access to the victim and growling at the aggressor.

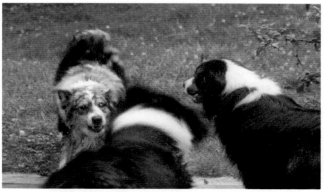

Fig. 6-7 A mediator dog (the black dog on the right) moving between and focusing on the victim of inter-dog aggression (the merle dog on the left) as a first step in moving her away from the aggressor. The black dog in the center is the aggressor. She has just tried to block the merle dog and snapped at her, and the merle dog turned and is threatening her back. The lack of acceptance of this response is shown in the shaking head. These dogs had not yet had a serious fight, but within 1 week of this one, the black dog in the center had seriously injured the merle dog even though the mediator dog had tried to bite the aggressor and pull her away.

-
  -
    - The mediator may physically position himself or herself so that the aggressor does not have access to the victim.
    - The mediator dog may physically bite the aggressor, should he or she gain access to the victim.
    - There may be more than one mediator dog in a household. If so, they work together to protect the victim.
  - If the clients review photos and video of the dogs, they will be able to identify mediators and relative victims and aggressions by these actions.
  - Dogs read dog signaling better than humans do. If the clients have one of these helpful and "supranormal" mediator dogs, they are lucky. This dog can help identify relative victims and aggressors and will provide guidance about whether the changes that are being made are helping.
  - Some mediator dogs are so good at what they do that no one may appreciate how hard they were working until they can no longer protect the victim. Do not be surprised if these dogs try to pull the aggressor from the victim if there is a true fight.
  - Clients must avoid aggressive events at all costs.
    - The aggressor can be placed in another room behind a locked door (hook and eye at the top to ensure no one can accidentally open the door).
    - Crates and gates can be used if the dogs cannot escape, see, or threaten each other (Fig. 6-8).
    - The victimized dog is always the dog given free range.

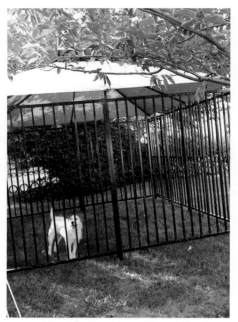

Fig. 6-8 An outdoor run/containment facility created for a dog who is aggressive to both other dogs in the household and who has seriously injured one dog and both humans. The other dogs have free run of the yard and because of the shrubs do not have to see this dog. (Photo courtesy of Dr. Donna Riddle.)

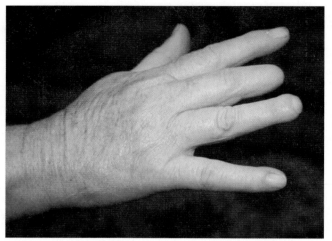

Fig. 6-9 Why one should never reach between two fighting dogs. This woman lost part of her finger and damaged another trying to separate two dogs who were fighting.

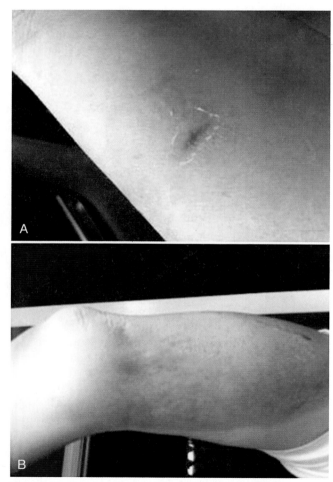

Fig. 6-10 Bites to one of the clients that occurred when trying to pull the dog in Figure 6-7 from his housemate. (Photos courtesy of Dr. Donna Riddle.)

- These dogs can *never* be left alone, unsupervised.
- Head collars may allow the dogs to be walked safely together, but separate walks may be necessary.
- If the dogs are in the car together, the aggressor should be locked in a crate or behind a metal grate, and he should not be able to see and stare at the victim.
- If the clients like to sleep with their dogs, they cannot have both dogs sleep with them. The victim should be the dog to sleep with the clients. If the clients wish to have the aggressor sleep with them, they should watch for an increased threat level on days after nights shared with the aggressor. If this happens, they cannot sleep with this dog.
- Clients *must* be disabused of the idea that they can have the peaceable kingdom and that love is enough. This attitude will lead only to risk and damage.
- Clients should not reach to separate these dogs. Most adults who are bitten are bitten when they get in the way of fighting dogs (Figs. 6-9 and 6-10).
  - Instead, keep blankets, brooms, or cardboard in each room to use to separate dogs. If the clients are truly avoiding contact, they will never need to use this as a fail-safe strategy.
  - Sealed bottles of club soda can be kept in each room. If they are shaken and then opened to

spray on the dogs, fighting dogs will often separate. This technique works only once or twice before most highly abnormal dogs learn to fight through it.

- Water from a hose under some pressure from a small nozzle can help separate fighting dogs, as can buckets of water.
- Air horns are sometimes helpful in startling dogs so that they separate, but they will go back to fighting if a plan to maintain the separation does not exist.
- Fights between dogs who are unknown and have no social history may be best terminated by devices that startle, such as air horns.
- Do not grab dogs by their back legs and upend them to pull them apart; most dogs just bite harder.
- Do not pull dogs to separate them. Most dogs will just bite harder, and tear injuries can cause serious damage.

- If the inter-dog aggression is toward unknown dogs only (and there are instances where these pathological dogs can live with other well-known dogs, who may be acting a way that minimizes the expression of the pathology, but they cannot encounter unknown dogs without reacting), treatment is going to be difficult because the aggressor always succeeds in chasing the victim away. Management becomes paramount.
  - Neighbors should know that the aggressor dog has a pathology and that they can help to avoid provocative interactions.
  - Aggressive dogs should be walked only in head collars (preferred if possible) or harnesses that can help control their movements and extract them from situations in which they might react.
  - Clients should know that restricting dog walks until very late at night and very early in the morning increases the risk of meeting other dogs with the same problem because everyone is trying to avoid meeting another dog.
  - These dogs cannot be free-ranging.
  - These dogs should not be left unattended behind fences where other dogs could pass.
  - If the dog's collar is fitted with bells, these will warn neighbors that the dog is present.
  - As soon as another dog is seen in the distance, these dogs should be turned around, asked to sit and calm, and then moved away from the dog.
- Behavior modification:
  - Clients often elect management only to avoid or minimize interactions between the dogs and medication to relieve each dog's anxiety.
    - It is fine to decide that desensitization and counter-conditioning of the dogs is too risky and that they will live separately.

- However, both dogs could still benefit from behavior modification designed to render them calmer and less reactive. This is a QoL decision for the dogs.
- For dogs who are aggressive to another dog in the household, the success of behavior modification will depend on the depth of the pathology of the aggressor and how early in the course of the violence the problem was recognized.
  - Once serious injury is done to the victim, the victim may become anxious and fearful.
  - Even in some cases of extremely early intervention, the aggressor is so reactive and dangerous that no behavior modification is done, and rehoming of the normal dog is chosen, or the dogs live completely separate lives. Clients should know that dogs can time and space share but will be injured if they accidentally get together.
  - In mild cases with relatively early intervention, behavior modification can teach each dog to relax, not react, and to take the cues about the appropriateness of their behaviors from the client.
  - In such cases, dogs can learn that inappropriate and reactive behaviors will not be tolerated or rewarded, but calm, non-threatening, delayed behaviors will be rewarded.
    - For this reason, the dog who is doing the best job of *behaving appropriately given the context, who can respond fluidly, and who can learn from his or her mistakes* should be rewarded and reinforced before the other, offensively aggressive dog (see Table 6-5).
    - Reinforcement can include feeding this dog first, walking her first, offering her a toy first, petting her first, et cetera. The clients are not creating or reinforcing a hierarchy or rank order. Instead, they are rewarding normal behaviors from each dog; one dog is rewarded for not causing the problem and the other is rewarded for being non-problematic and calmly tolerating a delay in response. If the problematic dog is improving with individual behavioral modification and medication, this delay may help the anxious dog to model her behaviors on her more appropriate housemate.
  - Both dogs will benefit from individual behavior modification designed to teach them to be calmer and less reactive and to have as their default behavior looking to the client for signals that will keep them safe.
- For dogs who act as aggressors to unknown dogs encountered on the streets, behavior modification should focus on teaching them to be calmer and less reactive and to have as their default behavior turning, sitting, and looking at the client for cues about the appropriateness of their behavior.

- Medication/dietary intervention:
  - Both the victim and the aggressor may need medication.
    - If the aggressor is explosive, the SSRI fluoxetine may be the best first-choice medication.
    - The victim needs to be treated with TCAs, SSRIs, et cetera, that are chosen on the basis of their behaviors.
    - If the victim has become hypervigilant, gabapentin may help.
    - If the victim has become withdrawn, a BZD such as alprazolam may help, and it may stimulate their appetite so that they are happier to work for treats.
    - If a fight occurs, both dogs should be given a BZD (e.g., alprazolam) as soon as possible in an attempt to interrupt molecular memory from being made.
    - No one has investigated the use of centrally acting alpha agonists or affiliative medications such as nasal oxytocin for dogs involved in inter-dog aggression, but both medications may have promise.
  - Neutering is often recommended for both dogs.
    - Neutering is unlikely to make things worse, and no one should be breeding these dogs.
    - Although there are no data, hormonal fluctuations that occur with heat cycles may help to make dogs more reactive and interactions more unpredictable. More males congregate around estrus females and so may joust for her attentions. There are also anecdotal reports that females who are intolerant of other dogs become more so during estrus.
    - Castration of male dogs seems to benefit most dogs who encounter other dogs in situations in which female access is an issue (Hopkins et al., 1976). There are no good data on effects of neutering on the development or treatment of this condition.
    - There are no data to support any contention that neutering dogs makes them more reactive to each other.
- Miscellaneous interventions:
  - Judiciously used doors, gates, and crates can keep these dogs living together safely in the household.
  - Clients should be cautioned that dogs who can see each other can threaten each other—it is not sufficient just to sequester one of the dogs.
  - The aggressor should wear bells on a breakaway collar at all times. If the victim always knows where the aggressor is, her anxiety level will decrease because she has control over avoiding the aggressor.

Helpful Handouts

- "Protocol for Generalized Discharge Instructions for Dogs with Behavioral Concerns"
- "Protocol for Handling and Surviving Aggressive Events"
- "Protocol for Deference"
- "Protocol for Teaching Your Dog to Take a Deep Breath and Use Other Biofeedback Methods as Part of Relaxation"
- "Protocol for Relaxation: Behavior Modification Tier 1"
- "Tier 2: Protocol for Desensitizing and Counter-Conditioning a Dog or Cat from Approaches from Unfamiliar Animals, including Humans"
- "Protocol for Understanding and Treating Dogs with Inter-Dog Aggression"
- "Protocol for Using Behavioral Medication Successfully"
- "Generalized Guidelines for Using Alprazolam for Noise and Storm Phobias, Panic, and Severe Distress"
- "Protocol for Choosing Collars, Head Collars, Harnesses, and Leads"
- "Protocol for Handling 'Special-Needs Pets' during Holidays and Other Special Occasions"

Last Words

- Calling this situation "sibling rivalry" is to do the dogs and their pathology a disservice. Such anthropocentric terminology minimizes risk where it may exist and provides the clients none of the tools needed to understand or manage changing relationships between dogs. To attribute uncritically what is treated as a "normal" human developmental stage or pattern to dogs who are truly aggressive and suffering is simply wrong. In fact, the blanket assumption that behaviors associated with "sibling rivalry" in humans are "normal" and not damaging likely allows bullies and sadists broad leeway. These types of terminologies are to be avoided at all costs.
- Inter-dog aggression between household dogs is one of the most severe and heartbreaking of canine behavioral conditions.
- These dogs can and do kill each other. Severe injury is most common.
- This is not a simple condition to manage for two reasons:
  - keeping dogs separated without accidental access and with QoL takes a lot of effort and forethought and a fail-safe plan and
  - people are sabotaged in this effort by their belief in and longing for a peaceable kingdom. Most people have at least one more severe fight after diagnosis that finally convinces them of the risks of association and the benefits of intervention and separation.
- If the clients decide to place one dog, it is easiest to find a home for the "normal" victimized dog.
- No other dogs can be introduced into the household while the aggressor is alive, unless this is done under extremely controlled conditions or the clients

absolutely know that the dog will not react to them (e.g., some dogs will accept having males brought in, but not females).

- Clients should *not* assume that if the aggressor gets along with another dog in the park that she would get along with that dog at home: she may not.
- Clients need to re-think any illusion that they might have that their household is a "pack."
  - The concept of "pack" implies that all the dogs were born into the family group and grow up knowing all the other dogs, who are in some way related to them.
  - Instead, in most households, unknown dogs of various ages are imposed on resident dogs without regard to their needs or behavioral profiles.
  - Few people have true "packs," and the assumption that everyone should get along as a family group is dangerous.

Redirected Aggression
Diagnostic Criteria and Description
- Redirected aggression (threat/challenge/contest) is aggression that is consistently directed toward a third party when the aggressor was thwarted in or interrupted from exhibiting aggressive behaviors to the primary target.
- This is not "accidental" aggression.
- The aggressor did not make a "mistake."
- The aggressor actively pursues the third party, particularly if they were associated directly with the interruption of the aggressor's behaviors. Redirected aggression is secondary to a primary diagnosis of concern.

Common Non-Specific Signs
- The behaviors most often seen are those associated with frank aggression.
  - If the dog is growling and lunging at another dog on the street and is pulled away, he redirects his aggression to the person manipulating him.
  - If a dog is lunging at a cat and another dog grabs him, he redirects his aggression to the dog who thwarted him.
- Dogs exhibiting redirected aggression often bite, although the bites do not usually break the skin. There is little to no warning.
- The redirected aggression occurs in response to being yelled at, physically punished, or otherwise thwarted from pursuing another aggressive behavior.

Rule Outs
- None.

Etiology, Epidemiology, and Risk Groups
- Redirected aggression involves a behavioral exchange "in kind" with the substitution of an identical activity, albeit with a different target, for the interrupted one.
- Only the focus of the aggression has changed.

- Redirected aggression is not to be confused with *displacement activity*, which is not an exchange "in kind."
  - In displacement activity, both the target and the behavior are altered as a result of a frustrated, thwarted, interrupted, or corrected behavior.
- A diagnosis of redirected aggression is very specific and is unassailably identified by discrete behavioral descriptions.
  - Dogs with redirected aggression usually go after the nearest individual, regardless of whether they were involved in the initial conflict.
  - In the absence of the interruption of the threat, these dogs are non-aggressive to the victim of their redirected bite.
  - The most common diagnostic error would be to call a behavior "redirected aggression" when the "aggression" was actually accidental.
  - When accidents happen, the bite is simply a function of lack of time and space for the aggressor to cease pursuit.
  - The most common accidental bite occurs when humans reach between two fighting dogs and are bitten because one dog was already in the process of biting the other and could not stop.
  - Dogs who are fighting could also redirect their aggression to humans.
  - In redirected aggression, the bite may be prolonged or repeated, and the dog may stare or growl at the human or other target.
  - In an accidental bite, the dog usually opens his mouth quickly, without growling and staring.

Common Myths That Can Get in the Way of Treatment or Diagnosis
- The dog did not "mean it."
  - Whether the dog "meant it" has no bearing on the issue. If a bite occurred, an injury may be sustained. Furthermore, the redirected event flags what could otherwise be another serious problem involving aggression. A full behavioral history and work-up is warranted.

Commonly Asked Client Questions
- Did the dog do this because he was jealous of the other dog's attentions to me?
  - No. We do not do a good job of evaluating labels such as "jealousy" in dogs, so we should be careful about assuming a motivation we cannot assess. It is important to remember that this diagnosis is really about another aggression, so the intervention of the human could be viewed—from the dog's viewpoint—as irrelevant and a nuisance.
- Didn't the dog know it was me?
  - It may not matter what the dog knew. That the dog was sufficiently aroused to engage in redirected aggression suggests that he was serious about the original focus of his aggression. It

is important to learn if this is an ongoing pattern reflective of a behavioral pathology.

Treatment
- Management:
  - The first step in management is to identify the behavioral situation under which the bite occurred.
  - If there is an ongoing problem, the clinician should assess whether there is sufficient evidence to make a diagnosis.
  - The incident could be an exceptional but usually is not.
- Behavior modification:
  - All dogs who become this aroused would benefit from behavior modification designed to teach them to relax, be calm, and become less reactive.
  - If there is a primary diagnosis, it must be addressed.
- Medication/dietary intervention:
  - Intervention for redirected aggression is not usually needed if the primary anxiety-related condition is addressed.
  - Once the primary condition resolves or is controlled, the redirected aggression also resolves.
  - Treatment for redirected aggression may be required if the victim is now anxious or fearful, and this is a change, and/or the aggressor is more vigilant and reactive, and this is a change.
- Miscellaneous interventions:
  - If there are certain circumstances under which the clients are reasonably certain they could see the behavior (e.g., when walking a dog who is reactive to other dogs on the street), a good harness or a head collar could help interrupt the behavior as it starts. Harnesses and head collars will also help the client to remove the dog from the situation to which he is reacting.

Helpful Handouts
- "Protocol for Teaching Cats and Dogs to 'Sit,' 'Stay,' and 'Come'"
- "Protocol for Deference"
- "Protocol for Teaching Your Dog to Take a Deep Breath and Use Other Biofeedback Methods as Part of Relaxation"
- "Protocol for Choosing Collars, Head Collars, Harnesses, and Leads"
- "Protocol for Handling and Surviving Aggressive Events"

Last Words
- This condition is a flag for other conditions and may co-occur with other conditions that have control as their focus (e.g., impulse-control aggression). Identify and treat the primary problem.

Food-Related Aggression
Diagnostic Criteria and Description
- Food-related aggression involves consistent aggression that is exhibited in the presence of, and only in the presence of, food (including dog food), bones, rawhides, biscuits, blood, treats, or table scraps in the absence of torture or starvation.
- Not all dogs who have food-related aggression care about all foods or care equally about all foods.
- Most affected dogs care only about a few types of highly desirable, valuable foods (e.g., Greenies, real bones, food-flavored nylon, or gummi bones).

Common Non-Specific Signs
- Affected dogs usually give a lot of warning and begin to growl as a human or another animal approaches the food they are eating or guarding.
- Food caching and guarding without ingestion is common, especially for items such as bones, and unless someone knows where the food being guarded is, this situation can be a challenge.

Rule Outs
- History of starvation or extreme food limitation.
- Chronic hunger, regardless of cause.

Etiology, Epidemiology, and Risk Groups
- This is a very restrictive and specific diagnosis.
- The number or range of items involved, although possibly reflecting danger and risk, do not affect the diagnosis, but all items must be some kind of food.
  - This is an important issue because many "chew toys" do not advertise that they may have gum or starch in them and so are not truly "chew toys" to dogs who become aggressive in the presence of valued food items but instead are viewed as "food."
- It is possible that aggressions that are stimulated by different classes of food indicate varying neurochemical modalities and that these differences may represent subclasses of this diagnosis.
- This diagnosis highlights that *food is not a possession* but rather something very different than a possession.
- A very good evolutionary case could be made for aggression related to food being potentially important, and we need to consider that for some dogs food-related aggression may be hardwired.
  - In feral or homeless dogs, the ability to protect food when needed may have been adaptive, although the ability to share food may have benefited the dog's continued residence in a social grouping of homeless or feral dogs.
- Although this type of aggression may be associated with impulse-control aggression, aggression to food is not a requirement for impulse-control aggression.
- If food-related aggression co-occurs with impulse-control aggression, it appears to precede it, which may suggest the development of some neurochemical propensity to shared reactivity (Box 6-3).
- Dogs who have non–food-related aggressive diagnoses may become more reactive in the presence of a highly valued food item *without* showing the

Aggressive Diagnoses That May Be Part of a "Control Complex"

- These diagnoses all may be associated by underlying reactivity and impulsivity
- Control complex diagnoses that are frequently co-morbid
  - Food-related aggression
  - Possessive aggression
  - Protective aggression
  - Territorial aggression
  - Redirected aggression
  - Impulse-control aggression

consistent pattern of aggression needed to make this diagnosis. This effect may be one of heightened general reactivity and/or hunger level, suggesting, again, that management of the environment includes the dog's internal environment. *Lowering overall reactivity is an essential step in any treatment.*

Common Myths That Can Get in the Way of Treatment or Diagnosis

- Protecting food is one variant of "resource guarding" and may or may not be normal. Other "resources" usually listed include toys, beds, attention from humans, et cetera.
  - The concept that "resource guarding" is a useful umbrella term for a range of bothersome dog behaviors that are a *variant of normal* prevents clients and veterinarians from evaluating how abnormal the dog is and how much risk is posed by the behavior. The "resource guarding" concept also encourages people to think that they can and should teach dogs not to guard "resources."
    - Most dogs have favored foods, toys, places, and people, but most do not guard them. Sometimes the dogs may take food or toys they do not wish to share away, but they need to be aggressive in their presence.
    - The context in which the behavior occurs and all relative risks are ignored by the "resource guarding" approach. With a careless assignment of "resource guarding," mildly and restrictively aggressive dogs are grouped with seriously and dangerously aggressive dogs, without any clear plan for mitigating risk.
      - Some dogs may be aggressive to other dogs at feeding time only if they are hungry. When these dogs are not hungry, they can be around even the most valued food item without showing any aggressive behavior. Mitigation and minimization of risk for these dogs may be as simple as ignoring them and/or asking them to go to a spot away from anyone else when they are

anticipating all meals so that their relative hunger level doesn't affect anyone else.
      - Risk assessment indicates that some dogs should be protected from sources that will provoke their aggression so as to minimize exposure to provocative and potentially dangerous situations. Risk assessment strategies for dogs who are seriously aggressive in the presence of some types of food (e.g., real bones, biscuits, pizzle sticks, rawhide, treats, table food) but not others (e.g., their dog food) will include removing these items from the dog's repertoire. If dogs are aggressive to other dogs, cats, or humans when fed their daily food, risk assessment and minimization argues that these dogs should be fed undisturbed in a controlled circumstance.
- Dogs are supposed to be protective of their food.
  - In fact, dogs are supposed to behave appropriately, in context, and if they have never been teased or threatened about food or starved, there is no valid reason for any aggressive behavior when food is present.

Commonly Asked Client Questions

- Does this mean that my dog cannot have treats?
  - Whether the dog can have treats depends on:
    - if the dog is aggressive before, during, or after being given the treat,
    - if the dog finishes the treat quickly or carries it around, and
    - how well the clients can control the behaviors of the humans and other animals in the household.
  - If the dog becomes increasingly aggressive as the time for the treat nears or as the treat appears, does not finish the treat relatively quickly at one time, or will be a potential risk to others because of their behavior or his own, he cannot have treats. This advice is primarily intended to mitigate any risk to children who may not be aware that the dog is sitting in front of a cushion because he buried a treat in it.
- Should I teach the dog to let me take food from his bowl or his mouth?
  - There are numerous behavior modification programs that are designed to teach dogs that you can take food from them. Almost all of them beg the question: why would you want to do this? We must be careful not to do things to dogs just because we can. The concern about being able to take something "in an emergency" likely either does not pertain at all here or pertains only rarely. Very few food items are fatal if ingested. When bones are too large to swallow, most people will be able to retrieve them unless the dog is so aggressive that gradually teaching him to allow

you to take food from his dish would not have mattered anyway.

- Normal dogs leave other dogs alone while eating or wait near them to check the dish when they are finished, or they sneak up to them and attempt to steal food while acting unobtrusive. Dogs who sneak up on other dogs are often snapped at. All of these behaviors are normal, and none of them resemble the notion that humans should be able to take food anytime.
- Dogs whose humans feel that they should always be able to take food may become more, not less, anxious because the humans are viewed as always at risk for taking something from the dog.
- Dogs who have been on the streets may have a very good reason for protecting their food, and teaching them that you can take food from them if they do not immediately accept that you should is likely to be a long and pointless process.
- People who are worried about accidentally giving the wrong medication in food should know that if the dog has been taught to take medication in food (cream cheese, peanut butter, brie, hot dogs, paté, butter, et cetera), he will likely have swallowed the food with the medication before they can even think of getting it back. Double-check medications before giving them to the dogs.

Treatment

- This is one condition that is either self-correcting or more trouble and risky to treat than it is worth.
- Management:
  - Dogs who are seriously aggressive around food of any kind should have it only under very clear, protected circumstances.
    - Such dogs may be fed behind a baby gate or a locked door. No one should pick up the food bowl until the dog is out of the room and sometimes out of sight.
    - Such dogs should be meal fed and never be left food *ad libitum.*
  - Even if these dogs do not require the protection of a gate or door, they should be fed out of the main traffic ways so that accidents are less likely to happen. These dogs can eat outside on the porch or deck or in a room other than the kitchen or dining room.
  - Anyone who has young children and a dog who is aggressive around food needs to know that toddlers and babies are food magnets: they almost always have some food with them or they smell like food. Separating the dog when the children have food and ensuring that the dog is locked out of the area where they are if they are going to carry around food are good and safe ideas.
- Behavior modification:
  - If the food-related aggression is mild and of recent origin, standard desensitization and counter-conditioning programs will work. Clients may wish to hire a certified dog trainer who uses only humane techniques to help them implement such a program.
  - If the food-related aggression is severe or long-standing, it may be easiest and safest to avoid it.
  - Rather than punishing dogs when they are aggressive with food or inadvertently rewarding them by luring them away with food, it is best if they can be ignored so that the situation is neutral.
  - All dogs should be asked to sit (or stand if sitting is painful) quietly, take a deep breath, be quiet, and wait until the food is put in front of them. The food should not be put down until all dogs are calm and quiet.
- Medication/dietary intervention:
  - For dogs who have historically been strays and/or starved, food is a serious issue. If there are no individuals in the house who could be at risk (e.g., young children or old, ill, infirm, incapacitated, or immune-compromised individuals), having food available *ad libitum* in each room may render these dogs less aggressive and more calm.
    - If the dogs begin to guard the food and/or their aggression worsens, the strategy failed.
  - Many dogs who are aggressive around food only when hungry could benefit from a diet rich in fiber and/or fats to delay passage and emptying times. Increasing fat can be done simply by adding fish oil that is reach in omega-3 and omega-9 fatty acids. Polyunsaturated fatty acids, including the omega fatty acids, can enhance a feeling of satiety.
  - Many dogs who are aggressive around food only when hungry may do better with multiple small meals a day than with one or two large meals a day.
  - Some medications alter the taste of foods, which could render dogs hungrier or more reactive. Some medications may cause nausea and gastrointestinal distress. Clients should be aware of these patterns.
  - BZDs, regardless of reason for use, make most patients hungrier. This side effect can be a benefit for some conditions but will cause problems for these patients.
  - SSRIs especially seem to cause changes in how foods taste. There are numerous reports of dogs treated with fluoxetine becoming anorectic.
  - The use of many SSRIs and newer nonselective serotonin reuptake inhibitors has been associated with weight gain. It is impossible to know whether the gain is due to the medication itself or changes in the patient's activity level, which can be profound.
- Miscellaneous interventions:
  - Some dogs who are aggressive around food gulp their food and become aerophagic. These dogs

may also eat so quickly that they drop food from their mouth.

- Use of food bowls that have pillars that slow consumption may help.
- Some sources recommend putting rocks in the food dish to slow consumption. If this is done, the rocks must be larger than the dog's throat so that they do not become a choking hazard.
- Food toys may be ideal ways to slow consumption in these dogs, but whether the food is moist or dry the toy now becomes a mobile food source. Dogs who are aggressive and use food toys should be sequestered and released only when done.
- Clients should understand the health risks of aerophagia (e.g., gas, bloat/gastric dilation, and volvulus).

Helpful Handouts
- "Protocol for Generalized Discharge Instructions for Dogs with Behavioral Concerns"
- "Protocol for Understanding and Managing Dogs with Aggression Involving Food, Rawhide, Biscuits, and Bones"
- "Protocol for Deference"
- "Protocol for Teaching Your Dog to Take a Deep Breath and Use Other Biofeedback Methods as Part of Relaxation"
- "Protocol for Teaching Cats and Dogs to 'Sit,' 'Stay,' and 'Come'"

Last Words
- A special case of potentially aggressive behavior involving an essential substance—water—is dealt with in the section on possessive aggression because clients comment on the guarding of the bowl.
- Food-related aggression is easy to manage and avoid but tough to treat reliably in complex social environments (e.g., environments with children). It may be wise always to use avoidance and management as a fail-safe—even if clients wish to work with dogs to help them become less aggressive in the presence of food.
- Unfortunately, most trainer manuals recommend teaching dogs that you can take their food. We would not tolerate anyone doing this to us. We should ask ourselves why we wish to teach our dogs we are unreliable and not worthy of their trust with respect to their sustenance.

Possessive Aggression
Diagnostic Criteria and Description
- Aggression (threat/challenge/contest) that is consistently directed toward another individual who approaches or attempts to obtain a non-food object or toy that the aggressor possesses or to which the aggressor controls access.
- The aggressor does not have to be using or near the object when he or she acts to protect it.

- The aggressor is unaggressive in the absence of the object associated with the contentious behavior.
- This diagnostic category includes only non-food, non-gustatory items. The stimuli and neurochemical changes associated with aggression toward objects versus food are likely very different (see preceding discussion of "resource guarding").
- Although this aggression may be correlated with the occurrence of canine impulse-control aggression (or feline impulse-control/status-related aggression), the latter is about control of activity or access—it is *not* about control of objects—and no diagnosis of impulse-control/status-related aggression should be made on the basis of a response to an object.
- For a diagnosis of possessive aggression to be made, the response to the object must be consistent, restrictive, and repeatable.
- If the patient *also* fulfills the criteria for impulse-control aggression and/or other diagnoses, those diagnoses should be made in addition to, not instead of, the diagnosis of possessive aggression.

Common Non-Specific Signs
- Affected dogs engage in:
  - guarding of objects,
  - carrying of objects, and
  - hiding and monitoring objects.
- Affected dogs will growl when another individual (canine/human) approaches the object (whether or not the aggressor is engaged with it).
- Some of these dogs will seem to present the object to another but threaten them if they try to take it.
- If a number of dogs in the household have toys, the aggressor may threaten them until they relinquish them and the aggressor "possesses" all of them.

Rule Outs
- Normal play behavior should be ruled out.
  - Normal play behavior between dogs and humans or dogs and dogs that involves toys and "stolen" objects that the dogs are treating like toys usually involves vocalizing, including "play growls."
  - Clients may not recognize normal play behavior and how fierce it can become.
  - Clients also may not recognize when behaviors change from "play" to true aggression.
  - Clients may inadvertently discipline dogs who are playing. The dogs learn that the client represents a risk to their games and will confiscate their toys. These dogs may learn to become aggressive to the clients as a way to keep their toys.
  - This version of this problem is a completely preventable problem. When the veterinary staff discusses puppy care with clients with puppies, one topic discussed should be recognizing play growls. By showing clients videos of real and play growls and by encouraging the clients to videotape play with their puppy for assessment at their

next visit, induction of possessive aggression can be avoided.

Etiology, Epidemiology, and Risk Groups

- True possessive aggression usually starts and becomes fully pronounced during social maturity.
- Many dogs who protect their toys from other dogs may be unreactive to humans and vice versa.
- Anyone who teases dogs using their toys could inadvertently teach dogs that they are a risk and encourage the dog to protect the toy.
- There are few data on the development of this condition, but it can be part of a "control complex" where dogs strive to control as many physical and social aspects of their world as possible.

Common Myths That Can Get in the Way of Treatment or Diagnosis

- People routinely believe that they "should" be able to take toys from dogs.
  - This is a subset of the belief that we "should" be able to do things to dogs because we are humans and they are dogs. Such thinking is outdated and dangerous and leads to inhumane treatment of all animals.
- Clients may have been told that they must be able to take toys from dogs to show the dog "who is the boss."
  - This is dangerous and outdated thinking that is a result of the unfortunate and wrong belief structure that we must "dominate" dogs.
- We must be able to take items from dogs in case the dog gets a "dangerous" item.
  - If the clients are worried about the dog's access to "dangerous" items, it is easier to ensure such items are not present. Most people do not leave knives on the sofa.
  - However, in a true emergency situation, dogs who are scared may bite because they are afraid, but most dogs will allow themselves to be helped.

Commonly Asked Client Questions

- I want to play with my dog but he never brings back the ball, Frisbee, stick, et cetera. If I try to take it from him, he growls. How do I get the toy?
  - If it is important to get that specific toy back (e.g., a squeaker that the dog will swallow is hanging from it), trade the dog for another toy. We need not teach dogs to relinquish items, no matter what, but teaching them to *"trade"* from early puppyhood is a *valuable relationship skill*.
  - For trading to work well and easily, the dog must know how to sit on request and be willing to do so. See the "Protocol for Teaching Cats and Dogs to 'Sit,' 'Stay,' and 'Come.' "
    - As soon as the dog is sitting calmly, the client can offer the dog a better toy or a desired treat. The client then moves away with the dog while providing treats and instructions

(and perhaps a lead), and someone else retrieves the toy.
    - This strategy should be reserved for situations with real risk.
  - However, you don't get the toy back if the risk in doing so is greater than the risk of the dog having the toy.
    - Simply, the dog can have the toy, and the client ends the game. The dog will usually abandon the toy, and it can be picked up and put away or the game started again.
  - If the dog really will play, the client needs to have a series of toys. This is one example of a preventive strategy that is also a treatment strategy. A bucket of balls or a stack of flying disks allows the client to avoid reaching for the dog's possession when he has it. Instead, once the dog has caught the toy, another is thrown. All of the toys are retrieved at the end of the play session when the dog is tired and elsewhere.
    - By throwing a second toy without trying to take the first, the client teaches the dog that the client is not a threat and that the dog is self-rewarded for relinquishing the first toy by catching a second. The reward pertains even for dogs who can carry multiple toys in their mouth at once because the dog is rewarded for not becoming aggressive.

Treatment

- Management:
  - See previous discussion in the section on commonly asked client questions.
  - This condition is most easily treated by managing the environment so that the dog cannot gain access to possessions he or she might want to control.
  - No one should reach for anything the dog is guarding.
  - Walking away from the dog and trading, when needed, are the preferred management strategies.
- Behavior modification:
  - There are very few dogs who are affected with possessive aggression alone. Accordingly, teaching dogs to sit calmly and rewarding them for being non-reactive when people reach toward them, if this can be done safely, will benefit a general treatment plan for reactive dogs.
  - If the clients have just noted that this condition is developing, teaching the dog to sit, take a deep breath, and then "trade" could prevent the condition from fully developing.
  - For dogs who have the constellation of aggressive diagnoses involved in a control complex, getting as many situations under control as possible matters. These dogs will benefit from full engagement in the behavior modification programs that

not only encourage them not to react but also teach them more appropriate behaviors (e.g., "Tier 2: Protocol for Desensitizing and Counter-Conditioning Dogs to Relinquish Objects").

- Medication/dietary intervention:
  - If dogs are highly reactive in the presence of certain objects or toys and patrol the environment seeking these items, they may benefit from treatment with a TCA and/or an SSRI plus active behavioral modification to teach them to relax and to take their cues about the appropriateness of their behavior from their people.
    - If the behaviors are ritualistic, a TCA such as clomipramine may be beneficial.
    - If the behaviors are explosive, a SSRI such as fluoxetine may be beneficial.
    - If a dog is worried all the time, consider a medication such as gabapentin, either alone or in combination with a TCA or a SSRI.
- Miscellaneous interventions:
  - Engaging these dogs in tasks where relinquishment is always rewarded (e.g., obedience training and trials; bringing you the remote control), especially if done early, may be helpful in changing the course of the condition.

Helpful Handouts
- "Protocol for Generalized Discharge Instructions for Dogs with Behavioral Concerns"
- "Protocol for Deference"
- "Protocol for Teaching Your Dog to Take a Deep Breath and Use Other Biofeedback Methods as Part of Relaxation"
- "Protocol for Relaxation: Behavior Modification Tier 1"
- "Protocol for Preventing and Treating Attention-Seeking Behavior"
- "Protocol for Teaching Kids—and Adults—to Play with Dogs and Cats"
- "Protocol for Teaching Cats and Dogs to 'Sit,' 'Stay,' and 'Come'"
- "Protocol for Choosing Toys for Your Pet"
- "Tier 2: Protocol for Desensitizing and Counter-Conditioning Dogs to Relinquish Objects"

Last Words
- The key to identifying correctly when there is a real threat involves watching the dog's behavior. Dogs who are affected with possessive aggression are not enjoying playing with the object. Rather than play and active engagement, these dogs worry and guard. If joy is rare and concern is common, the diagnosis is present and needs redress.
- Not all dogs who growl and take objects are aggressive: many of the dogs about whom clients worry are playing and engaging in attention-seeking behaviors that the clients cannot recognize. If there is doubt or concern and before any diagnosis can be made, the consulting veterinarian should observe the specific behaviors on video or in person.

- There is one category of behavior that is usually grouped with possessive aggression (see Table 6-7) but that may be more complex: guarding water bowls.
  - Sometimes truly aggressive dogs will guard empty or full water dishes simply because they represent an object over which it is possible to struggle with a human or another dog for access.
  - However, dogs who have been deprived of water at some point in their lives may huddle over and/or lie down with their forelimbs around a water dish even when they are not thirsty. These dogs may always choose to keep a water dish in sight. Sometimes they are aggressive to those who take or use the dish, but mostly they stop others from using it simply by their vigilance.
  - Although water is not food, it is essential to life. A dog who experienced profound thirst knows the pain that accompanies such thirst and may not be able to move from the dish.
  - By placing a water dish in each room and in places outside and keeping them full, clients will allow the dogs to recover from the fear of not having access to water. With time, dogs stop guarding and then stop checking some dishes. By removing one dish at a time over a very long period and seeing if the dog remains calm while not increasing his vigilance of other dishes, the clients will be able to reduce the number of dishes the dog needs to a manageable number.
  - Deprivation of water is a profound experience, however, and even a 1-day lapse of access to fresh water can cause these dogs to revert.

Predatory Aggression
Diagnostic Criteria and Description
- This diagnosis involves extremely quiet aggression or behaviors congruent with subsequent predatory behavior (staring, salivating, stalking, body lowering, tail twitching, et cetera) that are consistently exhibited in circumstances associated with predation or toward victims that usually include infants or young or ill animals.
- Neither death nor ingestion, should death ensue, is a necessary sequela. Serious injury is most common when the target is a human or another dog.
- Confirmed cases of predatory aggression are generally quiet, unheralded attacks, which involve at least one fierce bite and shake.
- Behaviors exhibited include staring, salivating, stalking, body lowering, and tail twitching.
- The classic behaviors are consistently exhibited toward species-contextual prey items (i.e., cats, birds) or toward individuals that exhibit uncoordinated movements and sudden sleep and wake cycles (i.e., human infants, young or ill animals, geriatric humans).

- When all of these conditions are met, this diagnosis is unassailable; however, there is leeway in interpretation, and one seldom knows if an actual attack *would occur*. Although acceptance of uncertainty minimizes the cost of tragedy, it does not contribute greatly to our knowledge about the condition.
- Discrete analyses of the behaviors involved (*sensu* de Meester et al., 2011) should elucidate different forms of this behavior and the role that the behavior of the victims plays in determining the form that the aggression will take.
- The form that the aggression takes is important because the term "predatory aggression" can also be used to describe aggression to joggers and bicyclists. There is little to no evidence that such behaviors are a form of or related to predatory aggression. Caution is urged in considering this circumstance predictive of or similar to occurrences of predatory aggression that do not involve the motion engendered by athletic endeavors.
  - Most canine aggression faced by joggers and bicyclists is likely territorial aggression where the dog begins to react only once the jogger or cyclist has approached within a certain distance of the property and then relents once the jogger or cyclist is a certain distance past the property. Dogs exhibiting territorial aggression are vocal and obvious and engage in no covert stalking behaviors.
  - Dogs from breeds that herd for a living may be triggered by the motion of bicycles, cars, skateboards, joggers, et cetera.
    - The behaviors of dogs from herding breeds or lines should be consistent with the herding form common in their breed(s), and their behaviors are most likely to focus on controlling the direction of the activity.
    - Rather than exhibiting silent, slow, intermittent stalking behaviors, herding dogs exhibit obvious, continuous, and sometimes vocal behaviors designed to collect or move the subject(s).
    - Dogs who are herding are obvious in their monitoring behaviors and re-adjust themselves in response to movement. Dogs with predatory aggression tend to freeze in this circumstance.
    - Some breeds and/or lines of herding dogs grab as part of their herding behaviors. No ethological analysis exists, but these types of herding moves are very different from moves used in predation, predatory aggression, and inter-dog aggression and should not be confounded with them.

Common Non-Specific Signs

- The most common signs are staring accompanied by mydriasis, salivation, silent intermittent stalking, and start and stop movements that are guided by the behavior of the victim.

- The predatory attack is usually triggered by movement of the victim after a period of stillness.
  - The stillness can be short. Normal dogs and humans who realize that they are about to be attacked by a predatory dog generally pause before trying to flee and are attacked as they flee.
    - For this reason, so many bite prevention programs, whether for domestic dogs or wildlife, recommend slowly backing away from the threatening carnivore while keeping the attacker in the peripheral visual field.

Rule Outs

- If the complete sequence of behaviors is understood and observed, there are no medical conditions that could be mistaken for predatory aggression.
- Dogs whose hearing, sight, or mobility is failing may be more reactive in any situation that they would view as provocative, but the initial sequences of observing and stalking are missing from their behavioral suites.

Etiology, Epidemiology, and Risk Groups

- Dogs who have dispatched neighborhood pets and wildlife may be more at risk for exhibiting predatory aggression than dogs who do not exhibit these behaviors, but predatory aggression is so rare that odds ratios and risk cannot be accurately calculated.
- Dogs who have exhibited true predatory aggression to humans appear to have had a history of at least one predatory aggressive event involving non-human animals.
- The condition of some humans and pets makes them look like "good victims." Sudden start and stop sleep cycles, such as those exhibited by babies, in coordination, and inconsistent movement all may play roles in triggering true predatory aggression.
- Young infants and older, debilitated individuals of any species may be most at risk.
- Dogs who are taught to fight other dogs exhibit stylized versions of the behaviors used in predatory aggression with resultant similar patterns in wounds (Figs. 6-11 and 6-12).
  - *Dogfighting is illegal in most Western countries and should be illegal in all countries.*
- It is especially important to remember with this diagnosis that any dog of any breed can exhibit predatory aggression and that most mastiff/bully breed dogs are wonderful (Figs. 6-13 and 6-14).
  - Dogs with this training or skill set will exhibit very different behaviors than dogs in the early phases of inter-dog aggression. As inter-dog aggression becomes more serious, the behaviors change, mirroring predatory attacks.
    - Predatory attacks involve grabbing the neck and holding onto and crushing the larynx, slashing at the neck and throat, and shaking the victimized dog by the throat (Figs. 6-15 and 6-16).

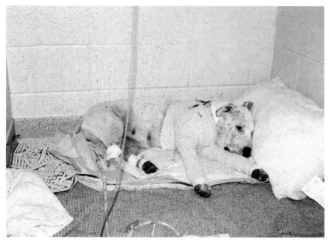

Fig. 6-11 This dog was used as a "bait" dog to train other dogs to fight. Notice that this dog's wounds are classic predatory wounds designed to subdue another animal. The wounds are to the neck and front legs and shoulders. Note also that this dog has not had her ears cropped, which makes it easier for the fighting dog to grab her, and that her face is extensively scarred, suggesting that she has been used in this capacity before.

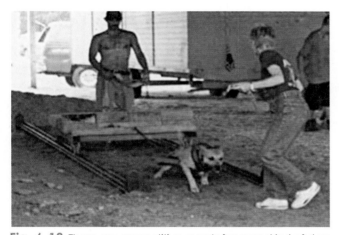

Fig. 6-13 There are competitive events for every kind of dog. Here, the dog is to pull as much weight over a track of known length as he can. Most dogs who are mastiff/bully breeds have no problem aggressions, but they are strong.

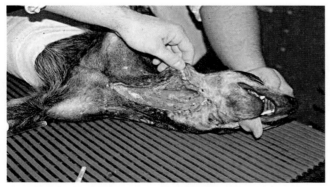

Fig. 6-15* One of two Australian cattle dogs (mother and son) attacked by another dog when they were fenced in their own yard. This predatory attack involved slashing of the throat (this dog is alive and physically recovered).

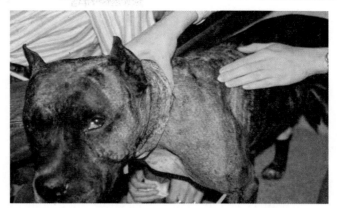

Fig. 6-12 The dog who caused the injuries in Figure 6-11. Notice that he has a few defensive wounds with drains. Once he was shaved, the numerous underlying scars indicated that this was not his first fight. Note that his ears are cropped.

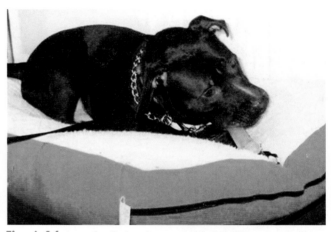

Fig. 6-14 A perfectly lovely, normal "pit bull" rescued after a seizure of fighting dogs. The dog had just been evaluated for potential placement and was settling down on soft beds with a gummi bone, two things he might never have had before.

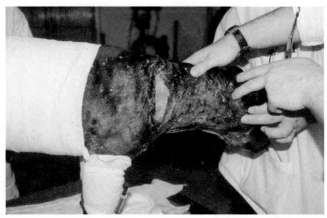

Fig. 6-16* Slashing style of neck wound on the second dog.

*Permission to use Figures 6-15 through 6-19 for educational purposes was given by the clients, whose dogs ultimately recovered physically from the attack. The Behavior Clinic Research Fund contributed $1000 to help offset the cost of treatment, which was greater than $20,000 (1990s dollars). Thanks to Dr. Art Jankowski for realizing the value of this case for behavioral medicine education and for his willingness to include a focus on behavior in the ongoing treatment of the case.

- Predatory attacks involve grabbing and tearing at the soft underbelly including either side of the chest (Fig. 6-17) and the groin area (Fig. 6-18).
- Predatory attacks involve deep wounds on the backs of the hind legs and serious punctures and crush injuries on forelegs (Fig. 6-19).

Common Myths That Can Get in the Way of Treatment or Diagnosis

- Dogs from Nordic or mastiff breeds are often maligned as being more "predatory" than other breeds.
  - There is no breed predisposition for predatory aggression. This is a pathological diagnosis that is about individual, not breed-associated behavior. Dogs of any size or breed can be affected.
  - Nordic breed dogs can be harder for some people to read because the thick hair of the face can obscure some facial expression. In fact, we do not know if these dogs exhibit the same facial expressions as do other dogs because selection for such expressions would have been relaxed if the information conveyed was slight or difficult to assimilate.
- Clients often think that because the dog has always been sweet for them that his or her behaviors do not pose a risk for their new baby or debilitated relative.
  - If there is any concern about any interaction, the dog should always be supervised (the cost of error is huge) and an informed third party (e.g., veterinary behavior specialist) should observe the dog's behaviors in the contexts in question.
  - There is absolutely no evidence that "temperament" tests with dolls can predict dogs' behaviors toward babies and small children. No validation study has been done, but this test is often inappropriately used as a test for predatory aggression.
- Clients often think that if their dog shows any signs of predatory aggression that they must euthanize or relinquish the dog.
  - This is not true. Babies to whom dogs may react with predatory aggression will grow out of the phase where the dogs view them as prey. These children can go on to have a perfectly normal and happy relationship with the dog. The pathology has nothing to do with the child and everything with how the dog views certain movements and attendant behaviors.

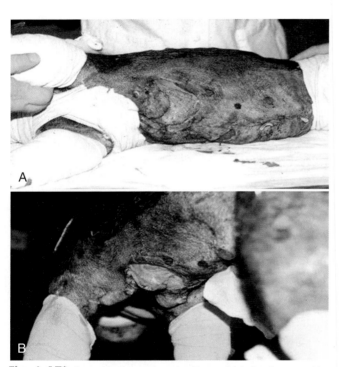

Fig. 6-17* **A** and **B**, Wound under the rostral chest caused by grabbing and tearing at the skin.

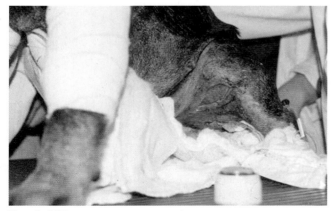

Fig. 6-18* Inguinal, full-thickness skin loss wounds caused by grabbing and tearing.

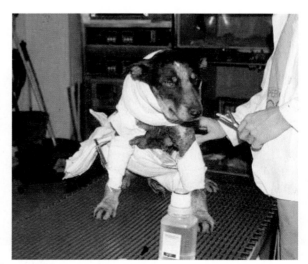

Fig. 6-19* Foreleg bandages cover deep puncture wounds that are classic for predatory events intended to hobble the victim.

- The baby must be protected from the dog for the first few months of life, which can easily be done with leads and locked doors.
- As soon as the child can sit up unsupported, the dog is no longer predatory.
- For this scenario to have a good outcome, the clients must have a realistic perception of risk and their role in determining it.
- As clients have children later in life and have dogs before human children, automatic relinquishment is not a popular choice. Fortunately, a safe choice that prevents relinquishment is available.
- Clients and children who can understand the need to protect such dogs may become more empathetic and humane.

Commonly Asked Client Questions
- Must I get rid of my dog?
  - No; see the preceding discussion. That said, a very detailed specific plan of protection needs to be agreed on and implemented by all involved, including the veterinary staff. Components of this plan should include:
    - A plan for ensuring that the child is never left alone with the dog until it is clear that the dog is reliable and not a concern. This means that the dog will not ever be close to the child in the first 6 months.
    - A way to lock the dog safely and humanely away from the child when the dog is not on a lead and head collar with a person guiding his or her behaviors. Crates, kennels (with roofs), and doors that lock are optimal. Flimsy gates and invisible fences do not provide adequate containment in this circumstance.
    - A way to have the dog with the child under extremely controlled circumstances.
      - Such co-habitation is desirable but can happen only if the dog is able to attend to the adults and not focus on the child.
      - The dog should be wearing a head collar and lead and should be maintained at least 1.5 body lengths from the child.
      - If the clients feel more comfortable with a muzzle and they can kindly and humanely condition the dog to enjoy wearing the muzzle, this is fine, but they should know that a muzzle provides no real protection for an infant if a dog lunges for the child.
      - Low-key interactions where no one fusses and the dog is rewarded for looking away and ignoring the child are best.
    - An early warning system that tells people when the dog is present. This could be a simple bell on a collar around the dog's neck or a security monitor worn on the dog's collar that beeps when the dog is within some predetermined distance of the child or other

victim (www.brickhousesecurity.com). These auditory cues are part of a fail-safe system and should not be relied on alone to keep anyone safe.
- Can/do affected dogs kill/maul people?
  - Yes. Fortunately this is rare.
- Can this dog go to another home?
  - Yes, if the other home does not have infants or incapacitated older humans or animals, the dog can do wonderfully and be happy and safe. The people taking the dog must understand the diagnosis.
- Will the dog grow out of this?
  - No, but babies will.
- My dog stalks neighborhood wildlife and kills bunnies. Will he stalk and kill human babies?
  - First, predatory aggression is rare.
  - Second, more often than not the answer is no, but you cannot be sure until the dog is observed under controlled circumstances. Predatory tendencies or behaviors to small animals do not guarantee that the dog will react inappropriately with infants; such behaviors *may* indicate that these dogs are at greater risk for such problems, but the data are few.
  - Predatory aggression does not increase the risk or precede the development of other problem aggressions, and it does not preclude the dog from doing well with the child as the child ages.

Treatment
- Management:
  - This is a diagnosis for which all treatment is management. See the previous discussions.
- Behavior modification:
  - If the dog is anxious because of the presence of the baby or debilitated human or pet, that anxiety should be treated, but pure predatory aggression is not going to respond to behavior modification. It is safer not to attempt it.
- Medication/dietary intervention:
  - If the dog is otherwise anxious, hypervigilant, and focused, TCAs or SSRIs may help, *but clients should be disabused of the idea that these or any other medication or diet will treat true predatory aggression.* Medication may be part of a QoL decision for the dog but should not be expected to "fix" this problem.
- Miscellaneous interventions:
  - Because these dogs will be spending considerable periods of time away from the objects of their focus, it is very important to ensure that they get the physical and mental exercise needed to ensure a good QoL. Food toys, other pets, outdoor runs, and behavior modification sessions that allow them to be rewarded for being well-behaved all are beneficial for them, although these interventions will not fix the *problem*.

Helpful Handouts

- In terms of improving dogs' QoL and ability to behave admirably once they are no longer focused on potential targets, the following may help:
  - "Protocol for Deference"
  - "Protocol for Teaching Your Dog to Take a Deep Breath and Use Other Biofeedback Methods as Part of Relaxation"
  - "Protocol for Relaxation: Behavior Modification Tier 1"
  - "Protocol for Introducing a New Baby and a Pet"
  - "Protocol for Choosing Collars, Head Collars, Harnesses, and Leads"
  - "Protocol for Teaching Cats and Dogs to 'Sit,' 'Stay,' and 'Come'"
  - "Protocol for Generalized Discharge Instructions for Dogs with Behavioral Concerns"
  - "Protocol for Handling and Surviving Aggressive Events"

Last Words

- These dogs are not engaging in predatory behavior because they are hungry.
  - This is not usually true predatory behavior.
  - These dogs are not usually hungry.
  - Most often, the dogs do not eat the individuals that they have killed.
- Analysis has shown that the damage done to dead humans by the dogs who live alone with them most often occurs post-mortem and is the result of true hunger (Maksymowicz et al., 2011). These events are not examples of predatory aggression and do not give dogs a "taste" for human flesh.
- Most dogs who react to cars passing, joggers, cyclists, skateboarders, et cetera, whether or not they are from a herding breed/line, are not exhibiting predatory aggression and can learn not to do this.
  - Clients need to work with these dogs to have an "emergency stop" signal ("Halt!" "Arrête!" "Cease!" "Stop!") for which they are rewarded at first in non-provocative circumstances and then in increasingly more provocative circumstances.
  - A lead and head collar or harness can help, and no dog should have free range without these until they are reliable (and this means that 99% of the time you know what they will do and it is something desired).
  - All dogs should have an emergency stop signal.
- If the clients are unwilling to adhere to the standards set forth in the "Protocol for Introducing a New Baby and a Pet," everyone would be better off with the dog placed in an infant-free home. These dogs can go to other homes and do not need to be euthanized.
- Dogs that are predatory to other animals should never be off lead, unsupervised, at large, or confined in a fence that other animals might cross (i.e., invisible fences). No unprovoked killing of any other species should be excused or tolerated because it can be controlled.

Impulse-Control Aggression
Diagnostic Criteria and Description

- Impulse-control aggression is best defined as an abnormal, inappropriate, out-of-context aggression (threat/challenge/attack) consistently exhibited by dogs toward people under any circumstance *involving passive or active control of the dog's behavior or the dog's access to the behavior.*
- Any intensification of any aggressive response from the dog on any passive or active correction or interruption of the dog's behavior or the dog's access to the behavior confirms the diagnosis.
- This is a *diagnosis that is about using control and controlling behaviors to gain information in what the dog perceives to be uncertain circumstances.*
- "Impulse-control aggression" has variously been called "dominance aggression" (Reisner et al., 1994), "impulsive aggression" (Amat et al., 2009; Fatjo et al., 2007; Våge et al., 2008, 2010), and "conflict aggression" (Luescher and Reisner, 2008). We have chosen the label of "impulse-control aggression" because it is the most informative descriptor for all variants of the condition, and it addresses the fact that the dog is using the aggression to get information from the environment while struggling with a postulated heightened neurochemical (likely glutamate) reactivity, factors that are unaddressed if we call this "conflict aggression."
  - The concerns about the other labels include that all aggressions can appear "impulsive," external "conflict" is at the heart of all aggressions, and internal "conflict" is rooted in anxiety and uncertainty, making these labels less clear and informative.
  - If the criteria are adhered to and the descriptors are understood, the terminology used here, which is also not ideal, will uniquely identify a diagnosis of a class of aggression that differs from others usually enumerated. It is important to understand that impulse-control aggression can be a primary diagnosis or *one secondary to another anxiety-related condition (e.g., generalized anxiety disorder).*
  - The label of "dominance aggression" allowed relatively easy recognition of the set of dogs that shared this diagnosis, but the concept of "dominance" as applied to pet dogs is flawed, and it has encouraged techniques that are dangerous to owners and dogs alike and unfair and often abusive to dogs. For more information on this issue, see the "Protocol for Generalized Discharge Instructions for Dogs with Behavioral Concerns," the American Veterinary Society of Animal Behavior (AVSAB) Dominance Position Statement (www.avsabonline.org/avsabonline/images/

stories/Position_Statements/dominance%20 statement.pdf), and the Dog Welfare Campaign position statement (www.dogwelfarecampaign. org/why-not-dominance.php).

- There are at least two broad forms of impulse-control aggression:
  - truly impulsive aggression and
  - aggression that can become seemingly impulsive when attempts by the dog to address his own anxiety by controlling people's actions fails.
- Considerations pertaining to the *second, more common group* of impulsive dogs:
  - Dogs with impulse-control aggression can be particularly dangerous because their problem is rooted in a struggle with people over control of all aspects of the social environment. *This struggle is not because most of these dogs are mean and malicious.* Instead, they struggle and provoke people *because this is the only way they can get information from and about the social environment and interactions.* These dogs become impulsive and overtly aggressive when they cannot get clear information or when the information received confirms a threat, from the dog's perspective. With treatment, the dog both broadens the types of interactions from which information can be obtained and has a greater lag time to an impulsive response. Both of these aspects are essential components of successful treatment.
    - Dogs with any form of this diagnosis are unable to sit back and take the cues about the appropriateness of their behavior from the contextual environment.
    - They also are unable to distance themselves from people about whom they are unreasonably concerned.
    - Most people with these dogs have not done anything malicious to them, are not deliberately provoking the dogs, and are usually not even aware that their behaviors may be provocative to the dogs.
    - Some of the behaviors to which the dogs are most reactive are behaviors that are similar to those seen in rough play or social challenges with other dogs (e.g., reaching over the dog's neck or back, standing over the dog), but affected dogs are usually good with other dogs, and no correlation has been shown between this diagnosis and those pertaining to other animals.
    - Because the pattern of the dog's reactivity may depend on that dog's relationship with individual people *plus* his threshold for reactivity at that time, people may view these dogs as "unpredictable." Once people understand the pattern of the dog's behaviors, these dogs no longer seem "unpredictable."

- These dogs are so uncertain of their relationships with humans that every time the human exhibits a behavior that *might* be construed to be a "challenge" or "threat," the dog pushes back to learn:
  - whether the human is a threat,
  - which human behaviors are offered in response to the dog's "threat," and
  - whether the human's response depends on context.
- Accordingly, dogs with this form of aggression may victimize only certain groups of people.
- Dogs with impulse-control aggression have a focus on control that is *abnormal* and *out of context.*
  - A normal and confident dog might stand in the way by the door because he wants attention or because he wants to accompany the person leaving. If that dog is not given attention or allowed to accompany someone, he is disappointed but accepting.
  - A dog with impulse-control aggression stands in the way at the door because he is anxious and realizes that doors can signal changes in social contexts or interactions, and he must monitor all potential changes. When he is uncertain about whether the change will affect him, he provokes the situation—by stiffening and blocking, by grabbing—in an attempt to get information. Part of the pathology often involves a further misunderstanding of the response received.
- Considerations pertaining to the first group of impulsive dogs:
  - Truly impulsive dogs are always anxious and always uncertain. Depending on other stimuli contributing to their arousal, they may be more or less likely to react at different times.
  - Dogs who are truly impulsive (the first group) may also use the rule structure discussed for the second group, but *the extent to which they react may depend on their overall response to all stimuli at that time, rather than on a specific behavior that caused them to react.*
    - For dogs in this first group, their impulsivity and reactivity shape the form that their control takes; for dogs in the second group, their controlling behaviors shape the form that their impulsivity takes.
    - The same classes of behaviors may provoke dogs in both groups, although the underlying neuropathology may likely differ between these two forms.
  - The dogs in this group of truly impulsive dogs seem more unpredictable than the dogs in the second group (although the same stimuli provoke

them) because there are times when they are better able to control their impulsivity and times when they are less able to control their impulsivity.

- The extent to which these dogs are able to control their impulsivity may depend on the effect of multiple stressors on their overall threshold level (see the discussion on reactivity and thresholds in Chapter 2).

- If clients pay attention to these dogs, they realize that they are never fully relaxed and always anxious, even if they are attempting to seek interactions with humans that are usually viewed as calming (e.g., petting).

- These dogs act as if they are always trying to control their reactivity and to find some way not to react, which is why the behavior modification discussed here works so well.

- Behavior modification allows the dog to lower her reactivity level and raise her threshold for reaction in response to signals that provide a clear set of expectations in circumstances that the dog would otherwise find provocative.
- When these dogs are unable to control their reactivity, we see the impulsive, aggressive explosions.

- This is a very discrete definition of impulse-control aggression and has the advantage of not coupling the challenge to food (food-related aggression), toys (possessive aggression), or space (territorial aggression).

- These aggressions all can be correlates of impulse-control aggression and when associated with it may be indicative of a more severe situation (see Box 6-3 and associated discussion for more information).

- Control and access are key. Most of the problems with diagnosing the condition arise from the human's misunderstanding of canine social systems, canine signaling, and canine anxieties associated with endogenous uncertainty about contextually appropriate responses.

- This diagnosis cannot be made on the basis of a single event. The behavior, once it begins, will become more visible and consistent, but data on early signs, patterns of change with experience, and changes in intensity are lacking.

- These diagnostic criteria are radically different from the common descriptions of impulse-control aggression that specify that the dog will often react to being pushed on, to being corrected with a leash, or to being pushed from a sofa or a person.

- *The number of situations in which the dog reacts inappropriately or the intensity with which he or she reacts does not affect the diagnostic criteria,* although these factors may affect ability to treat the condition, prognosis, and risk to people.

- These dogs are very different from dogs who are pushy or assertive.
  - Pushy and assertive dogs are usually confident and do a good job of reading contextual cues.
  - Many people prefer pushy, assertive dogs because they work well in competitive obedience and trial situations and because some people feel that these dogs are "personality plus."
  - Being pushy or assertive does not mean that a dog has impulse-control aggression.

- The feline version of this condition is likely status-related/assertion/impulse-control aggression. The behavioral manifestations are sufficiently phenotypically different between the species to warrant separate consideration, if not a separate diagnostic category.

Common Non-Specific Signs

- These dogs commonly stiffen, stare, become aroused, block and/or grab people when the dogs are:
  - pushed on,
  - handled about the head or muzzle,
  - toweled around the head, neck, or back,
  - handled about the feet,
  - "corrected" verbally,
  - "corrected" with a leash/collar,
  - reached over,
  - bumped into,
  - stepped over, especially if in a doorway or accessway or in front of a bed or sofa,
  - pushed from a sofa, a bed, or a person,
  - disturbed while sleeping or resting,
  - stared at, and
  - physically moved out of the way or through a door or accessway.

- Clients note that these dogs:
  - often push on people,
  - put their paws on people's heads, shoulder, and back,
  - straddle people but may not mount them,
  - block access to doorways and/or entryways,
  - block correctional opportunities (e.g., by grabbing the person's wrist),
  - stare at people,
  - dilate their pupils suddenly when staring at people,
  - "talk back,"
  - lean on people with their paws or backs,
  - "hug" people and give them "kisses" by licking them over their entire face and head (a purely deferential lick is usually placed at the side of the mouth),
  - "bill pop" by smacking the teeth of the upper and lower jaws together while licking their lips and moving their head away; this is invariably in response to something they have been asked to do and with which they do not want to comply,

- snorting when asked to comply with an instruction, and
  - stamping their feet when asked to comply with an instruction.
- Most of the aforementioned behaviors can also be exhibited by pushy dogs, but increased numbers and intensity of behaviors should raise the index of suspicion that a diagnosis of impulse-control aggression may be appropriate.

Rule Outs

- Some of the non-specific behaviors listed can be due to pain or general illness.
- Dogs who react only to having their feet handled may have had a painful and scary experience with nail trims.
  - All dogs and people should be taught humane, low-stress ways to trim nails because problematic nail trims are the trigger for so many aggressions.
- Because of their effects on "mood," endocrine conditions (primarily hypothyroidism, Cushing's disease, and Addison's disease) should be ruled out.
  - Note: Many behavioral conditions in dogs have been attributed to "hypothyroidism" and "borderline-low thyroidal measures." There are no data to support such attributions. While no one doubts that any medical illness, including one that affects global metabolism, can make dogs more reactive, which can manifest itself as aggression, and that hypothyroidism can occur co-morbidly with a behavioral condition (Fatjó et al., 2002), no data exist that support a therapeutic role for thyroidal supplementation in the absence of true thyroidal illness confirmed by physical and laboratory data. Studies comparing thyroid analytes in dogs who were aggressive to humans with those who were not aggressive to humans have found no difference in any measurable value (Carter et al., 2009; Radosta et al., 2011). In one study using a randomized, double-blinded, placebo-controlled study design, dogs treated with thyroxin were not significantly improved in their presentation of impulse-control aggression when compared to those treated with placebo (Dodman et al., 2013). Assertion and extensive data massage do not help us create prudent scientific approaches or successful treatment strategies. These studies strongly support treating behavioral conditions with medications for which excellent putative mechanisms of efficacy exist (e.g., TCAs, SSRIs, SARIs, et cetera, plus behavior modification programs designed to teach new ways of interacting and/or reacting), rather than delaying treatment by using hormonal supplementation for which there is no support. Treatment with thyroxin is not benign and can cause thyrotoxicosis (Overall, 1998). In humans, thyroxin supplementation of standard anti-depressant and anti-anxiety medication converts some proportion of non-responders to the psychotropic medication into responders (see Overall, 1997, Appendix E for a lengthy discussion and Cooper et al., 2007). Whether this conversion occurs in dogs has not been tested, and with newer medications of different mechanisms of action, it may or may not be relevant. However, anyone using TCAs, SSRIs, et cetera in dogs and cats who require thyroid testing should remember that these medications artificially lower assayed thyroid values.
- Heavy metal toxicosis can be associated with atypical aggressions.
- Seizure disorders have always been a concern because impulse-control aggression has been considered episodic. Once a good history is taken, it seldom appears episodic.

Etiology, Epidemiology, and Risk Groups

- Males are more commonly diagnosed with impulse-control aggression; however, when females are diagnosed, they are younger than males (8 months vs. 12 months) (Overall et al., 1999), and they exhibit a more explosive, fulminant form of the condition than males. Males often develop the condition more slowly. All affected patients fully demonstrate the condition by social maturity within their 2nd year of life.
- Both forms of impulse-control aggression may be rooted in some aspect of impaired glutamate and/or serotonin (5-HT) activity or metabolism.
  - Glutamate is an excitatory amino acid that contributes to arousal and neurocytotoxic states and that has receptor cross-reactivity for a number of neurotransmitters. Glutamate is metabolized into glutamine, which can be an excitatory neurotransmitter itself (Fonnum, 1984) and excreted in the urine.
  - Urine of canine aggressive or non-aggressive patients with behavior complaint was screened for abnormal metabolites (Giger and Jezyk, 1992). Aggressive dogs have abnormal metabolic screens, in the absence of any metabolic disease, statistically more frequently than dogs with a non-aggressive diagnosis.
    - The three most commonly identified amino acids were glutamine, taurine, and alanine, all excitatory neurotransmitters (Overall, Giger, and Jezyk, unpublished).
    - Glutamine anomalies have been reported to occur in familial aggregations of human aggression (Brunner et al., 1993; Cases et al., 1995; Coyle and Puttfarcken, 1993; Smirnova, 1993a, 1993b) and are associated with neuronal death and excitotoxicity (Olney, 1994).
    - For dogs with behavioral conditions other than impulse-control aggression, 65 of 84 dogs

excreted abnormal levels of amino acids, and 19 of 84 had normal levels.

- When only dogs with impulse-control aggression were examined, 185 of 210 had abnormal metabolic screens, and 25 of 210 were "normal." The most frequently detected abnormality for the dogs with impulse-control aggression was glutamine ($P < 0.05$; log-likelihood ratio test) (Overall, Giger, and Jezyk, unpublished).

- Mutations in monoamine genes and aberrancies in monoamine function have been demonstrated in humans and rodents and postulated in dogs.

- Numerous studies have found variations in factors affecting glutamate (Ogata et al., 2006) or low levels of circulating 5-HT or its metabolite, 5-hydroxyindoleacetic acid (5-HIAA), in the plasma and/or cerebrospinal fluid (CSF) (Çakiroglu et al., 2007; Mehlman et al., 1994; Peremans et al., 2003; Reisner et al., 1996; Rosado et al., 2010), although some of these results have proved difficult to confirm (Mertens, 2002).

- This condition appears to be heritable.
  - There are lines in which no generation is unaffected.
  - In some family lines, 50% of the dogs are reported to be affected.
  - Even in the absence of a multi-generation familial history, if numerous first-degree relatives (mother, father, brother, sister, daughter, son) are affected, the index of suspicion for a genetic basis must be raised.

- A pairwise comparison of behaviors exhibited in fear aggression, possessive aggression, and protective aggression with impulse-control aggression showed that:
  - Growling, baring teeth, biting, and staring occurred statistically more frequently in impulse-control aggression than in fear aggression ($G_{adj} = 18.62, 4.67, 11.22, 18.18$, respectively; all $P \leq 0.05$).
  - Barking, growling, biting, and staring all were statistically more common in impulse-control aggression than in possessive aggression ($G_{adj} = 9.41, 4.82, 9.65,$ and 14.08, respectively; all $P \leq 0.05$).
  - Barking, as expected given its warning function, is more commonly exhibited in protective aggression ($G_{adj} = 16.50, P \leq 0.05$), but growling, baring teeth, biting, and staring all are more common in impulse-control aggression than in protective aggression ($G_{adj} = 17.17, 12.69, 16.96, 14.08$, respectively; all $P \leq 0.05$).
  - In no pairwise comparison was snapping statistically more frequently represented, which suggests that *snapping and biting are not tightly coupled in impulse-control aggression. For people to expect aggression to occur in a strictly ordered chain of events, this pattern may make the dog seem "unpredictable"*

(from Overall, 1997, from a re-analysis of Voith and Borchelt, 1982).

- This analysis shows that growling, staring, and biting all are more common in dogs with impulse-control aggression than in dogs with other common aggressions. If clients are taught to watch for dogs who stare and growl, the vast majority of cases of impulse-control aggression or potential impulse-control aggression will be seen and treated early.

- These data further support the separate classification of the diagnoses as used here.

Common Myths That Can Get in the Way of Treatment or Diagnosis

- "Dominance" is a concept found in traditional ethology that pertains to an individual's ability, generally under controlled conditions, to maintain or regulate access to some resource (Hinde, 1967, 1970; Landau, 1951; Rowell, 1974). It is a description of the regularities of winning or losing staged contests over those resources (Archer, 1988). It is not to be confused with status and does not need to confer priority of access to resources (Archer, 1988; Rowell, 1974).

- In situations in which the concept of "dominance" has been used with regard to status, it is important to realize that it is not defined as aggression on the part of the "dominant" animal but rather as the withdrawal of the "subordinate" (Gartlan, 1968; Rowell, 1972, 1974).

- The behavior of the relatively "lower status" individual, not the relatively "higher ranking" one, is what determines the relative hierarchical rank.

- Rank itself is contextually relative. Truly "high-ranking" animals are tolerant of "lower ranking" ones (Barrette, 1993; Boyd and Silk, 1983; Kaufmann, 1967).

- "Dominance displays" infrequently lead to actual combat. Instead, combat ensues when such displays are not effective (Walther, 1977).

- If there is no assumption of a "dominance"-based system, one is seldom identified. When free-ranging baboon interactions were classified by behavioral types (e.g., friendly, approach-retreat) and then analyzed according to specific behaviors of the participants, no "dominance" system was noted (Rowell, 1967).

- The concept of dominance was originally developed for use in describing territorial interactions in birds (Hinde, 1956), and since then the concepts of both "dominance" and linear hierarchies have been grossly misunderstood and misapplied (Archer, 1988; Beaver 1981; Gartlan, 1968; Overall, 2011; Rowell, 1974).

- The concept of "dominance" seriously confused the issues pertaining to this diagnosis. There are three conceptual areas where harm was done.
  - "Dominance" was equated with social status or order in a rigid hierarchy, which was thought to develop through contests in young pups that would predict social relationships as adults.

Sequential possession of a bone was used as an assay for "dominance" in puppies (James, 1949; Pawlowski and Scott, 1956; Scott and Fuller, 1965).

- In reality, puppies are far more fluid in their relationships, which are changing as their brains continue to mature. The rank hierarchy achieved was a function of the experimental design, not of the behaviors. The design used would impose a rank hierarchy, whether or not one existed.

- Because of the forceful way in which this rigid rank hierarchy was "assumed" to develop, humans were encouraged to be at the "top" of the hierarchy and told to be "dominant" to their dog.

  - Our historic and evolutionary relationship with dogs is one of cooperative and collaborative work. A hierarchical relationship such as the type formerly recommended would not have allowed dogs to work with humans in the ways that they have because humans would have had to make all of the work decisions.
  - Social systems based on deferential behaviors and on gaining accurate information can look exactly like these "top down" systems, if they are not carefully observed. Deference and compliance in contextually appropriate situations removes the need for control whether or not someone thinks it is present and successful.

- Dogs exhibiting this diagnosis, which is based in pathological anxiety and not in use of inadequate force, were subjected to treatment involving physically and behaviorally forceful behaviors meant to "dominate" them.

  - The most devastating advice ever given to people with dogs is that they "dominate" their dogs and show the "problem" dogs "who is boss." Under this rubric, untold numbers of humans have been bitten by dogs they have betrayed, terrified, and given no choice.
  - For dogs who have an anxiety disorder that involves information processing and accurate risk assessment, the behaviors used to "dominate" a dog (e.g., hitting, hanging, subjecting the dog to "dominance downs," "alpha-rolls," and other punitive, coercive techniques) convince that troubled, needy, pathological dog that the human is a threat with the result that the dog's condition is worsened.

Commonly Asked Client Questions

- Can we "cure" this condition?
  - No. We likely "cure" no behavioral conditions because of complex brain chemical interactions and molecular learning. However, these dogs can improve to the point that no one would know that they had ever been affected.
- Is this condition environmental or genetic?

- All conditions have environmental and genetic components, even if the genetic component affects only how you recover from an assault.
- Is this condition heritable?
  - Yes. This condition runs in family lines, is more common in certain breeds than others, can affect 50% of the dogs in any line, and appears not to skip generations.
  - There are also sporadic versions of this condition, but some of these may be passed on if they are due to certain types of mutations.
- If my dog is affected, can I breed him?
  - No dog with this condition should be bred because affected dogs suffer and are often abused. This is one condition for which there is good evidence that genetics matter. Although there are sporadic and likely heritable versions, no one should wish to perpetuate this condition for any reason.
- Should I castrate my dog/neuter my bitch?
  - Testosterone acts as a behavioral modulator. Dogs exposed to testosterone *and* who have inappropriate, out-of-context behavior:
    - may be more reactive at any given time and may react more quickly to a stimulus,
    - may react to a more intense level,
    - may stay reactive for a longer period of time,
    - may have a longer and more protracted denouement phase, and
    - may stabilize at their pre-reaction levels only after a delayed time.
  - Although castration may provide an edge by decreasing the chemical impetus toward greater reactivity, it does nothing to diminish the learned component.
  - Most of the testosterone is out of the system within 6 hours after castration, with the bulk decreasing within 72 hours of castration (Hopkins et al., 1976).
  - Removal of one chemical component of the reaction can be beneficial and should be done, but the learned component of the behavior must still be addressed with treatment.
  - For very young bitches who are exhibiting impulse-control aggression before their first heat, a heat cycle may help to modulate the aggression, but no one should just wait for this to happen. Instead, environmental, behavioral, and pharmacological modifications should be ongoing.
  - Whether or not the dog is neutered, he/she should not be bred.
- Can dogs with this condition have a good QoL?
  - Dogs with this condition can have an excellent QoL, if they are provided lifelong treatment with appropriate environmental, behavioral, and pharmacological interventions. Because this condition is based in neurochemical dysfunction and

anxiety, lifelong management—which will become automatic with practice—should be expected.

- Can this condition be prevented?
  - Possibly, we can prevent the *display* of the condition. All of the tools that are used to treat behavioral problems can prevent them. If dogs are raised with the behavior modification programs recommended, they should display few to no signs of the condition, although they may have the genetic and neurochemical liability associated with it.
- Is this dog dangerous?
  - Danger assessment is a function of both human and dog behavior.
    - If the clients do not manage these dogs well by avoiding situations that trigger the dog, the risk increases as a function of the clients' behaviors.
    - If the clients ensure that the dog is not put in situations in which his or her particular behaviors are triggered, the risk decreases as a function of the clients' behaviors.
  - Predictability of both human and dog behaviors are essential for any assessment of danger.
    - Clients often come to a consultation thinking that the dog is unpredictable, but after completing the history forms and/or the consultation, the patterns of the dog's behaviors are clear. Clients need to believe that if faced with those patterns the dog will be reactive.
    - Clients need to assess how predictable their household is. Small children can make any environment more unpredictable.

Treatment

- Management:
  - The key to successful treatment of impulse-control aggression lies in avoiding triggering the aggressive response.
    - If possible, clients should avoid all situations identified during the consultation that are associated with any degree of agonistic arousal by the dog.
    - This is not the same as not interacting with the dog.
    - Clients should give the dog a set of expectations of appropriate behaviors by telling the dog he or she is good when the dog is not reactive and ignoring/withdrawing from the dog when the dog is reactive.
  - If the clients do not feel that they can monitor and manage the dog's interactions, they should feel comfortable putting the dog elsewhere until they can focus on the dog (e.g., in a crate, behind a sturdy gate, behind a locked door with a chew toy or something else interesting to the dog). It is easiest to do this before the dog is aroused.
  - No one should be allowed to interact with the dog unless the client is sure that all instructions will be followed. It is easy to make these dogs worse, even if the intentions were good.

- Behavior modification:
  - The essential behavior program for these dogs is the "Protocol for Deference." Most dogs innately defer to people (Netto et al., 1992), and dogs with impulse control will willingly do so if they understand the rules for interaction.
  - In this context, the "Protocol for Deference" acts as a humane and benign set of rules that decreases reactivity and provides instructions for the dog about expectations for his or her behavior.
  - The "Protocol for Relaxation: Behavior Modification Tier 1" will help clients teach the dog a new set of responses ("relax and take my cues about whether to worry from my people") that can replace the old rules ("react no matter what whenever worried"). If the clients wish for their dogs to improve to the extent possible, the protocol for relaxation is important.
  - The "Protocol for Teaching Your Dog to Take a Deep Breath and Use Other Biofeedback Methods as Part of Relaxation" can be key to improvement in these dogs, but unless the clients understand it and are good at reading dogs, they could make the dog more anxious. For clients for whom veterinarians have any concerns, the help of a good, humane, certified professional dog trainer (www.ccpdt.org) may render implementation of behavior modification programs more useful.
  - "Tier 2: Protocol for Desensitizing Dogs Affected with Impulse-Control Aggression" should be used only after the dog and human have completed tier 1 and the other programs successfully.
  - These dogs have spent their lives provoking situations to try to learn where risks lie and which behaviors are good and safe. Accordingly, telling them that they are good when they are is the most effective change clients can make. By helping the dog to identify behaviors that are rewarded, the dog learns where he or she is behaviorally safe, and improvement becomes rapid and dramatic.
- Medication/dietary intervention:
  - Serotonin has been postulated to decrease aggression in cats (Katz and Thomas, 1976) and humans (Linnoila and Virkkunen, 1992), whereas norepinephrine has been postulated to facilitate it (Eichelmann, 1977a, 1977b; Reis, 1971, 1974; Yudofsky et al., 1986, 1987).
  - Serenics, or specific 5-hydroxytryptamine (serotonin) agonists, have been shown to cause an experimental dose-dependent decrease in aggression in the standard rat model (Mos and Olivier, 1989; Mos et al., 1990).
  - Arginine vasopressin antagonists experimentally decrease offensive aggression in the rat model

(Ferris and Potegal, 1988; Ferris et al., 1995), possibly through enhancement of the neural network controlling agonistic behavior that is normally restricted by serotonin.

- All these data link aggression, anxiety, and the serotonin/glutamate complexes.
- Impulse-control aggression is one condition for which some putative data about mechanism are available, and these data can inform pharmacological treatment. Plasma serotonin and CSF serotonin (5-HT) have been shown to be lower in some dogs with impulse-control aggression compared with non-aggressive dogs (Çakiroglu et al., 2007; Reisner et al., 1996; Rosado et al., 2010). It has been suggested that increased activity of the serotonin transporter protein (5-HTT) may contribute to or cause these decreases in 5-HT (Rosado et al., 2010).
- There may also be a role for glutamate metabolism in this condition, and because both glutamate and 5-HT can affect NMDA receptors, their roles may not be independent.
- *The treatment of choice has been the SSRI, fluoxetine, which was developed for the treatment of impulsive conditions.*
- Other TCAs, SSRIs, or nonselective serotonin reuptake inhibitors, in combination or alone, may also be beneficial.
- *Because overall arousal and anxiety levels are also important, medications such as gabapentin can be helpful as part of a polypharmacy approach.*
- Excitatory amino acids can be cytotoxic, so supplements (e.g., omega-3 fatty acids) and diets that can limit their damage may also help (Re et al., 2009).
- *Rather than relying on one medication, supplement, or diet, a polypharmacy approach is encouraged.* Treatment outcomes do not correlate with blood levels of serotoninergic compounds, but side effects do, so combining medications with an understanding of expected effects, side effects, and cytochrome P-450 patterns (see Chapter 10) is recommended.
  - Dogs who may have cardiac conduction disturbances should be monitored by a cardiologist if treated with TCAs and SSRIs because in rare cases they have been postulated to cause heart block; however, the risk appears relatively low for dogs (Reich et al., 2000).
- Miscellaneous interventions:
  - Head collars and harnesses can greatly improve the amount of humane physical control that clients have over their dogs.
    - These are not just for big dogs. Dogs have four feet on the ground, and when they are aroused even small dogs can overpower a human.
    - Any dog who is aggressive for any reason or who might make a mistake and who can physically wear a head collar can have his or her head turned away from the focus of their intense behavior. Preventing and aborting aggressive events is essential, and well-fitted, humane head collars and harnesses can help clients to help the dog avoid problematic interactions.

Helpful Handouts
- "Protocol for Deference"
- "Protocol for Teaching Your Dog to Take a Deep Breath and Use Other Biofeedback Methods as Part of Relaxation"
- "Protocol for Relaxation: Behavior Modification Tier 1"
- "Protocol for Understanding, Managing, and Treating Dogs with Impulse-Control Aggression"
- "Protocol for Preventing and Treating Attention-Seeking Behavior (Primarily to Help Clients Distinguish between Pushy Behaviors and Problematic Ones)"
- "Protocol for Generalized Discharge Instructions for Dogs with Behavioral Concerns"
- "Protocol for Handling and Surviving Aggressive Events"
- "Tier 2: Protocol for Desensitizing Dogs Affected with Impulse-Control Aggression"
- "Protocol for Using Behavioral Medication Successfully"
- "Protocol for Choosing Collars, Head Collars, Harnesses, and Leads"
- "Protocol for Handling 'Special-Needs Pets' during Holidays and Other Special Occasions"

Last Words
- The most common mistake that clients make with affected dogs is inadvertently to reinforce anxiety-related behaviors. This is why it is so critical that clients understand normal dog behaviors and signals.
  - Because clients defer to the initial challenges that they perceive to be nonaggressive, such as the pressing of paws on the client's shoulders, frequently interpreted as a "hug," the appearance of aggression is viewed as having a "sudden onset."
  - Instead, if the clients ignore pushy behaviors, and instead ask dogs to defer to them by sitting before any kind of interaction with humans, the chances of inadvertently rewarding a behavior associated with uncertainty are minimized.
- These dogs worsen quickly and can become extremely dangerous if punished, threatened, shocked, or otherwise roughly treated.
- Clients often want prognoses assigned to conditions; this condition demonstrates that prognoses in many behavioral conditions should be assigned to interventions. If the client is willing to meet the humane needs of the dog, follow the treatment recommendations, and humanely minimize the chance that the dog can do harm (these dogs can learn to be more aggressive from "practicing" their aggressions), the

dog will improve, no matter how profoundly affected he or she is.

Idiopathic Aggression

Diagnostic Criteria and Description

- This is an aggression that occurs in an unpredictable, toggle-switch manner in contexts not associated with stimuli noted for any other behavioral aggressive diagnosis and in the absence of any underlying causal physical or physiological condition.
- This diagnosis must be distinguished from any neurological condition.
- Intensive characterization of attendant behaviors will be necessary to rule out the most common condition with which this is confused: undiagnosed or subtle impulse-control aggression.
- Idiopathic aggression is often called "rage," a term that should not be used because of our inability to define adequately the analogous emotional conditions in pets that are experienced and described by humans.
- In the vast majority of situations in which this diagnosis is a consideration, if a behavioral diagnosis can be considered, that diagnosis is almost always impulse-control aggression.
- Clients with pure-bred dogs may prefer a label of "rage" or "idiopathic aggression" because patterns in lines come under less scrutiny. Good familial histories of as many dogs as possible in the lines involved should be taken for all behavioral conditions.

Common Non-Specific Signs

- The entire range of behaviors associated with aggression could be displayed in the absence of a pattern that fits medical/somatic conditions or other behavioral conditions.

Rule Outs

- The primary rule outs are epileptiform seizure activity and central nervous system, generally brain, neoplasia.
- Acutely painful conditions can appear "idiopathic."
- Treatment with corticosteroids may cause heightened reactivity, which could conceivably appear as a manifestation of "idiopathic aggression."

Etiology, Epidemiology, and Risk Groups

- Idiopathic aggression seems to appear most often in dogs 1 to 3 years old, which may be a confounding factor in distinguishing it from impulse-control aggression.
- The age at which most idiopathic epilepsy develops is also 1 to 3 years.
- Idiopathic aggression cannot be behaviorally induced in a clinical setting.

Common Myths That Can Get in the Way of Treatment or Diagnosis

- This diagnosis may be mythological, given the insistence on lack of pattern.

Commonly Asked Client Questions

- Is this "rage"?

- Almost every aggressive behavior labeled as "rage" is consistent with impulse-control aggression.
- The exceptions are most often due to neurological conditions or to conditions such as REM sleep disorders.

Treatment

- Management:
  - Avoid any circumstances thought to be associated or provocative.
- Behavior modification:
  - As for other aggressions.
- Medication/dietary intervention:
  - Without a better diagnosis, competent treatment will be unlikely.
- Miscellaneous interventions:
  - Send clients home with instructions to video the dog and to keep a log of every behavior about which they are concerned and what preceded and followed those behaviors.
  - Have the clients watch the other pets in the household and see if there is any pattern to their responses. If there is, the condition is being misdiagnosed as "idiopathic."

Helpful Handouts

- As for other aggressions.

Last Words

- If the clients are really observant, they may actually notice the first instance of impulse-control aggression, and at that point it would look "idiopathic."

The most common contextual associations of aggression diagnoses discussed are outlined in Table 6-6. Table 6-7 contains an aggression screen that shows associations between specific behaviors and diagnoses.

Must All Dogs with Non–Management-Related Concerns That Involve Any Aggressive Response Be Assigned a Diagnosis of One of the Types of Pathological Aggression?

No. The list of diagnostic categories used here for clinically recognized pathological aggression may not be exhaustive. Different people select for different canine behaviors and preferred behaviors, and management of dogs varies culturally. Conditions requiring other diagnoses could exist, may exist in the future, or have existed in the past. Management of dogs also affects which behaviors are expressed and how they are expressed. Additionally, even if a diagnostic criterion is met, the form that diagnosis takes may vary across cultures, breeds, and individuals.

More importantly, for any of the diagnoses discussed here to be made, the behaviors must be consistent and meet the criteria.

- Isolated events do not permit assignment of a diagnosis.

TABLE 6-6

Classification of Canine Aggression: Sentinel Non-Specific Signs

Diagnosis	Signs
Maternal aggression	• Protects toys, bedding from people or dogs • Long-distance vocalization if puppies present • May nip if pup taken, usually vocal • If constantly threatened, may eat toy or pup • Dependent on hormonal state; passes with change in this
Play aggression	• Barking/growling/snapping while playing, usually with people or other dogs (not in solo play). • May start out with play vocalizations and change to serious growling in response to rougher play • Usually puppies or younger dogs • Dog may have never learned to play (early orphaned or rough play as a puppy); plays roughly and uses actual growls, rather than play growls, with other dogs • Uses teeth to grab people's hands, legs, clothing • Will grab arm even when playing tug with a toy
Fear aggression	• May bark, growl, or snarl while backing up • May shake and tremble during and after aggression • May bite from behind and then run away • May be associated with painful medical treatment or abuse • Can be induced by inappropriate punishment • Recipient can be canine or human • Dog will cower and look for escape route—dangerous if cornered
Pain aggression	• Usually in response to being manipulated or before manipulation of something the dog has learned is painful • Does not necessarily back up—will grab hands in an attempt to stop pain or anticipated pain • May be in response to rough play from children or other dogs, particularly if recipient is old and arthritic • Can progress to fear aggression
Territorial aggression	• Protects property by barking/growling/snarling/biting • Property can be stationary (house) or mobile (car) • Protects regardless of who is present • Made worse by any kind of fence or confinement (can tell exactly where boundaries are) • Aggression intensifies as approach distance decreases • Unaggressive in the absence of the territory, *but* may quickly re-define a territory (i.e., a kennel run) • May be part of the control complex that includes impulse-control aggression
Protective aggression	• Protects people from other people or dogs • May single out one person to protect • Stands between person being protected and others • Barks/growls/snarls/bites with likelihood for more aggressive behaviors to occur the closer the person is • May be stimulated to react by quick moves or embraces • Unaggressive in the absence of its people
Inter-dog aggression	• Most commonly male-male; female-female • May occur within sexual competition for mates (may be worse if female dog in heat is present with intact male dogs) • Usually starts at social maturity (18-24 months of age) • Challenges may start as stares, bumps, mounting, or exclusion by lateral body blocks from food, play, or attention • May be generalized or occur only in specific singular control/contest situations (e.g., access to a bed, access to doors, in a certain room) • May be made worse by endogenous hormones but is *social* and can occur in households with early neutered pets • Related to actual or perceived hierarchical relationships • Older or weaker dog may be victimized (*caution* for dogs temporarily ill if they have frequently been challenged as above) • May be best understood by watching a "mediator" dog

Continued

TABLE 6-6

Classification of Canine Aggression: Sentinel Non-Specific Signs—cont'd

Diagnosis	Signs
Re-directed aggression	• In response to a correction or thwarting of a desire • Correction could be physical or verbal • May be a growl or involve active inhibition of the person or animal doing the correction or thwarting (biting of hand or wrist); biting of a third dog that intervenes in a dog fight • May be more common with social maturity (18-24 months of age)—no data • Individual who is victimized (human or animal) was not part of original social interaction • Part of the control complex that includes impulse-control aggression
Food-related aggression	• Growling on eating when approached or in sight of other dogs or people • Tremendously long approach distances • Will bite if perceives threat (real or imagined) to food • Either turns and actively guards food or continues to eat in uncoordinated manner while growling, often dropping food • May be non-aggressive with dog food, but aggression escalates with rawhides, real bones, scraps, or treats • Part of control complex that involves impulse-control aggression • Best early indicator that impulse-control aggression may develop
Possessive aggression	• Will not relinquish toys or stolen objects; can be objects stolen in play from another human or dog • May present objects for play and then growl if someone tries to take them • May protect an object that they have been watching from across the room • Part of control complex involving impulse-control aggression
Predatory aggression	• Silently stalks small animals, birds • May also stalk infants and or stare at them silently, drooling • May track and stalk bicyclists or skateboarders • Pattern of high-pitched sounds, uncoordinated motion, and sudden silences may provoke • Dangerous
Impulse-control aggression	• Estimated to be 90% male • Usually occurs at social maturity (approximately 12-36 months of age) but usually becomes apparent to clients within the dog's 2nd year • If female may occur in very young puppy (8 weeks) • Mean age of onset for females approximately 8 months and for males approximately 11.5 months • Worsens with punishment and threats (hallmark) • Has familial and sporadic version • May be core part of any control complex
Idiopathic aggression	• Atypical, toggle switch aggression • No contextual association identifiable • Most commonly reported in dogs 1-3 years of age • Usually is misdiagnosed impulse-control aggression

• Normal, adaptive, sane, or reasonable responses to what may be trying conditions do not merit assignment of a diagnosis. Most of us would want a dog to bite if that bite saved our life.
• Behaviors that seem quirky but are contextually clear may not warrant a diagnosis because to make one would be trivial and adds nothing to our understanding of the behaviors or to our ability to improve them. This is the pattern for many *situational aggressions*.
  • For example, a number of dogs dislike being reached for over a gate or fence. Some dogs will growl and snap if reached for. These dogs do not retreat and do not appear fearful. These dogs do not attack everyone who comes to the fence, although they may show varying ranges of greeting and warning vocal behaviors. It's the "reaching over" the fence that is problematic. In this example, these dogs are otherwise completely unaggressive. You could reach for these dogs if the gate or fence wasn't there, you could pick them up, they don't care about food, are happy to have a lead put on, will meet other dogs, can be groomed, et cetera. Perhaps these dogs were hurt in some earlier experience with being reached for over a gate. Perhaps gates have fallen on them

TABLE 6-7

Aggression Screen

Activity	Diagnoses	NR*	S	L	B	G	SP	BT	WD+	NA✓
1. Take dog's food dish with food	●		←———————————————→						●	
2. Take dog's empty food dish	●		←———————————————→						●	
3. Take dog's water dish	●		←———————————————→						●	
4. Take food (human) that falls on floor	●		←———————————————→						●	
5. Take rawhide	●		←———————————————→						●	
6. Take real bone	●		←———————————————→						●	
7. Take biscuit	●		←———————————————→						●	
8. Take toy or toys	● ○ ● ●		←———————————————→						●	
9. Human approaches dog while eating	● ● ⊘		←———————————————→						●	
10. Dog approaches dog while eating	● ● ⊘		←———————————————→						⊘	
11. Human approaches dog while playing with toys	● ●		←———————————————→						●	
12. Dog approaches dog while playing with toys	● ●		←———————————————→						●	
13. Human approaches/disturbs dog while sleeping	● ●		←———————————————→						●	
14. Dog approaches/disturbs dog while sleeping	● ● ●		←———————————————→						●	
15. Step over dog	●		←———————————————→						●	
16. Push dog off bed/couch	● ●		←———————————————→						●	
17. Reach toward dog	●		←———————————————→						●	
18. Reach over head	●		←———————————————→						●	
19. Put on leash	● ● ●		←———————————————→						●	
20. Push on shoulders	● ●		←———————————————→						●	
21. Push on rump	● ●		←———————————————→						●	
22. Towel feet when wet	● ●		←———————————————→						●	
23. Bathe dog	● ●		←———————————————→						●	
24. Groom dog's head	● ●		←———————————————→						●	
25. Groom dog's body	● ●		←———————————————→						●	
26. Stare at	●		←———————————————→						●	

Types of agression:	● Fear	● Possessive	● Impulse control	● Predatory
	○ Pain	⊘ Territorial	○ Maternal	● Redirected
	● Food related	● Interdog	● Protective	● Play

Behavior key: NR = no reaction; S = snarl (noise); L = lift lip (can see corner teeth); B = bark (aggressive, not an alerting bark); G = growl (not a play growl); SP = snap (no connection with skin); BT = bite (connects with skin, regardless of damage); WD = withdraw or avoid; NA = not applicable (animal has never been in that situation)

*If the dog has no consistent problematic behaviors associated with situations in this list, the dog likely doesn't have or show the aggression associated with the context. Changes can occur.

+If the dog withdraws without any aggressive response consider that true fear, without aggression, may be involved. If the dog exhibits any of the noted behaviors and withdraws before, during or after exhibiting them, consider a diagnosis of fear aggression.

✓Remember that the dog who has not been in certain situations may react to them once exposed. You cannot know whether a dog will react if the dog has not been exposed. However, if the client is not exposing the dog because of concern or risk, you will want to know this.

Continued

TABLE 6-7

Aggression Screen—cont'd

Activity	Diagnoses	NR*	S	L	B	G	SP	BT	WD+	NA✓
27. Take muzzle in hands and shake	● ●		←————————————→						●	
28. Push dog over onto back	● ● ●		←————————————→						●	
29. Stranger knocks on door	● ⊘		←————————————→						●	
30. Stranger enters room	● ⊘		←————————————→						●	
31. Dog in car at toll booth	● ⊘		←————————————→						●	
32. Dog in car at gas station	● ⊘		←————————————→						●	
33. Dog on leash approached by dog on street	●		←————————————→						●	
34. Dog on leash approached by person on street	●		←————————————→						●	
35. Dog in yard - person passes	● ⊘		←————————————→						●	
36. Dog in yard - dog passes	● ⊘ ●		←————————————→						●	
37. Dog in vet's office	● ●		←————————————→						●	
38. Dog in boarding kennel	●		←————————————→						●	
39. Dog in groomers	● ●		←————————————→						●	
40. Dog yelled at	● ●		←————————————→						●	
41. Dog corrected with leash	● ● ● ●		←————————————→						●	
42. Dog physically punished - hit	● ● ●		←————————————→						●	
43. Someone raised voice to owner in presence of dog	●		←————————————→						●	
44. Someone hugs or touches owner in presence of dog	●		←————————————→						●	
45. Squirrels, cats, small animals approach	●		←————————————→						●	
46. Bicycles, skateboards	●		←————————————→						●	
47. Crying infant	●		←————————————→						●	
48. Playing with 2 year old children	● ●		←————————————→						●	
49. Playing with 5-7 year old children	●		←————————————→						●	
50. Playing with 8-11 year old children	● ●		←————————————→						●	
51. Playing with 12-16 year old children	● ●		←————————————→						●	

Types of agression:

● Fear	● Possessive	● Impulse control	● Predatory
○ Pain	⊘ Territorial	○ Maternal	● Redirected
● Food related	● Interdog	● Protective	● Play

Behavior key: NR = no reaction; S = snarl (noise); L = lift lip (can see corner teeth); B = bark (aggressive, not an alerting bark); G = growl (not a play growl); SP = snap (no connection with skin); BT = bite (connects with skin, regardless of damage); WD = withdraw or avoid; NA = not applicable (animal has never been in that situation)

*If the dog has no consistent problematic behaviors associated with situations in this list, the dog likely doesn't have or show the aggression associated with the context. Changes can occur.

+If the dog withdraws without any aggressive response consider that true fear, without aggression, may be involved. If the dog exhibits any of the noted behaviors and withdraws before, during or after exhibiting them, consider a diagnosis of fear aggression.

✓Remember that the dog who has not been in certain situations may react to them once exposed. You cannot know whether a dog will react if the dog has not been exposed. However, if the client is not exposing the dog because of concern or risk, you will want to know this.

when someone reached for them. Perhaps the fence is a dividing line that says to them that they are expected to warn people as part of their *completely normal* behavioral profile. If the last-mentioned is true, the behavior has either been self-reinforcing or people have helped to reinforce it. Perhaps the dog cannot see very well and when he looks up at the fence or gate he growls as part of a process to collect information that he can assess in the absence of that collected visually. We can make up anything we want, and it doesn't matter. The dog's behaviors in this example meet no diagnostic criteria. Even if you made the case for this behavior being part of territorial aggression, we gain nothing in terms of information that will help us to avoid, prevent, or intervene in the behavior than we already have when we say that "the dog will snap at you if you reach over the fence." In fact, we have no idea how common this behavior is and should consider that it might be a variant of normal.

- If the dog exhibits a very narrowly described reaction in a narrowly described situation, this reaction does not merit a diagnosis. It is safe to assume that the dog does not like that kind of interaction and is telling you he does not want to engage in that type of interaction. The dog is doing an excellent job of communicating these points and providing as much warning as is needed. *If we accept that dogs (and other species) are cognitive and that they have needs, we must also accept that their needs may not be ours and that they can have likes and dislikes that should be respected.* We should not assign them a diagnosis because they are telling us that they do not wish to do something. Instead, we should consider that we may wish to respect their desires (i.e., "let sleeping dogs lie"). In fact, by doing so, *we can test whether we missed a diagnosis.*
  - In the case of the dog who doesn't wish to be reached for over a gate, if we remove the gate completely or open the gate first and allow the dog to come to us before reaching for him, and he continues to be non-reactive, he was uneasy about some aspect of the situation. We cannot know what that was, and so it doesn't matter if the reasoning seems rational to us.
  - In contrast, if the dog now begins to growl if we pet him, or if we reach toward him to put down a dish, or when we shift him in bed, the growling involving the gate may involve more than a dislike. This dog now is showing a pattern that may warrant a diagnosis.
  - The first step in treatment of *any* diagnosis is to avoid "provoking" the dog. *We avoid repeating the behaviors that elicit the problematic response.* So, how can we know if we aborted a developing aggression by avoiding a behavior the dog disliked? We

cannot know. However, if the dog is developing a pathological anxiety involving aggression, avoidance will ultimately not be enough because the dog is abnormal: as the pathology progresses, even the most benign circumstances may ultimately be difficult for the dog to parse, and at that point the diagnosis becomes clear.
- For mild pathologies, avoidance of the provocative stimulus may be sufficient to prevent the dog from becoming worse, especially if the people who are engaged in avoidance are also providing a predictable, humane rule structure that encourages calm and safe behaviors through rewards. *It is likely that the same people who are willing to let a dog say that he doesn't like something are also providing excellent information for the dog about preferred behaviors that can minimize risk and anxiety.* In this case, the dog may improve because of the occurrence of/changes in co-morbid patterns of behaviors *in the humans* who live with the dog. The dogs who do best have people who meet their needs.

Not all dogs who exhibit behaviors associated with "aggression" are "aggressive." Dogs can growl, snarl, or bark as part of a normal social repertoire. It is extremely unfortunate that this concern has not been taken seriously by many of those seeking to understand "temperament" or otherwise assess behavioral patterns solely through the use of client questionnaires, which are often asserted to be validated but which, when fully examined, do not meet true validation criteria (Duffy et al., 2008; Hsu and Serpell, 2003; Serpell and Hsu, 2001).

Hsu and Serpell (2003) used clinical behavioral records and a clinical questionnaire that asked about dogs' responses to very specific circumstances and found that the questions asked mirrored the behaviors observed extremely well. These questions were then incorporated into the Serpell and Hsu (2001) questionnaire to produce the Canine Behavioral Assessment and Research Questionnaire (CBARQ) (Hsu and Serpell, 2003), which the authors then claimed was "validated." In fact, what was validated were the questions from the clinical questionnaires created by those acknowledged in the paper (K.L. Overall, S. Crowell-Davis) (Overall, 1997; updated in Overall et al., 2006). That such validation could occur was a function of the use of the discrete behavioral questionnaire in conjunction with direct and video observations of the dog and an in-person, real-time discussion with the owners about what their answers on the questionnaire actually represented in terms of the dog's behaviors. This detailed approach using standardized questionnaires, video, and in-person review avoids the common miscommunication and mistakes in labeling and interpretation most common with respect to canine aggression and play (Tami and Gallagher, 2009).

It is not surprising that owner information about *specific quantitative and qualitative reactions* from the clinical questionnaire provided the best distribution of behavioral classifications (Hsu and Serpell, 2003). Some of these classifications *may* represent true phenotypes. Responses to questions involved well-defined, objective categories of response and were verified by the clinicians during clinical evaluations of the dog. This ensured that both clinician and client agreed on the interpretation of the dog's behavior. In no case were clients asked if their dogs were "aggressive" to strangers. Discrete responses about specific behaviors (i.e., growl, bark, withdraw) in specific contexts (i.e., stranger approaches on the street) were solicited. These were interpreted in a clinical context that acknowledges that some responses may be "normal" given breed and context and that behavioral profiles of true pathologies differ from non-pathological situations (e.g., "growling" can be a normal, non-problematic behavior and need not indicate problematic "aggression"). This approach is a far cry from that taken in a number of articles that provide potentially misleading behaviors about breeds and/or behavioral patterns in situations such as shelters.

The best outcomes are obtained when questionnaires are used with direct behavioral observations, and the questionnaires published here and elsewhere (Overall, 1997; Overall et al., 2006) are not intended for use without direct observation, video, or other extensive information. The standard should be not to make determinations unless the assessments are found to be repeatable and reliable. When compared, such assessments are always superior to questionnaires alone (De Meester et al., 2008, 2011; van der Borg et al., 2010). The argument is clear for crisp diagnostic criteria, excellent, validated definitions of behaviors, and avoidance of terms and judgments that may allow us to think we know something that we do not.

When considering whether "aggressive behaviors" indicate a problem aggression for dogs interacting with other dogs, we must understand the range of "normal" behaviors. Not all dogs who live together are always ecstatic with each other. If you are a dog, a growl, snarl, or snap may keep another dog's mouth out of your dish or keep him from sitting on you in the car. These behaviors are used in normal signaling and can be adequately interpreted *only* given the *patterns and context*. These behaviors should not lead to a judgment of "aggressiveness" or a diagnosis of "inter-dog aggression."

Even certain types of recognized aggression may be variants of "normal." Many dogs who are utterly unaggressive in most situations are aggressive when left in cars. That these dogs do not need to exhibit such extreme threatening behavior to disperse potential thieves is not the issue. The issue is whether their response to being left in the car is rendering their behavior problematic in other circumstances. If the answer is "no," we may want to consider this extreme display is a repeatable variant of normal and encourage the clients to park where no one—however clueless—is likely to put their hands through car windows. If they wished, the clients could work extremely hard to modify this behavior, but such guarding behavior is an inordinately gratifying and self-rewarding one because no one enters the car and people who approach almost always move away. The effort to change such behavior might be extreme for *something that may not be a problem for the dog.*

Meeting the dog's needs also means respecting likes and dislikes, even if they are not what we would prefer, as long as the dog is not suffering or experiencing compromised welfare because of his or her behaviors or situations. This means that we should ask about and keep records of behavioral responses but understand that even quirky, unusual, or undesirable behaviors may be variants of non-pathological behaviors that will not benefit from a diagnostic label. This approach requires that we work hard at seeing the world from the dog's (or cat's, or horse's) viewpoint.

Are There Objective Ways for Clients to Monitor Their Pet's Progress with Diagnoses Involving Aggression?

Yes. This can be done using the *aggression screen* in the history forms. This screen was developed to separate the dog's behavior from how people interpreted it. In other words, it's not helpful from the diagnostic viewpoint to know if the client thinks that the dog is "aggressive," but it is useful to know if the dog growls when you take his food dish, how often this occurs, and whether any other behavioral responses occur with this one. This screen is best used by having the client complete it and then reviewing it with the client after watching video of the dog and observing the dog. Such observation allows the veterinarian to query, for example, whether the growl was a "play growl" or a "serious/offensive growl" and encourages meaningful education of the client.

Without such redundancies, questionnaire interpretation should be viewed with caution. In fact, without such assessment, global use of such questionnaires has produced conclusions about aggression and breeds that are likely not warranted and are not repeatable or reliable (Duffy et al., 2008). The aggression screen published here and in many other earlier incarnations (Overall, 1997, and in numerous notes and proceedings found online; Overall et al., 2006) has been validated by others by comparison of the client responses with the recorded behaviors (Serpell and Hsu, 2001).

The use of a standardized methodology and defining criteria removes the need to rely on non-specific signs and instead allows us to use the non-specific signs (e.g., response when pushed from the bed, response when verbally reprimanded) and the type of reaction within

Situation	No reaction	Snarl/lift lip	Bark/growl	Snap/bite	Withdraw	Not applicable
Take dog's dish with food	X					
Take rawhide		X				
Take real bone		X	X			
Pet dog		X				
Reprimand dog		X				
Put on a leash		X				
Push dog from bed		X				

A

Situation	No reaction	Snarl/lift lip	Bark/growl	Snap/bite	Withdraw	Not applicable
Take dog's dish with food	X					
Take rawhide		X				
Take real bone						
Pet dog						
Reprimand dog		X				
Put on a leash						
Push dog from bed		X				

B

Fig. 6-20 A, Sample subset of aggression screen assessing reactivity, severity, and intensity *before* treatment.
Reactivity (proportion of situations in which the dog reacts compared with the number possible): 6 situations of 7 total, = 6/7 = 0.86
Severity (point calculations for specific behaviors):
Specific behaviors are scored as:
Barking and growling: 1 point
Snarling and lifting the lip: 2 points
Snapping and biting: 4 points
So, this dog's severity score is calculated as follows:
1 at 1 point = 1
6 at 2 points = 12
2 at 4 points = 8
Total = 20 points (of 42 possible, were the dog to react to every category); 20/42 = 0.47
Intensity (number of points divided by the number of situations in which the dog reacts or the average number of points per reaction—this provides some estimate of how forceful the dog's behaviors are): 20/6 = 3.33
B, Sample subset of aggression screen assessing reactivity, severity, and intensity *after* treatment for the same dog.
Reactivity: 3 situations of 7 total = 3/7 = 0.43
Severity:
0 at 1 point = 0
3 at 2 points = 6
0 at 4 points = 0
Total = 6 points (of 42 possible, were the dog to react to every category); 20/42 = 0.14
Intensity: 6/3 = 2.0

each contextual category evaluated (e.g., bark/growl, snarl/lift lip, snap/bite) to gauge the reactivity, severity, and intensity of the reaction in an unambiguous manner (Overall and Dunham, 2002). Such knowledge can keep all of us safer. For the purposes of helping veterinarians and clients evaluate changing behavior in their dogs, reactivity, severity, and intensity can be defined and assigned a relative score based on responses to the aggression screen.

Here, *reactivity* is defined as the number of categories in which the dog reacts inappropriately as a proportion of the total number of categories, *severity* is the score of how much the dog reacts given the total number of points available if the dog exhibited all reactions in all categories, and *intensity* is the total number of points accrued for all reactions divided by the number of categories in which the dog reacts (Fig. 6-20). For ease of use, the six aggressive categories have been reduced to three by combining similar behaviors, but they could just as easily have been left as six categories. Barking and growling have been arbitrarily assigned 1 point; snarling and lifting the lip, 2 points; and snapping and biting, 4 points. This point distribution was selected simply because it spreads out the data, making patterns easy to see.

In the example in Figure 6-20, *A,* the dog has a reactivity of 0.86, a severity of 0.47, and an intensity of 3.33, as calculated in the legend. If this dog is treated and the same screen conducted 2 months later shows the changes in Figure 6-20, *B,* these calculations change. If the clients cease allowing the dog on the bed, so

that the dog is not pushed from the bed and reprimands cease, the dog stops reacting in the categories. Real bones are now not part of the repertoire. The clients have also been working with the dog, so they can now pet the dog and put the dog's lead on without difficulty. The reactivity, severity, and intensity all have decreased in a way that clients can assess objectively and graphically in addition to their subjective evaluations.

Such assessments can help encourage clients in their hard work and indicate areas where help is still needed. This approach also allows the use of repeated measures designs for treatment assessment and for comparisons within or across families, age groups, sexes, or breeds. In behavioral medicine, many of the data are the behaviors, so quantification of discrete behavioral responses is critical for accurate phenotype determination. The same quality of information cannot be obtained using only questionnaires that ask for owners' opinions of their dogs' behaviors (*sensu* Podberscek and Serpell, 1997). Instead, clear categorization and measurements of actual behaviors (Ohl et al., 2008; Overall et al., 2006) and the ability to assess repeatedly how suites of behaviors change with time, alterations in the social environment, and maturation of the dog, in combination with assessment of co-varying physiological traits, are likely to provide the best phenotypes for mapping. Responses for different populations of dogs can then be compared. This thoughtful, detailed approach largely eliminates the chance of spurious correlations based on unfounded myth.

Abnormal Canine Behaviors and Behavioral Pathologies *Not Primarily Involving* Pathological Aggression

CHAPTER

7

This chapter focuses on conditions, concerns, and diagnoses that do not have at their core aggressive behavior. Behavioral conditions are often co-morbid, however, and any one of these conditions may co-occur with a condition involving aggression as a primary or secondary diagnosis.

All of the conditions discussed in this chapter are or can become pathological. For dogs whose problematic behaviors involve elimination, the elimination behaviors may be the result of management practices or may be normal behaviors displayed in contexts clients find undesirable. The manner in which these problematic behaviors are addressed before veterinary intervention is sought can create anxiety (see Box 2-1 for a listing of non-specific signs of anxiety). Because of this and the risk of co-morbidity, concerns about elimination behaviors are addressed at the end of this chapter.

Fear/Fearful Behavior
Diagnostic Criteria and Description
- True fear involves responses to stimuli (social or physical) that are characterized by withdrawal and passive and active *avoidance behaviors* associated with the sympathetic branch of the autonomic nervous system (Hydbring-Sandberg et al., 2004) and in the absence of any aggressive behavior.
- Fear and anxiety have signs that overlap. Some non-specific signs, such as lowering of the back, shaking, and trembling, can be characteristic of both fear and anxiety.
- Truly fearful dogs lower their entire bodies, necks, head, ears, and tails and appear to fold into their limbs (Galac and Knol, 1997). Anxious dogs do not do this and exhibit a wide range of stances.
- The physiological signs of fear and anxiety probably differ at some very refined level, and the neurochemistries of each are probably very different in a way that is not addressed by the *relatively* non-specific medications we commonly use (see Table 10-5 for a summary of the complexity of the distribution of subtypes of serotonin receptors).

- Refinements in qualification and quantification of the observable behaviors will hopefully parallel these differences.
- True fear always involves avoidance, with an apparent intent to decrease the probability of social interaction. This is in contrast to anxiety, where avoidance is not the first choice. Dogs who are driven primarily by anxiety may put themselves into a social system, although it makes them uncomfortable and worried.

Common Non-Specific Signs
- Specific behavioral responses may include (Fig. 7-1):
  - tucking of neck, head, tail, and all limbs,
  - hunched back,
  - trembling,
  - salivating,
  - licking lips,
  - turning away (Fig. 7-2),
  - hiding (even if the only hiding possible is by curling into oneself, averted eyes, et cetera),
  - urination and defecation in extreme cases,
  - release of anal sacs,
  - dander may become apparent and fur/feet may feel damp, and
  - for puppies, small breed dogs when fearful appear to vocalize more frequently at the veterinary clinic than large breed dogs, but both pant (Godbout et al., 2007).

Rule Outs
- Endocrinopathies, including Cushing's disease and hypothyroidism, can result in many of the same signs, but the pattern is usually different.
  - There are periodic vogues for treating fear and a variety of anxiety-related conditions with thyroxine because the non-specific behavioral signs can occur with hypothyroidism. See the discussion in Chapter 6 on thyroidal involvement in aggression.
    - Unless the dog also has physical signs of hypothyroidism, this is unlikely to be the cause of fear.
    - Treatment with thyroxine is not benign and can cause iatrogenic thyrotoxicosis.

231

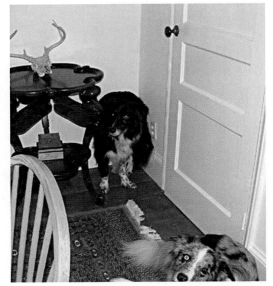

Fig. 7-1 Two border collies from the same household. Notice the merle dog is calm and watching the photographer. The black collie is backed into a corner, tail tucked, back hunched, head lowered a bit, gaze averted, and her lips and nose dripping. The black collie has true fear; the merle collie is normal.

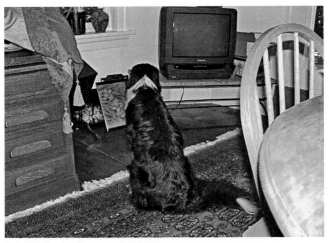

Fig. 7-2 The same collie in Figure 7-1 when she was not permitted to go into a corner. She turned her back on the humans, tensed her body, pulled her ears back and down, flush with her head, and hunched over a bit.

- ▪ If hypothyroidism may be a concern, laboratory evaluation should include a full thyroid (not just thyroxine [T_4]) panel using the dialysis method, and this evaluation should be performed before treating the patient with behavioral medications.
  - ▪ Tricyclic antidepressants (TCAs) and selective serotonin reuptake inhibitors (SSRIs) artificially lower the laboratory values of many parameters used to assess thyroid function, rendering the interpretation of the test difficult at best.

- • Any infectious or toxic agent that can affect the nervous system could potentially cause many of these non-specific signs, but the pattern is different. Fear can be insidious in the way that it is characteristic of infectious/toxic conditions, but a dog's behaviors are not usually dependent on the social or environmental context if he has a toxic or infectious condition.

Etiology, Epidemiology, and Risk Groups
- • There appear to be two main groups of fearful dogs:
  - • dogs who develop/display fear as very young puppies (5 to 8 weeks of age) and
  - • dogs who become increasingly fearful as they move through social maturity (1 to 3 years of age)
    - ▪ It is unclear whether this second group of dogs was ever truly "normal" because we lack contextual, early, standardized assessment.
- • For both groups of dogs, there appear to be sporadic and heritable forms, although the data are poor.
- • For very young puppies (5 to 8 weeks of age), fear can be due to lack of exposure or a heritable version of fear that appears to render the dogs averse to approaches of and interactions with strangers.
  - • These dogs may freeze when faced with unfamiliar humans, and if not completely problematic as puppies, they worsen as they move through social maturity.
  - • These dogs have consistent behavioral and physiological responses to unfamiliar people.
  - • These dogs are usually quite good with other dogs.
  - • Many lines of purpose-bred dogs have dogs who respond this way. Such behaviors may have been selected for during the process of trying to produce "tractable" laboratory dogs.
  - • This condition can be detected at the first veterinary visits. When tested using a series of behavioral provocations that are part of routine care, these puppies withdraw and become quiet, although they may pant (Godbout et al., 2007).
    - ▪ When examined using the same techniques at 18 months of age, the same dogs are fearful as young adults (Godbout and Frank, 2011).
  - • If protected, these dogs can live a good life as pets, but people have to understand that they are likely never to be outgoing.
    - ▪ Good, consistent treatment with sophisticated medications combined with behavior modification from an early age has not been tried in dogs, but it appears to help in mice.
- • For dogs who begin to show fear during social maturity or for dogs who worsen during this time, clients will often express concerns that they ignored about some behavior during puppyhood.
- • Dogs can become fearful with time, but when this happens, the fear is not usually global, and

identification of stimulus/stimuli that trigger the response will help in the process of treating it.

Common Myths That Can Get in the Way of Treatment or Diagnosis

- He's just "shy."
  - Being "shy" is fine if the dog is not actively unhappy or suffering a decrement in his quality of life (QoL), but these concerns need to be assessed. Being more or less outgoing are variants of normal. Quivering in fear, salivating, and hiding when approached by non-threatening strangers are not normal behaviors.
- This is "normal" in this breed.
  - Although some breeds do—deliberately or accidentally—select for pathologies, no one wants a breed to exhibit a pathological behavior where the dog suffers. If all other members of the family are like this—and this can and does happen—the client needs to seek a veterinary geneticist who will work with a behavioral specialist to counsel the client.
- He will "grow out of it."
  - These dogs do not "grow out" of their fear. In fact, their fear worsens with time. Clients especially notice the profound changes that occur at social maturity, yet the dog is easiest to treat and responds best if treated as early as possible. Clients should be given some objective criteria (e.g., behavioral tasks that can be videotaped) by which to evaluate young dogs or puppies for whom there is a concern. If the vet and the client cannot measure improvement over a few weeks to months and with increased humane exposure to target situations, treatment should be started.

Commonly Asked Client Questions

- Will he/she ever be normal?
  - Not completely, but with some protection and good treatment, these dogs can look like they are normal and be happier.
- Are drugs needed for the rest of his life?
  - If medication is helping, and if the medication is causing no untoward side effects, treatment may be for life because this may be what the dog needs. Emphasis must be on QoL.
- Could we have prevented this?
  - We do not know because while we know some forms of fear appear to be heritable, we do not know at what level or mechanism the pathology resides.
  - Too much early exposure may make the dog worse.
  - These dogs likely would benefit from extremely early treatment with medication and truly humane behavior modification. In fact, the earlier, the better.
- Should we have known this would happen?
  - Clients need to know what questions to ask and what behaviors to observe. When adopting a rescue or shelter dog, we attribute much to his or her current condition/surroundings and past trauma. It's possible that the fear contributed to relinquishment.
  - If clients are buying a dog from a breeder, they need to ask specifically about fears, anxieties, phobias, and genetic patterns, *and* they need to see other dogs in the line and speak to as many people as possible who have those dogs. If clients do all of this and can detect no hint of problems, either everyone thinks that the pathology is "normal" or this is truly rare.
- Are we to blame?
  - People often engage in behaviors that scare dogs and most dogs are recoverable. Fearful dogs, by definition, are not recoverable easily. If people subjected a dog to a set of behaviors they knew to be causal of fear for that dog or if they did not intervene when they saw this happen, they are to blame.
  - Most people are misinformed or uninformed. This is sad and may make them feel terrible, but intent matters, so they are not really to blame.
  - Once clients know what the problem is and that there is help available, they become responsible for that dog. If they continue to put the dog in untenable conditions (from the dog's perspective) or refuse to give it appropriate care, the balance of blame shifts in their direction.
  - *A more useful focus is assigning responsible roles for everyone in the dog's anticipated improvement.*

Treatment

- Management:
  - Part of the management of this condition involves screening for it at every single veterinary visit.
    - Veterinarians see dogs at a very young age, and given the data from Godbout et al. (2007), dogs at early risk for this condition are recognizable at all ages.
    - Normal puppies are outgoing and forgiving at vets' offices, especially if vets focus on them and play with them.
    - Very young puppies are more focused on humans at veterinary offices than are older puppies. We do not know if this pattern is due to age alone or to learning that vets' offices are scary places, but we can take advantage of it and play more with young puppies.
    - Any puppy who withdraws further the longer that he or she spends at the vet's, especially if nothing is done to him or her, needs immediate intervention (e.g., alprazolam, possibly) and a long-term treatment plan.
  - Dogs with this condition should be protected from stimuli known to trigger it until they are engaged in an active behavior modification plan,

combined with pharmacological treatment to facilitate the behavior modifications.

- Clients will need a detailed list of circumstances from which to protect the dog and a way in which to do so.
- Clients need to know that this is a QoL decision.

- Behavior modification:
  - Behavior modification is essential.
    - Dogs need to be taught to relax on cue and to offer a behavior that calms them and allows them to get their information from their people.
    - Clients may need help implementing such programs and could benefit from help from a certified pet dog trainer, applied animal behaviorist, or others trained in these techniques.
- Medication/dietary intervention:
  - Supplements containing omega-3 fatty acids and other polyunsaturated fatty acids (PUFAs) may have a beneficial effect on fearful behaviors by preventing damage to neurons that could inhibit the ability to recover from a fearful event.
  - Available nutriceuticals (alpha-casozepine [Zylkene], L-theanine [Anxitane], Calmex, and Harmonese) may benefit fearful dogs because they all have some effect on γ-aminobutyric acid and promote calmer behaviors through inhibition. Some of these may also have neuroprotectant effects (see Chapter 10).
  - Royal Canin's CALM diet contains alpha-casozepine, and studies to date have shown very mild but potentially promising effects on behavioral indicators of stress (Kato et al., 2012; Palestrini et al., 2010).
  - In all but the mildest circumstances, medication may be warranted because:
    - QoL matters,
    - these dogs tend to worsen with time, and this can happen quickly, and
    - medication affects pathways that govern molecular learning, permitting quicker, and likely better, implementation of behavior modification and the learning of new behaviors.
  - Medications that may help come from the following classes of drugs:
    - TCAs (amitriptyline, nortriptyline, clomipramine) may help dogs to be less anxious and more outgoing as they modulate neurochemical activity. Broad-spectrum TCAs affect many norepinephrine/noradrenaline (NE/NA) and 5-hydroxytryptamine (5-HT) receptors and so may address a variety of neurochemical variants of fear. If the fearful response involves any ritualistic components, clomipramine may be the first drug of choice.
    - SSRIs (fluoxetine, sertraline) have been shown to be helpful in some forms of panic, fear, and profound anxiety. Because they target specific 5-HT$_{1A}$ subtype receptors, they mostly affect

regions of the brain involved in learning and so may have their greatest effect in combination with behavior modification designed to teach patients more successful and less distressing behaviors.

- Benzodiazepines (BZDs; alprazolam, clonazepam) and related compounds (gabapentin) may be essential for alleviating fear and incipient panic and can be given daily or as needed.
- Alpha-2 agonists (clonidine) can be useful for extreme fear with enhanced reactivity because they alter the peripheral vascular tone that is part of the feedback coupled to reactive responses. These can be used daily or as needed.
- Serotonin-2 antagonist reuptake inhibitors (SARIs; trazodone) affect 5-HT$_{2A}$ receptors and given the distribution of these may modulate some activity/motion associated with fear. It is unlikely that in profound, non-situational fear, treatment with trazodone alone, will be helpful, but it is often used situationally because it is a sedative.

- Miscellaneous interventions:
  - *Protection is undervalued as a treatment strategy*, although people recognize its value as a coping strategy. Risk assessment is essential here. When nothing good is likely to come from the interaction, it's not necessary (e.g., the dog is not bleeding uncontrollably) and/or the clients will not have the patience or time to guide the dog through the interaction or experience in a way that could benefit the dog, avoiding the fearful situation will protect the dog from becoming worse and making more molecular changes at the neuronal level that will help him to be more reactive.

Helpful Handouts

- "Protocol for Generalized Discharge Instructions for Dogs with Behavioral Concerns"
- "Protocol for Deference"
- "Protocol for Teaching Your Dog to Take a Deep Breath and Use Other Biofeedback Methods as Part of Relaxation"
- "Protocol for Relaxation: Behavior Modification Tier 1"
- "Tier 2: Protocol for Desensitizing and Counter-Conditioning a Dog or Cat from Approaches from Unfamiliar Animals, Including Humans"
- "Protocol for Understanding and Treating Dogs with Fear/Fearful Aggression"
- "Protocol for Treating Fearful Behavior in Cats and Dogs"
- "Protocol for Using Behavioral Medication Successfully"

Last Words

- People become worried and scared when their dog is fearful and may delay seeking help in the hopes that the dog "will grow out of it." Truly fearful dogs do not "grow out of it," and the risks must be frequently and clearly explained because the earlier these dogs are treated, the more normal they become. When deciding whether to use medication on a very young dog, minimize the cost of error, which is that the dog will worsen, and consider early use of medication in combination with true behavior modification (not just training or obedience training).

- None of us are perfect, and no dog needs to be perfect. Clients who can adequately protect dogs from the objects of their fear may choose protection as a strategy, but they need to ensure that they can continuously implement the protection over a decade or more. Few clients have stable enough lives to guarantee this approach.
- There are lines within breeds where all or most of the dogs exhibit some form of fear. Genetic counseling can help breeders to make choices that can alter this pattern.
- Noise reactivity may enhance the risk for some types of fears and anxieties. Whether this is the case for true fear is currently unknown.
- Dogs who are fearful may be difficult to assess medically, especially for pain. The sympathetic response to fear will mask a number of non-specific signs of physical ailments and may ultimately worsen pain. If the dog is painful after the fearful event, chances are he was painful before it. Medication and rehabilitative therapy to alleviate the pain should be considered, especially because nociceptive perception and anxiety become neurochemically associated centrally.

Generalized Anxiety/Generalized Anxiety Disorder (GAD)

Diagnostic Criteria and Description

- Consistent exhibition of increased autonomic hyperactivity and hyper-reactivity, increased motor activity, and increased vigilance and scanning that interferes with a normal range of social interaction in the absolute *absence* of any specific provocative stimuli.
- This diagnosis is characterized by a heightened monitoring and attentiveness to environmental and social stimuli, which is accompanied by increased autonomic arousal (e.g., panting, increased heart rate and respiratory rates, mydriasis) when stimuli are present.

Common Non-Specific Signs

- These dogs are often identified by some combination of the following behaviors:
  - constant monitoring of the social and physical environment manifest as increased locomotion, attentiveness, vigilance, and scanning,
  - easy distractibility manifest as lack of focus or what clients often call an inability to concentrate or pay attention,

- hyper-reactivity involving a lower threshold for reacting, an out-of-context reaction, and a reaction that continues after the stimulus is gone,
- physical and physiological signs of increased autonomic arousal, including dilated pupils, increased respiratory rate, increased heart rate, and near constant pacing once aroused,
- sporadic or persistent diarrhea (this may be the most under-appreciated sign of this condition), and
- weight loss, which clients may not appreciate, associated with increased activity.
- Specific behavioral responses to stimuli can include pacing, barking, whining, and lunging, all of which are triggered at levels below which most dogs react and which persist for longer periods of time than would be true for normal dogs.
  - *The form of the specific behavioral response may be affected by breed.* For example, some border collies with GAD may exhibit parts of herding sequences or complete herding behavior (in the absence of true herding targets) as one of their manifestations of GAD.
- Most "normal" dogs will habituate to the triggers that provoke the vigilance and scanning and autonomic hyper-reactivity and hyperactivity that occurs in GAD.

Rule Outs

- The signs of GAD are sufficiently non-specific that they can be associated with pain, cardiac disease, or endocrinopathies.
- True hyperactivity may be a concern, but the attentiveness and monitoring that are characteristic of GAD are lacking.
- In elderly dogs, cognitive dysfunction (CD) can share signs with GAD, and *GAD may be a sequela to changes involved in early CD and/or "normal" aging in which visual and auditory capabilities change suddenly.*
- Inflammatory bowel disease/irritable bowel syndrome (IBD/IBS) is an often diagnosed but seldom verified condition. Any dog with IBD/IBS should undergo a complete behavioral history and evaluation. If IBD/IBS is not confirmed but the behavioral history is informative, the diarrhea may be a non-specific sign of heightened reactivity and autonomic arousal.

Etiology, Epidemiology, and Risk Groups

- As with most behavioral conditions, GAD becomes most apparent as dogs pass through social maturity, suggesting that shifts in neurochemistry and/or regional brain activity are contributory.
- There are no population-level data about prevalence and risk.
- GAD may run in family lines, but there are no conclusive data.
- GAD is often co-morbid with other anxiety-related conditions, especially noise reactivity/phobia.

- The extent to which altered auditory acuity could be involved has not been investigated.
- *Diagnoses involving aggression (e.g., true inter-dog aggression, impulse-control aggression) are often secondary to GAD.*
  - In such circumstances, *treating GAD often sufficiently raises the threshold for the aggression,* allowing it to resolve.
  - Clients and vets should be aware of co-morbidity and ask whether the reactivity leads to the concomitant anxiety disorder, or whether the anxiety would remain were the reactivity lessened.
    - Dogs who are less reactive may do a better job of attending to and understanding other dogs or people because they can relax and process the signals. Dogs with primary diagnoses involving aggression may not be able to read, process, plan, or act on the signals of others, regardless of whether they can take the time to observe and monitor them.
- Attention-seeking behavior must be a diagnostic rule out because some dogs can learn that they can encourage non-stop attention by constantly moving and engaging in similar behaviors.
  - Dogs with attention-seeking behavior do not engage in the behaviors when they are alone; dogs with GAD engage in them regardless of the presence of the clients or anyone else.
- Other dogs in the household appear to know that these dogs are abnormal and may avoid them when they are very reactive. If the client has another dog, the comparison of the behaviors of the two dogs can be dramatic and informative.

Common Myths That Can Get in the Way of Treatment or Diagnosis

- This breed is very vigilant.
  - There is adaptive, in-context vigilance and vigilance that occurs regardless of the context. If the dog exhibits the latter, a diagnosis of GAD should be considered.
- The dog will outgrow this behavior—he is so active just because he is young.
  - Normal activity has peaks and troughs. Dogs with GAD react profoundly to any perceived stimulus and instantly become aroused and distressed. Affected dogs would interrupt play with other young dogs if a new stimulus was sensed.
  - Clients should be encouraged to monitor such subtle differences in behavior early. Affected dogs will not outgrow the behavior with time but instead will learn to become more reactive and distressed, and react more quickly.

Commonly Asked Client Questions

- Is this the result of the dog's diet?
  - Diet is an unlikely cause of an anxiety disorder, although if the dog has any food-related allergies

these could contribute to making the dog more reactive.
- Is this the result of vaccinating the dog?
  - There is no evidence that vaccinations can cause any anxiety-related condition in healthy animals. Repeated trips to the vet, regardless of the reason, can be viewed by the dog as a series of frightening experiences (see earlier discussion on fear/fearful behavior).
- Does this mean the dog is not getting enough exercise?
  - Given the incidence of obesity, most dogs in the United States do not get enough exercise. Although increased exercise and aerobic scope can benefit most anxious dogs, exercise alone tends not to alter the behaviors of vigilance and scanning in these dogs.

Treatment

- Management:
  - Controlling exposure of triggers that elicit the most extreme responses may help to keep the dog's responses in a more manageable range. Curtains/drapes may help for dogs who respond to movement. Crating or gating the dog away from windows, doorways, letterboxes, et cetera, may help him not to react and so modulate the extent to which he becomes vigilant.
  - Clients have usually yelled at or reprimanded these dogs frequently. Yelling and reprimands don't work, and the risk is that dogs learn to tune out most of the client's requests. Teaching the client to talk to and interact with the dog only when the dog is sitting still and is quiet and attentive is a challenge but necessary if the client is to expand the extent of time in which the dog can focus on anything.
  - Clients should avoid as many circumstances as possible that trigger or worsen the behaviors. This may mean that the dogs have to stop going in the car or to the dog park, but such deprivations will be temporary, and the activities can be slowly resumed as the dog improves.
- Behavior modification:
  - Clients and trainers often find it extremely hard to work with behavior modification in dogs with GAD. The lack of focus and willingness to pay attention and the hyper-reactivity and distress are challenges. For dogs who are unable to work with basic behavior modification until they begin to respond to medication, simply teaching the dog to sit quietly, look at the client, and take a deep breath—even if the dog must get up after each iteration of this exercise—will lay the foundation for using improved communication for helping the dog as the medication renders him less reactive.
  - The protocols for deference, relaxation, and deep breathing all will help, and all are necessary, but

complete engagement in these may not be possible until the dog has begun to respond to medication.

- Medication/dietary intervention:
  - There is some weak evidence that extremely high protein levels may render some dogs more reactive if these dogs are not working hard physically. If the dog is eating a very high-protein diet (>25%), lowering the protein may help the dog improve.
  - Medication is usually the key first step in allowing the dog to be less vigilant, less distressed, and more attentive to the client and other dogs about whether there are legitimate reasons for arousal.
  - Medications to which these dogs best respond include:
    - Gabapentin, alone or in combination with TCAs and/or SSRIs. Gabapentin is ideally suited to decrease overall arousal and non-specific anxiety levels with very few potential side effects.
    - TCAs (clomipramine, amitriptyline if in combination with SSRI) will affect both NE/NA and 5-HT subtype receptors, and their ultimate effects may be determined by the overall distribution of those in the specific patient's brain. Generally, both NE/NA and 5-HT receptors are involved in the behaviors associated with most anxieties, although the relative contributions may vary among patients.
    - SSRIs (fluoxetine, sertraline, luvoxamine) primarily affect the 5-HT$_{1A}$ subtype receptor and so may exert their largest effects in the hippocampus and cortex in regions involved in learning. As such, they should speed the acquisition of new, more suitable coping behaviors taught through behavior modification and modulate arousal level.
    - SARIs (trazodone) affect 5-HT$_{2A}$ subtype receptors, which are commonly involved in anxiety-related conditions involving repetitive movement.
    - Central alpha agonists (clonidine) stimulate central NE/NA receptors and modulate NE/NA receptors in the peripheral vasculature decreasing the agonistic sympathetic response. Depending on the level of the arousal response, they may be helpful. When used with TCAs, which also potentially increase central NE/NA and/or the efficiency of receptor actions and turnover, clients should be asked to watch for side effects, including agitation, that can result from increased central NE.
    - BZDs (alprazolam, clonazepam) may be helpful if there is concomitant noise reactivity/phobia or the dog's reaction to a specific stimulus or set of stimuli is extreme. BZDs affect the reticular activating system and may help to engender a lower reactive state in general. BZDs can be used as outlined in the protocols for noise/storm phobias and panic.
      - Because diarrhea may be a non-specific sign of arousal combined with distress, treatment as needed with loperamide (Imodium) may be beneficial because it will decrease a physiological component of arousal.
  - As these dogs improve, clients note that they begin to gain weight despite the same diet. Clients can be instructed to watch for weight gain as a sign that the dog is no longer patrolling so much as part of his need to be hypervigilant.
  - Clients may also note that if there are multiple dogs in the house, all dogs seem calmer and may play more as the GAD resolves or is controlled.

Miscellaneous Interventions

- Some clients in desperation may have tried severe control techniques, including extensive and inappropriate crating, which usually makes the dog worse including non-jumping harnesses, which may injure active dogs; and electric shock to stop the dog. None of these are likely to be effective, but their discussion or use can be a gauge of the extent to which these dogs are disrupting the household.
- For dogs who are always monitoring the auditory environment, white noise may help, as may headphones (e.g., Muttmuffs) or ear plugs if the dogs will wear them.
- At first, the presence of other dogs is unlikely to help because these patients are too reactive and worried to focus on them. As affected dogs begin to improve, they may play more and become more able to use non-reactive dogs as models for calmer behaviors and sensors for true risk.

Helpful Handouts

- "Protocol for Generalized Discharge Instructions for Dogs with Behavioral Concerns"
- "Protocol for Deference"
- "Protocol for Teaching Your Dog to Take a Deep Breath and Use Other Biofeedback Methods as Part of Relaxation"
- "Protocol for Relaxation: Behavior Modification Tier 1"
- "Protocol for Preventing and Treating Attention-Seeking Behavior"
- "Protocol for Understanding and Treating Dogs with Noise and Storm Phobias"
- "Protocol for Understanding and Treating Generalized Anxiety Disorder (GAD)"
- "Protocol for Using Behavioral Medication Successfully"
- "Generalized Guidelines for Using Alprazolam for Noise and Storm Phobias, Panic and Severe Distress"

Last Words

- In contrast to the rare dog affected with true hyperactivity or hyper-reactivity alone, these dogs are responding to *perceived stimuli* and are distressed. They *can* lie down, relax, and sleep but are easily aroused and seldom seem to modulate their distressed, anxious response once they have become aroused.

- Dogs with true hyperactivity/hyper-reactivity *do not* require the presence of a stimulus to trigger their behaviors, they seldom completely relax and lie down unless exhausted and are then easily aroused, and are usually unresponsive to contextual cues about re-directing their activity.
- Dogs with GAD may take longer to calm down, lie down, and relax than unaffected dogs, but they can do so, and in the absence of stimuli that they monitor they can take contextual cues, relax, and sleep. As they become more normal and less worried, they engage more frequently in such behaviors.

- The danger with the diagnosis GAD is that it is very specific but could easily and carelessly be made in the absence of critical thought or a complete history. Accordingly, it should be *a diagnosis of last resort, not first*, and all of the signs should concomitantly be present under conditions where any of these signs would have subsided in a "normal" or asymptomatic animal.
- This does not mean that the condition may not be common. GAD is likely very common, especially in breeds or individuals that have been selected for faster response times.
- If we are interested in accurately describing phenotype so that we can understand mechanism, the ability to label and understand a condition discretely is nowhere more important than it is here.
- The most common non-specific sign that is likely to be overlooked and classified as a catch-all medical diagnostic category, IBS, is diarrhea. We would benefit from knowing how many animals displaying "IBS" have other behavioral signs of anxiety.
- Finally, this condition may be analogous to what has been called "generalized reactivity to environmental stress." The latter is a description, not a diagnosis.

Separation Anxiety
Diagnostic Criteria and Description
- Physical, physiological and/or behavioral signs of distress exhibited by the animal *only* in the absence of, or lack of access to, the client.
- The diagnosis is confirmed if there is consistent, intensive destruction, elimination, vocalization, or salivation exhibited *only* in the virtual *and/or* actual absence of the client. In virtual absences, the client is present, but the dog does not have access to the client (e.g., a door is closed).
- Signs of distress should be evaluated in currency and terminology that is meaningful to the dog.

- The most commonly reported behaviors (elimination, destruction, excessive vocalization) are *only* the most readily apparent signs of anxiety.
- Drooling, panting, freezing, withdrawal, and cognitive signs of anxiety will be less commonly diagnosed because they are *less apparent to people*, but they occur, and *dogs displaying them may be even more profoundly affected* than dogs who show more obvious signs.

Common Non-Specific Signs
- Specific behavioral signs may include:
  - urination,
  - defecation,*
  - salivation,
  - destruction* (Fig. 7-3),
  - panting,
  - pacing,
  - freezing/immobility,
  - trembling/shaking,
  - vocalization* (bark, whine, growl, howl) (Fig. 7-4), and
  - diarrhea.
- Some dogs may show suites of correlated behaviors. For example, salivation appears to occur more commonly in dogs who freeze and become immobile. Clients will wish to note which suites of behaviors their dogs exhibit so that they can monitor these non-specific signs for changes (hopefully, improvement) during treatment.

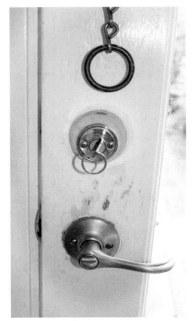

Fig. 7-3 Classic type of damage to a door that could indicate that a dog has or is developing separation anxiety. Notice that there are older and relatively more recent scratches.

---

*Signs that are those most readily recognized by clients because they are so apparent.

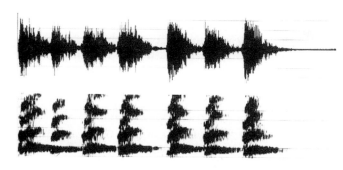

Fig. 7-4 Sonogram of a dog with separation anxiety. Note the atonal, repetitive nature of the barks that characterize distress.

BOX 7-1

Ease With Which Signs of Separation Anxiety Are Recognized

Clear, obvious, and easy to recognize
↓ Destruction
↓ Defecation
↓ Urination
↓ Loud, disruptive vocalization
↓ Licking with dermatological lesions
↓ Salivation with saliva staining
↓ Salivation without saliva staining
↓ Soft, non-disruptive vocalization
↓ Temporal, transient anorexia
↓ Pacing
↓ Withdrawal/freezing
Less clear and more difficult to recognize

- Not all signs are equally recognized, and many dogs with separation anxiety are undiagnosed or under-treated (Box 7-1).
  - Neighbors often complain of vocalization or clients can hear the dog vocalize as they leave.
  - Urination and saliva can evaporate during client absences. A black light can help locate urine, and salivation can be recognized in the absence of visible saliva staining—even in black dogs—by feeling the forelimbs for stiff, stuck together hair.
- When vocalization is involved, barking tends to be repetitive and atonal in nature, with characteristics of distress and isolation barks as identified by Yin and McCowan (2004).
- Non-specific signs other than those listed may occur in separation anxiety. If the criterion "distress only in the absence of the client(s) or access to the client(s)" is met, it doesn't matter whether the behavior is in the list of non-specific signs. If the dog moves apples from a basket on the kitchen counter to a basket by the fireplace all day whenever left alone and is distressed, this bizarre behavior is a sign of separation anxiety.

- Some dogs become distressed only when no one is home, some dogs become distressed when certain people are missing. Regardless, the best way to assess whether the dog is affected by separation anxiety is to video the dog from a few stationary locations (at least one should be the door by which people exit, and another should be the dog's favorite resting place) when the clients are home and when the dog is left alone (or left without access to the preferred person/people). The above-described behaviors will become apparent when the videos are compared.
- Everyone, whether or not they have concerns about their dog's behavior when alone, should video their dogs one to two times per year when left. This practice is part of the good monitoring that should be encouraged to ensure dogs the best possible QoL.
- All related diagnoses should be carefully considered because the complaints of elimination, destruction, and vocalization are non-specific in origin and occur in many behavioral conditions. For example, overactivity associated with greeting can also be a correlate of separation anxiety, but it is important to recognize that this may be an anxiety response designed to elicit reassurance, or it may be a behavior that the humans have inadvertently conditioned.
- For signs to be attributable to separation anxiety, they must occur *only* when the dog is separated or denied access to the client or clients (Table 7-1).
  - *Differential diagnoses for elimination* include separation anxiety, incomplete housetraining, access to appropriate elimination areas, fear, excitement, "submissive" elimination, marking, and incontinence.
  - *Differential diagnoses for destruction* include separation anxiety, play, normal puppy behavior, fear, over-reaction to arousing stimuli, overactivity, and inanimate play.
  - *Differential diagnoses for excessive vocalization* include separation anxiety; stimulation by bells, trucks, people talking, et cetera; social facilitation (other dogs); play; aggression; and fear.
  - When signs of separation anxiety appear in older dogs, they may be associated with anticipatory anxiety. Of 26 dogs 10 years old or older, 13 were diagnosed with separation anxiety (i.e., the behaviors occurred only in clients' absence) (Chapman and Voith, 1990), whereas signs in 6 were attributed to breakdown of housetraining (i.e., "cognitive dysfunction") that did not meet the necessary and sufficient conditions for separation anxiety.

Rule Outs
- The most common medical rule out is thyroidal illness.
  - Although it is true that hypothyroid dogs can be uncertain and that thyroidal hormones can affect behavior, it is important to remember that

TABLE 7-1

Alternative Diagnoses, Conditions, and Causes to Rule Out for Non-Specific Signs of "Elimination" and "Destruction"

Non-Specific Sign	Necessary to Rule Out before Making a Diagnosis of Separation Anxiety
Destruction	Play (e.g., soft pillows, cushions, plants, rolls of toilet paper, things that "play back") Puppy teething Rodent infestation Nesting/denning (e.g., pregnancy or pseudocyesis) Thermoregulation Separation anxiety Cognitive dysfunction (CD) Panic Noise/storm phobias
Urination	Upper or lower urinary tract disease (e.g., UTI) Endocrinopathy (e.g., diabetes, Cushing's disease) Incomplete housetraining Marking Insufficient access Treatment with corticosteroids Excitement or "submissive" urination Separation anxiety CD Hormonal incontinence Arthritis
Defecation	Dietary change or indiscretion Parasitemia Marking Incomplete housetraining CD Incontinence associated with age/arthritis IBS Panic

CD, Cognitive dysfunction; IBS, irritable bowel syndrome; UTI, urinary tract infection.

behavioral conditions are common, and hypothyroidism relatively rare. See the discussion in Chapter 6.

- Unless the dog also exhibits physical signs of thyroidal illness and extensive and multiple laboratory indications that confirm this (low T_4, low free T_4, *and* high thyroid-stimulating hormone), thyroidal illness is not the cause of the distress.
- Supplementation with thyroid hormone/thyroxine is not benign. Iatrogenic thyroidal toxicosis can result in signs or worsening of signs of separation anxiety.

- Treatment with TCAs, SSRIs, and related compounds falsely lowers thyroidal values, and so it is preferable to subject dogs to thyroidal profiles before treatment with these compounds.

Etiology, Epidemiology, and Risk Groups

- Separation anxiety has been postulated to be an outgrowth of a distress response from separation associated with a highly social state. Physiological signs such as anorexia, depression, diarrhea, vomiting, and excessive licking represent non-specific neuroendocrine correlates of anxiety.
- Numerous studies on "attachment" to humans have shown that dogs demonstrate true attachment (Palestrini et al., 2005), but the extent to which alterations in attachment behaviors affects re-homed or abandoned/relinquished dogs remains unclear. It is likely that dogs are variable in their resilience, and the studies to date have been too small and the conditions too variable to define the relative response surfaces. Few data exist, and there are ethical impediments to doing many of the studies that would be illuminating. That said, some patterns are believed to pertain, and many dogs diagnosed with separation anxiety who have been relinquished repeatedly may be quite anxious and clingy, suggesting that attachment and uncertainty about it lasting are issues for the dog. There is likely huge variability in resiliency that would affect the response surfaces for any attachment situation.
- Most of what is believed about the etiology, epidemiology, and risk groups for the development of separation anxiety is not proven, but there is evidence that if dogs react to or are phobic of noises in a repeatable manner, they may have an increased incidence of separation anxiety and/or other anxiety-related conditions. It is critical to screen for co-morbid conditions because unless all aspects of the dog's distress are treated, the dog will not improve. The most common and profoundly debilitating co-morbid conditions include panic disorder (PD) (Fig. 7-5) and noise/storm phobias.
  - In one study of 141 dogs who met the diagnostic criteria for separation anxiety and/or noise phobia during the course of a year in which all behavior clinic patients were screened using the same instrument, co-morbidity was significantly greater than would be expected by chance alone. This study suggests that being affected by one condition may predispose one, likely at the neurochemical level, to be affected by another.
    - The "risks" of co-morbidity in this population, based on the estimated conditional probabilities, were as follows (Overall et al., 2001). The notation "P[x/y] =" is read: "the probability having condition 'x' given that you have condition 'y' is." Probabilities range from zero (it never happens) to 1 (it always happens) but are

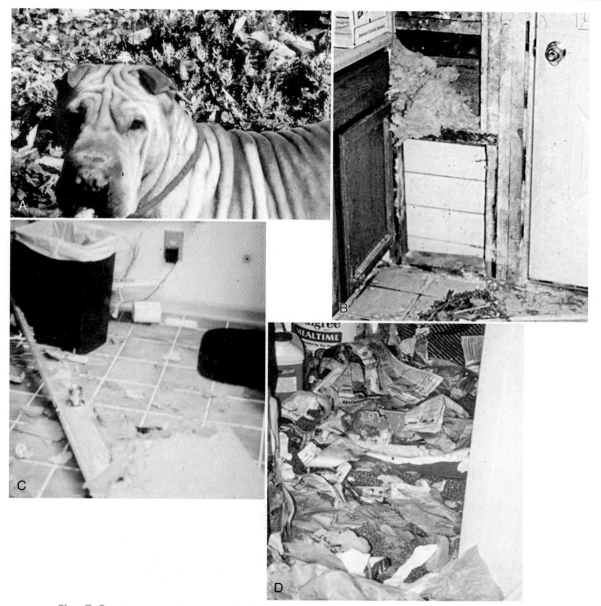

Fig. 7-5 A 5-year-old, male, castrated Shar pei patient diagnosed with separation anxiety and panic disorder and the damage he did when left alone for 2 hours. The dog destroyed the new addition to the house. He was not playing, or he would have played with the toilet paper, which was not destroyed (**C**). He did not eat the food in the pantry (**D**). The patient broke all of his nails (blood is visible where the door jamb would have been, **B**) and teeth and damaged his nose during the destruction. The photo of the patient shows his nose healing (**A**). (Photos courtesy of Jack McCann.)

often informally represented as percentages (the probability times 100). (SA indicates separation anxiety, TP indicates storm [thunder] phobia, and NP indicates noise phobia.)

- P [SA/TP] = 0.8701 (87%)
  P [TP/SA] = 0.6147 (61%)
  The probability that the dog had separation anxiety given that he had storm phobia was 0.87, or 87%. The probability of the reverse—that the dog had storm phobia given that he

had separation anxiety—was only 0.61, or 61%. That these are not identical suggests that these are different conditions.

- P [SA/NP] = 0.8804 (88%)
  P [NP/SA] = 0.7364 (74%)
  The probability that the dog had separation anxiety given that he had noise phobia—which was defined as any non-storm noise—was virtually the same as for storm phobia, 0.88, or 88%. The probability that a dog with

separation anxiety had noise phobia—a more generalized response—was greater than for storm phobia, 0.74, or 74%.

- P [TP/NP] = 0.7609 (76%)
  P [NP/TP] = 0.8974 (90%)
  For noise and storm phobias, the probability that you have one given that you have the other is not equal, suggesting that these are two different reactions in dogs. The chance of having a noise phobia, given that you have a storm phobia, was 0.89, or 90%, suggesting that the unpredictable nature of storms may play some role in how reactive dogs become across all noises.

- Some risk patterns are emerging in populations of dogs with separation anxiety (see Box 7-2 for a set of examples).
  - Dogs who have separation anxiety and are relinquished as a result are likely to have profound

---

BOX 7-2

Triggers for Display of Signs by Dogs Exhibiting Separation Anxiety

Associated with People
- Dog left totally alone but not problematic if at daycare or with a petsitter
- Dog left by one special person or a few people, so not helped by daycare or a petsitter
- Dog is home with person or people but denied access by doors/gates (i.e., a "virtual" absence)

Associated with Physical Environment
- Dog experiences schedule changes (e.g., daily schedule changes from fixed to erratic or early to late)
- Dog experiences the same or similar signs when exposed to a scary event (e.g., storm/thunderstorms—cues could be barometric pressure changes, ozone, lightning, darkness, wind, or rain)

Associated with Other Internal Factors
- Dog experiences signs with age regardless of stability of physical or social environment
- The behaviors are generally thought to be the most severe within the first 15 to 20 minutes of separation, but this may not be true, and many anxiety-related behaviors (autonomic hyperactivity and hyper-reactivity, increased motor activity, and increased vigilance and scanning) may become apparent as the client exhibits behaviors associated with leaving. With judicious use of video, the extent, duration, and onset of behaviors involved in this condition could be exhaustively identified. Some very panicky dogs may begin to be distressed when the alarm is set at night because the client sets the alarm only on days when she leaves.

---

separation anxiety in the new home. This is not the same as saying abandonment causes separation anxiety. In this situation, the dog is abandoned because of the behavior problem, and that abandonment subsequently adversely affects the cognitive and behavioral manifestations of extant separation anxiety. Abandonment itself furthers a worsening pathology.

- Dogs who have been re-homed, especially those with multiple re-homing experiences, may be at risk for developing separation anxiety because of enhanced uncertainty about their chances for staying in a home.
- Dogs who have been neglected and/or roughly treated may exhibit separation anxiety once they get a home where this is no longer the case when those with whom they associate the improved conditions are not present.
- Dogs who have been trapped alone during any traumatic event (e.g., earthquake, fire, robbery) or profound illness may have extreme, albeit justifiable worries about being left alone.
- Dogs who have had extremely impoverished or protected puppyhoods where they were not allowed to explore, make mistakes, meet other dogs or humans, get out of their run, or just be alone may have decreased behavioral flexibility to deal with the absences of humans when finally faced with them. Puppies first acquired at an age of 7 months were more likely to develop separation anxiety problems than puppies acquired at 10 to 15 weeks of age (Takeuchi et al., 2001), suggesting that lack of early exposure may have affected later flexibility.
- Dogs who are beginning to experience cognitive impairment and/or diminution in auditory, olfactory, or visual acuity may begin to show signs of separation anxiety, likely because they feel compromised in their ability to monitor and function in the social environment.
- Dogs who have relied on another dog or cat for their cues about how to react may experience separation anxiety if that animal is hospitalized or dies. In the case of death, true depression may be a sequela.

Common Myths That Can Get in the Way of Treatment or Diagnosis

- The dog is urinating, destroying, defecating, et cetera, because he is "angry" or "spiteful."
  - If the behaviors of concern occur in the contexts defined, they have nothing to do with "anger" or "spite." Concerns about anger and spite suggest that the client is seeing this only from his or her perspective. Seen from the dog's perspective, these behaviors are about distress. A video will convince even the most narcissistic client.
- The dog is "punishing" the client for his or her behavior/schedule/choice in boyfriends/girlfriends.

- See the previous answer. Although the dog may not like the new friend, dogs usually have more direct ways of showing this.
- The dog is exhibiting the problem behaviors because he loves me too much to be separated from me.
  - The dog may adore the client, but these behaviors are about distress. Love should not be pathological.
- People who work too much cause separation anxiety in their dog. Dogs are "pack" animals and need to be with their people.
  - Most dogs do not "need" to be with their people 24 hours per day. If the human is working so much that the dog's minimum needs of food, shelter, and protection are not being met, that person should not have a dog. In the case of such extreme deprivation, many behavioral conditions could begin to appear, but the myth always credits the absence of the human with the development of the separation anxiety. There is no evidence for this myth and lots to refute it. For example, most people who work do not have dogs that demonstrate signs of separation anxiety.
- The dog develops separation anxiety because the client is always home and never "taught" the dog how to be left alone.
  - Normal dogs will teach themselves about being left alone, given the chance (Cannas et al., 2010; Frank et al., 2007). By 2 to 4 weeks of age, pups start to follow each other, and by 5 weeks they will rush an opening in a run as a group (Scott and Fuller, 1965). By 5 weeks of age, if allowed to explore, dogs will begin to go off by themselves, honing exploration skills that continue to develop rapidly through 14 weeks of age. In fact, if not allowed freedom to explore and experience new people, new animals, and new environments on their own by 14 weeks of age, dogs acquire this ability only with difficulty.
- The dog develops separation anxiety because the clients "spoil" the dog by allowing the dog to sleep in their bed, lie on the sofa, et cetera.
  - No study has been able to demonstrate that separation anxiety is more common in dogs with very attentive owners compared with dogs of owners who do not fuss over their animals (Flannigan and Dodman, 2001; King et al., 2000a; Voith et al., 1992). Were this true, all the dogs in any household would have exactly the same problems, and no study has been able to show this. Also, clients who do not have children are no more likely to have dogs with separation anxiety than clients with children.
- The dog shrieks while the client is gone because he is an "only dog," and dogs need other dogs.
  - Studies have shown that dogs with separation anxiety come from both single-dog and multi-dog homes. In multi-dog homes, the other, unaffected dogs do not develop separation anxiety and are not a sufficient stimulus to stop the patient from developing or expressing it.
- The dog will not have a problem if you get him a companion dog.
  - See the previous response. For some dogs who like other dogs and are able to learn from them, once they begin to improve they may be able to learn to worry less by mirroring a "normal" dog. That dog could be outside of the home. For people who want another dog, realistic expectations are key. If the new dog is not completely normal, the first dog's distress may be scary and provoke behavioral concerns in that dog as well. Once the original dog is well along the path to recovery, a nurturing, normal dog from whom he can take his cues *may* be helpful, but clients need to attend to the "nurturing, normal" part of this recommendation (Figs. 7-6 and 7-7).
- The dog destroys because he is "bored" and needs a job or more things to occupy him (but he never plays with or eats the food from his food toys until you come home).
  - *The myth of boredom is particularly insidious.* Most dogs with separation anxiety are neither understimulated nor deprived. That most dogs start showing signs of distress within 10 minutes (Palestrini et al., 2010) refutes suggestions of "boredom." Video reveals that affected dogs ignore the invitations of other dogs to play with them and do not eat food toys that they would otherwise gobble.
  - In fact, distressed dogs *cannot* eat: the level of distress they exhibit is associated with the

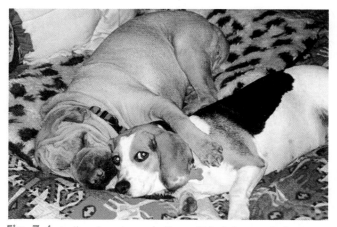

Fig. 7-6 As the dog shown in Figure 7-5, A, began to improve, it was clear that he liked other dogs and would follow and take his cues from other dogs with whom he had spent time (e.g., the neighbor's dogs, dogs at the veterinary hospital). The clients were able to rescue a laboratory beagle who was very sweet, calm, and normal. The clients were happy to have two dogs and knew that the adoption may not have a profound therapeutic effect. (Photo courtesy of Jack McCann.)

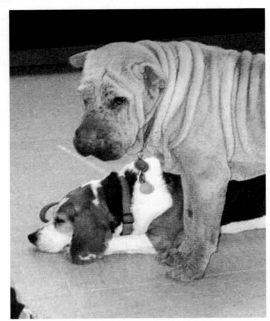

Fig. 7-7 In this case, the adoption was incredibly helpful, and the patient was happy to take cues about his behavior from his beagle companion, a trend that continued as the dogs aged.

sympathetic nervous system—the emergency system. No one wants food when sympathetic nervous system neurochemicals predominate.

- Dogs who dig their way through walls and doors or who escape by breaking a window not only injure themselves physically but also usually seek out someone—anyone—who is home or who will sit with them. The "stimulation" of their "escape" was neither the point nor sufficient to fix their distress.
- Most dogs will enjoy having a job whether it's to go to work with their people, scent work, agility, or herding. However, having a job does not stop them from being distressed when they are alone.
- Dogs need "limits." You should always "crate" your dog when you are gone.
    - This pathology is not about "limits." It's about distress. Some dogs feel more secure in crates, and some dogs feel trapped in them (see the discussion in the treatment section). No one should de facto put a dog into a crate because they are leaving and/or the dog is perceived to need "limits."
- Rescuers, shelters, and rescue sites often speak of dogs that are "Velcro" dogs. "Velcro" dogs are portrayed as dogs for people who really want attention from dogs: "She'll always be by your side and you'll always know where she is."
    - There is a difference between *a dog who wants and likes to be with people* and *a dog who must be with*

people—any people—to stay sane and not panic. The word "Velcro" should not be used to disguise or mask a problem or in an attempt to match a needy dog to a needy human. Needy humans may have less mental space—not more—for the special needs of a dog with a behavioral concern.

Commonly Asked Client Questions

- Can this condition be cured?
    - No, because treatment does not change any genetic component of the dog's response surface. At the heart of this condition, similar to all behavioral conditions, is an abnormal perception, abnormal information processing and/or an abnormal response to information perceived and processed. *The extent to which the dog can learn calm behaviors is key, and this ability is usually aided by medication.* We can do such a good job of controlling the dog's distressing behaviors and teaching him ways to avoid becoming more distressed that it would be very hard for most people to know that the dog had a problem. Clients should know that dogs who have had separation anxiety in the past may relapse in the presence of a profound stressor. Anticipation of such events should lead to adjustments in medication and other protective, prophylactic interventions.
- If medication is used, is it for life?
    - Maybe. The probability that long-term medication use is needed may be related to the duration of the condition and the severity of the signs. This is why screening for behavioral problems at each visit is so important. Even if long-term medication is needed, this is likely the healthier choice for the dog in terms of risk of injury and QoL. Annual laboratory and physical examinations can identify risks that may warrant changing medications or dosage reduction.
- Is this condition heritable, or are there liability genes?
    - We do not know the answer to this question. We do know that if the dog reacts profoundly to noises, he may have a co-morbid anxiety-related condition, including separation anxiety. In most breeds, noise reactivity/phobia runs in family lines as well as occurs sporadically. These patterns strongly suggest that liability genes for separation anxiety may exist and that we should seek to identify them for genetic counseling if for no other reason.
- Would this dog do better in another home?
    - *The best outcomes occur in families where the primary interest of the humans is to meet the dog's needs humanely and provide the best QoL.* Unless the clients know that they cannot meet the dog's needs *and* know of a home that can meet these needs that also wants the dog, *and* the home is familiar to the dog, *and* the dog is happy to go, they will do more harm than good in re-homing this dog.

Treatment
- Management:
  - *Questions about the presence and pattern or patterns of behaviors associated with separation anxiety should be included in all histories for all visits because the problem is one of the most common canine problems and yet is so often missed in its early stages. The long and short screening questionnaires in this text have sections that assess these complaints. Early intervention is important.*
  - Clients should be encouraged to keep a log of the dog's behaviors using the non-specific signs exhibited by the dog on the video (see Table 7-2 for an example). A client version of this log is found in the handouts: "Log for Dogs with Separation Anxiety." Monitoring non-specific signs allows the client and the veterinarian to recognize patient progress or lack thereof. The pattern of the signs can also be essential in helping the clinician decide if the patient meets the criteria for diagnosis in cases where multiple behavioral conditions may be ongoing.
    - If the client learns that the dog can be left for 4 hours without elimination but not 6 hours, the client knows that—for now—he or she needs to avoid longer absences. Avoidance is key in the treatment of all behavioral problems because every time the behavior—no matter how undesirable or abnormal—is repeated, the dog will be reinforced for the behavior. Practice reinforces learning at the molecular level. Logs are best used in combination with video surveillance because some signs are much easier for clients to note than others.
  - The dog should not be left alone unless there is no other choice. The dog may be able to go many places with the client.
  - Many dogs with separation anxiety are less distressed if left in cars because cars signal that clients always return. *Leaving a dog in a car is an*

TABLE 7-2

Daily/Weekly Schedule for Dogs with Separation Anxiety

Day/Date: _____

Absence No./Time Left	Maintenance Style	Amount of Time Left	Signs Noted
Absence 1 Time: ___	Left free Crated Confined in room Left outside—doghouse or run Left outside—fenced Outside—free/unrestrained Other—please note: ___	<5 minutes 5-10 minutes 10-20 minutes 20-30 minutes 30 minutes to 1 hour 1-2 hours 2-4 hours 4-6 hours 6-8 hours >8 hours	None Urination Defecation Destruction Vocalization Salivation Other—please note: ___
Absence 2 Time: ___	Left free Crated Confined in room Left outside—doghouse or run Left outside—fenced Outside—free/unrestrained Other—please note: ___	<5 minutes 5-10 minutes 10-20 minutes 20-30 minutes 30 minutes to 1 hour 1-2 hours 2-4 hours 4-6 hours 6-8 hours >8 hours	None Urination Defecation Destruction Vocalization Salivation Other—please note: ___
Absence 3 Time: ___	Left free Crated Confined in room Left outside—dog house or run Left outside—fenced Outside—free/unrestrained Other—please note: ___	<5 minutes 5-10 minutes 10-20 minutes 20-30 minutes 30 minutes to 1 hour 1-2 hours 2-4 hours 4-6 hours 6-8 hours >8 hours	None Urination Defecation Destruction Vocalization Salivation Other—please note: ___

emergency, short-term situation and is not appropriate in many climates or locations. There have been reports of the dog damaging the inside of the car.

- Dog sitters, dog walkers, daycare, boarding, and pet sitting by an older child who is not otherwise allowed to have a dog may all be options that could mitigate the dog's distress.
- If the dog likes crates, will go into a crate willingly, can sleep and eat in a crate, and is calm when in a closed and locked crate, crating or gating the dog may be part of the solution.
  - Not all dogs can be crated or gated. Many dogs will break their nails or teeth attempting to get out of the crate, and dogs have killed themselves by becoming entangled in or impaled on the crate if they panic. Clients should not even consider using a crate as a management strategy for dogs with separation anxiety unless they can video the dog responding as stated when they are home and not with the dog for hours at a time. The risk of gating or crating a dog who views this as entrapment rather than security is huge, and in such cases, it will always make the dog worse (Figs. 7-8 through 7-10).
  - No dog who is crated should wear a lead or collar of any kind because these pose strangulation hazards if the dog becomes distressed.
- No dog with separation anxiety should be tied. Tied dogs are at increased risk of injury or death from strangulation if they become distressed.
- Food toys *may be good indicators of when dogs start to improve* enough to eat, but *they are not a treatment* for separation anxiety. Dogs who are profoundly distressed cannot eat. If a fresh food toy is left for the dog daily, the day he starts to use it indicates that he was sufficiently less distressed to be able to take food, and so he is rewarded for less distress.
  - Dogs vary from less to more distressed during the time they are left, so thinking of the food toy

as a true reward for not reacting to an absence may not be accurate.

- Behavior modification:
  - All emphasis must be placed on ensuring that the dog does not panic and that she learns to be as calm as possible when left or as people signal that they might leave.
    - The cue that may trigger worry or panic for the dog may be one that occurred the night before. If clients set an alarm, lay out clothes, or pack a briefcase on the nights before they will leave, the dog could start to show signs of distress or panic the night before. Routines to teach the dog that she should calm and not worry need to address these triggers also.

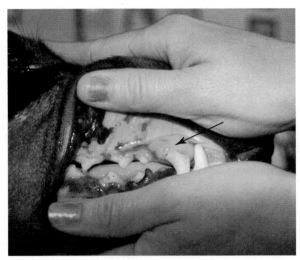

Fig. 7-9 The dog who did the damage shown in Figure 7-8. Note that she has a lesion on her gum above her right canine tooth because of the destruction in which she has engaged, including chewing on and through metal.

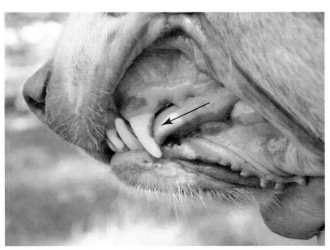

Fig. 7-10 This dog repeatedly chewed on the bars of his crate in an attempt to get out. Notice the deeply worn, grooved back surface of his left upper canine tooth. This is a classic lesion for dogs who chew on their crates. All of this dog's canines look like this, and he may eventually need to have crowns on his four canines.

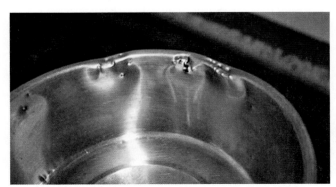

Fig. 7-8 Food bowl of a dog with separation anxiety who was crated to prevent destruction. The dog destroyed anything put in the crate as well as the crate itself. These holes were made by the dog shown in Figure 7-2. Note that the dog *chewed through and pierced stainless steel.*

- Clients inadvertently reward anxious behaviors for two common reasons:
  - They think the dog is just seeking their attention and they don't distinguish between *dogs who want attention* and *those who need it,* so the latter group of dogs is inadvertently rewarded for anxious, pesky behaviors.
  - They recognize that the dog is distressed, and they are seeking to reassure the dog. Unless the dog is rewarded only when calm, anxious behaviors are also being reinforced, resulting in a miscommunication.
- If clients use the "Protocol for Deference" for all interactions with their dogs—no matter how brief or benign—the dog will learn that he is rewarded for sitting calmly and looking at the client, and the client will be able to reinforce calm behaviors.
- Dogs who are globally anxious will benefit greatly from the "Protocol for Teaching Your Dog to Take a Deep Breath and Use Other Biofeedback Methods as Part of Relaxation." Deep breathing allows clients to use the physical signs of an underlying physiological state to help decide how much and what kind of attention to provide these dogs. Attention of the right sort will help these dogs improve at the most rapid rate possible. If the dog can learn that she is rewarded for physiological changes that indicate a lower reactive state, the dog will not only learn to calm down to get attention but will also learn that she feels better when she does so and so can and will repeat these behaviors (this is cognitive therapy for dogs).
- Please tell clients to *ignore all instructions to ignore these dogs* until they lie down and stop interacting with the clients. This is likely both counterproductive and cruel.
  - Co-morbidity is the rule with anxiety conditions, and lack of human input, especially when the human is available, may contribute to true clinical depression in these dogs.
  - Although we do not wish to reward the anxious behaviors, we also must avoid behaviors that provide the dogs with no useful information. Punishment—which is how the dog could interpret this tactic—does not provide information about which behaviors are rewarded.
  - It is far preferable to talk calmly to the dog, but not hug, kiss, fawn over, or otherwise interact in any way that provisions social attention until the dog is calm enough to ensure that anxious behaviors are not being inadvertently reinforced.
- Affected dogs can learn to be less anxious with a combination of behavior protocols.
  - There is no sense in even trying to teach the dog that he is rewarded for calm behavior when left unless he can learn that he is rewarded for calm behavior when in the presence of the client. One behavior modification program that does this is the "Protocol for Relaxation: Behavior Modification Tier 1." Until the dog can sit calmly and wait for the client's rewards and cues while separated *in the house* and under different types of stimulating circumstances, it is foolish to try to implement this plan with the client leaving the house.
- Recommendations for the treatment of separation anxiety usually include an instruction to teach the dog to ignore "departure cues." This text also has a handout about how to implement this recommendation ("Tier 2: Protocol for Teaching Your Dog to Uncouple Cues about Your Departures from the Departure").
  - The intent of these "departure cues" is to *de*-sensitize dogs—who are already sensitized to cues that signal the client's departure—to such cues. Common cues that cause dogs distress include packing or picking up a briefcase, putting on sunglasses, picking up the car keys, et cetera. *If* the clients can identify cues that cause the dog to begin to worry—including setting an alarm the night before a departure—*and if* they are successful in their initial behavior modification efforts (e.g., "Protocol for Relaxation: Behavior Modification Tier 1") they *may be* able to use desensitization and counter-conditioning techniques to help the dogs not react to these triggers.
    - Caution is urged for attempting a too-rapid progression by trying to fix everything at once. All behavior modification should be monitored for behaviors indicating progress and behaviors indicating trouble. It is easy to video any desensitization plan that uses departure cues. *Any clients seeking to desensitize dogs to events, behaviors, triggers, et cetera, associated with actually leaving the dog alone need to be aware that there is a huge risk that they will actually sensitize the dog and make him worse.* Video will allow the clients to see if their interventions are having the desired effect.
- Clients are often encouraged to teach the dog that he can be left alone for increasing amounts of time ("Tier 2: Protocol for Desensitization and Counter-Conditioning Using Gradual Departures") or that he need not be so concerned about activities that occur by the door ("Tier 2: Protocol for Desensitization and Counter-Conditioning to Noises and Activities That Occur by the Door"). Again, these behavior modification programs *may* be helpful if the client is good at basic behavior modification techniques and the client can monitor the dog's response using video. *Otherwise, these techniques can cause the dog to worsen and to become more sensitized and reactive to departures and activity at doors.*

- If there is any doubt, watch a video of the client's work with the dog with the client.
- If there is still a concern that the client may not executing the behavior modification well and correctly, encourage the client to enlist the help of a Certified Professional Dog Trainer (www.ccpdt.org), a trainer who is a Certified Dog Behavior Consultant (CDBC; www.iaabc.org), a Pat Miller Certified Trainer (PMCT; www.peaceablepaws.com), or any trainer who is excellent at operant conditioning and techniques used in behavior modification and who has the certification and ethical credentials that provide some comfort level that only positive techniques will be used.
- Medication/dietary intervention:
  - Diets such as the CALM Diet formulated by Royal Canin, which contains alpha-casozepine and an anti-oxidant complex of vitamin E, vitamin C, taurine, and lutein, are intended to be fed before and during stressful events. There are no specific, controlled data for the treatment of dogs with separation anxiety, and in the published literature the effects are mild.
  - Nutraceuticals, such as alpha-casozepine (Zylkene), L-theanine (Anxitane; Calmex, which includes other compounds), and Harmonese, have been reported to help distressed and anxious animals, but there are no specific, controlled data for separation anxiety.
  - Because the act of being distressed, anxious, and panicky can itself contribute to the production of reactive oxygen species and other neurochemical stressors, non-specific treatment with anti-oxidants and omega-3 fatty acids (Nordic Naturals) may provide an ancillary benefit for patients with many behavioral conditions, including separation anxiety.
  - Dogs with separation anxiety and/or other co-morbid anxieties may have periodic diarrhea. There have been suggestions that probiotic supplements or additions of food containing probiotics (e.g., all natural yogurt) to the diet may favor a "healthier" and less reactive gastrointestinal system and provide "immune support." Data for such interventions in behavioral conditions are lacking; however—and clients should know this—there are few to no risks to such approaches.
  - Medication is almost always an essential part of treatment of clinical separation anxiety. In the United States, two medications have veterinary labels and are licensed for use in dogs with separation anxiety: fluoxetine (Reconcile; Lilly) and clomipramine (Clomicalm; Novartis).
    - Based on the placebo-controlled, double-blind studies required to license these medications, we know that they substantively decrease distressed behaviors in dogs over a treatment period of 2 months (King et al., 2000a, 2000b; 2004a, 2004b; Landsberg et al., 2008; Simpson et al., 2007).
    - Clomipramine has been studied for long-term treatment of separation anxiety with favorable outcomes (King et al., 2004b).
- For both the clomipramine and the fluoxetine studies, *treatment with medication sped the rate at which dogs acquired calmer behaviors through behavior modification*, in addition to having direct effects on anxiety.
- Medications to which these dogs best respond include:
  - TCAs (clomipramine, amitriptyline, if in combination with SSRI). *If separation anxiety is primarily characterized by ritualistic components, clomipramine may be the drug of choice.*
  - SSRIs (fluoxetine, sertraline, luvoxamine). *If separation anxiety is primarily characterized by explosive components, fluoxetine may be the drug of choice.*
  - SARIs (trazodone). *Trazodone affects regions of the brain associated with motor activity and so may be a suitable ancillary medication for some affected dogs.*
  - Gabapentin, alone or in combination with TCAs and/or SSRIs, may be useful if reactivity is the primary concern. The side-effect profile of this medication is favorable, so clients may feel more confident when using it in combination with other medications. Because it affects BZD receptors, it may also augment BZDs without some of the more systemic potential side effects of BZDs (e.g., concerns about any of the hepatic metabolic pathways).
  - BZDs (alprazolam, clonazepam) may be helpful if there is concomitant noise reactivity/phobia or the dog's reaction to a specific stimulus or set of stimuli is extreme because they affect the reticular activating system. BZDs can be used as discussed in the protocols for noise/storm phobias and panic.
  - Central alpha agonists such as clonidine, depending on the level of the arousal response. For dogs who panic, clonidine is an option should the dog be unresponsive to or experience side effects of BZDs and be unresponsive to gabapentin. Because clonidine affects central NE/NA receptors, the peripheral sympathetic response is lessened, which helps some dogs who become quickly and profoundly distressed.
  - Because the diarrhea may be a non-specific sign of arousal, treatment as needed with loperamide may be beneficial because it will decrease a physiological component of arousal.
- Not all signs are equally controlled by all medications, a concern that may be addressed with polypharmacy.

- Miscellaneous interventions:
  - Synthetic analogues that are products of canine pheromones have been frequently suggested as an aid in the treatment of separation anxiety. There are no sufficiently controlled or reported studies that suggest a helpful effect (Frank et al., 2010). Some BZDs appear to affect both olfactory epithelia involved in pheromone detection and limbic regions on which ultimate projections may be made. By regulating Fos expression in these regions, BZDs may affect some regions involved in defensive behavior (e.g., the prelimbic cortex and the medial amygdala) but not affect defensive behavior and defensive aggression in the ventromedial hypothalamic nuclei. It's possible that the reported weak and variable pheromonal responses are due to effects on these and related pathways. If true, this could provide a putative mechanism that could be tested. No such mechanistic tests have been done to date.

Helpful Handouts

- "Protocol for Generalized Discharge Instructions for Dogs with Behavioral Concerns"
- "Protocol for Deference"
- "Protocol for Teaching Your Dog to Take a Deep Breath and Use Other Biofeedback Methods as Part of Relaxation"
- "Protocol for Relaxation: Behavior Modification Tier 1"
- "Protocol for Understanding and Treating Canine Panic Disorder (PD)"
- "Protocol for Understanding and Treating Dogs with Separation Anxiety"
- "Protocol for Using Behavioral Medication Successfully"
- "Generalized Guidelines for Using Alprazolam for Noise and Storm Phobias, Panic, and Severe Distress"
- "Tier 2: Protocol for Teaching Your Dog to Uncouple Cues About Your Departures from the Departure"
- "Tier 2: Protocol for Desensitization and Counter-Conditioning Using Gradual Departures"
- "Tier 2: Protocol for Desensitization and Counter-Conditioning to Noises and Activities That Occur by the Door"

Last Words

- Separation anxiety is a condition that is often *a problem for the client*, so it gets a lot of attention, and lucky dogs have people who seek help.
- Veterinarians would be wise to use the increasing awareness of separation anxiety to educate clients about the extent to which separation anxiety and other behavioral conditions are *problems for the dog and his QoL*. If clients understand that early intervention may prevent co-morbidity of behavioral problems and they understand which behaviors indicate problems, there is an increased chance that they will be better participants in the dog's behavioral and overall veterinary care.
  - Asking about elimination patterns is very important for assessing the presence of anxiety disorders, but even when this is routinely done, sporadic/periodic diarrhea or loose stool is often uncritically considered a sign of IBD/IBS. We need to be more critical in our thought process. *If the dog always has diarrhea or soft/loose stool when the client returns home but not on weekends when the client is home, the dog may have subclinical separation anxiety or separation anxiety that is undiagnosed.*
- Clients who have rescue dogs or have adopted dogs from shelters may be "pre-adapted" to watch for signs of separation anxiety. By ensuring that they know the history of dogs in their care, veterinarians can provide *anticipatory guidance.*
- Affiliations between veterinarians and shelter/rescue groups can help decrease the severity of separation anxiety experienced by the affected dogs.
- *All dogs should be screened for all behavioral conditions at all appointments.* The short history form found on the accompanying website can help all veterinarians do this. Dogs with separation anxiety worsen the longer they are untreated.

Quantifying Changes in Behavior for Dogs Treated for Noise Reactivity and/or Separation Anxiety—AIR and SAIR Scores

As we did with the *aggression screen*, where we created intensity, severity, and reactivity scores, we can use the results of the noise and separation anxiety screens to create an "anxiety score."

For the purposes of the *separation anxiety and noise phobia/reactivity screen (SANP)* section of the questionnaire, we can calculate separate separation anxiety and noise reactivity scores. For noise reactivity, we have created an anxiety intensity rank (AIR) score that allows us to compare reactive dogs and to compare individual dogs before and after treatment.

The AIR score is calculated as follows.

Step 1: Note the situations in which a distressed response of any kind is seen, and assign a score based on frequency of response.

1. Storms/thunderstorms
2. Gunshots
3. Fireworks
4. Other noises

For each of these situations, assign a score that correlates with the frequency with which the dog reacts when exposed in a way that matches the terminology used in the SANP section of the questionnaire (Table A).

Continued

Quantifying Changes in Behavior for Dogs Treated for Noise Reactivity and/or Separation Anxiety—
AIR and SAIR Scores—cont'd

TABLE A

Frequency Category of Dog's Reaction to Any Noise Once He Encounters It and Score Assigned to That Category of Frequency

Frequency of Occurrence of Any Signs of Noise Reactivity/Phobia Based on Percentage of Time That Dog Reacts Once Exposed	Score Assigned to Frequency
0%—reactions never occurs	0
>0% but <40%—reaction occurs more often than not	1
>40% but <60%—dog reacts or doesn't react about equally	1.5
>60% but <100%—reaction occurs less often than not	2.5
100% of the time—reaction always occurs	4.0

Step 2: Count the number of behavioral responses the dog exhibits when exposed to the situations. For noise reactions, there are 11 possible behaviors exhibited, not all of which are equally easy for clients to see, but when comparing dogs before and after treatment we can assume that clients will be see the same behaviors for comparison. The 11 listed behaviors are salivate, hide, defecate, tremble, urinate, destroy, escape, freeze, pant, will not eat food/treats, pace, pupil dilation, and vocalize (bark, whine, growl, howl). Clients can include a category of "other," if they wish.

Step 3: Multiply the number of signs by the frequency score for each trigger of the reactions, then sum these to provide the AIR score.

To see the utility in this approach, we can compare two dogs, both border collies. Table B shows the score calculations for border collie 1, and Table C shows the score calculations for border collie 2.

TABLE B

AIR Score Calculation for a Very Noise Reactive Dog

Noise Category	Frequency Weight	No. Signs	Score
Thunder	4	5	20
Fireworks	4	5	20
Gunshots	4	4	16
Other (weed whacker)	4	1	4
			Total score = 60

TABLE C

AIR Score Calculation for a Dog Who Is Not Noise Reactive

Noise Category	Frequency Weight	No. Signs	Score
Thunder	0	0	0
Fireworks	0	0	0
Gunshots	0	0	0
Other (people yelling—runs and hides; sirens—howls)*	1	3	3
			Total score = 3

*Both of these could be normal behaviors and may be because this dog's AIR score is so low.

Clients who have noise reactive/phobic dogs can re-calculate the AIR score at set times during treatment to obtain more objective measurement of behavioral change and determine which situations may need more help.

SAIR scores

A similar approach can be taken for dogs who are left when distressed. In the SANP section of the questionnaire, we ask about the following behaviors when left for real and in a "virtual" absence:

- Destructive behavior when separated from the client(s)
- Urination when separated from client(s)
- Defecation when separated from client(s)
- Vocalization when separated from client(s)
- Salivation when separated from client(s)
- Panting when separated from client(s)

Quantifying Changes in Behavior for Dogs Treated for Noise Reactivity and/or Separation Anxiety—AIR and SAIR Scores—cont'd

We use the same frequency categories that we did for noise reactivity and phobia. A separation anxiety intensity rank (SAIR) score can be calculated as shown in the following example (Table D).

This type of calculation will help provide both the clinician and the client with more objective assessment of improvements or relapses that the dog is experiencing during treatment.

TABLE D

SAIR Rank Calculations for a Dog Who Destroys Every Time He Is Really Left

Using the same frequency x score assignment as for AIR scores, we can compare dogs with separation anxiety with each other or across time to assess improvement with treatment or exposure.

- Vocalizes 40%-60% of the time he is really left and salivates <40% of the time he is really left (3 signs, total: 1 sign at a score of 4, 1 sign at a score of 1.5, and 1 sign at a score of 1)
- When his virtual absences are assessed, he destroys and vocalizes <40% of the time when he does not have access to his people for 2 scores of 1

SA Category	Frequency Weight	Score
Real Absence Signs		
Destruction	4	4
Urination		
Defecation		
Vocalization	1.5	1.5
Salivation	1	1.0
Panting		
		Subtotal score = 6.5
Virtual Absence Signs		
Destruction	1	1
Urination		
Defecation		
Vocalization	1	1
Salivation		
Panting		
		Subtotal score = 2
		Total score = 8.5

Phobia

Diagnostic Criteria and Description

- Profound, non-graded, extreme response to some consistent stimulus or set of stimuli manifest as intense, active avoidance, escape, or anxiety behaviors associated with the activities of the sympathetic branch of the autonomic nervous system.
- Behaviors can include catatonia or mania/panic concomitant with decreased sensitivity to pain or social stimuli.
- Phobias usually appear to develop quickly, with little change in their presentation between bouts. Fears may develop more gradually, and within a bout of fearful behavior, there may be more variation in response than would be seen in a phobic event.
- Once a phobic event has been experienced, any event associated with it or the memory of it may be sufficient to generate the response.
- Once fully developed, repeated exposure results in an invariant pattern of response.
- Phobic situations either are avoided at all costs or, if unavoidable, are endured with intense anxiety or distress.
- The criteria must apply only in the presumptive trigger/stimulus for the reaction or during a period signaling that exposure to the trigger/stimulus is possible or imminent.

Common Non-Specific Signs

- Specific behavioral signs may include:
  - urination,
  - defecation,

- salivation,
- destruction,
- panting,
- pacing,
- freezing/immobility,
- trembling/shaking,
- vocalization (bark, whine, growl, howl),
- escape behaviors,
- vomiting, and
- diarrhea.
- Some dogs may show suites of correlated behaviors. For example, salivation appears to occur more commonly in dogs who freeze and become immobile. Clients will wish to note which suites of behaviors their dogs exhibit so that they can monitor these non-specific signs for changes (hopefully, improvement) during treatment.

Rule Outs
- Medical rule outs will depend largely on the system involved. Many of these dogs will have prior diagnoses of IBD/IBS.
- Clients often have concerns about the dog's auditory and visual acuity because the behavior is confusing until the pattern is clear.
- If the behavior is very episodic, clients become concerned about brain tumors.
- Behavioral rule outs include fear/fearful behavior, GAD, PD, and storm/noise phobia, all of which could be co-morbid.

Etiology, Epidemiology, and Risk Groups
- Dogs with fears and/or related anxieties may be at increased risk for non–noise-related phobias, but there are no published data.
- Phobias are thought to develop when escape from the stimulus is impossible.
  - If the dog is unable to move because of crippling fear, he has no conscious cognitive ability to escape and so may become phobic. Dogs can become phobic of anything.
- The hallmark of a phobia is its sudden, profound development.
  - It is unclear whether the "suddenness" of development is a function of client attentiveness, but sudden, profound development is also reported for humans with phobias.
  - We know little about the development of phobias because early signs may be missed, but once fully developed, which appears to happen quickly and with relatively little exposure, each phobic episode is more like the others than they are different.
- Dogs experiencing entrapment in any injurious or potentially injurious situation may become phobic (e.g., dogs caught in fires may make an association with an apartment or a crate, dogs in car accidents may become phobic of cars or the restraint system in use when the accident occurred, dogs attacked and

profoundly frightened by one specific dog may become phobic of the breed, dogs used in illegal dog fighting may become phobic of all dogs or certain people, et cetera).
- Given that so many dogs exposed to terrible stimuli do not become phobic, it's likely that there is some genetic liability associated with the development of phobias. If noise/storm phobias are specific cases of phobias, in general, we know that these run in family lines.

Common Myths That Can Get in the Way of Treatment or Diagnosis
- The dog will grow out of it. Leave him alone.
  - Once fully developed, dogs do not worsen, but they tend to react to more stimuli and take progressively longer to recover from each phobic bout.
    - Do not ignore this.
    - Treat as early as possible.
    - Protect the dog when in the midst of a phobic event by getting him out of the context as soon as possible.
- A firm hand is needed. "Babying" the dog will just make him worse.
  - This is true for neither humans nor dogs but is still a prevalent view in many communities. At some point, the line to abuse will be crossed.

Commonly Asked Client Questions
- Is this preventable?
  - To the extent that the humane puppy raising and exposure conditions discussed here are used and early intervention is practiced, we may be able to prevent some dogs from becoming phobic, but there are two impediments to doing so: (1) We do not recognize early signs of phobia and so are usually dealing with a fully developed condition. (2) It is likely that not all phobias are the same behaviorally or neurochemically. Although we frequently lump noise phobia and storm phobia for ease of discussion and treatment, their clinical co-morbidity presentations suggest that they are different conditions. This pattern likely holds for other phobias, especially if they affect or are affected by different sensory modalities (e.g., sight, sound, smell, touch, vibration, et cetera).
- Is this heritable?
  - There are probably liability genes that increase risk for the development of phobias. We know nothing about this.
  - A major concern is the issue of shared environmental exposure, which could make phobias appear to be heritable when they are not. This is a particular concern for litters of puppies.

Treatment
- Management:
  - Avoiding any known triggers is essential.

- If the trigger cannot be avoided, removing the dog—physically, if need be—from the situation as soon as possible is important.
- Depending on how the dog responds to the phobia, enclosure in a crate may not be possible. See the discussion of the use of crates for dogs with separation anxiety.
- Behavior modification:
  - It is extremely difficult to desensitize and counter-condition dogs who are phobic because they respond so quickly and profoundly that, by definition, these methodologies may be impossible even to implement. To do so, some treatment with medication must usually succeed first, and the clients need to find creative ways to mimic the stimulus known to provoke the behavior.
  - Lowering the dog's overall reactivity level may help, so using the strategies in the "Protocol for Deference" and the "Protocol for Teaching Your Dog to Take a Deep Breath and Use Other Biofeedback Methods as Part of Relaxation" may help.
- Medication/dietary intervention:
  - Unless part of an overall program to reduce reactivity and protect neurons against the effects of the phobic experience, nutraceuticals and diet alone are unlikely to help phobic dogs.
  - This is a condition where medication is not negotiable—it is essential for the dog's welfare, well-being, and QoL.
  - Medications most likely to be effective are those that address panic:
    - BZDs, such as alprazolam or clonazepam, should a long-lasting medication be needed. BZDs can be used as for the protocols for noise/storm phobias and panic.
    - SSRIs, such as fluoxetine, sertraline, and paroxetine, which have been useful in similar situations in humans.
    - Gabapentin, alone or in combination with TCAs and/or SSRIs, if reactivity is the primary concern.
    - Central alpha agonists, such as clonidine, depending on the level of the arousal response. For dogs who panic or become quickly phobic, this medication is an option should the dog be unresponsive to or have side effects with BZDs.
- Miscellaneous interventions:
  - Clients frequently ask about pheromonal analogs and wraps.
  - The data on effects of pheromonal analogues, when any effect is shown, suggest that the effect is sufficiently mild and non-specific that these would not be useful in phobic dogs.
  - Wraps (Anxiety Wrap, Thunder Shirt) are gaining popularity.

- Wraps truly have no side effects if someone is present when they are worn. Panicky dogs could move around in these and cut off the circulation to some part of their body.
- Wraps may help by placing constant pressure on the body, which may help muscles to relax.
- Some wraps could contribute to overheating.
- In any study done to date, it's impossible to separate the effect of the wrap itself from the attention to the dog and her needs.
- Leaning or pressing on the dog using constant pressure or long, slow, deep strokes may cause the muscle bellies to relax and could help these dogs in the recovery from a phobic event.

Helpful Handouts
- "Protocol for Deference"
- "Protocol for Teaching Cats and Dogs to 'Sit,' 'Stay,' and 'Come'"
- "Protocol for Teaching Your Dog to Take a Deep Breath and Use Other Biofeedback Methods as Part of Relaxation"
- "Protocol for Relaxation: Behavior Modification Tier 1"
- "Protocol for Generalized Discharge Instructions for Dogs with Behavioral Concerns"
- "Protocol for Understanding and Treating Dogs with Fear/Fearful Aggression"
- "Protocol for Treating Fearful Behavior in Cats and Dogs"
- "Protocol for Using Behavioral Medication Successfully"
- "Generalized Guidelines for Using Alprazolam for Noise and Storm Phobias, Panic, and Severe Distress"
- "Protocol for Handling 'Special-Needs Pets' during Holidays and Other Special Occasions"

Last Words
- Regardless of whether clients can identify the triggering stimulus, these dogs need immediate help.

Neophobia
Diagnostic Criteria and Description
- Consistent, sustained, and extreme non-graded response to *completely novel, unfamiliar objects and circumstances* manifest as intense, active avoidance, escape, or anxiety behaviors.
- These behaviors are associated with arousal of the sympathetic branch of the autonomic nervous system.
- Behaviors noted include catatonia or mania concomitant with decreased sensitivity to pain or social stimuli.
- Repeated exposure results in an invariant pattern of response.
- For true "neophobia" to be diagnosed, it is implicit that the fear is due to a complete lack of exposure,

during the sensitive period and possibly beyond, to the stimuli eliciting the response.

- It is unusual, but not impossible, that young dogs and cats experience such an artificial and depauperate environment because most animals will explore most circumstances *given the chance*.
- The risk of true "neophobia" is high for puppy/kitten mill/farm raised animals and becomes more pronounced for dogs/cats sold after 3 months of age and those kept as breeders. *These commercial breeding conditions pose true welfare risks, and clients should be actively informed of them.*

- The stage at which a fear becomes a phobia is unknown but is epistemologically important. Patterns related to the development of fears and phobias involve evaluation of frequency, intensity, and qualification of actual behaviors.
- Risks associated with the development of related behaviors are generally unknown for animals already exhibiting some fear or anxiety and so may not be considered in the development of these extreme, early fears.
- A phobic response is difficult to miss but because of that is doubtless more complex than is commonly appreciated.

Common Non-Specific Signs

- As for other conditions involving phobia or panic, specific behavioral signs could include:
  - urination,
  - defecation,
  - salivation,
  - destruction,
  - panting,
  - pacing,
  - freezing/immobility,
  - trembling/shaking,
  - vocalization (bark, whine, growl, howl),
  - escape behaviors,
  - vomiting,
  - diarrhea, and
  - mydriasis.
- The most common client descriptions involve dogs who spent an extended amount of time at their breeders (at least through 3 months of age) in varying degrees of restricted circumstances.
  - Some very small dogs may never have been outdoors if the breeder lived in an apartment building.
  - Some dogs have never been out of the yard in which their runs were contained.
  - Some dogs have never experienced urban noise and bustle.
  - Some dogs may have only been carried when outdoors.
  - All of these dogs can experience neophobia even though they did not live in completely or extremely deprived environments. *The role of*

context in the development of the specific avoidance response is key.

Rule Outs

- Other fears and phobias not dependent on an absolute absence of exposure during a sensitive ontogenic stage are the main rule outs.
  - A diagnosis of neophobia requires absence of exposure to the triggering stimulus at least during the sensitive period.

Etiology, Epidemiology, and Risk Groups

- Scott and Fuller (1965) noted in their early experiments that if dogs did not have experience leaving their run before 14 weeks of age, they never chose to leave it, even if the door was open.
  - Forced departures caused extreme distress.
  - This pattern is supported by the responses of dogs in commercial breeding facilities.
- There is likely to be a strong genetic component for this condition, and the genetic risk is likely to interact with environmental exposure in some way. This assumption is derived from the observation that many animals experience extreme environments and can—or appear to—recover, albeit possibly incompletely. *Quite small amounts of early exposure may be sufficient to avoid this condition in many, but not all, dogs.*

Common Myths That Can Get in the Way of Treatment or Diagnosis

- These dogs will recover from their fear given time and exposure. This is a normal response to being adopted into a new home.
  - Neophobic dogs do not show any decrement in their response given time and exposure.
  - This is not a normal response to being adopted. Some hesitation and increased attention to new environments and the behaviors of dogs in them may be a normal response to being adopted.
- All dogs go through fear periods—usually at 9 to 10 weeks of age and 9 to 10 months of age. It's normal for puppies to have prolonged fear periods.
  - As previously discussed in Chapter 4, by 9 to 10 weeks, dogs are sufficiently cognitively sophisticated to appreciate that exploration of the world is not without risk. It is normal that they change their behaviors to become more cautious or less certain if, in the course of their explorations, something startled or scared them. This is not the same as a neophobic response and is completely unrelated to it functionally.
  - Dogs can enter social maturity at 9 to 10 months of age. It is postulated that at this time their brains undergo substantial neuronal remodeling leading to some dogs becoming more concerned and others becoming more boisterous. This is not the same as a neophobic response and is completely unrelated to it functionally.

Commonly Asked Client Questions

- Can these dogs get better, or must they be protected for the rest of their lives?
  - Some dogs can improve, and some dogs will need to be protected. Improvement may never be complete, but if there is a genetic component to how the dog reacts to the deprivation, we should expect that there is the rare dog who can completely overcome it. The more realistic the clients are, the earlier they intervene, and the more they are able to manage the dog's exposure to provocative stimuli, the more likely that the dog will improve to the extent possible for him.
- Could I have known that there was a risk that this dog would be affected by neophobia?
  - This question embodies the reason that clients should obtain puppies from reputable rescues or shelters who have made an effort to learn as much as possible about the dog's behaviors or from reputable breeders who insist that the clients see the dogs in person both on- and off-site with their human and canine family members. If the client is able only to view a video of the dog, they should require a Skype video in real time where they have an improved chance of seeing the dog's responses under real-world conditions.
  - As long as we have no agreed-on, enforceable, reliable standard of care and best practices for breeders of dogs, dogs and puppies will be subject to sub-optimal developmental conditions that contribute to and play a role in behavioral pathologies.

Treatment

- Management:
  - As with all phobic conditions, identification and avoidance of the provocative stimulus is essential. This prevents the dog from suffering and avoids learning to become more reactive and fearful that is associated with repeated exposure.
  - Avoidance of the stimulus that provokes the neophobic response may also interfere with any generalization of fearful responses that could occur (e.g., a form of stimulus response generalization).
  - Absolute avoidance may be impossible so anything that can be done to attenuate cues (e.g., eyeshades, ear plugs, walking the dog at traditionally less noisy/hectic times, knowing the garbage and delivery truck schedules and working with these to provoke the dog less) until the dog is actively engaged in and improving on a treatment program involving medication and behavior modification should be encouraged.
- Behavior modification:
  - Teaching the dog to sit, calm, and relax in non-provocative situations must be the first step. These dogs need to *learn that they do not have to react* to everything and can have control over

a number of activities, circumstances, and exposures where they can excel at and be rewarded for not reacting, staying calm, and breathing deeply.

- Medication/dietary intervention:
  - *The best hope for as complete recovery as possible may lie with early use of medication.* We now know that most medications recommended for such conditions encourage the processes of cellular and molecular learning (long-term potentiation) and the protein translation needed for these to occur. The earlier in the ontogeny of any pathological behavior that this occurs, the better for the patient.
  - Medications commonly recommended are those used in fears and phobias and may include:
    - Daily use medications to decrease overall reactivity and anxiety, which will also facilitate the learning of new, calmer behaviors:
      - TCAs:
        - Amitriptyline
        - Clomipramine
        - Nortriptyline
      - SSRIs:
        - Fluoxetine
        - Fluvoxamine
        - Paroxetine
        - Sertraline
      - SARIs (possibly, but untested):
        - Trazodone (preferentially with another medication)
      - Other:
        - Gabapentin
    - Medications to address or prevent acute outbursts of extreme fear, usually manifest as mania or acute behavioral paralysis:
      - BZDs
        - Alprazolam
        - Clonazepam
      - Central alpha-2 agonists
        - Clonidine
- Miscellaneous interventions:
  - If these dogs learn to have a good, reliable, and instructive relationship with other dogs, they may learn to take their cues about the appropriateness of their behaviors from the other dogs.
  - Anxiety Wraps may help some of these dogs as part of an integrated treatment plan. If they don't help, they also are unlikely to do harm in this situation. No data exist.

Helpful Handouts

- "Protocol for Generalized Discharge Instructions for Dogs with Behavioral Concerns"
- "Protocol for Deference"
- "Protocol for Teaching Your Dog to Take a Deep Breath and Use Other Biofeedback Methods as Part of Relaxation"
- "Protocol for Relaxation: Behavior Modification Tier 1"

- "Protocol for Understanding and Treating Dogs with Fear/Fearful Aggression"
- "Protocol for Treating Fearful Behavior in Cats and Dogs"
- "Protocol for Using Behavioral Medication Successfully"
- "Generalized Guidelines for Using Alprazolam for Noise and Storm Phobias, Panic, and Severe Distress"
- "Informed Consent Statements for the Most Commonly Used Medications"

Last Words
- Although it will not help the patient directly, encourage the client to learn as much as possible about the other dogs in this line and whether they suffer from this condition. Encourage the client to ask the breeder specific questions, and offer to talk with the breeder yourself. *There is no uniform "best practices" standard for breeders.* A discussion may help in distinguishing whether the problem is due to a lack of knowledge/education or to neglect and negligence (the latter being more common with puppy mills/farms). If you can identify which is involved, you may improve life for future generations, and your client may be able to use social media to help spread the message.

Noise and Storm Phobias
Diagnostic Criteria and Description for Noise Phobia
- Profound, non-graded, extreme response to noise manifest as intense avoidance, escape, or anxiety and associated with the sympathetic branch of the autonomic nervous system.

Diagnostic Criteria and Description for Storm Phobia
- Profound, non-graded, extreme response to some aspect of the storm (accompanying noise, wind, lightning, thunder, ozone levels, changes in barometric pressure, alterations in illumination, et cetera) manifest as intense avoidance, escape, or anxiety and associated with the sympathetic branch of the autonomic nervous system.

Diagnostic Criteria and Description for Noise/Storm Phobias
- Behaviors can include mania or catatonia concomitant with decreased sensitivity to pain or social stimuli.
- Once established, repeated exposure results in an invariant pattern of response.

Comment
- Noise/storm phobias may have overlapping pathologies, overlapping risk factors, and overlapping phenotypes, but they are not the same because many more stimuli are involved in storms than in most noises.
- Noises can be complex, and responses of dogs to various noises can be complex.

- The response of dogs to storms and gunshots appears to be similar (Hydbring-Sandberg et al., 2004).
- The response of dogs to fireworks is different than their response to storms and gunshots, possibly because of the extreme visual component to the stimulus.
- From the data collected on co-morbidity, which were previously discussed, we know that reactivity/phobia to general noises appears to be a different condition than reactivity/phobia to noises associated with storms.
- The extent to which these differences may matter for treatment is unclear, but they become important for phenotypic and genetic studies of reactivity/phobia in dogs.
- Dogs who are continuously and characteristically distressed when exposed to noises/storms but who do not meet the criteria for a "phobia" may best be classified as "reactive" and monitored, treating as warranted by signs.
- Predictability of the triggering stimulus, or lack thereof, may be responsible for the dog's reaction.

Common Non-Specific Signs
- Specific behavioral signs could include:
  - urination,
  - defecation,
  - salivation (Fig. 7-11),
  - destruction,
  - panting,
  - pacing,
  - freezing/immobility (see Fig. 7-11),
  - trembling/shaking,
  - vocalization (bark, whine, growl, howl),
  - escape behaviors,
  - vomiting,
  - diarrhea, and
  - mydriasis (Fig. 7-12).

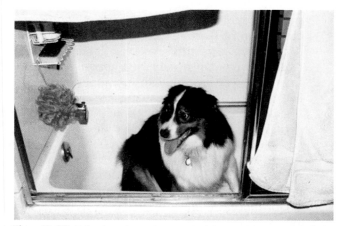

Fig. 7-11 This dog has storm phobia and becomes rigid, freezes, salivates, and tries to hide from the visual stimuli associated with storms, although his trigger is either noise or lightning.

- Clients are able to recognize mydriasis more easily in situations of noise phobia than they can for many other phobias or panicky situations and so it may be a useful sign to monitor.
- Some dogs may show suites of correlated behaviors. For example, salivation appears to occur more commonly in dogs who freeze and become immobile. Clients will wish to note which suites of behaviors their dogs exhibit so that they can monitor these non-specific signs for changes (hopefully, improvement) during treatment.

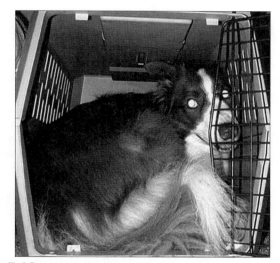

Fig. 7-12 A border collie hiding and panting during a storm. Note the extreme mydriasis. (Photo courtesy of Dr. Melanie Chang.)

Rule Outs

- Noise/storm phobias are fairly clear, but as they are developing clients often worry about the dog's ability to see or hear well and about whether physical pain is driving the behavior.
- Pain, poor hearing, and poor vision are easy to rule out.
- Extremely acute hearing is impossible to evaluate clinically, but the behavioral pattern should distinguish between a phobic response and a dog who has enhanced auditory skills.
- Early in the development of these conditions, clients recognize extreme fear but may not *correctly identify the stimulus, so the dog should be screened for all potential fears.*

Etiology, Epidemiology, and Risk Groups

- Noise/storm phobia/reactivity can affect any dog or breed, but it appears endemic in the herding breeds with some lines having half or more of the dogs affected, and no generation is skipped (Fig. 7-13).
- The distinction between "reactivity" and "phobia" is blurry. Well-controlled dogs can look "reactive." We do not know if all "reactive" dogs will go on to be "phobic," given time and exposure. Dogs who respond with concern to noise but lack the complete "phobic" criteria should be labeled as "reactive" and closely monitored.
- No data exist on very early development of the condition, but data show that it is fully pronounced by 4 years of age.
  - If dogs in affected lines were assessed and monitored from birth, it is likely that full development occurs much earlier than 4 years.

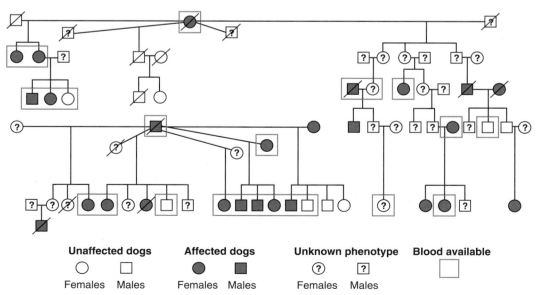

Border Collie pedigree for noise reactivity/phobia

Unaffected dogs		Affected dogs		Unknown phenotype		Blood available
○	□	●	■	⑦	?	□
Females	Males	Females	Males	Females	Males	

Fig. 7-13 Border collie pedigree for noise reactivity/phobia. (Pedigree courtesy of Dr. Melanie Chang.)

- If one relative of an affected dog is known to have noise/storm phobia/reactivity, chances are more relatives are affected.
- If a dog has noise/storm phobia/reactivity, the assumption should be made that his or her offspring have a high risk of being affected, and this should inform breeding decisions.
- Genome scans have revealed that no one gene, even within a breed, appears to be solely involved, and multiple gene involvement is likely and would make sense given the various presentations.
- All genes identified with increased risk affect neuronal information processing in some way, so it appears that auditory acuity is not the main cause of the reactivity.
- *Noise phobia/reactivity is a common co-morbid condition with other anxiety disorders, including GAD and separation anxiety.* The association with separation anxiety may be profound, as discussed earlier. Any dog that is diagnosed with noise phobia/reactivity should be screened for all other anxiety disorders.

Common Myths That Can Get in the Way of Treatment or Diagnosis

- This is normal behavior in herding dogs.
  - This is *not* normal behavior, and in many dogs noise/storm phobia/reactivity actually interferes with their ability to work.
- The dog will outgrow this.
  - Dogs *do not* outgrow this phobia/reactivity. Instead, they hone their suffering.
- You have to beat this out of the dog.
  - Beating any dog is abusive and will serve only to suppress their willingness to show that they are phobic.
- All border collies have this tendency because it's necessary for good herding ability. A firm hand and a willingness to discipline the dogs stops them from displaying the behavior.
  - Noise/storm phobia/reactivity is a pathology. Not all border collies are affected, but this type of attitude will ensure that those who are affected are bred and that the dogs who suffer silently are over-represented. This myth represents an abusive attitude that does not consider the welfare or well-being of the dog.
- Myths that pertain to other phobias are also applicable here.

Commonly Asked Client Questions

- Should I have been able to tell whether the puppy would have been affected?
  - It is likely that affected dogs were not completely normal as puppies, especially if the pathology is about processing information. Currently, we have identified no specific behavioral, metabolic, or genetic markers that would permit early identification. Identifying such markers, if they exist, should be a goal.

- Can I lessen how pronounced the condition can be by exposing the dog to noises or noise-desensitization CDs?
  - Working dogs who are raised and trained in the vicinity of military jets can still develop noise/storm phobia/reactivity. We do not have the data to assess whether any protective effect exists.
  - Noise-desensitization CDs may help dogs who are displaying early signs of the condition, but for impaired dogs they are of limited help. There are no data about whether they can confer a protective effect, but if they do, it may be one affecting threshold of response, not outcome.
- Should I breed this dog?
  - *The general advice given about any dogs with any behavioral problems is not to breed them because there is always a risk—and in some cases such as this one, a known pattern supporting the risk—that the condition is heritable.* Not breeding the dog will prevent another dog from suffering and potentially from being abused, abandoned, relinquished, or euthanized because of that problem. Noise/storm phobia/reactivity is one of the few conditions that can be truly sporadic, is exquisitely sensitive to the environment, some of which can be managed, and can be pharmacologically controlled/alleviated. In some parts of the world, storms are exceedingly rare. If the clients accept that the puppies will be affected *and* if the clients already have excellent homes for any dog who will be born with families who *know* that the dogs will be affected *and* will always adhere to state-of-the-art treatment, the puppies *could* have an excellent QoL.
    - Under no circumstances should anyone think that were this dog to be bred that they were not breeding for pathology—those who choose to breed these dogs *are* breeding for pathology, but if the dog is otherwise wonderful, the sporadic nature of the expression of the condition plus the ability to alleviate the suffering by early and effective intervention *may* mitigate breeding concerns. These breeders may also be excellent collaborators for scientists seeking markers and greater understanding of this condition.
  - If the dog is not flawless—physically and behaviorally—in all other ways, don't breed the dog.

Treatment

- Management:
  - Avoidance of the noises that trigger the responses are key. This can be done though the use of noise cancelling headphones (Fig. 7-14), acoustic tiles, competing noise (TV/radio), white noise, ear plugs, et cetera.
  - If the dog reacts to other correlates of storms (e.g., lightning), he must also be protected from those stimuli through eye shades or goggles (Figs. 7-15 and 7-16).

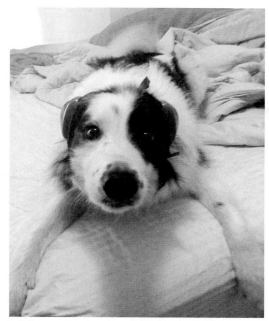

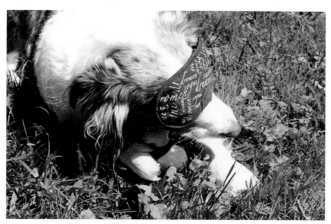

Fig. 7-16 The same dog shown in Figure 7-15 was conditioned to wear an eye shade in any conditions and to enjoy a chew toy while wearing the shade. This conditioning makes it easier to control the stimuli to which the dog is exposed.

Fig. 7-14 A border collie with noise phobia wearing Mutt Muffs, ear muffs designed for dogs who must ride in and be lowered from helicopters. (Photo courtesy of Angelica Steinker.)

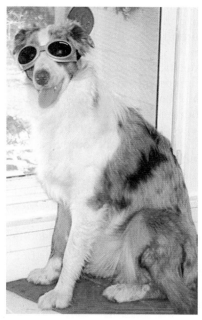

Fig. 7-15 Young Australian shepherd wearing Doggles to blunt visual stimuli.

- Behavior modification:
  - Clients should not tell these dogs that it is "okay." The clients are seeking to reassure the dog, but the dog knows it is not "okay," and the contradictory signal will not help.
  - Behavior modification should focus on teaching the dog to relax and not to react under normal circumstances and then not to react increasingly noisy circumstances.
    - In fully phobic dogs, the second half of this instruction may not be possible until medication has broken the cycle of their reactivity and they are not panicked.
  - Behavior modification can also be helpful for conditioning dogs not only to accept but also to associate any helpful devices or interventions with fun events.
  - These dogs must not be punished.
  - These dogs must not be forced to engage in any jobs or specific behaviors that contribute to scaring them if they are reacting or are known to react in such circumstances (e.g., no herding of sheep in thunderstorms).
  - Desensitization and counter-conditioning using CDs developed for this purpose is unlikely to be successful alone except in very mildly affected dogs or dogs who recently started to show signs.
    - Desensitization and counter-conditioning using specialty CDs may help some dogs, in combination with a program of other, daily behavior modification and relaxation and medication.
- Medication/dietary intervention:
  - Because noise/storm phobia/reactivity may predispose dogs to other anxiety-related conditions or increase the risk of developing a co-morbid condition (these are not the same), protection against cellular/neuronal stress using anti-oxidants and omega-3 fatty acids may have some benefit.
  - Once behavioral signs associated with a phobic response are present, humane intervention mandates medical treatment.
    - BZDs are most commonly used to abort panicky and phobic behaviors if given to the dog during

or after exposure to the stimulus, and they may prevent these behaviors from appearing if given before the dog is exposed to the stimulus.

- The most common BZDs used are alprazolam, clonazepam, and diazepam, in order of high effectiveness/low side effects to lesser effectiveness/more side effects.
- BZDs affect the reticular activating system and render the dog's ability to inhibit reaction greater.
- Alprazolam is considered a panicolytic BZD and similar to all BZDs enters the circulation within minutes of ingestion. Alprazolam can be used to abort an incipient or ongoing panic attack if the dog is susceptible to it.
- Some dogs appear not to respond at all to BZDs. This type of lack of response appears to be genetic in humans and is likely genetic in dogs. The reverse is also likely true, and dogs who have extreme and undesirable responses may also have different genetic variants of cytochrome P-450 (CYP) enzymes.

- If the dog does not respond to BZDs or only partially responds, central alpha-2 agonists such as clonidine may help. Clonidine acts to decrease the peripheral sympathetic response and may aid in learning new ways not to react. If the dog is also taking a TCA or serotonin norepinephrine reuptake inhibitor, the clinician should remember that both medications increase central NE/NA and its efficiency in stimulating second messenger systems. The predominant NE/NA nucleus is the *locus ceruleus*, which is in the amygdala, emphasizing the role for substances that affect NE/NA in fear.
- Noise/storm phobia/reactivity is a common co-morbid condition, and so any other anxiety-related condition should be treated with TCAs, SSRIs, or derivative classes of medications.
- Daily treatment with TCAs, SSRIs, and related classes of medications may help raise reactivity thresholds and alter the dog's response surface for dogs who are frequently exposed to provocative noises (e.g., dogs living in the southeastern United States in the summer) (Crowell-Davis et al., 2003).
- There is no evidence that homeopathic treatments provide any help.
- Miscellaneous interventions:
  - Work may help some mildly affected dogs learn that they have some control over whether to react, and it may help some dogs who are recovering also to learn to focus on and control their responses by managing things that they enjoy, but it is not a panacea for the average affected dog.

- Massage, slow, long, firm strokes, and leaning against the dog may help some dogs to relax their muscles.
  - Under no circumstances should these dogs be petted in the traditional sense. Petting is associated with arousal and rewards and is very different from being firmly held and protected.
- Storm capes have been recommended for dogs who react to storms.
  - These are based on the principle of the Faraday cage that interrupts static electrical charges.
  - For a Faraday cage to be effective, the dog must be completely surrounded by it, but the capes do not cover the dog's feet.
  - A placebo-controlled, pseudo-blinded study using client ratings showed no difference between a placebo cape and the "real" one, but both groups improved, suggesting attention may have some remedial benefit (Cottam and Dodman, 2009).
- Wraps (Anxiety Wrap, the Thunder Shirt) are gaining popularity.
  - Wraps truly have no side effects if someone is present when they are worn. Panicky dogs could move around in a wrap and cut off the circulation to some parts of their body.
  - Wraps may help by placing constant pressure on the body, which may help muscles to relax.
  - Some wraps could contribute to overheating.
  - It's impossible to separate the effect of the wrap itself from the attention to the dog (attending to her needs, et cetera) in any study done to date, especially when outcomes are evaluated by client ratings and opinions.

Helpful Handouts
- "Protocol for Deference"
- "Protocol for Teaching Your Dog to Take a Deep Breath and Use Other Biofeedback Methods as Part of Relaxation"
- "Protocol for Relaxation: Behavior Modification Tier 1"
- "Protocol for Understanding and Treating Canine Panic Disorder (PD)"
- "Protocol for Understanding and Treating Dogs with Noise and Storm Phobias"
- "Protocol for Using Behavioral Medication Successfully"
- "Generalized Guidelines for Using Alprazolam for Noise and Storm Phobias, Panic, and Severe Distress"
- "Informed Consent Statements for the Most Commonly Used Medications"

Last Words
- *Clients will assume that noises to which their dog reacts are restricted to loud sounds, such as guns, truck backfires, fireworks, and storms. This misconception may prohibit implementation of a needed intervention program. In fact, dogs with noise reactivity/phobia who do not*

seem to improve or who seem to experience recidivistic events frequently may react to noises that no one has considered as problematic. Turning the pages of a newspaper, clicking the snap latch on a lead, using a turn signal in the car, et cetera, all may adversely affect some noise reactive dogs. These observations suggest that the quality of the noise matters, that noise phobia/reactivity is variable, and that it may affect how information is obtained and processed.

- Noise/storm phobia/reactivity is the quintessential QoL condition. It can be managed, but early intervention is best. Time penetrance is likely a huge factor in the presentation of the neurochemical pathology underlying this condition.
- Any dog who reacts at all to noise should be screened regularly for other anxiety-related conditions.

Canine Post-Traumatic Stress Disorder (C-PTSD)

Diagnostic Criteria and Description

- Profound, non-graded, extreme response manifest as intense avoidance, escape, or anxiety and associated with the sympathetic branch of the autonomic nervous system in response to exposure to an identifiable, untenable (from the patient's perspective) stimulus or situation that the individual was unable to avoid or from which escape was impossible when these behavioral and physical signs were first felt.
- *Confirming behaviors can include mania or catatonia concomitant with decreased sensitivity/responsiveness to pain or social stimuli.*
- Once established, repeated exposure to any aspect of the original circumstance—including an endogenously or exogenously induced memory of the event—that triggers the original response or that triggers a memory of the original response results in an invariant pattern characteristic of that patient.
- The exhibition of this condition is dependent on a socially or environmentally contextual trigger. The cognitive component may mean that the trigger may not be obvious, but with good observations, it can be inferred when not obvious.

Common Non-Specific Signs

- Non-specific signs may include:
  - freezing, with or without trembling,
  - pacing and an inability to settle,
  - shaking/trembling,
  - licking at lips,
  - salivating,
  - heightened and constant vigilance,
  - inability to meet anyone's gaze,
  - inability to eat or engage in any other behaviors during an active event of C-PTSD,
  - unwillingness or inability to engage in behaviors in which the dog had previously, perhaps even joyously, engaged; for working dogs, this means that they cannot or will not work, although some

of them may go through the motions to get back to their kennel quickly,
  - hiding,
  - weight loss,
  - chronic or intermittent diarrhea,
  - adverse changes in skin and coat quality and texture,
  - social withdrawal,
  - loss of all joy and ability to enjoy anything, and
  - secondary stress and distress behaviors including destruction, self-mutilation, et cetera.

Rule Outs

- If these behaviors occur only during sleep, rule outs include nightmares and rapid eye movement (REM) sleep disorder. Dogs affected with C-PTSD may have bad nightmares and could have nocturnal episodes of panic, but the condition is recognized because of lack of function during activities that occur when awake.
  - Nightmares are easily disrupted, and dogs appear fine when they are awake.
  - REM sleep disorders are complex, and it may be difficult to tell when the dog is truly awake versus asleep. Dogs can behave very strangely during a REM sleep disorder event.
- As is true for humans, dogs who experience real physical trauma as part of the event leading to C-PTSD could have a traumatic brain injury (TBI), in which physical, generally compressive or concussive, damage to regions occurs, or neck injuries, including injuries that may affect the spine and/or have affected brain oxygenation.
- Endocrinopathies, including Cushing's disease and hypothyroidism, can result in many of the same signs, but the pattern is usually different.
- Any infectious or toxic agent that can affect the nervous system could potentially cause many of these non-specific signs, but the pattern is different. Although C-PTSD could be of sudden or gradual onset, it's not insidious in the manner that infectious/toxic conditions are, and the dog's behaviors are not dependent on the social or environmental context.

Etiology, Epidemiology, and Risk Groups

- We do not know enough about this condition to determine risk groups, but dogs who have been postulated to have the condition have fallen into the following groups:
  - dogs who have been extremely roughly treated/abused as part of training,
  - dogs who have been consistently threatened and/or injured as a function of their social conditions (e.g., dogs who live with a dog who is always trying to injure them, "bait" dogs for dog fights),
  - dogs who have experienced severe trauma/injury in a situation out of their control and for which they could have no context (e.g., being caught in a hurricane or earthquake), and
  - working dogs who experience profoundly traumatic and threatening conditions for which it was

impossible to train; the condition may be more likely in working dogs who—under these conditions—fail in their mission (e.g., the explosives detection dog errs and someone is killed).

- As with panic and noise and other phobias, it is likely that there is a genetic liability to this condition. Some dogs appear to be extremely resilient and recoverable, whereas others may appear to be fine until exposed to some series and level of stressors. If this is true, the ability to identify and use genetic markers for resilient/recoverable genotypes and more susceptible ones would be extremely useful.
  - As is true with noise phobia and impulse-control aggression, if this condition appears to run in family lines, or multiple first-degree (mother, father, brother, sister, daughter, son) relatives are affected, breeding this dog is not a good idea.
- It is unclear if reactivity to noise—or a familial reactivity to noise—increases the risk of C-PTSD, but this, along with problem-solving, coping, and training styles, has been considered as potentially playing a liability role.

Common Myths That Can Get in the Way of Treatment or Diagnosis

- The dog just has to work through this.
  - These dogs cannot "work" through anything and if forced to be in the situation will become more reactive.
    - Enhanced reactivity can be manifest as greater withdrawal or as offensive and defensive aggression.
- All dogs react in certain situations. You just have to force them to handle it, and then they will know that they can handle anything.
  - The idea that by surviving something that is profoundly distressing you will learn that you can survive such events is common, but it has been refuted by more recent data about learning. At some level of distress (and this likely varies by dog, to some extent), it is impossible to make the appropriate cytokines and neurotrophic agents that would permit the transcription of new protein that is the result of learning (see Chapter 10).
  - Repeated exposure risks more damage.

Commonly Asked Client Questions

- Will this dog ever be "normal" again?
  - We do not actually know if this dog was ever "normal," and this is part of the problem. We cannot verbally question dogs and so may confuse a number of dogs who are not expressing any behavioral concern but who are at risk for it with dogs who are not at risk for that concern (i.e., "normal").
- Can this dog be fixed?
  - Because we know little about the actual causal pathology, "fixing" the dog may mean different things to different people.

- We can alter neurochemistry and molecular responses with medication, and we may even change the shape and number of receptors and neurons.
- These changes may or may not fade if medication is discontinued.
- Behavioral recovery is possible, and dogs can look unaffected, but there may be some underlying dysfunction whose phenotype is being controlled or affected by behavioral, environmental, and pharmacological intervention. In this case, the risk is still present. See Figure 7-17 for a graphic example.

Treatment

- Management:
  - The primary management tool is removal from the situation that triggers the condition and protection from exposure to it in the future.
  - The earlier this is done, the more likely behavioral and pharmacological intervention are to help the dog recover.
  - If the dog recovers, he or she may be able to learn to return to the provocative environment, although everyone should be aware of the risk of relapse.
- Behavior modification:
  - If triggers associated with C-PTSD can be identified, structured programs of desensitization and counter-conditioning can be undertaken.
    - Before such programs can be implemented, dogs should be treated using techniques that

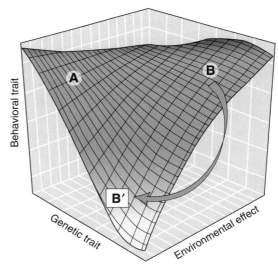

Fig. 7-17 In this drawing, A and B represent individuals who have the same behavioral phenotype but for whom the underlying factors driving the phenotype differ. In the case of A, environmental changes matter little. In the case of B, environmental changes are everything. While well regulated as a result of behavioral, environmental, and pharmacological interventions, B looks and behaves just like A. If B is put in an untenable environment, B becomes very different behaviorally (B'). Dogs who are well controlled with some combination of behavioral, environmental, and pharmacological interventions may look like B and revert to B' when such treatment is removed.

encourage relaxation and teach the dogs that they can have some positive control over some of their reactions. The following protocols will help.

- "Protocol for Deference"
- "Protocol for Teaching Your Dog to Take a Deep Breath and Use Other Biofeedback Methods as Part of Relaxation"
- "Protocol for Relaxation: Behavior Modification Tier 1"

- Exposure to desensitization and counter-conditioning programs before the dogs can effectively engage in and demonstrate the behaviors desired from these protocols may actually sensitize these dogs and make them worse.

- If it is not possible to identify triggers, the dogs may still benefit from learning the behavior modification programs and learning to relax, but desensitization and counter-conditioning will be difficult, if not impossible.

- Once dogs are taking a medication to which they are having a favorable response, they may be able to participate in behavior modification at the truly cognitive level by learning that they have control over some of their reactions and can engage in alternative behaviors that help them to calm.

- Medication/dietary intervention:
  - The BZD alprazolam is considered "panicolytic," and it is, if the patient is sensitive to it and experiences no side effects. We have no good population data indicating how common lack of an effect to this medication or true side effects are, but clients can test for each (see "Generalized Guidelines for Using Alprazolam for Noise and Storm Phobias, Panic, and Severe Distress"). Alprazolam can be given four to six times a day and has a huge efficacy range. It is usually best given with another medication that treats the underlying level of non-specific anxiety.
    - Alprazolam and other BZDs are controlled substances in the United States and so not suitable for some households.
  - Daily medication with a medication that affects serotonin (a specific TCA, SSRI, and less specific TCAs, serotonin norepinephrine reuptake inhibitor, et cetera) is needed. If the dog exhibits behaviors that are more ritualistic than impulsive/explosive, clomipramine may be a good choice. If the patient is explosive, the SSRI fluoxetine may help. If the patient is most concerned about social aspects of interactions, the SSRIs sertraline or paroxetine may be beneficial.
    - These medications vary in their affordability and availability by country. Such factors can and should inform treatment decisions.
  - Regardless of the medication chosen, ensure that the patient is treated long enough to know whether there is an effect (generally up to 8 weeks).

- Daily treatment with medications designed to raise reactivity threshold (gabapentin) or lower reactivity in general (clonidine) may help, and polypharmacy is common in these cases.
- In humans, intranasal oxytocin has helped in many of the social manifestations of this condition. If this proves useful for dogs, we will need to ensure that at-risk dogs learn to tolerate or even desire (through external and internal reward structures) intranasal medications.

- Miscellaneous interventions:
  - The roles for flexibility and cognitive stimulation are under-explored for such conditions.
    - If dogs have games that they can play and love, they may be able to use these as physical and behavioral outlets to recover from stressors. For this to work the dogs need to have some control over the choice of activity and the direction it takes.
    - There are now commercially available puzzle games for dogs and such games can be home-made and tailored to the dog's particular need; Figure 7-18 shows a puzzle box with a ball made for working detection dogs.
    - If it is possible to manage stimuli that the dog finds arousing using goggles, eye masks, ear plugs, et cetera, the dog may learn that these help and begin to relax when these appear.

Helpful Handouts

- "Protocol for Generalized Discharge Instructions for Dogs with Behavioral Concerns"
- "Protocol for Deference"
- "Protocol for Teaching Your Dog to Take a Deep Breath and Use Other Biofeedback Methods as Part of Relaxation"
- "Protocol for Understanding and Treating Canine Panic Disorder (PD)"

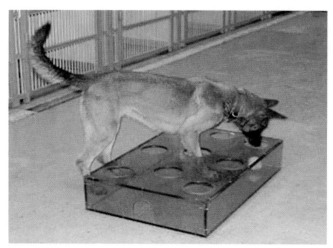

Fig. 7-18 A Belgian malinois who is a working detection dog using a puzzle box into which a tennis ball has been rolled. She can get the ball using her nose or paws through the one side hole or any of the top holes.

- "Protocol for Understanding and Treating Dogs with Noise and Storm Phobias"
- "Protocol for Understanding and Treating Generalized Anxiety Disorder (GAD)"
- "Protocol for Relaxation: Behavior Modification Tier 1"
- "Protocol for Using Behavioral Medication Successfully"

Last Words
- Screen for co-morbid conditions. Whether C-PTSD is primary or secondary, co-morbid conditions are likely to exist.
- Assess dogs who are at risk frequently using the survey in Fig. 7-19.

Cognitive Dysfunction (CD)/ Cognitive Dysfunction Syndrome (CDS)
Diagnostic Criteria and Description
- CD is defined by *changes* in interactive, elimination, sleep cycle, navigational behaviors, or related cognitive behaviors, attendant with aging, which are explicitly *not* due to primary failure of any organ system.
- *The changes must be ongoing* (this diagnosis cannot be made on the basis of a one-time event) and *progressive*.
- CD is a potential animal model for the age-dependent cognitive changes that occur in humans. The affiliated behaviors may be associated with Alzheimer's-like (senile dementia of the Alzheimer's type) lesions.
- It is unclear if this condition in dogs or cats is associated with age-dependent changes in dopaminergic (suggested because selegiline, a monoamine oxidase inhibitor with large effects on dopamine, is used to treat CD) or other neurotransmitter function or micro-embolic events.
- The main methods for evaluating CD in humans are not applicable to cats and dogs because they primarily rely on written and verbal responses for assessment. Refinements in cognitive tests based on learning, memory, problem solving, olfactory function (Overall and Arnold, 2007), and navigational skills should enhance our understanding of this condition, especially when combined with imaging and serum, plasma, urine, and cerebrospinal fluid biomarkers.
- *Not all dementias are the same in humans, and this is likely to be true in animals.* Neither dogs nor cats make neurofibrillary tangles, but they make β-amyloid plaques (Head et al., 2005, 2008). Whether the burden of plaque correlates with the burden of the CD is an open question in all species. Even when we make the relevant and necessary mechanistic refinements (e.g., characterization and tracking of amyloid load correlations with age and performance), we will likely have some populations with relatively large amyloid burdens but little impairment.
- Although we know that some genotypes of humans may render them more susceptible to certain types of or onset times for Alzheimer's disease, these data do not currently exist for dogs. Given the number of dog breeds, and the size range of these breeds, it would not be surprising if certain genotypes were not protective of such cognitive change or carried an increased risk of it.
- There are three main contributors to problematic, age-related brain aging changes, all of which interact to compromise brain function:
  - Oxidative changes associated with processes such as free radical formation.
  - Formation of lesions, including those composed of amyloid.
  - Shifts in oxygen and energy availability.
- Aging is associated with increased expression of *genes associated with stress and inflammation*, especially in the brain region primarily involved in associational learning, the hippocampus.
- This loss of neurons is associated with decreased expression of genes that are involved in the ability of neurons to send and receive signals.
  - Brain-derived neurotrophic factor (BDNF) is essential for the processes of making and repairing all components of neurons.
  - BDNF, which stimulates cytosolic response element binding protein, has three main functions:
    - enhances growth of serotoninergic (5-HT) and norepinphrinergic (NE) neurons,
    - protects these neurons from neurotoxic damage, and
    - helps in remodeling neuronal receptors, altering function by enhancing mRNA transcriptional changes in translated protein products (i.e., receptors).
- When amyloid deposition is sufficiently extensive, it physically disrupts communication between neurons worsening the above-mentioned processes.
- Because the canine and feline behaviors we evaluate to make the diagnosis of CD are so general, we must remember that these behaviors could be natural sequelae to a variety of organ system changes. *If so, the diagnostic criteria will lead to many false-positive diagnoses.*

Common Non-Specific Signs
- In this condition, the signs are extremely variable and non-specific and may include:
  - nocturnal vocalization,
  - disorientation, including getting stuck in corners or going to the wrong side of a door,
  - alterations in social/interactive behaviors; early in the condition, this may appear as a form of increased "neediness"; late in the condition, this appears as a truly disengaged dog,
  - changes in locomotor behavior,
  - changes in sleep cycles; dogs are sometimes more awake and active at night,
  - "loss of housetraining," and

Assessment and monitoring tool for C-PTSD for client and working dog

1. Client/Handler:	2. Date:
3. Dog/K9:	4a. Breed: 4b. Weight: _____ lbs/_____ kg 4c: Sex: ☐ M ☐ MC ☐ F ☐ FS
5. Do you have any concerns, complaints, or problems about your dog's/K9's urination behavior?	☐ Yes ☐ No If you answered **yes**, (a) What is your concern/complaint? (b) How often does the concern/complaint occur (how many times per week)? (c) Is the pattern different on days when you do different tasks, and if so how?
6. Do you have any concerns, complaints, or problems about your dog's/K9's defecation behavior?	☐ Yes ☐ No If you answered **yes**, (a) What is your concern/complaint? (b) How often does the concern/complaint occur (how many times per week)? (c) Is the pattern different on days when you do different tasks, and if so how?
6a. Does your dog experience periodic bouts of diarrhea?	☐ Yes ☐ No
6b. If so, are these associated with specific deployment tasks or with specific events or experiences?	☐ Yes ☐ No
7. Does your dog/K9 destroy its kennel or any other objects?	☐ Yes ☐ No If you answered **yes**, what objects–specifically–does the dog destroy?
8. Does your dog/K9 exhibit any vocalization about which you are concerned or that has changed or is new?	☐ Yes ☐ No If you answered **yes**, what is/are the vocalization(s) and when do they occur: **Vocalization** / **When does this occur** a. Barking b. Growling c. Howling d. Whining
9. Does your dog/K9 show any changes in any type of aggressive behavior, including trained, controlled biting?	☐ Yes ☐ No If you answered **yes**, what are the changes? To whom is the dog aggressive?

Fig. 7-19 Tool for repeat assessments for dogs with or at for developing C-PTSD. This tool can be used for pet or working dogs, and is best used as a repeated assessment when conditions contributing to risk are known to be present (e.g., working dogs in war zones, pet dogs who have been seized or relinquished due to abuse, neglect, or some other horrific circumstance).

Continued

10. Has your dog/K9 had any changes in sleep habits?	☐ Yes ☐ No If you answered **yes**, what are these, specifically?
11. Has your dog had any changes in eating habits or patterns?	☐ Yes ☐ No If you answered **yes**, what are these, specifically?
12. Has your dog/K9 had any changes in locomotor behaviors or its ability to get around or jump on the bed, et cetera?	☐ Yes ☐ No If you answered **yes**, what are these, specifically?
13. Has your dog/K9 gained weight?	☐ Yes ☐ No If you answered **yes**, how much?
14. Has your dog/K9 lost weight?	☐ Yes ☐ No If you answered **yes**, how much?
15. Has your dog/K9 lost muscle/tone?	☐ Yes ☐ No
16. Has your dog/K9 gained muscle/tone?	☐ Yes ☐ No
17. Is your dog/K9 exhibiting any behaviors about which you are concerned, worried or would like more information?	☐ Yes ☐ No If you answered **yes**, please list these behaviors below:

Fig. 7-19, cont'd

- increased anxiety in situations in which the dog was formerly comfortable; this may be the first sign clients notice if they are paying attention.
- The history questionnaire contains objective questions that can help clients and veterinarians decide if the pattern of these non-specific signs fits with a diagnosis of CD. See Fig. 7-20.

Rule Outs

- This is one condition where our ability to assess the cognitive component is confounded by age-associated changes and debility.
- Dogs who are arthritic may appear to interact less but may choose to move less because of pain.
- Dogs who are arthritic may have more elimination accidents because they cannot navigate as well as needed to get outside, and, once outside, they may be sufficiently painful that they interrupt urination or defecation.
- With pain, arthritis, and other degenerative physical changes, a dog's ability to digest food may change, necessitating a change in their elimination schedules and/or diet. If clients are unaware of these potential needs, they will not meet them, and it could look like the elimination indoors is associated with cognitive change when it is associated with physical change and unmet needs.
  - Dogs may be unable to smell their food and may be less stimulated to eat if they have dental disease. Behaviors associated with changes in olfactory ability could look like changes in cognitive function.
- Dogs who are experiencing decrements in visual and auditory capability may change the manner in which they interact because they are lacking social cues. These dogs may also become more reactive, which could appear as a social and interactive change to their people.
- Activity level can be directly affected by whether the dog can see and hear. If they are not sensing stimuli and no effort is made to expose them to such stimuli,

Behavior screen for age-associated changes that can be used at each visit to monitor physical and behavioral patterns that could be associated with cognitive dysfunction

1. Locomotory/ambulatory assessment (tick **only** 1)
   - ☐ a. No alterations or debilities noted
   - ☐ b. Modest slowness associated with change from youth to adult
   - ☐ c. Moderate slowness associated with geriatric aging
   - ☐ d. Moderate slowness associated with geriatric aging plus alteration or debility in gait
   - ☐ e. Moderate slowness associated with geriatric aging plus some loss of function (e.g., cannot climb stairs)
   - ☐ f. Severe slowness associated with extreme loss of function, particularly on slick surfaces (may need to be carried)
   - ☐ g. Severe slowness, extreme loss of function, and decreased willingness or interest in locomoting (spends most of time in bed)
   - ☐ h. Paralysed or refuses to move

2. Appetite assessment (may tick **more** than 1)
   - ☐ a. No alterations in appetite
   - ☐ b. Change in ability to physically handle food
   - ☐ c. Change in ability to retain food (vomits or regurgitates)
   - ☐ d. Change in ability to find food
   - ☐ e. Change in interest in food (may be olfactory, having to do with the ability to smell)
   - ☐ f. Change in rate of eating
   - ☐ g. Change in completion of eating
   - ☐ h. Change in timing of eating
   - ☐ i. Change in preferred textures

3. Assessment of elimination function (tick **only** 1 in **each** category)
   - a. Changes in frequencies and "accidents"
     - ☐ 1. No change in frequency and no "accidents"
     - ☐ 2. Increased frequency, no "accidents"
     - ☐ 3. Decreased frequency, no "accidents"
     - ☐ 4. Increased frequency with "accidents"
     - ☐ 5. Decreased frequency with "accidents"
     - ☐ 6. No change in frequency, but "accidents"

   - b. Bladder control
     - ☐ 1. Leaks urine when asleep, only
     - ☐ 2. Leaks urine when awake, only
     - ☐ 3. Leaks urine when awake or asleep
     - ☐ 4. Full-stream, uncontrolled urination when asleep, only
     - ☐ 5. Full-stream, uncontrolled urination when awake, only
     - ☐ 6. Full-stream, uncontrolled urination when awake or asleep
     - ☐ 7. No leakage or uncontrolled urination, all urination controlled, but in inappropriate or undesirable location
     - ☐ 8. No change in urination control or behavior

   - c. Bowel control (Circle appropriate answer, if this occurs, please)
     - ☐ 1. Defecates when asleep
       - Formed stool   Diarrhea   Mixed
     - ☐ 2. Defecates without apparent awareness
       - Formed stool   Diarrhea   Mixed
     - ☐ 3. Defecates when awake and aware of action, but in inappropriate or undesirable locations
       - Formed stool   Diarrhea   Mixed
     - ☐ 4. No changes in bowel control

4. Visual acuity–how well does the client think the dog sees? (tick **only** 1)
   - ☐ a. No change in visual acuity detected by behavior - appears to see as well as ever
   - ☐ b. Some change in acuity **not** dependent on ambient light conditions
   - ☐ c. Some change in acuity dependent on ambient light conditions
   - ☐ d. Extreme change in acuity **not** dependent on ambient light conditions
   - ☐ e. Extreme change in acuity dependent on ambient light conditions
   - ☐ f. Blind

5. Auditory acuity–how well does the client think the dog hears (tick **only** 1)
   - ☐ a. No apparent change in auditory acuity
   - ☐ b. Some decrement in hearing–not responding to sounds to which the dog used to respond
   - ☐ c. Extreme decrement in hearing–have to make sure the cat is paying attention or repeat signals or go get the cat when called
   - ☐ d. Deaf–no response to sounds of any kind

Fig. 7-20 Behavior screen for age-associated changes that can be used at each visit to monitor physical and behavioral patterns that could be associated with cognitive dysfunction.

Continued

6. Play interactions–if the dog plays with **toys** (other pets are addressed later), which situation best describes that play? (tick **only** 1)
   - ☐ a. No change in play with toys
   - ☐ b. Slightly decreased interest in toys, only
   - ☐ c. Slightly decreased ability to play with toys, only
   - ☐ d. Slightly decreased interest and ability to play with toys
   - ☐ e. Extreme decreased interest in toys, only
   - ☐ f. Extreme decreased ability to play with toys, only
   - ☐ g. Extreme decreased interest and ability to play with toys

7. Interactions with humans–which situation best describes that interaction? (tick **only** 1)
   - ☐ a. No change in interaction with people
   - ☐ b. Recognizes people but slightly decreased frequency of interaction
   - ☐ c. Recognizes people but greatly decreased frequency of interaction
   - ☐ d. Withdrawal but recognizes people
   - ☐ e. Does not recognize people

8. Interactions with other pets - which situation best describes that interaction? (tick **only** 1)
   - ☐ a. No change in interaction with other pets
   - ☐ b. Recognizes other pets but slightly decreased frequency of interaction
   - ☐ c. Recognizes other pets but greatly decreased frequency of interaction
   - ☐ d. Withdrawal but recognizes other pets
   - ☐ e. Does not recognize other pets
   - ☐ f. No other pets or animal companions in house or social environment

9. Changes in sleep / wake cycle (tick **only** 1)
   - ☐ a. No changes in sleep patterns
   - ☐ b. Sleeps more in day, only
   - ☐ c. Some change - awakens at night and sleeps more in day
   - ☐ d. Much change - profoundly erratic nocturnal pattern and irregular daytime pattern
   - ☐ e. Sleeps virtually all day, awake occasionally at night
   - ☐ f. Sleeps almost around the clock

10. Is there anything else you think we should know?

Fig. 7-20, cont'd

they may sleep at times when they would otherwise have been awake. This outcome can translate to sleep cycle changes.
- Old dogs, like old people, are often taking a variety of medications. These medications can have adverse interactions, including sedation and ataxia, which, especially when combined with arthritides, can *make a dog appear as if she has CD/CDS when she does not*. A good *medical* history is required to diagnose this condition.
- In exceptional circumstances, the nocturnal activity and vocalization could be mistaken for a REM sleep disorder.

Etiology, Epidemiology, and Risk Groups
- Estimates from numerous studies suggest that at least 25% of dogs older than 10 years show one of these signs associated with brain aging, and that by 15 years, more than 60% of dogs are affected to some extent (Neilson et al., 2001).

- Caution is urged in uncritical acceptance of these types of estimates. The data are taken primarily from phone surveys and client questionnaires that focus on presence or absence of certain predetermined categories and not on the reasons for the patterns noted.
- The best data come from a combined approach using client reporting and direct physical and behavioral examination. This approach is almost never taken.
- Some dogs diagnosed with CD may have an old-age onset version of separation anxiety.
  - In the latter case, alterations in visual, auditory, and olfactory acuity, combined with alterations in motor capability, may render animals more anxious about the presence of and social relationships with humans.
- To date, *dogs with established, severe impairment have been laboratory dogs*, and no matter how "enriched" any

laboratory environment is, it must be absolutely mind-numbing. In fact, dogs maintained in artificial, behaviorally and intellectually depauperate environments may be more at risk for cognitive change with aging.

Common Myths That Can Get in the Way of Treatment or Diagnosis

- Behavioral changes that occur with age are "normal," and there is nothing you can do about this.
  - There is a lot of variation in how well animals within any species age, and there is a lot of variation in how "successful aging" (i.e., aging without cognitive impairment) occurs.
  - There are a number of old animals who have few demonstrable cognitive changes.
  - Patient needs may change (e.g., the dog has to go out more frequently and stand on grass, not slate or tile), but if met, the dogs can do well.
  - Increased aerobic exercise of any kind (e.g., swimming, underwater treadmills), alterations in diet/supplements, and enhanced cognitive stimulation can help slow or derail behavioral changes associated with aging.
- Old dogs have had their time, there is no sense trying to treat them, things will just continue to go wrong, so the treatment of choice is euthanasia, and there are a lot of young dogs in shelters who need homes.
  - It is true that there are dogs in shelters who need homes, and anyone who can give a quality home to a homeless animal of any kind should be encouraged to do so.
  - Prevention and early intervention through diet, exercise, and cognitive stimulation matter for both behavioral and physical conditions. Aging, *per se*, is not a death sentence.
  - We cannot make dogs young again, but we can provide them a better QoL with such intervention.
  - Euthanasia is not a treatment.
  - Although it previously was commonly believed that old dogs should just be "put out of their misery," we have more options now, and people should visit their vets to avoid euthanasia in older dogs, not to implement it, unless there is absolutely no other choice.
    - Veterinarians should know that clients avoid or delay seeking treatment if they are afraid that the vet will recommend euthanasia. This pattern is ironic in that it increases the likelihood of serious pathology, which could *render euthanasia more likely.*

Commonly Asked Client Questions

- Can this condition be fixed?
  - We cannot reverse the dog's age, and we cannot rid them of any amyloid lesions, although there are promising experimental studies in rodents suggesting that amyloid burdens can be altered (Cramer et al., 2012). However, we can address the pathologies associated with these by addressing functional change using diet/supplement, exercise, medication, and cognitive stimulation.
- How long will the dog have left if he or she is treated?
  - We cannot know the answer to this question, but the earlier intervention is attempted, the greater the likelihood of a longer and happier life. Overall, the amount of life left will increase, but the QoL will increase even more.

Treatment

- Management:
  - Helpful management changes include the following:
    - Ensure that the dog is taken out as often as necessary.
    - If the dog is not getting a lot of exercise, stimulate his muscles with range-of-motion exercises and/or massage daily. See Jurek and McCauley (2011) for an excellent tutorial on range-of-motion exercises; books on massage for dogs and cats are becoming common.
    - Consider using swimming pools, heated baths, and underwater treadmills to help ameliorate alterations in mobility.
    - Dogs who liked to catch balls and Frisbees when young may not wish to jump, but they would be happy to chase and/or retrieve these same toys if they are rolled. Rolling food toys and puzzles also serves to enhance and maintain eye-paw coordination, and because the toys/puzzles make noise, even dogs who are losing visual and auditory acuity can benefit.
  - Ensure that the medications the dog is taking are the medications he or she needs, and review all potential and present side effects every 3 months or more often if needed.
  - Teach the client to signal clearly to the dog to address any deficits in vision or hearing common to aging dogs.
    - There are vibrating collars that can signal to deaf dogs. See www.deafdogs.org/resources/vibramakers.php for information and sources. Under no circumstances should an element of shock/e-stim/electric shock be used.
    - Dogs may benefit if clients signal to them using gentle taps/strokes.
    - Clients should stand where the dog can see and hear them, remembering that dogs see movement well.
    - Providing surfaces that have traction by using rubber mats or rugs can help dogs get more exercise and have fewer elimination accidents.
- Behavior modification:
  - Teaching the dog to take a deep breath and relax may help with enhancing cognition and may help the dog to control pain.

- Specific behavior modification protocols may be implemented if the dog is physically able to do them. To request that a very arthritic dog "sit" may be to cause pain. If clients wish to use these programs they can reward the dog for lying down and looking to the left or right, rather than enforcing the dog to engage in any motor activities.
- In addition to some scent work, other forms of cognitive stimulation may include basic obedience or clicker work or working to teach new or maintain old tricks. Devoting 5 minutes to such work three to four times a day can be priceless. Some of this work can be incorporated into daily life: if clients are getting up from the table, they can ask the dog to come with them and to sit or wait and offer a paw. There is nothing better than ongoing stimulation and interaction.
- Medication/dietary intervention:
  - This is the area where most work is being done and where we currently have so much help and hope. The best results appear to occur from an approach that combines behavioral and cognitive enrichment with supplements, foods, and medication (Head et al., 2009; Milgram et al., 2002, 2004, 2005; Pop et al., 2010).The best time to implement dietary or supplement intervention is before the dog is showing any signs of brain aging. This means that dietary/supplement changes should be made in middle age (4 to 5 years for large dogs, 5 to 8 years for medium dogs, and no later than 8 to 10 years for small dogs). This is also the time to begin supplementation with Ocu-GLO Rx for vision (www.animalnecessity.com).
  - PUFAs, especially arachidonic acid (ARA), docosahexanoic acid (DHA), and eicosahexanoic acid (EHA), play roles in maintaining neuronal integrity and enhancing energy use by neurons.
    - All of these PUFAs are essential for early brain development.
    - ARA is thought to maintain especially hippocampal cell membrane fluidity and protect cells in the hippocampus from oxidative stress.
    - DHA may encourage developmental stage–specific associational learning, although the data are mixed.
    - Supplementation with DHA and EPA affects concentration of these substances in rat brains, and their distribution is not uniform (see www.nordicnaturals.com for compounds specially formulated for dogs and cats, and note that cat and dog dosages and formulations differ).
    - Diets deficient in α-linoleic acid especially cause decreases of DHA in the frontal cortex—the part of the brain responsible for complex learning and integration of information and executive function.
    - In dogs, low concentrations of DHA during gestation and/or lactation depress the retinal sensitivity of puppies, which can have profound and complex behavioral outcomes. Current data support the need for DHA for optimal neurological development in puppies, and there are hints that it may improve both early and long-term cognitive abilities, but the data are scant.
    - Age-related cognitive decline in dogs may be associated with decreases in omega-3 PUFAs in the brain.
  - Medium-chain triglycerides (MCT) increase fatty acid oxidation and so may increase omega-3 PUFAs in the brain via metabolism of adipose tissue. MCT-enriched diets increase brain phospholipid and total lipid concentrations and may decrease levels of Alzheimer precursor protein in old dogs.
  - Foods:
    - New foods are being developed all the time, but two already exist.
      - Hills B/D is a diet formulated to redress the damage caused by oxidative stress. It does so by providing high levels of anti-oxidants including vitamins C and E and L-carnitine to facilitate energy availability and enhance neuronal signal transmission. The strongest data for an effect are in laboratory dogs, for whom the largest changes in learning ability occurred in dogs fed this prescription diet and simultaneously exposed to environmental stimulation. Effects of such an anti-oxidant diet are also apparent in levels of BDNF, which have been shown to be similar to levels found in young dogs.
      - Nestle Purina's EN is designed to use MCTs as an energy source and is high in omega-3 and omega-6 fatty acids, which may help maintain neuronal integrity. Both the B/D and EN diets take advantage of anti-oxidants in the hopes of decreasing the effects of oxidative stress.
      - Royal Canin's CALM Diet is meant to reduce non-specific oxidative stress. It contains alpha-casozepine and an anti-oxidant complex of vitamin E, vitamin C, taurine, and lutein.
  - Supplements:
    - Senelife (Ceva Santé Animale) uses anti-oxidants (resveratrol), structural enhancers of neuronal membranes (phosphatidylserine), and a co-enzyme of neurotransmitter function (pyroxidine) to address three factors that can affect brain aging.
    - Aktivait (Vet Plus, UK; available online only in the United States at this writing) also addresses

structural concerns by providing DHA, EPA, and phosphatidylserine, plus the antioxidants vitamins C and E, selenium, *N*-acetyl-L-cysteine, and α-lipoic acid.

- NOVIFIT (NoviSAMe, Virbac) is S-adenosylmethionine (SAMe). One study showed improvements in social interactions, disorientation, and changes in sleep-wake cycles in dogs with mild to moderate CD syndrome.
- *Supplementation with Ocu-GLO Rx (www.animal necessity.com) may slow, stop, or prevent age-related retinal/lenticular degeneration* that may accompany CD. Many of the compounds in this supplement also are used in some of the cognitive supplements because reactive oxygen species and other oxidative assaults affect all nervous tissue (grapeseed extract, lutein, omega-3 fatty acid, vitamin C, vitamin E, vitamin B_1, vitamin B_3, vitamin C B_6, folate, vitamin B_{12}, biotin, pantothenic acid, zinc, α-lipoic acid, co-enzyme Q10, lycopene, green tea extract).

- Medications:
  - Selegiline (Anipryl; Pfizer) is a monoamine oxidase B inhibitor licensed to treat CD. It works by inhibiting the degradation and recycling of the monoamine neurochemicals (i.e., norepinephrine, serotonin, dopamine), with its largest effect on dopamine. By providing increased neurochemical stimulation to neurons, their synapses are maintained, and the effects of BDNF are able to occur. This medication works best as a preventive and treatment if given when the first signs of CD begin. The most dramatic effect is noticed by clients if the dogs are moderately affected, but that's because the decline was so apparent. Treatment of CD with medication is another example of a situation when treating early and often is preferred.
  - For some dogs who exhibit non-specific signs of anxiety as their first behavioral changes with age, treatment with TCAs or SSRIs may help. The effects that the clients see are the ones on anxiety, but because these medications also cause their effects by increasing signal transduction efficiency, they help to keep neurons healthy and signaling effectively to other neurons. As a result, they may have protective and treatment roles for CD.
  - Dogs who are experiencing some sleep cycle changes may also benefit from treatment with a BZD because of their calming effects on the reticular activating system. Avoiding BZDs with sedative intermediate metabolites that could pose a risk for older dogs or make them groggy on awakening (e.g., diazepam) may be helpful. Because alprazolam is also helpful in reducing anxiety, it may be an excellent choice for a "before bed" medication. If the dog is having difficulty sleeping through the night, a longer acting BZD such as clonazepam may be helpful.
    - REM sleep disorders should be distinguished from conditions that appear to disturb the dog's sleep (e.g., very active dreams) and cognitive changes associated with alterations in sleep cycles with age. REM sleep disorders can be variable: some respond well to TCAs and SSRIs, and some are worsened by them. Clonazepam is the longest acting of the BZDs without highly sedative intermediate metabolites and so is often used for many sleep-related conditions, including REM sleep disorders.
  - Propentofylline—xanthine derivative with neuroprotectant effects and which helps to improve blood flow.
  - Nicergoline—ergot derivative that is a potent vasodilator that putatively works by improving blood flow.
- Miscellaneous interventions:
  - The most commonly omitted intervention is the cognitive one.
    - Even dogs who are bedridden could use the commercially available food puzzles.
    - Food toys can also be made using a bucket or small pool with water and some liver frozen in a 125-mL container of broth. The frozen treat will float, and the dog can work to get it.
    - We know from the human literature that all conditions involving cognitive impairment also involve decrements in olfactory ability. We also know that biopsy specimens of aged dogs' olfactory epithelium show depositions of amyloid among olfactory neurons (Overall and Arnold, 2007). These patterns suggest that olfactory stimulation may be one form of cognitive stimulation to which older dogs can be exposed.
      - Olfactory stimulation may be as simple as dragging a freshly cooked bone through grass and encouraging the dog to follow the path. The marrow from the bone can be the reward at the end.
      - There are in-house nose-work exercises that many dogs would find fascinating.
    - This association between decrements in cognition and olfactory function may also suggest that we need to pay attention to the volatile olfactory component of our dog's dinners. Warming food and providing warm broth allows odorant molecules to volatilize, stimulating the dog's brain and encouraging eating.
    - Smelling the air and all the information that it carries to dogs can be a huge benefit to a dog

whose ambulatory skills are compromised. A dog buggy may be the treatment of choice (Figs. 7-21 and 7-22).

- Social interaction and exposure to new stimuli are essential for keeping cognitive skills sharp. We often think that withdrawal from such social situations is normal for an older dog, when instead the older dog is just painful, unaware, or unable to get to where he or she can participate. Because they are slow and quiet, they are left out. This is a huge mistake, and every effort should be made to include these older dogs if we wish for them to maintain neurons that can

"talk" to each other. Pet strollers are an under-used option for older arthritic pets. As is shown in Figures 7-21 and 7-22, a stroller allows this very old Australian shepherd to accompany her people and the other dogs on the regular 3-mile walks that she would otherwise be unable to do. Although she is not getting aerobic exercise, she is using muscles involved in balance and attentiveness, while getting much-needed social and olfactory stimulation. Also, she knows she is included in the family's activities and loved.

- For dogs who do not need buggies but who may wander, a locator system can be invaluable. Good locator systems allow the dog to go variable distances (programmed by the client) before a beep alerts the client (Fig. 7-23).

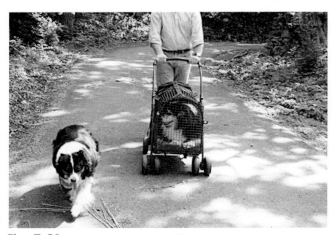

Fig. 7-21 Tess, 14 years old and in the buggy, was unable to go on the long walks the other dogs would take multiple times a week. Rather than leave her alone for hours at a time, the buggy allowed her to experience novel and complex stimuli, use different muscles, have the company of the other dogs (here accompanied by Flash), and smell the world as she passed through it.

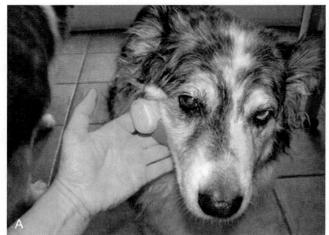

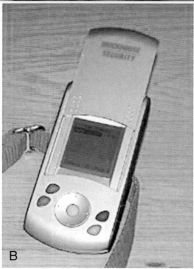

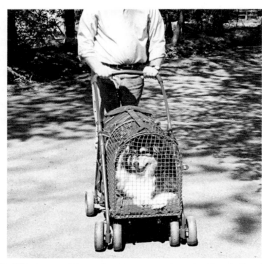

Fig. 7-22 The positive effect on Tess of such stimulation is clear in her engaged and relaxed facial expression. Dogs of her age and debility are too often left alone, and they resort to sleep in the absence of cognitive stimulation.

Fig. 7-23 This 13-year-old dog is cognitively intact but beginning to lose hearing and visual acuity and some flexibility. The locator beacon on her collar (**A**) communicates with a hand-held unit (**B**) that alerts her people that she is more than 10 feet away (the settings are variable). This particular system is from Brickhouse Security.

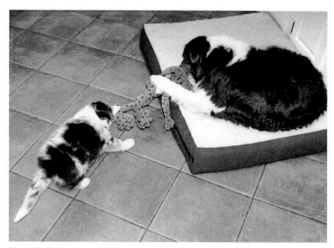

Fig. 7-24 Flash, on the right, was 12 years old when Toby (at 9 weeks), on the left, was adopted in the household. Raising this puppy became part of Flash's legacy, but the positive effects on his cognition and social and motor skills are clear in this photo.

- Teaching a younger dog how to do something is a cognitive enhancer. Groups of dogs of different ages who get along is wonderful cognitive enhancement (Fig. 7-24).

Helpful Handouts
- "Protocol for Teaching Your Dog to Take a Deep Breath and Use Other Biofeedback Methods as Part of Relaxation"
- "Protocol for Understanding and Helping Geriatric Animals"
- "Protocol for Preventing and Treating Attention-Seeking Behavior"
- "Protocol for Understanding and Treating Canine Panic Disorder (PD)"

Last Words
- People who have fed, exercised, and cared for their dogs well and who have sought behavior-centered veterinary practices, do not wish to hear that their dogs are "just getting old." They no longer have to hear this. Veterinarians should prepare patients and clients for age-based and stage-based care and evaluate whether supplements and dietary change is warranted as dogs move into middle age.
- We and our dogs will age and die, but none of us have to go gently into that good night.

Depression
Diagnostic Criteria and Description
- There is debate about whether the term "depression" should be used for non-humans. We lack the data that exist in human medicine for population-wide descriptions and determinations of animals affected with depression.
- A reasonable set of diagnostic criteria could include a prolonged (>1 to 2 weeks) endogenous or reactive pattern of behavior that may include withdrawal from social stimuli, withdrawal from activities that were previously engaging and enjoyable, alterations in appetite, and alterations in sleep-wake cycles that are not incidental.
- The condition is likely confirmed if the patient also expresses decreased locomotor/motor activity and actual physical removal from normal social and environmental stimuli in the absence of any neurological or physiological condition.
- The reactive form of depression will be easiest to recognize and acknowledge in dogs.
  - Some forms of reactive depression in dogs may be comparable to "adjustment disorder" in humans.
  - In an "adjustment disorder" type of depression, the behaviors are those enumerated here but are a *response* to a drastically altered environment over which the patient had no control (e.g., relinquishment, abandonment, re-homing, death of a close human or another pet). *Bereavement and grief can be the essential triggers for this type of depression.*

Common Non-Specific Signs
- Some signs seen in human depression may be applicable to dogs, but they are non-specific and must be interpreted in the context of the definition for canine depression.
  - The definition used here allows individuals sensitized to watching for the signs to recognize the following in a context that should be meaningful to the dog:
    - loss of appetite,
    - disruptions in sleep cycles, including sleeping a lot when normally awake,
    - weight loss (occasionally, weight gain),
    - loss of range of behavioral and emotional expression, loss of interest in formerly enjoyable activities (playing ball, going for a walk, being groomed or massaged),
    - decrease in energy and activity levels,
    - social withdrawal,
    - unexplained, non-specific and transient pain and stiffness, and
    - gastrointestinal distress (sporadic diarrhea, tenesmus, mucus in feces).
  - These behaviors are recognizable and could be noted on a daily log that allows clients to record time of day, circumstance, and response. A sample log entry might look like this: "*8:30 A.M. Picked up leash for walk, called dog, no response, lay in corner with head down. Called three more times. Went over to dog, encouraged him to get up, and dog finally rose and went for a walk, but listless, did not sniff environment.*"
  - Note that in this example the client highlights behaviors that could be monitored and measured before and after treatment: responding to a lead and sniffing while on a walk.
    - We could also measure time to get to door, steps taken per unit time, et cetera.

- Measures that could be objective can be developed based on the specific nature of the dog's behaviors and the client's concerns.
  - Clients can be provided with tick sheets to note the occurrence and frequency of certain behaviors.
    - The behaviors assessed would have to be relevant to the patient and the patient's household.
      - For example, the complaint of "not chewing on rawhides" is irrelevant in a household where dogs do not get rawhides, and "not playing with toys" is irrelevant to dogs who did not play with toys before they began exhibiting the signs about which their humans are concerned.
  - Any assessment measure used must matter *to the dog* and specifically to *that dog.*

Rule Outs
- The non-specific signs of depression are common ones that can be associated with "malaise" resulting from almost any illness.
- Common conditions that should be ruled out include:
  - infectious diseases, especially tick-borne disease,
  - endocrine conditions, especially hypothyroidism,
  - early renal or hepatic failure, and
  - neoplasia; the first signs of hemangiosarcoma can look just like the signs of depression.

Etiology, Epidemiology, and Risk Groups
- We do not know which dogs are at risk for this condition, but profound life changes resulting in loss (e.g., the loss of a human, companion animal, home) can put dogs at risk for the reactive form of depression.

Common Myths That Can Get in the Way of Treatment or Diagnosis
- There is a common belief that dogs accept and survive tragedy much better than humans do and that they will—and should—just "snap out of it."
  - This myth may have developed because humans realize that the number of dogs abandoned and/or in shelters is truly appalling. By believing that dogs are good survivors and can handle such abandonment better than we can, we relieve ourselves of guilt.
  - Dogs do not just "snap out of it." In fact, dogs who survive earthquakes, hurricanes, and similar trauma may never be completely normal, and their rates of relinquishment are high.

Commonly Asked Client Questions
- Is it possible that my dog is depressed?
  - Clients have been told dogs don't get depressed. If you query them, they will tell you that something may have happened that seemed to cause the dog to lose all joy. Such a description meets the criteria for depression.
- Can the depression my dog is experiencing be treated?

- Yes. Use of SSRIs, such as fluoxetine, plus planned work with dogs that includes them but begins to give them some structured tools for attending to and having some control over the world around them can successfully treat these dogs.
- "Work with dogs that begins to give them some structured tools for attending to and having some control over the world around them" is another way of defining behavior modification.

Treatment
- Management:
  - Dogs should be encouraged—not forced—to engage in behaviors that they previously found pleasurable.
  - Dogs should be protected from interactions that clearly distress or frighten them.
  - As long as the dog is maintaining his weight, dietary intervention isn't necessary, but if the dog stops eating his normal diet, ensure that the food he gets is something he would have formerly loved and ensure that it is served warm so that the olfactory component of eating is emphasized. Stimulating his olfactory neurons may protect them from damage and may help peak his interest.
  - Try to keep the dog on a regular schedule, especially as far as exercise is concerned. If he will walk, exercise him as much as possible. Increasing his aerobic scope may help.
- Behavior modification:
  - If the dog can work with a set of exercises he has enjoyed with which he has succeeded, the rhythm of these exercises may help in re-engaging with the dog.
  - It will be difficult to teach the dog new behavior modification exercises when the dog is depressed.
- Medication/dietary intervention:
  - PUFA supplements, including omega-3 fatty acids, may help prevent the dog from worsening by helping to combat inflammation and oxidative stress.
  - Medication is key to helping these dogs regain joy in their lives.
    - Most dogs will need a SSRI or one of the newer derivatives. Fluoxetine, sertraline, and paroxetine all have been used in these conditions. Decrements in serotonin and studies of knockout genes affecting 5-HT_{1A} receptors have been implicated in animal models of depression.
      - The distribution of the 5-HT neurons, especially 5-HT_{1A} neurons, the density of receptors, and the rate at which receptors are regulated and form part of a signal transduction path all likely factor into efficacy of these substances. The molecular shape of each SSRI molecule varies, to which one might attribute differential response within

a diagnosis. Such response could also be due to vagaries of neuronal density, distribution, et cetera.

- The monoamine oxidase inhibitor selegiline has been used in Europe for similar conditions but is not widely used in the United States except for CD. The primary effect of selegiline is as a monoamine oxidase inhibitor whose main target is dopamine, although all other monoamines (e.g., serotonin, norepinephrine, phenylethylamine) are affected to some extent. The effects of the medication will be determined, in part, by the distribution of central dopaminergic neurons.
- BZDs may help because they stimulate appetite as a fortuitous side effect and so may facilitate working with and rewarding the dog. BZDs have been postulated to disinhibit inhibited behaviors, so some recovery of appetite may be attributable to this effect on the hypothalamus.
- If the dog does not respond to other medications, stimulants may be an option. They are used to help move humans from nonresponsiveness toward a more responsive form of depression where medication may help.
- Because depression affects social interaction, use of oxytocin via nasal spray may have potential, but there are no reports of such use.

• Miscellaneous interventions:
  - Massage and any other actions that may make the dog happy (e.g., swimming, hiking in a place that stimulates his olfactory system) may help.
  - In this condition, time matters. If tincture of time and behavior modification has not helped in a week or so, do not delay treatment with medication further.
  - For dogs who are very close to specific people or other animals and/or who rely on them, death of the companion/friend can be devastating.
    - Dogs and cats should be given the chance to visit with their dying human companions and to see them after death.
    - They should also be able to visit with their ill and dying canine and feline companions and to spend time with them after death.
      - This last recommendation is especially important for dogs and cats who are rescues.
      - Dogs and cats can understand death but may not understand absence.
      - Given their own relinquishment history, uncertainty could contribute to anxiety and depression in rescued patients.
      - If end of life involves euthanasia, the other dogs and cats should be given the opportunity to be present. As we move more toward humane home hospice care for terminally ill animals, it will be easier for the other dogs and cats in the family to be present, which may greatly comfort the dying animal if the dogs/cats were close.
        - If signs of unremitting depression appear at any stage of the hospice care for or after the death of the companion, treatment as soon as possible may shorten the treatment course.

Helpful Handouts
- "Protocol for Teaching Your Dog to Take a Deep Breath and Use Other Biofeedback Methods as Part of Relaxation"
- "Protocol for Using Behavioral Medication Successfully"
- "Protocol for Handling 'Special-Needs Pets' during Holidays and Other Special Occasions"
- "Protocol for Teaching Cats and Dogs to 'Sit,' 'Stay,' and 'Come'" (for dogs who may not know these requests)
- "Protocol for Teaching Kids—and Adults—to Play with Dogs and Cats"
- "Protocol for Choosing Toys for Your Pet"

Last Words
- The definition of depression in humans does not adapt easily to dogs (or other animals). Because of the variable relationships we share with animals, *it is important that any definition of depression be relevant from the animal's viewpoint and that assessment takes into account the evolutionary history of the animal, roles played, and the context in which the diagnosis is being made.*
- In humans, depression can be defined as "an illness that involves the body, mood, and thoughts, that affects the way a person eats and sleeps, the way one feels about oneself, and the way one thinks about things" (www.medterms.com/script/main/art.asp?articlekey=2947). It has also been termed "a clinical mood disorder associated with low mood or loss of interest and other symptoms that prevents a person from leading a normal life" (www.webmd.com/depression/depression-glossary?page=2). Depression has been termed by the World Health Organization as a "common mental disorder that presents with depressed mood, loss of interest or pleasure, feelings of guilt or low self-worth, disturbed sleep or appetite, low energy, and poor concentration" (www.who.int/mental_health/management/depression/definition/en).
- A diagnosis of depression in humans is made on the basis of meeting the definitional criteria and on the types, duration, and frequency of the signs. We must remember that most human conditions that use such information pertaining to signs are able to do so because of large prospective or retrospective studies seldom possible or available in veterinary medicine.

Obsessive-Compulsive Disorder (OCD)/ Compulsive Disorder

Diagnostic Criteria and Description

- Repetitive, stereotypic motor, locomotor, grooming, ingestive, or hallucinogenic behaviors that occur out of context to their "normal" occurrence or in a frequency or duration that is *in excess of that required to accomplish the ostensible goal.*
- As the condition progresses, the behaviors are manifest in a manner that interferes with the animal's ability otherwise to function in his or her social environment.
- When fully manifest, the dog is unresponsive to human or animal intervention and to pain.
- This diagnosis is sometimes called only compulsive disorder in the veterinary literature because we cannot directly assess the obsessive component in dogs and cats.
    - In humans, the behaviors are abnormal ones that have as characteristics recurrent, frequent thoughts or actions that are out of context to the situations in which they occur.
    - These behaviors in humans can involve cognitive or physical rituals and are deemed excessive (given the context) in duration, frequency, and intensity of the behavior.
    - It would be a mistake to believe that this condition does not have cognitive components or forms in animals. In fact, one could argue that the compulsive behaviors are the result of obsessive "thoughts."
    - There is now ample evidence that dogs are cognitive and that they mirror assays of human performance when adapted to a species that is non-verbal.
    - We should remember that the ways we assess whether humans "obsess" involves asking about them and observing patterns of speech and behavior. Independent assays of obsession (e.g., imaging) are seldom done.

- For dogs and cats, direct observation, especially under a variety of conditions, can confirm that this condition has cognitive aspects involving intense, unremitting focus (e.g., obsession).
- Given the responses of non-affected dogs to the manifestations of OCD in affected dogs, it appears that dogs perceive and experience concern, rendering it more likely that they can obsess. Such discussions about diagnostic terminology need to account for divergent evolutionary histories for animals that rely heavily on structured language and those that do not.
- Separate from the obsession issue is the issue of relative intensity: whether a behavior is excessive or a manifestation of OCD may be a determination of degree. *Careful description and recording of behaviors and their durations could provide data that would permit evaluation of the extent to which such behaviors may lie on a continuum.*
- Good histories and observation are important because in some peculiar forms OCD could resemble seizure-like activity. However, we should remember that "seizure-like" activity is more poorly defined than most behavioral conditions. By definition, some epileptic or seizure-like activity is stereotypic, which is one reason why this very explicit and specific diagnosis category is preferable to that of stereotypy.
- In both humans and dogs/cats, a hallmark of OCD that distinguishes it from neurological conditions involving motor tics, et cetera, is that OCD behaviors follow a set of rules created by the patient. This condition is likely to be mechanistically heterogeneous (e.g., multi-factorial). *Regardless of the type of behavior in which the dog engages, it must be sufficiently pronounced to interfere with normal functioning to make this diagnosis.*
- OCD can be primary (truly endogenous) or secondary and likely associated with thresholds for stimulation (Fig. 7-25).

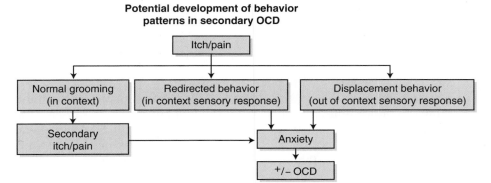

Fig. 7-25 Schematic for how OCD can develop as a secondary condition to dermatological concerns involving pruritus and/or pain.

Common Non-Specific Signs

- Depending on the form the OCD takes, the dog will exhibit the repeated behavior in a manner consistent with some internal and unforgiving rule structure. For example, dogs who "hallucinate" will have a rule governing the repetitive manner in which that dog "chases" the "invisible mouse" or "catches" the "fly."

- Dogs may seek out opportunities to engage in the OCD behavior, especially if they have been reprimanded or disciplined for engaging in them. As a result, clients may insist that they never see the dog lick, but the lesion is evidence that profound licking occurred.

- The most commonly noted behaviors include (Fig. 7-26):
  - chasing and/or biting at provocateurs that do not exist and/or associated indirect signs, such as shadows,
  - licking/barbering/chewing/plucking/sucking at or on various body parts,
    - The individual dog tends to focus on one or a few body parts and consistently attend to these; another affected dog of the same breed may choose other regions (Figs. 7-27 and 7-28).
  - repetitive, atonal vocalizations,
  - ritualistic activity including spinning/circling/pacing/chasing, and
  - stalking and subsequent ingestion or other oral behaviors (e.g., licking, sucking) of non-food objects in a way that is characteristic of the dog,
    - Dogs who ingest items like stones or rocks swallow them whole and may have learned to grab quickly and swallow all at once in a way that is associated with aerophagia (Fig. 7-29).

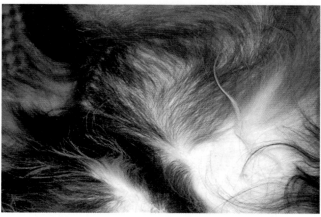

Fig. 7-27 Sparse hair in the inguinal region of a Bernese mountain dog who sucks, plucks, chases, and snaps at moving objects not present. (Photo courtesy of the client.)

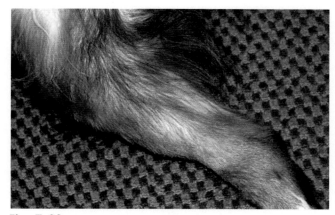

Fig. 7-28 The area of the medial hind leg where much of the plucking behavior is concentrated. Notice the absence of dermatological lesions. The dog appears not to disrupt the skin, and the client confirms the absence of papules and pustules. (Photo courtesy of the client.)

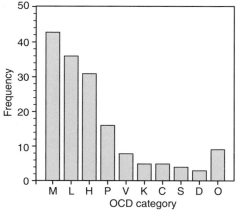

Fig. 7-26 Relative frequencies of types of OCD behaviors for the patients described in Overall and Dunham (2002). *M,* Self-mutilation; *L,* locomotor behavior; *S,* spinning/chasing; *H,* hallucination; *P,* pica; *V,* vocalization; *K,* licking; *C,* coprophagy; *S,* sucking; *D,* digging; *O,* other. (From Overall and Dunham, 2002.)

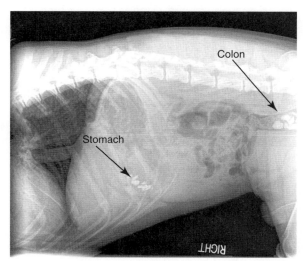

Fig. 7-29 Radiograph of a 2-year-old, male, castrated golden retriever who seeks out and swallows rocks and air. (Photo courtesy of Cheryl Taylor.)

■ That such dogs appear always to be on patrol for targets confirms the role for obsessions in this diagnosis.

Rule Outs

- Depending on the form the OCD takes, medical rule outs can be numerous.
- The most common conditions to rule out are:
  - hormonal conditions (e.g., hypothyroidism),
  - primary neurological disease (especially if the dog engages in motor or locomotor activity),
    - ■ Tics, licking, and sudden head movements all are common "seizure signs."
    - ■ Although status epilepticus and profound epileptiform seizures clearly differ in behavioral presentation, some authors have argued that "temporal" or "frontal lobe epilepsy" may be causal of or confused with OCD (Dodman et al., 1996). Such conditions should be ruled out.
      - ■ Phenobarbital is a sedative, an effect that may appear therapeutic at first. If OCD is involved, this condition usually outpaces any of the effects of barbiturates, and the non-specific signs re-emerge and progress.
      - ■ At the neurochemical level, behavioral and neurological conditions are on some complex continuum. It is likely that some forms of "motor seizures" share a neurochemical signature with behavioral conditions and, depending on brain region, may share behavioral effects. Quantitative electroencephalograms (EEGs) and sophisticated imaging hold promise for understanding such interactions.
      - ■ Dogs who respond best to seizure medication are those who have altered consciousness. Dogs with OCD are completely present, although incredibly focused. Although dogs with OCD might experience temporary relief from the sedative effects of classic medications for seizures, they ultimately require TCAs, SSRIs, et cetera. Dogs with OCD may also benefit from other medications now used for some types of seizure disorders, including *N*-methyl-D-aspartate (NMDA) blockers (Schneider et al., 2009) and gabapentin, which further supports the lack of independence between behavioral and neurological conditions.
  - toxicity (including heavy metals such as lead),
  - infectious diseases including, but not restricted to, tick-borne diseases,
  - undiagnosed or untreated pain secondary to another condition; see Zulch et al. (2012) for an excellent case report of licking associated with pain caused by tail injury, and
  - other behavioral conditions including attention-seeking behavior.

- The diagnosis may be difficult to confirm, but most of the rule outs can be dismissed on the basis of radiology, imaging, laboratory evaluation (which may include a cerebrospinal fluid analysis), and some toxicology panels.
- Video is essential for correct diagnosis: the pattern of the behaviors involved in OCD tends to separate this diagnosis from other conditions with causal and possibly confusing behavioral shifts.

Etiology, Epidemiology, and Risk Groups

- OCD runs in family lines—careful questioning reveals no generations are skipped (Dodman et al., 2010; Moon-Fanelli and Dodman, 1998; Moon-Fanelli et al., 2007). This is also true for cats (Overall and Dunham, 2002).
- The form the OCD takes depends on breed (e.g., the jobs for which the dog was selected affects at least the type or pattern of OCD) (Figs. 7-30 and 7-31). We have no good data on incidence rates in breeds, although spinning in bull terriers is often reported in certain lines of bull terriers (Moon-Fanelli and Dodman, 1998) and sucking on flanks or objects is common in certain lines of Doberman pinschers (Moon-Fanelli et al., 2007).
- The extent to which OCD may be expressed can depend on the physical and social environment. There is likely variation in response surfaces in dogs from different lines, and so some dogs require extreme stress to develop OCD, whereas others may display signs consistent with OCD under less stressful conditions (Fig. 7-32).

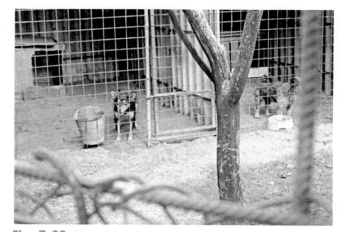

Fig. 7-30 This kelpie is kept in a kennel under extremely poor conditions. Many herding dogs spin or chase their tails when stressed or when affected by OCD. Not all cases of OCD are endogenous. Some, such as this case, are profoundly affected by kenneling and social conditions. Water is present, and he has a plywood doghouse, but the husbandry and social situation is depauperate and deplorable, although legal where this dog lives. Here he rests between bouts of spinning, which occur almost continuously unless he is otherwise stimulated. He is almost never taken from his run.

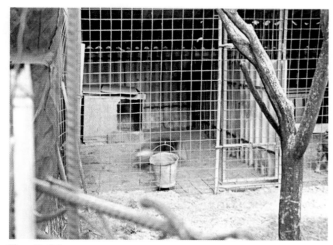

Fig. 7-31 The kelpie spins until he is exhausted or has something else on which to focus.

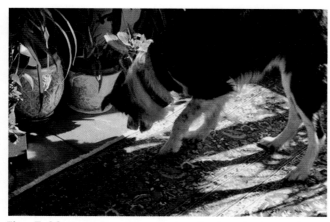

Fig. 7-32 A border collie chasing shadows he is causing as part of his OCD. Note the attentive stance, raised left forepaw, and open mouth. This dog chases and interacts with reflections caused by light and shadows and is exhausted by them. He is never able to "chase away" or "hold" these reflections.

- One study (Overall and Dunham, 2002) that looked at roles for breeds found the following associations:
  - German shepherds: hallucinations, tail chasing,
  - Dalmatians: hallucinations,
  - Rottweilers: hallucinations,
  - soft-coated Wheatons: self-mutilation,
  - Labrador retrievers: licking, self-mutilation,
  - Golden retrievers: licking, self-mutilation, and
  - Bull terriers: tail chasing and spinning.
- Forms may vary among relatives (e.g., if the patient sucks or licks herself, a sister may circle, et cetera). This pattern has not been demonstrated for cats.
- Heritability appears to be complex; one locus has been postulated to confer increased susceptibility in Doberman pinschers (Dodman et al., 2010).

- Age of onset appears to be 1 to 3 years (median age of onset, 12 months; mean age of onset, 20.3 months) (Overall and Dunham, 2002), as is true for most behavioral conditions, suggesting that the neuronal remodeling associated with social maturity is involved in the pathology.
- Density of neurons in the amygdala and the head of the caudate nucleus has been shown to be decreased in humans, but similar data do not yet exist for dogs.
- An inability to inhibit behavior has been proposed as an endophenotype in human OCD (Chamberlain et al., 2005).
  - This aspect also appears to be relevant for dogs, but we lack any type of assessment tool that allows all dogs to be uniformly evaluated for most aspects of behavior. However, ease of inhibition could be more easily gauged than many other behaviors and likely has applications here.
- OCD spectrum conditions in humans are thought to include attention-deficit/hyperactivity disorder (ADHD), Tourette's syndrome, and trichotillomania (compulsive hair pulling) (Chamberlain et al., 2005). We lack the data to use such an approach in veterinary behavioral medicine, but it could doubtless identify diagnostic subgroups that are important.
- Once OCD is diagnosed, lifetime medication is required, although you may be able to decrease or taper it; this depends in part on behavior modification, concomitant/co-morbid conditions, and rate of onset/improvement.
- *Especially when dermatological conditions are co-morbid, all aspects of roles for anxiety, pain, and pruritus must be addressed because we now know that pain, anxiety, and pruritus are related at both the central level and the level of the dorsal horn of the spinal ganglion* (Fig. 7-33) (Lagerström et al., 2010).

Common Myths That Can Get in the Way of Treatment or Diagnosis

- The most common myth pertaining to OCD is that it is a variant of normal behavior. Pathologies may have been deliberately or accidentally selected for in the breed, but they are hardly "normal."
  - Herding dogs are often implicated in this myth of normalcy. Comments such as "All Shelties spin" need to be addressed with fact. Not all spinning is the same, some dogs who spin do so because they are suffering, and all Shelties, in fact, do not spin.
  - By accepting/asserting a pathological behavior as normal, we do the following things:
    - We fail to address that the dog may be suffering and that the behavior is a non-specific sign of stress or pathology.
    - We relinquish the chance to intervene early when intervention will be most simple and helpful.
    - We tacitly approve breeding for the pathology.
    - We fail to acknowledge that something associated with this concern must have been desirable

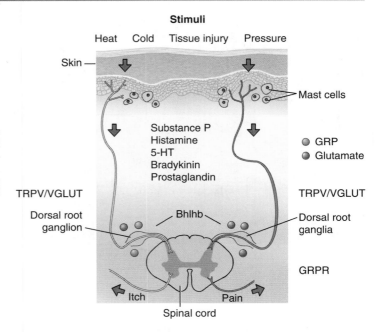

Fig. 7-33 Pain, anxiety, and pruritus are related at both the central level and at the level of the dorsal horn of the spinal ganglion. *TRPV,* Vanilloid receptor; *VGLUT,* vesicular glutamate transporter; *GRP,* gastrin-releasing peptide; *GRPR,* gastrin-releasing peptide receptor; *Bhlhb,* a transcription factor; *5-HT,* 5-hydroxytryptamine. (Adapted from Patel and Dong, 2010, and Rang et al., 2012.)

at some point if a large proportion of any line or breed is affected. If we fail to acknowledge this pattern, we will be unable to understand the genetic variance-covariance matrix that is operating and so cannot know if it is possible to select for desirable traits without carrying along those that are injurious.

- We pass on the misery to the next generation.

Commonly Asked Client Questions

- Can this dog improve/become normal?
  - This is two different questions.
    - In answer to the first question, all affected dogs can improve—we are discussing the matter of the degree to which they can improve. Some dogs will need medication for an extended period just to break through their distress long enough to render them susceptible to learning an alternate way to live.
    - In regard to the second question, some dogs will become so happy and so free of their nonspecific signs that people will think that they are "cured" or "normal." Unfortunately, these dogs never become "normal." If we think about treatment in terms of the response surface for the individual dog, behavioral, environmental, and genetic factors all contribute to the outcome.
    - Some dogs exhibit less profoundly affected behaviors, some have greater space for environmental intervention, and some have a greater degree of genetically based plasticity for learning new ways to cope and make their lives more predictable. This trifecta will help the dog look "normal." He will never be normal, and the clients must understand what this means.

- Stressors could have profound effects on these dogs, so if there is a social or physical disruption that affects the dog, the client should expect to see some backsliding. The good news is that dogs appear to be like humans: the greatest predictor of potential for recovery is that the dog recovered before. Resiliency likely has genetic components, but we can teach resiliency using behavior modification by rewarding a range of alternative, acceptable responses.

- Will medication be lifelong?
  - Yes, unless the problem just started and responded almost instantly to treatment, it is far safer to treat the dog for life. Once established, the plan for OCD is to stay the course and manage minor setbacks. In almost all cases, continuous medication makes these plans possible.

Treatment

- Management:
  - Recognizing, understanding, planning for, and managing stimuli that provoke an OCD burst in the dog are essential steps in recovery. For example, if the dog spins when unfamiliar people come visit, not having the dog present or introducing the dog when everyone is calm and the visitors have been schooled in specific behavior modification exercises in which they should engage in with the dog can help.
  - This is a condition that is about patterns. The dogs are using a failed rule structure to—ostensibly—help them cope with situations that, regardless of the level of the pathology, the dog finds distressing. We help the dog by replacing rules that cause them to react and become distressed with rules associated with relaxation and non-reactivity. The clients

should be able to recognize the patterns that appear in the dog's behaviors when the rules begin to slip. By staying the course, not over-reacting, not punishing the dog, and recognizing backslides for what they are—annoying but not tragic—clients will be able to manage the dog's behaviors by keeping the patterns as stable and helpful as possible.

- Behavior modification:
  - In extreme cases where the behaviors are unremitting, it may be exceedingly difficult to engage in any behavior modification until the dog has experienced some relief from medication. This may mean that clients cannot begin to engage in active behavior modification for 3 to 5 weeks.
    - In such cases, clients should not think that they can do nothing. Instead, they should focus intensely on any possible form of passive behavior modification.
      - Having the dog defer to them by sitting (or lying down) and looking at them for a cue will help clients to teach the dog another source for his focus. Once the dog can calmly and immediately sit and attend to them, clients can very slowly stretch the time that the dog stays in the sit (or down). If the dog begins to lick his lips, looks around, cannot focus, or otherwise shows any signs of decreased attention or of distress, the clients have pushed the dog too far. Let him get up, encourage him to get some exercise or engage in some other task that competes with his ability to perform the OCD, and then repeatedly come back to the passive behavior modification exercises as discussed in the "Protocol for Deference."
      - After clients have been able to make some progress with the "Protocol for Deference," they can start on teaching the dog to take and hold a deep breath, rewarding the dog for the calmness that accompanies exhalation ("Protocol for Teaching Your Dog to Take a Deep Breath and Use Other Biofeedback Methods as Part of Relaxation").
  - As soon as the dog is able, true behavior modification in terms of the "Protocol for Relaxation: Tier 1" should occur. The goal here is twofold:
    - We want to teach the dog a behavior that competes with the OCD in a manner that not only inhibits the performance of the OCD, but that also helps the dog to relax and learn that he has some control over his behavior.
    - We want to provide the dog with a successful set of rules that can be used to replace the rules that govern his OCD. That OCD is a rule structure, albeit a failed one that makes the dog more, not less anxious, is helpful because the dog already understands and uses rule structures.

If we can change the focus to a rule structure that focuses more on interaction with the external world and on relaxed, enjoyable activities at times when the dog would have engaged in the OCD, we can make real progress.

- Medication/dietary intervention:
  - Medications that can be helpful in controlling the anxiety that drives OCD may include:
    - BZDs:
      - Alprazolam is especially useful if there are explosive components to the OCD and/or ones that are provoked by known triggers.
      - Clonazepam is extremely useful if calming effects over a longer period of time provided by other BZDs are needed.
    - TCAs:
      - Amitriptyline
      - Clomipramine was developed for the treatment of OCD and may be the medication of choice if the manifestation of the condition can be characterized by ritualistic activity.
      - Doxepin is an H_1 antagonist, which is especially useful if there are dermatologic manifestations of OCD; it can be used in combination with other medications with care and reduced dosages.
      - Nortriptyline
    - SSRIs:
      - Fluoxetine is generally preferred if OCD has explosive components or an explosive start to the bout. If the entire form of the OCD can be characterized by its impulsivity, fluoxetine may be a more efficacious medication.
      - Fluvoxamine
      - Paroxetine
      - Sertraline
    - SARIs:
      - Trazodone may be best used as an adjuvant medication with others that are more specific for other receptor classes. Its associated effect on movement affected by 5-HT_{2A} receptors suggests that its addition may be helpful in some situations.
    - Other:
      - Gabapentin may be especially useful if neuropathic pain is involved and may be extremely helpful as a second or third medication to help address arousal and more global anxieties.
      - Memantine (an NMDA antagonist) has been efficacious as an adjuvant in OCD that resolves incompletely, suggesting that regulation of signal transduction pathways to more general levels may be useful.
      - Clonidine is a centrally acting alpha agonist that can be especially useful if there are explosive components to the OCD and/or

ones that are provoked by known triggers. By decreasing arousal through lowering peripheral sympathetic responses, clonidine may help the dog be able to make cognitive associations over which he or she has some control and that had previously been blurred.

- Some dogs with OCD, especially if there is a self-mutilation component, do themselves considerable damage. Under no circumstances, unless used as a last resort to spare the remaining limb, should digits or limbs be amputated as a "treatment" for OCD. The pathology that is in the dog's head will not be addressed by the removal of a limb or tail, and dogs with true OCD will continue to mutilate more proximal body areas. Instead, these dogs should be treated with the above-mentioned medications that will treat pain and pruritus and possibly long-term antibiotics to control any residual infection. If needed, fentanyl patches and butorphenol injections may help. Some of these dogs need to be sedated while the SSRIs, TCAs, et cetera, are taking effect.
  - In such cases, acepromazine should be avoided for long-term use or in high dosages because of problematic changes in perception and potential adverse effects on the extrapyramidal system.
  - Acepromazine should be avoided in dogs who are noise sensitive or phobic because it makes dogs more sensitive to noise, while scrambling their ability to understand the noise or their reaction to it (acepromazine is used as a dissociative agent).
  - Acepromazine *can* be used at very low dosages in combination with other sedative agents and in combination with narcotics for pain control (Grint et al., 2010; Hofmeister et al., 2010; McConnell et al., 2007; Sano et al., 2003).
  - TCAs and SSRIs may also have some anti-pruritic effects, and the most potent H_1 antagonist, doxepin, may also be slightly sedative. Clever polypharmacy, including use of the newer agents such as NMDA inhibitors, can help most of these dogs through crisis periods.
  - The use of topical lidocaine, either as a slow, sustained-release patch or as a gel, has been under-explored for dogs but may hold promise for some of these dogs who have a form of OCD involving mutilation. Such medications may render dogs less worried about bandages and dressing as has been the case in humans and may alter the perception of the stimulus sufficiently to help break cycles of licking and/or chewing.
- Miscellaneous interventions:
  - Re-directing the dog to a more suitable outlet for the particular behaviors that the dog is exhibiting may help (e.g., encourage the dog to chew on the freshly cooked beef bone, not herself), but these are stopgaps. The ease with which such re-direction is accomplished can serve as an index of improvement.
  - Massage may help because it is incompatible with virtually all OCDs and may be able to be worked into the behavior modification plan as a way of teaching the dog that he can have some control over his own behaviors.
  - Aerobic exercise that achieves true aerobic scope may help modulate the intensity and frequency of the behaviors and so act as part of an integrated treatment plan.
  - Elizabethan collars likely will distress these dogs more because of the difficulty they can cause for navigation. Any collar that prevents self-injury is going to be a long-term tactic for OCD dogs and so would need to be comfortable. Inflatable donut collars may be the best choices, but many dogs resist any collar. Dogs wearing such devices should be supervised.
  - For dogs who self-injure, bandages and wraps should be avoided when possible because they may serve as foci for more licking and chewing. If the wrap sufficiently changes the stimulus so that it is less noticeable, they may help, so some cast or splint designs may help lesions to heal. Such interventions are not often used but may be most successful in combination with topical anesthetics.
  - Dogs who self-injure may have a particular sensitivity to sutures. If they recover from their OCD and require any surgery, this concern should be noted and factor into decisions made. Knowing that some intervention may be problematic for the dog causes the humans charged with his care to watch that dog differently and so makes early intervention possible. This is a form of anticipatory guidance.

Helpful Handouts
- "Protocol for Deference"
- "Protocol for Teaching Your Dog to Take a Deep Breath and Use Other Biofeedback Methods as Part of Relaxation"
- "Protocol for Relaxation: Behavior Modification Tier 1"
- "Protocol for Understanding and Treating Obsessive-Compulsive Disorder (OCD)"
- "Protocol for Preventing and Treating Attention-Seeking Behavior"
- "Generalized Guidelines for Using Alprazolam for Noise and Storm Phobias, Panic, and Severe Distress" (for dogs who have explosive components with known triggers for their OCD)
- "Informed Consent Statements for the Most Commonly Used Medications"

Last Words
- Co-morbidity is the rule with OCD. Screen all dogs for other anxiety-related conditions, and treat all of them.

- Other conditions that may be neurodevelopmental (e.g., blindness, deafness, epilepsy, "seizure" activity) often co-occur in families where OCD (and other anxiety-related conditions, such as noise phobia) has been identified. Although the behavioral condition always appears to be inherited separately from the other conditions, including when these may be due to inborn errors of metabolism (Uchida et al., 1997), it is possible that in polygenic conditions there may be shared liability genes that could affect how profoundly ill the patient can become. Anyone interested in understanding the molecular genetics and neurobiology of these conditions may wish to consider these associations.
- We don't know what the early stages of OCD look like. Encourage all clients, especially clients with breeds or breed groups in which OCD is either relatively common or may have been directly or indirectly selected for, to monitor puppies for odd, ritualistic behaviors and to interrupt them. Ease of interruption is a good indicator of how severe the problem may be.

Panic Disorder (PD)
Diagnostic Criteria and Description
- A sudden, all-or-nothing, profound, abnormal response that results in extremely fearful behaviors (catatonia, mania, escape) where the provocative stimulus may be unknown/unclear, situational, internal, or generalized.
- PD differs from conditions involving phobias, where the provocative stimulus is more discrete and identifiable and where the level of distress characteristic of panic may not be achieved.
- The term *panic disorder* should be restricted to a described pattern of similar events. A *panic event* is a singular or infrequent event where the patient exhibits these behaviors, but the data are insufficient to determine if the consistent pattern exists as required for *panic disorder*.
- Once a patient has experienced one panic event, the patient is more likely to have another, but there are no data in domestic animals that show that experiencing one or more panic events leads to the consistent pattern necessary to make a diagnosis of PD.

Common Non-Specific Signs
- As for other related conditions, specific behavioral signs could include:
  - urination,
  - defecation,
  - salivation,
  - destruction,
  - panting,
  - pacing,
  - freezing/immobility,
  - trembling/shaking,
  - vocalization (bark, whine, growl, howl),
  - escape behaviors,
  - vomiting,
  - diarrhea, and
  - mydriasis.

Rule Outs
- Other conditions involving fears and phobias. It would be very easy to use a non-specific label such as PD to disguise an incomplete or less than helpful history.
  - Once the concern of specificity is discussed with the clients, they are usually quite good at recognizing associations that may trigger or co-vary with a phobic or fearful outburst. In such cases, a diagnosis of PD can be a diagnosis of exclusion.
- Dogs who are undergoing profound changes in sensory function or who have a poorly controlled (or undiagnosed) endocrine condition can look like they have PD.

Etiology, Epidemiology, and Risk Groups
- We do not know enough about this condition to comment on the epidemiology. Dogs who have been severely stressed and distressed may be more at risk for PD, but there is likely a large underlying genetic component for sensitivity and for resilience.
- Clients are better at recognizing situational PD involving dogs who panic during storms, when compelled to go to the vet's office, et cetera.
- Approximately 20% to 30% of human patients with major depressive disorder have panic attacks. The role of panic has been investigated in dogs only more recently. Panic attacks share many of the attributes of noise and storm/thunderstorm phobia. In one clinic population, when the diagnoses of separation anxiety, storm/thunderstorm phobia, and noise phobia co-occurred, the signs of each appeared worse and more intense than when either occurred alone (Overall et al., 2001). If such dogs follow the pattern common for co-morbid diagnoses in humans, longer persistence of the signs and a less favorable overall outcome may one outcome of co-morbidity.
- In human medicine, childhood separation anxiety is seen as an important antecedent in adult PD and is prevalent as an undercurrent in the dreams of human patients with PD. This suggests, in humans as in pets, that although separation anxiety can occur separate from PD and other phobia-related conditions, when the two co-occur the interaction is an important factor in the assessment and treatment of either.
- If phobic reactions to noise and storms are related to panic in dogs, such interactions are important.

Common Myths That Can Get in the Way of Treatment or Diagnosis
- The dog would be just fine if the people left him alone and stopped spoiling him.
  - None of these pathological behavioral conditions is caused by "spoiling" the dog, although people

who are more vested in their dog's well-being and QoL may more easily recognize atypical deviations from normal. This sensitivity could give the appearance of an association with attention (e.g., spoiling) to the dog's needs to someone with a more anthropocentric mindset.

- If "spoiling" were the issue, puppies would be at high risk for separation anxiety. Instead, a study that followed puppies over the first few months of life found that when pups were left, very few of them showed true signs of distress, and the few that did adapted relatively quickly to absences and ceased showing distress when left (Cannas et al., 2010).

Commonly Asked Client Questions

- Can these dogs get better, or do I just have to accept that the dog has periods where he completely breaks down?
  - With the appropriate medication, virtually all dogs should improve to some extent. Unfortunately, without being able to recognize external triggers, we have a very limited ability to protect the dog, although it is possible that we can protect him while he is exhibiting the panic.
    - Panicolytic medications (alprazolam, clonidine, and, under some circumstances, clonazepam) should be administered as soon as possible when the dog begins to panic to break the cycle.
    - The dog should be kept calm and safe from any behaviors that could pose a risk. A secure, comfortable, quiet room with low levels of illumination may help.
    - The clients should refrain from telling the dog that it is okay but should use any means that they know can truly calm the dog (e.g., press on him, take him into bed with them).
  - It is critical that we accept that the impetus for most panic and for PD may have an internal, not external, trigger. Improvement may never be complete. It is likely that there are liability genes for conditions such as PD, and so family history is important. This condition is so little understood in dogs that it would be inappropriate to guess the extent to which cases are heritable or sporadic.
  - The more realistic the clients are, the earlier they intervene, and the more they are able to manage the dog's distress, the more likely that the dog will improve to the extent possible for him.
- Could I have known that there was a risk that this dog would be affected by PD?
  - Too little is known about this condition to answer this question.

Treatment

- Management:
  - In contrast to phobias, we cannot identify provocative stimuli in PD and so cannot avoid them. If the stimuli are internal, all we can do is learn to identify the behaviors that indicate that the dog is becoming distressed as early in the sequence as possible. Our goal must be to prevent the dog from suffering, while also preventing him from learning to become more reactive with practice.
  - Truncating any panicky reactions may also interfere with any generalization of fearful responses that could occur (e.g., a form of stimulus response generalization).
  - Anything that can be done to calm the dog (e.g., massage, holding him without petting him, leaning or pressing on him) should be encouraged.
- Behavior modification:
  - Teaching the dog to sit, calm, and relax in nonprovocative situations must be the first step. These dogs need to learn that they can have some control over their internal reactivity and be rewarded for not reacting, staying calm, and breathing deeply.
- Medication/dietary intervention:
  - The best hope for as complete recovery as possible may lie with early use of medication. We now know that most medications recommended for such conditions encourage the processes of cellular and molecular learning (long-term potentiation) and the protein translation needed for these to occur. The earlier in the ontogeny of any pathological behavior that this occurs, the better for the patient.
  - Medications commonly recommended are agents used in fears and phobias and may include:
    - TCAs, all of which affect 5-HT and NE/NA to varying extents. Choice of a TCA may be predicated on the relative effects on these neurochemicals (see Chapter 10 for an in-depth discussion) and the potential side effects that could result.
      - Amitriptyline
      - Clomipramine
      - Nortriptyline
    - SSRIs—the literature in humans suggests that SSRIs are superior for treating PD, especially paroxetine and sertraline, but we do not know if this is also true for dogs because we lack the large-scale studies possible in human psychiatry. Regardless, when TCAs and SSRIs are effective in such situations, it is because they enhance efficiency of the signal transduction pathway and facilitate the translation of new proteins by doing so. This process allows for more efficient transfer of neuronal information and "learning" at the molecular level, both of which have neurotrophic effects.
      - Fluoxetine
      - Fluvoxamine
      - Paroxetine
      - Sertraline

- SARIs:
  - Trazodone (preferentially with another medication) appears to exert some of its effects through effects on motor activity. Whether it is a useful adjuvant for PD is unknown.
- Other:
  - Gabapentin acts to calm arousal and so may be a useful addition to other PD treatment.
- Medications to address or prevent acute outbursts of extreme fear, usually manifest as mania or acute behavioral paralysis, include:
  - BZDs (alprazolam, clonazepam)
  - The effect of BZDs in any condition involving panic, profound fear, or a profound reactive anxiety may be partially attributable to regulation of the hypothalamic-pituitary-adrenocortical (HPA) axis, especially in the paraventricular nucleus (PVN) through effects of vasopressin (AVP). Temazepam has been shown to blunt in a dose-dependent manner secretion of adrenocorticotropin hormone owing to a known stressor, while enhancing the release of AVP into the PVN. Taken together, these effects of BZDs modulate central nervous system regulation of the HPA axis (Welt et al., 2006).
- Midazolam has been shown through studies of Fos expression to affect activity in limbic regions, including regions involved in pheromone detection (olfactory epithelium) and transduction (medial amygdala and bed nucleus of the stria terminalis), and to increase defensive behavior, especially in the prelimbic cortex, lateral septum, lateral and medial preoptic areas, and dorsal premammillary nucleus of rodents. Other sites involved in defensive behavior and defensive aggression (ventromedial hypothalamic nucleus, paraventricular nucleus of the hypothalamus, periaqueductal gray, and cuneiform nucleus) are unaffected by the BZD midazolam (McGregor et al., 2004).
  - Central alpha-2 agonists (clonidine) decrease peripheral sympathetic arousal and can form part of a learned feedback loop that connects blocking of physical effects and non-specific signs of PD in situations previously known to provoke them. With behavior modification, this can be a potent effect.
- Miscellaneous interventions:
  - If these dogs learn to have a good, reliable, and instructive relationship with other dogs, the other dogs may be helpful in calming them when they panic.
    - Anxiety Wraps may help some of these dogs as part of an integrated treatment plan.
    - *No collars, harnesses, wraps, et cetera, should ever be left on a dog, especially a dog who may panic, when that dog is home alone.*

Helpful Handouts
- "Protocol for Deference"
- "Protocol for Teaching Your Dog to Take a Deep Breath and Use Other Biofeedback Methods as Part of Relaxation"
- "Protocol for Relaxation: Behavior Modification Tier 1"
- "Protocol for Preventing and Treating Attention-Seeking Behavior"
- "Protocol for Understanding and Treating Canine Panic Disorder (PD)"
- "Protocol for Using Behavioral Medication Successfully"
- "Generalized Guidelines for Using Alprazolam for Noise and Storm Phobias, Panic, and Severe Distress"
- "Informed Consent Statements for the Most Commonly Used Medication"

Last Words
- This condition is likely under-recognized except in older animals who panic because of encroaching debilities pertaining to auditory, visual, and olfactory acuity and locomotor capabilities. Endogenous panic is hard for clients to understand.
- This condition is often common as a co-morbid condition:
  - Separation anxiety and PD
  - Inter-dog aggression and PD
  - Inter-dog aggression secondary to PD
  - OCD and PD
  - Noise/storm phobias and PD
  - GAD and PD
  - GAD and PD with impulse-control aggression secondary to PD
- It is critical that dogs with anxiety-related conditions are fully worked up and screened for any co-morbid medical or behavioral condition.
- There is one context in which dogs who panic should be recognizable by veterinarians: dogs who panic at veterinary visits. Veterinarians would do well to learn to use preventive (before coming to the vet's) and interventional (given while at the vet's) panicolytic medication.
- Finally, clients need to remember that dogs who panic can injure themselves, and the first sign of panic may be unexplained injury.

Overactivity
Diagnostic Criteria and Description
- Motor activity that is in excess of that exhibited when the animal experiences a regular exercise and interaction schedule and that occurs in the absence of any signs of organic disease or true hyperactivity.
- *Overactivity resolves with increased aerobic activity and interaction.*
- Overactivity is a management-related "diagnosis" that is contingent on contexts that include the age of the dog, the age of the client, the breed of the dog, and the dog's social and physical environment.

- Overactivity must be distinguished from attention-seeking behavior, hyperactivity, and hyper-reactivity.
- Overactivity is a diagnosis that is not divorced from either the environment (the context in which the determination must be made) or from the client's understanding of "normal" behavior for the dog's breed and age.

Common Non-Specific Signs

- The most common signs reported are the signs that the clients find annoying:
  - lack of attentiveness to the client on walks,
  - pulling, non-linear walking with lots of starts, stops, and changes of direction when on a lead,
  - pacing and "getting into things" when at home regardless of whether people are present,
  - lunging at the door, bolting through the door, escape attempts, and jumping on dogs and people who are met regardless of their response, and
  - clients report that these dogs "never settle."
- Puppies are expected to be highly active and rambunctious. Many overactive dogs maintain or increase that level of activity throughout adulthood until they are quite old. From the research standpoint, it would be interesting to know if these dogs experience brain aging in a way that differs from calmer dogs.

Rule Outs

- Endocrine disease and treatment with steroids could cause some similar behaviors.
- For intact male dogs, the presence of females in season could cause similar activity, but it would be directed toward the female or her residence.
- If any of these reasons were implicated, the behavior noted should be a change. Instead, people with overactive dogs report that the dog is always like this. They usually comment that they thought this would pass once the dog was no longer a puppy, but in many cases the dog just gets more active.
- Overactivity must be distinguished from hyperactivity and hyper-reactivity.

Etiology, Epidemiology, and Risk Groups

- This is one condition where breed, lineage, and age all can matter. Dogs from breeds asked to engage in the type of work that involves extensive or near-continuous physical effort (most carting and herding breeds) and for which periods of calm have no value may be over-represented in the group of dogs thought to be "overactive."
- Dogs from working lines versus pet or show lines within a breed may have a completely different behavioral profile compared with the pet/show dogs. If this is the case, the dogs from working lines are generally more active and more inquisitive. These are desirable traits for working dogs but may be less desirable in pet dogs.
- Especially in dogs selected for "high drive," overactivity may be a big concern if that "drive" is not

appropriately engaged. A border collie who looks for explosives all day is suitably engaged in intellectual and physical activity in a way that she would not were she to live in an apartment as a pet.
- Perception of "overactivity" may change with human age. People who have "always had" Dalmatians or German shepherds may not have had a puppy or a young dog for a decade or more and may have forgotten that they, too, aged in that decade and may not have the tolerance for or ability to deal with a very rambunctious young dog.

Common Myths That Can Get in the Way of Treatment or Diagnosis

- The clients have had this breed their entire life and have never had this problem.
  - It's possible that this dog is no different than any of the other dogs, but the clients are now older and have other interests or altered mobility, or they forget that the kids are gone and the dogs were always with the kids, et cetera.
    - We often speak of pets of appropriate age and size for babies and young children, but we should also discuss how *human aging* affects the appropriateness of pet size, activity, and other aspects of "temperament."
    - Space and access to it matters. A rambunctious dog *appears* very different if you can let him out into a 4-hectare, fenced yard (whether or not he uses it) than he would if you lived in an apartment.
  - Veterinarians should help clients to appreciate life-stage and lifestyle changes that could affect their dogs and cats.
- The dog is just bored.
  - These dogs often have very stimulating environments with chew toys, but they need activity with true aerobic scope. These dogs are seldom bored but may be under-exercised. Unfortunately, a common response to the annoying behaviors is to lock the dog in a pen, kennel, or crate. The pen/kennel/crate is usually much more limited in interest and options than the house, so this "solution" must be extremely behaviorally painful for the dog.
- These dogs "should" grow up and behave.
  - The tyranny of the "shoulds" litters the veterinary behavioral literature. *This concern has nothing to do with "should" and everything to do with "can't."* Some dogs are easy keepers and very happy to adjust their activity level to that around them. Some dogs just cannot sit still no matter how much people want them to do so, but there are creative ways of meeting these dogs' needs.
- If the dog is a bitch, breeding her young will slow her down.
  - This may be the worst reason for breeding a dog. Babies should not have babies. Repeatedly

breeding a dog to exhaustion is unspeakable cruelty to that dog.

- No one should even think of breeding any dog if they do not already have sufficient excellent homes waiting for any puppies that are born.
- Anyone who is distressed by overactivity and is unwilling to meet the dog's behavioral needs to address it certainly does not have the patience and skill to raise puppies successfully through at least 8.5 weeks in an environment that best prepares them for future challenges.
- Finally, if the tendency to need more, not less, aerobic exercise has any heritable components (and it likely does) and this is a complaint, why breed more of these dogs?

Commonly Asked Client Questions

- Will the dog ever grow out of this?
  - If the dog is 2 years old and his or her activity level hasn't decreased (it may stay the same or increase), the dog is unlikely to grow out of this. Very active 9- or 10-year-old dogs can be behaviorally like normally active 2-year-olds.
- Will neutering/ovariohysterectomy (OHE)/spaying/castration help?
  - Dogs who are neutered do experience some changes in metabolism and may gain weight more easily. However, unless all of the dog's high activity is addressed at members of the opposite sex, for the purposes of true overactivity, neutering is likely to have a relatively small effect. It may help to remember that most dogs engaged in agility in the United States are neutered.

Treatment

- Management:
  - Management is key here. Clients need to learn about the dog's aerobic scope needs and try to meet them. Suggestions include:
    - dog walkers.
    - Consider doggie daycare, but ensure that the caretakers know that this is a special needs dog and may play roughly and not focus well at first.
    - Training the dog to use an in-house treadmill (with complete supervision and possibly the human on another treadmill at the same time); clients contemplating this option may wish to consult a rehabilitation specialist for training instructions.
    - Swimming is an ideal exercise for these dogs.
    - Flyball may be preferred by clients to agility because the dog does all the running in flyball. Clients who are also active or committed to becoming active may wish to consider agility.
    - If the dog is structurally sound, see if anyone in the neighborhood who jogs wants a canine running partner.
    - Many children who would love to have pets and who would be good for pets may not be allowed to have them because of style. Consider recommending such a child to play and work with tive dog.
    - Work. Most people think of physical work such as herding for overactive dogs, but intellectual work can be as or more important. Nose work is becoming popular (www.k9nosework.com; www.funnosework.com) and requires time but relatively little physical effort on the human's part. Taking the dog to work and asking him to work by coming everywhere with you, sitting every time you stop, taking a deep breath before standing, et cetera, is a cognitive and social workout that most dogs can only fantasize about. This is one of the best solutions for clients who may have age, lifestyle or life-stage mismatches with the dog. The dog does not have to go everywhere or go all the time for the value of this type of approach to be appreciated.
- *Behavior modification:*
  - All dogs can benefit from the basic behavior modification protocols listed.
    - For overactive dogs, behavior modification provides structure, information, and attention.
    - These programs alone can make these dogs much more manageable because they meet some of the dog's needs for cognitive stimulation.
- *Medication/dietary intervention:*
  - None unless the dog is otherwise distressed. It would be inappropriate to medicate a normal behavior, and it is wrong to sedate these dogs.
  - Some dogs may respond to the protein level in their food. If dogs are not working regularly, they are unlikely to need the high protein and fat levels that are in many diets and may do better on lower protein diets (see the discussion in Chapter 10). If the amount of protein in a dog's diet is to be decreased, considerations for quality of the protein become more important. Clients will need guidance about this.
  - Some of these dogs may benefit from PUFA supplementation (especially with omega-3 fatty acids). Such supplementation may make it easier for the dogs to learn calmer behaviors because of the mitigating effect on neuronal oxidants generated by overactivity and its impediments.
- Miscellaneous interventions:
  - These dogs are often so obnoxious to walk that they are just turned out into yards where they get *less* of what they need socially, aerobically, and intellectually. Good harnesses and head collars—along with training on how to use them—can make walking these dogs pleasurable (see the "Protocol for Choosing Collars, Head Collars, Harnesses, and Leads").

- Play with other playful and active dogs wears out dogs like no other activity. Clients should be encouraged to find or start play groups. Groups of dogs should be made with attention to size, age, and style of play (chase vs. rough and tumble) and with an eye to avoiding problematic behaviors.
  - Taking the dog to the "dog park" has become common. However, this is not a panacea for any canine behavioral problem. Dogs with true behavioral pathologies as well as dogs without decent manners training (including an excellent recall) should not be taken to dog parks, especially as a "solution" to their perceived problem. Before taking their dog to a dog park, clients should pay a visit to understand the rules and dynamics of the park.
    - Good parks practice safe play.
    - The best parks are double-fenced and/or double-gated. Such practices prevent tragic accidents and allow dogs to be segregated if intense situations develop.
    - All dog runs should be double-gated to provide a buffer and to prevent escapes.
    - Dogs should be temperamentally suited to their play groups.
    - Unless the dogs are relatively inactive, likely to stay right next to their people, and flawlessly behaved, there should be a person for every dog. One person can monitor two of their own active dogs without interference, but other dogs constitute interference.
    - Small dog runs should be provided and kept for small dogs.
    - Shrubbery should provide natural buffers.
    - The park should be clean and provide cleaning supplies (even if these are limited to only "poo" bags and a garbage can that is emptied at least daily when the weather is warm). Off-lead and on-lead rules should be posted, and there should be times posted for group play and solitary play for dogs who need to play ball or Frisbee alone.
    - There should be a plan for how to manage humans and dogs who do not play well with others.
    - The best parks provide water for the dogs (and humans) through dog fountains (very common in Europe), water coolers, or just taps of various heights and some metal bowls that can be washed between uses. Failing this, everyone should carry their own water and collapsible bowls.
    - For parks that allow free play, there should be a posted plan for injuries to dogs and humans.
    - Most parks don't have first aid kits, but clients may wish to consider having a first aid kit, if just to deal with wasp and bee stings.

Helpful Handouts
- "Protocol for Deference"
- "Protocol for Teaching Your Dog to Take a Deep Breath and Use Other Biofeedback Methods as Part of Relaxation"
- "Protocol for Relaxation: Behavior Modification Tier 1"
- "Protocol for Choosing Collars, Head Collars, Harnesses, and Leads"
- "Protocol for Teaching Kids—and Adults—to Play with Dogs and Cats"
- "Protocol for Choosing Toys for Your Pet"

Last Words
- Overactive dogs are over-represented in shelters. Unmannered, overactive dogs can knock over adults and seriously injure them. Such dogs pose a real risk to children. People tolerate a worsening of this condition in dogs that they think are otherwise sweet (e.g., Labrador retrievers) or in dogs for whom they think such frenetic behavior is "normal" (e.g., "high-drive" dogs). Both of these attitudes are problematic and lead to killing dogs.
- Overactivity is a completely manageable condition. With early, appropriate management, these dogs can have lovely social manners and be a problem to no one. For this to occur, two things need to happen.
  - Veterinarians need to step up and engage in *anticipatory guidance*. Veterinarians need to provide realistic interventions and accurate, data-based risk assessment that will convince clients to allow the veterinary and training teams to help them.
  - People have to let go of the concept that these behaviors are "normal" for "high-drive" dogs. Everyone should have an "off switch." If we have encouraged breeding for dogs with whom people find it difficult to live under normal circumstances, we must reverse that trend. Breeders need to be involved in considering the behavioral liabilities of the "product" that they produce. People have to lower their tolerance for behaviors that are difficult while concomitantly look for every conceivable way to meet the dog's needs. It is entirely conceivable that we lack the will and are not sufficiently good and compassionate people to render this recommendation a reality.
  - We need to consider the role that increasing human obesity may play in the preferences that people have for "styles" of dogs. Any dog of a normal activity level could appear "overactive" if his or her humans are obese and do not or cannot get exercise. In such cases, dogs may act as flags for worsening public health concerns in humans. The role for veterinarians in this case is undefined, but as we more closely approach a "one

health" approach, which unites and integrates shared risk factors for human and veterinary medicine, such considerations should matter.

Hyperactivity/Hyperkinesis
Diagnostic Criteria and Description
- Motor activity in excess to that warranted by the animal's age and stimulation level that occurs in a consistent manner and that does not respond to "correction," re-direction, or restraint.
- For *true hyperkinesis* to be diagnosed, there is the *additional requirement of sympathetic signs (increased heart rate, increased respiratory rate, vasodilation) even when at rest.* These signs, when present, should occur in the absence of other signs or significant laboratory data associated with thyroid or other somatic disease.
- For *true hyperkinesis* as defined in the original literature to be diagnosed, the dog must respond to treatment with amphetamine or methylphenidate by displaying a paradoxical decrease in motor activity.
- Most dogs that clients call hyperactive—a diagnosis that does *not* depend on the dog's exercise level compared with his or her needs—are actually *overactive*—a diagnosis that *does* depend on the dog's exercise level compared with his or her needs.
- Hyperactivity is a very specific diagnosis for which specific behavioral signs have been poorly elucidated. *Unfortunately, this term is used a lot but seldom truly defined.*
- In the original literature, "hyperkinesis/hyperactivity" in dogs focused on laboratory dogs as a potential animal model for a very restrictive variant of hyperactivity in humans ("hyperkinesis") (Corson et al., 1971).
- Truly *hyperkinetic* human patients were defined as displaying physiological signs of hyperactivity (increases in heart rate and respiratory rate) in addition to congruent behavioral signs.
  - Dogs were defined by Corson as being *"hyperkinetic/hyperactive" only* if they responded to treatment with *0.2 to 1.0 mg/kg methylphenidate with a 15% decrease in heart rate and respiratory rate 75 to 90 minutes after treatment* (Corson and Corson, 1976; Corson et al., 1971, 1980).
- Stimulants such as dextroamphetamine (Dexedrine), methylphenidate (Ritalin), and pemoline (Cylert) were expected to have paradoxical effects in truly "hyperkinetic/hyperactive" animals, including humans. These medications were thought to produce excitement in "normal" individuals and *paradoxical calm in "hyperkinetic/hyperactive" individuals.*
- Dogs who become more aroused when given amphetamines are not considered to meet the criteria for "hyperkinesis/hyperactivity."
- *Truly hyperactive states that meet these conditions are rare in canine and feline patients* (see review in Marder, 1991) and may not be common in humans.

- In the past 20 years, the focus in humans has shifted to attention deficits, inattentiveness, and related high activity levels (ADHD). This loose constellation of non-specific signs/client complaints has been increasingly used to describe a "hyper-active" dog, in the absence of the criteria or tests that may justify such descriptions in humans. *We need to define dogs better on the overactive/hyperactive/hyper-reactive spectrum.*

Common Non-Specific Signs
- These dogs never seem to sit down or settle.
- These dogs always have some signs of sympathetic arousal: slightly elevated baseline heart rates and temperatures, dilated pupils.
- Affected dogs arouse easily and appear to sleep less and less deeply, although this has not been measured.
- Affected dogs change their focus frequently, but possibly because they encountered a lot of stimuli that affected their sympathetic arousal. Their altered focus does not have to be due to an inability to pay sustained attention. *The hallmark of this condition is not attentional focus but sympathetic arousal.*
- We have failed to develop valid, repeatable, and broadly applicable tests of attentiveness and focus. Such tests are actually not that hard to develop and would be the first step in truly assessing the morass and complaints that form the overactivity/hyperactivity/hyper-reactivity spectrum. Tests fall into two broad categories: functional assays that can be profoundly affected by culture, environment, and training/learning/previous experience (both in terms of attending to cues and learning to ignore them) and biobehavioral/neurophysiological measures that are more independent of experience, culture, and environment.
  - The amount of time that a dog will spend searching for a ball is one test of focus used in working dogs. As a caveat, the dog in question must be extremely interested in balls and playing with them, and the ball should be a preferred reward for the dogs for whom this is a suitable test.
  - The amount of time that a dog requires to learn certain requests (e.g., "sit," "down," et cetera) could be standardized for testing conditions, age, and breed and provide some baseline data on how variable the breed is and how breeds vary.
  - The amount of time any dog will sit and look at you for a treat that the dog knows you are holding can be one measure of attentiveness or focus in a dog who is highly motivated for food.
  - The amount of time that a dog will sit and look at a person's face searching for cues about

what is expected could evaluate an extreme form of focus, were the conditions under which the test was done controlled (which would include posture, tone, et cetera) and were data on the dogs recorded and evaluated in a way meaningful to the dogs. Implicit in this is an understanding that human culture matters and dogs who are raised in apartments may not be the same as dogs who are raised on farms.

- Increasingly, responses to passing dogs or cues on computer screens have been used to assess variation in attentional focus in dogs in experimental studies concerning learning, but in terms of evaluating whether dogs on the overactivity/hyperactivity/hyper-reactivity spectrum have some reliable deficits in attention or behaviors indicative of these is unknown.
- Neurobehavioral measures such as papillary flickers or eye movements are under-explored in dogs but may hold great promise.

- Affected dogs do not actually seem distressed by their behavior, in contrast to dogs who have GAD. Instead, they seem to ricochet from one behavior to the next without undue concern.
- Affected dogs do not seem to respond to aerobic exercise the way overactive dogs do. Although they may calm a bit, the effect is minimal because exercise cannot over-ride the sympathetic system.

Rule Outs

- It is important to remember that the way this condition was originally defined may not match current usage and we know very little about the condition.
- The key rule outs are behavioral conditions (overactivity, hyper-reactivity, and GAD) and any physiological condition that causes sympathetic arousal (tumors affecting sympathetic activity via hypothalamic, pituitary, or adrenal function, especially pheochromocytoma).

Etiology, Epidemiology, and Risk Groups

- Our knowledge of this condition is too incomplete for any meaningful statements to be made. If the sympathetic patterns identified by Corson et al. (1971, 1980) are real and are the defining characteristics of this condition, it is likely that there is some heritable component. The prevalence may be sufficiently low to preclude evaluation.

Common Myths That Can Get in the Way of Treatment or Diagnosis

- These dogs have just been spoiled or ill-managed. These dogs need discipline, and this behavior will stop.
  - This logic is often applied to any dog who does not respond as the humans wish, whether or not the human's wishes are reasonable or in the best interests of the dog.
  - This type of explanation is often code for "use shock to stop the dog's behavior." If this condition

exists as defined, shock would be particularly cruel here because if it succeeded in stopping the undesirable behaviors, it would do so in contravention to the stimulation of the sympathetic nervous system. The distress that this duality would cause in the dog would be extreme.

- Any time people state that applying shock in any form to the dog (e-stim, zaps, pulses, stimulation, or any other happy misnomer) stops the undesired behavior, they should also *measure* the other behaviors. Shocked dogs—similar to shocked rodents—should offer fewer and fewer behaviors with time. Shock is not selective and *not behaving* is not the same from the dog's perspective as exhibiting improved behavior or improved or even adequate QoL.

Commonly Asked Client Questions

- Will this behavior ever improve?
  - We do not understand this condition sufficiently to offer any answer other than that we do not know. If we can find the right combination of medication and behavior modification, these dogs can improve, but they are always going to need to be managed with respect to all modalities of treatment.
- Is this behavior the result of additives or colorings in their food?
  - This is an interesting question. It is almost impossible to conduct a well-designed study to evaluate the effects of additives and coloring agents on behavior. Baseline behaviors would need to be measured, and the sample size of participants would have to be huge to include adequate numbers of dogs at the extremes of the spectrum. If people think that these substances might be affecting their pet's behaviors, they can select a diet that eliminates them and feed that diet only for at least 3 and preferably 6 months, as for hypoallergenic diets. Some objective measure (video in set circumstances) before and after would be desirable and would be required were this type of study to be done across many patients. However, if the client is willing to rely on his or her own opinion about effects and to take no measures, then if the client thinks the dog is better, that's all that matters. It doesn't matter if the dog is really better if the clients are happy and the dog has a good QoL. But please do not call this a scientific experiment.

Treatment

- Management:
  - Any actions that decrease sympathetic arousal should be practiced.
    - This may mean that heavy drapes must cover the windows if a road is visible.
    - Limited interactions with other dogs or novel people may be required.

- Decibel levels may need to be controlled precluding loud parties.
  - Strict schedules may help.
- Behavior modification:
  - All dogs benefit from basic behavior modification programs. These dogs may benefit more than most because these programs provide them with a set of rules that will allow them to govern their sympathetic responses.
    - To attain this outcome, the dog/client duo must reach the point when behavior modification becomes true cognitive therapy for dogs. This can happen, but it requires extraordinary efforts on the part of the client and talented dogs who learn that they can rely on and completely trust their humans.
      - The opinions expressed here about cognitive therapy for dogs are singular, and many people do not believe this is possible.
- Medication/dietary intervention:
  - Stimulants, TCAs, SSRIs and many other medication groups have been prescribed as treatments.
  - Methylphenidate and other related compounds became commonly used in humans to decrease inattention and to increase self-control (Gadow et al., 1990) and to increase motivation for and compliance with attendant behavior modification (Arnold et al., 1973).
  - The number of indications and conditions for which sympathomimetic amines are now used has grown, *not because more humans and dogs are recognized as truly "hyperkinetic/hyperactive" using the original criteria but because we now recognize that these compounds also affect neurotransmitters and receptors that affect anxiety, attentiveness, and memory.*
  - *Dogs who are treated with sympathomimetic amines and respond in the desired manner should not be assumed to be truly hyperkinetic or hyperactive or to have a canine version of ADHD* (see Chapter 10 for a detailed discussion of how these medications work). It is difficult to find diagnostic criteria for dogs for any of these conditions with the exception of the original derivative definition from Corson (Marder, 1991; Overall, 1997). *Assessment of attention is seldom done in dogs,* and we may wish to consider whether the dogs who might be good candidates for the attentional benefits of these medications are *hyper-reactive,* rather than truly hyperactive. This approach more clearly defines the clients' concerns and behaviors that we can actually assess, while avoiding the historical confusion that arose as a result of a search for a laboratory dog model for a human condition. *Accordingly, some hyper-reactive dogs may benefit from sympathomimetic amines, in combination with or instead of SSRIs, TCAs, BZDs, and related*

medications such as gabapentin, all of which are now also used to enhance learning and decrease anxiety and reactivity. Additionally, clonidine has been used to treat autonomic hyperarousal in human PTSD and so may be useful in conditions in dogs involving hyperarousal and *hyper-reactivity.*

- Miscellaneous interventions:
  - The extent to which massage, pressure, using an underwater treadmill, which can provide constant, mild compression, Anxiety Wraps, et cetera, may help is unknown. Clients often feel that anything is worth trying. The caveat to be added here is that this is true as long as the dog's QoL is maintained or improved.
  - Re-homing these dogs to a place where their activities are not disturbing to humans—a farm or a home where people are not bothered by the dog—may be a humane choice because if these behaviors are accepted, no one will be engaging in interventions that are inhumane or injurious to the dog. The problem is that the availability of such homes is low.
  - Sometimes people with special needs family members feel that they can provide good homes for special needs dogs. This is a kind and generous thought, but it often does not work because the dogs speak another language and become another stress. Normal, calm dogs may be therapeutic to humans with special needs.

Helpful Handouts

- "Protocol for Deference"
- "Protocol for Teaching Your Dog to Take a Deep Breath and Use Other Biofeedback Methods as Part of Relaxation"
- "Protocol for Relaxation: Behavior Modification Tier 1"
- "Protocol for Preventing and Treating Attention-Seeking Behavior"
- "Protocol for Choosing Collars, Head Collars, Harnesses, and Leads"
- "Protocol for Teaching Cats and Dogs to 'Sit,' 'Stay,' and 'Come'"
- "Protocol for Teaching Kids—and Adults—to Play with Dogs and Cats"
- "Protocol for Choosing Toys for Your Pet"
- "Protocol for Using Behavioral Medication Successfully"
- "Informed Consent Statements for the Most Commonly Used Medications"

Last Words

- When dealing with conditions where diagnostic criteria appear to drift, we should adequately represent what we know and don't know to the client.
- With such diagnoses, the roles for logical thought, putative mechanisms, and the use of a diagnosis as a hypothesis to be tested cannot be overstated.

Hyper-Reactivity

Diagnostic Criteria and Description

- Physical and behavioral response to an external stimulus (e.g., a sound or smell), activity, or social stimulus that is out of context, given the stimulus, and/or extreme in form, frequency, intensity, or duration.
- Affected dogs usually have a low threshold for reactivity and extremely rapid arousal.
- Signs may include vocalization, extreme motor activity, inattention to signals, lack of focus, and sympathetic arousal in response to extreme activity, but these dogs do not meet the hyperkinetic criteria of true, aberrant, sympathetic arousal and aberrant baseline sympathetic functioning.
- Before making this diagnosis, it is important to ensure that the dog is not overactive (inadequately exercised or stimulated) and that he or she does not have GAD, in which the dog is anxious across classes of stimuli and *motor activity is a failed response for dealing with the anxiety.*
- *Dogs who are truly hyper-reactive may not be distressed.* Instead, they appear hypersensitive to anything that arouses them and behave with a motor energy and lack of focus that is annoying to humans. The humans may complain that they cannot train the dog without the dog becoming aroused, so the question of lack of focus is usually raised but seldom quantified (see discussion in the section on hyperactivity).
- It's important to ensure that exhibition of hyper-reactivity is not a learned response to attempting to force a dog with GAD to function in complex, stimulating environments.
- Hyper-reactive dogs may not start out as anxious, but *anxiety can develop as a sequela.* The reactivity becomes reinforced and learned at the molecular and neurochemical levels. This is the logic behind treating hyper-reactivity with TCAs, SSRIs, and some stimulants that broadly affect multiple classes of receptors.

Common Non-Specific Signs

- Signs may include vocalization, extreme motor activity, inattention to signals, lack of focus.
- These dogs may destroy parts of the house or items in the house but not just when left alone. They destroy secondary to their extreme motor activity and apparent lack of focus.
- These dogs may injure people by jumping on them, grabbing at them, and bowling them over because they do not seem to be able to stop long enough to realize that these events are occurring and may be a problem for the people. In fact, these dogs appear to become more aroused the more such interactions occur.
- Clients will often note that these dogs become "overexcited" very easily and then are unable to relax or focus.
- These dogs are often described as having a lot of "environmental sensitivity," which can cause them either to shut down completely and respond to very little (except escape) or to become aroused in excess of what is appropriate given the context.

Rule Outs

- Hyperactivity, GAD, and endocrine and neurological conditions that can affect perception and arousal.

Etiology, Epidemiology, and Risk Groups

- The roles played by arousal and reactivity cannot be ignored if we are to understand dogs with anxiety-related conditions, such as separation anxiety, noise phobia, and storm/thunderstorm phobia.
- We should expect that problems with arousal and reactivity could occur without primary anxiety.
- Some dogs either respond more quickly to a stimulus or react more intensely to a given stimulus than other dogs.
- At some level, this "hyper-reactivity" is probably truly pathological and represents yet another phenotypical manifestation of some neurochemical variation associated with anxiety. If so, the more frequently the dog reacts to the anxiety-provoking stimulus, the worse and more rapid the response.
- At some point, any exposure can result in a full-blown, non-graduated anxious reaction in which true panic may be involved, but dogs with hyper-reactivity may achieve profound arousal without anxiety.
- Anticipation and early treatment is critical for all groups of individuals, supporting the concept that behavioral phenotype and underlying neurochemical response are linked in a dynamic way. Early intervention can be accomplished only by understanding the spectrum of signs exhibited in related conditions.
- Data support the concept that altering the underlying neurochemical response of a substrate associated with affect and learning has profound implications for outcome and severity of signs in co-morbid diagnoses. The extent to which reactions to noise may predispose dogs to other anxiety-related conditions, whether the number of non-specific signs may affect time penetrance, and whether there's a role for duration of illness in wosening the condition can be best addressed in prospective studies (Overall et al., 2001).
- This condition could have both heritable and neuro-developmental components. We do not pay sufficient attention to the *in utero* environment of dogs. We must begin to do so (Overall, 2011).
- It is possible that in selecting for very quickly responsive dogs we overshot and selected for a pathology in many breeds in which hyper-reactivity seems to be "common." We have no numbers to support any assertions of "commonness," and the time has long passed when we should have been collecting these.

Common Myths That Can Get in the Way of Treatment or Diagnosis

- These dogs have just been spoiled or ill-managed. These dogs need discipline, and this will stop.
  - This logic is often applied to any dog who does not respond as the humans wish, whether or not the human's wishes are reasonable or in the best interests of the dog.
  - This type of explanation is often code for "use shock to stop the dog's behavior." If this condition exists as defined, shock would be particularly cruel here because if it succeeded in stopping the undesirable behaviors, it would do so in contravention to the stimulation of the sympathetic nervous system. The distress that this duality would cause in the dog would be extreme.
  - Any time people state that applying shock in any form to the dog (e-stim, stim, zaps, pulses, stimulation, or any other happy misnomer) stops the undesired behavior, they should also *measure* the other behaviors. Shocked dogs—similar to shocked rodents—should offer fewer and fewer behaviors with time. Shock is not selective, and *not behaving* is not the same from the dog's perspective as exhibiting improved behavior or improved or even adequate QoL.

Commonly Asked Client Questions

- *Is it possible that this dog has ADHD?*
  - We do not have an equivalent diagnosis in dogs, and the diagnosis in humans now lacks sufficient specificity that its use has been called into question. That said, a diagnosis of hyper-reactivity may be as close as the dog version can get because the client's question is prompted by what they perceive to be the dog's lack of focus and attention.
- *Could my dog have a form of canine autism?* It seems like he cannot learn.
  - Dogs often have conditions that are homologous or analogous to the human condition. They may even be affected by conditions that we cannot recognize as the same as the ones in humans because we cannot evaluate conditions in dogs the way many are evaluated in humans. Autism is a condition in humans that is incredibly variable and for which the diagnostic criteria are being continually defined. If we enlarge the discussion to autism spectrum disorder, it's probably safe to say that dogs could have some of the genetic and neurodevelopmental deficits that affect humans with an autism spectrum disorder, but given the types of verbal and cognitive testing that are necessary, we may never know if dogs experience a canine version of the conditions.
- *Does my dog have a canine version of sensory integration dysfunction/sensory processing disorder?*
  - See the discussion on the constraints of diagnosing autism/autism spectrum disorder in dogs.
  - Humans with sensory processing disorder may have fairly dramatic swings in their responsiveness—from hypersensitive to hyposensitive—to a number of classes of stimuli responsiveness and functions for which they are dysfunctional: tactile, vestibular, proprioceptive, olfactory, auditory, oral input, visual input, language processing, social/emotional/self-regulation. Establishing baselines for these functions/stimuli responsiveness and evaluating deviations from these baselines will be difficult in dogs. Auditory, olfactory, tactile, vestibular, and visual functionality may be promising for assessment. However, not all dogs are the same, and such differences may affect how they perceive and react to the world.
    - McGreevy et al. (2004) found that *dolicocephalic dogs* have strong visual streaks and relatively low densities of ganglion cells in the area centralis, and *brachycephalic dogs* have the reverse: concentrated ganglion cells in the area centralis and low to no concentrations in a visual streak.
    - Red/green cones (medium to long wave) were denser in the temporal region than in the area centralis in *brachycephalic dogs* and less concentrated in the temporal retina in *dolichocephalic dogs*.
  - A hypersensitivity to touch to which dogs do not habituate quickly has long been associated with dismissal from working dog programs (e.g., "touch sensitivity"), but we lack the quantitative assays that allow such data to be collected in a valid and repeatable (i.e., useful) manner. However, there is some promise on the horizon for evaluating auditory function and reactivity (Kemper et al., 2011; Scheifele et al., 2012; Schemera et al., 2011) using awake brainstem auditory evoked response testing to determine baseline and subsequent changes in auditory threshold and frequency sensitivity, P300 auditory cognition testing, and otoacoustic emissions testing of canine cochlear function.
- Will the dog ever improve?
  - We do not understand this condition sufficiently to offer any answer other than that we do not know. If we can find the right combination of medication and behavior modification, these dogs can improve, but they are always going to need to be managed with respect to all modalities of treatment.
- Is this the result of additives or colorings in their food?
  - This is an interesting question. See the discussion in the section on hyperactivity.
- Why does this dog sometimes shut down and then sometimes explode when a stimulus affects him? Why does he have two such different responses?

- These responses appear to be two ends of a continuum, so clients are confused. Instead, if we think of these responses as being locations on a Mobius strip of possible responses, the dog's response makes more sense (Fig. 7-34). The response that the client is witnessing is a function of what came before that and what the dog perceives could come after or as a result of the triggering stimulus.
- The more predictive information that the clients can provide the dog, the better. A script where the client asks the dog to "sit," "look," "look around," return focus to "look" at the client, "walk," "sit," "look," et cetera, gives the dog a tone, cadence, and activity level that functions to provide a reliable set of rules that render the world and the dog's responses to it more predictable. This is what true behavior modification does when done correctly.

Treatment

- Management:
  - The use of harnesses and head collars may help minimize the damage that these dogs can do in interacting with humans and animals.
  - Anything that appears to help the dog (eye shades, ear muffs) attend more to her people can be employed as long as it does not hurt, punish, or scare the dog.
    - This criterion rules out the use of shock for the treatment of this or any other behavioral condition.
- Behavior modification:
  - All dogs benefit from basic behavior modification programs. These dogs may benefit more than most because these programs provide them with a set of rules that allow them to govern their sympathetic responses.
    - To attain this outcome, the dog/client duo must reach the point when behavior modification becomes true cognitive therapy for dogs.

This can happen, but it requires extraordinary efforts on the part of the client and talented dogs who learn that they can rely on and completely trust their humans.
  - The opinions expressed here about cognitive therapy for dogs are singular, and many people do not believe this is possible.
- When these dogs are aroused, they can be oblivious to most distractions, "corrections," and competing stimuli. Only when their arousal level begins to drop can they focus on something external. That shift in focus can be used to ease the dog from profoundly reactive and potentially dangerous behaviors to calmer and more secure responses.
  - The use of a toy or blanket that the dog can carry and the ability to use a set of cues/signals that they have fast-mapped act as safety signals and can be important steps in recovery (see Chapter 2 for more information).
- Medication/dietary intervention:
  - Medications commonly recommended are agents used in fears and phobias, and the rationale for these is discussed in previous sections. These medications may include:
    - TCAs:
      - Amitriptyline
      - Clomipramine
      - Nortriptyline
    - SSRIs—the human literature suggests that SSRIs are helpful for improving attentional state:
      - Fluoxetine
      - Fluvoxamine
      - Paroxetine
      - Sertraline
    - SARIs:
      - Trazodone (preferentially with another medication; while trazodone is being prescribed for many conditions, there are no controlled studies as of this writing)

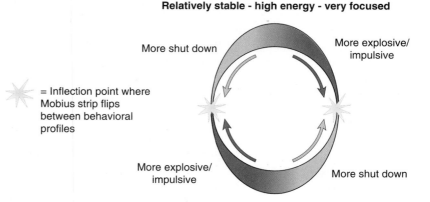

Fig. 7-34 Mobius strip model of a response surface to understand cycling/alternating of behaviors of a hyper-reactive dog. The dog can be unresponsive and shut down or responsive but more explosive as the extremes of the response. This dog has high-energy and low-energy phases, and his behaviors decay from relatively stable ones, given these phases, to very extreme ones, the presentation of which depends on where the dog was on his response surface when he began to react. The twist of the Mobius strip affects sudden shifts in behavior.

= Inflection point where Mobius strip flips between behavioral profiles

Relatively stable - high energy - very focused

More shut down

More explosive/impulsive

More explosive/impulsive

More shut down

Relatively stable - low energy - less focused

- Other:
  - Gabapentin
- Medications to address or prevent acute outbursts, as discussed for noise/storm phobias and PD:
  - BZDs:
    - Alprazolam
    - Clonazepam
  - Central alpha-2 agonists
    - Clonidine
  - Stimulants:
    - Dextroamphetamine
    - Methylphenidate
    - Pemoline
  - Some newer seizure medications may have helpful effects on attentiveness.
- Because of the amount of neurocytotoxic damage that constant arousal may facilitate, supplementation with PUFAs (especially omega-3 fatty acids) is recommended.
- Miscellaneous interventions:
  - The extent to which massage, pressure, using an underwater treadmill that can provide constant, mild compression, Anxiety Wraps, et cetera, may help these dogs is not known. Clients often feel that anything is worth trying. The caveat to be added here is that this is true as long as the dog's QoL is maintained or improved. Clients should note that active dogs wearing wraps need constant monitoring.
  - Re-homing these dogs to a place where their activities are not disturbing to humans—a farm where the dog may work or a home where people are not bothered by the dog—may be a humane choice because if these behaviors are accepted, no one will be engaging in interventions that are inhumane or injurious to the dog. If the rules for work allow these highly active dogs to use their unique qualities everyone will be happy, but watchful care of stock is essential to ensure that hyper-reactive dogs do not grab and damage others. Such homes are not common. Focusing only on containment (crates, runs) as a strategy does not meet these dogs' needs and will likely make them worse.
  - Very active humans who also need a lot of stimulation may be able to do quite well with these dogs if the dog is a relatively constant companion.

Helpful Handouts
- "Protocol for Deference"
- "Protocol for Teaching Your Dog to Take a Deep Breath and Use Other Biofeedback Methods as Part of Relaxation"
- "Protocol for Relaxation: Behavior Modification Tier 1"
- "Protocol for Preventing and Treating Attention-Seeking Behavior"

- "Protocol for Using Behavioral Medication Successfully"
- "Informed Consent Statements for the Most Commonly Used Medications"
- "Protocol for Choosing Collars, Head Collars, Harnesses, and Leads"
- "Protocol for Teaching Kids—and Adults—to Play with Dogs and Cats"
- "Protocol for Handling 'Special-Needs Pets' during Holidays and Other Special Occasions"

Last Words
- Our lack of knowledge should be made clear to the client. In this way, we may hope to learn enough about this condition to begin to understand what interventions can help these dogs.
- Clients should feel that they can have short holidays from trying to fix these dogs and instead just keep them safe and maybe enjoy the dog. If clients feel every single thing that they do could make the dog worse or better, they will be exhausted. Sometimes, the clients just need a little time off.

Incomplete Housetraining
Diagnostic Criteria and Description
- Consistent, age-*in*appropriate elimination in the house/apartment in areas not suitable/preferred for elimination.
  - Some dogs are purposely trained to use litterboxes, showers, drains, or other areas within the house/apartment for elimination.
- The location and times at which elimination occurs are not associated with lack of an appropriate place to eliminate, opportunity to eliminate, other behavioral conditions (e.g., separation anxiety), or any medical condition (e.g., urinary tract infection).
- This diagnosis is confirmed if the dog is older than 6 months of age and has never consistently avoided eliminating in the house/apartment or in indoor areas specifically not designated for elimination.
- Although housetraining is relatively straightforward, and normal dogs develop the ability to inhibit elimination physically in certain areas by 8.5 weeks of age, an exhaustive history coupled with an excellent description of the elimination behaviors is often the only way to determine that a dog may never have been housetrained.
  - A map of all soiled areas will be informative.
  - Video of the dog eliminating will be informative.

Common Non-Specific Signs
- Dogs urinate or defecate indoors in areas not set aside for elimination.
- Other dogs may live in the household and restrict their elimination to areas acceptable for them and acceptable to the clients.
  - Not all dogs prefer the same substrates or locations for elimination. Some dogs are quite fussy.

Incomplete housetraining may be easiest to recognize when compared with this range of normal preferences.

Rule Outs

- Common behavioral conditions in which elimination indoors could occur include:
  - separation anxiety
  - marking behavior
  - PD
  - storm/noise phobia
  - fear
    - The dogs may be too fearful of the location intended for elimination or the associated stimuli to eliminate; they later eliminate indoors because they must; this fear may be transient, seasonal, or associated with a schedule (e.g., school bus arrival).
    - Dogs may also have been so rigidly trained with punishment that part of their elimination routine involves postures that stopped the punishment (e.g., "submissive" behaviors); any dog who routinely exhibits this type of "submissive" urination should be screened for a history of harsh punishment or the presence of concomitant anxiety/fear-related conditions.
      - "Submissive" behaviors can also be exhibited by dogs who are generally uncertain/anxious/fearful in social situations involving humans; the humans mistakenly think that these are desirable behaviors because dogs should "submit" and humans should "dominate" and so fail to realize that the dog is extremely worried and asking for information about what types of behavioral responses are preferred.
  - CD.
- Box 7-3 lists the common conditions in which complaints about elimination most frequently factor.

BOX 7-3

Common Conditions in Which Complaints about Elimination Most Frequently Factor

1. Medical conditions
2. Incomplete housetraining
   a. Insufficient access to appropriate areas
   b. Development of an inappropriate substrate preference
3. Separation anxiety, profound fear, panic disorder, and other related conditions
4. Marking behavior
5. Submissive urination
6. Excitement urination
7. Geriatric incontinence

- Common management-related conditions in which elimination indoors could occur include:
  - Changes in mobility associated with age, illness, injury, or social threats from other animals; in such cases, affected dogs may simply be experiencing impaired or incomplete access to a location acceptable for elimination.
  - Leakage after ovariohysterectomy (OHE) in females, especially if neutered after multiple heat cycles, can be common, especially when sleeping or if asked to wait long periods of time between opportunities to urinate; clients can smell urine on the dog, the dog may be damp, or urine staining around the vulva, feathers, and hind legs may be common.
    - Providing frequent opportunities for elimination helps.
    - Regular administration of phenylpropanolamine (PPA) usually has the side effect of increasing urinary sphincter tone, and the problem largely abates.
- Common medical conditions in which elimination indoors could occur include:
  - dietary indiscretion,
  - parasitemia,
  - gastrointestinal bacteremia (e.g., *Campylobacter, Salmonella*),
  - viral conditions (e.g., parvo),
  - foreign bodies or gastrointestinal obstruction,
  - anal sac disease,
  - toxicosis (e.g., lead [plumbism] or garbage),
  - food allergies,
  - rapid dietary shifts,
  - maldigestion/malabsorption syndrome,
  - urinary tract disease,
  - neurodevelopmental conditions (e.g., lissencephaly, reflex dyssynergia),
  - neurodegenerative conditions (e.g., disk disease),
  - endocrine conditions (e.g., Cushing's disease, diabetes), and
  - treatment for medical conditions/iatrogenic causes (e.g., administration of antibiotics).

Etiology, Epidemiology, and Risk Groups

- Dogs small enough to be picked up and carried may be over-represented in the population of dogs who are incompletely housetrained.
  - Tiny dogs have relatively high metabolisms that co-vary with small bladders, so they may need to go out extremely frequently.
  - Tiny dogs may be more common in apartments, and it is difficult in apartments to get a desperate dog out the door quickly.
  - It is easier to clean up after a tiny dog than a large one.
  - It is easy to miss urine, especially if it has evaporated, if the dog and the amount are quite small. In this case, the dog learns to continue eliminating in the inappropriate areas.

- Hounds are reported to be difficult to housetrain because they are so focused on odor; however, the hounds that people insist cannot be housetrained are all small but not tiny (e.g., beagles) suggesting that motivation levels of the client may increase with the size of the hound.
- Some breeds are reported to be difficult/impossible to housetrain (e.g., Yorkshire terriers), so people may put little or no effort into the process.
- Dogs who do not have access to appropriate elimination areas will use inappropriate ones and may learn to prefer these.
  - Factors contributing to insufficient access or that deprive dogs of safe substrates and locations for elimination can include:
    - changes in the client's schedule, a particular risk for older dogs,
    - arthritides, if the dog is expected to use a dog door or get into a tall litterbox,
    - snow and ice may prevent all but the most hardy and sure-footed dogs from eliminating outside, and
    - social environments that are threatening (e.g., a neighbor's dog whose run or fence is up against the client's).

Common Myths That Can Get in the Way of Treatment or Diagnosis

- This dog is a breed/sex/type that cannot be housetrained.
  - Unless the dog has an anatomical abnormality or neurological pathology, all dogs can be housetrained. The limiting steps are the frequency with which they need to get outside and the ease with which they can do so.
    - By 8.5 weeks of age, dogs have the neuromuscular development needed to inhibit spontaneous elimination.
    - By 8.5 weeks of age, dogs have the cognitive development needed to learn preferences for specific substrates and locations for elimination.
    - By 8.5 weeks of age, dogs can begin to learn signals that will tell people they need to go outside if the people reinforce associated signals and behaviors.
- The dog is eliminating in the house because of "spite."
  - Dogs and cats do not eliminate for spiteful reasons. Not everything is about the human. Yes, it is inconvenient to have to clean up after the dog, but the dog is not focused on the cleanup unless it acts as a flag for harsh and scary punishment to follow.
- I was told to crate the dog to housetrain him. I crate him, but he still eliminates in the crate.
  - Time matters. When awake, puppies cannot go more than an hour, if active, and 2 to 3 hours, if relatively inactive, without eliminating.

- Adult dogs should not be expected to last more than 6 hours without having a chance to eliminate in an appropriate area. Failing this, elimination in a crate may be a sign of panic or fear.

Commonly Asked Client Questions

- Why is he/she doing this? He/she gets to go out/ has a litterbox, et cetera?
  - Is the area where the dog is expected to eliminate clean? If not, he or she will not use it.
  - Is the area where the dog is expected to eliminate accessible in all senses of the word? If not, that dog does not have access to a suitable place to eliminate.
  - Is the area where the dog is expected to eliminate scary, risky, or distracting in any way? If so, the dog cannot or will not eliminate in the designated area.
  - If the dog is to eliminate outdoors, is the only time the dog is allowed to experience the sounds, smells, and other sensations of the outdoors when he or she is taken to eliminate? If so, the dog will learn to delay elimination to have access to this rich sensory and cognitive environment.
- We got an adult dog specifically because we did not want to housetrain a pup. Why is she/he doing this?
  - Clients often assume that adult dogs adopted from the streets or from a humane shelter will be housetrained because of their age. This is a faulty assumption.
    - Dogs who have been allowed free range do not know that they are to eliminate outside: they eliminate outside without inhibition because this is where they are.
    - When brought inside, these dogs exhibit the same lack of inhibition about substrate, although they may not soil their sleeping areas.
    - These dogs are not stupid, spiteful, or malicious, although the clients often believe that they are. Adopted, formerly free-ranging, or re-homed adult incompletely housebroken dogs will require work on the client's part to *shift* their substrate preference to a more appropriate one or to help them develop a suitable substrate preference.
    - These dogs may never prefer a particular substrate such as grass, sawdust, or cement, but *they can learn that there are substrates to be avoided.*
  - Clients requiring that their new dog already be housebroken may do better by adopting an animal from a shelter that can provide an accurate history, from a person they know who wishes to relocate a dog with known propensities, or from a rescue group where the dogs had lived with a reliable foster family.
    - Stress, unpredictable or changing environments, too much time in crates, and dietary changes associated with re-homing all can cause dogs to have indiscretions during the

first few days in their new home. If managed as discussed, housetraining issues will resolve within 3 to 4 days for these dogs.

Treatment

- Management:
  - All dogs should be taken to the desired area for elimination:
    - on awakening,
    - within 15 to 20 minutes of eating,
    - immediately after playing,
    - immediately if they slow down while playing, and
    - at least every hour when awake up to 12 weeks of age, every 2 to 3 hours when awake up to 6 months of age, and at least three to four times a day for an adult dog.
      - Put a bell on the dog's collar (preferably a collar that will come off or apart if the dog hooks it on something). Bell the dog or use an "umbilical cord" leash to aid in supervision.
  - If clients are not doing these things, they are not managing the dog's physical needs.
  - Client must understand the relationships between physical size, age, activity, metabolism, and bladder size.
    - Clients need some meaningful reference to understand the association between glomerular filtration rate and the puddle on the floor. If veterinarians describe bladder size when full in terms of fruit (e.g., a young Yorkie is a small grape or cherry and he grows into a small apricot), clients will begin to understand these associations and will be able to time access for elimination appropriately.
    - Dogs develop the ability to inhibit elimination and the cognitive level to learn to prefer substrates or locations by about 8.5 weeks of age. If elimination in an appropriate spot is clearly and properly reinforced by clients or breeders when dogs are 8 to 9 weeks of age, virtually all puppies can be housetrained in a few days.
  - The paradigm described here requires that someone is available to take the dog out when needed. If no one is home, housetraining is likely going to be delayed.
  - Clients can learn when puppies' bladders are full by watching them: puppies who need to eliminate slow down and may look around or hesitate and squat.
  - Puppies can be better "followed" if they have a bell on their collar (if the bell stops, get them out immediately) or if they have a bungee cord–type lead tied to the client (they can play, but clients are aware of changes).
  - Because dogs innately attempt not to soil bedding and resting areas, enclosing puppies in small

places can help with housetraining if other needs are met.
  - If the dog is to be enclosed and left alone on a schedule that does not meet his or her physiological needs, an area specifically recognizable for elimination (e.g., a "wee pad") must be provided.
  - Dogs should not be allowed to explore, play, and socialize first but should be encouraged to do this after they eliminate.
  - Because of odor associations, choose a few restricted areas for elimination at first and return to those.
  - If the dog is leash-walked, shorten the leash to encourage walking in a small area to mimic elimination behavior.
  - If the dog is not leash-walked, the client should stand relatively still and not stroll or play with the dog until he or she has eliminated.
  - Permit cautious sniffing.
  - If the pup has to go down stairs to eliminate, carry him/her and press a towel to his/her crotch.
  - Young pups who are just developing neuromuscular control may be jolted by stairs and distance, thwarting any attempt to help the dog to inhibit elimination.
  - Do not worry that pups who are carried will never learn to go outside at their own initiative. They know how to walk. They need to know that they are rewarded for inhibiting elimination in inappropriate areas, and this strategy permits that.
  - Clients should be cautioned *not* to reward *only* a very narrow set of substrates for elimination.
    - Were they training themselves, dogs would choice a variety of substrates and locations for elimination and be able to use the variety, even if they had a preference. Humans may not allow dogs the same amount of sampling that they allow themselves.
    - If dogs are taught to eliminate only on grass or cement, they may find a change of season, a trip, a stay at the vet's, or any indoor dog show painful.
    - Dogs with such narrow preferences also are often very rigidly trained and tightly controlled, and so they will make themselves ill—even to the point of not eating and drinking—to avoid eliminating on any but their preferred substrate.
- Behavior modification:
  - Both client and patient behavior modification is involved in addressing incomplete housetraining.
  - Punishment has absolutely no role in housetraining. In fact, dogs who are very rigidly trained where and when to eliminate by use of severe punishment (and sometimes shock is involved) may develop "submissive" urination because the

clients may think "submission" is the preferred behavior. It is not.

- As soon as the dog squats or assumes any posture associated with elimination (and these are varied and can appear odd to clients), he or she should be praised.
  - If clients wish for the dog to like using a less common particular substrate (e.g., grass, cement, a "wee pad" in a box), they should immediately reward the dog with praise and a treat when he or she finishes eliminating.
- The client must be physically present, within touching distance, to help the dog to focus and to reward the dog when elimination is completed. If the dog is outdoors, this generally means that the dog is on a lead. If the client cannot touch the dog, the client cannot take advantage of the window of time in which rewards will work best.
- Dogs should not be allowed free play or exploration before elimination but should be encouraged to exercise/explore/sniff/play after elimination.
- Dogs are good observational learners. Watching another dog eliminate in a preferred spot can help.
- Medication/dietary intervention:
  - None
- Miscellaneous interventions:
  - Odor is important to dogs. Dogs use odor to tell them whether anyone has visited the spots where they have eliminated and eliminated on those spots. Urine and feces contain information that will allow dogs to identify who left the urine or feces, identify sex, identify diet, et cetera. In short, dogs use the olfactory information gained from sniffing urine and feces to get information about issues ranging from social interaction to foraging. Odor matters.
    - If a sample of the dog's urine or feces can be taken to a place where the client desires the dog to eliminate, the dog may be able to use the associated olfactory cues to reinforce preferred behaviors. This assumes that the area is not filthy and that the urine/feces is used as a cue.
    - If the dog has eliminated anywhere the client does not desire, the client must remove the odor cue. Just washing the area may not be sufficient.
      - Remove feces and as much urine as possible by blotting.
      - Use club soda to bubble up and dilute odorants. Repeat many times.
      - Finish with an odor eliminator that both renders odorants too heavy to volatilize and uses enzymes to degrade components of urine, feces and odorants.

Helpful Handouts
- "Protocol for Generalized Discharge Instructions for Dogs with Behavioral Concerns"
- "Protocol for Deference"
- "Protocol for Teaching Your Dog to Take a Deep Breath and Use Other Biofeedback Methods as Part of Relaxation"
- "Protocol for Basic Manners Training and House-training for New Dogs and Puppies"
- "Protocol for the Introduction of a New Pet to Other Household Pets"
- "Protocol for Teaching Cats and Dogs to 'Sit,' 'Stay,' and 'Come'"
- "Protocol for Teaching Kids—and Adults—to Play with Dogs and Cats"

Last Words
- This is the quintessential problem that requires the clients to meet the dog's needs. Few needs are more basic than the need to eliminate when your bladder or bowel are full.
- Veterinarians should monitor dogs for signs of fear that may occur during housetraining. The first time dogs are harshly punished or abused often occurs in the context of eliminating in the house.
- Dog abuse and child abuse are tightly coupled. Children, too, are often first abused because of urine or feces laden diapers or clothing.

Marking Behavior Involving Urine or Feces
Diagnostic Criteria and Description
- Urination or defecation that occurs in frequencies and/or locations inconsistent solely with evacuation of bladder and bowel but consistent with social and olfactory stimuli.
- It is more certain that marking occurred if, in addition, the urination or defecation is:
  - repeated,
  - associated with species-typical postures distinct from postures used in simple elimination, and
  - consistent with limited and identifiable social and olfactory stimuli.
- Social and olfactory stimuli can be difficult to evaluate. Determining how they are perceived by the dog or cat is even more difficult.
- Postures and associated behaviors should be sufficiently well described in a circumscribed manner that is not consistent with anxiety, excitement, or incomplete housetraining.
- Marking functions can also be part of normal elimination that does not involve behavior that is distasteful to the client. As such, they would never be called in to question under this category, illustrating the problem with the diagnostic label.
- Marking is usually normal behavior and so becomes a management issue.
- When marking behavior begins to occur in contexts, frequencies, and durations that are extreme, the underlying anxiety associated with the marking should be identified and treated.
  - For example, dogs who live in houses overlooking a street may be very interested in the urine

and feces deposited along the curb and may eliminate there. If such a dog began to pace in front of the overlooking window, depositing urine and feces in front of the window at every opportunity, this is not a normal marking behavior.

- This behavior is not in direct response to an olfactory cue.
- This behavior is not occurring in the appropriate location (e.g., where other dogs have eliminated or walked).
- This behavior is occurring in a frequency or intensity that is excessive.

Common Non-Specific Signs

- Urine/feces are found in relatively smaller amounts than would be associated with full evacuation of the bladder or bowel.
- Urine/feces more frequently than has been the elimination pattern in the past.
- Urine/feces are deposited in areas that have some social association. The association could be with another animal living in the house or with an animal that can be seen from the house.
- Many dogs who are exhibiting marking associated with anxiety also display increased vigilance and scanning, increased arousal, and increased monitoring of the behaviors of the provocateur(s) of the marking.

Rule Outs

- See earlier under incomplete housetraining.

Etiology, Epidemiology, and Risk Groups

- Dogs exhibiting this behavior appear to be entering social maturity or are socially mature. There are no good data.
- Intact male dogs are reported to urine mark more frequently than neutered dogs, although there is a large learning component to marking (Dunbar and Buehler, 1980; Dunbar and Carmichael, 1981; Hopkins et al., 1976).
- If intact bitches are present and in estrus and intact males, especially those who are experienced in mating, are present, the males may mark anything the females have touched or passed. This is normal behavior.

Common Myths That Can Get in the Way of Treatment or Diagnosis

- See earlier under incomplete housetraining.

Commonly Asked Client Questions

- Why is the dog doing this?
  - Dogs use urine to communicate information about their identity, sex, health and reproductive status, last visit, recent diet and, likely, neurochemical status (metabolites of neurotransmitters are excreted in the urine).
    - Dogs may be marking as part of a contextually normal suite of these communication behaviors, and the marking is occurring in a location that is undesirable to the clients.

- Dogs who are distressed or anxious may focus to an abnormal extent on the types of information conveyed by the urine marks. If the primary anxiety is addressed, the marking resolves.
- Some dogs mark with feces, especially at edges of their property where other canids visit, as part of a normal behavior. Occasionally, marking associated with anxiety or distress may include fecal marking.
- Anxious dogs may mark their own people, their clothes, possessions, and favored spots as a way to "claim" or highlight their relationship with the people about whom they care.

- Will neutering stop this behavior?
  - Although the study has never been replicated or expanded, older research (Hopkins et al., 1976) found that castration prevented or decreased the frequency of urine marking by males by about two thirds. Lesser effects were found for non-specific fighting/agonistic behavior between dogs, roaming, and mounting. If the behavior has not been ongoing for a long time, neutering may help, and the effects should be seen relatively quickly. Virtually all of the testicular testosterone is absent from the dog's circulation in 24 to 48 hours. If weeks have gone by and the dog is still marking, the behavior is not due to hormonal facilitation. Such marking could still be normal, or it could be due to anxiety.

- Can females mark?
  - Females can and do mark with urine and/or feces. Cocking the leg is not necessary for urine marking, but many females cock their legs or use front leg handstands. Many males mark by squatting or moving while in a modified cock.
  - Fecal marking can use similar postural patterns. Feces leave long-lasting visual signals and likely contain different volatile compounds that may communicate different classes of information. The amount of area covered by the feces or urine may matter in canine communication, which may help explain some of the behaviors that elevate legs or rumps.

Treatment

- Management:
  - Cleaning must have as its focus removal of the odor cue. Just washing the area may not be sufficient.
    - Remove as much urine/feces as possible by blotting.
    - Use club soda to bubble up and dilute odorants. Repeat many times.
    - Finish with an odor eliminator that both renders odorants too heavy to volatilize and uses enzymes to degrade components of urine, feces, and odorants.

- If the stimulus that is triggering normal marking behavior can be identified and removed/avoided, this may help.
- For anxious/distressed dogs, avoidance is key but will likely be insufficient alone.
- Behavior modification:
  - As with all anxiety-related concerns, teaching dogs to sit, relax, and not react to the stimulus can help them learn that they have control over whether to react.
  - Any agonistic relationship with any other animal or human must be treated. Marking usually resolves as the treatment progresses.
- Medication/dietary intervention:
  - If the marking is frequent, anti-anxiety medications are likely an essential component of the treatment plan.
  - Medications commonly recommended are those used in fears and phobias and may include:
    - TCAs:
      - Amitriptyline
      - Clomipramine
      - Nortriptyline
    - SSRIs—the human literature suggests that SSRIs are helpful for improving attentional state:
      - Fluoxetine
      - Fluvoxamine
      - Paroxetine
      - Sertraline
    - SARIs:
      - Trazodone (preferentially with another medication since there are no blinded, controlled studies using trazodone in dogs)
    - Other:
      - Gabapentin
- Miscellaneous interventions:
  - Belly bands (Fig. 7-35) will not stop the dog from engaging in the behavior of lifting his leg and

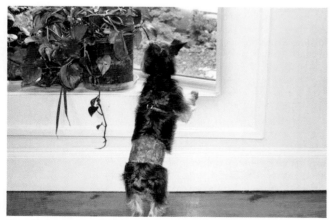

Fig. 7-35 Yorkie who marks indoors wearing a belly band. He is not as comfortable lifting his leg to mark when wearing the band but still marks, based on the urine found on the pad in the band.

urinating, but they can prevent soiling of the target area and provide what may be unpleasant feedback to the dog. By preventing repeated soiling, the olfactory stimulus to return to the same area to mark is lessened.
- Any humane barriers that prevent the dog from experiencing or reacting to the stimulus may be helpful.
- If the dog is intact, neutering may help but only to the extent that the behavior is facilitated by circulating hormones. Learned behaviors will not disappear, but the interest in exhibiting may be altered.

Helpful Handouts
- "Protocol for Deference"
- "Protocol for Teaching Your Dog to Take a Deep Breath and Use Other Biofeedback Methods as Part of Relaxation"
- "Protocol for Relaxation: Behavior Modification Tier 1"
- "Protocol for Generalized Discharge Instructions for Dogs with Behavioral Concerns"
- "Protocol for Understanding and Treating Dogs with Inter-Dog Aggression"
- "Protocol for Basic Manners Training and House-training for New Dogs and Puppies"

Last Words
- Clients and vets can usually figure out the extent to which marking of any kind is driven by normal behavior or by anxiety by asking themselves one questions: Is the dog doing this because he/she *wants* to do it, or is the dog doing this because he/she *must* do this? Dogs who want to mark but are not compelled to do so are usually normal, but dogs who feel they must cover another dog's urine or they must mark in a certain spot are likely anxious and would benefit from treatment.
- Clients should realize that very confident dogs can mark to advertise but that dogs who are being victimized by other dogs may fight back using marking because they cannot fight back physically. If clients note changes in elimination patterns, they should also look at the general social relationships in the household and ask if there is a problem (Fig. 7-36).

Submissive Urination
Diagnostic Criteria and Description
- Urination that occurs as the dog is approached/reached toward and that occurs when the dog is in a posture that ranges from incomplete squatting or sitting to a full-fledged grovel, with rolling on the back, tucking the tail, retracting the flexed forelimbs, turning the head.
- Dogs who reach the full-fledged grovel stage are often salivating and/or shaking, suggesting that this behavior has components of fear and/or anxiety.

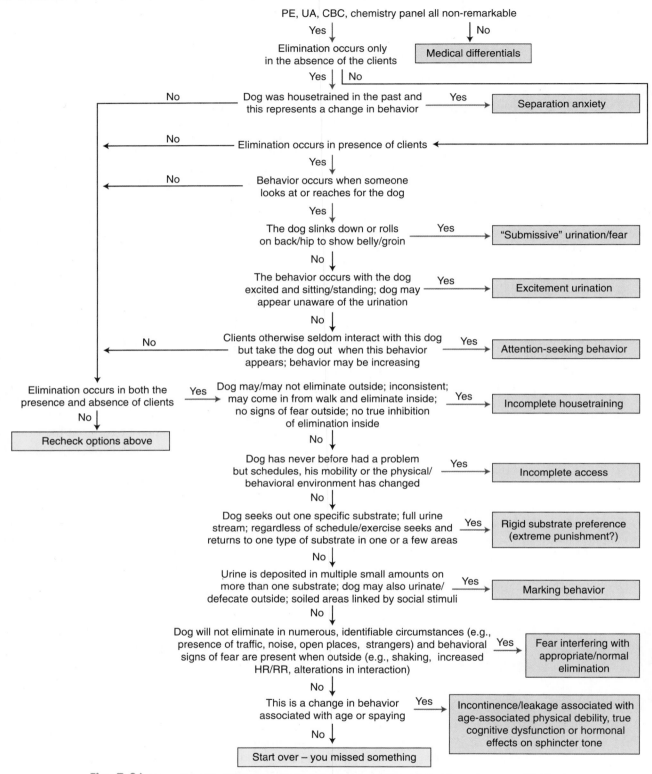

Fig. 7-36 Flow chart/decision algorithm diagnosing canine elimination concerns. *PE*, Physical examination; *UA*, urinalysis; *CBC*, complete blood count; *HR*, heart rate; *RR*, respiratory rate.

- Dogs need not have been harshly disciplined or abused for them to assume this posture, although it is important to know whether this was or is the case. Humane considerations are paramount for these dogs.
- As an arm is moved over the dog, the dog may assume a more "submissive" posture and urinate. The submissive posture can range from sitting, hanging the head, and exposing the groin to a full-fledged grovel, with rolling on the back, tucking the tail, retracting the flexed forelimbs, turning the head, and salivating and urinating. Dogs do not have to have been beaten to assume this extreme posture.

Common Non-Specific Signs

- crouching,
- slinking,
- lowering of head and neck,
- aversion of eyes,
- licking of lips,
- salivating,
- nose running,
- trembling,
- arched back, and
- all associated with urination from this posture when addressed, looked at, reached toward, touched, or otherwise interacted with.

Rule Outs

- neuromuscular pain, including subluxated/luxated disks, and
- renal/urinary tract infection/pain.

Etiology, Epidemiology, and Risk Groups

- Female dogs are more frequently diagnosed with submissive urination.
- It is unclear if this becomes a learned behavior after being disciplined for leaking—which is more common in young females than in males—or if there is some true association with sex.

Common Myths That Can Get in the Way of Treatment or Diagnosis

- "Submissive" behavior is normal.
  - "Submission"—defined as extreme deferential, appeasement, and disengagement behaviors designed to signal lack of any threat and interference—may be a variant of normal behavior; however, it is seen so rarely, even in true fights between dogs, that to say this behavior is a variant of normal may be to miss the point.
  - In the absence of a provocative—albeit rare—stimulus, submissive urination is out of context and so may be a non-specific sign of anxious and/or fearful behavior exhibited by a dog who potentially worries about many things.

Commonly Asked Client Questions

- Did I do something to cause this?
  - Unless the dog was treated roughly, the answer is no. Clients should know that most puppy mill/

farm puppies duck and don't make eye contact and may cringe when reached for, but they do not urinate when doing so.
- Will this stop if we let her have a heat cycle?
  - This condition is not hormonal, but if the dog is older, she may have some urinary incontinence, which could exacerbate the situation. Treatment with phenylpropanolamine (PPA) for the neuromuscular aspect of the incontinence may speed the rate at which the "submissive" urination responds to treatment.
- Is this because we spayed her young?
  - No, see previous answer.
- She looks like I beat her. Is she that miserable?
  - Possibly. The key to helping dogs with this condition rests in accurate assessment of the extent of their anxieties. If this is truly the only situation about which she worries, changing modes of greeting will help, but an exhaustive history is needed to ensure that the dog is not affected by any other anxiety-related conditions.

Treatment

- Management:
  - Dogs with submissive urinating can be well managed in a way that also helps them to improve.
    - These dogs should keep their bladders as empty as possible.
      - These dogs should have a chance to urinate before every interaction of any kind. This means greeting them with no fuss (and for some dogs that may mean no eye contact or tactile or verbal communication) and immediately guiding them to an area where they can safely urinate (a fenced yard or pen).
        - If the dog does not have an enclosed, safe area for off-lead urination, gently use a slip lead and collar as she moves through the door to restrain and guide her to the appropriate spot.
    - Reward the dog verbally when she has completed urination and is attentive. The dog should not be reached for until she has been taught which behaviors are rewarded when this occurs and which are neglected or ignored.
    - These dogs should never be reached for, even to put on a lead. Instead, they should be taught to sit and look—with their head up—at anyone making a request of them for a treat.
      - If the dog begins to shift posture or leak when handed the treat, the treat can be tossed on the floor on the far side of the dog so that none of the associations with the submissive urination postures are maintained.
    - As soon as the dog shows any of the signs associated with submissive urination, the client

should ignore the dog and walk away. No punishment should be used. Soiled areas can be treated with club soda/seltzer/sparkling water and blotted when the dog is not present.

- Behavior modification:
  - All anxiety-related conditions must be treated, but treatment for all of them will involve starting with teaching the dog to sit calmly and look at the client for a treat without exhibiting any signs of the submissive urination.
  - The standard behavior modification protocols, if practiced slowly and using the technique of shaping, are usually sufficient to treat submissive urination within a long weekend if there is no other affiliated anxiety-based condition.
  - Classic desensitization/counter-conditioning can be used to treat submissive urination.
    - The dog should start with an empty bladder.
    - The dog is asked to sit while the food is held over her head and moved backward over the head.
    - The dog continues to sit while tracking the food, but she need not meet the eyes of the client.
    - As soon as the dog's rump touches the ground without any leakage, the treat is released.
    - If the dog rolls, grovels, or leaks, she does not get the food. The client can gently move away.
    - Once the dog has returned to a less concerned state, the client tries again. Sooner or later the dog will be without residual urine and will be able to get the treat. The treat has to be released quickly and another treat instituted.
- Medication/dietary intervention:
  - If the dog leaks easily, daily treatment with PPA may help render behavior modification and learning new ways to respond to human approaches easier.
  - If a long weekend of gradually shaping more relaxed and appropriate greeting behaviors, combined with frequent opportunities to empty the dog's bladder, is not sufficient to resolve the situation, the anxiety driving the submissive urination is profound and/or the dog has other anxiety-related conditions. In such circumstances, anti-anxiety medications may help. The first tier of medication can include:
    - TCAs—these medications have increased sphincter tone and anti-cholinergic effects, which are usually undesirable outcomes of treatment. In this case, such an effect is desirable.
      - Amitriptyline—which has large anti-cholinergic effects
      - Nortriptyline
      - Clomipramine (e.g., Clomicalm)
    - SSRIs:
      - Fluoxetine (e.g., Reconcile)
    - BZDs:
      - Alprazolam
      - Clonazepam
- Miscellaneous interventions:
  - Diapering the dog may help the dog to associate the submissive behaviors with the urination, if she is not already doing so.
  - For clients whose patience is limited, diapering also prevents soiling.
    - Briefs and pads for dogs in season /in heat/in estrus can be used or diapers can be fitted from creative reconfiguring of diapers available for children.
    - Clients who elect to diaper their dogs must know to wash and rinse the dog carefully and often and to keep her dry.
  - For dogs who are very sensitive to any attention but who like toys, the toy can act as a safety signal or secondary reinforcement that indicates that the dog can and will walk calmly to his or her area for elimination without submissively urinating. This way, rather than talking to or reaching for the dog, if the client holds out a toy, the dog's focus can be re-directed, and the dog can be rewarded for not crouching and emptying her bladder normally.

Helpful Handouts

- "Protocol for Generalized Discharge Instructions for Dogs with Behavioral Concerns"
- "Protocol for Deference"
- "Protocol for Teaching Cats and Dogs to 'Sit,' 'Stay,' and 'Come'"
- "Protocol for Basic Manners Training and House-training for New Dogs and Puppies"
- "Protocol for Preventing and Treating Attention-Seeking Behavior"
- "Protocol for Teaching Your Dog to Take a Deep Breath and Use Other Biofeedback Methods as Part of Relaxation"
- "Protocol for Relaxation: Behavior Modification Tier 1"
- "Protocol for Using Behavioral Medication Successfully"

Last Words

- Patience is of paramount importance in treating this condition. Verbal reassurance can accompany the good behavior, but some of these submissively urinating dogs will cringe and leak at very loud and exuberant words, even if the words are positive. Clients must be alert to full manifestations of the dog's excessively deferential behavior and avoid providing any of the cues that could provoke it. As the dog's behavior improves, the clients can gradually add all the behaviors that provoke the elimination but must do so in a manner that does not elicit relapse. This means that clients must proceed slowly and pay attention to the dog's signals.

- Some clients may need the help of a dog trainer who uses only humane techniques and who can implement true behavior modification.
- Vets should screen these dogs for any signs of abuse, rough treatment, and other anxiety-related conditions as part of this assessment and future assessments.

Excitement Urination
Diagnostic Criteria and Description
- Urination by dogs who are generally young, exuberant, and who do not have complete neuromuscular control when stimulated by anything.
- The urine can drip, leak, or pour from the dog, but the dog is often completely unaware of the urination unless he or she calms.

Common Non-Specific Signs
- These dogs engage in enthusiastic greeting and interactive behaviors without attending to the concomitant urination.
- The amount of urine spilled is associated with how full the bladder is.
- Dogs can exhibit excitement urination even though they have recently urinated during a leash-walk.
- Excitement urination may be worse if the dogs are awakened or startled and then become very excited.
- Affected dogs do not assume normal urination postures when excited and may urinate while walking, standing, or jumping up and down.
- The dogs often outgrow this behavior.

Rule Outs
- Urinary tract infections
- Renal pathology (infection, neoplastic, developmental)
- Endocrine conditions including diabetes and Cushing's disease
- Polydipsia and high activity levels
  - This is common in very young puppies who play with their water and the reflections in it. They then seem to leak whenever they change behavior.
  - Smaller amounts of water doled out more frequently and after walks will usually resolve urination associated with juvenile polydipsia.
- Polydipsia associated with behavioral concerns, including a history of water deprivation
  - Some dogs who have been deprived of water guard water bowls and drink whatever is offered, even if this causes their bladder to overflow.
  - Placement of numerous filled smaller water dishes throughout the house usually allows them to realize that they will not be deprived of water, and so they drink and urinate less. Once this behavior is stable, water dishes can be removed gradually.
- Neurological deficits
- Hypothalamic neoplasia

Etiology, Epidemiology, and Risk Groups
- Except for being young and very excitable, there appear to be no risk groups.

Common Myths That Can Get in the Way of Treatment or Diagnosis
- The dog cannot be housetrained.
  - Age, tincture of time, and a bit of work by the client can resolve this issue. Only the exceptional dog (e.g., one with lissencephaly) cannot be housetrained to some extent.
- This behavior is spiteful.
  - The dog is largely unaware of urinating. No dog would choose to exhibit a behavior that gets him punished or renders the client angry as a way of "getting back" at the client.
- The dog is "dirty."
  - The only dogs who would choose to be soiled by their own excrement are those who have learned that they have no choice (e.g., puppy mill/farm dogs). These dogs are unaware of the urination.

Commonly Asked Client Questions
- Will the dog ever grow out of this?
  - Usually, yes, but clients can hasten the process by keeping the dog's excitement level below that which is associated with urination. By teaching the dog to be calm and attentive at a very young age, the client will only engender a better mannered dog.

Treatment
- Management:
  - As for dogs with "submissive" urination, these dogs should keep their bladders as empty as possible.
    - These dogs should have a chance to urinate before every interaction of any kind. This means greeting them with no fuss (and for some dogs that may mean no eye contact or tactile or verbal communication) and immediately guiding them to an area where they can safely urinate (a fenced yard or pen).
      - If the dog does not have an enclosed, safe area for off-lead urination, gently use a slip lead and collar as he moves through the door to restrain and guide him to the appropriate spot.
    - Reward the dog verbally when he has completed urination and is attentive. The dog should not be reached for until he has been taught which behaviors are rewarded when this occurs and which are neglected or ignored.
  - These dogs should never be reached for, even to put on a lead. Instead, they should be taught to sit and calmly look at anyone making a request of them for a treat.
    - If the dog begins to shift posture or leak when handed the treat, the treat can be tossed on the floor on the far side of the dog so that none of

the associations with the excitement urination postures are maintained.

- Behavior modification:
  - The standard behavior modification protocols, if practiced slowly and using the technique of shaping, will aid in treatment of the excitement urination.
  - Consistency is key and is difficult because these dogs are so excitable.
  - By not accidentally rewarding overly exuberant behaviors clients will encourage the dogs to offer calmer, more quiet behaviors.
  - Classic desensitization/counter-conditioning can be used to treat excitement urination.
- Medication/dietary intervention:
  - For some dogs, the addition of PPA or anti-anxiety medications may make it more difficult for them to leak.
  - Before using medication, ensure that the clients are adequately addressing the excitement behaviors using good, humane behavior modification.
- Miscellaneous interventions:
  - Diapering the dog may help the dog to associate his enthusiastic responses with the output of urine. This may be an essential step in helping the dog to make the connection.

Helpful Handouts

- "Protocol for Generalized Discharge Instructions for Dogs with Behavioral Concerns"
- "Protocol for Deference"
- "Protocol for Teaching Cats and Dogs to 'Sit,' 'Stay,' and Come'"
- "Protocol for Basic Manners Training and House-training for New Dogs and Puppies"
- "Protocol for Preventing and Treating Attention-Seeking Behavior"
- "Protocol for Teaching Your Dog to Take a Deep Breath and Use Other Biofeedback Methods as Part of Relaxation"
- "Protocol for Relaxation: Behavior Modification Tier 1"
- "Protocol for Using Behavioral Medication Successfully"

Last Words

- Treating the excitability is the key to treating the urination.
  - Keys to controlling the excitability include:
    - frequent walks so that the bladder is always as empty as possible,
    - teaching the dog to relax and to ignore excitable circumstances, and
    - once the clients are sure that the dog is house-trained and *does* have neuromuscular control, not interacting with the dog when he exhibits excitement urination.
  - The clients may do well by requesting that the dog perform an activity that is incompatible with

the excitement (lying down with the neck and chin fully extended).

- Very excitable, exuberant dogs often need more daily aerobic exercise. This can be provided by playing with Frisbees, agility training, high-jumping, or running with other dogs off lead in a safe, protected environment.

Attention-Seeking Behavior
Diagnostic Criteria and Description

- Use of vocal or physical behaviors to obtain passive or active attention from people when the people are engaged in passive or active activities not directly involving the dog.
- If needed, the intensity of the behaviors exhibited increase until the human activity is interrupted and attention is re-focused on the dog.
- Attention-seeking behavior may be the label used for what is simply an undesirable but potentially normal behavior. The key is to distinguish between *wanting* the attention versus *needing* the attention, regardless of context. If the latter, the attention-seeking behavior is not only abnormal, but also it is probably a correlate, sign, or subclass/endophenotype of another anxiety disorder.
- The key to understanding this behavior is that the specific behaviors exhibited are simply a means to engender human attention of any kind, whether or not that attention redresses concerns raised by the dog's behavior.
  - For example, a dog who appears to be choking may "recover" simply by being talked to and picked up, if the choking was symptomatic of attention-seeking behavior. Were the dog really choking it's unlikely that this intervention would be effective.

Common Non-Specific Signs

- vocalizing (barking, whining, crying, howling, et cetera),
- jumping on,
- pawing at,
- grabbing at,
- chewing on,
- eliminating in front of,
- exhibiting any other behavior in a context solely designed to re-direct people's attention to the dog, and
- dogs can learn to sneeze, cough, vomit, fall over, twitch, et cetera, if they have this condition and people rush to their side offering all kinds of inducements to encourage them to cease engaging in the behavior.

Rule Outs

- Medical rule outs include any somatic condition that could be a correlate of the behavior.
  - For example, if the dog is coughing and sneezing, it is important to rule out a respiratory tract infection.

- Attention-seeking behavior is a common co-morbid diagnosis. Any affected dog should be screened for other behavioral conditions.
  - Hyperactivity, hyper-reactivity, GAD, and impulse-control aggression are common conditions in which attention-seeking behavior may play a profound role.

Etiology, Epidemiology, and Risk Groups

- It's unclear if there are risk groups. People are quick to attribute many annoying "small dog" behaviors to attention-seeking behavior, but no rigorous studies have been done.

Common Myths That Can Get in the Way of Treatment or Diagnosis

- The dog is very fragile and needs constant attention.
  - Few dogs are sufficiently fragile to require nonstop attention.

Commonly Asked Client Questions

- Is he doing this to get back at me?
  - The appropriate response should be "for what"? Why would a client think that they had done something to engender an attention-seeking behavior? The answer to that question will likely allow the veterinarian to assess many aspects of behavioral care and husbandry.
- Is this because I spoiled him?
  - Many dogs do not live a depauperate life and never develop truly pathological attention-seeking behavior. Dogs can learn behaviors that get them attention that they want without this being pathological. Most of these dogs will be as creative as their humans tolerate. If we are discussing dogs who truly need to go through such gyrations because they always need attention, this is not due to anyone's interpretation of spoiling.

Treatment

- Management:
  - If the attention-seeking behavior is pesky but not pathological, it's best addressed with management. If people simply stop responding to the annoying behaviors, the dog will stop exhibiting them. This process is called *extinction*. Extinction is an extremely easy process to overcome because it is exposure-dependent. Please read the section on resistance to extinction in Chapter 3.
    - Resistance to extinction is powerful, so clients need to be aware of their behaviors and the dog's responses at all time.
      - The easiest way for a client to do this is to videotape themselves interacting with their dog in a number of contexts. The problematic scenarios and human responses will jump out at them.
  - If the attention-seeking behavior is pathological, the above pertains, but active behavior modification needed to teach the dog to become

calm and learn an entirely new way of communicating and interacting is needed.
- Behavior modification:
  - All behavior modification should focus on teaching the dog to be calm, to look to his humans for all the cues about the appropriateness of his behavior, and to modulate his response to any attention.
    - Classic desensitization and counter-conditioning exercises are useful in teaching the dog to react less effusively and to prolong the interval between seeing the stimulus (e.g., his person) and reacting. The key to addressing truly pathological attention-seeking behavior is to address the dog's overall reactivity. See the section on the role of reactivity in many behavioral diagnoses in Chapter 2.
  - Clients need to understand that much attention-seeking behavior is about asking questions and getting information. Accordingly, they should reward behaviors that they find acceptable with clear actions that convey helpful information and ignore any behaviors for which they cannot do this.
    - *This does not mean that clients should ignore the dog for any prolonged time until the dog ceases to note their existence. This very cruel advice is found in a number of places. Not only are most clients incapable of doing this, but this intervention could induce profound depression and learned helplessness. We do not need to break something to fix it.*
- Medication/dietary intervention:
  - Many newer nutraceuticals may help dogs who seek attention when mildly anxious. Because of the amount of neurocytotoxic damage that constant arousal may facilitate, supplementation with PUFAs (especially omega-3 fatty acids) is recommended.
  - If the attention-seeking behavior is truly pathological, it must be pharmacologically treated as a QoL issue. Additionally, this likely is a co-morbid diagnosis, and the other condition would also benefit from pharmacological intervention.
  - Common medications that may prove helpful include:
    - TCAs:
      - Amitriptyline
      - Clomipramine
      - Nortriptyline
    - SSRIs—the human literature suggests that SSRIs are helpful for improving attentional state:
      - Fluoxetine
      - Fluvoxamine
      - Paroxetine
      - Sertraline
    - SARIs:
      - Trazodone (preferentially with another medication since no controlled studies on trazodone use in dogs exist)

- Other:
  - Gabapentin
- BZDs:
  - Alprazolam
  - Clonazepam
- Central alpha-2 agonists
  - Clonidine
- Miscellaneous interventions:
  - Increased aerobic exercise may be a real boon to these animals, especially if it interferes with their ability to exhibit the attention-seeking behavior and involves an activity that the dog likes.
  - Having another dog who is normal to whom to compare the dog with attention-seeking behavior can help the client understand how odd the dog's behaviors are. Furthermore, if the client learns to work with a normal dog, they will be better able to help the problematic dog learn that only calm, contextual behaviors will be reinforced.
  - Many of these dogs do well in some form of structured class *if they enjoy the task*. Note that work and agility training can be self-rewarding and teach the dog other, calmer behaviors that are more suitable to reward.

Helpful Handouts

- "Protocol for Preventing and Treating Attention-Seeking Behavior"
- "Protocol for Generalized Discharge Instructions for Dogs with Behavioral Concerns"
- "Protocol for Deference"
- "Protocol for Teaching Your Dog to Take a Deep Breath and Use Other Biofeedback Methods as Part of Relaxation"
- "Protocol for Relaxation: Behavior Modification Tier 1"
- "Protocol for Teaching Cats and Dogs to 'Sit,' 'Stay,' and Come'"
- "Protocol for Teaching Kids—and Adults—to Play with Dogs and Cats"
- "Protocol for Choosing Toys for Your Pet"
- "Protocol for Using Behavioral Medication Successfully"

Last Words

- Because we assume that these dogs are being annoying to get attention, we may fail to see how truly distressed many of these dogs are. Truly pathological attention-seeking behavior may be an early warning sign that other anxiety-related conditions are on the horizon.

Rem Sleep/Rem Sleep Behavior Disorder

Diagnostic Criteria and Description

- REM sleep/sleep behavior disorder is a condition where the paralysis characteristic of REM sleep is absent or only partially penetrant, allowing action choreographed by dreams to occur.
- In both humans and dogs, common behaviors seen during REM sleep/sleep behavior disorder can be scary and fairly violent involving flailing, kicking, running, grabbing, biting, chasing, and loud vocalization.

Common Non-Specific Signs

- Dogs with REM sleep/REM sleep behavior disorder may exhibit any or all of the following behaviors:
  - vocalization including growling, snarling and snapping,
  - locomotion including running in place, running throughout the house, threatening, chasing, and "pinning" someone (canine or human), and
  - pawing, grabbing, biting, and shaking.

Rule Outs

- seizure activity of any kind,
- attention-seeking behavior,
- brain infarcts,
- neoplasia,
- encephalitis resulting from any cause,
- depression,
- C-PTSD, and
- true narcolepsy.
  - Narcolepsy involves deficits in orexins, the hypothalamic peptides involved in regulating wakefulness.
  - Narcolepsy in Labrador retrievers and Doberman pinschers studied to date involves lack of function of the orexin/hypocretin 2 receptor (Taheri et al., 2002).

Etiology, Epidemiology, and Risk Groups

- In humans, REM sleep/sleep behavior disorder is associated with neurodegenerative disease and may precede its diagnosis by a few years. No such data are available for dogs.
- Withdrawal from TCAs, especially imipramine, has been implicated in humans.
- Use of SSRIs may also be implicated for some percentage of affected humans, although as a percentage of those taking such medication, the risk should be small. We lack any of the data that would make even a comparable guess in dogs possible.
- In one case of idiopathic canine REM sleep/sleep behavior disorder (Bush et al., 2004), within 2 minutes of REM sleep the first sleep-associated behavioral event occurred. Because the dog was undergoing video EEG and recorded EEG, it's known that this dog was not having a seizure.
- The mesopontine area of the brainstem is thought to be relatively inactive during REM sleep, and decreases in 5-HT and NE/NA levels in the pontine tegmentum are thought to induce REM sleep and associated muscle relaxation. Any aspect of this pathway could be impaired in this condition (Lu et al., 2006).

Common Myths That Can Get in the Way of Treatment or Diagnosis

- The dog is acting out during sleep what he cannot do during the day.

- No. As hard as it is to believe, not everything our dogs do is about us. These dogs have a treatable pathology that is independent of us or the other pets in the household.

Commonly Asked Client Questions

- Is this dog dangerous?
  - This is an excellent question. Few cases of this condition have been reported (but see Bush et al., 2004), but injuries to humans and other dogs have been reported. Other dogs in the household have a lot of trouble understanding what is happening to their housemate and may be injured when they approach to see what's ongoing. Sometimes dogs who sleep next to or intertwined with the patient can be injured. Fear can become a sequela for them. Dogs who have this condition have been known to show re-directed aggression, only when thwarted during one of these events.

Treatment

- Management:
  - The dog must be protected from any damage he could do to himself, and others must be protected from any damage the dog could do to them.
    - This generally means that these dogs sleep separately in a padded area where striking, biting, or crashing into something is not going to hurt them.
  - If the dog can be safely awakened, it may be helpful to do so. If the dog is then walked or massaged, he may be able to go back to sleep without a return to the episodes.
- Behavior modification:
  - Pharmacological response is essential for full implementation of behavior modification, all of which is focused on teaching the dog to lower his arousal level generally and to be calm.
- Medication/dietary intervention:
  - Medication is an essential part of treatment of this condition. Helpful medications include:
    - BZDs:
      - Clonazepam is preferred over alprazolam because of the longer half-life.
    - TCAs may lower anxiety and help in some dogs but may further dysregulate the pontine system in other dogs.
      - Amitriptyline
      - Clomipramine
      - Nortriptyline
    - SSRIs may lower anxiety and help in some dogs but further dysregulate the pontine system in

other dogs. If the BZDs are not helpful, other medication choices should be rational but will involve trial and error.
- Fluoxetine
- Fluvoxamine
- Paroxetine
- Sertraline
- Other:
  - Gabapentin may help stimulate inhibitory pathways.
- Central alpha-2 agonists
- Clonidine has not been used for this condition, but it may decrease central arousal and so be beneficial in dogs who are otherwise unresponsive.

- Miscellaneous interventions:
  - Increased aerobic exercise may be helpful for these dogs, although it is not curative.
  - Clients often comment on their dog's dreams. Distinguishing between a very active dream and a REM sleep/sleep behavior disorder may be facilitated by gentle attempts to awaken the dog. If the dog does not stretch and return to sleep fairly quickly after having their dream disrupted and/or if the dog is impossible to awaken or becomes more forceful, assessment and putative treatment for a REM sleep/sleep behavior disorder should be sought.

Helpful Handouts

- "Protocol for Preventing and Treating Attention-Seeking Behavior"
- "Protocol for Deference"
- "Protocol for Teaching Your Dog to Take a Deep Breath and Use Other Biofeedback Methods as Part of Relaxation"
- "Protocol for Relaxation: Behavior Modification Tier 1"
- "Protocol for Using Behavioral Medication Successfully"
- "Protocol for Understanding, Managing, and Treating Dogs with Impulse-control Aggression"
- "Protocol for Understanding and Treating Re-Directed Aggression in Cats and Dogs"

Last Words

- Dogs who have had truly awful and scary experiences may have very bad nightmares. These outbursts are more likely to be associated with C-PTSD than with a REM sleep/sleep behavior disorder. Pursue an exhaustive history and treat accordingly.

Feline Behavior

Normal Feline Behavior and Ontogeny: Neurological and Social Development, Signaling, and Normal Feline Behaviors

OVERVIEW OF NORMAL CAT BEHAVIOR

Evolutionary History and the Cat's Relationship with People

If the story of dogs is the story of collaborative work with humans, *the story of cats is one of disease and theft-of-food control.* The domestic cat, *Felis catus,* is derived from *Felis libyca,* the African wildcat that is said to "tame" when taken into a household. Genomic cladistic analysis has grouped together a cluster of small cats— *F. catus* with *Felis silvestris* (the European wildcat), *F. libyca* (the African wildcat), *Felis bieti* (the Chinese desert cat), *Felis margarita* (desert cat), *Felis nigripes* (the black-footed cat), and *Felis chaus* (the jungle cat) (Johnson et al., 2006)—but *Felis silvestris lybica* wildcats from Israel, the United Arab Emirates, and Saudi Arabia are alone among those in the wildcat lineage because *they are genetically indistinguishable from domestic cats* (Driscoll et al., 2009). This means that *domestic cats must have arisen from a single location, the Middle East.* None of the cats we now recognize as "domestic" are derived from wildcats in any other locations.

The data suggest that approximately 6.2 million years ago, during the Miocene, movements between North America and Asia were facilitated by lower sea levels, several glaciations, and more temperate climate changes. At this time, ancestral cats could have moved into Africa and to the Middle East along with humans and microtene rodents—a food source for the ancestral cats.

This juxtaposition of cats, rodents, and humans likely allowed feline "domestication" about 10,000 years ago, which is 5000 to 25,000 years *later than for dogs,* using conservative estimates of domestic dog development. The cohabitation of these small, tamable cats and humans occurred at a time when agriculture was beginning to become established in the Middle East. *The establishment of agriculture may have been the key that united cats and humans, and both genetic and archeological data support this time period as the one when cats and humans began to live together in an exceptional form of "domestication"* (Driscoll et al., 2009).

As humans changed their behavior from a wholly nomadic/hunter gatherer lifestyle to one that was agrarian, they began to *store food that attracted rodents, and the rodents brought the cats with them.* The modern house mouse, *Mus musculus domesticus,* was among the species that emerged in these settlements 9000 to 10,000 years ago. Rodents carry disease and "steal" and foul food, but they also are just the right size to provide a meal for *F. catus,* who often acts as a sit-and-wait predator along rodent trails.

Cats were tolerated and/or encouraged—or at least not molested—because their foraging mode and food preferences benefited humans without risk and without requiring any effort by humans to get the cats to do their "job." The symbiotic/mutualistic relationship between cats and humans did *not* require that humans expand or modify innate feline behavior, and the force of that pattern is seen in the behavior of cats today.

- Feline predatory behavior and most of the other attendant social behaviors that cats exhibit in human households have been only slightly changed in their structure and behavioral elements since the cat was "domesticated."
- Because cats have had little direct influence on human economics (e.g., compared with that of hunting or herding dogs), there has been little intervention in their behavior by humans in the past hundred years (Young, 1985).
- Lack of selection for specific suites of behaviors ("behavioral domestication") also may be reflected in the range of body sizes for present-day cats. In the wild, the range of body sizes of wild cat species *greatly* exceeds the range of size of wild dog species, and the *range of body sizes* of domesticated dogs far surpasses that reported for wild canids. In contrast, the size range of domestic cats is relatively small and well within the range of body sizes reported for their wild counterparts. Even large domestic cats are relatively small compared with their wild relatives.

- The lack of human intervention is supported by coat color patterns. One of the most common feline coat colors, the tabby, has radiated worldwide, yet this color is extremely similar to that of the European wildcat and Norwegian forest cat.

The concept of the "domestication" of cats seems oxymoronic to many who share their lives with cats. People frequently joke that "we have dogs, but cats have us." It may help to consider that the word "domestication" is used to mean different things for the different groups of animals for which it is used:

- Dogs, with whom we evolutionarily first formed *true collaborative partnerships based on work*
- Stock, animals such as sheep, goats, cows, chickens, and horses, *who work for—not with—and/or serve us in the most utilitarian of contexts* (i.e., providing food, fiber, compelled labor, et cetera)

In the case of dogs and stock, it is clear that the animals involved had the behavioral and physiological qualities that met Galton's (1865) six conditions for domestication:

- hardy,
- easy to tend,
- inborn liking of humans,
- comfort-loving,
- useful to people, and
- breed freely.

These conditions ensured that artificial selection would allow humans to *alter physique, behaviors, and physiologies* in ways that helped or were desired by humans and that the *resultant derivative changes, as much as any of the conditions enumerated by Galton, are responsible for the condition of the domesticated species that we see today.*

For stock, we have altered looks, physiology, and some aspects of behavior, such as flight distance and tractability. For dogs, where we may well have a true co-evolutionary relationship, as part of selecting dogs for specific tasks and working with them in those tasks, we have facilitated neuromolecular changes that mirror those of humans (Saetre et al., 2004). This process of choosing desirable behaviors and physiologies and altering them in ways favorable to humans is at the core of the process of "domestication," and *it has not been traditionally involved in our relationship with cats until the most recent few hundred years.* The process of domesticating cats is *actively ongoing* and can be seen in the breeds developed in the past 50 years and in changes in coat length and texture, ear shape, social preferences, and physical and vocal behaviors.

F. catus lives in family groups and must have been present in sufficient density and proximity to *allow humans to observe aspects of their social systems and so to develop a relative level of comfort about feline behavior.* This proximity would not have been possible with larger, more muscular and powerful, more solitary, and more reclusive cats who would have posed a risk to humans because of their size, their dietary breadth, *and the* inability to observe all aspects of their behaviors. *This last part is important because, in contrast to dogs, cats do not have social systems that are readily identifiable as being analogues or homologues of human social systems.* Given the difference between human social systems and cat social systems, humans may be less able to extrapolate their signals to the cat and to communicate their desires to cats directly in a communal working relationship. Both cats and humans would have been—and still are—at risk for miscommunication. Cats are model carnivores. A truly symbiotic or collaborative relationship with a cat species larger than *F. silvestris libyca* would simply have been too risky.

The misunderstanding of cats is a serious humane concern. Cats continue to rise in popularity as pets worldwide. Cats are now the most popular pet in the world, with a third of U.S. households having at least 1 cat and 600 million cats living with humans worldwide (Driscoll et al., 2009).

BEHAVIORAL ONTOGENY IN CATS

Domestic Cat Social Grouping and Reproduction

The focus of feline social groups is invariably the female and her kittens. Most studies have concentrated on matrilineal relationships as the focus of the social grouping. Similar to lion prides, domestic cat groups are often composed of related females and their juvenile offspring. It has been postulated that this social pattern is driven by the reproductive pattern of female cats. See Table 8-1 for a summary of reproductive hallmarks.

TABLE 8-1

Hallmarks of Feline Reproductive Biology

Event	Time/Age
Males reach puberty	10 months
Females reach puberty	10 months—if born in late spring may delay cycle until following year
Minimum cycling frequency	3 weeks
Length of estrus with copulation	4 days
Length of estrus without copulation	9-10 days
Gestation	63 days—3-7 days longer than *F. silvestris libyca*
Capacitance period for sperm	24 hours
Time when ovulation occurs after copulation	24 hours
Re-entry into estrus if kittens die	15 days after their death

- Domestic cats reach puberty at about 10 months of age, although females born in the late spring may not cycle until the following year.
- Peaks in sexual activity occur from mid-January through March and from May to June in the Northern Hemisphere.
- Domestic cats are seasonally polyestrous and generally experience two cycles per year if not bred. *Domestic cats can cycle every 3 weeks for several months—a fact that may help the most reluctant client to consider neutering the cat.* Estrus in cats lasts 9 to 10 days in the absence of copulation but only 4 days if copulation occurs because cats are induced ovulators.
- Gestation in female domestic cats is approximately 63 days. This is longer, by 3 to 7 days, than the gestation period for *F. sylvestris libyca* (Hemmer, 1979; Schmidt et al., 1983). Litter sizes vary from 1 to 10 kittens with a mean of 4.5 kittens per litter. Most domestic cats allowed to do so have two litters per year (Liberg and Sandell, 1988), so *one cat may produce an average of nine kittens a year.* It is easy to understand how cities or neighborhoods with feral or semi-feral stray cat populations can be overwhelmed within a few years if the cats are left intact and have some access to shelter and food.
  - In one cohort study on the effect of trap-neuter-release (TNR) programs designed to decrease the number of unowned/feral cats for humane, public health, and conservation reasons, the mean number of kittens per litter was three (range, one to six). Fetus counts indicated a median litter size of 4, with a range of 1 to 10 kittens as reported (Liberg and Sandell, 1988). Before 6 months of age, 127 of 169 (75%) kittens born to the unneutered cohort died or disappeared, with trauma as the most common cause of death (Nutter et al., 2004).
- Cats usually have eight nipples. Only three pairs of these nipples may produce sufficient milk to provide nourishment for a kitten, and the back nipples are preferred by kittens (Rosenblatt, 1976). Teat preference is established by 1 to 3 days, when present, and 80% of all kittens develop a teat preference (Rosenblatt et al., 1961). Kittens identify their mother and their preferred nipple using innate and learned olfactory cues (Raihani et al., 2009). The effects of such patterns on early nutrition and neurodevelopment have not been investigated, but for cats who may be compromised, this pattern may lead to some kittens being under-nourished, a pattern that contributes to increased reactivity and later problematic behaviors (Carola and Gross, 2010; Green et al., 2011).
- Females form stable matriarchal groups and may join in communal nests and engage in shared care and nursing (Macdonald and Apps, 1978;

Macdonald et al., 1987). The queen moves the kittens if (1) the nest is fouled by feces, (2) undigested prey remains as the kittens get older, or (3) the site is disturbed by a strange male cat (Leyhausen, 1979).
- Queens stimulate kittens to eliminate by the ano-genital reflex until 23 to 39 days, and kittens can usually eliminate voluntarily by 3 weeks. This developmental change may be associated with the queen's mobile behaviors. Cats move kittens most frequently between 25 and 35 days (Schneirla et al., 1963).
- A familiar male may be such an integral part of the social group that he will guard against disturbances of foreign males (Macdonald et al., 1987). Communal nests may function in part to repel intruder males; however, they may also function to ensure that all kittens receive nourishment, should the number of nipples or the production of the milk be insufficient to support large litters. In a large farm study, males would provide care and succor for the kittens, if these males were residents within the larger social group (Macdonald et al., 1987).
- The presence of several reproductive males may facilitate communal care, including communal care provided by males (Kerby and Macdonald, 1988; Turner and Mertens, 1986). In such cases, no "dominant" male monopolizes all the matings (Natoli and de Vito, 1988). If males can neither monopolize all matings nor guarantee paternity, it might be advantageous for them to contribute to communal care. Many studies have shown that they are close to and will collaborate with females who are sisters and mothers (and possibly grandmothers) (Curtis et al., 2003). Males seldom provide lactating females with food or bring food directly to the kittens (Liberg, 1980), but they may care for the kittens, washing, guarding, and "nursing" them in non-nutritive relationships. It is now established that cats have "preferred associates" (Curtis et al., 2003), but these relationships go beyond the purported genetic ones.
- Females may further add to the stability of such social systems through their behavior during proestrus. During proestrus, females are attracted to males but are not receptive to their courtship behavior and reject attempts at copulation.
- It has been postulated that this is a device to enhance male-male competition (Bradshaw, 1992).
- *This proestrus behavior also provides females with the opportunity to assess the staying power and abilities of males.* In colonies that are sufficiently large, a proestrus that allows the females to evaluate males that are attracted to them would be one mechanism by which they could identify resident males and males with skills that may contribute to the best outcomes for the young.
- Finally, if the females are attractive to a number of males and all those males are part of the colony, that behavioral interaction could help facilitate

communal care. In such cases, there may be an element of uncertainty of paternity, but copulation could then act to solidify social relationships where individuals "within" the group are treated differently than individuals considered "outside" the group. There are no data on whether animals known to the group are less likely to practice infanticide or more likely to provide communal care; there are even fewer data on whether the extent of a genetic or social relationship makes a difference for either of these factors. It has been postulated that males within colonies could be related. If this were the case, *infanticide would not be an appropriate genetic strategy* and would likely not enhance any single male cat's genetic contribution because insemination by a brother would also be genetically advantageous.

- Relatedness has become a fascinating issue because ovulation is induced and estrus for any queen lasts only about 4 to 5 days (Natoli and de Vito, 1988, 1991; Paape et al., 1975; Schmidt et al., 1983).
  - Liberg (1983) noted that at the peak of fertilization the queen was monopolized by the "dominant" male in the group. Females can thwart this guarding by allowing younger, lighter males to mate before mating with the older, heavier male, resulting in some mixed paternity litters, and colonies where almost half the kittens are not fathered by the putative "dominant" male (Yamane, 1998).
  - A 24-hour capacitance period is necessary for cat sperm, and the female ovulates 24 hours after copulation (Hamner et al., 1970), so a solitary copulation may not be sufficient to induce females to ovulate and to ensure that sperm capacitance occurs at the time of ovulation.
  - This physiological pattern could argue strongly for either the guarding effect noted by Liberg (1983) or the effect hinted at by Bradshaw (1992) and found by Yamane (1998) in which multiple males might possibly contribute to insemination and, indirectly, to the stability of the social group in groups where males provide a portion of the communal care for the young. *It is conceivable that both modes function depending on the demography of the group and the resources available to it.* Social structure is influenced by both the age and the sex structure of the group and will interact with the resource, predation, and physical and biophysical environments to affect behaviors.
- The issue of infanticide may be a concern in free-ranging groups and in breeding catteries. In domestic cats, weaning normally starts at approximately day 30 and continues through day 60 of the kitten's life. If kittens die, regardless of the cause of death, the queen enters estrus approximately 15 days later (Liberg and Sandell, 1988). *Under normal circumstances, cats might have two litters a year; if there is a litter death, the inter-birth interval can be only 133 days.* Infanticide in domestic cats has been rarely observed directly (for exceptions see Dards [1983] and Liberg [1983]). An evolutionary argument can be made for the occurrence of infanticide in *unstable groups* or in *groups that experience a cataclysmic change in the social structure.* Females are induced ovulators, and the basis of social communal relationships may be influenced by the relatedness of the colony (Packer et al., 1991). There are no hard data to support this view of infanticide, and *it would be inappropriate to assume that all of the social relationships within feline groups are driven by direct genetic relationships.*

In summary, cats are social, their social relationships are complex and incompletely understood, and their patterns of group sociality differ from those of dogs and humans.

Weaning Period

Weaning is complete at approximately 60 days, and by week 12, milk quality has substantially changed. The kittens begin to accompany their mother on hunting expeditions with increasing frequency between 8 and 16 weeks of age.

Kittens in wild groupings often stay with their mother until at least 6 months or 1 year of age and then disperse. During this intermediate period, should they stay with the mother or with the mother's social group, the kittens often form independent social associations (Leyhausen, 1979; Macdonald et al., 1987). After approximately 10 to 14 months of close association with the mother and her social coterie, the kittens experience what has been described as a "social" weaning from the group (Wolski, 1982).

It has been postulated that this extended "weaning" period provides protection from harassment from the breeding tom or toms in the group. This explanation appears simple given the complexity of the social and breeding groups already described. It is more likely that dispersal is regulated by the same factors that govern dispersal in other free-ranging populations of non-domestic animals—the interaction of the demographic, predation, resource, and physical and biophysical environments. As cats enter and move through the period of "social maturity," they may experience the brain chemistry changes that allow them to become increasingly independent.

Early Neurobehavioral Development

For cats, we lack many of the detailed ontogenetic data available for dogs, but the landmarks that are well established are included here and summarized in Table 8-2.
- The tactile sense is present early in gestation.
- Kittens are born unable to see but locomote freely.

TABLE 8-2

Developmental Hallmarks and Periods, including Sensitive Periods and Associated Neurodevelopmental and Behavioral Landmarks*

Developmental Hallmark or Ability	Period/Age
Tactile sensitivity fully developed	Day 24 *of gestation*
Vestibular righting reflex developed	Day 54 *of gestation*
Teat preference established	1-3 days
Purring begins	2 days
Eyes open	10-14 days
High-pitched calls by kittens to summon queen peak	1 week
Age at which separation from mother leads to fearful and aggressive behavior to cats and humans	2 weeks
Age at which exposure to low temperature influences the rate of temperature regulation development	2 weeks
Periods of quiescence found in EEG activity	2 weeks
Age at which ultrasonic calls are given by kittens when exploring the nest	Through 3 weeks
Age at which exposure to low temperature ceases to influence the rate of temperature regulation development	4 weeks
Closeness of other kittens has a calming effect	2-4 weeks
Kittens able to recognize mothers by sight and smell	End of 3 weeks
Queen begins to teach predatory behavior	3 weeks
Queen stimulates elimination via anogenital reflex	23-29 days
Kittens eliminate voluntarily	3 weeks
Age at which singleton kittens emerge from nest box	3-7 weeks
Queen starts to bring kittens solid food	4 weeks
Free-ranging cats bring kittens live prey	By ~4 weeks
Normal social play behavior starts	3-4 weeks
Age at which if kittens are exposed to another species (e.g., Chihuahua dog), they will show no fear at 12 weeks	4 weeks
Age through which kittens cannot retract their claws	4 weeks
Age at which kittens will use scratching material if it is provided	5 weeks
Kittens can kill mice on their own	~5 weeks
Kittens moved by queen most frequently	25-35 days
Early period for social play	2-5 weeks
Defensive response toward large and difficult prey develops	During month 2
Kittens independent in their ability to eliminate and find substrates suitable for elimination (the appropriate materials should be provided)	5-6 weeks
Adult-like response to visual and olfactory stimuli, including to silhouettes of adult cats and adult cat urine	~6 weeks
Middle period for social play	5-7 weeks
Gape/flehmen response appears	~6 weeks
Gape/flehmen response fully developed	7 weeks
Age by which if kittens are handled regularly, they will approach unfamiliar objects rapidly and spend more time with them at 4-7 months	Birth to 45 days
Age at which if kittens are handled by numerous people (five people in the study), they will show less fear and more interest in people later	5.5-9.5 weeks
Peak in EEG activity	6-8 weeks
Kittens can respond to an olfactory challenge	7 weeks
Kittens begin to cover their urine or feces if they are going to do so	7 weeks
Queen ceases to bring kittens solid food	7 weeks

TABLE 8-2

Developmental Hallmarks and Periods, including Sensitive Periods and Associated Neurodevelopmental and Behavioral Landmarks—cont'd

Developmental Hallmark or Ability	Period/Age
Male kittens engage in twice the object play as females	By 7 weeks
Eye-paw coordination honed/object play	7-8 weeks
Late period for social play	7-10 weeks
Kittens completely weaned	60 days
Male and female kittens similar in mass and behavior	Until ~8 weeks
Male kittens become larger than females	Beginning at ~8 weeks
Social relationships that provide the context for future communal suckling	During first 2 months
Object play increases	By 60 days
Complex motor activity fully functional	10-12 weeks
Milk quality changes	12 weeks
No sex differences in social play behavior	4-12 weeks
Pounce, belly-up, and stand-up displays 90% effective in obtaining a play response from another kitten	6-12 weeks
Social play patterns become more associated with predatory behavior and social fighting	By 12 weeks
Handling kittens for only 15 minutes a day produces kittens more solicitous of people	Birth to 12-14 weeks
Post–social play period	14 weeks
Social fighting may start	14 weeks
Sex differences appear in social play behavior	12-16 weeks
Litters composed entirely of females are less aggressive in their play than all-male litters	12-16 weeks
Social play behavior begins to decline	12-14 weeks
Feral cats abandon kittens	As early as 4 months
Free-ranging males demonstrate sexual behavior	19 weeks
Amplitude and absolute power of EEGs decrease to adult levels	20-24 weeks
Free-ranging females demonstrate sexual behavior	23 weeks
Male cats reach adult weight	3 years
Female cats reach adult weight	2 years
Age at which male cats will stop squatting and start spraying unless inhibited from doing so by the social environment	8-10 months
Puberty	10 months
"Social weaning" from maternal group may occur	10-14 months

*Note: These periods indicate when cats are first most receptive to the noted stimuli. There is no implication that cats ever stop learning from their experience. See text for references.
EEG, Electroencephalogram.*

- Kittens 2 to 4 weeks old exhibit plasticity physiologically and behaviorally. Exposure to low temperature can influence the rate of temperature regulation development at 2 weeks of age, but this effect is lost by 4 weeks (Jensen et al., 1980). This observation reinforces the extent to which early ontogeny is important in cats.
- Eye opening, between 10 and 14 days, is affected both by the environment and by genetics. Kittens of young mothers appear to open their eyes earlier than kittens of older mothers. Female kittens tend to open their eyes slightly earlier than males, but there also appears to be a strong paternal genetic effect on timing of eye opening (Bateson and Turner, 1988; Turner et al., 1986). This is probably not independent of the paternal effect on "boldness" (McCune, 1992).
- Electroencephalogram (EEG) activity in cats has periods of quiescence at 2 weeks, but EEG activity is continuous by 4 weeks. A peak in EEG activity occurs between 6 and 8 weeks, suggesting a

neurodevelopmental shift, but amplitude and absolute power of EEGs do not reach approximate adult values until 20 to 24 weeks of age (Lewis et al., 2011).

- Kittens can recognize their mothers by sight and smell by the end of the third week of age (Martin and Bateson, 1988).
- By about 6 weeks of age, kittens demonstrate an adult-like response to visual and olfactory social stimuli, including silhouettes of adult cats and the scent of adult cat urine (Kolb and Nonneman, 1975). At about this time, the gape (flehmen) response to cat urine appears; this becomes fully expressed by 7 weeks of age. It has been postulated that the gape response, in its full adult form, is an indication of the maturation of the vomeronasal organ.
- The classic adult threat posture of tail down, arched back, and erect ears is often seen concomitant with the development of the gape/flehmen response and appears at about the same time (Kolb and Nonneman, 1975).
- Kittens can learn from firsthand, trial-and-error experience and by watching other cats. They are quicker at observational learning if they are watching their mother (Chesler, 1969; John et al., 1968), suggesting that there may be a role for very elegant, complex, and detailed signaling behaviors that have not been studied.
- The role of early social exposure in learning is also suggested by experimental results derived from maze problem-solving tests (Hebb-Williams closed field test). Alley cats achieve much higher scores than housecats, but they also make more errors (Pollard et al., 1971).

Effect of Deprivation on Ontogeny

- Cats isolated from other cats from birth until 7 months of age are slow to accept introduced cats (Kolb and Nonneman, 1975; Konrad and Bagshaw, 1970).
- Kittens who are isolated from other kittens until late in their first year of life display exaggerated autonomic responses characterized by galvanic skin responses and disruption of regular sleep rhythms (Wenzel, 1959).
- Neonatal isolation leads to changes in normal pain response in dogs (Melzack and Scott, 1957), but it is correlated *with increased aggression in cats and rats* (Guyot et al., 1983).
- Kittens artificially *separated from their mothers at about 2 weeks of age become fearful and aggressive toward both other cats and people,* demonstrate random locomotion, and learn poorly (Bacon, 1973; Seitz, 1959).

Effects of Litter Size on Ontogeny

- Singleton kittens are quicker to emerge from nest boxes, between 3 and 7 weeks (Mendl, 1988), and appear to show little distress when left alone.

- Two kittens, when left by their mother, appear all right while together, but if the kittens are separated and then left by their mother, they appear more distressed than a singleton kitten that is left alone (Mendl, 1988). Most variation in individual behavior is probably not attributable to litter composition (Deag et al., 1988).

Factors Affecting Ontogeny of Feeding Behaviors

- By the time the kittens are about 4 weeks of age, the queen starts to bring them solid food, representing the beginning of the weaning phase (Ewer, 1961; Kovach and Kling, 1967; Martin and Bateson, 1988). This phase is completed by 7 weeks of age.
- *Kittens who are nursed on a breeder nipple* nurse normally but will not be permitted to nurse on a lactating queen because they give inappropriate social responses to her (Rosenblatt et al., 1961). These kittens can *form social attachments to other kittens, but they do so slowly.* The extent to which these slow social attachments and inappropriate social responses to lactating queens may affect their own ability to raise kittens has not been investigated. Such scenarios might be an important factor in the abandoned, feral cat population in which a decreased plane of nutrition and early abandonment may be common.
- *Kittens who are weaned early also develop predatory behavior far earlier* than do normally weaned kittens and are more likely to be mouse killers (Tan and Counsilman, 1985; Warren and Levy, 1979). Late weaning of kittens appears to delay predatory behavior and decreases the propensity to kill mice. This association may be indicative of nonspecific learning in response to the most common prey (mice), but the implications of this are important for people who are going to hand-rear cats. People who hand-raise early-weaned kittens might experience problems with earlier predatory behavior.

Ontogeny of Elimination Behaviors

- By about 5 to 6 weeks of age, kittens are totally independent in their ability both to eliminate and to start to find substrates resembling the ancestral substrate for elimination.
  - For the first 3 to 5 weeks, the queen stimulates the kittens to eliminate and cleans up after them.
  - By 3 to 5 or 6 weeks of age, kittens begin to seek open, well-drained substrates and use them for both urination and defecation (Fox, 1975).
  - Covering of urine or feces may not occur—the ancestral condition is to spray urine a large percentage of the time, and feces may not be covered in many arid environments. Feces are often used

as signposts for territorial delineation (Wemmer and Scow, 1977), but it may also be possible to make a case for disease control when feces are left exposed. When feces are exposed, disease transmission is decreased, and parasites are killed in arid environments.

- If the cats are going to cover their urine and feces, they appear to start to do so about the same time they are able to respond fully to an olfactory challenge, at approximately 7 weeks of age. No quantitative data exist for age-specific elimination behaviors in cats.

- As late as 13 to 18 months of age, young males may only squat to urinate (Wolski, 1982), suggesting a strong social component for spraying. It is rare for free-ranging males to show urine marking in paternal areas. Housecats who are not interacting in these social environments usually stop solely squatting at about 8 to 10 months of age.

ONTOGENY OF SOCIAL BEHAVIOR AND ROLE FOR NUTRITION

- The most significant side effect of early weaning might be on play behavior. Under normal conditions, object play increases by the second month (Bateson, 1978; Dumas, 1992), but under early-weaning conditions generated by gradual separation, the administration of bromocriptine (a dopamine antagonist that stops lactation) (Bateson and Young, 1981), or decrease in the maternal food supply, certain types of play show an early increase (Bateson and Young, 1981; Martin, 1984; Martin and Bateson, 1985). These changes may be adaptive responses to forced independence.

- *Queens fed 50% of their* ad libitum *intake during the second half of gestation and for the first 6 weeks postpartum* produce kittens with abnormal play behavior. Afflicted *kittens have more accidents during play, the males demonstrate increased aggression during social play, and the females demonstrate less climbing and more running behavior; also, the cerebrum, cerebellum, and brainstem do not appear to grow at the same rate as the rest of the brain.* The brain and body appear to achieve normal size once rehabilitated with food, but the extent to which there might be long-lasting effects on attachment has not been fully explored (Smith and Jansen, 1977a, 1977b, 1977c).

- *When maternal food intake at gestation is 50% of normal,* this produces *kittens with delays in postural corrections, crawling, suckling, eye opening, running and walking, and play and climbing* (Simonson, 1979). These kittens also have *delayed predatory and exploratory behaviors* and experience the growth stunting that becomes apparent only after weaning. The greatest behavioral delays appear in behaviors that regulate coordination, and these kittens have *poor learning ability,* *increased reactivity, abnormal fear and aggression, and a decreased responsiveness to normal environments.*

- *Low-protein diets late in gestation and during lactation* correlate with delayed development; kittens that experienced these restricted diets are *uncoordinated and exhibit fewer social interactions with their mothers and poorer attachment responses to their mothers* (Gallo et al., 1980, 1984).

- Social relationships that provide the context for future communal suckling develop within the first 2 months after birth (Macdonald and Apps, 1978). These relationships are adversely affected by these nutritional situations.

- Cats who are abandoned and may become feral or cats born to mothers that are abandoned and possibly feral develop abnormal social behaviors. *The combination of poor learning, increased reactivity, out-of-context and more intense than normal reaction in any foreign circumstance, abnormal fear accompanied by aggression, and decreased ability to respond in normal situations may render these animals poor candidates for both rehabilitation and for pets.* "Good Samaritans" should be aware of these associations and have realistic expectations.

- Well-nourished male and female kittens are similar in mass and behavior until about 8 weeks of age. Thereafter, males are larger than females (Liberg, 1983). Males take 3 years to reach their adult weight, whereas females take only 2 years. This occurrence is associated with the period during which cats mature socially.

- Under normal conditions, feline tactile sensitivity is fully developed by the 24th day of gestation, and the vestibular righting reflex is developed by the 54th day of gestation. It is unknown how early in gestation the effects of dietary restriction are manifest.

These findings are in line with findings from research showing that early and *in utero* deprivation cause long-lasting detrimental effects on behavior, promoting hyper-reactivity and anxiety (Carola and Gross, 2010; Green et al., 2011). We do not know whether there are epigenetic effects that shape behavior transgenerationally as has been found in other species (Radtke et al., 2011), but there is no reason why cats should be exempt. Such risks may be most profound for feral and/or homeless cats.

The effects of weaning on behavior are summarized in Table 8-3.

Ontogeny of Play and Predatory Behavior

The play behavior of kittens has been extensively studied, in part because of the potential association between play and predatory behavior in cats. The rich, imaginative type of play in which kittens engage is one of the appeals of having a kitten. Although play changes with age (Table 8-4), cats do not stop playing as they

TABLE 8-3

Effects of Early Weaning

Event	Effects
Early weaning	Object and other types of play appear before 2 months
Queen fed 50% of *ad libitum* intake during second half of gestation and 6 weeks postpartum	Abnormal play that includes more accidents; more aggression from males during social play; more climbing and running behavior by females; slowed growth of the cerebrum, cerebellum, and brainstem
Queen fed 50% of intake at gestation	Kittens experience delays in postural corrections, crawling, suckling, eye opening, running and walking, play and climbing Delayed predatory and exploratory behaviors Growth stunting in kittens that is apparent only after weaning Delays in behaviors associated with coordination Poor learning ability, increased reactivity, abnormal fear and aggression, decreased responsiveness to normal environments
Low-protein diets late in gestation and during lactation	Delayed development Uncoordinated and fewer social interactions with mothers Poorer attachment response to mothers

Note: See text for references.

TABLE 8-4

Developmental Hallmarks in Play and Predatory Behavior

Age	Hallmark Behaviors
3-4 weeks	Social play begins
4 weeks	Free-ranging queens begin to bring kittens live prey as weaning begins
5 weeks	Kittens can start to kill mice on their own
5-8 weeks	Predisposition to respond defensively toward large and difficult prey develops
6 weeks	Vertical stance elicits play from a littermate 8% of time
7 weeks	Males engage in twice the object play that females do
7-8 weeks	Real honing of social play associated with development of eye-paw coordination
4-12 weeks	No sex differences in social play
12-16 weeks	Sex differences in social play appear
12-16 weeks	Litters comprising only females play differently than all-male litters
10-11 weeks	Complex motor activity fully functional
12-16 weeks	Social play declines
≥12 weeks	Social play patterns change into social fighting and predatory behavior
6 weeks	Side-step posture elicits play 20% of the time
12 weeks	Side-step posture elicits play 3% of the time
6-12 weeks	Pounce, belly-up, and stand-up behaviors are 90% effective in eliciting play from another kitten
12 weeks	Vertical stance elicits play from a littermate 24% of the time
4 months	Age at which feral cats may abandon their kittens
6 months	Age at which cats that did and did not play with small objects as kittens were tested for differences in predatory skills; no difference was found

age if they have someone with whom to play. *The character of the play alters, but cats can continue to be playful given the appropriate stimulation.*

- Sex differences in social play appear by weeks 12 to 16 but are not present between weeks 4 and 12 (Barrett and Bateson, 1978).
- *Females who play with males become more male-like in their play behavior than females who play with females*

(Caro, 1981a, 1981b). Whether this factor affects later aggressive play behavior for females raised with male siblings only has not been investigated.

- Normal social play starts at approximately 3 to 4 weeks of age when the kitten can ambulate. It is honed when eye-paw coordination is developed at approximately 7 to 8 weeks of age (Barrett and Bateson, 1978; Martin and Bateson, 1985).

- Complex motor activity is fully functional by 10 to 11 weeks (Villablanca and Olmstead, 1979).
- Social play begins to decline at about 12 to 14 weeks of age (Caro, 1981a; West, 1974, 1979).
- Social play patterns become more associated with predatory behavior and social fighting by the third month, possibly concomitant with a change in systems that control motor behavior (Caro, 1980b, 1981b; Pellis et al., 1988; West, 1979).
- Many motor patterns in play resemble motor patterns for hunting (Caro, 1979, 1980a, 1980c), but there is no definitive link with play as "practice" behavior for predatory skills and the development of those skills later in life except to the extent that we all learn from experience in any social situation in which we are placed (Martin, 1984).
- Cats deprived of play still develop predatory behavior (Baerends-van Roon and Baerends, 1979).
- Cats who did not or could not play with small objects as kittens appear to be no different than other cats when examined with regard to predatory skills at 6 months of age (Caro, 1980b), but *cats are still more likely to kill the types of prey that they had known since kittenhood* (Caro, 1980a).
- The predisposition to respond defensively toward large and difficult prey develops some time during the second month (Adamec et al., 1983).
- Free-ranging domestic cats start to bring their kittens live prey about 4 weeks of age, coincident with the beginning of the weaning.
- Kittens can start to kill mice on their own at approximately 5 weeks of age (Baerends-van Roon and Baerends, 1979).
- *It is not inevitable that cats will hunt, especially if they are not weaned early and if they are not taught to do so by their mothers.* The presentation of *palatable food starting at kittenhood may inhibit hunting,* although the behaviors of killing and eating are separately, centrally controlled (Adamec, 1975b, 1976a, 1976b).
- Although individually controlled, there is some interaction between killing and eating, which is substantiated by interactions between areas of the lateral and ventromedial hypothalamus. The ability to inhibit hunting through the presentation of palatable foods early in life and throughout life may be important for clients who do not wish their cats to hunt.
- *The tendency to kill when hunting or to exhibit hunting behavior increases with hunger* (Biben, 1979) and decreases when prey is more difficult to capture.
- Population control at the community level plays a role in hunting behaviors. Females with kittens to feed tend to be far more adept hunters than females who do not have kittens (Turner and Meister, 1988). It has been postulated that this facilitation is a dopaminergic/prolactin response.

- *Weanling kittens eat food preferred by their mother* even though that food may not be a common food in cat diets (Wyrwicka, 1978).
- *Kittens appear to be able to learn to kill a rat by watching another cat do so* (Kuo, 1930). They also learn a preference at this stage and restrict their preference to the strain of rat with which they are familiar.
- Competition within litters may also hone some predatory skills (Caro, 1980a, 1980b, 1980c), and some cats appear to be able to "catch up" to more skilled littermates during ontogeny (Caro, 1980b).
- *Cats can learn about a variety of tasks through observation and may learn more quickly if it is their mother they are observing. This finding has profound and helpful applications for clients adopting kittens who may also be able to adopt the mother.*
- The tendency for cats to retrieve their young in response to high-pitched vocalization peaks at 1 week after parturition (Schneirla et al., 1963). Early in life (during the first 3 weeks), kittens use ultrasonic calls as they explore their nest (cited in Deag et al., 1988). These calls may function in helping their caretakers locate them and keep them together.
- Eight kitten play postures have been identified (West, 1974):
  - belly-up,
  - stand-up,
  - side-step,
  - pounce,
  - vertical stance,
  - chase,
  - horizontal leap, and
  - face-off.
- Behaviors, some of which are associated with later predatory behavior, that are most successful in eliciting play from another kitten are the pounce (39% of all play-eliciting behaviors), the belly-up display (14% of all play-eliciting behaviors), and the stand-up (16% of all play-eliciting behaviors). These behaviors are 90% effective in obtaining a response from another kitten between 6 and 12 weeks of age.
- As the cat matures, other behaviors become important in the play elicitation communication repertoire. The vertical stance elicits play behavior only 8% of the time at 6 weeks of age, but by 12 weeks of age it elicits play response from another littermate 24% of the time. In contrast, the side-step posture elicits play 20% of the time at 6 weeks of age but only 3% of the time at 12 weeks of age (West, 1979). It is important to emphasize these normal changes in communicatory and play behavior to clients because potential problems in communication could arise when people play too roughly with their kittens. Clients need to know appropriate, age-specific play behaviors.
- In his study of singleton litters, Mendl (1988) found that *singleton kittens did not engage more frequently in*

self-play or object play than kittens in litters of two. This finding suggests that social and object play should be separately driven.

- Solitary kittens directed all of their play toward the mother; given that the mother is more likely to be absent from the nest than a sibling would, singleton kittens might experience less social play.
- *Between 2 and 4 weeks of age, the particular closeness experienced by kittens to other kittens has a calming effect* (Rosenblatt et al., 1962).
- *Physical contact with the queen, particularly nuzzling of the face, has a calming effect on kittens* (Beaver, 1992). These observations have implications for early weaning.
- *Kittens are weaned* early if the queen cannot provide enough food; this *results in stimulation of the early development of both object and social play* (Bateson et al., 1990).
- In the case of early weaning, the siblings and the mother are still present; their presence could have a significant effect on the extent to which rough play might be modulated. In the usual, non-experimental situation involving early weaning, the mother is no longer present. No studies have been done on whether these two types of early weaning have different effects on inappropriate play behavior or the early development of predatory aggression in cats. It is likely that early weaning that also precludes the social interaction of an older, experienced cat could foster more inappropriate play behavior and play aggression.
- Feral cats often abandon kittens by about 4 months of age. At this time, the kittens increase their environmental exploration.
- Barrett and Bateson (1978) noted *that males engage in twice the object play as females by 7 weeks of age,* and by 19 weeks of age these free-ranging males are demonstrating sexual behavior.
- Female kittens usually do not demonstrate sexual behavior until 23 weeks of age. Litters composed solely of females appear to be less aggressive in their play than all-male litters; this difference is recognizable by weeks 12 to 16.
- West (1979) postulated that the function of play, rather than teaching cats to be better predators later in life, might be to keep litters together when the litter is vulnerable; this would enhance their ability to develop good social relationships that might serve to redress vulnerability later in life. No studies have directly addressed this issue, but the work of Macdonald et al. (1987) suggests that this might be so.

FACTORS AFFECTING FEEDING BEHAVIORS

- *Odor* is sufficiently important for feline feeding behavior that the odor of a palatable food (cooked rabbit) *can initiate feeding in the absence of any change in food offered* (Robinson, 1992a).
- *Moisture determines meal size and eating speed* (Robinson, 1992a). If a cat's diet is diluted with water, the cat compensates by eating more (Castonguay, 1981; Mugford, 1977). This effect is not found if inert substances such as kaolin or cellulose are added to the diet (Hirsch et al., 1978; Kanarek, 1975)—hence the basis for low-calorie cat foods.
- Wet food is initially consumed quickly, followed by a subsequent decrease in feeding rate. Dry, calorically dense food is consumed at a slower, more consistent rate. It is unclear whether the costs of handling affect this comparison.
- The preferred food temperature is 35° C—this may be the temperature that most effectively releases volatile fatty acids.
- Cats gain and lose mass cyclically (Randall and Lasko, 1968). This pattern may be associated with their annual cycles of corticosteroid, thyroxine, and epinephrine, which peak in the winter (Anderson, 1973; Randall et al., 1975). Regardless, cats appear to regulate the intake of energy, not volume or mass (Robinson, 1992a). For commercial dry foods (360 kcal/100 g), an average meal contains 22.7 to 31.3 kcal. Cats eat an average meal of 35.5 kcal from fresh meat (136 kcal/100 g), 30.2 to 44.8 kcal from canned meat (80 to 90 kcal/100 g), 19.8 to 32.5 kcal from canned meat and cereal (115 kcal/100 g), and 30.1 kcal from semi-moist food (320 kcal/g) (Robinson, 1992a).
- *One unpleasant food experience can lead to rejection of that food for months* (Houpt, 1982; Macdonald et al., 1984, 1985). Cats have a requirement for thiamine (particularly with a carbohydrate-rich diet). The first symptom of thiamine deficiency could be anorexia. A single arginine-deficient meal can lead to ammonium intoxication, causing emesis and lethargy. Such factors are usually redressed by commercial cat foods, but young animals with abnormal eating patterns may not ingest sufficient food to modulate these concerns. A thorough investigation is warranted in the case of any young kitten that does not eat and thrive.

EARLY SOCIAL DEVELOPMENT AND AGE-SPECIFIC EFFECTS ON FRIENDLINESS AND EXPLORATORY BEHAVIOR

In 1937, Lorenz defined a "critical period" with regard to imprinting. Implicit in the definition was a definitive onset and offset. During these critical periods, animals were postulated to be able to learn to respond to certain stimuli, and before and after these periods animals were unable to respond to the stimuli. The concept of a critical period was modified by Bateson (1979). Instead, Bateson defined a *"sensitive period"* as an age *range during which particular events are especially likely to have long-term effects on individual development.* A sensitive period may *best be defined as the period of time when you are best able to attend to and be affected by the relevant stimuli, which, when missed, puts you at risk for concerns pertaining to those stimuli.* This concept is particularly relevant for developing parts of the nervous system (i.e., visual cortex) that rely on stimuli to direct their development (Rauschecker and Marler, 1987). For example, exposure to contours of only one orientation can have long-term effects on the visual system. Whether any period is "critical" versus "sensitive" may be a matter of our scale of measurement. We should be mindful that there is almost always more variation and plasticity in any behavior and its development than is commonly thought.

Although the concept of a sensitive period can be useful when applied to the ontogeny of neural development, it has been grossly misapplied in discussing the development of kitten and puppy behavior. *The concept of a "sensitive period" has been transferred, almost without critical thought, to be synonymous with a "socialization period."* It is most valuable to use the concept of a sensitive period in terms of risk assessment.

- Animals are not behaviorally or developmentally able to respond to all stimuli when they are born.
- They can begin to respond to certain stimuli within certain broad periods.
- There is a considerable amount of variability in response to specific stimuli both within and between litters.
- Missing the appropriate stimuli (those to which the individual is now capable of responding) during these periods does not guarantee a "poorly socialized" animal; however, the *risk of inappropriate contextual responses* increases with increased deprivation.
- Animals should *be exposed to all relevant social stimuli early and in a non-traumatic manner.* When the individual animal is developmentally ready to learn from the stimulus, it will do so.
- No harm results from the presence of any stimulus (i.e., other cats, humans) before the time that the animal is best able to attend to it, *if no undue trauma or fear is involved.*
- Animals experiencing all of the appropriate "socialization" may still have behavioral problems.
- Although sensitive periods have been less emphasized in the importance of the development of good pet cat behavior than have sensitive periods in the importance of good pet dog behavior, *feline sensitive periods may be shorter, more discreet, and more frequently legitimately implicated in the development of behavioral problems such as play aggression, inappropriate play behavior, and fear aggression.*
- Karsh (1983a, 1983b, 1984) provided baseline data about "sensitive" periods and defined the specific behavioral changes that can occur within the above-outlined time frames for kittens reared in a laboratory situation.
  - Kittens that were handled by people for only 15 minutes a day from birth through 12 to 14 weeks of age spent more time exploring the person and giving head rubs and would leave and return several times.
  - Kittens in home-reared litters that were held 1 to 2 hours a day, if brought to the laboratory, would go directly to people and climb onto their lap, purr, and go to sleep. These behaviors were not seen in the laboratory kittens, although laboratory kittens were not fearful of people. The home-reared kittens were *handled four to eight times longer* than the laboratory kittens, but they were *also exposed to a more varied and unpredictable environment than the laboratory kittens.*
  - It would be inappropriate to over-interpret these results, but it is probably fair to say that the earlier the kittens are handled and the more they are handled, the more friendly they are likely to be.
- The number of handlers that each kitten experiences appears to influence the extent to which it is "friendly" (Collard, 1967). This finding may have implications for the social development of cats in small or very large litters.
- When kittens are handled regularly for the *first 45 days of their life, they approach unfamiliar objects more rapidly and spend more time with them at 4 to 7 months of age* than kittens who are not handled (Wilson et al., 1965). This is an important finding because it suggests that *early social stimulation also affects how cats will later interact with the non-social environment.*
- Handling also appears to affect developmental rate: The age at eye opening, the age at which the nest box was left, and the rate at which Siamese kittens develop the classic Siamese coloration are earlier or faster for kittens that are handled (Meier, 1961; Meier and Stuart, 1959).
- The effect of handling on developmental rate is enhanced when the litter size is smaller. Karsh and Turner (1988) postulate that these developmental effects could be due in part to increased maternal attention.
- Kittens handled by five people compared with one or none from 5.5 to 9.5 weeks of age show less fear toward people, play more with people, and are more affectionate to them. These kittens purr more, rub more, and mouth the people with whom they are playing.
- The effects of early handling appear to be generalizable to species other than humans. Kittens are more likely to attach to conspecifics and more likely to accept dogs and other animals in the absence of conspecifics if introduced early (Kuo, 1930, 1960). Fox (1969) demonstrated that kittens exposed to

TABLE 8-5

Latency to Approach Novel Humans and Duration of Stay with Humans for Kittens of Different Age Groups That Were Exposed to 15 Minutes of Petting and Handling per Day Compared with Kittens That Had No Handling

	Group 1 (Petted/Handled from 3-14 Weeks)	Group 2 (Petted/Handled from 7-14 Weeks)	Group 3 (No Petting/Handling)
Duration of stay	41 seconds[a,b]	24 seconds[a,c]	15 seconds[b,c]
Approach latency	11 seconds[a,b]	42 seconds[a]	39 seconds[b]

Note: Letters refer to statistical comparisons between groups discussed in the text. a = P < 0.025; b = P < 0.001; c = P < 0.075.

Chihuahua pups from 4 weeks of age showed no fear of them at 12 weeks of age. Kittens with no exposure to the puppies avoided them and behaved defensively when they were approached by them at 12 weeks of age.

- Three rigorous experiments elucidate the time periods within the first few months of life in which kittens are most susceptible to learning specific sets of behaviors and the effects for these periods of varying amounts of exposure to and handling by people (Table 8-5) (Karsh and Turner, 1988).
  - In a comparison of cats kept in maternity cages and exposed to different amounts of attention, kittens were assigned to one of three petting groups:
    - kittens petted for 15 minutes a day from 3 to 14 weeks of age (group 1),
    - kittens petted for 15 minutes a day from 7 to 14 weeks of age (group 2), and
    - kittens who received no handling at all for the entire period, from 3 to 14 weeks of age (group 3).
  - Cats were evaluated first at 14 weeks of age and every 2 to 4 weeks thereafter until the cats were a year of age. "Holding time" and "approach time" were used as measures of willingness to interact with humans. "Holding time" was defined as the amount of time an unfamiliar experimenter could hold and lightly restrain the cat before the cat squirmed and tried to leave. "Approach time" was the amount of time that it took the cat to approach the novel person sitting in the room to which the cat was introduced.
    - Cats with early handling stayed twice as long as cats that were not handled (41 seconds vs. 15 seconds; P < 0.001 (a)) and longer than the cats with late handling (24 seconds; P < 0.025 (b)).
    - Cats with early handling approached within 11 seconds, whereas cats that were not handled approached within 39 seconds (P < 0.025 (b)).
    - There was no statistically significant difference between the cats with late handling and the cats that were not handled in terms of latency

TABLE 8-6

Effects for Groups 1 and 2 (in Table 8-5) if Period of Handling Was Expanded from 15 Minutes per Day to 40 Minutes per Day

	Group 1 (Petted/Handled from 3-14 Weeks)	Group 2 (Petted/Handled from 7-14 Weeks)
Duration of stay	77 seconds	70 seconds
Approach latency	9 seconds	13 seconds

of approach (42 seconds vs. 39 seconds; P < 0.75 (c)). A larger study would be required to determine whether the direction (cats with late handling have a longer latency than cats that were not handled) is significant and indicative of age-dependent learning about avoidance. Regardless, the results suggest that if the effect is reflective of reality, it is not insurmountable.

- When exposure time per day was increased from 15 minutes to 40 minutes for cats handled between weeks 3 and 14, the cats permitted holding for 77 seconds compared with 41 seconds when they were handled only for 15 minutes a day. Cats handled from 7 to 14 weeks of age (group 2) permitted holding for 70 seconds compared with 15 seconds when they were handled only for 15 minutes a day (Table 8-6).
- *The greatest effect of increased handling time appears to occur between 7 and 14 weeks of age.*
- The same pattern is apparent for approach latency (11 seconds vs. 9 seconds) for cats handled between 3 and 14 weeks of age, but the difference is not statistically significant (see Tables 8-5 and 8-6). For cats handled from 7 to 14 weeks of age, increased exposure decreases approach latency from 42 seconds to 13 seconds. This change is statistically indistinguishable from the change found in cats handled very early. Two age groups—cats handled from

TABLE 8-7

Mean Holding Scores (in Number of Seconds)
That Kittens Are Content to Be Held without
Struggle by a Novel Person, Given the Age at
Which They Were Handled

	Weeks 1-5	Weeks 2-6	Weeks 3-7	Weeks 4-8
All cats	87[a,b]	109[a,c]	108[b,d]	87[c,d]
Sample size (n)	18	21	19	17
Non-timid cats	110[a,b]	126[a,c]	120[b,c]	104[a,c]
Sample size (n)	13	17	16	13
Timid cats	27	36	42	35
Sample size (n)	5	4	3	4

Note: The time handled is in seconds; the group "all cats" was analyzed as a unit and then reanalyzed when segregated into its two component groups, "non-timid cats" and "timid cats"; letters refer to statistical comparisons and levels discussed in the text.

3 to 14 weeks of age and cats handled from 7 to 14 weeks of age—spent approximately the same amount of time (1.5 minutes) with an unknown individual.

- These results emphasize that early handling is important and that increasing the amount of time handled has the greatest effect for slightly older and more coordinated kittens.

- Kittens handled only during the discrete periods of weeks 1 to 5, 2 to 6, 3 to 7, and 4 to 8 most definitely demonstrate the age-specific effects of handling (Table 8-7).
  - The mean holding scores of cats handled from 2 to 6 weeks of age and 3 to 7 weeks are significantly greater than mean holding scores for cats handled at 1 to 5 weeks (a, b) and 4 to 8 weeks (c, d).

- There are no statistically significant differences between the handling scores for weeks 2 to 6 and 3 to 7 or for handling scores for weeks 1 to 5 and 4 to 8, but the handling scores for the former versus the latter groups are statistically significantly different from each other.

- These differences are exaggerated for cats classified as non-timid cats, with the same statistical patterns apparent.

- The data are particularly interesting for cats classified as genetically timid or unfriendly. Although the general pattern of the changes is similar to that for both the non-timid cats and the group composed of all cats, there are no statistically significant differences for the handling scores between any of the four periods; this is partly because the sample sizes are quite small.

- These data indicate that even were the curve not relatively flat, the magnitude of the differences in handling scores for any of the periods in comparisons of the timid cats with either of the other cats for those periods is large, and timidity is a significant factor ($P = 0.001$) (a-d) that does not interact with handling periods (Karsh and Turner, 1988). This pattern suggests a gene by environment ($G \times E$) effect. *These data strongly suggest that not only should cats be handled early and often but also that if the cat is genetically predisposed to being timid or less friendly, handling may modulate the behavior to some extent, although that such cats may never respond to the same extent as non-timid cats.* This finding has profound implications for people wishing to choose cats as excellent pets and should help good Samaritans with risk assessment. These results have been confirmed by McCune (1992). No data exist for any effects of intensive and early supplementation of diet or other interventions.

- Karsh's studies *suggest that adverse effects of early weaning could be modulated by the human environment.* She postulates that one-person cats (a common correlation of early weaning) might be held longer and get more quality of attention (Karsh, 1984).

- Early weaning in a cattery situation can be part of a well-designed program to prevent the transmission of coronavirus. In combination with Karsh's work, this suggests that *breeders in cattery situations can produce not only healthy cats but also behaviorally well-adjusted cats if they are able to combine early weaning with intensive handling of the young kittens, starting at 2 weeks of age.*

- Clients and breeders should be encouraged to learn to understand the types of behaviors associated with play so that they can recognize when the cats are deviating from normal, age-specific play behavior. Of particular interest are early weaned kittens who may show earlier predatory and rough play behavior. Early intervention will lead to more suitable pets and fewer relinquishments, abandonments, and euthanasias.

- The $G \times E$ interaction is further emphasized in comparisons of "shy" versus "non-shy" animals (Martin and Bateson, 1985). *Cats who used the top of a complex climbing apparatus had mothers that spent the most time on the frame in the first sessions* (John et al., 1968). There is much variation both within and among litters, but this result suggests that further work is needed on both maternal genetic effects *and* the effects of the mothers' skills on observational learning in kittens.
  - If litters stay with the queen for a protracted time in a social setting, the queen continues to show maternal behavior, even when her offspring are adults (Deag et al., 1988).

- This pattern is more apparent if offspring are daughters. Again, this may be indicative of a G × E interaction that can serve as a mechanism for facilitating the structure of female social groups. No studies have examined this possibility.
- Kittens who are totally hand-reared from birth may have problems with successful reproduction when they are adults (Mellen, 1988).
- Hand-rearing may contribute to later, non-specific social problems even if such rearing occurs in the presence of the queen (Baerends-van Roon and Baerends, 1979).
- Finally, all of these data should be considered within the context of the foraging mode of "domestic" cats. Domestic cats have traditionally been defined as "sit-and-wait" predators, meaning that they hide from their prey and sit and wait by trails, dens, nests, et cetera, as indicated by physical, olfactory, and vocal cues about prey activity. Among mammals, cats are really the only "sit-and-wait" predators, and domestic cats are the quintessential mammalian species using this strategy. Coat color patterns in ancestral cats acted as disrupted coloration and aided the cat in hiding. As a condition of this hunting strategy, cats are compelled to sit quietly hidden and then react almost instantly with a heightened level of arousal. The behavioral and neurochemical difference between sitting quietly hidden and the profound arousal and reactivity required for successful hunting may have placed constraints on feline brain development with respect to cognitive and social strategies. Cats have "normal" arousal patterns that are unlike other species, an observation that likely has implications for how they develop problematic or pathological behaviors.
- Combine the outcomes of foraging mode on brain development and behavior with the lack of any active, overt, and intentional efforts to alter feline behavior in ways that permitted collaborative work with humans, and the constraints on social development discussed previously may be more easily understood and more profound.

ROLE FOR "PERSONALITY TYPE" IN FELINE BEHAVIOR

Personality types have been identified for domestic felines.

- Feaver et al. (1986) described some cats as "sociable, confident, and easy-going." This designation is equivalent to Karsh's (1983a, 1983b) "confident" cat and to Meier and Turner's (1985) "trusting" cat.
- Feaver et al. (1986) also characterized some cats as "timid/nervous," which is equivalent to Karsh's (1983a, 1983b, 1984) "timid" cat and Meier and Turner's "shy, unfriendly" cat (1985).

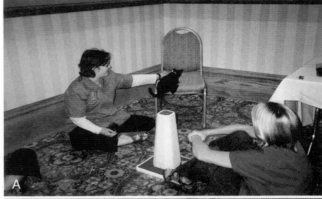
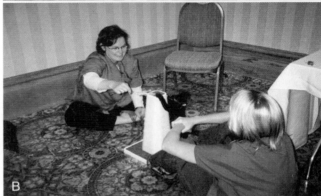

Fig. 8-1 **A** and **B**, A very bold, 8.5-week-old cat is shown participating in a teaching lab for veterinarians. In just a few minutes he was trained to jump from the scratching post to the chair and back. "Boldness," in cats as in dogs, likely facilitates object and social learning and problem-solving ability. These are almost always unmet needs in pets, especially cats. This cat was adopted by someone in the course and named Harry, for the non-feline wizard.

- Feaver et al.'s (1986) classification of "active, aggressive" cats is analogous to Karsh's (1983a, 1983b, 1984) "active" and Pavlov's (1927) "excitatory temperament."
- Turner (1991) reported two types of "friendly" personalities in housecats. He characterized these as the "play" type versus the "petting" type.
- McCune (1992) has re-characterized friendliness as boldness (Fig. 8-1). No associations between age, sex, client, or household type and "personality type" have been noted, but some of these factors may be relevant for some types of feline aggressions, including play-related aggression. "Boldness" appears to be one personality style for cats for which some consistent data exist (Lowe and Bradshaw, 2001; Reisner et al., 2004). "Bold" cats are more likely able to experience and learn from a wider variety of experiences than are "shy" or "timid" cats.
- In a controlled experimental study, cats fathered by "friendly" or outgoing cats were more likely to explore unfamiliar people *and* inanimate objects when tested at 1 year of age. These effects were

enhanced by early handling (McCune, 1992), which confirm earlier observational findings that patterns of behaviors within and between litters suggested that temperament of kittens is largely paternally determined (Beaver, 1992).

- Coat-color effects have been noted for both mink and foxes with regard to heritable tendencies toward fear and aggression (Bradshaw, 1992), and coat pelage characteristics have been associated with tractability and startle responses in cattle (Grandin et al., 1995). The full extent of the interaction between coat characteristics and behavior is not understood but may be important given the fate of neuroectoderm in ontogeny (Smith and Gong, 1974).

HOW CATS COMMUNICATE

Four main modes of communication used by all species have special resonance for cats.

1. Visual signals are most useful over short to intermediate distances and for information that is to be used and acted on immediately.
2. Auditory signals, including signals involving vocalization, are longer distance signals. Because of the manner in which sound moves, they can coordinate group movements over distances where a visual signal would be lost. These signals work best in the present.
3. Olfactory signals are complex because they can be used by animals separated in time and space, in contrast to the other classes of signals. Because of the manner in which odorant molecules disperse, olfactory signals can contain information that speaks to the passage of time and so may render understanding some social interactions more difficult. Olfactory signals are most pronounced in the first 24 to 48 hours.
4. Tactile signals are seldom examined or considered for dogs and cats, but they are an essential part of social signaling that may act as an early warning system for the group or as an assay of risk or comfort for individuals.

None of these modes of communication operate in a vacuum. If anything, these signals will reinforce each other. *Information that is redundant is always important information. For very important information, redundancy reduces risk.* By observing redundancy, we can appreciate what matters to the individual cat. When these four signaling modalities are not congruent, we should pay attention because the cat is uncertain and may be stressed.

Understanding Visual Communication

Cats have acute visual capabilities.
- Cats can discriminate elimination at one fifth the threshold of humans, but their resolution is only one tenth that of humans (Ewer, 1973).

- Siamese cats appear to have decreased stereoscopic vision compared with other feline breeds (Packwood and Gordon, 1975).
- Felines, similar to astronauts, Arctic explorers, and seafarers, may experience an environmental training effect on their vision: free-ranging cats are hypermetropic, whereas caged cats are myopic (Belkin et al., 1977).
- Cats are capable of color discrimination (Sechzer and Brown, 1964).
  - The extent to which this ability factors into intraspecific signaling is unexplored, but the contrast between the color of pupil and iris must be apparent to cats.
  - Because so much information about immediate intent in fearful and agonistic situations is communicated by pupil size and shape, color and the relative abundance detected may be important.
    - Completely round pupils are associated with fear, full oblong pupils are associated with offensive aggression, and slightly off-round/undilated oblong pupils are associated with a relaxed state.
    - Size of pupil correlates with intensity of underlying state.
- Visual communication in domestic pet felines involves the use of the eyes, ears, mouth, tail, and coat (pelage) (Fig. 8-2).
  - Facial signals change far more quickly than postural signals and may contain the most up-to-date contextual information that is derived from the response of the receiver of the signal.
  - Ears are fluid and move quickly in domestic pet felines.
    - Erect ears are apparent when the cat is alert and focusing on a stimulus.
    - Slightly relaxed ears are indicative of a calm cat who is not focusing on any stimulus but could focus instantly.
    - Ears that are swiveled, displaying the inner pinnae sideways, are indicative of increased passive aggression or of offensive or actively assertive activity.
    - Ears that are swiveled downward and sideways or that are rotated downward are associated with more deferential signaling or associated with increasing defensive aggression.
    - Ears that are pulled all the way down and to the back/rear of the cat so that the inner pinnae are not at all visible are indicative of extreme, defensive postures and active, overt, defensive aggression as a last resort, after all other choices have failed. For such cats, the outer pinnae are flattened in a mask-like molding against the head.
    - If the inner pinna is visible and flat against the head, as if sculpted in a mask, this is indicative

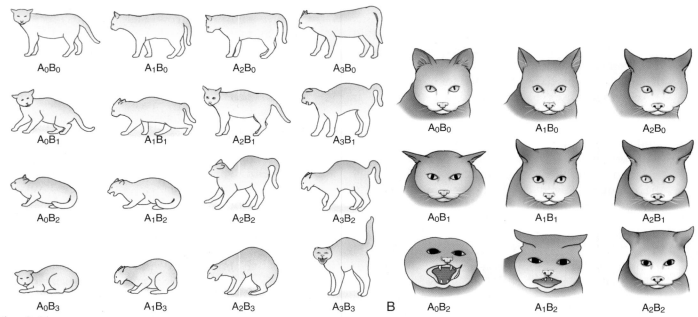

Fig. 8-2 A, A classic illustration of feline agonistic behavior as described by Leyhausen (1979) and Overall (1997).

- A_0B_0 represents the basic relaxed, copacetic cat who is monitoring the environment. As one moves from A_0B_0 to A_3B_0 (across the x-axis), the cat is becoming more assertive, more confident, and more offensively aggressive. The offensive aggression here is passive and is related more to eliciting deferential behavior from another than it is about engaging in actual combat. Factors to note include the fully extended hind legs, the elevated rump and piloerected tail, the set of the head and neck, and the ears that are slightly pulled back.
- Moving from A_0B_0 to A_0B_3 (down the y-axis), the cat is becoming more withdrawn, more avoidant of interaction, potentially more fearful, and more defensively aggressive. Aggression will ensue only when this cat can no longer escape.
- The cat represented in A_3B_3 is exhibiting mixed signals and is in an extremely heightened state of reactivity. The tail is elevated, indicating that interaction is a possibility. The back is arched in a classic fearful posture (note that the back is also arched in A_0B_3, but the cat is lying down). The neck is tucked and the underside of the neck and all teeth are exposed. A signal that uses full disclosure is one used to diffuse an undesirable situation. This cat is signaling that he will stand his ground but will not actively and overtly seek aggression unless pursued. It would be inappropriate to call either this posture or that portrayed in A_0B_3 as "fear/fearful aggression." Both of these cats want their antagonist to leave. One cat (A_0B_3) has invoked withdrawal from the interaction as his first choice and as such is not meeting the criteria for "fear/fearful aggression," although he could meet the criteria for fearful behavior. The problem is that if this cat is approached and cornered, he will become extremely reactive and aggressive, whereas a dog might freeze. In contrast to the cat in A_3B_3, the cat in A_3B_0 is confident. The cat in A_3B_0 will back down any challengers and will pursue them if they do not back down; the cat in A_2B_3 would neither seek nor choose to interact with a challenger, given the choice, again not quite meeting the criteria for "fear/fearful aggression" as it is often used for dogs because this cat will not face the opponent down hoping to increase the distance between them. He also would not then pursue and nip anyone who backed up and turned away, as a dog might. These differences are important because they go to the heart of how cat behaviors have not been truly modified as part of "domestication." Cats may be fearful, but we are best served using illustrations such as this chart in a manner that allows us to classify cats with respect to risk for offensive aggression (x-axis) or defensive aggression (y-axis), rather than using the classifications common for dogs, who appear to have very different reactivity profiles.

B, The position of the ears, neck, and head; plane of the shoulders; posture of the mouth and nares; and shape and size of the pupils all are important in feline communication.

- A_0B_0 represents a relaxed cat who is monitoring the environment.
- A_2B_2 represents a cat that is more offensively and assertively aggressive as represented by body posture A_3B_0 (**A**). Note the set neck and shoulders, slightly lowered head, movement of the pinnae, dilation of the nares, and clamping of mouth. This is a very confident and serious cat.
- A_2B_0 represents a cat that is fearful and attempting to withdraw. This cat will avoid interactions if possible. Note the positioning of the eyes and the oblique (non-direct) gaze. The cat's ears are back but up, and his neck and head are more withdrawn than set and pushed forward as in A_2B_2. This is the facial expression of the cat in A_0B_3 in **A**.
- A_0B_2 represents a cat that will pursue aggression but only as the last resort. The neck, inside of the throat, and teeth all are exposed, in contrast to A_2B_2. Also, the pinnae are fully swiveled and everted. This is the facial expression of the cat in A_3B_3 in **A**. (Classic feline facial expressions are from Leyhausen [1979]. Interpretations differ from the original, as noted.) (Adapted from Leyhausen, 1979, and Overall, 1997.)

of extremely offensive behavior and active, overt, offensive aggression should the target of this aggression fail to defer or leave.

- Pupillary changes can be extremely informative, but clients will not watch for the useful changes unless taught how to do so. Cats read cat behavior better than people read cat behavior and so may use these signals to modulate their own behaviors.
  - Miotic pupils are correlated with autonomic parasympathetic responses.
  - Mydriatic pupils are correlated with sympathetic, fight-or-flight response.
  - It is important to evaluate pupil size in conjunction with ambient light conditions because many pupils could dilate even in a relaxed cat if the room is dark.
  - Regardless, a direct stare is a challenge or threat in cats and is usually exhibited by assertive, forceful, confident cats, including cats exhibiting offensive aggression (Fig. 8-3; also see posture A_2B_2 in Fig. 8-2, *B*). Note that pupils usually maintain some of their ovoid shape.
  - The more defensive the cat, the more round and dilated the pupils (see posture A_0B_2 in Fig. 8-2, *B*). The expression in A_0B_2 in Figure 8-2, *B* goes with the body posture A_3B_3 in Figure 8-2, *A*.
- Nares expand as cats experience any sympathetic response (all postures except A_0B_0 in Fig. 8-2, *B*). This expansion is accompanied by a tightening of the jaw muscles and prominent vibrissae in offensively aggressive cats (see posture A_2B_2 in Fig. 8-2, *B*, which goes with posture A_3B_0 in Fig. 8-2, *A*).
- Overall body posture in cats communicates a lot of information. Facets that can be addressed should include the overall resting body posture, the head carriage, the back position (arched or level posture), leg positioning, and tail posture and activity. Leyhausen (1979) has illustrated variations in all of these postures in a classic set of illustrations from his book on predatory behavior (see Fig. 8-2). The interpretation of these behaviors presented here benefits from additional information about social and signaling behavior that was not available to Leyhausen. As is true with all good science, historical interpretations that are solid are always built on.
  - All historical cat breeds have had tails, and so one would expect that tail signaling is important.
    - Tails that are kept out and behind usually signal that the cat is alert, confident, relaxed, and friendly—the basic copacetic, "willing-to-explore-the-environment" state.
    - Tails that are erect but slightly curled can also indicate a relaxed and friendly cat. They further indicate a cat who is outgoing and willing to solicit or receive interaction. The curl of the tail is often facing the individual with whom

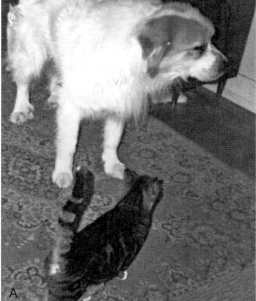

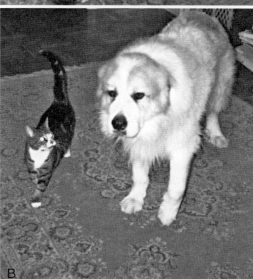

Fig. 8-3 **A** and **B**, Note the direct stare and the assertive carriage of the tail in this cat interacting with a great Pyrenees. The dog is correctly responding with a deferential turn of the neck while not making eye contact. This dog and cat live together companionably, but the cat defines the limits of their interaction. (Photos by N. Rosenberg and E. Elliot.)

the cat is willing to interact in a non-agonistic manner (Bradshaw and Cameron-Beaumont, 2000; Cafazzo and Natoli, 2009).
- Cats who are walking or trotting may hold their tails at 40-degree angles to the horizon of the back; the tail lowers as the pace increases (Kiley-Worthington, 1976, 1984). This altered posture may be functional, not communicatory.
- Offensive postures use tails that are straight down or that are held perpendicular to the ground.

TABLE 8-8

Feline Tail Postures

Posture	Interpretation of Signal/Context in Which It Occurs
Vertical	Play Greeting, often with motion Sexual approaches by females Willingness to interact, but movement and other congruent signals determine whether the interaction is to be friendly Affiliative gesture in a confident cat "Frustration"—denial of access or behavioral opportunity—if the tail is whipped
Half-raised	Sexual approaches by females
Horizontal	Amicable approach Sexual approach by females
Concave	Defensive behavior
Lower	Offensive aggression (if rigid and flicking) Defensive aggression (if more flaccid)
Between the legs	"Submission" (caution with this label) Fear Withdrawal from social interaction Hiding

Adapted from Bradshaw, 1992.

- Erect, bristled tails are associated with a combination of offensive and defensive behaviors. Any animal with an erect, bristled tail is in a heightened state of reactivity and will react in a context that is indicated by its facial signals.
- Bradshaw (1992) has combined the classic tail signaling as described by Leyhausen (1979) with updated data to classify tail positions as vertical, half-raised, horizontal, concave, lower, and between legs (Table 8-8).
  - The vertical tail position has been associated with greeting. The cat may be walking, trotting, standing, engaging in social play or object play or in a sexual approach, if female.
  - The half-raised tail appears to be solely associated with sexual approaches by females.
  - Horizontally held tails can indicate an amicable approach or a sexual approach by a female.
  - Concave tails are indicative of defensive aggression, whereas lowered tails are indicative of offensive aggression.
  - Tails found between the legs are indicative of "submission," which may be better described as withdrawal and a profound unwillingness to interact.

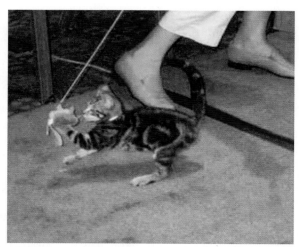

Fig. 8-4 A kitten exhibiting the classic inverted "U" over the dorsum in a chase with a toy, where the second step—with distance increasing—never occurs.

- Some cats, particularly young cats, often carry their tails in a U-shaped, concave position. (See the ethogram in Table 8-9 for examples.)
  - If the tail is concave in an inverted "U" over the dorsum, the cat usually alters the distance between herself and another animal by chasing the other cat. At first, the distance between the cats is *decreased*, but when using this signal the distance is *ultimately increased* between the two cats, usually because of a chase. The concave inverted U-shaped tail angled over the dorsum serves as a distance-increasing measure, emphasizing the role of context and timing in the understanding of any signal function (Fig. 8-4).
  - Tails that are concave away from the back in an inverted "U" shape usually are associated with cats who are willing to interact—the interaction can be aggressive or not—but who are a little unsure about taking the lead. This tail posture is often accompanied by sitting on the hind feet. Cats displaying the U-shaped tail away from the back generally decrease the distance between themselves and another individual but do so by soliciting the other individual so that *they reverse the previous pattern:* they back up and then approach.
- Bernstein and Strack (1996) have identified a five-posture tail classification that is a variant of that already discussed.
  - In position 1, the tail is slightly down and behind the cat.
  - In position 2, the tail is slightly curved above the horizon of the back, with or without movement.

Text continued on p. 344

TABLE 8-9

Ethogram for Visual/Tactile Behaviors Based on Cats Who Are *Not Domestic**

Behavior/Signal	Description/Characterization
Watch	Direct observation of the focus and circumstances by moving the head and the eyes; the cat can be distracted and attend to activity elsewhere because there is no strict focus on any one individual or object 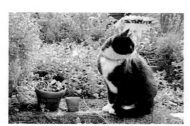 Note that although the cat is looking over his shoulder, his body is relaxed—his back, neck, and feet are clearly not tense and his tail is curved but not actually wrapped around his feet
Stare	Watchful gaze where the cat is not easily distracted; blinking and head movements decrease and face tenses; gaze may follow the individual who is the focus of the gaze as that individual moves 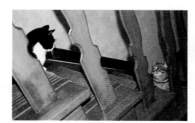
Pupils are vertical ovals	Normal, attentive state; size affected by ambient light 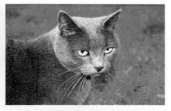 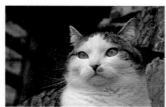 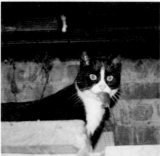 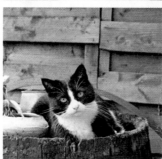

Continued

TABLE 8-9

Ethogram for Visual/Tactile Behaviors Based on Cats Who Are *Not Domestic*—cont'd

Behavior/Signal	Description/Characterization
Pupils are round	Reactive, agitated state; both level of reactivity and ambient light affect size

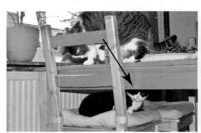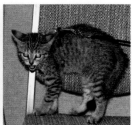

| Ears back | Pinnae pulled against skull; if ears are also pulled down, the inner pinna may not be visible (see the cat on the left) |

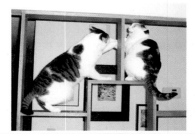

| Ears flat | This is a more extreme version of ears back with pinnae flush with the skull; ears may lie close to the top of the head; if pulled close to the top of the head, the inner pinna may be visible (see the cat on the right) |

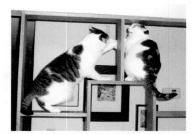

| *Ears erect and forward* | Pinnae vertical in the classic cupped feline triangular shape rotated and moved directly forward; may flick and move to orient to sound |

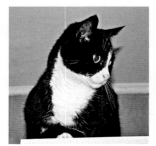

TABLE 8-9

Ethogram for Visual/Tactile Behaviors Based on Cats Who Are *Not Domestic*—cont'd

Behavior/Signal	Description/Characterization
Tail up	Tail is vertical to the cat's spine and may be still, wave gently, or just wave at the tip. If the tip only waves, movement can be gentle or agitated. This is an affiliative signal, and cats use it only when they wish to interact (and not all interactions are friendly) and are confident

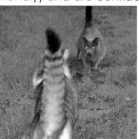

Tail quiver	Tail rhythmically agitates, vibrates, or flickers in small waves; seen when cats are engaged in the spraying posture, whether or not urine is released

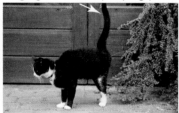 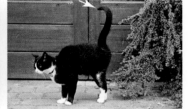

Tail under	Tail is tucked tightly under the body against the abdomen; generally accompanied by crouching; seen in fearful or defensively aggressive contexts

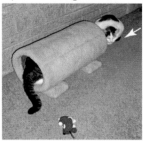

Tail wrap	Tail is wrapped around the feet and/or legs of the cat; this posture is commonly seen when cats are wary and cannot escape but are not open to interaction

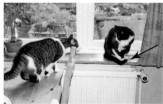 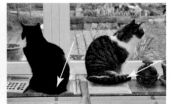

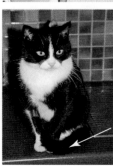 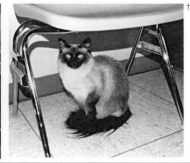

Continued

TABLE 8-9

Ethogram for Visual/Tactile Behaviors Based on Cats Who Are *Not Domestic*—cont'd

Behavior/Signal	Description/Characterization
Tail twined	Tail is wrapped with and around another cat's (or a dog's) tail in an alternating pattern

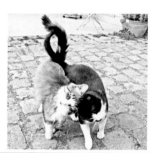

Behavior/Signal	Description/Characterization
Stand	Upright posture where all four legs bear equal/normal weight distribution in an untensed manner
Hind quarters stand	Stand only on back legs to reach or sniff at focus

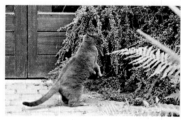 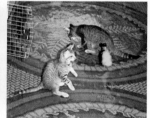

Behavior/Signal	Description/Characterization
Sit	Hind legs folded and hind end flush with the surface while front legs are extended

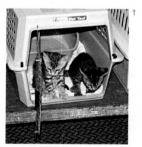

Behavior/Signal	Description/Characterization
Sit with	Sitting close to (within one cat length or within touching distance) to another cat, a human, or other animal

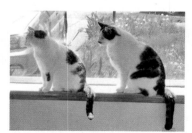

TABLE 8-9

Ethogram for Visual/Tactile Behaviors Based on Cats Who Are *Not Domestic*—cont'd

Behavior/Signal	Description/Characterization
Lie	Cat's body is flush with and supported by the surface; a variety of postures possible depending on how secure the cat feels, the social situation, and the thermal environment

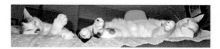

Follow	One cat travels closely behind another cat, human, or other animal and takes directional cues from that individual

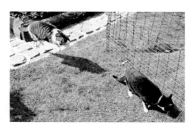

Knead/tread	Alternating movements, by hind feet for treading and front feet for kneading, against some object, surface, or individual; claws may be in or out

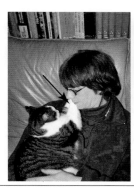 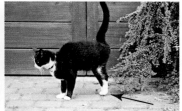

Social rub	Cat rubs another cat, human, or other animal using his or her: Head—rubs dorsum of head/ears/side of cheeks/chin over focus of attention Flank—rubs side of body against or over focus of attention Tail—rubs tail against or over focus of attention

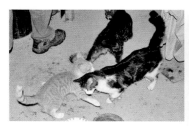 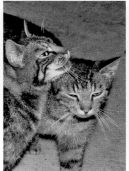 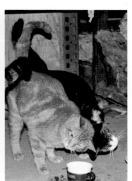

Continued

TABLE 8-9

Ethogram for Visual/Tactile Behaviors Based on Cats Who Are *Not Domestic*—cont'd

Behavior/Signal	Description/Characterization

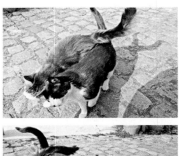
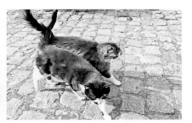
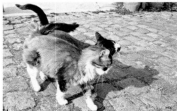
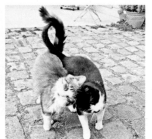
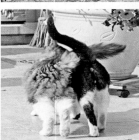

There can also be social rubbing not associated with direct social interaction where cats exhibit these same behaviors against a sofa, a corner of a wall, a tree, et cetera, as part of scent and visual marking. As with all scent marks, the behaviors are sufficiently characteristic that if a conspecific (or one who knows that cat well) observes the behavior they know that a scent mark may accompany the visual display. The visual display itself is also important

TABLE 8-9

Ethogram for Visual/Tactile Behaviors Based on Cats Who Are *Not Domestic*—cont'd

Behavior/Signal	Description/Characterization
Object rub	Movement of head/neck/body along any horizontal or vertical surface or object. Note that the cat can show all the behaviors associated with spraying and not spray. The cat rubbing the cedar bench did so with his tail base as he moved back and forth. At the time, he was eyeing another male cat many meters away across a garden. Females who are sexually receptive will also rub objects, accompanied by plaintive vocalization including yowls and howls

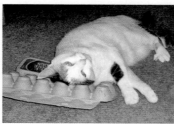 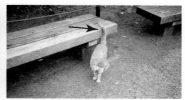 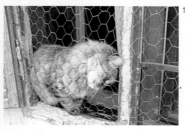 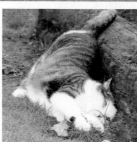

Social roll	Cat moves around on his or her back on the ground/surface, moving back and forth, exposing the neck and belly, and possibly moving limbs and tail against or in the close presence of another cat or any other individual with whom the cat is socially comfortable

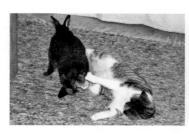 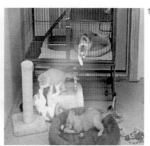

Continued

TABLE 8-9

Ethogram for Visual/Tactile Behaviors Based on Cats Who Are *Not Domestic*—cont'd

Behavior/Signal	Description/Characterization
Social play	Chasing, pouncing, grabbing, batting, sucking, and pushing against another individual involved in similar behaviors. It's not unusual for participants alternately to pull and push at each other using their paws 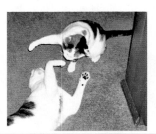
Arch back	Back formed into a curved, upside-down "U" while the cat stands rigidly; often accompanied by piloerection; tail may also be piloerected and moving briskly or held straight up 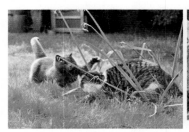 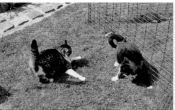 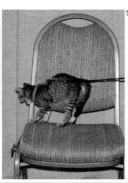
Crouch	Defensive posture where cat lowers body so that only feet, not legs, may be visible; cat folds inward on itself and may become small in a self-protective manner or in a covert, attentive manner (remember, cats are sit-and-wait predators and are also small enough to be prey in some environments) 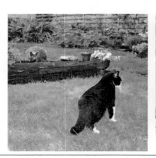 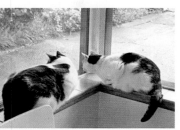

TABLE 8-9

Ethogram for Visual/Tactile Behaviors Based on Cats Who Are *Not Domestic*—cont'd

Behavior/Signal	Description/Characterization
Lordosis	Mating behavior in a female cat where she crouches down and then raises her hind quarters, while pressing her belly to the ground and turning her tail as part of the solicitation for mating
Mount	Cat climbs over the back of another cat while aligned in the same direction; forefeet of the mounting cat are in front of the mounted cat's hind legs, and hind feet of mounting cat are behind the hind feet of the mounted cat. Cats may also mount pillows or non-feline individuals. Thrusting may or may not occur. If this behavior occurs during mating or masturbation, the mouthing cat will grab the other cat by the nape of the neck, or an object, and hold firmly with the teeth while treading with the back legs. Intromission of the penis may or may not occur 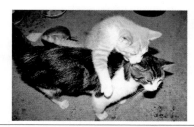
Sniff	Movement of air during inspiration through nostrils as cat moves over the surface of interest. When interacting with other cats, cats frequently and carefully examine by sniffing each others' noses; anal, perianal, and tail base areas; and bodies 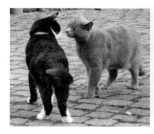 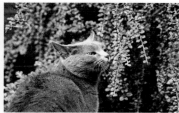 Notice the closed nostrils associated with beginning of inspiration cycle and the forward movement of the whiskers, both characteristic of the process for obtaining olfactory information
Lick	Movement of the cat's tongue over his or her own body area, a surface, or his or her own nose and mouth area 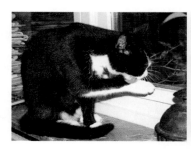 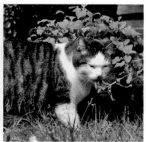

Continued

TABLE 8-9

Ethogram for Visual/Tactile Behaviors Based on Cats Who Are *Not Domestic*—cont'd

Behavior/Signal	Description/Characterization
Touch nose	Touching of a cat's nose to any object or another cat's nose. Cats tend to touch with their nose objects sticking out and directed toward them (like a human finger or another cat's nose)

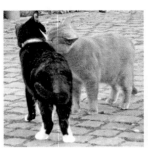 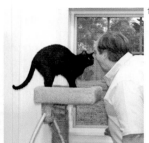

Nuzzle	Pushing of one cat's head against the head or body of another; this behavior involves pushing without rubbing
Paw/pat	Using forepaw, repeated touching of another individual or object; claws are retracted

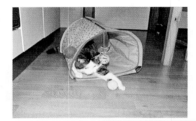

Pounce	Leaping of one cat onto another or onto a toy; the cat need not stay attached

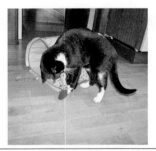

Cuff	Strike at one cat by another using a curved or angled forepaw with claws extended

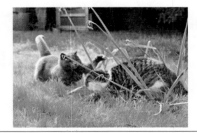

TABLE 8-9

Ethogram for Visual/Tactile Behaviors Based on Cats Who Are *Not Domestic*—cont'd

Behavior/Signal	Description/Characterization
Swat	Very forceful version of the cuff, where the claws are clearly visible and the cat is tensed and positioned to get the most force from reaching for and hitting another individual with his or her foot and claws; also used in play with objects and predatory behavior 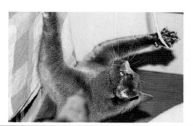
Stalk	Slow following of individual or object with front of body lowered while attentively watching/staring at the focus of the activity; activity may start and stop; may but does not need to be part of predatory behavior and can occur in play and predation; precedes pouncing; the lower the front of the body, the closer the cat is to pouncing 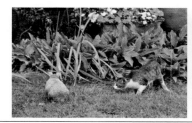 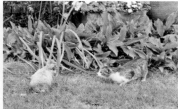
Scratch/rake	Using extended forelegs and stretched body, the claws are drawn backward simultaneously or in an alternating manner; speed, distance, and focus can vary greatly; acts as both a visual and an olfactory signal 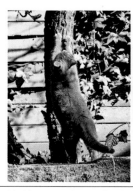 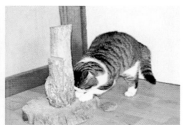
Social grooming/ allogrooming	Licking and manipulation of the fur of another cat using teeth and tongue 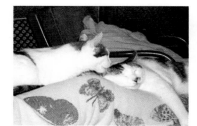

Continued

TABLE 8-9

Ethogram for Visual/Tactile Behaviors Based on Cats Who Are *Not Domestic*—cont'd

Behavior/Signal	Description/Characterization
Gape/flehmen	Opening and cupping of mouth as an odor is inhaled that provides odorant molecules to the vomeronasal organ and to the olfactory epithelium; the flehmen response is shown in a young, captive cheetah in a breeding sanctuary after he sniffed the urine that the cheetah on the other side of the fence had just deposited 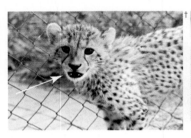 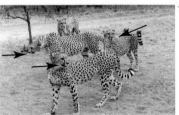 Note the adult cheetahs engaged in the flehmen response; a dead antelope is in a truck approaching these cheetahs on a preserve. Also note how much more visible these cheetahs are if their tails are seen and moving
Mouth threat	Threat delivered with a gaped mouth without hissing; ears are often back to some extent, cat stares and pupils are dilated; tongue may be rolled as in hissing 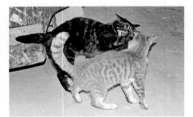
Hiss	Sound delivered with rolled tongue and mouth opened approximately midway; agonist signal usually delivered as part of defensive aggression 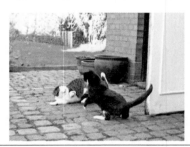
Yawn	Full open mouth movement where teeth may show, tongue may curl and protrude, eyes close, and body is relaxed; this distinguishes from hissing and from panting where the mouth can be open and be accompanied by yawning, but the cat is watchful; the latter is seen in anxiety 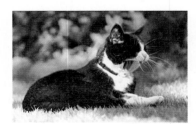

TABLE 8-9

Ethogram for Visual/Tactile Behaviors Based on Cats Who Are *Not Domestic*—cont'd

Behavior/Signal	Description/Characterization
Snapbite	Cat opens and shuts mouth without grabbing anything or anyone during an interaction with or visualization of another cat
Napebite	Grabbing of the female cat's neck by the male cat during mounting and mating; the posture ensures that the female cannot turn her head and grab the male
Bite	Grabbing of another individual using the teeth and mouth

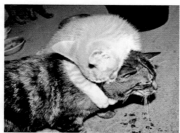

Squat urination	Urine is voiding when the cat is almost sitting; hind quarters are held up and a bit forward and forequarters are held a bit back so that the cat balances in a "V" shape while urinating on a horizontal surface
Spray urination	Cat stands while urinating and forcefully expels urine; cat is usually treading and waving tail while doing so; urine is expelled in an arch and usually hits a vertical surface from which it may drip; if the cat is standing in an open area, a streak of urine will fall onto the horizontal surface, the shape of which depends on the force with which the urine was expelled and the amount of urine expelled

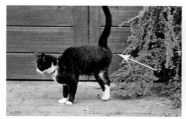 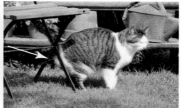

Defecate	Deposition of feces, usually while in a crouched position
Scratch/scrape/rake associated with areas for elimination	Movement of feet, with or without claws retracted, over the area around, over, or near which the cat has eliminated or where the cat has detected another scent; alternating front paws are used, in variable patterns; soil or substrate is moved but may not cover the urine or feces; scratch marks are apparent, and the rearrangement of the substrate acts as visual signal, in addition to an olfactory one
Scratch and cover	Movement of the forepaws across substrate to bury or cover urine and/or feces; some cats who cover urine may not cover feces and vice versa
Defecate on landmark or surface	Placement of feces in the open on a prominent object or location, generally one that has some topographic or visual elevation; feces can also be deposited and fall or be smeared across a vertical surface

*Note: Ethograms are catalogs of behaviors with clearly enunciated descriptions, definitions, characterizations, and requirements. No universally accepted ethograms exist for dogs or cats. Italicized terms were not included in the source document. A more extensive ethogram that has overlap with this one was created by Wedl et al. (2011) for the evaluation of dyadic play in cats. The Wedl et al. ethogram further divides behaviors into state (e.g., posture) or event (e.g., activity) variables. Citations can be found in Bradshaw and Cameron-Beaumont unless otherwise indicated. *Developed by Bradshaw and Cameron-Beaumont (2000), adapted for domestic cats. Photos except as noted are courtesy of Anne Marie Dossche, with thanks. †Photo by K.L. Overall.*

- In position 3, the tail is high above the back with the tip slightly back and curved or up.
- These positions are associated, respectively, with information gathering, monitoring approaches, and beginning a non-aggressive interaction.
- In position 4, the tail is curved down and between the legs. This is a defensive posture that indicates that escape is a possible option.
- In position 5, the entire tail is whipped rapidly back and forth. This movement is associated with an incipient and active aggressive behavior (biting and scratching) or is a precursor to active, defensive escape. This posture and activity has also been associated with an unattainable object of focus (e.g., birds outside a window), which may be accompanied by chattering teeth and vocalization.

- It has been suggested that some of these tail postures, particularly in very aggressive or defensive situations, are less clear than might otherwise be expected for an appendage so important to signaling because the cat is protecting the tail from injury. Disruptive coloration is another explanation (Orotolani, 1999). In a grassland environment, the domestic cat's ancestral environment, a tail can be an excellent long-distance signal because it is best seen when moved (Fig. 8-5).

- Descriptions of body posture should include the position of the head, the back, and the legs, usually in combination with each other.
  - *A head-up, straight-back posture*, where the topline of the dorsum is parallel to the ground, accompanied by a *tail that is out and behind*, is generally indicative of a *relaxed, alert cat* (see posture A_0B_0 in Fig. 8-2, *A*).
  - *Straight legs, particularly if they are accompanied by elevated hindquarters,* are indicative of an *offensive posture.* Cats' hind legs are slightly longer than their front legs, so this posture is achieved by muscular contraction that straightens the legs (see posture A_3B_0).
    - *Straightening the legs* contributes to the classic appearance of the *"rump hump"/elevated rump* where the base of the tail and the slightly elevated hips become very apparent. Piloerection of the tail may be prominent, but the tail is held down, tightly clamped against the hindquarters.
  - An *elevated rump* is easily visible from a distance. A cat who is successful in controlling an agonistic interaction generally is also a cat who can elevate his rump first and maintain this posture. Cats who are very as-

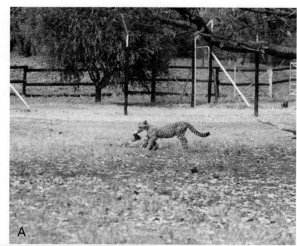
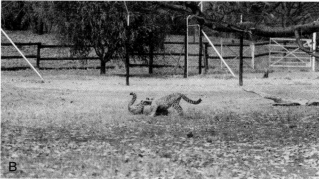

Fig. 8-5 A and **B**, Two young cheetahs are playing in a cheetah sanctuary and breeding facility in South Africa. Notice how much more visible the cheetah who is rolling on the ground is when his tail is moving (**B**).

sertive often use this posture to signal to cats who may challenge them.

- The *sternal crouch* posture is defensive. It is usually accompanied by placing the tail on the ground and then tucking it around some part of the cat. Such actions not only signal withdrawal to other cats, but protect the tail, which is so important for signaling (see posture A_0B_2, A_0B_3 and A_1B_3).
- The *belly-up* display involves displaying the ventrum.
  - This is the classic play posture of kittens, but it can also be seen in some fights because it signals a lack of offensive behavior and a sense of vulnerability. A belly-up display could indicate an unwillingness to pursue a more overt, direct, agonistic behavior. When a cat displays its underbelly, it indicates, by exposing one of its most vulnerable areas, that it is exhibiting deferential behavior, much in the same way that canids do when they display the side of their neck and then their abdomen to the individual with whom they are interacting. This signal indicates

that the cat displaying it is not willing to initiate and pursue an overtly aggressive act.

- Cats who display the belly-up posture in a protective, defensive context also tend to bring their back feet up, with their claws unsheathed, to protect the softest, most vulnerable area of their abdomen. These additional signals confirm the congruent belly-up signal indicating a lack of willingness to initiate the aggression but providing additional information about the potential cost of pursuit. Cats who position their feet in this manner and display their claws are willing to engage in active defensive aggression. If the aggressor backs off, the cat displaying the protective belly-up posture will not pursue the aggression or the aggressor. As such, this signal indicates more about pursuit than it does about deference and we should consider that such behaviors do not fit neatly with the concept of "submission."
- The classic "Halloween cat" exhibits the *arched back posture*. This posture indicates a high degree of reactivity (see posture A₃B₃).
  - Reactivity can be either offensive or defensive. The rest of the cat's postures and behaviors will indicate in which capacity the arched back is functioning.
  - A cat exhibiting the arched back is informing the individual with whom the interaction is occurring that, depending on that individual's behavior, the cat is prepared to act in either modality, although he would not seek active aggression. Such signals provide all of the participants with the option of stopping the interaction.
- Vibrissae position is important. Whiskers rotate forward with offensive aggression, overt threats, or keen interest.
- Body positions used by a queen with her kittens have been discussed separately.
  - The postures that have been elucidated for females caring for their young include sit, sit-nurse, half-sit, on-side-lie, half-sit and on-side-lie, crouch, lie, crouch and lie, and shift.
    - On-side-lie, half-sit, and shift posture all occur very early in the caretaking of kittens.
    - Sit-nurse peaks at about 4 weeks, concomitant with the beginning of weaning.
    - Sit, crouch, and lie all are behaviors that are seen later in the weaning period more frequently than earlier.
    - With the exception of the half-sit, all of these behaviors are influenced by both the mother and the stage of the development.
    - Occurrence of the half-sit is not a significant function of age.

Some more commonly informative behaviors for clients are included in the ethogram in Table 8-9.

Being able to read cat signals and understanding the implications of certain body postures is essential for both clinicians and clients, but few clients or veterinarians are taught how to do this. Some progress has been made by individuals who are concerned about stress behaviors associated with veterinary care, including care that generates pain, and with relinquishment. The stress score in Table 8-10 was developed for the assessment of shelter cats, but it can readily be adapted to use in veterinary practices and in clients' homes.

For clients, the best use of this "Cat-Assessment-Score" or "Cat-Stress-Score" is for quality of life assessments when there has been a physical or social change in the household or when the client perceives there has been an intrinsic and unexplained change in the cat's behavior. By encouraging clients to complete such assessments routinely and repeatedly, we train them to observe feline body postures and we ask them to make objective assessments that can be tracked across time to learn if the cat's stress level is increasing, decreasing, or fluctuating depending on the context.

The original Cat-Assessment-Score was created by McCune (1992) and adapted by Kessler and Turner (1997) for use in shelter assessments. Using a pre-defined scale ranging from 1 (fully relaxed) through 7 (terrorized), 11 aspects of the cat's behavior can be scored. The aspects of feline communication assessed include:

- general body posture,
- positioning of the belly,
- positioning of the legs,
- tail posture,
- head posture,
- eye movement and opening,
- pupil size,
- ear position,
- whisker orientation,
- type of vocalization, and
- assessment of activity that depends on objective descriptors.

The value in such an approach is its clear descriptors, ability to assess congruence between different body regions and signaling repertoires, and an objective standard that suggests there may be high inter-rater reliability (a measure of how likely different observers are to agree) and intra-rater reliability (a measure of how likely the same person is to rate the same behaviors in the same way during at least two different evaluations), two measures of validity that are too often ignored. A similar scale for dogs is presented in Chapter 1 and in the handout and questionnaire section. A similar approach has been taken by McCobb et al. (2005), who simplified the scale to be broadly

TABLE 8-10

Seven-Level Cat-Stress-Score

Score	Body	Belly	Legs	Tail	Head
1—Fully relaxed	I: Laid out on side or on back A: NA	Exposed, slow ventilation	I: Fully extended A: NA	I: Extended or loosely wrapped A: NA	Laid on surface with chin upward or on surface
2—Weakly relaxed	I: Laid ventrally or half on side or sitting A: Standing or moving, back horizontal	Exposed or not exposed, slow or normal ventilation	I: Bent, hind legs may be laid out A: When standing extended	I: Extended or loosely wrapped A: Tail up or loosely downward	Laid on surface or over body, some movement
3—Weakly tense	I: Laid ventrally or sitting A: Standing or moving, back horizontal	Not exposed, normal ventilation	I: Bent A: While standing extended	I: On body or curved backward, may be twitching A: Up or tense downward, may be twitching	Over body, some movement
4—Very tense	I: Laid ventral, rolled or sitting A: Standing or moving, body behind lower than in front	Not exposed, normal ventilation	I: Bent A: When standing hind legs bent, in front extended	I: Close to body A: Tense downward or curled forward, may be twitching	Over body or pressed to body, little to no movement
5—Fearful, stiff	I: Laid ventrally or sitting A: Standing or moving, body behind, lower than in front	Not exposed, normal or fast ventilation	I: Bent A: Bent near the surface	I: Close to body A: Curled forward, close to body	On plane of body, less or no movement
6—Very fearful	I: Laid ventrally or crouched directly on top of all paws, may be shaking A: Whole body near to ground, crawling, may be shaking	Not exposed, fast ventilation	I: Bent A: Bent near surface	I: Close to body A: Curled forward, close to body	Near to surface, motionless
7—Terrorized	I: Crouched directly on top of all fours, shaking A: NA	Not exposed, fast ventilation	I: Bent A: NA	I: Close to body A: NA	Lower than body, motionless

Score	Eyes	Pupils	Ears	Whiskers	Vocalization	Activity
1—Fully relaxed	Closed or half open, may be slowly blinking	Normal (consider ambient light)	Normal (half back)	Normal (lateral)	None or soft purr	Sleeping or resting
2—Weakly relaxed	Closed, half opened, or fully/ normally opened	Normal (consider ambient light)	Normal (half back) or erect and moved to front	Normal (lateral or forward)	None	Sleeping, resting, alert, or active, may be playing

TABLE 8-10

Seven-Level Cat-Stress-Score—cont'd

Score	Eyes	Pupils	Ears	Whiskers	Vocalization	Activity
3—Weakly tense	Normally opened	Normal (consider ambient light)	Normal (half back) or erect and moved to front or back and forward on head	Normal (lateral) or forward with small amount of tension	Meow or quiet	Resting, awake, or actively exploring
4—Very tense	Widely opened or pressed together	Normal or partially dilated	Erect to front or back or back and forward on head	Normal (lateral) or forward with tension	Meow, plaintive meow, or quiet	Cramped sleeping, resting, or alert, may be actively exploring, trying to escape
5—Fearful, stiff	Widely opened	Dilated	Partially flattened	Lateral (normal) or forward and back	Plaintive meow, yowling, growling, or quiet	Alert, may be actively trying to escape
6—Very fearful	Fully opened	Fully dilated	Fully flattened	Back	Plaintive meow, yowling, growling, or quiet	Motionless, alert, or actively prowling
7—Terrorized	Fully opened	Fully dilated	Fully flattened back on head	Back	Plaintive meow, yowling, growling, hissing, or quiet	Motionless, alert

Note: A further development of the Cat-Assessment-Score by McCune (1992).
A, Active; I, inactive; NA, not applicable. From Kessler and Turner, 1997.

categorical and narrative for the purpose of assessing shelter cats (Box 8-1).

Veterinarians would benefit from using such scores at visits and with hospitalized cats. A similar approach has been taken for cats who are painful or distressed (Table 8-11) with respect to assessment of pain. This assessment could also be used to evaluate aspects of stress and comfort level in hospitalized cats. The behavioral assessment through score 3 could be used for pet cats in people's homes, cats in shelters, and cats in free-ranging situations to help make decisions about preferred social affiliations (Table 8-12).

Feline Vocal Communication—What Can Cats Hear and What Are They Saying?

Vocal Communication

Moelk's (1944, 1979) classification of vocal communication involved five categories of vocal display: purr, chirr, call, meow, and growl/snarl/hiss.

- The *purr* is the classic feline sound associated with a contented cat. Nursing kittens purr, and occasionally older cats purr when slightly anxious. Little sonographic information is available about cat calls (McKinley, 1982), but it is conceivable that the purr that is elicited in the slightly anxious situation is considerably different from one elicited in other situations and that it communicates different information than the purr that is elicited in very relaxed situations.
- The *chirr* is like a meow that has been rolled on the tongue. Queens chirr when calling the kittens from the nest. If cats are friendly with each other, the chirr is a sound that one might make in eliciting the approach of another.
- The *call* is a very loud murmur that is produced with the mouth closed. It is primarily associated with a female who is solicitous of mating. The same signal has been reported to occur in males who are fighting with each other (Wolski, 1982).
- The *meow* is probably the most variable of the feline vocal signals. Cats use this signal to announce their presence, to solicit attention from others (epimeletic), or when they are thwarted in their ability to attain something they wanted. Meows produced by

BOX 8-1

Cat Stress Score

Score 1.0—Fully Relaxed
- Body laid on side or back
- Belly exposed and slow ventilation
- Legs fully extended
- Tail extended or loosely wrapped
- Head laid on the surface with chin upward or on the surface
- Eyes closed or half open and may be blinking slowly
- Pupils normal
- Ears half back (normal)
- Whiskers lateral (normal)
- No vocalization
- Sleeping or resting

Score 2.0—Weakly Relaxed
- Body laid ventrally or half on side, sitting, standing, or moving with back horizontal
- Belly exposed or not exposed and slow or normal ventilation
- Legs bent, hind legs may be laid out, and legs extended when standing
- Tail extended or loosely wrapped and may be up or loosely downward
- Head laid on the surface or over body and some movement
- Eyes closed, half opened, or normally opened
- Pupils normal
- Ears half back or erected to front
- Whiskers lateral or forward
- No vocalization
- Sleeping, resting, alert, or active, and may be playing

Score 3.0—Weakly Tense
- Body laid ventrally, sitting, standing or moving, and back horizontal
- Belly not exposed and normal ventilation
- Legs bent and legs extended when standing
- Tail on the body or curved backward, up or tense downward, and may be twitching
- Head over the body and some movement
- Eyes opened normally
- Pupils normal
- Ears half back (normal), erect to front or back and forward on head
- Whiskers lateral (normal) or forward
- Meowing or quiet
- Resting, awake, or actively exploring

Score 4.0—Very Tense
- Body laid ventrally, rolled or sitting, standing or moving, and body behind lower than in front
- Belly not exposed and normal ventilation
- Legs bent, hind legs bent when standing, and extended in front
- Tail close to the body, tense downward or curled forward, and may be twitching

- Head over the body or pressed to body and little or no movement
- Eyes widely opened or pressed together
- Pupils normal or partially dilated
- Ears erect to front or back or back and forward on head
- Whiskers lateral or forward
- Meow, plaintive meow, or quiet
- Cramped sleeping, resting, or alert, may be actively exploring, and trying to escape

Score 5.0—Fearful, Stiff
- Body laid ventrally, sitting, standing, or moving, and body behind lower than in front
- Belly not exposed and normal or fast ventilation
- Legs bent or bent near to surface
- Tail close to the body, curled forward
- Head on the plane of the body and less or no movement
- Eyes widely opened
- Pupils dilated
- Ears partially flattened
- Whiskers lateral, forward, or back
- Plaintive meow or yowling, growling, or quiet
- Alert and may be actively trying to escape

Score 6.0—Very Fearful
- Body laid ventrally or crouched directly on top of all paws, may be shaking, and whole body near to ground
- Belly not exposed and fast ventilation
- Legs bent or bent near to surface
- Tail close to the body and curled forward close to the body
- Head near to surface and motionless
- Eyes fully opened
- Pupils fully dilated
- Ears fully flattened
- Whiskers back
- Plaintive meow, yowling, growling, or quiet
- Motionless, alert, or actively prowling

Score 7.0—Terrorized
- Body crouched directly on all fours and shaking
- Belly not exposed and fast ventilation
- Legs bent
- Tail close to the body
- Head lower than the body and motionless
- Eyes fully opened
- Pupils fully dilated
- Ears fully flattened back on head
- Whiskers back
- Plaintive meow, yowling, growling, or quiet
- Motionless, alert

From McCobb et al. (2005), adapted from McCune (1992).

TABLE 8-11

Pain Scale

Pain Score	Behavior	Response to Palpation	Body Tension
0	• Content and quiet when unattended • Comfortable when resting • Interested in or curious about surroundings	• Not bothered by palpation of wound or surgery site or to palpation elsewhere	• Minimal
1	• Signs are often subtle and not easily detected in the hospital setting; more likely to be detected by the owner(s) at home • Earliest signs at home may be withdrawal from surroundings or change in normal routine • In the hospital, may be content or slightly unsettled • Less interested in surroundings but will look around to see what is going on	• May or may not react to palpation of wound or surgery site	• Mild
2	• Decreased responsiveness, seeks solitude • Quiet, loss of brightness in eyes • Lays curled up or sits tucked up (all four feet under body, shoulders hunched, head held slightly lower than shoulders, tail curled tightly around body) with eyes partially or mostly closed • Hair coat appears rough or fluffed up • May intensively groom an area that is painful or irritating • Decreased appetite, not interested in food	• Responds aggressively or tries to escape if painful area is palpated or approached • Tolerates attention, may even perk up when petted as long as painful area is avoided	• Mild to moderate • Re-assess analgesic plan
3	• Constantly yowling, growling, or hissing when unattended • May bite or chew at wound but unlikely to move if left alone	• Growls or hisses at non-painful palpation (may be experiencing allodynia, wind-up, or fearful that pain could be made worse) • Reacts aggressively to palpation, adamantly pulls away to avoid any contact	• Moderate • Re-assess analgesic plan
4	• Prostrate • Potentially unresponsive to or unaware of surroundings, difficult to distract from pain • Receptive to care (even aggressive or feral cats will be more tolerant to contact)	• May not respond to palpation • May be rigid to avoid painful movement	• Moderate to severe • May be rigid to avoid painful movement • Re-assess analgesic plan

Produced by Hellyer PW, Uhrig SR, Robinson NG, 2006, Colorado State University.

domestic cats are shorter in mean duration than meows produced by true wild cats (0.84 second vs. 1.50 seconds), have higher mean fundamental frequencies (609 Hz vs. 255 Hz), and have higher mean formant frequencies (1458 Hz vs. 1055 Hz) (Nicastro, 2004), suggesting that these vocal factors could have been shaped by living with people.

• The *growl/snarl/hiss* sounds are open-mouthed calls that are given in both offensive and defensive agonistic situations. These sounds may function to warn about subsequent behaviors should the aggressor pursue the interaction. There may also be a component of intimidation to these sounds that is associated with sex and body size. An element of vocal surprise may accompany these signals, which could be beneficial in an agonistic situation.

• Kiley-Worthington (1984) noted that cats also *chatter* their teeth when watching unattainable play. The chatter was called a displacement activity, although it may be indicative of underlying anxiety.

TABLE 8-12

Adapted Scale for Use in Homes, Shelters, or Free-Ranging Social Situations

Score	Behavior
0	• Content and quiet when unattended • Comfortable when resting • Interested in or curious about surroundings
1	• Signs often subtle and not easily detected; more likely to be detected by owner(s) at home • Earliest signs at home may be withdrawal from surroundings or change in normal routine • May seem unsettled • Less interested in surroundings but will look around to see what is going on
2	• Decreased responsiveness, seeks solitude • Quiet, loss of brightness in eyes • Lays curled up or sits tucked up (all four feet under body, shoulders hunched, head held slightly lower than shoulders, tail curled tightly around body) with eyes partially or mostly closed • Hair coat appears rough or fluffed up • May intensively groom an area that is painful or irritating • Decreased appetite, not interested in food
3	• Constantly yowling, growling, or hissing when unattended • Unlikely to move if left alone

Note: This scale sorts cats into those who are within their comfort zone and those who are not, regardless of the cause.

McKinley (1982) performed sonographic analysis of feline vocalizations and classified them into two broad groups on the basis of spectral characteristics: homogeneous, or pure, calls, and complex calls involving two or more pure types. *Pure calls include murmurs, growls, squeaks, shrieks, hisses, spits, and chatters. Complex calls include mews, moans, and meows.*

Table 8-13 presents a summary of the combined classifications of feline vocal signals.

The vocalization of kittens may differ from vocalizations of adult cats.

- Kittens can recognize a familiar voice by 4 weeks but do not generally take special notice of *each other's vocalizations until 9 weeks* (Moelk, 1944).
- Brown et al. (1978) describe a variety of cries given by kittens. Their type A cry often is given by kittens who awaken hungry, cold, or trapped (Haskins, 1979).
- Kittens may purr and tread while suckling.
- Purring can start at 2 days of age (Frazer-Sisson et al., 1991; Remmer and Gautier, 1972; Stogdale and Delack, 1985).
- Grunts are common at birth but disappear at maturity unless the cat is engaged in a particularly difficult task.
- Moelk describes an "acknowledgment" vocalization that starts at about 12 weeks of age and occurs when the kitten visualizes something he or she is about to receive.
- Mothers approach kittens with a variation of the chirr call that has been called a "brrp" or a "mhrn" (Moelk, 1979); this call is probably equivalent to the "chirp." These calls may function to stimulate kittens to nurse or to urinate or defecate.

- Very young kittens give an ultrasonic call if they are distressed so that their mother can locate them.
- By 3 weeks of age, calls of deaf kittens were louder and lower pitched than normal (Romand and Ehret, 1984). This may be part of the reason that deaf kittens may appear abnormal to others. It is not clear whether these kittens are shunned early and may have abnormal social development as a sequela to deafness.

Humans are able to recognize, appropriately interpret, and respond to a range of feline vocalizations, especially with respect to contextual effects on the "meow" vocalization.

- Humans can group meows as urgent or pleasant (Nicastro and Owren, 2003).
- The *meow is the most common cat-to-human vocalization* (Bradshaw and Cameron-Beaumont, 2000), but it is not a common cat-to-cat vocalization. This vocalization is rare in feral cats (Nicastro and Owren, 2003).
- Cat meows may act as referential signals, communicating specific information that is reliably correlated with behavioral context (Nicastro and Owren, 2003; Nicastro, 2004) based on the characteristics of the sounds coupled with the perceptions of the humans evaluating them.
  - Meows were recorded from five behavioral contexts common to human-cat interaction, including food-related calls (made before regular feeding), agonistic calls (calls made when the cats were antagonized by their owners, such as during vigorous brushing), affiliative calls (made when the cat solicited affection from their owners), obstacle calls (made when cats solicited help to negotiate

TABLE 8-13

Interpretation of Feline Vocalizations

Call	Description/Interpretation/Characteristics
Murmur	Rhythmically pulsed vocalization; exhalation; social interactions, solicitation, non-threatening; possibly due to dyssynchronous contraction of muscles in larynx and diaphragm (Remmers and Gautier, 1972)
Growl (MO)	Low-pitched, harsh, agonistic; lengthy—lasts 0.5-4 seconds with a fundamental pitch of 100-225 Hz
Yowl (MO)	Variable, higher pitched, rising threat, agonistic, offensive threat; can appear later in overtly defensive response to offensive aggression; lasts 3-10 seconds with a fundamental pitch of 200-600 Hz
Howl (MM)	Loud, plaintive call, location signal, uncertain, agonistic; lasts 0.8-15 seconds with a fundamental pitch of 700 Hz
Squeak	High-pitched, raspy; anticipation of feeding, females post-copulation
Shriek	Loud, high-pitched; pain, fear, aggression
Hiss (MO)	Agonistic, mouth open, teeth visible; overtly defensive aggression (cat usually avoids frank aggression at first); lasts 0.6-1 second and is atonal
Spit (MO)	Soft sound before or after hiss; overt defensive aggression; lasts ~0.02 second and is atonal
Snarl (MO)	Offensive aggressive signal, threat; lasts 0.5-0.8 second with a fundamental pitch of 225-250 Hz
Chatter	Anticipatory, frustration
Purr (MC)	Contact, contentment, nursing, mild conflicting anxiety; lasts >2 seconds at a fundamental pitch of 25-30 Hz
Chirr/trill/chirrup (MC)	Queen's call to kittens, greeting; lasts 0.4-0.7 second with a fundamental pitch of 250-800 Hz
Mew	High-pitched, medium amplitude; mother-kitten interaction for location, identification, encouragement
Moan	Low frequency/long duration; epimeletic; regurgitation, solicitation
Meow (MM)	Greeting, epimeletic, willingness to interact; lasts 0.5-1.5 seconds with a fundamental pitch of 700-800 Hz
Shriek	Pain, release signal, escape, fear of manipulation; lasts 1-2.5 seconds at a fundamental pitch of 900 Hz

Note: Does not include sexual calls.
MC, Mouth closed; MM, mouth moving from open to closed; MO, mouth held open. Data from Bradshaw and Cameron-Beaumont, 2000; Kiley-Worthington, 1984; McKinley, 1982; and Moelk, 1944.

a barrier, such as a closed door or window), and distress calls (made when the cats were placed in an unfamiliar environment, which was a car in this study). Specific behavioral profiles were noted to accompany these call types (Table 8-14), demonstrating the importance of understanding integrated signal modalities.

- All cats gave at least some single calls, mostly meows with short duration, limited frequency modulation, and less acute spectral tilt. Humans found these sounds relatively pleasant.
- Some calls had long duration, more acute spectral tilt, and more variety in vibration modes (the number of discrete segments) and appeared more urgent. Humans found these sounds less pleasant.

- The fundamental frequencies and first formant frequencies of housecats are shorter in duration than are those of feral cats, and all acoustic parameters of meows of housecats were higher in frequency than were those of their feral counterparts (Yeon et al., 2011).

Given these outcomes, and the differences in formant and fundamental frequencies and meow duration in domestic cats versus feral cats, one could hypothesize that the cat meow vocalization is an adaptation to human auditory preference. It is equally likely that this signal is the result of a reward structure where—regardless of reason—cats who meowed were provided with a resource they sought or liked. Humans may have also obtained additional, confirming, or redundant information from the non-vocal signals given by the cat.

TABLE 8-14

Context Category in Which Meows Were Noted and Accompanying Behavioral Descriptions

Context Category	Behavioral Description
Food related	Cat orients toward owner and/or food; eyes open, looking alternately from owner to food; ears up; tail up
Agonistic*	Cat orients toward offending object (e.g., hand or hairbrush) spitting; growling; ears back; eyes wide open; tail down and mobile
Affiliative*	Cat orients toward owner; leg rubbing; purring; eyes closed or half open; tail up
Obstacle	Cat orients toward obstacle (e.g., window or door); eyes open, looking alternately from owner to obstacle; tail up
Distress (being placed in a car)	No specific orientation, with repetitive movement such as pacing; eyes wide open; ears up but slightly back; tail down and mobile

Contexts in which pair-wise comparisons were always statistically significantly different. From Nicastro and Owren, 2003.

FELINE OLFACTORY SIGNALS—SIGNALS USING SMELL

As is true for dogs, cats have larger amounts of olfactory epithelium than humans. Domestic cats have 20 cm² of olfactory epithelium compared with 2 to 4 cm² in humans. This surface area is less than the maxilloturbinal development seen in dogs, for whom rapid respirations during exercise bring more air over the olfactory apparatus.

The difference between the olfactory epithelium distribution of the cat and the dog could be an adaptation to differences in hunting styles (Radinsky, 1975).

- Canids tend to hunt prey much larger than themselves and follow the prey over an extensive distance and time period.
- Most cats are solitary hunters and hunt and consume prey that requires a burst of, but not sustained, activity.

It is possible that the development of the olfactory apparatus is an adaptation to, or a corollary of, these differences in hunting styles.

Dogs can detect some volatile compounds at extremely low concentrations that are thousands of times lower than humans could detect (Davis, 1973; Walker et al., 2006). It is likely that cats are similar.

Cats exhibit a true gape/flehmen response and possess a vomeronasal organ/fluid pump. The vomeronasal duct opens into the incisive duct, rather than into the nasal cavity, as is the case for mice, and some vomeronasal nerve fibers extend past the accessory olfactory bulb, likely helping to integrate the main olfactory system and vomeronasal system information (Salazar and Sánchez-Quinteiro, 2011). Both the main olfactory system and the vomeronasal organ system are used to detect odorants and pheromones.

The cat has sebaceous glands on the tail (caudal glands), the forehead (temporal glands), the lips (perioral glands), the chin, and the pads (pedal glands) and glands associated with the whiskers. All of these areas can leave waxy secretions when rubbed.

- Rubbing of the tail and lips occurs most commonly on inanimate objects (Fox, 1975). Rubbing can leave and transfer scent.
- *It has been hypothesized that rubbing makes it easier to transfer and carry a scent rather than to deposit one* (Rieger, 1979). Such behaviors could alter the quality of a "colony scent" and may benefit the group.

Cheeks, ears, and flanks may also produce odorous secretions (Wolski, 1982). "Bunting," the process of rubbing on people, especially with the head and side of the face, is associated with scent deposition. Bunting is also associated with stimuli that inspire a gape/flehmen response; urine that is 3 days old can elicit bunting (Verberne and deBoer, 1976).

- Bunting is also a social behavior and may be an indication of a cat's confidence, comfort level, or relative social status or role in a group. More confident cats may bunt less confident cats and cats of lower status (Macdonald et al., 1987).
- It is unclear if the social rules governing this type of combined tactile and olfactory display are dependent on age, degree of familiarity, circumstance, et cetera.
- The form that head rubbing takes depends on topography (Verbene and deBoer, 1976). Cats who rub at the level of the cheek usually form a line from the corner of the mouth to the ear; if the cat is rubbing a higher object, he or she usually rubs the undersurface of the object using his or her forehead and ears followed by the side of the throat.
- Inanimate objects are rubbed by the flanks and tail. Males do not appear to rub more than females, but they may have more active sebaceous glands (Verbene and deBoer, 1976).
- If no other cats are present when a new cat is introduced into the environment, the new cat will sniff the room and rub the boundaries of it using the

submandibular gland. If other cats are present, this sequence is omitted.

- If two cats are introduced into a room, the one that is familiar with the room initially may follow the new cat, attempting to smell his or her anal region. Any rebuff usually takes the form of swatting and hissing, illustrating that all signaling modalities interact.
- Higher ranking and/or more confident male cats may scent-mark more by rubbing their cheeks than cats who rank lower/are less confident, so it has been postulated that males unable to communicate through olfaction using rubbing may instead spray urine (Ralls, 1971). This observation suggests that spraying can be a response to more forceful, overt signaling and play a role as a more passive signal of status that allows the cat to avoid physical conflict. The interaction between status and the deposition of urine or feces is complicated and poorly investigated.
- Wolski (1982) and Macdonald et al. (1987) found that males spray as they patrol the edges of a hunting range, and females most commonly spray only when entering a hunting range and intermittently while foraging.
- If a new male or female comes into an area, the first approach may involve marking with urine.
- If a new male entered and his scent is not a group scent, no female permits approach within 4 to 5 m without exhibiting a defensive posture.
- Avoidance of conflict was correlated with urine marks and ability to induce withdrawal of intruders in response to these (de Boer, 1977).
- Males spray more frequently than females (62.6 times per hour compared with 6 times per hour) (Apps, 1986).
- Females have been reported to mark by spraying *only* when they enter a hunting range and then intermittently while foraging (Fox, 1975).
- Estrous females spray more frequently than nonestrous females, regardless of whether they are hunting (Macdonald et al., 1987).
- Both sexes exhibit a flehmen response to unfamiliar urine.
- DeBoer (1977a) estimated that urine loses most of its attraction after 24 hours.
- In free-ranging cats, feces are usually covered in core areas of farms but are not often covered on pathways (peripheral areas), suggesting that leaving a clear visual and olfactory signal conveys information about the area that is unambiguous (Macdonald et al., 1987).
- The rate of scent marking using urine and/or feces has been said to correlate with status or rank (Ralls, 1971).
- Natoli (1985) reported that adult cats of both sexes distinguish the urine of strange males from familiar males, and males investigate odors longer than females.
- Frequency of spraying depends on whether cats are traveling and on their sex, reproductive status, and *level of social maturity.*

- Cats spray once every 5.4 minutes at rabbit burrows when traveling (Corbett, 1979).
- Non-breeding males spray 12.9 times per hour during travel, whereas breeding males spray 22 times per hour (Liberg, 1980; Liberg and Sandell, 1988).
- Hunting females spray once every 16.7 minutes or every 70 m (Panaman, 1981).
- Urine marking is less commonly exhibited by transient males; only five of nine "occasional" males urine mark (Natoli and de Vito, 1991).
- For "regular" (non-transient) males, *urine spraying is positively correlated not with the threats they give but with the threats they receive* ($P < 0.05$), including:
  - interference with copulation ($P < 0.01$),
  - rubbing of the chin ($P < 0.05$), and
  - vocal threats ($P < 0.02$).
- Urine spraying is *not correlated with threats given*, with interference with copulation, or with true or false mounts (Natoli and de Vito, 1991).
- For occasional/*transient males, spraying correlates with rubbing behavior* ($P < 0.01$), but *chin rubbing does not differ among regular/nontransient males*, where it is correlated with both giving ($P < 0.02$) and receiving ($P < 0.01$) threats and vocal duets ($P < 0.01$).
- Bateson and Bateson (1988) report that *confident males spray.* This makes sense because spraying has a profound visual component that would be instantly recognized by any cat watching.
- It logically follows that spraying can be a more passive form of aggression or an assertive behavior designed to inform other known, neighboring cats in a manner that decreases or diffuses conflict.
- Males stop squatting by about 8 to 10 months of age and will spray to urinate unless socially suppressed from doing so. If they are not reproductive, they may squat only to urinate as late as 13 to 18 months of age (Wolski, 1982). It is rare for free-ranging males to show urine marking in paternal areas.

The extent to which anal sac secretions are involved in olfactory communication or scent marking is under-explored.

- Urine that is sprayed may be more oily and viscous than urine that is eliminated by squatting and may contain anal sac secretions (Wolski, 1982).
- Feral cats spend more time sniffing sprayed urine of unknown cats than they do urine excreted by squatting, but the surface covered may also differ (Natoli, 1985).
- In experimental situations, cats can distinguish between urine that has been deposited by spraying and squatting (Passanisi and Macdonald, 1990).

Olfactory responsiveness to catnip is genetic (Hart and Leedy, 1985; Tucker and Tucker, 1988; Wolski, 1982).

- Cis-trans-nepetalactone-monoterpene can be detected in concentrations of 1 part in 10^{10} (Waller et al., 1969).

- Cats who respond to catnip experience an intense combination of face rubbing and body rolling and may lick, chew, or eat the catnip; shake their heads; gape; roll; rub; and twitch (Hatch, 1972).
- These induced behaviors are exhibited in a context and style that sets them apart from species typical sex or hunting behaviors.
- Catnip-induced behaviors may resemble obsessive-compulsive behaviors, possibly suggesting an area of shared mechanism. No data exist.

FELINE TACTILE SIGNALING—SIGNALS USING TOUCH

The cutaneous response in cats relies on both type 1 slow-adapting (SA) epidermal units, and type 2 SA dermal units.
- The type 1 SA units are grouped in "touch corpuscles" and terminate in specialized structures called Merkel cells (Iggo, 1966). *The resting rate of the discharge is proportional to the amount of the displacement of hair/indentation of skin.* Accordingly, cats are very sensitive to stroking.
- The type 2 SA dermal units are far more widely distributed and terminate in Ruffini endings, which are exquisitely sensitive to touch. Cats have an abundance of both type 1 and 2 SA units. A good map of the SA units and the accompanying rapidly adapting mechanoreceptors can be obtained by locating the areas of the skin that result in a scratch response.
- The scratch response is a complete reflex, requiring no input from the brain.
- The extent to which the cat's type 1 and 2 SA receptors may factor into the development of self-mutilation (over-grooming, "psychogenic" alopecia, obsessive-compulsive disorder) is unknown but worthy of investigation.
  SA cells are also found in the soft tissue at the base of claws.
- These SA cells affect degree of extension and sideways displacement of the claw (Gordon and Jukes, 1964), an aspect that is completely overlooked in discussions of onchyectomy (declawing).
- This anatomy suggests that "phantom pain" may have a true sensory component and that *tactile sensory function should be part of a welfare assessment.*
- Cats are extremely manually dexterous. Hairs on the ventrum of the carpus have both SA and rapidly adapting (RA) receptors and vibration-detecting pacinian corpuscles (Burgess and Perl, 1973).
- These hairs play roles in the pawing motions seen in play and the pouncing motions seen in predatory behavior.

The somatosensory area of the muzzle of cats is larger than that of dogs. Sensory hairs (vibrissae) are found on the cheeks (whiskers/mystacials), above the eyes (superciliary vibrissae), and on the side of the face (genal vibrissae). Cats do not have inter-ramal (between the rami of the mandible) vibrissae associated with their submandibular glands, but dogs do. Leyhausen (1979) proposed that this distribution is a correlate of differences in social investigation patterns. Dogs sniff the anal region of other dogs as a first step in the investigatory sequence. Cats start nose-to-nose, proceed to neck-to-flank, and then move on to anal sniffing (Leyhausen, 1979).

All vibrissae are supplied with RA mechanoreceptors and SA receptors. These *receptors signal the central nervous system about the amplitude, direction, and rate of the displacement of the vibrissae.* Cats possess short, stiff hairs around the base of the lips that connect to similar receptors. Among wildcats, those who hunt at night have more prominent vibrissae than those who hunt primarily during the day.
- With the mechanoreceptors at the base of the canines, these vibrissae allow exquisite control over adjustment of position for predatory strikes. Considered with the *laterally compressed canines that connect to and that hold prey, permitting dislocation of vertebrae in one bite,* cats are uniquely adapted to their form of predation (Bradshaw, 1992).
- Biting in cats has been studied as part of agonistic and predatory behaviors (Adamec, 1975a; Adamec et al., 1980a, 1980b, 1980c). *The "quiet biting attack" is controlled by groups of neurons in the hypothalamus and midbrain that mediate the effects of learned behavior* (Bernston et al., 1973, 1976a, 1976b; Kolgan, 1989). This type of bite involves trigger zones around the face, lips, and mouth and the tactile stimuli of the guard hairs in the forepaw and is facilitated by interactions between the RA and SA receptors at the base of the vibrissae.
  - This may be why cats who self-mutilate do more chewing than licking. In contrast, dogs who self-mutilate do more licking.
- *Persistent biting in cats requires the stimulus of the trigeminal receptors* around the mouth, plus all the touch receptors already discussed (Siegal and Potts, 1988).
  - This association could also function in grooming abnormalities and potential obsessive-compulsive disorders.

UNDERSTANDING SOCIAL AND GROUP BEHAVIOR IN CATS

Types of Behaviors Involved

Leyhausen (1979) classified friendly behaviors into six groups:
1. sleeping together,
2. grooming,
3. rubbing against each other and sharing olfactory marks (this has been postulated to be very important in group situations and *may be one of the factors that irritates other cats in the household when one cat has visited the veterinarian*),

4. friendly greeting after a prolonged absence (although "friendly" is left undefined),
5. running beside each other and purring, while rubbing with the tail raised, and
6. play behavior.

Social cohesion is promoted by murmuring, purring, rubbing, and rolling. Behaviors such as rubbing and rolling are visual but may impart olfactory information. Cats who rub acquire odor from an individual or substrate. Individual cats who live in a group situation may rub together frequently and create a *colony* odor, which provides a fast assessment toll for recognizing whether an individual is an intruder.

Rubbing/allorubbing (rubbing another cat) is a key behavior that acts as social cement.

- If animals are well known to each other, they may rub bodies more frequently than animals that are not known (see photos accompanying the definition of "social rub" in Table 8-9).
- Allorubbing may involve foreheads, cheeks, flanks, and tails.
- If two animals that are known to each other approach and raise their tails, it may mean that they intend to rub (Bradshaw, 1992).
- The tail may specify the form of rubbing. If a second cat raises her tail, the cats might simultaneously rub each other. If the second cat does not raise her tail, the recipient may rub after the initiator has rubbed, or the recipient may not rub.
- The cat who is able to elicit the first rub is generally viewed as the higher status cat, or the one to whom the others will defer. Clients can use such information to understand social relationships in their own household.

Laboratory colonies of cats often provide an opportunity to observe cats who are relatively nonaggressive to each other in a confined, controlled situation. Podberscek et al. (1991b) studied a colony of cats composed of seven castrated males and one intact male. *Agonistic behaviors constituted less than 1% of the total interactions, indicating how rare such behaviors are in situations when the social "rules"—likely the result of long-term knowledge and exposure—are apparent. Such findings act as a cautionary tale for rankings of cats based on staged contest outcomes or interactions within novel situations.* Clearly, agonistic behavior is not the normal mode of behavior among known cats. A study of only female laboratory cats Hurni and Rossbach (1987) found that all the cats would sleep together and were quite companionable.

Maintenance behaviors *also* have value as signals.
- Turner (1988) noted that feral cats performed claw sharpening more often in the presence of conspecifics than when alone.
- The sole function of scratching is not to remove sheaths, although excess sheath material may increase the frequency of actual scratching.

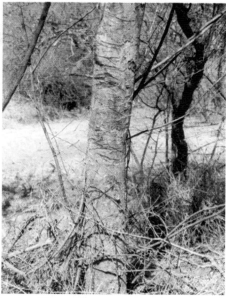

Fig. 8-6 Tree in the interstices of two lion prides showing old and new scratch marks.

- Scratching is also an olfactory signal. The timing of the visit by the scratching cat can be gauged by intensity of odorants and texture/color of the scratches (Fig. 8-6).
- Cats scratch new or old objects, but the *longer the object is scratched, the more significant it is to the cat.*

Social living provides any animal with the following:
1. a defense against predators,
2. an ability to exploit food resources that might not be exploitable were one asocial,
3. reproductive access to conspecifics,
4. facilitation of learning about the environment, and
5. a collective resistance to harsh environments.

All research on cat colonies supports that cats benefit from and use all of these factors as part of their complex social relationships within what are usually extended family groups.

What Rule Organizes Cats?

As noted by Liberg et al. (2000), there is great variability and flexibility in feline social systems. This variability is likely attributable to the shared demands of the demographic, social, biophysical, and resource environments in which they find themselves by virtue of being a species of almost infinite opportunism.

Discussions of the social nature of cats have been couched in "dominance-submission" terminology (Fonberg, 1985; Natoli and De Vito, 1988, 1991; Natoli et al., 2001), and terminology pertaining to "linear hierarchies." We should ask whether this approach is valid.

The *classic definition of "dominance" emphasizes both the minimization of fighting and that a truly "dominant" animal can aggress against another rarely and with impunity*

(Immelmann and Beer, 1989). *In this use of the concept of "dominance," "dominant" animals seldom actually aggress against others*, although they engage in much posturing and signaling behavior that encourages the other animal, or the recipient, *to initiate a deferential behavior.* This signaling or posturing can be very subtle and can be as simple as standing and blocking access to an entryway or to a desired area. *"Dominance" as defined in this manner is a correlate of some special skill, asset, or ability, which enhances overall social order and risk minimization.* The defining characteristic could be age, and in studies done by Feldman (1993, 1994), juvenile males were shown to roll over preferentially for older males, and older males were the recipients of most of the "belly-up" displays. *For the concept of "dominance" to add more to the social system that mere age does,* the aforementioned criteria must be met: *appropriateness of the behavior and risk minimization in service of more efficient social order.* Unfortunately, *this type of detailed care in establishing external referent and roles for behavioral sequences and outcomes is seldom observed, suggesting that we'd do best to let go of this concept.*

As now commonly used, the concept of "dominance" is seldom defined separately from scoring which cat is "dominant" and which cat is "submissive." There is almost never an external, independent referent that defines the condition in a way that allows it to be evaluated separately from the label. If cats exhibit "dominant" behaviors, they have higher "dominance" scores, and behaviors that are not "dominant" must be "submissive." Because so many of these evaluations are conducted in either staged or *de facto* contests (e.g., access to a food bowl, access to mates), "winning" is always confounded with the definition of "dominant" behaviors, whereas "losing" is confounded with the definition of "submissive" behaviors. Little thought is given to whether the labels "dominant" and "submissive" add anything to our understanding of cat behavior. In fact, they may obscure more than they add.

The fields of veterinary behavior and behavioral medicine has largely moved away from the concept of dominance in dogs for three reasons pertaining to advances in our knowledge and understanding:

1. The concept has been seen as epistemologically insufficient for understanding interactive dog behavior.
2. The use of the concept of "dominance" has occurred in a manner that causes clients to view their dogs within an adversarial context where every interaction is structured by some level of aggression.
3. As a result, the recommendation to redress such issues was to "dominate" the dog. The latter almost always involves punitive physical struggles in the guise of "training practices" that are risky for both parties and often abusive to the dogs.

As used, the application of this concept is injurious to an animal's welfare and quality of life. Because of the different relationship we have with cats, *cats have at least escaped the forceful and often abusive redress to which dogs so characterized have been subjected.* Unfortunately, the literature is rife with examples of epistemological insufficiencies for understanding cat behavior and the view that all relationships are about dominion.

Linear hierarchies are hierarchies determined by sequential "wins" in "contests" where the lower cats lose or lose to all of those above and the higher cats win or win over all those lower on a strict ladder. Transitivity is usually assumed, and dyadic relationships (interactions between pairs) are the rule. Transitivity means that if cat A "wins" over cat B and cat B "wins" over cat C, cat A would "win" over cat C.

All arguments of "dominance," "submission," dyadic (paired) "wins" and "losses," and transitivity are subject to how these terms are defined (because definitions are far from universal) and how outcomes were defined and evaluated. Even if the terms are discretely defined, it is almost always assumed that these are real properties and apply to the social relationships of the animals in question. Whether these properties are real and apply to the group studied is seldom evaluated or questioned.

When such consideration has occurred (Rowell, 1974), *relationships are better defined by non-aggressive interactions and by deferential behaviors designed to avoid conflict.* True aggressive encounters are exceptional in any social system, including those involving cat colonies (Natoli and De Vito, 1991). Of 1,066 interactions between cats classified as "agonistic" (e.g., the sum of the "aggressive" and "submissive" behaviors), only 1 involved frank aggression (Knowles et al., 2004). Overt fights are more likely if there is no difference in social stature between the individuals and if the cats view each other as equals (Wolski, 1982). Cats with "high status" may decline to fight their antagonist actively. These cats will often just walk away, sit, groom, and look away. Only a very confident cat (i.e., a cat who could elicit deference) would be able to do this.

This is *not* the same as saying relationships are defined by submissive behaviors. *Instead, we should consider that no concept of dominance is required to achieve social relationships organized by avoidance of unnecessary conflict and relationship status, determined by knowledge of or familiarity with the participants and their ability or skill levels.* The latter is a definition of *deference.*

When a dominance-submissive system is used to classify cat behavior and when the behaviors used for assessment are noted, three broad behavioral groups are recognized (Cafazzo and Natoli, 2009; Knowles et al., 2004; Natoli and De Vito, 1991; Natoli et al., 2001): *aggressive behaviors, submissive behaviors* (the two poles of "agonistic behavior"), and *affiliative behaviors.*

Aggressive behaviors generally include:
- threats—striking with a paw, biting, assuming a threatening posture, pointing, staring at, baring of the canines,

- chasing,
- ritualized vocal duels, and
- actual fighting.

Interference of copulation by blocking a male from mounting another female or by mounting the male himself may be included.

Submissive behaviors usually include:

- crouching with flattened ears,
- avoidance,
- retreat,
- fleeing, and
- hissing at.

Spraying and marking using chin rubs may be included.

Affiliative behaviors include:

- sniffing noses,
- rubbing, and
- tail up.

Given this classification system, one wonders how much actual behavior is not discussed. For example, this classification system would be wholly inadequate to discuss the behaviors of the cats in Figure 8-7, which represent the type of snapshot in time many sampling methods employ.

Cats forced to share a room developed a linear hierarchical relationship with an identifiable "dominant"/"alpha" male, independent of food resources Winslow (1938, 1944). "Dominance relationships" in these studies were estimated by using mounting behavior as an indication of status: Individuals who permitted themselves to be mounted were classified as having lower status, and individuals doing most of the mounting were classified as having higher status. Winslow ascertained that if you removed the most aggressive animal, the "next most aggressive" took over. In Winslow's system, the highest ranking animal mounted all newcomers regardless of their sex.

No other study has demonstrated this type of rigid, linear dominance hierarchy. Given the strikingly low frequency of agonistic interactions reported in other studies, we should ask whether some other factor contributed to this outcome.

Masserman and Siever (1944) and Baerends et al. (1957) found that stable "dominance hierarchies" were

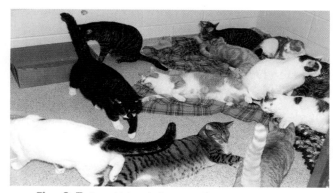

Fig. 8-7 A cat blood donor colony at a university.

apparent *if the group size was limited to four* and if the measurement of "hierarchy" was taken *at a feeding station*. It should be remembered that the evolutionary history of the domestic cat is as a solitary predator who eats multiple small meals during the day: concentrated, *ad libitum* feeding would be extraordinary. Never discussed in such designs is the extent to which clumped resources and forced social groupings can contribute to *pathological behavior.* Without such a discussion and evaluation, caution is urged in assuming that such studies are unequivocal portrayals of social behavior among cats.

- Artifact also played a role in the determination of rank in the study Knowles et al. (2004) where access to a single food bowl structured the "relationships" between the 28 cats studied. This study was complicated by the genealogical relationships between some but not all of the cats and a criterion of "displacement" for a determination of "dominant" versus "submissive."
- The artifact can be compounded by feeding cats periodically rather than *ad libitum* and in multiple areas. Cats in the former design are less cooperative and more aggressive than cats in the latter design (Finco et al., 1986).
- Clear, linear dominance hierarchies appear to be artifacts of provisioning (Baerends et al., 1957) and are stable over time *only* in experiments that are driven by food. "Dominant" animals may be able to announce or enforce their status by occupying specific spaces (Bernstein and Strack, 1993, 1996), although their preferred occupation of shelf and sleeping boxes appears driven by the responses of others, not by aggressive encounters (Podberscek et al., 1991b).
- Studies on colony cats generally involve cats in a relatively narrow age group. In Podberscek et al. (1991b), all cats were 2 to 3 years of age. Cats mature socially somewhere in this age range, with most cats maturing between 2.5 to 3.5 and 4 years of age (sexual maturity occurs by 6 to 10 months). The extent to which variation in age and maturity structure influences social behaviors in colony cats has not been investigated.
- Hierarchical relationships can be influenced by colony management. Laboratory cats with free access to food eat several small meals a day (7 to 16 meals) randomly without developing a hierarchical relationship and, when given the opportunity, will sleep alone (Thorne, 1982). Given that most laboratory cats sleep more in the day than during the night (Kuwabara et al., 1986), it would be interesting to know if most of the observations would change throughout a diel cycle.
- Natoli and de Vito (1991) describe shifting, linear "dominance hierarchies" that are based on the outcome of agonistic encounters. These hierarchies were not associated with any measure of copulatory success, and all of the males in the Natoli and de Vito

study marked regularly. Yet there was no difference between the type and frequency of marking among males.

- Yamane (1998) found that heavier males courted females both within their own group and in other groups. Lighter males courted only females in their own group. Heavier males almost always bested lighter males in any kind of contest, and mass varied with age—heavier males were older. None of this predicted male reproductive success. Based on DNA paternity analysis, almost half of the kittens produced in the group were fathered by extra-group males, suggesting that females prefer something other than he who appears to "win" a contest.

- Regardless of the study, within these experimental designs, any study that evaluated differences in the reliability of the hierarchy when using "aggressive" versus "submissive" behaviors were used found that ranks based on more "submissive" behaviors were more reliable than ranks based on "aggressive" behaviors (Curtis et al., 2003; Natoli et al., 2001). We should consider that avoidance of odd aggressive behaviors may be adaptive, whether those behaviors occur in natural or manipulated circumstances. Cats have preferred associates—cats who choose to sit within 1 m of another cat and possibly engage in grooming. Conflict is low among these associates (Curtis et al., 2003). We may be advised to conclude that any natural hierarchy is most likely to be fluid, dependent on knowledge of other cats and their skill sets, and self-reinforcing of appropriate social behaviors that minimize risk.

- If cats are rendered anxious, *the less anxious animals become higher ranking*. This finding has broad applicability for all animals and social systems, especially for those in which *inappropriate, out-of-context aggression is an outgrowth of anxiety*. Animals who are less anxious are more able to interact normally in an appropriate social context and provide the basis for a fluid social hierarchy to be determined by contextual response and maintained by deference.

- In his study of free-ranging cat populations, Leyhausen (1979) found that individual cats defer to others by sitting, moving to the side, or looking away.

- Deference systems based on knowledge of individual animals in the group are one characteristic of sociality.

Marking (feces and/or urine) may be important in the maintenance of complex, social hierarchies. Unless such subtle communicatory signals are noticed, one could assert that the social system is maintained by a far simpler mechanism, such as "linear dominance."

Roles for Spatial Structure

Social distance may affect the type and intensity of signaling behavior and so affect all aspects of relationships. Common ethological categories of distances include, from the largest to the smallest area affected:

- flight distance—the distance at which one will flee a potentially threatening situation,
- home range—the area in which one spends the most time (95% of all activities occur here), daily or seasonally,
- territory—an actively defended area (*sensu* Burt, 1943),
- critical distance—the interpersonal area in the center of use of the territory's core area,
- social distance, and
- personal distance (Hinde, 1970).

All of these distances can be identified within households of cats, and clients are usually able to do so as well as identify preferred associates, if asked, but we seldom ask for this information. Given the complexity of the feline social system and the extent to which it is so much more subtle than that for dogs, veterinarians would benefit from asking about these relationships and patterns and encouraging clients to report on them.

Much of the research on social relationships, "hierarchy," and spatial use focuses on who gets to meet whom. Within a population, one issue has been whether central locations differ from peripheral ones.

- Toms mate sequentially with the same female, rather than monopolizing her, regardless of core use location (Liberg, 1983).

- Multiple males are frequently reported to be in attendance of one estrous female (Dards, 1983), and under certain demographic situations there may be no competition for females because the females are unlikely to reject known males.

- Regardless of colony size, most amicable social relationships occur between females at the rate of 0.5 to 0.9 interactions per hour. Most aggressive social interactions occur toward intruders, regardless of location (Macdonald et al., 1987).

These findings suggest that the interaction of many environments, not just location with the colony, affects who interacts with whom.

Central and peripheral individuals may not have the same success in reproduction.

- When the number of kittens produced per female per year is examined with regard to location in colony, more litters fail per year in the periphery of large colonies than in small and medium colonies, but central areas of small colonies have failure rates greater than those of the periphery (Kerby and Macdonald, 1988; Macdonald et al., 1987).

- Female cats with peripheral locations have a greater distance between their den and food sites, and after 7 years, these individuals have no surviving descendants.

- More males disperse during their second or third year (correlated with the attainment of social maturity), if they are not protected from harassment by conspecifics. The extent of colony size on this buffer effect is unclear but merits further study.

These findings have a direct application for individuals who allow their cats to roam outdoors. One of the most commonly given reasons for the loss of pet cats is that the cat "left." Lack of refugia within complex, free-ranging cat social systems can contribute to feline emigration or death (Clancy et al., 2003).

Cat density has also been examined with respect to factors affecting colony size.

- In free-ranging situations, cat population densities range from 0.9 to 2350/km.
- Colony sizes can range from 1 to 52 cats (Jones and Coman, 1982; Rees, 1981), and home-range size is equally as variable.
- Densities of greater than 100 cats/km^2 are associated with plentiful resources, and densities of fewer than 5 cats/km^2 are associated with scarce, dispersed resources (Liberg and Sandell, 1988).
- Cats in dense populations (23.5 cats/ha) have *separate memberships in feeding groups that do not reflect their other interactions* (Izawa et al., 1982).
- Home ranges for both males and females (male home range, 620 ha; female home range, 170 ha) overlap minimally, but there is a greater overlap under conditions of patchy resources.
- In one study of cats in a dockyard that has been enclosed by a high wall since 1711, family groups range from 2 to 11 individuals, and all adult females are related (Dards, 1983). Mature males have freely overlapping home ranges that average 8.4 ha. Other males and females share group home ranges, ranging in size from 0.03 to 4.2 ha.
- Male home ranges can be two to four times larger than those of females and juveniles, and *males can travel 4 km per night* in the course of monitoring their home range (Wolski, 1982).
- Male interactions with females are most common in small colonies, but male interactions with males are most common in medium colonies.
- Female interactions with females are most common in medium-sized colonies; in these colonies, females spend 40% of their time with another cat, usually touching it.
- Groupings of cats are non-random; social groups are highly structured. In small colonies, males spend 31% of their time in the area that is the focus of most

activities, whereas females spend 65% to 85% of their time in this area.

- Home-range size is affected by social and physiological factors, such as queens in estrus. Males range farther than usual at such times (Bradshaw, 1992).
- Males in free-ranging groups usually have home ranges that are 3.5 times larger than those of females, and they range up to 10 km^2 (Liberg and Sandell, 1988).
- Males 2 to 4 years of age may challenge resident males, but they are not able to succeed in these challenges until they are approximately 3 to 5 years of age and have attained adult mass and are socially mature.
- Female home ranges overlap with those of males, *but the breeding lives of most females are short and do not last more than 6 years.* Under normal free-ranging conditions, domestic felines may not bear their first litter until they are socially mature, at approximately 2 to 3 years of age (Wolski, 1982).

Most of these data are from free-ranging domestic cats. Very few data are available for pet cats in true household groupings. Early data from longitudinal studies on domestic cats indicate that most people can identify a "dominant cat" on the basis of *responses that the cat receives from other cats* in the household (Bernstein and Strack, 1993). *Frank aggression is exceptional.* Hierarchies appear to be associated with assertive cat behavior *and* with the locations and subgroups in which the cats are found. One cat might elicit deference in one group situation, whereas another elicits deference in a more solitary situation involving a perch site. Data such as these are rare but essential if we are to understand the complexity and elegance driving social behavior in domestic cats.

When such data are collected, we would do well also to attend to how cats interact with humans. Wedl et al. (2011) found that the more active the cat, the fewer non-overlapping behavior patterns and the higher the event complexity of the cat's behavior. The older the cat, the lower the "dyadic complexity" for interactions between human-cat pairs. Finally, the more extraverted the human, the higher the number of non-overlapping behavioral patterns exhibited by cats. Redress of behavioral concerns for cats requires an understanding of all environmental contributions. For cats who are pets, the main interactive environment may not be that of conspecifics.

Undesirable, Problematic, and Abnormal Feline Behavior and Behavioral Pathologies

OVERVIEW OF FELINE BEHAVIORAL CONCERNS

People misunderstand cats, and to some extent *people expect to misunderstand cats*. In part, much of the confusion about feline behavior is a function of their atypical, opportunistic "domestic" status.

We have not worked with cats historically to shape their behaviors for collaborative work with us in the ways we have for dogs, horses, and stock.

- Dogs, as a species separate from wolves, likely co-evolved with humans over thousands or tens of thousands of years, during which time they may not have been fully "domesticated."

- "Domestication" may have occurred when we began to develop breed groups intended for specific tasks, which happened 3000 or more years ago. In contrast to wolves, which require handling by humans early in their ontogeny (beginning by at least 14 days of age) if they are not to be fearful and reactive to humans, *most dogs can adapt to delays in handling and exposure, and their normal, innate sensitive periods are greatly expanded from those of wolves*. When dogs cannot adapt or when they seem to have short sensitive periods, such patterns are indicative of pathology.

- In dogs, it is likely that this *sensitive period expansion* occurred concomitantly with changes in molecular and neurochemical function and gene expression (Saetre et al., 2004), which may represent some of the *true outcomes of active "domestication."* In contrast to dogs but similar to other, non-domesticated species, *cats have a relatively short and truncated sensitive period for exposure to humans* (Karsh, 1983a, 1984), *which may be associated with or evidence of lack of tampering associated with "domestication."* Combined with a remarkable neurology that allows for extremely rapid and pronounced arousal and reactivity (discussed later), this shortened sensitive period of cats may suggest why true domestication may be only ongoing now, while also shedding light on the potential etiology of some common feline behavioral patterns and pathologies (i.e., inter-cat aggression, impulse-control aggression, re-directed aggression).

- We have not selected cats to "please" us or to be easily handled by us, attributes that Galton (1865) stated were necessary for successful domestication to occur (see Chapter 8). No cat has been selected to work actively with us in a collaborative partnership, and although we lack extensive global data, the sensitive periods of cats who have been housecats for generations do not seem to differ from cats who have been free-ranging or feral for generations. Because of how cats may become feral, there may also be contributory genetic factors that influence the heritability of fear, which may influence how effects of social exposure are manifest or mitigated. There is scant research on this topic, but the implications for behaviors and interactions with humans are profound.

- Domestic cats have traditionally been defined as "sit-and-wait" predators, meaning that they hide from their prey and sit and wait by trails, dens, nests, et cetera, as indicated by physical, olfactory, and vocal cues about prey activity. Among mammals, cats are really the only "sit-and-wait" predators, and domestic cats are the quintessential mammalian species using this strategy. Coat color patterns in ancestral cats and many extant cat types/breeds act as disruptive coloration and aid the cat in hiding. As a condition of the "sit-and-wait" hunting strategy, cats are compelled to sit quietly hidden and then react almost instantly with a heightened level of arousal. The behavioral and neurochemical difference between sitting quietly hidden and the profound arousal and reactivity required for successful hunting *may have placed constraints on feline brain development with respect to cognitive and social strategies*. Cats have "normal" arousal patterns that are different from other species, an observation that likely has implications for how they develop problematic or pathological behaviors.

- As we have moved with cats to more urban lifestyles many of the behaviors that are normal for cats could be and frequently are problematic for their humans (i.e., eliminating and digging in gardens, especially if those gardens belong to others).

- Behaviors that people might find distressing (e.g., hiding, spraying, fighting with another cat) may be a *fairly normal cat's response to an environment that is confusing, stressful, or distressing to the cat.*
- Left to themselves, cats range widely. When they are constrained to live within a house or an apartment, that spatial constraint may alter and/or intensify a number of behaviors other than behaviors associated with mobility.
- We have no idea how often we see the types of extreme behavioral pathologies in "domestic" cats that we now know appear endogenously in dogs. We *do* know that when such profoundly abnormal behavior reaches the level of true pathology, as is the case in feline obsessive-compulsive disorder (OCD), the manifestation of the condition always appears to have *a component of environmental change or disruption.* In other words, although it is possible that the cat may be exhibiting pathological OCD (or other truly abnormal behaviors) at some very low level, and/or the cat may have a risk/liability to develop OCD, the abnormality is not seen or fully manifest *until the additional social or environmental stressor* is supplied (Overall and Dunham, 2002). *That the intersection of innate feline reactivity with other social/physical environments so consistently seems to be involved in some aspect of pathology may be further evidence that cats have not yet been "domesticated."*

The extent to which all of these patterns are attributable to the differences in our evolutionary history with cats compared with dogs or the extent to which these patterns are attributable to the uniqueness of a small, "sit-and-wait" predator who hides as a response to stress, is unknown. Because of the clear interplay of social and environmental effects in determining the manifestation or extent of abnormal feline behavior, and because *so many normal feline behaviors are often considered undesirable or "abnormal,"* no attempt to separate groups of problematic behaviors rigidly by class has been made here as was done for dogs. Instead, historical, social, environmental, endogenous, and evolutionary factors are discussed, when relevant, for each condition, as is *the importance of client knowledge and expectations.* It is hoped that this approach will allow the clinician to identify when behavioral pathologies and troublesome environments intersect in client complaints and so encourage the clinician to address and treat the whole cat and the cat-client relationship.

ZOONOTIC CONCERNS RELEVANT TO PATTERNS OF FELINE BEHAVIOR

There are four main zoonotic concerns that are germane to cat behavior: rabies, cat-scratch disease (CSD), toxoplasmosis, and toxocariasis. Both cats and dogs are subject to rabies. In rabies-endemic countries, good vaccination programs are an essential part of rabies control and eradication. Rabies is such a commonly discussed public health concern that the average reader will be aware of it. The same may not be true for *Bartonella* infections (commonly called "cat-scratch disease/CSD/cat-scratch fever"), toxoplasmosis, and toxocariasis. These are the conditions about which clients may have some information that they find confusing. Because so many behavioral problems involve complaints about the cat's elimination behaviors or rough treatment of humans by cats, it is imperative that we have an accurate assessment of zoonotic risk. Clients are often willing to tolerate some behavioral inconsistencies on the part of the cat (e.g., not always using the litterbox), and clients may adjust to some undesirable behaviors that the cat exhibits (e.g., never playing with the cat when he is on his back). However, *these minor behavioral issues become major ones when any human health concern is raised and will become the reason that the cat is relinquished or euthanized.* Especially in difficult economic times, cat behaviors—whether they are normal but undesirable or truly abnormal and damaging to the cat—must be viewed as one set of stressors in an interacting list of lifestyle stressors that can result in the client's decision to remove the cat from the household. Most relinquished cats are never re-homed. Relinquished cats are most often killed.

Cat-Scratch Disease

- Each year in the United States, 22,000 cases (1.8 to 10 cases/100,000 people) of CSD have historically been reported. There have been 2,200 people hospitalized annually (Jackson et al., 1993).
- The presumptive agent in CSD is the rickettsial organism, *Bartonella* (formerly *Rochalimaea*) *hensalae.* An occasional contributory role has been postulated for the bacteria *Afipia felis.* Of 45 human patients with CSD, 38 had titers of at least 1:64 for *B. hensalae. B. hensalae* is likely the predominant, but not the only, cause of CSD, and other *Bartonella* species have been implicated in infection (Breitschwerdt, 2011).
- CSD is most commonly seen in the late summer and fall everywhere it has been studied and coincides with seasonality in births of kittens (spring) and the entry of these kittens into the house in the fall/winter (Sanguinetti-Morelli et al., 2011).
- Flea infestations may be associated with a higher incidence of *Bartonella* infections, and it has been reported that most human patients with CSD have at least one kitten that has fleas (Zangwill et al., 1993). Patients with CSD are more likely to have a kitten 1 year of age or younger or to have been scratched by a kitten, than are non-patients (Zangwill et al., 1993). Although human patients diagnosed with CSD and living in households *with* kittens are more likely to have been scratched

or bitten than humans living in households *without* kittens, there appears to be no association, other than age, with patients' cats and cats of controls when indoor/outdoor status, litterbox use, and hunting behaviors are examined (Zangwill et al., 1993).

- Infection with *Bartonella* can occur *without* any history of bites or scratches by cats or exposure to cats. Coupled with the extremely complex relationship that the *Bartonella* organism has with vectors and reservoir hosts, it is not surprising that feline bartonellosis need not always manifest in the same manner across patients (Breitschwerdt, 2008).
- Cats transmitting *Bartonella* appear healthy, although they may have long-lasting, active *B. hensalae* infections (Regnery et al., 1992). People with what is viewed as traditionally conceived CSD tend to have localized skin lesions and regional lymph node involvement 3 weeks after exposure. Lymph nodes remain enlarged for several months. Systemic illness is rare, but fever, headache, splenomegaly, and malaise are common. These symptoms are usually self-resolving; however, arthritis, neuroretinitis, pleurisy, pneumonia, osteolytic lesions, granulomatous hepatitis, and encephalitis with coma and seizure can be unusual sequelae (Tompkins and Steigbigel, 1993). Individuals with immunocompromise or immunosuppression are at risk for more severe disease. Treatment ranges from outpatient care comprising relatively short courses of antibiotics to detailed, extended inpatient care.
- *Bartonella* species infections are increasingly implicated as a potential contributory factor in many immune diseases, including rheumatoid arthritis, and in vector-mediated chronic bacteremias (Maggi et al., 2012).

Because of the public health aspects of infection, fractious kittens should be sensibly and safely managed, and veterinarians should discuss the signs of *Bartonella* with the clients of such kittens. *Any feline aggression should be treated as soon as it is recognized, which is also humane for the cat.*

Toxoplasmosis

Toxoplasmosis, caused by *Toxoplasma gondii*, is an infection that may be mild or asymptomatic in adult humans but can be congenitally induced when pregnant females become infected with *T. gondii.* In adult humans, infection is usually, but not always, mild and may result in malaise, joint and muscle pain, transiently enlarged lymph nodes, and other non-specific signs of inflammation. Infants born with toxoplasmosis may have a range of profound problems primarily affecting the nervous system. For individuals infected in utero, pathology may include enlarged liver and spleen, gastrointestinal illness, hearing and/or vision loss or debility, seizures and cognitive impairments. For untreated infants, these conditions may become most pronounced as the nervous system matures when they pass through their teens. Maternal and fetal infections are treatable, but from the standpoint of the behavior of cats, most of these infections are preventable.

- *T. gondii* oocytes are shed in feces.
- Because cats are the final host and reservoir for *T. gondii,* cats are blamed for human infection. However, humans likely contact *T. gondii* most frequently through exposure to raw meat that has been infected because of poor hygiene (Torda, 2001).
- Human infection is rare and usually asymptomatic, *unless* the human is pregnant or immunosuppressed.
  - Pregnant woman can pass *T. gondii* to the fetus during pregnancy, resulting in abortion, stillbirth, or neurological complications for the infant (Tenter et al., 2000).
  - Immunosuppressed individuals may develop fulminant forms of the disease.
  - Pregnant and immunosuppressed humans should not handle raw meat, cat feces, or cat litter; should cook all meat thoroughly to ensure that cysts are killed before consumption; and should wash their hands thoroughly after interacting with their cats.
- Information for clients is available on the following websites: www.petsandparasites.org./cat-owners and www.cdc.gov/parasites/toxoplasmosis/gen_info/pregnant.html (both accessed April 24, 2012).

Toxocariasis

- Toxocariasis is a zoonosis caused by accidental human ingestion of the embryonated eggs of the roundworms *Toxocara canis* and *Toxocara cati,* which routinely affect dogs and cats.
- Especially in urban areas, cats with large—and likely untreated—worm burdens may use the same sandboxes and grassy areas in which human children play as areas to eliminate.
- If children ingest the eggs, the larvae hatch and migrate through the lungs and liver, causing inflammatory responses and clinical signs (visceral larval migrans), and/or the nervous system, potentially becoming stranded in the eye (ocular larval migrans) and causing blindness.
- Cats and dogs should be controlled in public spaces, and their feces should be picked up and disposed of hygienically. Children playing in public parks should be encouraged to wash their hands frequently. Clean water and cleansing agents should be provided in parks to facilitate hand washing. All cats and dogs who are at risk should be treated with anthelmintic agents, especially after giving birth. Because free-ranging and/or feral cats and dogs may be most at risk for contributing to this condition in the poorest neighborhoods, anthelmintic administration becomes a public health issue, requiring

creative approaches (Hotez and Wilkins, 2009). Trap/neuter/release programs in cities with large numbers of cases of toxocariasis may wish to incorporate de-worming.

VETERINARIANS AS GUARDIANS OF FELINE WELFARE

Many shelters *consider cats relinquished for elimination complaints or other behavioral concerns unadoptable.* This is unfortunate because often simply re-homing the cat may redress the concern, highlighting the extent to which physical and social stress affects manifestations of feline behaviors. Elimination and other behaviors that are *problems for the client* can become *life-threatening problems for the cat.*

Conversely, *behaviors that are truly problematic for the cat may go unaddressed if they are not also problematic for the client.* To protect the welfare of cats, veterinarians need to be objective observers and good educators about feline behavior.

Veterinarians should encourage behavioral observation at each veterinary visit and can facilitate discussions about behavior by using a short tick sheet that clients can complete on arrival at each appointment (see the following survey questionnaire about general cat behaviors; see also the short survey questionnaires to be used at all visits to monitor behavioral change in cats at the end of the text and on the accompanying website). History tick sheets not only allow veterinarians to assess behavior in a consistent manner at each visit and note potentially worrisome changes as early as possible, but also such tools teach clients which behaviors are important for them to monitor to provide the best care possible for their cats.

Clients should also be encouraged to maintain a library of videos of their cat's basic behaviors so that when something changes, they can show the veterinarian video of the cat and environment before and after the change. Remember, *in veterinary behavioral medicine, behaviors are the data.* Once we can see the behaviors, we are best able to understand what they mean.

FELINE BEHAVIORAL CONCERNS INVOLVING PLACEMENT OF URINE/FECES AS PART OF INAPPROPRIATE OR UNDESIRABLE ELIMINATION BEHAVIOR

It doesn't matter whether you call it a toileting problem, a litterbox problem, or undesirable litterbox use, *the most common behavioral concerns reported by clients about their cats involve elimination.* Complaints about litterbox use can often be anticipated and can usually be successfully treated if the client becomes good at observing the cat's behavior.

The most common behavioral complaint that clients have about their cats involves the location where the cat urinates or defecates. Some veterinary behaviorists divide complaints into those involving concerns with litterboxes (e.g., "toileting") versus those involving some form of marking. From the standpoint of identifying the global behavioral concern, this is a fine way to conceptualize the issue. If we can also understand the variability of responses within these groups, we can best meet the cat's needs from the cat's viewpoint.

The key to resolving *all* elimination concerns—even those involved in marking—is to recognize and be able to identify *the pattern in the choices the cat makes about elimination. The pattern involved in the cat's behavior tells us what the cat's needs are.* If clients can meet the cat's needs, the problem will resolve. Otherwise, the *biggest reason why cats are relinquished or euthanized involves elimination that the clients view as problematic.* Clients will keep cats about whom they have complaints pertaining to elimination behaviors 2 years before relinquishing, abandoning, or euthanizing them. This is sufficient time to resolve even tough elimination problems, but problems can be resolved only if veterinarians screen every cat at each visit (Fig. 9-1).

Specific diagnoses pertaining to lack of litterbox use and marking are individually discussed. An accompanying flow chart is provided in Figure 9-2.

Cats Who Do Not Use Their Litterbox

Concerns about litterbox use generally involve one or more of the following client complaints:
- The cat doesn't use the box at all.
- The cat uses the box for either urine or feces but not both.
- The cat eliminates right next to or on the box but not in it.
- The cat uses the box but doesn't cover urine or feces.

All of these *could* be normal behaviors, but when they represent a change in former behavior, they generally flag a behavioral problem.

Covering Urine and Feces

Ancestral cats, their wild relatives, and their feral counterparts may never cover their urine or feces. Not covering urine or feces may act to inhibit disease transmission if ova of parasites dry, but this behavior also acts to provide a visual and olfactory statement of feline presence and identity. *In such cases, urine and feces are currency,* not just elimination products. Some cats will never cover their urine and/or feces but may still vigorously scratch in the box. *If the cat's behavior changes* and previously covered urine and/or feces is now *not* covered, clients should also be alert to changes in scratching behaviors. Cats who like their litterboxes scratch a lot, whether or not they cover urine and/or feces (Sung and Crowell-Davis, 2006).

Text continued on p. 369

Survey questionnaire about general cat behaviors—to be used at all visits:

1. Client(s):	2a. Today's date: ___ / ___ / ___ 2b. Cat's date of birth: ___ / ___ / ___ ☐ Estimated ☐ Known
3. Patient's name:	4a. Breed: _____ 4b. Weight: _____ lbs/_____ kg 4c: Sex: ☐ M ☐ MC ☐ F ☐ FS 4d: If your cat is castrated or spayed [neutered] at what age was this done?_____ weeks/months (circle)
5a. Age in weeks at which your cat was adopted? 5b. How many owners has your cat had? 5c. How long have you had this cat?	a. _____ weeks/months (circle) b. ☐ 0 ☐ 1 ☐ 2 ☐ 3 ☐ 4 ☐ 5+ ☐ unknown c. _____ months

6. Is your cat (please circle):
   a. Indoor, only
   b. Outdoor, only
   c. Indoor/outdoor
	6b. How many litterboxes does your cat have:
	    ☐ 0 ☐ 1 ☐ 2 ☐ 3 ☐ 4 ☐ 5+
	6c. What types of litter do you use? _____
	    _____
	6d. How often do you change the litterbox completely?
	    _____ times weekly/monthly (circle)
	6e. How often do you scoop the box?
	    _____ times daily/weekly (circle)

7a. Does your cat leave urine or feces outside the litterbox?
 	
7b. Does your cat "spray"?
	☐ Yes ☐ No ☐ Don't know
	If you answered **yes**,
	   a. Urine—where specifically? _____
	   b. Feces—where specifically? _____
	   c. Both—where specifically? _____
	☐ Yes ☐ No ☐ Don't know
	If you answered **yes**, where specifically? _____
	_____
	_____

8. Do you have any concerns, complaints, or problems with urination in the house now?	☐ Yes ☐ No
	If you answered **yes**,
	(a) Where is the cat urinating that you find undesirable (list
	    all areas)? _____
	    _____
	(b) How many times per week is the cat urinating in places
	    you find undesirable? _____
	(c) At what time of day is the urination occurring? _____
	    _____
	(d) Is the pattern different on days when you are home and
	    days you are not home?_____
	    _____
	(e) Are you at work during the hours when the cat urinates?
	    _____
	(f) How many times per day does your cat usually urinate
	    when he or she is not urinating in places you find
	    undesirable? _____

9. Do you have any concerns, complaints, or problems with defecation in the house now?	☐ Yes ☐ No If you answered **yes**,

Fig. 9-1 Survey questionnaire about general cat behaviors.

	(a) Where is the cat defecating that you find undesirable (list all areas)? _____ _____ _____
	(b) How many times per week is the cat defecating in places you find undesirable? _____
	(c) At what time of day is the defecation occurring? _____
	(d) Is the pattern different on days when you are home and days you are not home? _____ _____
	(e) Are you at work during the hours when the cat defecates? _____
	(f) How many times per day does your cat usually defecate when he or she is not defecating in places you find undesirable? _____
10. Does your cat destroy any objects or anything else by chewing, sucking, or eliminating on them (e.g., furniture, rugs, clothes, et cetera) now?	☐ Yes ☐ No If you answered **yes**, what objects–specifically–does the cat destroy? Please list all of them and note which are destroyed when you are home or not home–please note that if they destroy at both times–tick both columns:

Object	When home	When gone
	☐	☐
	☐	☐
	☐	☐
	☐	☐

11. Does your cat mouth, bite, suck, or nip anything or anyone?	a. ☐ Yes ☐ No If you answered **yes**, to whom is this behavior directed? _____ _____ b. Is this a problem for you? ☐ Yes ☐ No

12. Does your cat exhibit any vocalization about which you are concerned?	☐ Yes ☐ No If you answered **yes**, what is/are the vocalization(s) and when do they occur:

Vocalization	Situation in which it occurs
a. Yowling	
b. Growling	
c. Meowing	
d. Hissing	

13. Does your cat show any signs of hissing, growling, or biting?	☐ Yes ☐ No If you answered **yes**, what does the cat do and when does he or she do it?

Sign	Situation in which it occurs
a. Hissing	
b. Growling	
c. Biting	

Fig. 9-1, cont'd

Continued

14. Have you ever been concerned that your cat is "aggressive" *to people*?	☐ Yes ☐ No If you answered **yes**, why?
15. Have you ever been concerned that your cat is "aggressive" *to cats*?	☐ Yes ☐ No If you answered **yes**, why?
16. Have you ever been concerned that your cat is "aggressive" *to animals other than cats*? Does your cat hunt or prey on other animals?	☐ Yes ☐ No If you answered **yes**, why? ☐ Yes ☐ No If you answered **yes**, which animals and where?
17. Has your cat ever bitten or clawed anyone, regardless of the circumstances?	☐ Yes ☐ No If you answered **yes**, what happened?
18. Has your cat had any changes in sleep habits?	☐ Yes ☐ No If you answered **yes**, what are these changes
19. Has your cat had any changes in eating habits?	☐ Yes ☐ No If you answered **yes**, what changes have occurred?
20. Has your cat had any changes in locomotory behaviors or ability to get around or jump on the bed, et cetera?	☐ Yes ☐ No If you answered **yes**, what changes have occurred?
21. Has anyone ever told you that they were afraid of your cat?	☐ Yes ☐ No If you answered **yes**, what did they say?
22. Has anyone every told you that your cat was ill-mannered?	☐ Yes ☐ No If you answered **yes**, why–what did the cat do that made them say this?
23. Do you have any concerns about your cat's grooming behaviors?	☐ Yes ☐ No If you answered **yes**, ☐ a. Little to no grooming ☐ b. Sucking ☐ c. Chewing ☐ d. Licking ☐ e. Self-mutilation/sores ☐ f. Barbering/trimming ☐ g. Plucking out clumps of hair
24. Is the cat exhibiting any behaviors about which you are concerned, worried or would like more information?	☐ Yes ☐ No If you answered **yes**, please list these behaviors below:

Fig. 9-1, cont'd

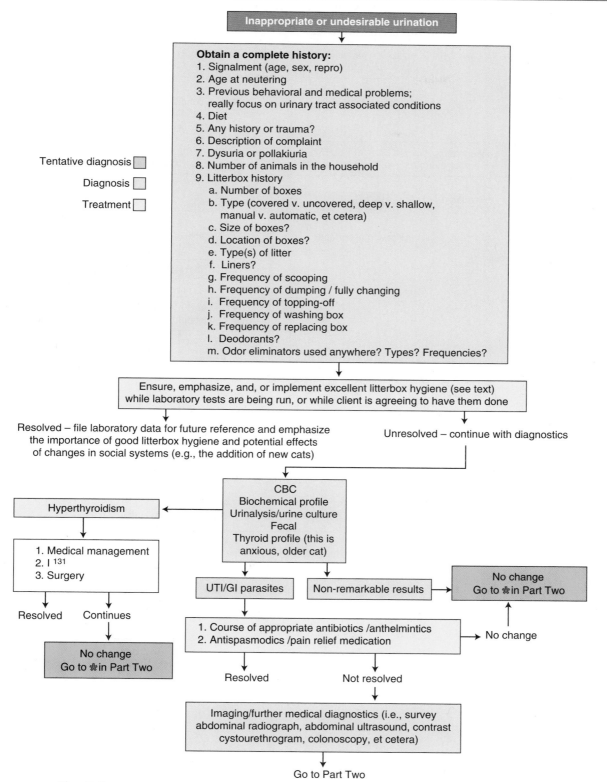

Fig. 9-2 Flow chart for treatment and diagnosis of feline elimination complaints. (Thanks to Mary Anna Labato, DVM, DACVIM, for input into a very early version of this flow chart.)

Continued

Part Two

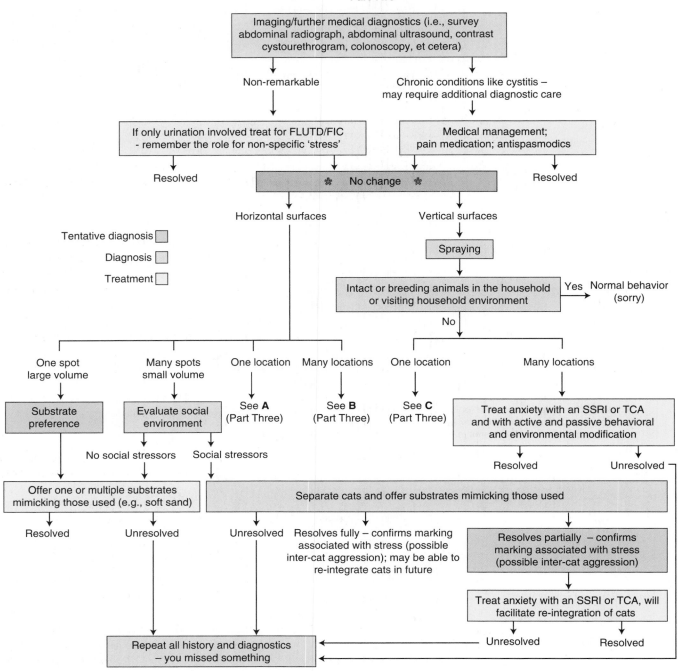

Fig. 9-2, cont'd

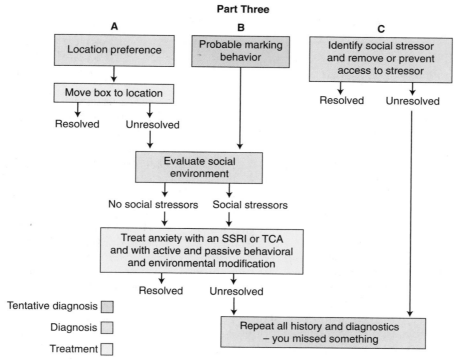

Fig. 9-2, cont'd

Complaints about litterbox use are almost always related to one of four diagnostic categories:
- substrate preference for elimination,
- substrate aversion for elimination,
- location preference for elimination, and
- location aversion for elimination.

These four diagnostic categories are represented by the heuristic scheme in Table 9-1.

Preferences for locations or substrates used for elimination are *"diagnoses" that may not represent abnormal feline behavior.* Cats have different innate preferences, and they likely have different aversion thresholds. Cats who may have endogenously expressed one preference may develop a secondary preference subsequent to developing an aversion. Cats may demonstrate preferences and aversions for all elimination or only for eliminating urine or feces. The extent to which (1) *distress and anxiety are expressed by the cat as part of these aversions and preferences,* (2) *the problematic elimination behaviors represent changes in behavior from former behaviors that the clients found acceptable,* and (3) *resolution of the concern becomes difficult* all likely reflect the *extent to which the cat may be exhibiting abnormal behaviors that are a function of underlying anxiety.* In such cases, diagnoses pertaining to elimination behaviors reflect true behavioral pathologies.

Feline Marking Behaviors Using Urine or Feces

Marking behaviors that use elimination include spraying and non-spraying marking. *Both spraying and non-spraying marking can be part of the normal signaling repertoire in cats.*

- *Non-spraying marking*: The *pattern* of deposition of urine or feces distinguishes non-spraying marking behavior from substrate or location aversions/ preferences. When *non-spraying marking is a consideration, the amounts of urine or feces are small and distributed over areas associated with social stimuli,* not with substrates or locations (Table 9-2).
- *Marking behavior involving spraying*: In marking involving sprayed urine (spraying), the cat treads on its front feet, raises its tail, quivering the tip, and sprays urine vertically (Fig. 9-3). If the cat is not backed against a vertical surface, sprayed urine makes a linear pattern on horizontal surfaces. Urine sprayed against a vertical surface drips and puddles (Fig. 9-4). Regardless, sprayed urine covers a larger surface area with urine than does squatting and so likely communicates different information than urine voided in a squat. The information communicated could simply be that the cat was confident enough to engage in the very visual behaviors that accompany spraying. Both male and female cats can and will spray, as will neutered/desexed cats. Neutering can decrease or stop spraying if it has been occurring for only a short while or it is related solely to estrus cycles or responses to them, and neutered cats spray less frequently than do cats who have not been neutered.

Risk factors for aversions, preferences, and marking are found in Box 9-1.

TABLE 9-1

Scheme for Thinking about the Most Common Reasons Why Cats Do Not Use Their Litterboxes

	Substrate	Location
Preference	• Deposition of normal amounts of urine or feces • Frequency of elimination may be unchanged • Substrates chosen linked by texture but not by location • Preferred substrates share some tactile association, which becomes clearer to clients on thoughtful examination • Common classes of substrate preferences include very soft substrates (clothing, bath mats, fireplace ashes) and smooth, reflective, cool surfaces (tile floors, sinks, granite countertops) • Cats who prefer cool surfaces may avoid soft ones • Preferences can develop innately—because the cat truly prefers some substrate other than the litter in the box—or they can develop after cats learn to hate their litter or box (an aversion)	• Deposition of normal amounts of urine or feces • Frequency of elimination may be unchanged • Regions chosen linked by region/location where urine/feces are found, not substrate • Changing substrates appears to have little effect on behavior of cats with location preferences • If a location preference is suspected and a litterbox is placed in the spot or spots chosen, the cat usually uses it • In contrast to *de novo* preferences, *aversions may have powerful anxiety components that must be addressed as part of treatment*
Aversion	• Deposition of normal amounts of urine or feces • Frequency of elimination may change in aversions because the cat must avoid so many substrates • Avoided substrates linked by texture, not by location • *True aversions develop when accustomed substrate changes in a way that is repugnant to the cat* • Hygiene is the most common reason for a substrate aversion • Litter feels different when soiled • Soiled litter creates a very different olfactory and chemical environment for the cat • Cats who find their litter aversive undergo a process of *sampling* and will find *another substrate* that *they* consider acceptable • Clients usually do not find these new substrates acceptable, which is what leads to veterinary consultation and a diagnosis of an aversion • *The extent to which simply providing a cleaner environment will help depends on both the strength of the cat's preference and on how distressed soiled environments render the cat*	• Deposition of normal amounts of urine or feces • Frequency of elimination may change in aversions because the cat must avoid so many locations • Avoided regions linked by region/location where urine/feces are found, not substrate • In this case the region may be broad or narrow, but the cat is averse to the region where the litterbox is placed • Cats can learn to loathe certain areas no matter how good the box, the litter, or the hygiene routine • Aversions to locations usually develop because of some stimulus that the cat associates with threatening, disruptive, or injurious stimuli (e.g., the box is behind the entry door, which can crash into the cat and box when opened) • In contrast to *de novo* preferences, aversions may have powerful anxiety components that must be addressed as part of treatment • *The extent to which gradually shifting the cat to a preferred spot will be successful depends on the amount of distress that the cat felt that led him/her to choose a new location*

DIAGNOSTIC CATEGORIES FOR ELIMINATION COMPLAINTS

Substrate Preference for Elimination

Diagnostic Criteria and Description

• Consistent elimination in an area or areas that are linked by some common sensory aspect.
• Common sensory aspects may include:

• open, smooth, reflective surfaces (e.g., tile floors, bathtubs, kitchen counters),
• soft, silky substrates (e.g., some silicacious litters, pearlized litters, clothes, towels, bath mats, plastic trash bags),
• soft, thick, absorptive surfaces (e.g., thick silk and wool rugs),
• soils, sands (e.g., houseplants), and

TABLE 9-2

Patterns That Separate Non-Spraying Marking from a Substrate or Location Preference or Aversion

	Location Preference/Aversion	Substrate Preference/Aversion	Non-Spraying Marking
Number of urine puddles or mounds of feces	1 large per elimination event	1 large per elimination event	Multiple small
Cat behavior	Covert only if punished or threatened by another animal in the household	Overt	Covert, difficult to see cat engage in behavior
Directly related social stimuli	Only if avoidance is involved	No	Yes
Other behaviors	Scratches and digs if normal for that cat and non-averse	Scratches and digs if normal for that cat and non-averse	Repeated sniffing and moving, much olfactory and visual assessment of area, if scratches, scratching most likely associated with additional olfactory signal, not with the type of scratching done before and after routine elimination

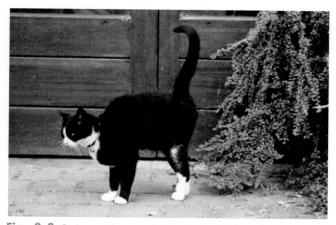

Fig. 9-3 Cat spraying against a bush. Notice the elevated, curled, and moving tail; the arched back; the movement of the ears; the stare; and the treading and movement of the hind legs. (Photo courtesy of Anne Marie Dossche.)

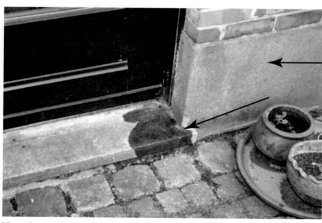

Fig. 9-4 Urine sprayed against a vertical surface (*small arrow* indicates outline of old urine stains) that then puddles (*big arrow*). (Photo courtesy of Anne Marie Dossche.)

BOX 9-1

Risk Factors for Aversions and Preferences

- Risk factors for elimination preferences and aversions include:
  - Dirty litter and/or litterbox
  - Litterbox too small and discourages active digging and exploration
  - Litterbox too high for cat to enter readily
  - Style (covered) and placement (in closets) that allow the cat using the litterbox to be trapped by a child, another cat, a dog, et cetera
  - Placement of litterbox in location that the cat cannot reach because of pain (arthritis), access (doors closed), or social factors (being chased by a new puppy)
  - Entrapment of odors by lid of covered litterbox placed in an area without adequate ventilation
  - Illness of any cat in the household that causes changes in bladder/bowel function
- Risk factors for marking are based on social stress and distress; stressors include:
  - Addition of another pet
  - Loss of a pet
  - Change in the composition of the human household
  - Change in the "stress" level of the household (e.g., illness, job change)
  - Visitation by an outside cat
  - Illness or change in relationships between cats in the household (e.g., that which may occur concomitant with social maturity)
  - True inter-cat aggression

- soft, non-particulate, absorbent materials (e.g., paper towels, newspapers).
- Cats who use their litterboxes consistently and who scratch and dig in them are using a preferred substrate. The clients agree that this substrate is one suitable for elimination.
- Cats who may be identifying preferred non-litter substrates to clients may be exhibiting completely normal behavior, but clients find it offensive. The diagnosis is made only when there is a client-pet preference mismatch.
- Cats who develop aversions to litter substrates or locations will usually develop a secondary preference for another substrate or location.
- As substrate preferences become more narrow and restrictive, the greater the risk that truly abnormal behavior may be involved.

Common Non-Specific Signs

- Clients find urine and/or feces on non-litter substrates.
  - When the clients can list every substrate ever used, these substrates are usually linked by some shared sensory—often tactile—characteristic.
- Finding urine and/or feces on non-litter substrates may be preceded by changes in litter (clients changed brands) and/or litterbox hygiene (e.g., change in frequency and quality of cleaning).
- Clients may not realize that the cat is eliminating elsewhere unless they monitor the litter for changes in use (e.g., changes in volume of urine/feces).
- In the case of a substrate preference, cats may be seen scratching around but not in the litterbox.
- Cats with substrate preferences may sniff and scratch a series of areas before beginning to eliminate on them, so clients should use these behaviors to watch for changes in litterbox use.

Rule Outs

- Cats with urinary tract infections (UTIs) may not be able to make it to the litterbox or be too painful to get into and out of the box as needed and may eliminate on any substrate available or near the litterbox.
- Older and arthritic cats may develop new preferences if they are unable to get into and out of the litterbox without pain.
  - If the cat is eliminating in a pattern that does not seem to be associated with how something feels, or where the substrate is, and the social environment appears to contain minimal stressors, a medical problem may be involved. The most common medical conditions that are associated with complaints about elimination are feline lower urinary tract signs/disease (FLUTD), bacterial cystitis, urethral obstruction, diabetes mellitus, cognitive dysfunction (CD), hyperthyroidism, lower motor neuron disease, enteritis/colitis, parasitemia.
  - The standard database for inappropriate elimination involving urination includes a physical exam,

complete blood count (CBC), serum biochemistry profile, urinalysis with culture, and thyroid profile (if the cat is >6 years old). For complaints involving defecation, a fecal flotation and direct smear should be included.

Etiology, Epidemiology, and Risk Groups

- Substrate preferences for elimination are extremely common, particularly among long-haired cats. Long, soft hair may collect more odor and/or pieces of litter, and so cats may learn early to prefer a substrate that allows them to remain free of material and odor.
- Histories for many affected cats may contain information about an extended period where the clients were ill, busy, or away and not changing the litter as often as before.
  - The "substrate preference" in this case may be as simple as *clean* litter. If the client reports that the cat gets into the box and enthusiastically uses it every time it is cleaned and changed, it is likely that the cat has a preference for very clean litter.
  - If the cat cannot escape filthy litter, he may start to sample other substrates and learn that he likes these as well or better than the litter he had previously been using. In such cases, a change in substrate type may be needed.
    - Some cats will use filthy litter and full litterboxes, but *no one should count on this*.
- The illness of one cat in the household may alter the perception of the litter for the other cats and cause them to sample other substrates. If any cat in the household is taking medication or has hepatic, renal, or gastrointestinal illness, clients should be advised to provide additional litterboxes for the well cats and/or observe them to learn if the illness is a problem for them.
- Cats who have been ill and either been forced to or had the experience of eliminating on a non-litter substrate can learn to prefer the new substrate.
- Cats who have undergone any surgery, including onychectomy (declaw), may find traditional litters painful and learn to prefer things like fabric, plastic, paper, and smooth surfaces that cannot get caught in or abrade their wounds. This preference may persist after recovery.

Common Myths That Can Get in the Way of Treatment or Diagnosis

- The common myth about elimination concerns is that the cat is doing this to "get even" with the client, for "spite" because the cat is "angry," and/or as a way to show displeasure about some aspect of the client's choices.
  - This is among the most anthropocentric of myths about cat behavior. If the client can be convinced to understand the cat's needs, the client usually understands that the cat is being put in a situation that is uncomfortable or untenable.

- Humans will seldom use filthy toilets unless there is no other option. Noting this may result in some understanding of the cat's concerns.

Commonly Asked Client Questions

- Will the cat return to using her litter if we clean more frequently?
  - Not necessarily. If this is a true preference, the litter offered will need to reflect the cat's preference.
    - What cats preferred before they learned of other textures may no longer be preferred by them once they have sampled something else. This is the best argument for encouraging clients to keep litterboxes and areas clean and pleasing to the cat.
- Can we switch the cat back to her original litter, gradually and over time?
  - Possibly, but the cat needs to be using an identified substrate 100% of the time for a prolonged period of time (weeks to months, depending on how long the problem had been ongoing before treatment) before this is even attempted. Once the clients are sure that the cat is eliminating in the litterbox using one substrate, the clients can gradually change the ratio of that substrate to the one they wish the cat to use. Very gradual changes over 1 or 2 months may provide the best outcome.
  - *If there is an accompanying aversion to the old litter, switching the cat back to his or her old litter will not work.* The extent to which a cat becomes averse may depend considerably on the cat.
    - Clients who have had cats who were not fussy can become very confused and angry when they have a cat who requires a very clean litterbox and surroundings. These clients will need help in understanding that the fussy cat is completely normal.
- Why does the cat seem to prefer the bathroom floor/hardwood floor/tile floor/bathtub/shower?
  - All of these surfaces share in common that they are reflective, cool, and well drained. This is the ancestral condition that cats sought for elimination. The cat may be making an innate choice, and that choice may be hard to shift. Mimic the substrate to the extent possible, up to and including lining a litterbox with tiles. These types of litterboxes can be washed, and if the tiles are not glued to the litterbox, they can go in the dishwasher.
  - If the cat is using the shower or tub and does not use a box placed in that area with a similar substrate available, it is going to be very hard to shift that preference, and the client may wish to settle for a situation that is at least easy to clean.
- How do we know which cat is doing this?
  - Cats who potentially defecate on inappropriate substrates can be given colored wax—which is what most non-toxic crayons are—by grating it into their food. Clients can use different colors

simultaneously for different cats if they can guarantee that each cat eats only his food. The wax passes through the cat's gastrointestinal tract with the color intact.
  - Red beets also are detectable in feces and can be fed to cats (one cat at a time).
  - Fluorescein can be given to cats to learn who is responsible for the urination. A detailed explanation is found in the section on spraying.

Treatment

- Management:
  - Clients should try to identify the types of substrates that the cat uses and mimic those.
    - Some silicacious, clumpable litters are extremely soft and may be palatable to cats who like soft substrates.
    - Some natural product litters (e.g., shredded corncobs, pelleted paper, wheat, buckwheat, pine, and other plant materials) appeal to cats who like soft litter; many of these are good at absorbing scent but do not clump.
    - Clay litters vary in size of particles, whether they clump, the extent to which they hold water and odor, et cetera, and clients will need to identify the specific type of clay litter that their cat likes.
    - Sawdust does not absorb odor, stays wet, and can be tracked from the box but for cats who like soft substrates it may be suitable for use if thrown away daily.
    - Number 3 blasting sand is known for its evenness of grain. Although it doesn't absorb as do modern litters, it drains well and may provide an alternative for some cats.
    - Litterboxes can be tiled or covered in impermeable surfaces that cats like.
    - Empty litterboxes or a cookie tray may be used by cats who prefer flooring.
  - Clients should be encouraged to watch cats use litter. If the cat scratches and digs in the litter and gets into it to do so, the cat likes the litter.
    - If the cat likes a very soft, trackable litter, clients can put the box on a mat that attracts dust and litter to limit tracking.
  - Litterboxes also matter and may not be separate from the litter preference for cats.
    - Litterbox condition matters. Deeply scored boxes feel rough and hold odor. Boxes should be well washed, rinsed, and dried as needed but at least once a week.
      - Any residual bleach smell may deter use because bleach kills olfactory neurons, which alters the cat's ability to assay his or her sensory environment.
    - Linear dimensions of boxes matter.
      - Arthritic cats and young kittens may be unable to get into tall boxes and so will not use them.

- If the litterbox is at least 1.5 times the body length of the cat, the cat is much more likely to use it (Sung et al., 2006).
  - The box must be large enough for the cat to dig, turn around comfortably, and sample a second area for digging without encountering the sides of the box or having to engage in unnatural and uncomfortable tail positions when squatting.
  - For some cats, commercially available boxes may not be sufficiently large, but under-bed sweater boxes may work.
- Liners should not be used. They affect the way the cat detects the substrate and invariably are linked with decreased use of the litter by cats.
  - Liners are useful to clients, not cats.
  - When cats like litter with liners, they often just like the liner because they can shred it. This may not be what the client intended, but it is useful information to have.
  - The very rare cat prefers boxes that have only liners. This behavior provides considerable information about preferences that may not be palatable to clients.
- Litter must be kept clean.
  - If one cat is using the box, the clients *may* be able to go 2 to 3 days without completely emptying the litterbox *if the litter is scooped multiple times a day.*
    - *Some cats will do best if the box is scooped as needed and emptied and washed daily.*
  - If multiple cats are using any box, the box will need to be completely emptied daily.
  - There should be one more box than there are cats in case some cats have separate preferences for urination and defecation.
    - This recommendation is predicated on having a small household of cats. What is "small" depends on how the cats get along, whether the cat group contains any family members, the size of the dwelling, the health of the cats, and the number of floors available to the cats.
    - Large numbers of cats within households may have social issues that override simple substrate preference issues, but if space permits, it is always helpful to provide one more box than there are cats. If this box is not used, it can be taken away, but non-use will be exceptional.
    - Litterboxes should be arranged in a way that allows clients to learn what the cat needs and wants.
      - Litterboxes should be placed on each floor.
      - Some litterboxes should be in more public places and some in more private places.
  - If clients wish to compare the use of two litters, they can do so in side-by-side litterbox comparisons, but otherwise separating the boxes will provide the client with the best chance of meeting the cat's preferences.
  - If older cats are in the household, clients should consider multiple boxes on the floor on which the cat spends most of his or her time and offering boxes of different heights or with entryways cut into the box.
  - If clients are modifying litterboxes, they should ensure all cut areas are smooth and/or protected and non-injurious.
- If there is more than one litterbox, all boxes should be scooped whenever used and changed at least every 2 to 3 days or more depending on use.
  - Clients may like litterboxes with lids, but cats generally may not.
  - Individual cats may have individual preferences with respect to type of box (Grigg et al., 2013), despite no reported statistically significant group preferences for cats offered open vs. covered litter boxes in a small study.
  - However, cats can become trapped and easily victimized by other animals in the household when in an enclosed box.
  - Enclosed boxes concentrate odor and ammonia vapor.
  - If cats spray against the back of the box, a shield can be made that does not enclose the entire box.
- Because cats are so good at smelling and identifying odor, the clients must clean well and thoroughly any affected area.
- Behavior modification:
  - If the problem involves a strong, innate preference, behavior modification is not likely to be successful.
  - If the cat has engaged in a sampling process after an illness, a vacation, or other inducements not to use the box without developing an aversion, and if the cat is social and will use the box in the client's preference, the client may be able to reward the cat with praise and a treat for getting into and using the box. There are no data to suggest the extent to which this can help, but it cannot hurt.
- Medication/dietary intervention:
  - If the cat has developed an aversion or a concern about any aspect of the litter or box, he or she may be difficult to convince to use a litter everyone can agree on without using an anti-anxiety medication. Medications that may help include:
    - Tricyclic antidepressants (TCAs):
      - Amitriptyline

- Nortriptyline (if sedated by amitriptyline)
- Clomipramine (Clomicalm)
  - Selective serotonin reuptake inhibitors (SSRIs):
    - Fluoxetine (Reconcile)
    - Paroxetine
- Before using medication, a laboratory evaluation (CBC, serum biochemistry profile) and at least a lead II electrocardiogram (ECG), especially if considering TCA/SSRI use, should be performed. Most of these medications are metabolized through renal and hepatic pathways, and clearance may be altered if renal or hepatic disease is a concern. Additionally, these medications will interact with other medications that share the same cytochrome P-450 system enzyme pathways, so a good medical history is important. TCAs and SSRIs may be more arrhythmogenic in cats than in other species.
- Cats older than 6 years should also have a thyroid profile as part of their baseline laboratory evaluation.
- Cats treated with monoamine oxidase (MAO) inhibitors (some flea and tick collars) should not be treated with TCAs or SSRIs.
- Medication use will need to continue for at least a few months until the clients are certain that the cat is always using the litter and is not distressed.
- Withdrawal should be gradual (see the "Protocol for Using Behavioral Medication Successfully").
- Full withdrawal of medication may not be possible for all cats.
- If the cat is painful, the aversion may be related to the pain. Treatment of pain is essential for the cat's quality of life (QoL).
  - Tramadol, a synthetic opioid that stimulates mu receptors, also affects serotonin receptors and may provide some very mild anti-anxiety effects. If tramadol is given with TCAs or SSRIs, clients should be advised that there is a very small risk of serotonin syndrome. If the client is taught how to monitor the cat, the risks are minimal.
- Miscellaneous interventions:
  - Some clients resort to atypical litters (e.g., dry beans, shredded paper towels, shredded rags, fake lawns, indoor/outdoor carpet, indoor garden patches, potting soil, et cetera) or allow the cats to become indoor/outdoor cats.
    - Clients should understand that the risk of death or injury to cats who are allowed outdoors is not trivial and that outdoor cats have a much shorter life expectancy than indoor cats.
  - Good, frequent, and ongoing cleaning of soiled areas is essential.
    - All urine and feces that can be removed should be removed.
    - Clients should crawl around on their hands and knees feeling and sniffing any potentially

soiled areas. If there is carpeting, walking barefoot may help.
- Urine fluoresces under black light and handheld, battery-operated black lights are readily available.
- Areas should be repeatedly washed with water and a fabric/color-friendly detergent.
- Areas should be rinsed and mopped up repeatedly.
- If there is wall-to-wall carpeting or a subfloor, the carpeting may need to be removed to clean well.
- Occasionally flooring needs to be removed.
- Vapor barriers should be installed if flooring is replaced.
- For very absorbent surfaces, the clients should soak the areas with club soda, which will help bubble urine to the surface; this should be blotted and repeated until everything appears and smells clean.
- Cats have superior olfactory abilities compared with humans: if the cat sniffs the area and is interested in it, it must be cleaned again.
- When everyone is convinced the area is clean, a good odor eliminator must be used. The best odor eliminators both enzymatically degrade the elimination products and prevent the odorant molecules from being aerosolized (Beaver et al., 1989). Products designed to eliminate hospital, mortuary, and disaster odors are available and appropriate for use.
- Prevention of repeated soiling is important. If the clients cover affected areas with plastics, rubberized matting or sheets, plastic carpet protectors, et cetera, the cat may no longer find the substrate appealing.
  - Unless the cat is truly in love with the new substrates provided, removing these barriers will result in a return of the cat and the undesirable behavior.
  - Clients should be reminded that such barriers can be removed for special events and the cat sequestered away from the area to minimize recidivistic events.

Helpful Handouts
- "Protocol for Understanding and Treating Cats with Elimination Disorders and Elimination Behaviors That Concern Clients"

Last Words
- Many clients complain about new substrate preferences that develop after an extended vacation when someone fed their cat but would not change the litter. The cat is repulsed by the filthy litter, seeks another area from desperation, and discovers that he prefers this substrate.
  - Clients would do well to avoid the problem by providing a new litterbox for each day they will

be gone. If they pre-fill it with litter and place it in a trash bag, the boxes will stack, and all the petsitter has to do is take out a clean box, put the dirty one in the bag, and seal it. The clients can then empty and clean boxes in a way that meets the cat's needs.

- Illness can also be implicated in the development of a preference; a cat with cystitis or diarrhea may not be able to make it to the litterbox and in the process of covering up the urine or feces on the carpet discovers that she likes the feel of carpeting.
- *A physical exam is essential.* This must include a complete urinalysis/fecal analysis, depending on the nature of the problem, and a CBC and serum biochemistry profile. Approximately one third of cats with substrate preferences who either do not respond or start to respond to environmental and behavioral modification and then relapse have apparent or occult UTIs.
  - Increasingly, FLUTD (Lekcharoensuk et al., 2001) and feline interstitial cystitis (FIC) (Westropp et al., 2006) are being identified because cats changed their elimination behaviors.
  - Diagnostic kitty litters are available (e.g., Perfect Litter Alert Specialty Cat Litter; www. perfectlitteralert.com) that change color to indicate pH in the range of 5.0 to 8.0; these can be mixed with other litters.
  - Advanced diagnostics may be required to identify FLUTD or FIC if all other tests appear unremarkable and there is no response to behavioral intervention.
- If the urinalysis/fecal analysis is positive, treat and suggest environmental/behavioral modifications also because the cat could have shifted his preference as a result of the illness.
- Given the amount of damage a client can do by scaring a cat, clients should not punish cats who do not use their litterboxes. *Punishment after the fact is useless anyway, and physical punishment, including rubbing the cat's nose in the soiled area, should be avoided at all costs because it teaches cats to avoid their people and may lead to physical or behavioral injury of the cat.*

Location Preference for Elimination
Diagnostic Criteria and Description
- Consistent elimination in one or a few areas where there is no litterbox.
- Changing the substrates appears to have little effect on the behavior of these cats, but if a location preference is suspected, and a litterbox is placed in the spot or spots chosen, the cat usually uses it.
- Common patterns for location preferences include:
  - a location away from doors, which may open, or equipment such as washing machines or heaters, which may turn on,
  - a location away from where other animals or people spend most of their time, and
  - a location where people or other animals are often reliably present (e.g., bathroom, kitchen, mudroom).
- Cats who are identifying preferred locations to clients may be exhibiting completely normal behavior, but clients find it offensive. The diagnosis is made only when there is a client-pet preference mismatch.
- Cats who develop aversions to certain locations (e.g., where their litterbox is constantly hit by a door opening) will usually develop a secondary preference for another location.

Common Non-Specific Signs
- Clients find urine and/or feces in one or a few linked areas, possibly on a variety of substrates but not in the litterbox.
  - The cat usually returns to the same general area, and if something is placed over the spot to obstruct elimination (e.g., a large box), the cat will often eliminate next to it.
  - If an object is removed that changes the sensory aspects of the location, the cat still uses the location (e.g., a bathmat is removed, and the cat eliminates where the bathmat was).
- This behavior is not usually associated with hygiene or brands of litter. Instead, it is associated with some aspect of the physical and/or social environment.
  - Some cats have a preference for litterboxes placed in busy and/or social places.
  - Some cats have a preference for litterbox placed in undisturbed/quiet places.
- Clients may not realize that the cat is eliminating elsewhere, especially if the cat is choosing a quiet, isolated area, unless they monitor the litter for changes in use (e.g., changes in volume of urine/feces). With a location preference for elimination, clients usually discover that the litter is not being used and so hasn't been changed.
  - *Any time the need to change a litterbox alters dramatically, attention must be paid to the cat.*
- Cats with location preferences exhibit the same elimination behaviors that they would in the litterbox but in their chosen area. They may sniff and scratch, even if the substrate prevents any covering.
  - If the clients are able to observe the cat, it is clear that the cat is using postures associated with elimination, not marking behaviors.

Rule Outs
- Cats with UTIs may be unable to make it to the litterbox or it may be too painful to get into and out of the box as needed and may eliminate in random areas.
- Older and arthritic cats may develop new preferences if they are unable to get into and out of the litterbox without pain. Pain may be a common reason why cats choose a new location for

elimination, and it should be suspected if a change in floor is involved.

- If the cat is eliminating in a pattern that does not seem to be associated with how something feels or where it is, and the social environment appears to contain minimal stressors, a medical problem may be involved. The most common medical conditions that are associated with complaints about elimination are FLUTD, bacterial cystitis, urethral obstruction, diabetes mellitus, CD, hyperthyroidism, lower motor neuron disease, enteritis/colitis, and parasitemia.
- The standard database for inappropriate elimination involving urination includes a physical exam, CBC, serum biochemistry profile, urinalysis with culture, and thyroid profile (if the cat is >6 years old). For complaints involving defecation, a fecal flotation and direct smear should be included.

Etiology, Epidemiology, and Risk Groups

- Location preferences either appear to be innate or develop because something happened that hurt or disrupted the cats.
  - Cats who are social may behave differently from shy cats when in litterboxes.
  - Cats who are painful or ill may find a more easily reached area in which to eliminate if getting to their litterbox makes them feel worse.
  - Cats who are scared or startled when in the litterbox will find another place to eliminate, secondary to their learned avoidance of the original location.

Common Myths That Can Get in the Way of Treatment or Diagnosis

- The common myth about elimination concerns is that the cat is doing this to "get even" with the client, for "spite" because the cat is "angry," and/or as a way to show displeasure about some aspect of the client's choices.
  - This is among the most anthropocentric of myths about cat behavior. If the client can be convinced to understand the cat's needs, the client usually understands that the cat is being put in a situation that is uncomfortable or untenable.
  - Clients should be able to understand that some locations make them more comfortable for elimination than others. Perhaps they can also understand that cats will vary in their preferences for privacy and stimulation.

Commonly Asked Client Questions

- Will the cat return to using her litterbox if we clean it more frequently?
  - The cat may like a cleaner box, but if she has this condition, she is really telling the client that she prefers another location.
- If we move the box to the area where the cat is eliminating and she uses it, can we move it back to her original spot?

- Maybe, but the cat needs to be using the box in the chosen area 100% of the time for a period of weeks or months before this is even attempted.
  - The longer the cat has been displaying the location preference, the longer it will take the client to be confident that the cat will use the litterbox as it is gradually moved.
  - Once clients are sure that the cat is always eliminating in the litterbox, the clients can gradually start to move the box by a few centimeters/inches a day to the location that the clients prefer.
  - If the cat returns to the area she chose, the clients will need to re-think the situation no matter how much they dislike the cat's chosen area.
  - If the clients can identify why the cat likes that location, perhaps they can identify a new area similar to it that the cat will also like and make the change gradually.
    - To make this work, the client would identify the area and put a litterbox there also. If the cat uses it, excellent. If not, the client can gradually move the litterbox being used toward the additional box in the newly chosen area, and the cat may use it. Very gradual changes over 1 or 2 months may provide the best outcome.
  - Generally, it is easiest to place the box where the cat will use it and live with this; however, if this is in the middle of the dining room or living room, clients will not find such choices acceptable. If the cat is very rigid in her choice, and the chosen rooms are not used often, the cat and her litterbox can be placed in another room or bathroom temporarily when the rooms are need to be used if this is what's needed to make the decision palatable to clients. This is not common, but it happens.
- *If there is an accompanying aversion to a location, the cat will not return to it.*
  - Clients will have to identify the exact factors causing the aversion and see if there are areas where they are able to accommodate the cat.
- How do we know which cat is responsible?
  - Cats who potentially defecate in inappropriate places can be given colored wax—which is what most non-toxic crayons are—by grating it into their food. Clients can simultaneously use different colors for different cats if they can guarantee that each cat eats only his food. The wax passes through the cat's gastrointestinal tract with the color intact.
  - Red beets are detectable in feces and can be fed to cats (one cat at a time).
  - Fluorescein can be given to cats to learn who is responsible for the urination. A detailed explanation is found in the section on spraying.

Treatment

- Management:
  - Clients should try to identify the location that the cat is willing to use and put a litterbox in that location.
  - Clients may like litterboxes with lids, but cats generally do not.
    - Cats can become trapped and easily victimized by other animals in the household when in an enclosed box, and one of their aversive associations may be with where the covered box was placed.
  - Covering the area that the cat has used with substrates that they do not prefer may discourage some cats to returning to their chosen locations as treatment progresses.
  - *Good cleaning is essential.*
- Behavior modification:
  - If the problem involves a strong, innate preference, behavior modification to alter that preference is not likely to be successful. Finding a way to accommodate the cat's preference will be more successful.
  - If the client can identify an area similar to the one the cat has chosen but that will require the cat to move areas, rewarding the cat with praise and/or treats for approaching and/or using the litterbox may help.
  - Sometimes some relative confinement within an acceptable area, combined with more attention and rewards for good behavior, can help a cat to switch to a litterbox within that area.
- Medication/dietary intervention:
  - Most clients and cats can work out solutions to location preferences relatively easily and without the aid of medication. The occasional cat exhibits real distress with change and so for that cat, medication is the humane choice.
  - If the cat has developed an aversion about where the litterbox is located or a concern about anything that happens because of where it's located (e.g., that a heater will turn on or a door will crash into him), anti-anxiety medication may help.
  - If the cat sometimes uses a new area that the clients have identified but still sometimes uses one with similar characteristics that the cat identified, medication may help the cat to worry less about the switch.
  - Medications that may help include:
    - TCAs:
      - Amitriptyline
      - Nortriptyline (if sedated by amitriptyline)
      - Clomipramine)
    - SSRIs:
      - Fluoxetine
      - Paroxetine
    - Benzodiazepines (BZDs)—may be most useful if combined with food rewards to try to shift a preference
      - Alprazolam
      - Oxazepam
  - Before using medication, a laboratory evaluation (CBC, serum biochemistry profile) and at least a lead II ECG, especially if considering TCA/SSRI use, should be performed. Most of these medications are metabolized through renal and hepatic pathways, and clearance may be altered if renal or hepatic disease is a concern. Additionally, these medications will interact with other medications that share the same cytochrome P-450 system enzyme pathways, so a good medical history is important. TCAs and SSRIs may be more arrhythmogenic in cats than in other species.
  - Cats older than 6 years should also have a thyroid profile as part of their baseline laboratory evaluation.
  - BZDs have been associated with rare hyperexcitability, rare profound sedation, and rare severe hepatotoxicity, but this story is more complex than just BZD use (see Chapter 10 for the entire discussion). BZDs can be abused by humans and are not suitable for use in all households.
  - Cats treated with MAO inhibitors (some flea and tick collars) should not be treated with TCAs or SSRIs.
  - Medication use will need to continue for at least a few months until the clients are certain that the cat is always using the litter and is not distressed.
  - Withdrawal should be gradual (see the "Protocol for Using Behavioral Medication Successfully").
  - Full withdrawal of medication may not be possible for all cats.
- Miscellaneous interventions:
  - Good, frequent, and ongoing cleaning of soiled areas is essential.
    - All urine and feces that can be removed should be removed.
    - Clients should crawl around on their hands and knees feeling and sniffing any potentially soiled areas. If there is carpeting, walking barefoot may help.
    - Urine fluoresces under black lights, and handheld, battery-operated black lights are readily available.
    - Areas should be repeatedly washed with water and a fabric/color-friendly detergent.
    - Areas should be rinsed and mopped up repeatedly.
    - If there is wall-to-wall carpeting or a subfloor, the carpeting may need to be removed to clean well.
    - Occasionally flooring needs to be removed.

- Vapor barriers should be installed if flooring is replaced.
- For very absorbent surfaces, the clients should soak the areas with club soda, which will help bubble urine to the surface. This should then be blotted and repeated until everything appears and smells clean.
- Cats have superior olfactory abilities compared with humans: if the cat sniffs the area and is interested in it, it must be cleaned again.
- When everyone is convinced the area is clean, a good odor eliminator must be used. The best odor eliminators both enzymatically degrade the elimination products and prevent the odorant molecules from being aerosolized. Products designed to eliminate hospital, mortuary, and disaster odors are available and appropriate for use.

Helpful Handouts
- "Protocol for Understanding and Treating Cats with Elimination Disorders and Elimination Behaviors That Concern Clients"
- "Protocol for Understanding and Treating Feline Aggressions with an Emphasis on Inter-Cat Aggression"
- "Protocol for Understanding and Helping Geriatric Animals"
- "Protocol for Treating Fearful Behavior in Cats and Dogs"

Last Words
- The development of a new location preference for elimination may be the first clue that the clients have that *all is not well in the pet household.* If cats learn to fear or loathe activities that occur when they are getting in or getting out of the litterbox, they will link their response to the location. Any client whose cat makes such a change needs to examine closely— and video—the interactions between animals and/ or other people in their household. A location preference, secondary to an aversive experience, may represent the beginning of profound problem interactions. Early treatment ensures the best outcomes.
- If the location chosen is one where the cat is more protected and/or hidden (e.g., the back of a closet in a little used spare room), the client should monitor other behaviors for this cat to assess whether the cat is truly hiding and withdrawing from interaction. *If so, none of the issues associated with elimination will resolve until the social issues are addressed.*
- A physical exam is essential. This must include a complete urinalysis/fecal analysis, depending on the nature of the problem, and a CBC and serum biochemistry profile. If the urinalysis/fecal analysis is positive, treat and suggest environmental/ behavioral modifications also because the cat could have shifted his preference as a result of the illness. Other illnesses (e.g., cardiac disease,

hyperthyroidism, arthritis) can affect how cats view where they eliminate and what they have to do to get to that location. *Behavioral change is the first sign most clients will have of serious physical illness.*
- Finally, as noted for substrate preferences, punishment will not help this situation and could damage the cat behaviorally and physically.

Substrate/Location Aversions
Diagnostic Criteria and Description
- Consistent avoidance of locations or substrates formerly used for elimination, often involving behaviors that indicate active or passive avoidance or distaste that is amplified if the cat is confined to the area or on the substrate that he or she finds so distasteful.
- The difficulty in assessing these conditions is that "aversion" is a very specific term, and we may be evaluating the extent to which the behavior is a true change.
- This diagnosis is not appropriate for cats who exhibit casual disuse of their litterbox. True avoidance of some aspect of location or substrate is necessary for this diagnosis to be made.
- Other elimination complaints/diagnoses can be secondary to this one and may not resolve until this diagnosis is made and addressed.
- It is possible to confuse location aversions and preferences with non-spraying urine or fecal marking.

Common Non-Specific Signs
- Complete disuse of litter and box.
  - Cats with substrate aversions but who are fine with the location of the box may use an area near the box, exhibiting the same elimination behaviors they did before the aversion developed but with whatever changes are dictated by the new substrate (i.e., they will dig on the tile but be unable to cover their urine/feces).
- Location aversions involve deposition of normal amounts of urine or feces in some specific place or similar places that have the same attributes.
  - If the substrate is changed, there is little to no effect on the behavior of these cats, which may help confirm a location aversion.
  - All places used by the cat will be linked by region or specific regional avoidance.
- Disuse restricted to litter
  - If the cat has a substrate aversion, he may perch on the box but not touch the litter, instead scratching outside the box.
- Secondary exhibition of "sampling behaviors" to find a new, preferred substrate or locations
  - The types of substrates or locations used over time will help inform the client about the character of the aversion: Was the aversion only to dirty litter or was the texture of the litter the issue? Was

the location too public or too private? Was the reaction to closed versus open litterboxes? Was the aversion to a pattern of behavior that occurred in that location (e.g., being chased by a puppy, being trapped by a bully cat, being hit by a door that opened unpredictably)?

- We have done a poor job of evaluating the olfactory effects of altered or soiled substrates, but given the sensitivity of the feline nose and how quickly olfactory associations are consolidated in the frontal cortex, we must believe that olfactory concerns are non-trivial.

Rule Outs

- Aversions can be difficult to distinguish from some medical issues, including UTIs, idiopathic cystitis, hyperthyroidism, et cetera.
  - Hyperthyroid cats may defecate more, and so the litterbox may need to be cleaned more often.
  - Cats with UTIs and cystitis usually eliminate small amounts in multiple locations and often show non-specific signs of pain (e.g., hunching, vocalizing, hiding).
    - The first sign of many UTIs or cystitis is a prolonged amount of time spent in the litterbox or repeated visits to the litterbox. These are not consistent with an aversion.
- If cats are noticed by the clients only during the sampling phase of the aversion, the clients may think that the cat is "not litter trained" or "losing his litter training."
  - The question that needs to be asked is whether the cat *ever consistently used* any substrate or location. If the answer is yes, these are not valid rule outs.
  - If a cat who previously had no difficulty stops using the litterbox, clients should be prompted to ask "What changed?"
    - Clients may not know how to tell if a cat loves her litter and box or whether she was just tolerating it and then some other stressor occurred. Clients must be educated about normal cat behavior and should be able to describe what behaviors their cat exhibits in the litterbox.
      - If the cat gets completely into the box, sniffs and turns and scratches before and after elimination (whether or not covering occurs), she finds this box/substrate acceptable.
- Aging can cause cats to change their litterbox usage patterns. In addition to an increasing probability of developing age-related medical problems that may affect metabolism, bladders, and bowels, *mobility changes with age.*
- Doors that may have been easy to open for a young cat are difficult for older cats.
- Stairs that once resembled a simplified agility course for the cat are now an impediment for litterbox access.

- For cats with hip or shoulder pain, litterboxes (or substituted sweater boxes) may have prohibitively high walls, requiring that they are safely re-engineered or replaced with short boxes or baking sheets.
- If long-haired cats develop balance problems, their hair may need to be washed or trimmed so that they are kept clean and don't develop an aversion to litter.
- Small amounts of forethought can provide much-needed help for life-stage changes that will affect our patients.

Etiology, Epidemiology, and Risk Groups

- Cats who are ill. If cats associate diarrhea, pain, vomiting, or other unpleasant signs of illness or debility with the litterbox or litter, they may be at risk for developing an aversion.
- Cats who have companion cats who are ill.
- Entrapment in the litterbox (either by a door or by another animal) or in the area where the litterbox is located (a closet whose door is closed).
- Filth and poor litter and litterbox hygiene.
- The addition of new cats or dogs to the household.
- Repeated changes of litter brands and types (e.g., clients who use the litter with the cheapest coupon of the week).
- Long-haired cats have been suggested to be more at risk for substrate aversions because their fine coats hold odors and particulate matter more readily than do short-hair coats. There are few reliable data.

Common Myths That Can Get in the Way of Treatment or Diagnosis

- Cats should not care about the type of litter they use or where their litterbox is.
  - Cats eliminate outside, when given the chance, and have an almost endless array of substrate and location choices when they do so. Clients do not realize that the cat is actually making choices if the cat is free-ranging. Given the roles that olfaction and elimination play in the feline social system, clients should realize *how restrictive and discordant their offerings of litterboxes and litters could be to their cats.* By watching what the cat avoids and what she chooses, the client can help address the cat's aversions.
- The common myth about elimination concerns is that the cat is doing this to "get even" with the client, for "spite" because the cat is "angry," and/or as a way to show displeasure about some aspect of the client's choices.
  - This is among the most anthropocentric of myths about cat behavior. If the client can be convinced to understand the cat's needs, the client usually understands that the cat is being put in a situation that is uncomfortable or untenable.

Commonly Asked Client Questions

- Will the cat ever again use a litterbox/location that the client finds acceptable?

- The answer to this question depends on the type and extent of the aversion and the ability of the client to adapt to any apparent alternative choices that the cat has identified.
- If fear or phobia is part of the aversion, the clients will be unlikely to shift the cat to something that the clients find acceptable without redress of the fear/phobia.
- If the cat is averse to a scented litter, what can the clients do to control odor?
  - (1) Scoop the litter multiple times per day; (2) dump the litter daily; and (3) wash the litterbox with hot water, and rinse and dry well every day.
  - Baking soda, activated charcoal, and other compounds that adsorb odor can be found in some litters and may help, but the clients should remember two things:
    - These may also be substances to which cats can become averse.
    - Aversions may be linked. *If the cat learns to loathe scented litter, he may also associate the scent with a specific texture and now have a much more complex aversion to address.*
    - There are areas where they are able to accommodate the cat.
- How do we know which cat is responsible?
  - Cats who potentially defecate in inappropriate places can be given colored wax—which is what most non-toxic crayons are—by grating it into their food. Clients can simultaneously use different colors for different cats if they can guarantee that each cat eats only his food. The wax passes through the cat's gastrointestinal tract with the color intact.
  - Red beets are detectable in feces and can be fed to cats (one cat at a time).
  - Fluorescein can be given to cats to learn who is responsible for the urination. A detailed explanation is found in the section on spraying.

Treatment

- Management:
  - Excellent litter hygiene, as noted, will help to prevent many substrate aversions.
  - Observing what the cat likes and where he likes it can help any client meet the cat's needs.
  - Clients must know what normal elimination behavior for that cat looks like. *If the cat is shy, the clients can use a video camera on a tripod and learn what the cat does in and/or near the litterbox.*
  - Assessment of the social relationships among animals, including humans, in the household can help the client to recognize and understand some aversions.
  - If a litterbox is unused or under-used, if the client videotapes the box over a few days, he or she may learn why no cat is using it (e.g., a door crashes into it three times a day, no one ever comes down

to the basement, the closet door is closed by the client's partner in the morning).
- Behavior modification:
  - The easiest and best form of behavior modification will be to reinforce substrates or locations that the cat likes or will at least use.
  - Elimination is a self-rewarding behavior. The reward of relief will be difficult to compete with if one is considering attempting to modify behavior involved in an aversion.
  - If the cat has become completely aversive to all aspects of litterboxes and cannot or will not go outside or is not allowed outside, rewarding cats for using any acceptable location and substrate *may be successful only if the cat is being treated with an anti-anxiety medication. True aversions are extremely problematic, which is why it is so important to practice appropriate care and hygiene routinely.*
  - If all else fails, clients can consider allowing the cat to be an indoor/outdoor cat. There are now creative and safer ways to allow cats outside (including onto an apartment terrace) by using cat enclosures and fences (www.purrfectfence.com; www.purrfectfence.com/outdoor_cat_enclosures.asp). Even if the cat is at little risk from vehicles and predators in the environment, enclosures and fences can help the cats to be good neighbors by preventing them from sharing their elimination products and patterns with the entire neighborhood. In this way, we address inter-specifies welfare concerns, which may have unappreciated and far-reaching consequences for all of us.
- Medication/dietary intervention:
  - Any concomitant pain or illness must be treated.
  - Cats who have had a history of constipation can learn to fear the litterbox if defecation hurts. Diets and supplements can help prevent or control constipation.
  - Anti-anxiety medications are often needed in the case of long-standing aversions.
  - Before using medication, a laboratory evaluation (CBC, serum biochemistry profile) and at least a lead II ECG, especially if considering TCA/SSRI use, should be performed. Most of these medications are metabolized through renal and hepatic pathways, and clearance may be altered if renal or hepatic disease is a concern. Additionally, these medications will interact with other medications that share the same cytochrome P-450 system enzyme pathways, so a good medical history is important. TCAs and SSRIs may be more arrhythmogenic in cats than in other species.
  - Cats older than 6 years should also have a thyroid profile as part of their baseline laboratory evaluation.
  - Medications may include:
    - TCAs:

- ▪ Amitriptyline
- ▪ Nortriptyline
- ▪ Clomipramine
- ▪ SSRIs:
  - ▪ Fluoxetine
  - ▪ Paroxetine
- ▪ BZDs—can be extremely useful if using food treats as part of a behavior modification program to reinforce appropriate substrates/locations or entry into areas where the cat can explore appropriate substrates/locations.
  - ▪ Alprazolam
  - ▪ Oxazepam
- ▪ Other:
  - ▪ Gabapentin
  - ▪ Buspirone—this is a partial 5-hydroxytryptamine 1A ($5\text{-}HT_{1A}$) agonist that can be helpful for cats who have aversions secondary to social conflicts with other cats. Only the cat who is "victimized" should be treated with buspirone (see the section on inter-cat aggression).
- • BZDs have been associated with rare hyperexcitability, rare profound sedation, and rare severe hepatotoxicity, but this story is more complex than just BZD use (see Chapter 10).
- • BZDs have abuse potential in humans and are not suitable for use in all households.
- • Cats treated with MAO inhibitors (some flea and tick collars) should not be treated with TCAs or SSRIs.
- • Miscellaneous interventions:
  - • Some cats will not eliminate where they are fed, so placement of food dishes may, but does not always, have a role in convincing the cat *not* to use one area.
  - • Closing doors, moving furniture, covering soiled areas with heavy gauge plastic (so that it cannot continue to be soiled), and replacing carpeting and/or flooring in soiled areas all can discourage a cat from eliminating in a chosen area, but they do nothing to address the original aversion. Success relies on such redress and identifying a suitable substrate/location that the cat will at least reliably use.
  - • If cats have known elimination times or passage rates, clients may be able to take advantage of these to follow the cat and to reward him for using an appropriate substrate. This strategy does not work for fearful cats.
    - ▪ Use of pheromonal analogue products has been suggested to "calm" animals, but they, or their vehicles/dispensers, may make some animals more reactive. Their efficacy is in doubt because most studies are poor and show, at best, a weak contributory effect. No controlled study on the use of pheromonal analogues

has demonstrated efficacy to the extent seen when the underlying anxiety is treated with medication.

Helpful Handouts

- • "Protocol for Understanding and Treating Cats with Elimination Disorders and Elimination Behaviors That Concern Clients"
- • "Protocol for Understanding and Treating Feline Aggressions with an Emphasis on Inter-Cat Aggression"
- • "Protocol for Understanding and Helping Geriatric Animals"
- • "Protocol for Treating Fearful Behavior in Cats and Dogs"
- • "Protocol for Using Behavioral Medication Successfully"

Last Words

- • Some cats may benefit from being confined to a restricted area at first. Clients need to ensure that the cat has a selection of litterboxes and litters and that the cat receives sufficient attention during confinement.
  - • If this was a very social cat before confinement, confinement has to be arranged to meet the cat's social needs.
  - • If the behavior of the other cats in the household changes when one is isolated, this hints to a social problem that may need to be addressed as part of the therapy for the elimination disorder.
  - • Access to the rest of the house can be expanded once the cat is using litterboxes and litter appropriately in the confined area. It is important that the expanded access be closely supervised because of the potential for relapses and potential social problems that may not have been previously recognized.
  - • A bell sewn or attached to the cat's collar can act as a reminder that supervision is necessary (Bear Bells; www.rei.com).
  - • Access should be gradually expanded. If the cat has truly learned and demonstrated a preference for a litter and/or litterbox style, this preference will generalize to the rest of the house if the re-introductions are gradual.
- • Clients often wait to seek veterinary help for an elimination concern—especially aversions—until they are moving, replacing the rugs, buying new furniture, having visitors, et cetera. *Aversions and preferences that are long-standing will not resolve quickly.* The veterinary staff needs to educate every client about cat elimination behaviors early and often *and emphasize the extent to which cats are good at hiding their concerns, with the expectation that aversions may be more common than appreciated.*
- • *Punishment is counter-productive and may enhance aversions.*

Common Myths That Can Get in the Way of Treatment or Diagnosis

- Spraying is the classic behavior for which clients readily assign to the cat some malicious motive. They assume that the cat is "mad" at them for something and that the urine is sprayed to get back at them.
  - Spraying that is not about identifying mates (and most owned cats in the United States are neutered) either may be a normal behavior indicating a cat-typical concern or may be due to underlying anxiety that the cat is experiencing because of some element of the social system or interactions within it.
  - A good history, complete with both video and still photos of all cats potentially involved, including any who may be outdoors, will determine whether this is normal but undesirable behavior that can be shifted through behavioral and environmental interventions or whether it is a problem for the cat requiring true interventional treatment.
  - Cats may also mark areas where the client frequents (the client's side of the bed, pillows), but this is more about establishing a close link with the client than it is about punishing them. Clients will not see the spraying this way, but they must be encouraged to do so if they are to understand what could be contributing to the cat's reason for spraying.

Commonly Asked Client Questions

- When cats spray people, clients commonly ask if the cat has better taste in partners/associates/dates/spouses than does the client.
  - It is unlikely that the cat and the client are using the same criteria to evaluate the client's personal relationships; however, any time animals appear to be concerned about one individual or one set of individuals, the clients may wish to take a more objective look and ask if the cat's or dog's concern is merited.
  - Spraying of a person by a cat may say more about the person's interaction with the cat than about that person's interactions with other people.
  - A cat who could identify a perfect mate would be worth a fortune.
- Can the cat be encouraged to cease spraying or to do it only in situations that the client finds acceptable (e.g., against the back of a litter box)?
  - Whether this will happen depends on the reason that the cat is spraying. If the cat is spraying in a certain place as a social signal, sometimes placing a litterbox with a shield in the area will encourage the cat to use the shield instead. If the cat is engaging in spraying as a way to be seen, a shield will also be a barrier and so might not help.
- Can spraying be treated?
  - Yes, but *the reason for the spraying must be understood and addressed.* In some cases, this will involve changes in social relationships between cats in the household or in creating visual or real barriers between some cats.
- How can we tell which cat is spraying in a multi-cat household?
  - Seeing one cat spray confirms *only* that *that* cat sprays. It does not confirm that the other cats *do not* spray.
    - Spraying by one cat can be an important facilitator for spraying by another cat.
  - If cats are individually confined and spray when confined, one can confirm that the isolated cat will spray and may contribute the spraying in the household.
    - The frequency and location of spraying may change once this focal cat is no longer isolated.
  - Cats can be given oral fluorescein, and then the environment can be checked for urine that fluoresces in the manner of fluorescein when exposed to a black light.
    - Fluorescein may be visualized as a yellow/orange/green stain. *Clients should know that fluorescein is a relatively inert compound that readily diffuses into tissues. It has been associated only occasionally with any side effects* (Davidson and Baty, 1991).
    - *Fluorescein can permanently stain many fabrics.*
    - Urine itself fluoresces under black light, but here the colors should be different.
    - Fluorescein can be obtained from solution (0.5 mL), ophthalmologic drops, tiny pieces of ophthalmic strips placed in capsules, or capsules or droppers of the stain rinsed from the strips (distillate from six fluorescein strips) in capsules and used at a dose of 50 mg/cat (Neilson, 2003).
    - Fluorescein can be injected subcutaneously (0.3 mL of 10% injectable solution) (Hart and Leedy, 1982).
    - Injectable fluorescein (250 μg/kg) can also be used, but this must be given intravenously by a veterinarian (Westropp et al., 2006).
    - For this method to be informative, only *one cat can be given fluorescein at a time,* and there should be a 7- to 10-day washout period between cats to ensure that the spraying cat can be identified.
    - Hand-held, battery-operated black lights are cheap, and any client with cats should consider the purchase of black lights early on.

Treatment

- Management:
  - The first steps in managing spraying involve identifying the cat or cats engaged in the spraying and understanding the pattern of the spraying behavior (Pryor et al., 2001).
  - Management-related treatment will focus on changing the pattern of the spraying behavior by altering stimuli.

- If the cat who is triggering the response is an outdoor cat, visual barriers (e.g., drapes, curtains, shutters, opaque coverings) may decrease the ability of the affected cat to monitor the behavior of outdoor cats.
- Regardless, the indoor cat still may smell the outdoor cat. *The use of good odor eliminators, discussed earlier in this chapter, is an essential part of a coherent plan to treat problematic spraying.*
- For cats for whom visual barriers and odor eliminators are not sufficient, removal of one cat from the immediate location may be necessary.
  - If the outdoor cat is owned, the clients should discuss with the neighbors containing him in a humane way so that the client's cat is not interacting with him.
  - Cat fencing can be used to keep a client's cats in or to keep others' cats out. Fencing is under-used in these situations and could at least provide a buffer zone around relevant windows and doors.
  - The indoor cat can be excluded from the room or section of the house to which the other cat has external access.
    - This strategy may compound anxiety in some cats who are accustomed to patrolling larger parts of the house.
- Occasionally, creating an area with litterboxes and a back splash or with plastic where the indoor cat can spray may help.
  - Such areas may be easier to clean, but cats often do not restrict their activities to this chosen area.
  - If the cat will spray in a litterbox, creating a backsplash for the box may help.
- Covering the soiled areas prevents them from becoming more soiled and alters the cat's olfactory cue, but the cover may also interact with any of the cat's innate tactile preferences to shift the location of the behavior.
- If the cat sprays people, controlled access to the people or areas in which they or their belongings are sprayed is essential.
- Behavior modification:
  - There are no studies on the effects of behavior modification on spraying, and one would expect, given the underlying social signaling that is driving spraying, that behavior modification by itself may have limited use.
  - Rewarding the cat for coming away from an area or for not focusing on it may be more helpful than is initially apparent, especially if this represents an opportunity for the cat to have calm attention and for being reinforced for being calm.
    - In this scenario, one is *rewarding the cat for a change in his reaction to some aspect about the stimulus.* This technique can be powerful.
    - If the cat sprays someone because the cat is worried about that person, having that person feed the cat and provide treats, grooming, and play may sufficiently alter the cat's concerns that she no longer has a stimulus to spray.
- *There is no role for punishment in treating spraying.* This condition is about social stimuli and their perception, so there is no context in which true punishment could work.
- A stimulus that interrupts an event of spraying (clapping hands, calling to the cat) may interrupt that bout of spraying, but because this isn't about choices for locations or substrates, the social interaction will continue somehow. What interruption may buy clients is the time to move the cat to an area to spray that is more palatable to the client.
- Sometimes, especially if the cat can be protected from the risks of being an outdoor cat, allowing the cat outside to spray changes the behavior from one that the clients cannot tolerate to one about which they no longer care. *The cat's behavior has not changed, but now the clients tolerate it.*
- Medication/dietary intervention:
  - Although we use medication as an aid in helping clients to manage spraying behavior that they may find offensive, the best use of medication is for cats who are spraying because they are concerned and anxious. In this latter situation, *treatment becomes a welfare issue for the cat.*
  - Medications used to treat spraying are those used to treat anxiety in cats. All cats involved in the spraying may need to be treated, but if the most anxious and distressed cat can be identified and treated, sometimes the other cats stop spraying, too, because the focal cat altered other social behaviors, in addition to spraying.
  - Medications have an important role to play if the cat is truly anxious and concerned. A pre-medication laboratory evaluation (minimally a CBC and a serum biochemistry profile plus at least a lead II ECG if using TCAs or SSRIs) should be done.
  - Medications commonly used include:
    - TCAs:
      - Amitriptyline—which is also commonly used for FIC or FLUTD and may be a helpful medication if pain is also involved
      - Nortriptyline—which is very similar in properties and usage to amitriptyline but may be less sedative because it is the active intermediate metabolite of amitriptyline
      - Clomipramine—which has a label for treating urine spraying in cats in some countries (Hart et al., 2005; Landsberg and Wilson, 2005; Lainesse et al., 2006, 2007a, 2007b; Seksel and Lindemann, 1998)
    - SSRIs:
      - Fluoxetine (Hart et al., 2005; Pryor et al., 2001)

- Paroxetine
- Sertraline
  - BZD—these may facilitate behavior modification that involves food treats.
    - Alprazolam
    - Oxazepam
  - Miscellaneous compounds:
    - Buspirone—especially if one cat involved is the victim in a situation involving inter-cat aggression (see the discussion on inter-cat aggression)
    - Progestins—the use of progestins has fallen out of favor because of the potentially profound physical and physiological side effects (e.g., diabetes, hair loss, bone marrow suppression); all of the newer medications are as or more efficacious than progestins.
- Miscellaneous interventions:
  - Electronic solutions, such as indoor invisible fences and/or mats that give the cats shocks, are likely to render cats more, not less, anxious and may increase the types of patrol and marking along the boundaries.
  - Some cats will not spray if they are diapered. Some cats will still spray but are now no longer soiling the environment. Diapers for small dogs experiencing heat cycles will fit many cats.
    - Many cats are not sufficiently compliant to allow this intervention.
  - Olfactory tractotomies and ischiocavernosus myectomies have been occasionally recommended for treatment of spraying in cats (Hart 1981; Komtebedde and Hauptman, 1990). Newer medications and understanding of feline social systems have rendered these approaches extreme and outdated. These surgical interventions may pose a welfare concern.

Helpful Handouts
- "Protocol for Understanding and Treating Re-Directed Aggression in Cats and Dogs"
- "Protocol for Preventing and Treating Attention-Seeking Behavior"
- "Protocol for Using Behavioral Medication Successfully"
- "Protocol for Understanding and Treating Cats with Elimination Disorders and Elimination Behaviors That Concern Clients"

Last Words
- The key to addressing feline spraying is to understand when it is normal but an issue for the client and when it is pathological and a welfare/QoL issue for the cat. Both of these issues can result in the death or relinquishment of the cat, but the treatment and educational approaches will differ.
- As soon as clients obtain cats or kittens, normal olfactory communication and the roles of elimination must be explained to them. *Whether the cat is*

exhibiting any undesirable elimination behaviors must be assayed at each visit.
- Because social factors play such a significant role in spraying, if all else fails, turning the cat into an outdoor cat may be able to be managed with lots of forethought and modern, humane cat fencing, but re-homing the cat may also make all the difference.

Non-Spraying Marking
Diagnostic Criteria and Description
- Non-spraying marking involves marking with feces or with urine that is voided during squatting.
- The determination that marking and not inappropriate urination (periuria) or defecation (perichezia) (i.e., a substrate/location aversion/preference) occurred is based on social criteria.
  - The events must occur in frequencies and/or locations that are inconsistent solely with evacuation of bladder and bowel but consistent with social and olfactory stimuli.
  - The behaviors must be repeated simply because it is almost impossible to make a diagnosis based on an exceptional incident.
  - The elimination event must be associated with species-typical postures distinct from postures used in simple elimination.
- Social and olfactory stimuli can be difficult to evaluate, and determining how they are perceived to the cat is difficult.
- Postures and associated behaviors should be sufficiently well described in a circumscribed manner that is not consistent with aversions or preferences.
- We often forget that sometimes cats are using their litterboxes for more than one function. Marking functions may also be part of normal elimination in areas and on substrates that are not distasteful to the client. As such, they would never be commented on, so we really have no idea how common non-spraying marking is.

Common Non-Specific Signs
- The cat will often mark using relatively small amounts of urine or feces in numerous but related places after sniffing and actively exploring the surrounding area. Sniffing and flehmen behaviors often punctuate the bouts of defecation.
- The placement of the urine or feces is linked by social cues but not necessarily by those associated with substrates or locations.
- Cats may scratch various areas and then sniff them before leaving a small amount of urine or feces.

Rule Outs
- The major medical rule outs are the same as for spraying and include UTI, FLUTD, and FIC. Cats who have any of these conditions may void relatively small amounts of urine frequently, but the

substrates and locations chosen are not associated with social stimuli.

- For cats who are marking with feces, hyperthyroidism should be on the list of diagnostic concerns.
- If there are multiple small puddles of urine, diabetes should be ruled out. Generally, puddles caused by marking are much smaller than puddles associated with diabetes.
- Location preferences tend not to involve multiple small pools of urine or multiple small piles of feces. Instead, the amount and style of feces or urine deposited in a location preference tends to be what has historically been the case for that cat.

Etiology, Epidemiology, and Risk Groups

- Non-spraying marking is one presentation of the ancestral condition in cats. There is no evidence that we have exerted any selective pressure to eliminate the tendency to squat and mark in the domestic cat.

Common Myths That Can Get in the Way of Treatment or Diagnosis

- As with all elimination concerns, clients think that the cat is angry with them, punishing them, deliberately making their life miserable, and in all ways being deliberately obnoxious.
  - Although an emotionally appealing argument, it is one that is completely anthropocentric. Urine and feces don't mean the same thing to humans as they do to cats, and clients can start collecting data that will lead to *the solution* once they understand this.

Commonly Asked Client Questions

- Can the cat be encouraged to cease doing this or to do it only in situations that the client finds acceptable (e.g., in litterbox)?
- Depending on the size of the area the cat is using, it may be possible to place litterboxes in the locations that will allow her to continue marking. Part of the issue from the cat's viewpoint may be the presence of her own scent, so this may not be a perfect solution.
- Can non-spraying marking be treated?
  - Yes, but the reason for the marking must be understood and addressed. In some cases, this will involve changes in social relationships between cats in the household or in creating visual or real barriers between some cats.
- How can we tell which cat is engaging in the marking in a multi-cat household?
  - Seeing one cat mark confirms *only* that *that* cat marks. It does not confirm that the other cats *do not* mark.
    - Marking using urine or feces by one cat can be an important facilitator for spraying and/or non-spraying marking by another cat.
  - If cats are individually confined and mark when confined, one can confirm that the isolated cat will

mark and may contribute to the olfactory complexity of the household.
  - The frequency and location of non-spraying marking may change once this focal cat is no longer isolated.
- Cats can be given oral fluorescein to learn who is engaged in the non-spraying marking with urine, as discussed in the section on spraying.
- Cats can be given colored wax—which is what most non-toxic crayons are—by grating it into their food. Passage of the wax will allow the client to determine who is marking with feces. Clients can simultaneously use different colors for different cats if they can guarantee that each cat eats only his food. The wax passes through the cat's gastrointestinal tract with the color intact.
- Red beets are detectable in feces and can be fed to cats (one cat at a time).

Treatment

- Management:
  - The first steps in managing non-spraying marking involve identifying the cat or cats engaged in the marking and understanding the pattern of the marking behavior.
  - Management-related treatment will focus on changing the pattern of the non-spraying marking behavior by altering stimuli.
    - If the cat who is triggering the response is an outdoor cat, visual barriers (e.g., drapes, curtains, shutters, opaque coverings) may decrease the ability of the affected cat to monitor the behavior of outdoor cats.
    - Regardless, the indoor cat may smell the outdoor cat. *The use of good odor eliminators, discussed earlier in this chapter, is essential as part of a coherent plan.*
  - For cats for whom visual barriers and odor eliminators are not sufficient, removal of one cat from the immediate location may be necessary.
    - If the outdoor cat is owned, the clients should discuss with the owners containing him in a humane way so that the client's cat is not interacting with him.
    - Cat fencing can be used to keep a client's cats in or to keep others' cats out. It is under-used in these situations and could at least provide a buffer zone around relevant windows and doors.
    - The indoor cat can be excluded from the room or section of the house to which the other cat has external access.
      - This strategy may compound anxiety in some cats who are accustomed to patrolling larger parts of the house.
  - Occasionally, creating an area with large, low litterboxes may help.
    - Such areas may be easier to clean, but cats often do not restrict their activities to this chosen area.

- Covering the soiled areas prevents them from becoming more soiled and so alters the cat's olfactory cue, but the cover may also interact with any of the cat's innate tactile preferences to shift the location of the behavior.
- Behavior modification:
  - There are no studies on the effects of behavior modification on non-spraying marking, and one would expect, given the underlying social signaling, that behavior modification by itself may have limited use.
  - Rewarding the cat for coming away from an area or for not focusing on it may be more helpful than is initially apparent, especially if this represents an opportunity for the cat to have calm attention and for being reinforced for being calm.
    - In this case, one is rewarding the cat for a change in his reaction to some aspect about the stimulus. This technique can be powerful.
  - *There is no role for punishment in treating non-spraying marking.* This condition is about social stimuli and their perception, so there is no context in which true punishment could work.
  - A stimulus that interrupts an episode of marking (clapping hands, calling to the cat) may interrupt that bout, but because this isn't about choices for locations or substrates, the social interaction will continue somehow. Interruption may buy clients the time to move the cat to an area that is more palatable to the client.
  - Sometimes, especially if the cat can be protected from the risks of being an outdoor cat, allowing the cat outside changes the behavior from one that the clients cannot tolerate to one about which they no longer care. *The cat's behavior has not changed, but now the clients tolerate it.*
- Medication/dietary intervention:
  - Although we use medication as an aid in helping clients to manage behavior that they may find offensive, the best use of medication is for cats who are marking because they are concerned and anxious. In this latter situation, *treatment becomes a welfare issue for the cat.*
  - Medications used to treat non-spraying marking are those used to treat anxiety in cats. All cats involved may need to be treated, but sometimes if the most anxious and distressed cat can be identified and treated, the other cats stop marking, too, because the focal cat altered other social behaviors, in addition to spraying.
  - Medications have an important role to play if the cat is truly anxious and concerned. Pre-medication laboratory evaluation (minimally a CBC and a serum biochemistry profile plus at least a lead II ECG if using TCAs or SSRIs) should be done.
  - Medications commonly used include:
    - TCAs:

- Amitriptyline—which is also commonly used for FIC or FLUTD and may be a helpful medication if pain is also involved
- Nortriptyline—which is very similar in properties and usage to amitriptyline but may be less sedative because it is the active intermediate metabolite of amitriptyline
- Clomipramine—which has a label for treating urine spraying and/or OCD in cats in some countries (Hart et al., 2005; Landsberg and Wilson, 2005; Lainesse et al., 2007a, 2007b; Seksel and Lindemann, 1998)
  - SSRIs:
    - Fluoxetine
    - Paroxetine
    - Sertraline
  - BZDs—these may facilitate behavior modification that involves food treats
    - Alprazolam
    - Oxazepam
  - Miscellaneous compounds:
    - Buspirone—especially if one cat involved is the victim in a situation involving inter-cat aggression (see the discussion on inter-cat aggression)
- Miscellaneous interventions:
  - Electronic solutions, such as indoor invisible fences and/or mats that give the cats shocks, are likely to render cats more, not less, anxious and may increase the types of patrol and marking along the boundaries.
  - Some cats will not mark if they are diapered. Some cats will still mark but are now no longer soiling the environment. Diapers for small dogs in heat/season/estrus will fit many cats.
    - Many cats are not sufficiently compliant to allow this intervention, and clients should consider risk assessment and whether they will do more harm than good.

Helpful Handouts
- "Protocol for Understanding and Treating Re-Directed Aggression in Cats and Dogs"
- "Protocol for Preventing and Treating Attention-Seeking Behavior"
- "Protocol for Using Behavioral Medication Successfully"
- "Protocol for Understanding and Treating Cats with Elimination Disorders and Elimination Behaviors That Concern Clients"
- "Protocol for Understanding Odd, Curious, and Annoying Feline Behaviors"

Last Words
- The key to addressing any type of marking behavior is to understand when it is normal but an issue for the client and when it is pathological and a welfare/QoL issue for the cat. Both of these issues can result in the death or relinquishment of the cat,

but the treatment and educational approaches will differ.

- As soon as clients obtain cats or kittens, normal olfactory communication and the roles elimination play in this must be explained to them. *Whether the cat is exhibiting any undesirable elimination behaviors must be assayed at each visit.*

- Because social factors play such a role in all marking, if all else fails, turning the cat into an outdoor cat may be able to be managed with lots of forethought and modern, humane cat fencing, but re-homing the cat may also make all the difference.

- The extent to which scratching with the feet and claws plays a role in either off-setting or augmenting urine or fecal marking is completely unaddressed. Considering that we often recommend cutting of the last phalanges of cats in the United States, we may wish to consider and redress what we do not know about the role of claws, pads, and accompanying glandular secretions in social behaviors.

CONCERNS INVOLVING AGGRESSIVE BEHAVIOR IN CATS

Our view of aggressive behavior in cats is tightly bound to our complex opportunistic "domestication" relationship with them. As unique "sit-and-wait" predators, cats must be able to go from prolonged periods of quiet, hidden, inactive behavior involving covert monitoring to sudden and profound arousal with accompanying reactive behavior. This is an exceptional suite of behaviors for most mammals to exhibit. We would also expect this very different style of foraging behavior in cats to affect social relationships between them, just as cooperative foraging has affected and been affected by social relationships in dogs, albeit in very different ways than cats experience. Likewise, their unique experience of "opportunistic domestication" will have affected not just cats' relationships with humans but likely also affected their molecular and neurochemical function and gene expression. The type of aggression witnessed by clients likely differs from aggressive behaviors clients see and recognize in dogs. If clients understand the differences in feline evolutionary history, social systems, and factors affecting sensitive periods, clients will likely be able to interact with and help cats in ways in which everyone benefits.

Attention has been focused on the extent to which feline aggression is covert rather than overt (Wolski, 1982), and defensive rather than offensive (Young, 1988).

- Offensive aggression generally involves behaviors that decrease the distance between the individuals, including approach (as a threat with subsequent flight of the other individual) and attack. The aggressor controls the interaction through the use of threat or the escalation of violence.

- Defensive aggression involves more passive behaviors that encourage avoidance and withdrawal, and the recipient to, or respondent of the aggression, controls the interaction, removing the stimulus for further aggression. Spraying can act as a defensively aggressive behavior when it serves this purpose.

Clients may not recognize aggression in their feline household because they focus only on overt forms of aggression seen commonly in dogs. The most common form of aggression in cats is subtle, covert aggression that involves posturing on the part of the aggressor and deference on the part of the recipient of the aggression. Misguided assertions that cats are not social have interfered with our ability to understand these types of aggressions when they occur between cats and when they are directed toward humans.

Cats are more likely to exhibit *overt aggression when they do not know each other or when they do know each other but perceive each other as equals and neither cat defers to the other. Covert aggression is more likely to occur if cats know each other well but do not see each other as equals.* This dichotomy of offensive (including predatory) versus defensive aggression has been well explored for cats in the neuroanatomic literature, especially for responses produced by the ventromedial hypothalamus (VMH) and the amygdala. These detailed neuromodulatory findings may be derived from the evolution of cats as "sit-and-wait" predators, and the profound swings in arousal and reactivity such a strategy demands.

- Excitation of the VMH leads to a *defensive response* in cats (Maeda, 1978).

- Both the amygdala and the VMH play a role in the defensive response to threats in cats (Adamec, 1990a, 1990b; Adamec et al., 1980a, 1980b, 1980c).

- The amygdala has monosynaptic, efferent projections to the ventrolateral aspects of the VMH and to the bed nucleus of the stria terminalis (BNST).

- The amygdala also has entorhinal cortical inputs to the ventral hippocampus (VHP) (Krettek and Price, 1978), suggesting roles for associational learning in any stimulation of the amygdala.

- Stimulation of the *lateral amygdala facilitates predatory attack and defensiveness in cats* (Adamec et al., 1980b, 1980c, 1983; Siegal and Pott, 1988; Siegal et al., 1977), but stimulation of the lateral amygdala using high intensity also recruits the VHP in these behaviors. This is potentially important because although cats seldom display food-related aggression, when they react in the presence of food, the reaction is profound and may be mediated by these neural circuits (Mongillo et al., 2012).

The medial amygdaloid nucleus is involved in:

- social behavior, including intra-specific (within species) aggression (Vochteloo and Koolhaas, 1987),

- avoidance (Bolhuis et al., 1984; Luiten et al., 1985), and

- sexual behavior (Harris and Sachs, 1975; Lehman and Winans, 1982).

Testosterone-binding sites in the medial amygdaloid nucleus may interact with vasopressinergic neurons within the amygdala (Roselli et al., 1989).

Associations between neuroanatomical stimulation and aggressive behavior have implications for underlying mechanisms of normal *and* abnormal cat behavior.

- Cats who are *more defensive* exhibit *less predatory aggression* than less defensive cats (Adamec, 1975b; Adamec et al., 1980a, 1980c; Anand and Brobeck, 1951).
- *Threatening stimuli recruit a larger population of cells in the amygdala of defensive cats* than in less defensive cats (Adamec, 1975b).
- *VMH cells are more responsive in defensive cats* (Adamec, 1990b).
- The extent to which the amygdala modifies social behavior can be predicated on previous social experience (Luiten et al., 1985; Sarter and Markowitsch, 1985).
- Activity in the amygdaloid nuclei and pyriform cortex is correlated with the feline estrous behaviors of rolling and vocalization. It has been postulated that the electroencephalographic changes noted in the amygdala during post-coital reactions are involved in ovulation (Hart, 1974d; Hart and Leedy, 1983; Hart and Voith, 1978).
- Lesions of the lateral amygdala or lateral midbrain induce the copulatory cry and subsequent response in cats, although queens with such lesions still tolerate mounting (Kling et al., 1960).
- Leyhausen (1979) described what he called *affective defense behavior* associated with affective signs: piloerection, retraction of ears, arching of back, pupillary dilation, vocalization, unsheathing of claws, and hissing (Shaikh et al., 1990). These behaviors can be produced by physical/electrical or chemical stimulation of the medial hypothalamus or brainstem periaqueductal gray matter (PAG).
- Leyhausen's (1979) *quiet biting attack* is elicited by electrical or chemical stimulation of the lateral perifornical hypothalamus, the ventral aspect of the midbrain PAG, *or* lower brainstem tegmentum (i.e., the region of BNST) (Bernston and Leibowitz, 1973; Bernston et al., 1976a, 1976b; Shaikh et al., 1990).
- Naloxone causes a dose-dependent and time-dependent *decrease in affective defense thresholds* and *an increase in the predatory response threshold. Opioid peptide systems* appear to act as a selective and potent modulator of affective defense systems in cats by *suppressing affective defense behavior within the limbic midbrain* (e.g., midbrain PAG, BNST, nucleus accumbens) (Shaikh et al., 1990).

Understanding some of these basic neurological patterns can help us to understand the manifestation of

some of the feline aggressions and suggest possible treatments.

Diagnoses Involving Feline Aggression

Because of the unique evolutionary history of cats, including their unique status as small "sit-and-wait" predators, and because of our interesting opportunistic "domesticated" relationship with them, we should realize that many aspects of feline aggression may be less obvious than we would otherwise expect. If we compare feline aggressions with canine aggressions, the extent to which subtlety and covert behaviors factor into both normal and problematic feline aggressions is impressive. When we assess pathological aggression in cats, *it is not sufficient to consider only the events that have caused the clients to pay attention.* A complete history, especially focusing on the patterns of the behaviors leading up to the aggressive event, is needed if we are to understand and possibly to help cats with pathological behavior that manifests itself as aggression. To help with this, clients should complete the aggression screen for cats. This tick sheet should help identify situations in which the cat is reactive, permitting not only evaluation of the diagnostic criteria discussed but also *some degree of risk assessment given the heightened level of arousal* so common in aggressive cats.

The diagnoses with an aggressive focus that affect dogs are not necessarily the same diagnoses that affect cats, and we should not expect them to be the same, given our very different evolutionary histories with these species. The most common of the feline diagnoses focusing on aggression are discussed here. The aggression screen for cats may indicate concerns that do not appear to meet the criteria for these diagnoses. At such times, one could ask whether the canine criteria could be helpful, understanding the limitations imposed by a species that evolved in the course of collaborative work with humans. Certainly, the occasional cat is fierce about having access to or controlling access for food, and the criteria for food-related aggression in dogs may be helpful. *However, the manifestation of the aggression is shaped by feline neurobiology,* which as discussed earlier is unique, and may produce behaviors *far more extreme than the behaviors seen in dogs* (Mongillo et al., 2012). Such thoughtful use of assessment tools and diagnostic criteria can benefit our patients and minimize risk for individuals who care for them (Fig. 9-8).

Aggression Caused by Lack of Socialization

Diagnostic Criteria and Description

- The effect of social exposure of cats to other cats and other species during sensitive periods (Bateson, 1979) is best viewed in the context of risk assessment. Animals for whom all sensitive period requirements are met can still have problems, and animals who miss "socialization" for, or exposure to, the

Aggression screen for cats:
This screen can be used in three ways: (1) to note the presence or absence, at any time, of any of the behaviors, (2) to keep as a log about the baseline behavior, noting how many times the behavior occurs, given the number of times it is attempted, per unit time (i.e., per week), and (3) to keep a log about frequencies of the occurrence behaviors, given the number of times the circumstance has been encountered, during treatment so that these numbers can be compared with (2). Please note if the reaction is consistent in style, or only directed towards one person, or only present in one restricted circumstance. If using this screen only for the first use, note if the cat has been worsening in intensity or frequency in any category.

Please note—we want to know what your cat does when you routinely interact with it—if you don't know how your cat would react in the following circumstances, please do not try to find out because you may provoke the cat.

KEY: NR = No reaction; S = Stare; B = Bite; H = Hiss, howl, growl, vocalize (not purr); SW = Swat/scratch; P = Piloerect/arch/puff up; TS = Switch or twitch tail; WD = Withdraw; NA = Not applicable

	NR	S	B	H	SW	P	TS	WD	NA
1. Take cat's food dish with food									
2. Take cat's empty food dish									
3. Take cat's water dish									
4. Take food (human) that falls on floor									
5. Take real bone									
6. Take food treat									
7. Take toy									
8. Human approaches cat while eating									
9. Another cat approaches cat while eating									
10. Human approaches cat while playing with toys									
11. Another cat approaches cat while playing with toys									
12. Dog approaches cat while eating									
13. Dog approaches cat while playing with toys									
14. Human walks past cat in doorways									
15. Human approaches/disturbs cat while sleeping									
16. Cat approaches/disturbs cat while sleeping									
17. Step over cat									
18. Push cat off bed/couch									
19. Reach toward cat									
20. Reach over head									
21. Put on harness or collar									
22. Push on shoulders or rump									
23. Pet cat when in lap									
24. Pet cat when not in lap									
25. Towel when wet									
26. Bathe cat									
27. Groom cat's head									
28. Groom cat's body									

Fig. 9-8 Aggression screen for cats.

	NR	S	B	H	SW	P	TS	WD	NA
29. Trim cat's nails									
30. Put on nail caps									
31. Stare at									
32. Stranger enters room									
33. Cat in yard - person passes									
34. Cat in yard - dog passes									
35. Dog enters room where cat is									
36 Human physically carries cat									
37. Cat in vet's office									
38. Cat in boarding kennel									
39. Cat in groomers									
40. Cat yelled at									
41. Cat physically punished - hit									
42. Squirrels, cats, small animals approach									
43. Cat sees another cat through window									
44. Cat sees squirrels, birds, dogs through window									
45. Human approaches cat who is at top of stairs									
46. Cat removed from hiding place									
47. Human body parts move under covers on bed									
48. Crying infant									
49. Playing with 2-year-old children									
50. Playing with 5-7-year-old children									
51. Playing with 8-11-year-old children									
52. Playing with 12-16-year-old children									

Fig. 9-8, cont'd

relevant periods can do well; however, *the risk of having problems attendant with the respective sensitive period increases if exposure during that period is missed.*
- Cats who have not had contact with humans before 6 to 12 weeks of age have missed sensitive periods important for the development of normal approach responses to people.
- If forced into a situation involving restraint, confinement, or intimate contact, these animals may become extremely aggressive.

Common Non-Specific Signs
- Even if these cats learn to accommodate some specific people, if a stranger appears, these cats usually disappear.

- If approached and unable to escape, these cats become extremely aggressive using their claws and teeth to avoid or escape handling.
- Approach distances tend to be extremely long.

Rule Outs
- Numerous conditions, including brain neoplasia, infections, and toxicity, could result in this type of profoundly aggressive response; however, this response is present in an affected cat virtually unchanged since very early kittenhood. For none of these other conditions could that be true.
- Rabies is not a trivial concern in cats. Knowing the source of the cat and the pattern of the behavior may help humans assign relative risk.

Etiology, Epidemiology, and Risk Groups

- Karsh (1983a, 1984), Karsh and Turner (1988), and McCune (1995) have examined the extent to which the social environment experienced by cats affected their ability to interact with people.
  - Cats who were not handled until 14 weeks of age were fearful and aggressive to people, regardless of the circumstances. These cats would not voluntarily approach humans and were aggressive if they could not escape.
  - In contrast, cats handled for 5 minutes per day from the day they were born until they were 7 weeks of age were quicker to approach and solicit people for interaction and gentle play, were quicker to approach inanimate objects, and were quicker to play with toys.
  - These findings suggest that there are complex, far-reaching consequences of early interaction with people. Lack of such social interaction with other cats may result in the same lack of normal inquisitive response to other cats.
- Total isolation from cats can have negative consequences for future interaction with humans.
- This constellation of deprivation scenarios may contribute to many of the aggressions seen in urban, feral cats. Without a lot of luck and inordinate amounts of intensive intervention, these cats will never be normal, cuddly pets, although they may attach to one person or a small group of people over a period of time.
- Lack of exposure likely interacts with suboptimal nutritional environments for the pregnant queen.
  - Kittens born to such queens generally have delayed developmental skills in addition to a decreased ability to learn, an increased (and usually inappropriate) reactivity to novel situations and stimuli, and an inappropriate response to other cats.
  - The chance that such cats will respond normally to most situations involving any interaction is diminishingly small.
  - Abnormal cats and cats with genetic tendencies toward decreased "friendliness" may be overrepresented in the feral cat population. These cats are aggressive at an early age and may be "dumped into" or returned to the stray population before neutering.

Common Myths That Can Get in the Way of Treatment or Diagnosis

- These cats simply require love and affection.
  - The impression that love and affection can fix anything can be extremely injurious to humans when faced with these cats and is manifestly unfair to the cats. Affected cats experienced altered neurodevelopment because of lack of exposure and possibly because of poor in utero and nursing nutritional environments. People who are willing to provide these cats with love and affection would be better served humanely sequestering the pregnant queen and providing early intervention in the form of supplemental nutrition and early handling of the kittens.
  - Because of the concerns with these cats, trap, neuter, and release (TNR) programs could greatly decrease the number of affected animals.
- These cats can improve with adequate handling and intervention.
  - There are many good Samaritans who view themselves as expert kitten raisers. *Age at which kittens are raised by humans matters.* Hand-reared kittens—those orphaned early—are often much more social with humans than would otherwise be the case because their early handling begins before week 2 and proceeds through week 9, the range of periods where exposure to humans is most productive. *These hand-reared kittens are not the kittens who are being discussed here.* The focus here is on older kittens (>8 to 12 weeks) who have missed all or most of their sensitive periods. With extraordinary amounts of effort and time, some of these kittens may learn to respond with less aggression and reactivity to a small number of people who have worked intensively with them.
  - This type of intensive rehabilitation effort is *not* an argument against the caution that these cats will never be normal and that they will always be reactive. To think that it is and that certain people or formulas could "fix" these cats is pure hubris and unfair to the cats.
  - If we truly understand and respect early brain development, we instead should take all possible measures to prevent this type of aggression from occurring by ensuring that all cats are wanted, regardless of their lifestyle, and have their social and nutritional needs met.
  - Nutritional needs may be more important than we think. In experimental studies, the amount of protein and fat in the queen's milk is directly related to her diet. Kittens fed diets low in protein and fat have relatively high mortality (Jacobsen et al., 2004). We can hypothesize that kittens who survive sub-optimal diets may not have the best physical and/or neurobehavioral development.
  - Emphasizing only the partial and very special exceptions of cats with this diagnosis who do better than expected removes the much-needed emphasis from how manifestly *these cats suffer.*

Commonly Asked Client Questions

- Can I fix this? Can't I just teach this cat to be social?
  - No, see the previous discussion. We can protect these cats from the worst of the stimuli that will provoke their aggressions and should do so, but we need to know that this also means that they may always get sub-optimal veterinary care.

Clients should be encouraged to think through how they can most humanely tackle routine care and to make a plan with their veterinary practice for emergency care. Anti-anxiety medications and/or sedation will likely figure into full veterinary evaluations

Treatment

- These cats will never be normal, cuddly pets, although they may attach to one person or to a small group of people over a period of time. Avoidance of the aggression is best. Gestures that would be considered solicitous by normal cats may be considered provocative by these cats. Passive attention should be encouraged through the provision of food and shelter and the use of kind words.
- If the cat is good with one person or a few people, the humans must be realistic and understand that the cat's behavior is also dependent on the environment and external stimuli. Clients should be calm but vigilant of any signs that the situation is becoming overwhelming for the cat.
- Management:
  - If forced into a situation involving restraint, confinement, or intimate contact, these animals may become extremely aggressive. Management should focus on avoiding such circumstances while minimizing risks to nutrition and physical safety.
  - These cats require protection that minimizes the chance of their victimization by humans and other animals.
- Behavior modification:
  - With time and in a very protected environment, these cats may learn some patterned behaviors that can be reinforced positively through desensitization and counter-conditioning.
  - The expectations for these cats must be extremely generous and realistic.
  - Clicker training may provide a uniquely suitable reward system for these cats and may allow a number of people to interact safely and happily with the cat in a way that benefits the cat.
- Medication/dietary intervention:
  - Medication (e.g., TCAs, SSRIs, serotonin norepinephrine reuptake inhibitors) designed to minimize anxiety and that could facilitate rapid learning and the acquisition of new skills and memories may help these cats to the limited extent possible.
  - The rate-limiting step is to get this medication into the cat. All TCAs and SSRIs are extremely bitter and so generally cannot be added to food.
  - Pilling these cats is almost without exception out of the question, and repository forms of most of these medications do not exist.
  - Compounding medication in topical gels/ ointments generally lacks efficacy because these medications are compounded with the anticipation of passage through the gastrointestinal system in mind. As such, these compounds are transformed in the liver, and those transformation processes often produce the active compound. Mere absorption through the skin cannot mimic this process, and it does not produce sufficient blood levels of the compounds to exert an effect (Ciribassi et al., 2003).
  - Because polyunsaturated fatty acids (PUFAs) may protect against oxidative damage and/or repair extant damage, one practical solution for these cats may be supplementation of cold water fish oils and diets that contain large amounts of these and other compounds designed to retard the development of reactive oxygen species (ROS).
- Miscellaneous interventions:
  - Modern cat fences may provide these cats with enclosures that do not feel like enclosures but that could keep them safe from cars and marauding animals.

Helpful Handouts

- "Protocol for Understanding and Treating Feline Aggressions with an Emphasis on Inter-Cat Aggression"

Last Words

- Most of these cats who are free-ranging may not be vaccinated. In countries where rabies is endemic, this means that in the event of a bite this is a dead cat.
- Accordingly, if these cats require any type of treatment, full sedation is recommended.
- Handling these cats may place humans at profound risk for bites and scratches and attendant conditions such as CSD. No one who is immunocompromised for any reason or who is pregnant should handle or interact with these cats.
- It is important to remember that this condition is largely preventable.
- Anyone focusing on rescuing feral cats needs to ensure that newborn kittens are handled from birth.
- Any breeder who wishes to produce the most tractable cat possible should do the same.

Play Aggression

Diagnostic Criteria and Description

- Consistent aggression that occurs in contexts where play behaviors (chases, pounces, grabs using feet, et cetera) could normally be the appropriate response in the social interaction.
- The hallmark of the condition that makes this a diagnosis is that the behaviors are out of context with the stimulation and/or cues received.
  - In true play, if one cat shrieks or freezes, the other cat stops. In play aggression, the normal "stop" signals are insufficient to stop the play and may even induce rougher play.

- The normal, accepted, or in-context range of social play behaviors are relatively well defined compared with abnormal, unacceptable, or out-of-context behaviors. The difficulty here will be to distinguish rough play that the animals have learned in their interactions from other animals or people from truly abnormal behavior. Analysis of discrete behaviors should also distinguish this type of behavior from behavior involved in attention-seeking behavior.

Common Non-Specific Signs

- Kittens and young cats generally stalk the objects of their focus (which could be human or animal) and stare, pounce, grab, and bite, and/or scratch.
- The grabbing, biting, and scratching intensify throughout the bout regardless of disengagement signals.
- Rather than exhibiting the classic bounce-and-flee behaviors common in social play in cats, the behaviors exhibited here have more in common with social fighting, but the object of focus and the stimuli that initiated the bout are not contextual.
- Movement of any kind can be sufficient to elicit the pounce if the cat is already exhibiting the related behaviors.

Rule Outs

- Predatory aggression involves more subtlety and true stalking. The bite involved in predatory attacks is also different and resembles that seen in classic biting and killing attacks and may involve shaking.
- Cats with attention-seeking behavior may grab at, bite, bat at, pummel, and throw themselves at the human whose attention they are seeking. Although partial or intermittent reinforcement can make these cats more forceful, they respond to attention given and can contextually re-direct their behaviors. Such re-direction does not occur in play aggression.
- Play behavior in cats can be quite rough, and inappropriate play behavior may inadvertently be encouraged by clients who play too roughly with kittens and cats. However, in contrast to full-fledged play aggression, true play is variable in its presentation, can be re-directed to inanimate objects, and can be modulated in response to cues from the recipient.
- Hyperthyroidism can cause cats to be extremely active and reactive, but two things usually distinguish hyperthyroidism from play aggression: (1) hyperthyroid cats are usually older, and (2) at some point hyperthyroid cats were normal in their play, and the roughness is a true change.

Etiology, Epidemiology, and Risk Groups

- Cats who are weaned early and then hand-raised by humans may never have learned to temper their play responses. This does not have to be the case, but the humans who raise them need to know how to avoid accidentally reinforcing untempered responses (e.g., always play with a wand toy or a toy that drags).
- Social play in cats peaks early and is replaced by more predatory activities by weeks 10 to 12 and by social fighting by week 14.
- Cats who never learned to modulate their responses as kittens may play too aggressively with clients.
    - These cats may not have learned that they have control over sheathing their claws in play (the ability to sheath claws volitionally is present by 4 weeks).
    - Cats may learn best about bite inhibition from another cat who has the same sensory and mechanical capabilities. Humans do not bite like cats do, do not have claws, and have differences in skin thickness and texture that may affect perceptions.
- Some humans routinely play too roughly with any animal. If they do so with a cat with play aggression, possibly thinking that such aggressive behavior is "normal" play for that cat, the aggression aspect of the play intensifies quickly as the cat becomes aroused. These cats may arouse more easily than cats who simply are exhibiting inappropriate play behavior.
    - Clients who swat at, toss, roll, poke, and prod their cats and kittens as part of play need to re-direct their own behaviors to toys or risk encouraging these cats and kittens to develop increasingly dangerous play aggression.

Common Myths That Can Get in the Way of Treatment or Diagnosis

- If you flick the cat on the nose with your finger or bite her back, the behavior will stop.
    - No. If you flick the cat on the nose with your finger you may hurt her (physically or mentally), which now convinces her you are a threat. You could also just have encouraged her to return your behavior with a more forceful one. Cycles of reactivity and aggression are perpetuated by reactivity and aggression. The goal of treatment should be to ameliorate this condition, not refine it. Injuring the kitten during a "correction" remains a valid concern. Clients are unlikely to be able to mimic successfully feline behaviors such as neck bites, growls, or hisses, which could help the kitten inhibit his play aggression.

Commonly Asked Client Questions

- Is this behavior due to bottle-feeding orphaned or early-weaned kittens?
    - It is unclear if there is an oral response component associated with play aggression or inappropriate play and bottle-feeding by clients. Were the kitten to nurse too hard on the queen or to hurt her in play, the queen would have swiftly corrected the kitten. Clients playing the nursing role correct

cats less frequently and are unable to provide the other species-specific behaviors attendant with nursing.

- Queens may also interact with kittens during lactation and nursing in a manner that would encourage other, more desirable behavioral responses (e.g., licking and massaging the kitten while nursing). It's also possible that there is a calming olfactory signal available to the kitten when nursing naturally that is missed when bottle-feeding. The data are few, but bottle-feeding deprives the kitten of the social response and environment that otherwise accompanies nursing. Although other cats cannot nurse kittens who require supplementation, they may be able to provide all of these other nurturing stimuli and can help kittens develop normal behaviors. Every bottle-fed kitten should be fostered by another cat; sex and reproductive status do not matter if the other cat likes kittens and is nurturing.

Treatment

- Management:
  - The best treatment for play aggression is management and early intervention.
  - Any cat who plays too roughly or exhibits play aggression should be stopped from doing so by blocking them with a blanket, broom, piece of cardboard, baby gate, or cardboard box—all of which can quickly be put between the cat and the human if they are available.
  - Clients must be vigilant for the first signs of any inappropriate behavior (pupils dilating, claws unsheathed, ears back, legs and shoulders stiffening, tail twitching) and interrupt or re-direct the cat as early in the sequence of his increasing reactivity as possible.
  - If the cat has already grabbed the person or animal, the victim should get up and let the cat fall, if possible, so that the cat can then be manipulated into another area until he calms. Brooms, boxes, thick blankets, cardboard, et cetera, all are helpful here.
  - If the cat will not let go of the person or animal, it is important to stay as calm as possible.
    - Cats arouse very easily thanks to their hypothalamic and amygdalic responses.
    - Aroused cats are more forceful.
    - If the cat cannot be dislodged using calm but firm pressure while wrapping as much of the cat in a blanket as possible, an aversive stimulus may be needed to disrupt the behavior. Any aversive stimulus used should be the minimum required.
    - If the clients have been paying attention and have sought help as soon as they noticed this behavior, a loud noise (a whistle) may be a sufficient disruptive stimulus. Failing this, a bottle of seltzer shaken and then emptied onto the cat will usually dislodge most cats, but no one should count on this working more than a few times.
  - Clients should not play roughly, and they should not tolerate rough play from their cats. Cats should not be allowed to play roughly with humans or other animals once the other animal begins to look uncomfortable. It is a good idea to interrupt any play that even looks like it could become rough by re-directing the cat's focus to a long-distance toy: a thrown ball, a feather on a stick, a piece of fabric that can be dragged a distance from the human, a remote controlled toy, or a ball made from wadded up paper that moves unpredictably when thrown.
  - One of the problems with play aggression is avoidance of the cat—the cat appears and grabs the person before the person was paying attention. If the cat wears a loud bell on a breakaway collar (so that the cat cannot get caught on something and hang himself), everyone in the household can be prepared not to interact with the cat unless the cat first sits calmly and directs his behaviors to a toy.
  - Cats who use their feet a lot may benefit from food toys that require that they "hunt" their food by manipulating the toy. There are many commercially available food toys, and clients can make their own. If these cats can be switched from meal feeding—where they can meet their caloric needs in minutes—to feeding using food toys and/or disseminated tiny caches of hidden food that the cat must find—which require that they spend a considerable time finding and/or manipulating something to get food—the cat's dexterity and activity will become more appropriately focused.
- Behavior modification:
  - The most commonly omitted step in "fixing" these cats is to tell them that they are good when they are not doing anything involving arousal. If these cats are sleeping or lying down calmly they should be told they are good. If they will tolerate slow, deep pets, they should receive them. If the cat will not tolerate physical handling without becoming aroused, he may be able to be rewarded for being quiet with a food treat or a toy tossed to him.
  - These cats respond wonderfully to behavior modification. They can learn to sit when requested for a treat (which can be offered on a long spatula or paddle).
  - If the clients are worried about reaching toward the cat, these cats clicker train well. The cat sits and is rewarded with a paired "click-and-treat."

- Once the cat is calm and his arousal level is lower, a toy can be thrown—assuming the throwing does not elicit a grab—or a toy on a stick can be engaged (Figs. 9-9 and 9-10).
- Medication/dietary intervention:
  - One would hope that most cats do not reach the stage where medication is needed, but treatment with some TCAs and/or SSRIs may render the cat less reactive and more able to learn other behaviors.
  - Some cats may be so abnormal in the threshold that triggers their arousal, the rate at which they become aroused, and the ultimate level of arousal that they attain that medication is necessary. In such cases, medication that addresses impulsive/explosive behaviors (e.g., fluoxetine, memantine) may be the best choice.
    - TCAs:
      - Amitriptyline
      - Nortriptyline
      - Clomipramine
    - SSRIs:
      - Fluoxetine
      - Paroxetine
- Miscellaneous interventions:
  - Remote-controlled treat dispensers that also make a sound (see the food dispensing *Treat and Train* by Sophia Yin) may have a role in rewarding the cat for ceasing to exhibit these behaviors, but clients would have to work with it when the cat is not showing these behaviors and at a point on the trajectory of the development of the aggression that is relatively early.

Helpful Handouts

- "Protocol for Deference"
- "Protocol for Understanding and Treating Play Aggression in Cats"
- "Protocol for Preventing and Treating Attention-Seeking Behavior"
- "Protocol for Teaching Kids—and Adults—to Play with Dogs and Cats"
- "Protocol for Choosing Toys for Your Pet"

Last Words

- These cats can learn to pick good victims for their "play." Victims who are unable to read the cat well or who cannot act accurately and swiftly to avoid the cat need to be protected from the cat through doors, gates, crates, and indoor screen doors. Individuals with debilitating physical or cognitive compromise, individuals who are seriously ill, children, et cetera, must be protected from these cats.

  It is important to distinguish between true play aggression and inappropriate play behavior (discussed later). One is always serious; the other need not be. If clients follow all instructions with their kittens and cats to play only with toys chosen for the style of the cat's play and the cat quickly becomes calmer and happy, the client has likely confirmed a diagnosis of inappropriate play behavior. If the cat continues to be forceful and scary in play, the risk for play aggression increases.
- Kittens with either play aggression that is recognized early or inappropriate play behavior can grow into lovely adult cats.

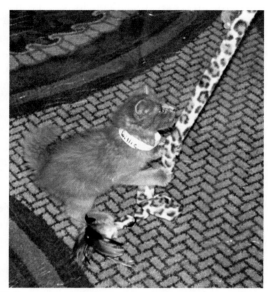

Fig. 9-9 A kitten who plays fiercely with his teeth and claws is ideally matched with a toy that can be grabbed in many places.

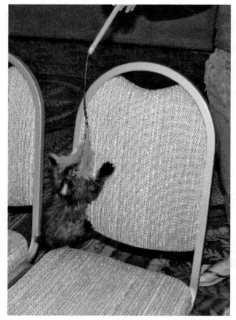

Fig. 9-10 A kitten who plays mostly with her claws is suitably matched with a feather toy.

Fear Aggression
Diagnostic Criteria and Description
- Aggression that consistently occurs concomitant with behavioral and physiological signs of fear as identified by withdrawal and passive and active avoidance behaviors associated with the sympathetic branch of the autonomic nervous system.
- Fearfully aggressive cats choose avoidance first. Failing this, they will become more overtly aggressive and will hiss, spit, and arch their backs, and piloerect.
- Cats with fear aggression exhibit a combination of offensive and defensive postures and overt and covert aggressive behaviors (Leyhausen, 1979).
- Flight, a defensive activity, is virtually always a component of fearful aggression in cats.

Common Non-Specific Signs
- Cats will hiss, yowl, arch their backs, put their ears back, piloerect, and attempt to back up or leave as they become fearfully aggressive.
- As the cat is pursued with increasingly fewer escape opportunities, he will stop, draw his head in, crouch, growl, roll onto his back, with his feet over his belly and paw at whomever is threatening him.
- If the approacher continues pursuit, the fearfully aggressive cat will attempt to strike, using the forepaws, and hold the approacher while kicking with the back feet and biting (Young, 1988).

Rule Outs
- The postural signals associated with fear aggression (the classic "Halloween cat") are so classic that few people could misinterpret it. What people miss is the cat's absence. People tend not to notice cats who are not there and they are often unable to say when one cat started avoiding another, the dog, or a human.
- Any medical condition that can cause withdrawal and/or pain may look like fear aggression.
- Fear aggression can be a sequela to veterinary treatment and/or concomitant with any condition requiring treatment.

Etiology, Epidemiology, and Risk Groups
- When fearful aggression involves other cats, the cats who are fearfully aggressive will actively avoid the other cats. Fearfully aggressive cats monitor for the presence of other cats and at the first indication (noise, odor) that the cat may approach they withdraw to the extent possible.
- Fear aggression is a common sequela to introducing new cats into a household. This outcome is not surprising given the evolutionary history of cats, where cats lived in extended, matrilineal family groups.
- Hiding is an adaptive response in a cat, an animal sufficiently small to be both predator and prey. Corticosteroid levels decrease in cats allowed to hide but increase in cats who are prevented from doing so. This common feline adaptation of hiding has profound implications for arousal levels, reactivity, and the learning that occurs when these cats are threatened.
- There are genetically friendly cats and genetically shy/timid cats. We do not know the extent to which shy/timid cats have the potential to become fearfully aggressive, but there are cats that, despite the best exposure possible, become aggressive whenever fearful. These cats also may become fearful with minimal provocation, suggesting a link between arousal levels and inappropriate responses.
- Any cat will defend himself if threatened. Whereas dogs will curl up into a ball and withdraw into themselves, this response is so rare as to be remarkable in cats.
- Depending on the type of threat, any cat can learn to become fearfully aggressive. *This phenomenon is particularly important when small children are involved because they may not know how to respond appropriately to a cat who is crouching and attempting to hide at their eye level. Any animal who is cornered and cannot escape has the potential to attack.*
- It is imperative that the cat *not learn* that his only recourse is aggression because this could lead to aggression in response to any approach.

Common Myths That Can Get in the Way of Treatment or Diagnosis
- Cats who are rolled onto their back and in a ball, with their feet pulled over their abdomen are being "submissive."
  - No animal in this posture is "submitting." This posture is indicative of a complete desire to withdraw from further interaction. In contrast to dogs, cats will always react if physically approached when in this position, and the reaction can be very explosive, aggressive, and dangerous.
  - Animals exhibiting this posture are doing their best to avoid further interaction. We should consider why they are doing this and allow that discussion to inform our next action. Any action taken by humans should involve assessment and mitigation of all risks. This includes the risks to the animal of being unable to escape something that causes him profound fear.

Commonly Asked Client Questions
- Will these cats bite?
  - Yes.
- How do we handle and/or separate fearfully aggressive cats from whatever is scaring them?
  - Sometimes, by providing a place to hide (e.g., cardboard box, crate, cat carrier), the fearful cat can be safely contained and removed to recover in a calm, non-threatening area.
  - Failing this, consider keeping a barrier between the human and the cat (e.g., a heavy blanket) if the cat must be moved.

- Removing the stimulus that is frightening the cat may be preferable, if possible, because this option gives the cat some control over his behavior. Having control over behavioral responses minimizes fear and panic.
- Hospitalized cats can also benefit from boxes and blankets that allow them to hide and render them safer. There are restraint bags and methods, when used correctly, that permit examination of one body region at a time, while allowing the rest of the cat to remain hidden.
  - Anyone can learn to do this with a good cat carrier and blankets. Veterinarians and technicians can and should practice on very compliant cats and dogs and/or stuffed animals.

Treatment

- Management:
  - Avoidance is key. Environments should be designed to avoid startling these cats and to allow them to hide.
    - Bells or chimes can announce the approach of people through a door or another animal through the house.
    - Boxes, especially ones to which other animals may not have access, can be helpful for these cats.
    - Keyed cat entry systems can be fitted in doors indoors and out, giving cats who are victimized and becoming fearfully aggressive wide range and space that is not also used by those who scare them.
  - If the fear aggression is restricted only to grooming and/or veterinary care, as soon as this behavior is noticed, efforts should be made to teach the cat to offer body parts for examination and care. Giving animals choices over when to offer a behavior or a body part can mitigate their fear and panic.
- Treatment options:
  - Behavior modification can be very effective early in the development of fear aggression. Emphasis should be placed on desensitizing and counter-conditioning the cat to the circumstances that induce the fear. To make this successful, cats have to learn some basic behavior modification—sitting, staying, and not reacting—at home and in a variety of novel circumstances. The place as much as the activity can become a fearful stimulus for the cat.
  - Clients should remember that cats can remain reactive for quite a long time after an aggressive event. Caution may be urged for clients seeking to provide solace. Cats should be neither rewarded nor told that "it's okay" for anxious or fearful behaviors. Clients are seeking to calm the cat, but instead the client may be reinforcing the inappropriate behavior.
  - Cats who are calm enough to accept a food treat can be helped with behavior modification.

- Pharmacological intervention designed to decrease the fear and facilitate the behavior modification can be a useful adjuvant. It is unclear whether any intervention can be successful if the condition has a genetic basis.
- Behavior modification:
  - Many of these cats respond quite well to clicker training because no one has to manipulate them.
  - Teaching fearful and fearfully aggressive cats to offer body parts for manipulation or examination can be done as part of routine desensitization and counter-conditioning. Because the level of fear and arousal may be difficult to assess, coupling this approach to clicker training is beneficial.
  - All of the behavior modification that is used to treat this condition can also be used *to prevent it:* all dogs and cats should be taught to offer regional areas for visual examination; to open their mouth on request; to show their belly, back, and butt; and to offer a vein for venipuncture.
- Medication/dietary intervention:
  - The most humane intervention for most of these cats is pharmacological, regardless of the trigger engendering the fear aggression.
  - For cats who are afraid of veterinary exams, well-thought-out preventive medication (e.g., alprazolam, a BZD, 2 hours before the visit and repeated 30 minutes before the visit) will stop the cat from panicking and allow her to learn that she does not need to be afraid and can have some control over her reactions. By using medication at the first sign of distress at veterinary visits and for subsequent visits, the cat may learn over time that she is comfortable enough that she does not need the medication.
  - Veterinarians who realize that cats are panicking or becoming progressively more distressed throughout the exam may wish to consider the use of a BZD to abort the increasingly fearful and panicky response in the hopes of relieving the cat's immediate distress and minimizing the chance that such distress will be repeated at future visits.
  - BZDs are fast-acting, need not be given daily, and generally help to facilitate behavior modification programs using food. TCAs and SSRIs are given daily and can be used with BZDs, if needed. TCAs/SSRIs are preferred if the cat's level of distress and anxiety is ongoing (e.g., they live with a cat who victimized them), whereas BZDs may be sufficient if the cat reacts fearfully with aggression to a specific and predictable stimulus.
    - The biggest concern about BZDs for cats is the potential for sedation, which can render the cat's behaviors more unpredictable.
    - Some cats also experience profound arousal when given a BZD, so before one is used therapeutically, a test dose is needed (see Chapter 10).

- There has been one cluster of cats in the United States that had atypical hepatic reactions to treatment with BZD, but this has not been reported anywhere else (see Chapter 10).
  - BZDs:
    - Alprazolam
    - Oxazepam
    - Lorazepam
    - Triazolam
    - Gabapentin (BZD analogue)
  - TCAs:
    - Amitriptyline
    - Nortriptyline
    - Clomipramine
  - SSRIs:
    - Fluoxetine
    - Paroxetine
- Miscellaneous interventions:
  - Cats can time and space share, and so by providing private and separate space many incidents of *fear aggression within the cat's own household* can be mitigated.
  - Left untreated, this condition always worsens quickly in cats.

Helpful Handouts
- "Protocol for the Introduction of a New Pet to Other Household Pets"
- "Protocol for Using Behavioral Medication Successfully"
- "Protocol for Treating Fearful Behavior in Cats and Dogs"
- "Protocol for Understanding and Treating Re-Directed Aggression in Cats and Dogs"
- "Protocol for Understanding and Treating Feline Aggressions with an Emphasis on Inter-Cat Aggression"
- "Protocol for Teaching Cats and Dogs to 'Sit,' 'Stay,' and 'Come'" for clients who wish to actively work with their cats

Last Words
- Because of the unique neurochemistry and responsiveness of the feline hypothalamus and amygdala, one of the major concerns about cats who become reactive is how long they stay aroused. Cats who are profoundly fearfully aggressive may not experience a "normal" arousal level for 24 to 48 hours, at a minimum. During the time that they are aroused, they should be left alone to the extent possible.
- It's possible that these cats are always overtly aroused to some extent and that such a condition may be one of those stimulated by lack of early handling. Specific mechanistic data are lacking.
- If cats must be handled when they are aroused, sedation and/or treatment with panicolytic medications are the humane choice.
- Finally, any intervention that makes a particular cat feel trapped will worsen fear aggression. People often think that they should try "flooding" the cat by placing him in a crate and exposing him to the stimulus that scares him—whether it is a place, event, or individual—until he ceases to be fearful. This is a terrible technique to use for any serious condition, and for a species that hides as a coping strategy it is abusive. The technique of "flooding" is one that constrains an animal to be exposed to what it most fears without the possibility of physical or behavioral escape. "Flooding" will always make a very frightened cat worse and any pathology in any species worse.

Pain-Related Aggression
Diagnostic Criteria and Description
- Aggression (threat, challenge, or contest) exhibited in contexts associated with injury, illness, or treatment/intervention that could potentially cause adaptive (nociceptive and inflammatory) pain or exacerbate maladaptive (neuropathic, functional, and central) pain (*sensu* Hellyer et al., 2007).
- The aggression exhibited is in excess of that required to indicate concern and to effect cessation of the offending stimulus.
- Because all aggressions have a learned component, if a cat has learned that he is made painful for a specific treatment/manipulation, he may exhibit signs of pain-related aggression *before* the actual treatment/manipulation. For example, the cat may splint and guard his abdomen before he is actually touched or reached for (Table 9-3).
- Evaluation of pain is difficult but increasingly possible (see Table 9-3).
  - Common signs of pain in cats include guarding/protecting body parts, withdrawal from social and physical interactions, growling, hissing, and anorexia.
  - Pain scales suggest that these behaviors may move from intermittent to more continuous behaviors as pain worsens (Hellyer et al., 2006), and aggression may be part of a normal progression until the cat is quite ill, at which point aggression may diminish.
  - We need to remember that domestic animals do not have opposable thumbs and so may use their mouths to grasp and restrain.
- For this diagnosis to be made, fear must not be primary (although anticipation of pain and the attendant anxiety may be involved), and *the behaviors must be in excess of those required to indicate the animal's concern and may precede manipulation.*
- Although this aggression occurs in the absence of behavioral and physiological signs of fear and avoidance behaviors, fear, fear aggression, and avoidance may become sequelae.

Common Non-Specific Signs
- Cats routinely have decreased activity as one of the signs of pain and pain aggression. If the cat is also

TABLE 9-3

Cat Pain Assessment Scale

Pain Score	Behavioral Patterns	Response to Palpation	Body Tension
0	Content and quiet when unattended Comfortable when resting Interested in or curious about surroundings	Not bothered about palpation anywhere	Minimal
1	Signs are often subtle and not easily detected in a hospital setting but are more likely to be detected at home by clients (if the clients are asked to monitor cat and schooled in how to do so) Earliest signs at home may be withdrawal from surroundings or change in cat's normal routine In the hospital, cat may be content or slightly unsettled Cat is less interested in surroundings but will look around to see what is going on	May or may not react to palpation of wound or surgery site	Mild
2	Decreased responsiveness, seeks solitude Quiet, loss of brightness in eyes Lies in curled-up posture or sits tucked up with all four feet under body, shoulders hunched, head held slightly lower than shoulders, tail curled tightly around body; eyes partially or mostly closed for either posture Hair coat appears rough or fluffed up May intensively groom an area that is painful, sensitive, or irritated Decreased appetite, not interested in food	Responds aggressively or tries to escape if painful area is palpated or if that area is approached Tolerates attention, may perk up with petting if painful area is avoided	Mild to moderate: Reassess analgesic plan
3	Constantly yowling, growling, or hissing when unattended May bite or chew at wound but unlikely to move if left alone	Growls or hisses at non-painful palpation; the concern is that the cat may be experiencing allodynia,* "wind-up,"† or fear that the pain could be made worse	Moderate: Reassess analgesic plan
4	Prostrate Potentially unresponsive to or unaware of surroundings; difficult to distract from pain Receptive to care—even aggressive or feral cats will be more tolerant to contact	May not respond to palpation May be rigid to avoid pain induced by movement	Moderate to severe: Reassess analgesic plan

*Allodynia—pain caused by a stimulus that does not normally result in pain (Hellyer et al., 2007).
†Wind-up pain—heightened sensitivity that results in altered pain thresholds both peripherally and centrally (consider using anti-anxiety agents) (Hellyer et al., 2007).
From Hellyer et al., 2006.

exhibiting decreased grooming and becomes more reactive (e.g., vocalizing, tensing, increased heart and respiratory rate, pupil dilation) when approached or when the intent to treat or manipulate is clear, pain aggression should be a consideration.

- An aggressive response to the slightest touch is abnormal.
- Biting should be a last, not the first, resort. By learning how the cat behaves when not painful and not being manipulated, it is easy to evaluate signs of aggression and decide whether they are directly or secondarily (pain aggression) related to the pain.

Rule Outs

- Primary neurological disease including blindness and/or deafness. Inability to anticipate an approach can lead to fear and heightened pain sensitivity.

Etiology, Epidemiology, and Risk Groups

- The experience and expression of pain are highly variable and individual.
- Clinicians must remember that the intensity of the pain experienced may be much greater than would be predicted on the basis of behavior alone.
- No one should assume that because animals are not complaining they are not hurting. Absence of patient complaints and dramatic behavioral displays can lead to under-treatment.
- In such cases, by treating the inapparent pain, the presence of pain may be confirmed by the display of more normal, happier behaviors and the abatement of pain aggression.
- Arthritis can also stimulate pain-related aggression. Arthritis is under-appreciated and often undiagnosed in cats because their response may be just to stay still.
  - Cats should be watched for their ability to get into and out of litterboxes as they age.
  - A push on the shoulders or the rump or a small child petting a cat too roughly could cause a cat with arthritis to experience pain and could cause pain aggression.
- Interactions with other cats and dogs can also cause pain aggression, especially if the individual with whom the cat is interacting is boisterous and young.
- Cats who have had an injury (e.g., a tail caught in a door, onychectomy) may become more sensitive to manipulation. Full examinations, including radiography, usually reveal no detectable abnormality, leading to discussions of "phantom" pain. Pain is a complex issue and probably under-appreciated in such circumstances. These cats also often respond well to behavior modification designed to teach them to relax and to anti-anxiety medication, but this phenomenon argues strongly against automatically encouraging prophylactic or therapeutic onychectomy.

Common Myths That Can Get in the Way of Treatment or Diagnosis

- All of the following are wrong and inhumane:
  - Cats don't feel pain the way we do.
  - Pain is a great immobilizer.
  - Pain is nature's way of telling you something is healing.
  - It will feel much better when the pain stops if the pain is allowed to occur.

Commonly Asked Client Questions

- Isn't it normal for an animal to bite when painful?
  - Not at first and not for relatively minor interventions. We become concerned when any animal's first response to attempted treatment is to bite. Knowing the behavioral and physical history may help. A cat who has had a lot of surgery and not a lot of good pain management may be more likely to have developed pain-related aggression and possibly fear aggression. We need to understand patterns of responses surrounding potentially painful events so that we can relieve the cat's pain and fear as early in the sequence of any fear/pain/anxiety as possible. One concern here is a hypersensitivity to touch (e.g., allodynia, neuropathic pain, functional pain) or "wind-up" pain, in which the cat becomes so worried that she actually makes herself more physically sensitive to pain.
- Must we control the pain to control this response?
  - We should assess the primary pain and its perception and treat both the pain and the anxiety. Pain must be assessed in a consistent manner. One tool is the pain scale presented in Table 9-3. Another is the stress scale presented in Table 9-4. (Similar scales for dogs are presented in Chapter 1.) By watching the cat and evaluating both scales on a routine basis, we should be able to intervene early in any painful, anxious event that risks becoming pain aggression or secondary fear aggression.

Treatment

- Management:
  - Behavioral assessments of pain may be more helpful than pain assessment scores or physiological measures in terms of possible interventions (Hansen et al., 1997; Hellyer et al., 2007; Holton et al., 1998a, 1998b; 2001).
  - Investing in a practice standard that encourages calm, humane, behavior-centered care may minimize the likelihood of this condition developing because of associations made.
  - Environments that are less noisy and where movement can be anticipated may have an effect on this condition. There are no data.
- Behavior modification:
  - If clients teach cats to be manipulated and offer body parts for manipulations, they may decrease the probability of pain aggression developing.

TABLE 9-4

Seven-Level Cat-Stress-Score*

Score	Body	Belly	Legs	Tail	Head
1—Fully relaxed	I: Laid out on side or on back	Exposed, slow ventilation	I: Fully extended	I: Extended or loosely wrapped	Laid on the surface with chin upward or on the surface
	A: NA		A: NA	A: NA	
2—Weakly relaxed	I: Laid ventrally or half on side or sitting	Exposed or not exposed, slow or normal ventilation	I: Bent, hind legs may be laid out	I: Extended or loosely wrapped	Laid on the surface or over the body, some movement
	A: Standing or moving, back horizontal		A: When standing extended	A: Tail up or loosely downward	
3—Weakly tense	I: Laid ventrally or sitting	Not exposed, normal ventilation	I: Bent	I: On the body or curved backward, may be twitching	Over the body, some movement
	A: Standing or moving, back horizontal		A: While standing extended	A: Up or tense downward, may be twitching	
4—Very tense	I: Laid ventral, rolled or sitting	Not exposed, normal ventilation	I: Bent	I: Close to the body	Over the body or pressed to the body, little to no movement
	A: Standing or moving, body behind lower than in front		A: When standing hind legs bent, in front extended	A: Tense downward or curled forward, may be twitching	
5—Fearful, stiff	I: Laid ventrally or sitting	Not exposed, normal or fast ventilation	I: Bent	I: Close to the body	On the plane of the body, less or no movement
	A: Standing or moving, body behind lower than in front		A: Bent near the surface	A: Curled forward, close to the body	
6—Very fearful	I: Laid ventrally or crouched directly on top of all paws, may be shaking	Not exposed, fast ventilation	I: Bent	I: Close to the body	Near to surface, motionless
	A: Whole body near to ground, crawling, may be shaking		A: Bent near the surface	A: Curled forward, close to the body	
7—Terrorized	I: Crouched directly on top of all fours, shaking	Not exposed, fast ventilation	I: Bent	I: Close to the body	Lower than the body, motionless
	A: NA		A: NA	A: NA	

Score	Eyes	Pupils	Ears	Whiskers	Vocalization	Activity
1—Fully relaxed	Closed or half open, may be slowly blinking	Normal (consider ambient light)	Normal (half back)	Normal (lateral)	None or soft purr	Sleeping or resting

TABLE 9-4

Seven-Level Cat-Stress-Score—cont'd

Score	Eyes	Pupils	Ears	Whiskers	Vocalization	Activity
2—Weakly relaxed	Closed, half opened or fully/ normally opened	Normal (consider ambient light)	Normal (half back) or erect and moved to front	Normal (lateral or forward)	None	Sleeping, resting, alert or active, may be playing
3—Weakly tense	Normally opened	Normal (consider ambient light)	Normal (half back) or erect and moved to front or back and forward on head	Normal (lateral) or forward with small amount of tension	Meow or quiet	Resting, awake or actively exploring
4—Very tense	Widely opened or pressed together	Normal or partially dilated	Erected to front or back, or back and forward on head	Normal (lateral) or forward with tension	Meow, plaintive meow, or quiet	Cramped sleeping, resting or alert, may be actively exploring, trying to escape
5—Fearful, stiff	Widely opened	Dilated	Partially flattened	Lateral (normal) or forward and back	Plaintive meow, yowling, growling, or quiet	Alert, may be actively trying to escape
6—Very fearful	Fully opened	Fully dilated	Fully flattened	Back	Plaintive meow, yowling, growling, or quiet	Motionless, alert, or actively prowling
7—Terrorized	Fully opened	Fully dilated	Fully flattened back on head	Back	Plaintive meow, yowling, growling, hissing. or quiet	Motionless alert

*Note: A further development of the Cat-Assessment-Score by McCune (1992). Both of these scales are contained in a client handout to encourage clients to evaluate all the cats in the household repeatedly using objective measures. See the "Protocol for Assessing Pain and Stress in Cats."
I, Inactive; A, active; NA, not applicable.
From Kessler and Turner, 1997.

- The manipulations most important to learn include offering nails for trimming, having teeth brushed, offering bellies for inspection and palpation, offering limbs and/or necks for venipuncture, and offering hind ends for temperatures.
- Desensitization and counter-conditioning to the veterinary practice, the clinician, the treatment room or ward, or any aspects of the procedures may be needed once pain aggression develops.

Such behavior modification will help with future veterinary care.
- Medication/dietary intervention:
  - We must treat the pain that precedes this condition. Opioids can be beneficial; mu opioid agonists such as morphine and hydromorphone are longer acting, but butorphanol is shorter acting. These may be especially effective in combination with other medications (Hellyer et al., 2007).

- Anxiety associated with the potential to experience pain can be treated with BZDs and/or other related compounds such as gabapentin.
  - Gabapentin was developed to treat neurogenic and myogenic pain and may have widespread use in pain aggression.
  - Midazolam has sedative, muscle relaxant, and hypnotic effects.
- Alpha-2 agonists may be extremely useful for treating *both the pain and the anxiety* associated with it and are reversible (dexmedetomidine feline dose, 0.02 to 0.04 mg/kg [20 to 40 μg/kg] intramuscularly; for reversal, atipamezole feline dose, 0.025 to 0.1 mg/kg intravenously or intramuscularly).
- N-methyl-D-aspartate (NMDA) receptor antagonists such as amantadine (3 to 5 mg/kg orally every 24 hours) are extremely useful for *both the type of pain worsened by anxiety and the anxiety itself.*
- TCAs and SSRIs are often used to treat *neuropathic and myogenic pain and the anxiety that may co-occur and/or augment the pain.* These agents will potentiate the effects of opioids. For these to work as well as possible, treatment needs to be continuous and daily.
- Miscellaneous interventions:
  - Cat muzzles are available, but most cats can be manipulated more humanely using a number of wrap techniques with blankets (Rodan et al., 2011).
    - If the cat is sufficiently distressed that she needs special handling and a wrap, she would benefit from anti-anxiety medication and some behavior modification.

Helpful Handouts
- "Protocol for Teaching Cats and Dogs to 'Sit,' 'Stay,' and 'Come'"
- "Protocol for Using Behavioral Medication Successfully"

Last Words
- Veterinary staff often think that pain aggression is normal when animals are badly injured or have undergone painful procedures. This need not be true, and the assumption that it is true subjects the patient to physical and behavioral suffering.
- Treating each possible episode of pain is essential. For animals with pain aggression, any procedure may be cause for anxiety, which heightens their already elevated response to pain. Use of topical analgesics such as lidocaine gel may help with vaccinations, venipuncture, and anal sac expression and may facilitate desensitization to these manipulations as discussed in Chapters 1 and 3.

Territorial Aggression
Diagnostic Criteria and Description
- Cats may defend areas from other cats and/or other animals, including humans. Defended areas may include foraging trails, and cats will mark burrows of animals they hunt (Corbett, 1979).
- Such cats may delineate their turf by patrol, chin rubbing, or spraying or non-spraying marking. Chin rubbing in males who are passing through someone else's territory correlates with their spraying behaviors (Natoli and de Vito, 1991).
- *Territorial concerns are attributed to feline aggressions far more often than the data support.*
  - Because of complex, transitive, feline social, possibly matrilineal hierarchies, a cat that is aggressive to one housemate may not be aggressive to another, and all of this occurs within the same "turf."
- Territorial aggression can be defined as aggression (threat, challenge, or contest) that is consistently demonstrated in the vicinity of a circumscribed area, when that area is approached, in the absence of an actual, contextual threat from those approaching.
- The aggression intensifies with decreasing distance, regardless of attempts at intervention, correction, or the desire to interact on the part of the approaching individual(s).
- This diagnosis should be made only after the relevance of the context in which it occurs has been evaluated.
  - If the cat is defending and/or marking a turf, and the perceived offender crosses into it, threats and a fight may ensue.
  - If part of the struggle involves social hierarchy, cats may lure or seek out their challengers and attack after the "territory" has been "invaded." *Because of the over-riding social component, territorial aggression can be difficult to treat without also treating the inter-cat aggression, which is usually the main problem, particularly if there is a marking component.*
  - Any appearance, change in, or alteration of a marking problem should act as a red flag for a possible underlying aggressive situation. Environmental modification (including resource and space sharing—Figs. 9-11 and 9-12), behavioral modification (including setting non-overlapping times to share space), and pharmacological intervention all are treatment options; however, aggressions involving strong, underlying social strife are notoriously difficult to treat once they become pronounced. Ultimately, one cat may have to be placed in another home or be banished to another region of the property.

Common Non-Specific Signs
- Heightened attentiveness and vigilance as the object of the aggression approaches. In cats, such vigilance is often manifest as staring and stillness, followed by quick attack as the cat becomes aroused.
- Cats may flick their tails and exhibit changing body postures while they are determining if a physical threshold has been crossed.
- The form of aggression intensifies with proximity.

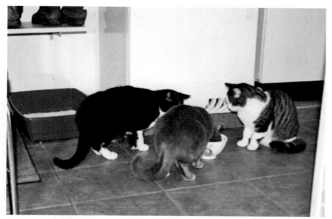

Fig. 9-11 Cats who are owned and part of a social grouping within a household sharing a resource—a food bowl—by waiting turns. (Photo courtesy of Anne Marie Dossche.)

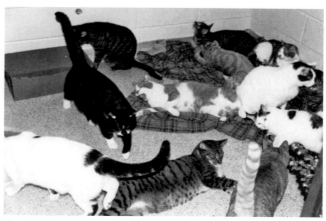

Fig. 9-13 In this group of blood donor cats, the empty cardboard box is a shared resource for which cats queue.

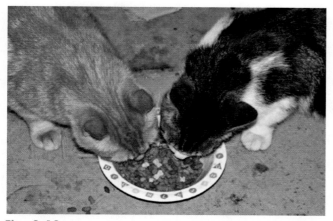

Fig. 9-12 Stray cats in a colony sharing a resource—a food bowl—simultaneously. (Photo courtesy of Anne Marie Dossche.)

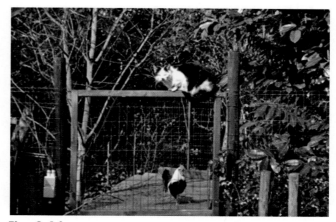

Fig. 9-14 Cat using a fence gate as a perch from which to survey the physical and social environment. (Photo courtesy of Anne Marie Dossche.)

Rule Outs
- The main rule outs are aggressions that are about social relationships and arousal and not about turf—inter-cat aggression and impulse control/assertion aggression.

Etiology, Epidemiology, and Risk Groups
- Territories can be floating, transient, or seasonal, or more permanent.
- Cats can patrol areas inside of the house or outside, but because cats are sit-and-wait predators, outdoor cats may be just as likely to be patrolling potential prey trails. The patterns of behavior related to turf are much more complex and subtle in cats than they are in dogs.
- Some cats may become territorial about their perching or hiding spots, their food dishes, or their bedding, but this is rare. Because of the manner in which cats cluster in familial and social groups, such areas are often shared, and cats time and space share well. When such sharing does not occur smoothly,

the aggression is far more likely to be due to relationships than to turf or objects in certain space. See Figure 9-13 for an example.
- Confined spaces, such as cars, crates, or fences, may provoke or intensify territorial aggression in dogs, but *in cats true confinement is more likely to provoke arousal because of an inability to escape and/or hide (their first choice for managing concern), resulting in aggression that is more likely due to fear or impulse-control issues.*
- The hallmark of any territorial aggression is that the animal is *not* aggressive when he is *removed from the territory*. If cats are removed from a circumscribed region but still fiercely follow an individual, their arousal is about the individual, not the turf.
- Fences may remove any ambiguity about boundaries for dogs but often act as perches for better viewing (Fig. 9-14) or vertical signposts for marking for cats, suggesting that we need to evaluate the complete social system when attributing aggression to specific diagnoses in cats.

Common Myths That Can Get in the Way of Treatment or Diagnosis

- Territorial aggression is about access to resources, and social animals are supposed to protect resources.
  - The definition of a "territory" requires that the animal actively defend its boundaries. In a home range—which is defined as the region where animals spend at least 95% of their time—defense of turf is not the rule except for the core area that may meet the criteria for a territory. It is extremely difficult to use these criteria in most putative cases of territorial aggression in cats once the social complexity of the situation is considered. Too many exceptions appear, usually involving difficulties in social relationships between specific individuals. Those problematic relationships occur wherever the individuals are, even if they are moved or they move to different spaces.
  - Defense of access to those spaces in cats may be an excellent example of territorial aggression, but this most commonly involves more passive, covert aggression using marking of all types.

Commonly Asked Client Questions

- If the issue of cat relationships is really at the core here, how do we tell which cat is the aggressor if we do not see who marks?
  - The cat who stares directly at the other is almost always the aggressor. The victim tends ultimately to look away. If one cat leaves the room when another cat enters, the cat leaving is the victim of the aggression.

Treatment

- Management:
  - If clients provide lots of three-dimensional space in visually complex environments (Figs. 9-15 and 9-16), cats will usually be able to share turf in a way that also allows them to manage their social concerns, unless one cat is a true bully and truly pathological (see the section on inter-cat aggression). Even in situations that are especially visually and olfactorily complex, given the opportunity cats will sort themselves according to social preferences (e.g., "preferred associates") and personality type (e.g., bolder and more outgoing versus more shy and less outgoing) (Fig. 9-17).
  - In an attempt to control access to turf, clients may consider an indoor or outdoor invisible fence system that relies on shock. Animals who are shocked become more reactive, not less reactive. Given the unique neuroanatomical reactivity that characterizes arousal in cats, this can be an especially dangerous and bad idea.
  - If the cat becomes highly aroused in one area, the cat may come to associate that area with such arousal. No one should reach for or interact with the cat; instead, blankets, boxes, et cetera, as already discussed, should be used to move the cat

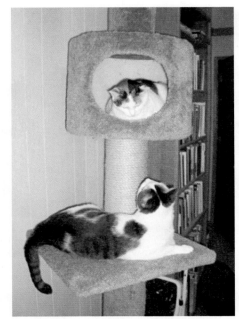

Fig. 9-15 Two vigilant cats sharing three-dimensional resources for perching. (Photo courtesy of Anne Marie Dossche.)

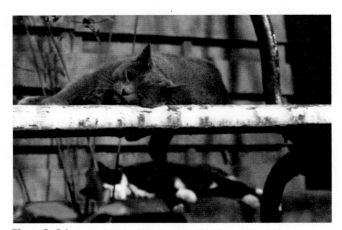

Fig. 9-16 Two non-vigilant cats sharing three-dimensional resources for perching and resting. (Photo courtesy of Anne Marie Dossche.)

to a safe and less arousing region when the cat can be humanely sequestered until she calms. Clients should be encouraged to remember that decreases in arousal to safe levels can take at least 24 to 48 hours.

- Behavior modification:
  - Behavior modification should focus on addressing the cat's heightened vigilance and arousal. Cats should be encouraged to attend to verbal cues and to look away from situations, on request, to keep arousal levels below that individual cat's threshold.
  - Until the cat is absolutely reliable, maintaining a safe room may be a good alternative.

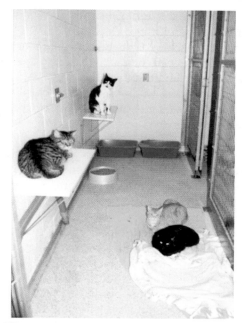

Fig. 9-17 Cats who are part of a blood donor colony and who are less social than the cats shown in Figure 9-11. All of the cats are in the same ward. By providing runs with open doors and shelf space, more reticent cats, such as those seen here, can find space where they are socially comfortable. This environment works if none of the cats have pathological aggression.

- Prohibiting access to areas that may trigger the cat's reactivity cascade or limiting the time spent there to small amounts insufficient to allow the cat to become more reactive may help, but these cats can react so quickly that many clients may not be able to do this or feel confident enough to try it.
- Frank inter-cat aggression in various social situations may render the cats more likely to patrol and protect turf.
- Cats can benefit from rule structures that ameliorate and contain anxiety by using a clear and humane rule structure (desensitization and counter-conditioning). If the rules change suddenly—the approach of very rowdy unpredictable kids or adults, guests, illness, a surprising seasonal change—the cat may not have a rule that helps him to cope with such change.
- Regardless of whether or not it is rational, if anyone is going to worry about the cat's behavior during any social gathering, the cat should be protected in a room away from everyone. Client uncertainty and anxiety will trigger the same in susceptible cats and dogs.
- Medication/dietary intervention:
  - There is anecdotal evidence, but little hard data, to suggest that some diets high in docosahexanoic acid (DHA) and eicosahexanoic acid (EHA) or

nutraceutical supplements containing high levels of PUFAs may render these cats less reactive. Such compounds may help to repair the damage done to neurons by ROS characteristic of highly aroused, reactive, and agonistic states.
- Use of nutraceuticals alone has been reported to lower activity levels, and heightened activity is one of the behaviors associated with these aggressions (e.g., Zylkene [alpha-casozepine], Anxitane [L-theanine], Calmex [L-theanine, L-tryptophan, and other ingredients], Harmonease). The data are usually weak for these compounds, and the effects may be relatively minor, but side effects are rare. Such agents may help as part of an integrated treatment program.
- Pheromonal analogue products (which are not pheromones and do not act like them) appear to decrease activity slightly in some situations that may provoke reactivity, but they do not appear to alter overall reactivity or aggression in any situation tested (Kronen et al., 2006).
- Medications should be chosen on the basis of their expected effects on anxiety.
  - SSRIs:
    - Fluoxetine—best if the cat is fairly explosive
    - Paroxetine
  - TCAs:
    - Amitriptyline
    - Nortriptyline—especially if the cat experiences any sedation with amitriptyline
  - BZDs and analogues
    - Gabapentin—although it is rarely used in cats, if the cat is constantly vigilant, gabapentin may help (it will need to be recompounded).
- Miscellaneous interventions:
  - There is no substitute for vigilance and environmental management for these cats.

Helpful Handouts
- "Protocol for Understanding and Treating Feline Aggressions with an Emphasis on Inter-Cat Aggression"
- "Protocol for Using Behavioral Medication Successfully"
- "Protocol for Teaching Cats and Dogs to 'Sit,' 'Stay,' and 'Come'"
- "Tier 2: Protocol for Desensitization and Counter-Conditioning to Noises and Activities That Occur by the Door"

Last Words
- The value of clicker training kittens (there are numerous books and YouTube videos that can help most clients) is that the client learns how to move the cat from place to place safely and for a reward. That type of ability and the relationship it engenders can be magical for treating these types of aggressions.

Maternal Aggression
Diagnostic Criteria and Description
- Consistent aggression (threat, challenge, or contest) directed toward people or other animals by a queen who has kittens, is about to have kittens, or who is experiencing pseudocyesis (false pregnancy).
- Threats and attacks are unprovoked by the approaching individual and may occur as a result of any near movement, not just that associated with an approach to the queen or kittens.
- Injury of the kittens is almost always accidental.

Common Non-Specific Signs
- Cats will hiss, snarl, growl, spit, et cetera, in response to being approached by humans or other animals when "nesting."
- Some very reactive cats may move quickly and grab at, scratch, and/or bite the passing individual.
- Most approaching individuals are able to avoid the queen at the first signs of arousal.
- Intensity of the threat is generally related to proximity of the approacher: the closer the individual, the more intense the aggression.
- Maternal aggression may be normal behavior. When aggression appropriate for protecting nest and kittens occurs, threats are intended to thwart further approach. Full attacks are rare for normal cats and appear to be directed toward unfamiliar or provocative individuals.
- As the kittens mature, the aggression—whether appropriate or not—usually resolves.
- There have been occasional reports of lines of cats who kill and may eat parts of their young when disturbed in even benign contexts. This is an extreme form of pathology.

Rule Outs
- This condition is likely a medical condition and related in part to reproductive hormones.

Etiology, Epidemiology, and Risk Groups
- *If the queen is continually annoyed (from her perspective) she may injure the kittens in the process of continually moving and hiding them.* Clients should watch for signs of increasing reactivity on the part of the queen and avoid stimuli associated with such reactivity.
- The role for arousal of cats who may already be prone to be reactive cannot be overemphasized in this situation.

Common Myths That Can Get in the Way of Treatment or Diagnosis
- This is a normal behavior.
  - Although some inexperienced or worried queens may occasionally be uncertain, if the queen is reacting this way routinely, either she is overly/pathologically concerned or she is being continuously harassed by the focus of her aggression. *Abuse and inappropriate treatment should be on the rule-out list.*

Commonly Asked Client Questions
- Will this happen if the cat is bred again?
  - It often does. Some cats become less reactive with mothering experience.
- Should the queen be spayed?
  - If this aggression is associated with repeated pseudocyetic events, not breeding or spaying the queen may be the most humane choice for the cat because her QoL may suffer.
  - If the queen kills the kittens without cause, she should not be bred again, given the reports of this extreme behavior running in family lines.

Treatment
- Management:
  - Provide a truly secure location for the queen and her kittens. Cats usually choose their own nesting areas, but they consider suggestions.
  - The provided area should be secure and not overly exposed but should also provide an unobstructed view of anyone who could approach.
  - Provide warning of an approach by talking to the cat. Anxiety worsens when dogs have incomplete information or must monitor the environment. Early warning can relieve related anxiety.
  - Quiet rooms or room with classical music, white noise, and/or dimmed light may help, but there are no data.
  - Provocation of the queen can be avoided by cleaning bedding and providing food and fresh water when she is elsewhere.
  - Restrict visitation to the queen until she starts letting the kittens roam a bit. Encourage this. If the queen is still reactive by week 6, if possible, encourage her to go away to do something she can enjoy (having a treat while lying in a window in the sun) while the kittens learn to explore new social and physical environments.
  - Remember that the queen's protective behaviors could restrict interactions of the kittens at a time when the kittens can most benefit from exposure. All kittens should be calmly handled by humans starting at about 2 weeks of age. Studies have shown an increase in willingness to approach people that increases when cats are held for 40 minutes compared with 15 minutes per day. The more time kittens can calmly spend around people and being comfortably handled by them, the better.
  - There are no data on whether queens who are overly protective have less outgoing kittens and/or whether this tendency could magnify an already extant genetic tendency to be less outgoing.
- Behavior modification:
  - All cats can benefit from learning to relax in response to calm stroking. If there is a known risk that this condition could occur, relaxation and handling behaviors taught before pregnancy and used throughout nursing should help.

- Medication/dietary intervention:
  - Although this condition likely has hormonal components, no interventions are recommended beyond spaying 2 months after the pseudocyetic event or after the kittens are weaned.
  - Non-surgical, post-weaning, hormonal treatments for pseudocyesis are not usually recommended because animals will usually cycle out of the condition, and if the cat does not have kittens but is lactating, the lactation will stop soon.
  - Any medications used could pass into the mother's milk.
- Miscellaneous interventions:
  - Breeders should inform anyone who has a cat from this line about this concern.
  - An honest appraisal of any patterns in the pedigree will help determine whether the occurrence of this behavior in one pregnancy may be exceptional. Cats from any pedigree with recurrences of maternal aggression would benefit from early genetic and behavioral counseling, especially if any killing of kittens has occurred.

Helpful Handouts
- "Protocol for Teaching Cats and Dogs to 'Sit,' 'Stay,' and 'Come'"
- "Protocol for Understanding and Treating Feline Aggressions with an Emphasis on Inter-Cat Aggression"

Last Words
- Most behavior specialists now recommend adopting cats as social units, if adoption of homeless cats is desired. This means that the kitten is adopted with his or her mother and/or possibly a sister or an aunt. There is no doubt that family units and communal care could mitigate pathological maternal aggression. However, this type of aggression is rare, so we are unlikely to know whether the support of the social unit could make a difference.

Re-Directed Aggression
Diagnostic Criteria and Description
- Re-directed aggression (threat, challenge, or contest) is aggression that is consistently directed toward a third party when the aggressor is thwarted in/interrupted from exhibiting aggressive behaviors to the primary target.
- This is not "accidental" aggression.
- The aggressor did not make a "mistake."
- The aggressor actively pursues the third party, particularly if they were associated directly with the interruption of the aggressor's behaviors. Accordingly, re-directed aggression is secondary to a primary diagnosis of concern.
- Re-directed aggression is always severe in cats but can be difficult to recognize in cats because it is often viewed as incidental to another form of aggression.

- In re-directed aggression, any interruption of an aggressive event between two parties by a third party results in re-direction of the aggressive behavior to the third party or to another, uninvolved individual. People often fail to realize that, especially in cats, the "interruption" may only be a threat: a stare, a posture, moving between two animals, et cetera.
- People may even see the behaviors of the interrupting cat as "incidental." Few behaviors between cats are truly "incidental."

Common Non-Specific Signs
- The behaviors most often seen are behaviors associated with frank aggression.
  - The cat may swat and hiss at the individual (human, dog, or cat) who interrupted them.
  - If the individual who interrupted the cat's behavior then responds to aggression with aggression, the original aggressor often intensifies his attack to both the interrupter and the original focus of his threats.
  - Because cats may become aroused so easily and to such a profound level, cats who were not involved in any part of the original interaction may be savagely attacked if the aggressor cannot gain access to the individual who aroused his or her ire.
    - This is the common situation for cats who may be lying near each other on a windowsill and one cat sees and reacts to an outside cat. The reactive cat cannot get to the outside cat which actually causes his arousal level to increase. As he becomes more aroused and reactive (which happens quickly), he lashes out at whomever is near, often another cat who is sleeping. Because *the attack is so savage and viewed as so unpredictable and out of context by the other cat, she may become profoundly fearful and suffer greatly from the event.*
    - *This is a diagnosis that always has more than one victim, and they all need treatment.*
- Individuals who are victimized by feline re-directed aggression are often bitten and scratched. Because of the rapid arousal process, there is little to no warning.
- Re-directed aggression can occur in response to being yelled at, physically punished, restrained, or thwarted by a cage, door, or window from pursuing another aggressive behavior.

Rule Outs
- None. Hyperthyroid cats may be more reactive, but the context in re-directed aggression is classic.

Etiology, Epidemiology, and Risk Groups
- Re-directed aggression involves a behavioral exchange "in kind" with the substitution of an identical activity, albeit with a different target, for the interrupted one.

- Only the focus of the aggression has changed.
- Re-directed aggression is not to be confused with *displacement activity*, which is not an exchange "in kind."
  - In displacement activity, both the target and the behavior are altered as a result of a frustrated, thwarted, interrupted, or corrected behavior.
  - A diagnosis of re-directed aggression is very specific and is unassailably identified by discrete behavioral descriptions.
  - Cats with re-directed aggression usually go after the nearest individual, regardless of whether they were involved in the initial conflict.
  - In the absence of the interruption of the threat, these cats may have been non-aggressive to the victim of their re-directed bite; however, this may no longer be true in the future. One incidence of re-directed aggression in a cat can shift the relationship of the two cats involved and others in the household. From this perspective, re-directed aggression is a treatment emergency.
  - The most common diagnostic error would be to call a behavior "re-directed aggression" when the "aggression" was actually accidental.
  - Cats who are fighting could also re-direct their aggression to humans, and the bites can be profound. Children, the elderly, and/or the infirm need to be protected from these situations because they make great victims for overly aroused cats.
  - In re-directed aggression, the bite may be prolonged or repeated.

Common Myths That Can Get in the Way of Treatment or Diagnosis
- "The cat did not mean it."
  - Whether the cat "meant" it has no bearing on the issue. If a bite occurred, an injury may be sustained. The re-directed event flags what could otherwise be another serious problem involving aggression. A full behavioral history and work-up is warranted, especially if the victim of the aggression was another animal in the household because these attacks are so severe they often cause profoundly fearful behavior.

Commonly Asked Client Questions
- Did the cat do this because he was jealous of someone else's attentions to me?
  - No. We do not do a good job of evaluating labels such as "jealousy" in any animal, so we should be careful about assuming a motivation we cannot assess. It is important to remember that this diagnosis is really about another aggression, so the intervention of the human could be viewed—from the cat's viewpoint—as irrelevant and a nuisance.
- Didn't the cat know it was me (or his feline/canine companion)?

- Again, it may not matter what the cat knew. That the cat was sufficiently aroused to engage in re-directed aggression suggests that he was serious about the original focus of his aggression. It is important to learn if this is an ongoing pattern reflective of a behavioral pathology.
- Did the cat do this because he was angry that we keep him inside?
  - Keeping him inside did not cause the event: his reaction to an individual to which he could not have access triggered the event. Many cats can watch outside cats pass by and not react. If the cat becomes so profoundly aroused in such situations, he is extreme, and his QoL would be improved by intervention.
  - Letting this cat out after such an event may not have the desired effect and may put this cat and other neighborhood cats at risk of injury.

Treatment
- Management:
  - The first step in management is to identify the behavioral situation under which the bite occurred.
  - If there is an ongoing problem, the clinician should assess whether there is sufficient evidence to make a diagnosis.
  - The incident could be an exception but usually is not.
- Behavior modification:
  - All cats who become this aroused would benefit from behavior modification designed to teach them to sit, attend to an external stimulus, be calm, and become less reactive. Clicker training cats to engage in a variety of behaviors for which they are rewarded while maintaining a subthreshold arousal level may help.
  - If there is a primary diagnosis, it must be addressed.
- Medication/dietary intervention:
  - When the primary condition resolves or is controlled, the re-directed aggression may also resolve, but with cats, there are many victims of the cat's explosive outburst.
    - It is essential that any cat or dog who is now avoidant or afraid of or reactive to the cat is treated.
    - The cat responsible for the re-directed event also needs treatment because he has now entrained his neurochemistry so that he will react more quickly and to a lower level of perceived threat in the future.
  - Medications may include:
    - SSRIs:
      - Fluoxetine is an excellent medication for explosive outbursts, and both the victim of the re-directed aggression and the aggressor may benefit if they now seem keen to challenge and fight each other.

- Paroxetine is an excellent SSRI to use in fearful or anxious cats, as is the case with some victims.
- TCAs:
  - Amitriptyline can be an excellent all-around anti-anxiety medication and may have palliative properties for cats who are painful.
  - Nortriptyline acts in a similar way to amitriptyline but may be preferred because it is less likely to cause sedation.
- Serotonin 2A antagonist/reuptake inhibitors (SARIs):
  - Trazodone may act as a mild anxiolytic and decrease motor activity associated with anxiety. There are no controlled studies on appropriate dosage in cats.
- BZDs and analogues—may help cats who are victimized be less anxious; may help in desensitization and counter-conditioning programs that use food rewards because they stimulate appetite
  - Alprazolam—can be used as needed or given every 12 hours
  - Oxazepam—very few sedation risks (will need to be recompounded)
  - Gabapentin—relatively low risk because this is a γ-aminobutyric acid (GABA) analogue that is not metabolized (will need to be recompounded)
- Miscellaneous interventions:
  - If there are certain circumstances under which the clients are reasonably certain they could see the behavior (e.g., a window overlooks an area where cats roam), a good harness could help interrupt the behavior as it starts, but it is preferable to change the cat's window or alter his ability to monitor outdoor cats (e.g., blinds or films on the windows).
  - Clients should be reminded that cats appear to remain reactive for an extended period of time after being thwarted in an aggressive interaction, and if they continue to be reactive, they can be quite hostile and potentially dangerous. Anyone who has a cat with re-directed aggression needs to understand the potential risk and be aware of the subtle behaviors signaling the cat's increasing arousal and hostile intent. Because re-directed aggression is often precipitated by another inappropriate behavior, it is essential to treat that behavior as well.
  - If there is a socially mediated conflict among the household cats, some environmental modification may be necessary to decrease the extent to which the involved cats are capable of interacting.
  - Clients should be encouraged to use inanimate objects (blankets, large pieces of cardboard, et cetera) to intervene between fighting animals. Use

of objects minimizes danger to the clients and may have the benefit of aborting the behavior while teaching the cat that there are consistent, undesirable consequences to his inappropriate behavior.

Helpful Handouts
- "Protocol for Understanding and Treating Feline Aggressions with an Emphasis on Inter-Cat Aggression"
- "Protocol for Understanding and Treating Re-Directed Aggression in Cats and Dogs"
- "Protocol for Treating Fearful Behavior in Cats and Dogs (for the Victim)"
- "Protocol for Teaching Cats and Dogs to 'Sit,' 'Stay,' and 'Come'"
- "Tier 2: Protocol for Desensitization and Counter-Conditioning to Noises and Activities That Occur by the Door"
- "Tier 2: Protocol for Desensitizing and Counter-Conditioning a Dog or Cat from Approaches from Unfamiliar Animals, Including Humans"
- "Protocol for Using Behavioral Medication Successfully"

Last Words
- This condition is a red flag for other conditions and may co-vary with other conditions that have control as their focus (e.g., impulse-control aggression). Identify and treat the primary problem.
- In cats, so many of these aggressions are accompanied by alterations in marking patterns and behavior that clients should be encouraged to monitor litter-box use and to check for signs of marking in the vicinity of the initial event.
- If the cat continues to be vigilant, the clients should monitor areas to which the cat attends for signs of urine or fecal marking or deposition. The sooner that such secondary issues are treated, the easier it will be to treat primary and re-directed aggressions.

Predatory Aggression
Diagnostic Criteria and Description
- This diagnosis involves extremely quiet aggression or behaviors congruent with subsequent predatory behavior (stealth, silence, heightened attentiveness, body postures associated with hunting—slinking, head lowering, tail twitching, and pounce postures—and lunging or springing at a "prey" item that exhibits sudden movement after a period of quiescence) that are consistently exhibited in circumstances associated with predation or toward victims that usually include infants, young or ill animals.
- Death is not a necessary sequela, and ingestion does not necessarily occur, should death ensue. Serious injury may occur.
- Confirmed cases of predatory aggression are generally quiet, unheralded attacks, which involve at least one fierce bite and shake.

- Behaviors exhibited include staring, salivating, stalking, body lowering, and tail twitching.
- The classic behaviors are consistently exhibited toward species-contextual prey items (i.e., rodents and birds) or toward individuals that exhibit uncoordinated movements and sudden sleep and wake cycles (especially human infants, young or ill animals, elderly humans).
- When all of these conditions are met, this diagnosis is unassailable; however, there is leeway in interpretation, and one seldom knows if an actual attack *would occur*. Although such an approach minimizes the cost of tragedy, it does not contribute greatly to our knowledge about the condition.
- Discrete analyses of the behaviors involved should elucidate different forms of this behavior and the role that the behavior of the victims plays in determining the form that the aggression will take.
- Solitary predatory behavior develops quite young in kittens (5 to 7 weeks of age), and cats can become proficient hunters by 14 weeks of age, especially if they are hungry. It is important to remember that cats are not small dogs.

Common Non-Specific Signs

- The most common signs are staring accompanied by mydriasis; salivation; silent, intermittent stalking; and start and stop movements that are guided by the behavior of the victim.
- The predatory attack is usually triggered by movement of the victim after a period of stillness.
  - The stillness can be brief. Normal individuals who realize that they are about to be attacked by a predatory cat generally pause before trying to flee and are attacked as they flee.

Rule Outs

- If the complete sequence of behaviors is understood and observed, there are no medical conditions that could be mistaken for predatory aggression.
- Cats whose hearing, sight, or mobility is failing or cats who are hyperthyroid *may* be more reactive in any situation that they would view as provocative, but the initial sequences of observing and stalking are missing from their behavioral suites.
- It is important to distinguish *predatory aggression*—a diagnosis and abnormal manifestation of behavior—from *predatory behavior*—usually normal feline behavior and contextually appropriate, if undesirable.
  - There is a lot of variability in feline temperament regarding predatory inclinations. Some cats have no interest in hunting, whereas other cats make *inappropriate context distinctions about prey items*.
  - *Cats learn to hunt and how to kill prey from their mother. Clients who do not wish for their cats to hunt should not allow the mothers to hunt.*
- Contextual distinctions matter if the prey item is the owner's foot or hand or a young infant. *Any cat who exhibits the above-described pre-pounce behaviors in these contexts may be at risk for inappropriate predatory aggression.*

Etiology, Epidemiology, and Risk Groups

- Cats who have dispatched neighborhood pets and wildlife may or may not exhibit such behaviors in other contexts. Good data are lacking.
- The condition of some humans and pets makes them look like "good victims." Sudden start and stop sleep cycles such as those exhibited by infants, coordination, and inconsistent movement all may play roles in triggering true predatory aggression.
- Young infants and older, debilitated individuals of any species may be most at risk. Individuals who are dressing, which involves start and stop movements, may also be good victims for cats with predatory aggression.
- Predatory attacks involve grabbing the neck and holding onto and crushing the larynx, slashing at the neck and throat, and shaking the victim by the throat, if the victim is small. Limbs often are treated like throats, and cats who attack people while dressing often treat moving clothing as they would prey.

Common Myths That Can Get in the Way of Treatment or Diagnosis

- Clients often think that because the cat has always been sweet for them that his or her behaviors do not pose a risk for their new baby or debilitated relative.
  - If there is any concern about any interaction, the cat should always be supervised (the cost of error is huge) and an informed third party (e.g., veterinary behavior specialist) should observe the cat's behaviors in the contexts in question.
- Clients often think they must euthanize or relinquish their cat if the cat shows any signs of predatory aggression.
  - This is not true if the cat reacts this way only to babies. Babies grow out of the phase where they are viewed as prey. These children can go on to have a perfectly normal and happy relationship with the cat. The pathology has nothing to do with the child and everything to do with how the cat views certain movements and attendant behaviors.
  - The baby must be protected from the cat for the first few months of life, which can easily be done with leads and locked doors.
  - The risk is greater with cats who direct their behaviors toward elderly individuals or individuals who are ill or incapacitated.

Commonly Asked Client Questions

- Must I get rid of my cat?
  - No, see the preceding discussion. A very detailed specific plan of protection needs to be agreed on and implemented by all involved, including the

veterinary staff. Components of this plan should include:

- A plan for ensuring that the potential victim is never, ever left alone with the cat until it is clear that the cat is reliable and not a concern.
- A way to lock the cat away from the child safely and humanely when the cat cannot be directly supervised. Crates, kennels (with roofs), enclosed sun porches, and doors that lock are optimal.
- An early warning system that tells people when the cat is present. This could be as simple as a bell on a collar around the cat's neck or a security monitor worn on a collar that beeps when the cat is within some predetermined distance of the potential victim (www.brickhousesecurity.com). These auditory cues are part of a failsafe system and should not be relied on alone to keep anyone safe.

- Can/do affected cats kill/maul people?
  - Yes. Fortunately this is very, very rare.
- Can this cat go to another home?
  - Yes, if the other home does not have infants or incapacitated older humans or animals, the cat can do wonderfully and be happy and safe. The people taking the cat must understand the diagnosis.
- Will the cat grow out of this?
  - No, but babies will.
- My cat stalks neighborhood wildlife and kills bunnies. Will he stalk and kill human babies?
  - First, predatory aggression is rare.
  - Second, more often than not the answer is no, but we have no data. Clients can collect their own data by watching the cat with guidance from their veterinarian.
  - Predatory aggression does not increase the risk or precede the development of other problem aggressions.

Treatment

- Management:
  - This is a diagnosis for which all treatment is management. See the aforementioned discussions.
- Behavior modification:
  - If the cat is anxious because of the presence of the baby or debilitated human or pet, that anxiety should be treated, but pure predatory aggression is not going to respond to behavior modification. And, it is safer not to even attempt it.
- Medication/dietary intervention:
  - If the cat is otherwise anxious, hypervigilant, and focused, TCAs or SSRIs may help, *but clients should be disabused of the idea that these or any other medication or diet will treat true predatory aggression.* Medication may be part of a QoL decision for the cat but should not be expected to "fix" this problem.

- Miscellaneous interventions:
  - Because these cats will be spending considerable periods of time away from the objects of their focus it is very, very important to ensure that they get the physical and mental exercise needed to ensure a good QoL. Food toys, other pets, fenced-in porches, kitty runs, clicker training sessions, play sessions, et cetera, that allow them to be rewarded for being a well-behaved focus of attention are all beneficial for them, although these interventions will not fix the *problem.*
  - Belling cats (Bear Bells) can give some advance warning to small prey but is not usually sufficient to avoid predation because of the element of stealth.
  - Scat mats and indoor invisible fences are usually insufficient to deter a focused cat. No one should rely on such devices for protection. *Aversive "treatments" such as electronic mats can often make a reactive or aggressive cat more reactive or aggressive. There are welfare and humane care issues involved in using these treatments, and they are not recommended.*
  - Finally, if the client is concerned only about *predatory behavior* directed toward outside wildlife, the best insurance for outdoor wildlife is to deny the cat access to them. In many parts of the world, this is becoming law as part of a strategy to protect endangered wildlife. Cat fences can fence either the cats in or the wildlife out, giving both some ability to coexist safely (www.purrfectfence.com, www.catfencein.com, www.catterydesign.com).
  - Cats kept indoors live longer than outdoor cats and are healthier than are outdoor cats. However, intellectual stimulation is often missing in the life of an indoor cat. This does not have to be the case; there are many clever ways to avoid having an under-stimulated, overweight, unengaged cat.

Helpful Handouts
- "Protocol for Introducing a New Baby and a Pet"
- "Protocol for Teaching Cats and Dogs to 'Sit,' 'Stay,' and 'Come'"
- "Protocol for Understanding and Managing Odd, Curious, and Annoying Feline Behaviors"

Last Words
- These cats are not engaging in predatory behavior because they are hungry.
  - This is not usually *true predatory behavior.*
  - These cats are not usually hungry.
- If the clients are unwilling to adhere to the standards set forth in the "Protocol for Introducing a New Baby and a Pet," everyone would be better off with the cat placed in an infant-free home.
- Cats have recurved teeth and claws, so bites or scratches should always be taken seriously. If the injured human is very old, very young, ill, or

immunocompromised, scratches and bites from cats must be viewed as serious risks for infection and be medically attended.

Impulse-Control Aggression
Diagnostic Criteria and Description

- Impulse-control aggression is best defined as an abnormal, inappropriate, out-of-context aggression (threat, challenge, or attack) consistently exhibited by cats toward people under any circumstance *involving passive or active control of the cat's behavior or the cat's access to the behavior.*
- Any intensification of any aggressive response from the cat on any passive or active correction or interruption of the cat's behavior or the cat's access to the behavior confirms the diagnosis.
- *This diagnosis has also been labeled as assertion or status-related aggression and has been described as the "leave me alone bite,"* identifying the circumstance in which people most often recognize it: petting the cat.
- This is a *diagnosis that is about using control and controlling behaviors in response to arousal that the cat experiences endogenously. In this aroused state, the cat is apparently unable to gain information from the social environment and becomes more globally anxious and reactive within a very short time.*
  - Because feline arousal stimulates brain regions associated with different types of biting, the cat's response to such stimulation is to bite fiercely and often repeatedly as the arousal peaks. This all can happen quickly, so it is critical that clients learn to watch for the earliest signs of agitation.
  - Impulse-control aggression is manifested differently for cats and dogs. For dogs, the anxiety comes first, and the reactivity represents one way of managing it by getting information that may help the dog to assign risk. To gain information, these dogs may solicit and provoke people, but they vary in their response across individual humans, depending on the response received. Some dogs are so anxious that they unable to engage even in this provocative manner and instead attempt to control their anxiety in a failed way that raises their arousal levels until they react explosively by grabbing someone. Although this latter mode more closely resembles the feline version, the mechanisms are likely very different, and dogs do not appear to go through this very forceful arousal phase. People report that they are surprised when it becomes clear that the dog is going to react quite suddenly. Once clients learn to watch these cats, they are able to recognize the entire arousal and solicitation sequence.
- The divergent evolutionary history of canine and feline social systems argues that this condition may not be homologous at all mechanistic levels, but

investigation into differences should shed light on a shared mechanism.
- These cats share with dogs a similar problem—the need for control of the situation during a time of heightened reactivity. However, given their different evolutionary histories, the mechanisms underlying the heightened reactivity likely differ.
  - *Dogs become more aroused the more uncertain they become.* The *anxiety is primary for dogs.* Normal behaviors may provoke the anxiety, but the pattern of the behaviors differs considerably between dogs and cats.
    - As noted, one subclass of affected dogs uses challenges to gain information about potential threats and social rules and reacts according to human response received.
    - A second class of dogs is sufficiently anxious that they cannot even solicit and use information and instead are constrained simply to attempt to control the reactivity that develops associated with increasing anxiety in situations over which they have no control. These dogs finally erupt aggressively in a manner that controls and stops all interactions, addressing—albeit completely pathologically—the anxiety → reactivity → heightened anxiety and subsequent reactivity cycle.
  - Affected cats may be provoked by *normal human behaviors that they solicit* simply because they are aroused. That arousal causes them to pursue the human interaction, whether or not it makes contextual sense. These cats can appear uncertain about why they want the attention, and the signs of arousal that they display conflict with the type of attention they appear to be seeking. Any attention given to them causes an increase in arousal and reactivity and may result in profound, impulsive aggression and damage.
    - These cats appear to need to control when the attention starts and when it ceases.
    - Some cats bite quickly and leave, some cats take the human into their mouth but do not bite, and some cats bite fiercely and repeatedly causing severe injury.
    - If clients can watch for and note the early signs of the arousal, they can avoid or re-direct the cat. If these cats have not reached their threshold for reactivity, they can calm over a considerable period, but clients should know that it then takes very little for them to become aroused again.
  - Given the reactivity shifts required by the cat's "sit-and-wait" foraging mode and their unique patterns of neuronal recruitment and brain reactivity, impulse-control aggression may be the pathological outgrowth of the ancestral reactivity condition in cats. We have no way of knowing whether this is true, but it suggests a

hypothesis that could be tested across populations of cats.

- If the diagnostic criteria are adhered to and the descriptors understood, this terminology will uniquely identify a diagnosis of a class of aggression that differs from others usually enumerated.
- Cats with impulse-control aggression have a focus on control that is *abnormal* and *out of context*. A normal and confident cat might stand in your way by the door because he wants attention or because he wants to go with you. If you do not give him attention or take him with you, he is disappointed but accepting. A cat with impulse-control aggression stands in your way at the door because *he is aroused and any changes in social contexts or interactions can cause him to become more reactive.* Part of the pathology involves a further misunderstanding of the response received, likely because arousal renders the cats too anxious to read accurately and respond to signaling behavior.
- The keys are control and access and response of any kind, suggesting that *movement matters in this condition for cats.*
- This diagnosis cannot be made on the basis of a one-time event. The behavior, once it begins, will become more visible and consistent, but data on early signs, patterns of change with experience, and changes in intensity are lacking.
- *The number of situations in which the cat reacts inappropriately and the intensity with which he or she reacts do not affect the diagnostic criteria,* although these factors may affect ability to treat the condition, prognosis, and risk to people.
- These cats are very different from cats who are pushy or assertive.
  - Pushy and assertive cats are usually confident and do a good job of reading contextual cues.
  - Many people like pushy, assertive cats because they have a lot of "personality."
  - Being pushy or assertive does not mean that the cat has impulse-control aggression.

Common Non-Specific Signs

- Clients who learn to watch for the behaviors that precede the attack become good at avoiding injury and calming the cat. The signs of impending aggression include:
  - staring,
  - tail flicking,
  - ears flat,
  - papillary dilation,
  - stiffening of body, but especially the head and neck,
  - unsheathed claws,
  - stillness or tenseness, and
  - low growls.
- Any movement, reaction, or interaction can cause what may be the clinical equivalent of the "active biting attack."

Rule Outs

- Some of the non-specific behaviors listed can be due to pain or general illness.
- Because of their effects on "mood," endocrine conditions (primarily hyperthyroidism) should be ruled out.
- Heavy metal toxicosis can be associated with atypical aggressions.

Etiology, Epidemiology, and Risk Groups

- There is almost no epidemiological information about this condition in cats.
- Most of the cats reported to be affected are in the midst of social maturity (2 to 4 years of age), which may suggest that some alterations in neurochemistry contribute to the development of the condition, but good data do not exist.
- Impulse-control aggression may be rooted in some aspect of impaired glutamate and/or serotonin (5-hydroxytryptamine [5-HT]) activity or metabolism.
  - Glutamate is an excitatory amino acid that contributes to arousal and neurocytotoxic states and that has receptor cross-reactivity for a number of neurotransmitters. Glutamate is metabolized into glutamine, which can be an excitatory neurotransmitter itself (Fonnum, 1984) and excreted in the urine.
  - Mutations in monoamine genes and aberrancies in monoamine function have been demonstrated in humans and rodents.
  - Numerous studies have found variation in factors affecting glutamate in dogs who have this condition (Ogata et al., 2006) or low levels of circulating 5-HT or its metabolite, 5-hydroxyindoleacetic acid, in the plasma and/or cerebrospinal fluid (Çakiroglu et al., 2007; Peremans et al., 2003; Reisner et al., 1996; Rosado et al., 2010). Similar data are lacking in cats.
  - If this condition is rooted in neurochemical response patterns of active biting attack, the amygdala, hypothalamus, hippocampus, and frontal cortex all should be involved. These regions are rich in 5-HT and glutamate receptors.
- Based on client and breeder reports, this condition may have heritable and episodic versions, but the data are poor.
- If clients are taught to watch for cats who stare (Kendall and Ley, 2006), dilate their pupils, and stiffen while the clients are approaching, they may be able to avoid being bitten, while re-directing the cat.

Common Myths That Can Get in the Way of Treatment or Diagnosis

- Some cats just don't like to be touched.
  - Although this is a true statement, it has nothing to do with what is going on here. The clients are confused because the cat appears to be seeking

attention and then violently responding to it. This diagnosis has nothing to do with "like" or "dislike."

Commonly Asked Client Questions

- Can we "cure" this condition?
  - No. We likely "cure" no behavioral conditions because of complex brain chemical interactions and molecular learning. However, these cats can improve to the point that no one would know that they had ever been affected.
- Is this condition environmental or genetic?
  - All conditions have environmental and genetic components, even if the genetic component affects only how you recover from an assault.
- If my cat is affected, can I breed him?
  - No cat with this condition should be bred just in case it is heritable. This is a potentially extremely dangerous condition.
- Will or does neutering help?
  - Almost all of the cats with this diagnosis have been neutered, but we know nothing about the inter-play of sex hormones and brain chemistry that occurs in this condition.
- Can cats with this condition have a good QoL?
  - Cats with this condition can have an excellent QoL if they are treated in an ongoing, lifelong manner with appropriate environmental, behavioral, and pharmacological interventions. Clients will need to agree to lifelong treatment and management and take precautions to remain safe. This may not be the cat they take to bed with them.
- Can this condition be prevented?
  - We don't know.
- Is this cat dangerous?
  - Yes, these cats are potentially very dangerous because of the arousal levels and willingness to bite. Cats have recurved teeth and may become hung on the skin or clothing of humans and become even more aroused. Any treatment must have a zero tolerance policy about circumstances associated with bites. If the circumstances cannot be avoided, the danger level may be considerable. Clients should remember that any danger assessment is a function of both human and cat behavior.
    - If the clients do not manage these cats well by avoiding situations that trigger the cat, the risk increases as a function of the clients' behaviors.
    - If the clients ensure that the cat is not put in situations in which his or her particular behaviors are triggered, the risk decreases as a function of the clients' behaviors.
  - Predictability of both human and cat behaviors are essential for any assessment of danger.
    - Clients often come to a consultation thinking that the cat is unpredictable, but after completing the history forms and/or the consultation,

the patterns of the cat's behaviors are clear. Clients need to believe that if faced with those patterns the cat will be reactive.
    - Clients need to assess how predictable their household is. Small children and debilitated or incapacitated family members may not be able to comply with management in a way that keeps them safe.

Treatment

- Management:
  - The key to successful treatment of impulse-control aggression lies in avoiding triggering the aggressive response. Clients must avoid and/or interrupt and re-direct these cats as soon as the arousal level begins to increase.
    - The first step in monitoring and modifying arousal levels is to control attention that the cat receives so that it occurs only when everyone is attentive to the potential risks.
    - These cats should not be allowed to sit on people's laps or sleep with them because of the rate at which they can become aroused and the level of human vulnerability such situations engender.
    - If the client chooses to interact physically and lovingly with the cat, the client should always provide the cat with an amount of attention via petting or brushing that has always been below the level at which the cat reacts.
    - The client would be safer giving three 1-minute petting sessions rather than one 3-minute petting session.
    - If the cat solicits attention by jumping onto the client, the client should stand up and gently allow the cat to tumble from his or her lap. The client should then refuse to interact with the cat until she can sit on request (assuming she has been taught to do so) and show all outward signs of being calm. Clients should remember that arousal levels in cats decay slowly, and the cat may react more easily when attempts to interact as noted are closer together.
  - If possible, clients should avoid all situations identified during the consultation that are associated with any degree of agonistic arousal by the cat.
    - This is not the same as not interacting with the cat.
    - Clients should give the cat a set of expectations of appropriate behaviors by telling the cat he or she is good when the cat is not reactive and ignoring/withdrawing from the cat when the cat is reactive.
  - If the clients do not feel that they can monitor and manage the cat's interactions, they should feel comfortable putting the cat elsewhere until

they can focus on the cat (e.g., behind a locked door).

- No one should be allowed to interact with the cat unless the client is sure that all instructions will be followed. It is easy to make these cats worse, even if the intentions were good.
- Behavior modification:
  - The essential behavior program for these cats is the "Protocol for Deference." Clients are unused to thinking of asking cats to sit and wait for attention, but almost all cats can be clicker trained to do this. By asking the cat to sit and be calm, clients are actually decreasing arousal levels.
- Medication/dietary intervention:
  - Both 5-HT and glutamate are hypothesized to be involved in conditions such as this one, and both may affect NMDA receptors. This information, plus the pattern of arousal that involves the amygdala, the hypothalamus, the hippocampus, and the frontal cortex, makes the suggested choices for medication straightforward.
  - SSRIs:
    - Fluoxetine—this is the medication of choice for *impulsive conditions*.
    - Paroxetine—if the cat cannot take fluoxetine for any reason, paroxetine may be another choice.
  - TCAs:
    - Amitriptyline
    - Nortriptyline
  - SARIs:
    - Trazodone
  - BZD or BZD analogues:
    - Gabapentin—because overall arousal and anxiety levels are also important, medications such as gabapentin can be helpful as part of a polypharmacy approach
  - NMDA receptor antagonists:
    - Memantine—the dosage range is not established for cats.
  - Omega-3 fatty acids—excitatory amino acids can be cytotoxic, so supplements (e.g., omega-3 fatty acids) and diets that can limit their damage may also help (www.nordicnaturals.com for cat-sized capsules).
  - Treatment outcomes do not correlate with blood levels of serotoninergic compounds, but side effects do, so combining medications with an understanding of expected effects, side effects, and CYP 450 patterns is recommended.
    - Cats who may have cardiac conduction disturbances should be monitored by a cardiologist if treated with TCAs and SSRIs because in rare cases they have been postulated to cause heart block. Cardiac evaluation may require sedation.
- Miscellaneous interventions:
  - Some clients have success in maintaining controlled access between cats and humans using key coded cat doors both inside and out. This method reminds them to be watchful of the cat's behaviors.
  - Clients need to think of safe areas as places where the cats can be left for at least 24 to 48 hours while they are aroused and make preparations for such stays. It may be easiest to have a room that can be locked that always has water and clean litter. If the clients cannot safely get food into the cat, they should know that most cats can go 1 or 2 days without food.
  - Clients should have blankets, brooms, cardboard boxes, et cetera, available and within easy reach in the areas of the house where the cat is most likely to accost them. These will allow the client to get the cat to the safe room without injury.
  - Clients should watch for re-directed aggression to others in the household, including other cats and dogs.
  - These cats do not belong at dinner parties, and guests do not have to meet them.

Helpful Handouts
- "Protocol for Deference"
- "Protocol for Understanding, Managing, and Treating Impulse-Control/Status-Related Aggression in Cats"
- "Protocol for Using Behavioral Medication Successfully"

Last Words
- These cats worsen quickly and can become extremely dangerous if punished, threatened, shocked, or otherwise roughly treated. There is no role for physical punishment or electrical shock in aborting the cat's behaviors, and such interventions will make the cat worse.
- Clients often ask about removing the cat's teeth and claws. There are ethical and QoL concerns involved in such decisions. Even cats who are declawed and have their canines removed can do clients serious damage. If emphasis is on treating the cats, tremendous shifts in pathological reactivity—which must be awful for the cat—and in keeping everyone safe, these interventions will never be considered.
  - It may be very difficult to trim these cat's claws, so good scratching posts are important.
  - If the cat becomes aroused when scratching and such arousal is due to the feedback received from the act, an exceptional justification for onychectomy *may* be made, but the decision has to be made on the basis of the well-being of the cat.
- Clients often want prognoses assigned to conditions, and this is the condition that demonstrates that prognoses in many behavioral conditions should be assigned to interventions. If the client is willing to meet the humane needs of the cat, follow the treatment recommendations, and minimize humanely the chance that the cat can do harm (these cats can learn to be more aggressive from "practicing" their

aggressions), the cat will generally improve, no matter how profoundly affected he or she is. Medication plays a large role in the cat's improvement in this condition.

- If clients do not understand the above-mentioned considerations and do not feel safe and/or if none of the above-mentioned recommendations improve the QoL for the cat, euthanasia is going to be a consideration because of the potential danger to the humans and the misery of the cat.

Inter-Cat Aggression

Diagnostic Criteria and Description

- "Normal," non-pathological aggression between cats is common only if the cats are toms. In most wild, feline social systems, a few males mate with most of the females. The skewed sex ratio in the breeding population is induced and maintained by vigilance and aggression on the part of the males. *This is not the type of inter-cat aggression discussed here; here we are talking about inter-cat aggression that is most likely pathological and problematic.*
- *Cats who fight with other cats outdoors also are not usually included in this diagnostic category if the cats are not living together or if the outdoor cats are from other households.* This distinction may or may not be correct, but it is assumed that many cats who do not know each other well and/or who do not live as part of the same social grouping may spar as part of "normal" behavior. The type of dogged pursuit that is seen by aggressors in inter-cat aggression between cats within households is not usually reported for non-household cats seen in agonistic encounters out of doors.
  - One pattern that suggests fights with outdoor, non-household cats may differ from fights with household cats is the incidence of abscesses. Abscesses are almost wholly seen in cats who fought with an outdoor cat who is not part of the daily social grouping.
- *True inter-cat aggression*—which is far more common and more likely than territorial aggression—is pathological and is more commonly based on *conflicts within social relationships/hierarchies than it is with sex.*
- Inter-cat aggression involves consistent, volitional, proactive aggression that is not contextual given the social signals, threat circumstances, or response received. If there is no provocative signal or interaction from the animal that is attacked, the attack should not have occurred.
  - *Cats who react as if there is a challenge about social status when there is none are reacting inappropriately and out of context.*
  - If there is a challenge (staring, blocking, hackles up, hissing, swatting, growling, et cetera) of any kind, a reaction might be appropriate, but it is important to remember that, as is true for people, many normal social behaviors in cats have rules.
    - If one cat responds to another cat's stare or approach by leaving, it would be an inappropriate social response for the staring cat to track down the cat who, appropriately, turned and left and subject that cat to more aggression and more overt aggression.
    - When this happens you know you have a problem.
    - Most aggression in cats is far more subtle than it is in dogs and because of this may be more damaging to household situations.
- At some level, the behaviors involved with aggression are normal behaviors. This diagnostic category, although usually associated with changes in social hierarchy that are often related to the development of social maturity in one of the involved parties, *does not depend on either hierarchy or social maturity: it depends on the contextual response.* This is a subtle but important distinction that supports the contention that social shifts and occasional threats can be normal.
- Problems arise when one cat will not accept lack of engagement by another cat.
- Inter-cat aggression is extremely complex, often subtle, and under-appreciated.

Common Non-Specific Signs

- Responses include passive aggression (staring and posturing), active aggression (hissing, swatting, pouncing, biting), and marking. Cats who consider themselves as more equal are less likely to participate in overt and active aggression—expect covert and more passive aggression. (See Box 9-2 for a heuristic model to use to understand the variants of this form of aggression.)
- Cats may start by staring at the other cat and then escalate to overt aggression with time.
- The common non-specific signs seen depend on whether the cat being observed is the aggressor or the recipient of the aggression (often called the victim).
- Cats who are aggressors often:
  - stare at the other cat,
  - block access to preferred (a sofa) or needed (a litterbox) locations by the recipient/victim of the aggression,
  - may raise their hackles, hiss or growl, and swat at the victim,
  - pursue the victim whenever he withdraws, and
  - almost continuously monitor the location and movement of the victim, while repeatedly blocking the target cat from engaging in many activities. Once alerted to it, the clients are able to recognize easily the dogged pursuit of one cat by another.
- When clients are uncertain whether any true aggression is occurring, they need only watch: if one cat entered a room and looked at or toward a second cat,

and the second cat left the room, that was an aggressive event.

- The response of the recipient of the aggression/victim depends on the relationship that the cats have had before the aggression started and on the basic temperament of the cat to whom the aggression is directed.
  - Shy cats make good victims and will avoid and/or hide from bullies at all costs even if this means having restricted access to food, water, litterboxes, and/or human attention.
  - Cats who had a fairly equitable relationship with the aggressor may hiss or growl back and posture extensively while holding their ground. Although these cats seldom start any of the aggressive events with the other cat, they do not back down from them. Clients may see paired threats when evenly matched and known cats are engaged in fighting.
    - In such situations cats can experience a prolonged period of near-constant fighting, possibly accompanied by any form of marking behavior.
- In multi-cat households, aggression on the part of one cat can change the relationships between the other cats. Shifting coalitions can form that depend on outcomes of daily interactions.
- Inter-cat aggression can be variable in its effect on eating and sleeping orders or arrangements and relationships with humans.

Rule Outs
- This condition may first become apparent to the client because one cat begins to mark or one cat ceases to use the litterbox.

BOX 9-2

Heuristic Model for Thinking about Phenotypic Patterns of Feline Aggression

Potential Axes
- Overt versus covert aggression
- Active versus passive aggression
- Offensive versus defensive aggression

Sample Scenarios
- Overt, passive, offensive aggression: confident cat stares when another enters the room (Fig. 9-18, A)
- Overt, passive, defensive aggression: less confident cat leaves the room or backs up and withdraws into smaller space, tail tucked, possibly while vocalizing (Fig. 9-18, B)
- Covert, passive, defensive aggression: vanquished or less confident cat marks with mystacial glands in boundary areas or areas from which the cat had been displaced
- Covert, active, offensive aggression: vanquished or less confident cat marks with urine or feces in boundary areas or with other glandular secretions in areas from which the cat had been displaced
- Overt, active, offensive aggression: chase and attack using claws and/or teeth and accompanied by vocalization by resident cat toward a new cat in the environment or toward a fairly evenly matched known cat (Fig. 9-19, A-C, and 9-20, A-C)
- Overt, active, defensive aggression: attack or response using hitting and/or swatting while leaning back or avoiding further pursuit (Fig. 9-19, D-F).
- Covert, active, defensive aggression: withdrawal and marking (urine, feces, glandular secretions) of restricted area by the victim cat (Fig. 9-20, D)
- Covert, passive, offensive aggression: displacement or theft of objects or situations associated with the "bully" or aggressor's ranking—toys, bed, food, or hidden copulations—accompanied by non-elimination marking

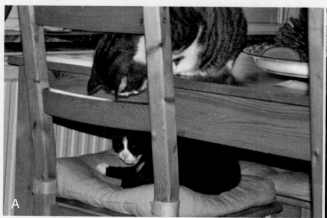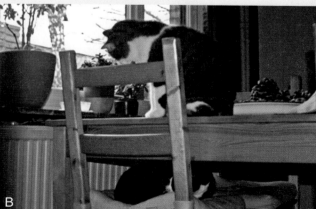

Fig. 9-18 **A** and **B**, The tabby cat is the aggressor. (See text for interpretation.) (Photos courtesy of Anne Marie Dossche.)

Continued

BOX 9-2

Heuristic Model for Thinking about Phenotypic Patterns of Feline Aggression—cont'd

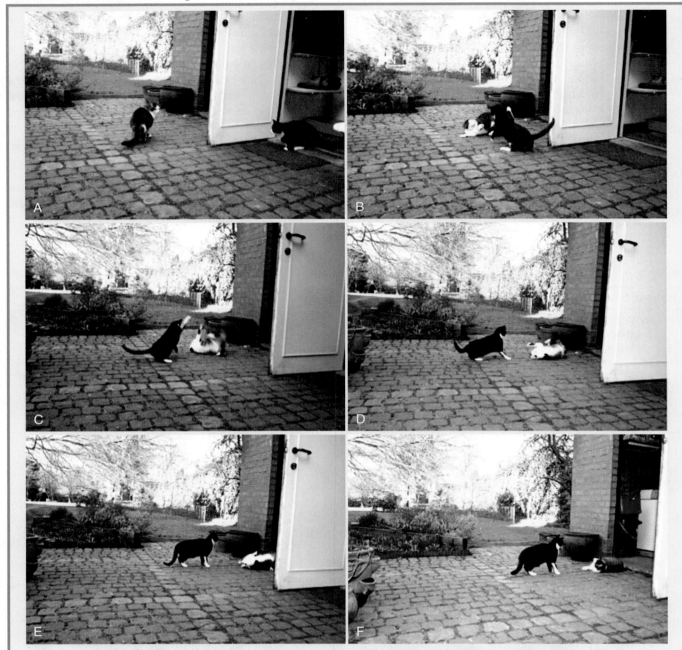

Fig. 9-19 **A-F,** The black cat is the aggressor. (See text for interpretation.) (Photos courtesy of Anne Marie Dossche.)

- Clients often think that one of their cats is physically ill because the cat is so withdrawn. Fear can mimic illness.

Etiology, Epidemiology, and Risk Groups

- Most inter-cat aggression occurs between housemates, and it may occur more commonly between different-sex housemates, in contrast to dogs.

- Because feline systems are matrilineal, aggression may become apparent only after the loss of a "matriarch" or cat fulfilling this role. It is not unusual for cats to have lived in relative harmony together for 2 years before there are problems because the development of these problems reflects the intrinsic change that all social animals experience when they become socially mature.

BOX 9-2

Heuristic Model for Thinking about Phenotypic Patterns of Feline Aggression—cont'd

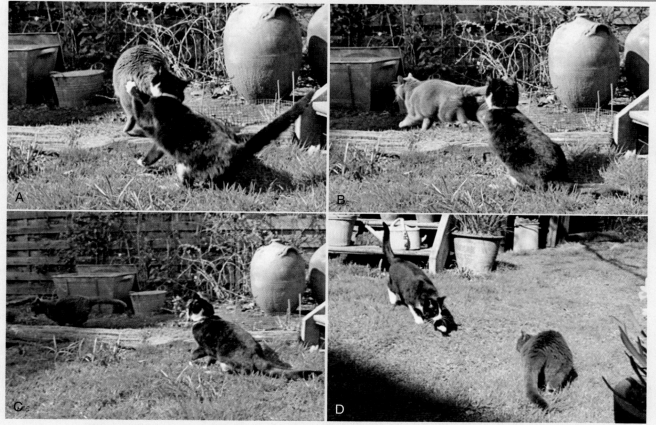

Fig. 9-20 **A-D,** The aggressor is the black and white cat. (See text for interpretation.) (Photos courtesy of Anne Marie Dossche.)

- Cats begin to become socially mature between 2 and 4 years of age. At this time, some cats may begin to challenge others and will not accept lack of engagement from the other cat and instead may repeatedly attack the other cat.
- Coalitions of cats are unstable, and clients may first report a problem with cats after introducing a new cat to the household. The new cat can be the trigger where cats may align by personality style, with some cats bullying others.
- Cats who are afraid of other cats can be afraid because they have been attacked and may develop fearful behavior or fear aggression as sequela. Fear can also develop without attack. Co-occurrence of diagnoses should alert clients and veterinarians to ask which came first.
  - Clients should be encouraged to apply the stress ratings in Table 9-4 to these cats. Such a comparison will allow them to recognize the extent of the fear experienced by the cat receiving the

aggression and to understand how behaviorally different the cats are.

Common Myths That Can Get in the Way of Treatment or Diagnosis
- The cats will work this out.
  - If this concern were simply a disagreement between two cats who were behaving normally, they would work it out, but invariably one cat is molesting another and affecting her ability to move and interact as she would otherwise choose to do.
- Cats are supposed to fight because they are not social.
  - Both parts of this supposition are wrong.

Commonly Asked Client Questions
- Will I have to get rid of one of the cats?
  - Re-homing cats is not the easiest plan, but with this condition, depending on the response of the victim and/or the fierceness of the aggressor, re-homing may be an option. The usual

preference is to re-home the victim because no one wants the aggressor. If the aggressor is re-homed, he should go to a single-cat home.

- Would making these cats into indoor/outdoor cats help?
  - Orchestrating safe ways for one of the cats to be able to spend much of his or her time outside may be part of a treatment plan because it may allow the cats to divide the area they have by temperament and interest. Allowing an aggressor outside, without a full treatment plan in effect, is not likely to alter any of his behaviors of concern.

Treatment

- Management:
  - Management is key in this situation. Cats can and will time and space share, but bullies think that they should determine to what extent such "sharing" occurs. The victims will comply with most strategies that keep them safe and remove the constant fear of attack.
  - If the clients realize that the cats are engaging in over-aggression and fighting, they should be cautioned never to reach between two fighting animals. Most people have good intentions and want to separate fighting animals to prevent injury to them, but this is the situation in which humans are most often injured.
  - Clients may wish to consider totally separating the cats for a few weeks to see what the response is and to see if they wish to try to have them together while closely monitored. If clients decide to separate the cats, they will need separate rooms, litterboxes, and water dishes as well as separate attention from humans. This separation is most easily accomplished by having one area of the house or apartment for one cat and one area for another. Clients with small living spaces may wish to rotate the cats.
  - If the situation has reached the stage where behavioral or physical injury is an outcome, the cats should never be left alone together unsupervised. Instead, they must be separated by physical barriers, and the cat left with free reign or in the most desirable area (e.g., the room with the window rather than the bathroom) should be the cat who is being victimized.
  - When/if the cats are together, the clients should watch them closely. Clients should be prepared to intervene in any threats by moving the aggressor into another room. To do this safely may require the use of cardboard, a broom, blanket, et cetera, to help in safely moving the aggressor. These are all "remote control" items that can help separate the cats safely.
  - If the cats are actively engaged in fighting, it may be difficult to get them apart.
    - Sometimes a bucket of water or a shaken bottle of seltzer aimed directly at them will be sufficient to get them apart, after which the aggressor can be covered by a blanket and moved to a safe area. The clients should not pick up either cat and should control the aggressor first. If the clients move to pick up the victim, they may experience re-directed aggression by the aggressor.
    - If no small children, high-strung humans, or nervous animals are in the house, a loud noise, such as that generated by a foghorn, can also help to separate the animals for whom nothing else works, but this should be a last resort. If clients must engage in such extreme behaviors, the cats' aggression is seriously out of control. *Screaming by humans, particularly young children, will worsen the situation.*
  - Clients should remember that cats can remain aroused for 24 to 48 hours and so should be kept separated and calm.
  - If the clients do not think the cats are to the point where total separation is needed, they should bell the cats with different-sounding bells (Bear Bells), or bell at least the aggressor.
    - Breakaway collars that will come apart if they snag on furniture or other objects are now widely available and are a safe option for attachment of bells in all environments.
  - The bell tells both the client and the victim when the aggressor is approaching. If the cats remain in the same room (the victim may choose to leave), the cats can have a chance to approach each other *if and only if* the client is certain that he or she can control the cats from a distance and prevent any injury. *Injury can be physical or behavioral.* Of these, *the behavioral injury may be worse for many cats who learn to live in constant terror.*
- Behavior modification:
  - Behavior modification is possible and will work best as part of an integrated treatment program that manages the cats' access to each other. Whether behavior modification can be attempted without medication depends entirely on the cats' behaviors.
  - There is no role for punishment in any behavior modification program with cats. The risk for re-directed aggression is enormous.
  - Clients will need to work with the cats separately and subsequently together to encourage them to be in each other's presence without reacting.
  - The cat who is victimized may be very fearful. Medication is necessary if this happens, and it will facilitate teaching the cat that he is rewarded with treats, attention, grooming, access to sunny resting spots flecks, et cetera, whenever he is calm.
  - The aggressor can also learn to sit and be calm in response to requests by clients who adequately reward favored outcomes.

- If the clients are going to work with the cats to try to get them back together with each other, some basic guidelines may help.
  - The cat whose right to exist is being reinforced should always get the attention first, in the presence of the other cat if this can be done quietly and without threats or overt aggression.
  - It may be safest to have both cats on harnesses and long leads. Harnesses provide a way to abort an interaction while allowing the cats to be together without a strict set of requests and rewards being given. Clients can sit quietly, with the cats secured at a distance where they can see each other but not lunge and connect.
  - Because staring is a threat in feline aggression, if the clients can reward the aggressor for looking away from the other cat, and he can calmly do so, they may succeed at teaching the cat to be less reactive. However, success is determined by the behavior of the cat who has received the aggression. The cats should remain together only if it is not behaviorally painful for the victim to do so.
  - If the behavior modification is working, both cats should be content to remain in each other's presence without threats and be able to look away from each other on request. This is very hard to accomplish.
- Medication/dietary intervention:
  - Medication is likely essential in most cases of true inter-cat aggression. Clients should be reminded that humane care and QoL concerns are paramount.
  - Choice of medication depends on whether the cat is the aggressor or victim.
  - SSRIs—these are appropriate for the aggressor and the victim, should the victim be withdrawn and/or overtly anxious and concerned.
    - Fluoxetine—especially if the aggressor is explosive in his aggression
    - Paroxetine.
  - TCAs—although seldom used in aggressors, they may be helpful for victims with relatively mild anxiety.
    - Amitriptyline
    - Nortriptyline—useful for cats benefiting from amitriptyline but who are a bit sedated by it; as the intermediate metabolite, this medication is less sedative.
    - Clomipramine—this medication is especially helpful for victims if they are engaged in any pathologically ritualized behaviors in response to the aggression (e.g., self-mutilation, barbering).
  - BZDs and analogues—for the victim *only*; BZDs render cats more outgoing and hungrier and so may facilitate work with food rewards.
    - Alprazolam
    - Oxazepam
    - Diazepam—*caution*—this is highly sedative and is metabolized into two additional active compounds.
    - Lorazepam
    - Triazolam
  - Other:
    - Partial 5-HT$_{1A}$ agonists
      - Buspirone—this is a medication for the victim *only* because—if it works—it will render the victim more outgoing and forceful. Clients should understand that this means that the victim may stand up for herself more and so may engage in active aggression that had not previously been present. This response has been misinterpreted as making an animal "more aggressive." Instead, it allows animals to be more assertive and they then may find themselves in situations where an agonist response makes sense contextually.
- Miscellaneous interventions:
  - Clients are increasingly becoming aware of cat fences and cat enclosures (www.purrfectfence.com, www.catfencein.com, www.catterydesign.com). Smart use of either or both of these where clients have yards can give cats large amounts of space where they cannot injure each other. However, the role of staring as a threat cannot be overlooked. Cats are not truly "separated" if one can stare at another.

Helpful Handouts
- "Protocol for Understanding and Treating Cats with Elimination Disorders and Elimination Behaviors That Concern Clients"
- "Protocol for Understanding and Treating Feline Aggressions with an Emphasis on Inter-Cat Aggression"
- "Protocol for Teaching Cats and Dogs to 'Sit,' 'Stay,' and 'Come'"
- "Tier 2: Protocol for Desensitizing and Counter-Conditioning a Dog or Cat from Approaches from Unfamiliar Animals, Including Humans"
- "Protocol for Using Behavioral Medication Successfully"

Last Words
- Clients do not watch cats the way they watch dogs and so usually think that the same type of loud, physical, and bloody display that dogs engage in is needed for cats to be termed "aggressive." Cats are different, and the fights are more subtle. Clients must be taught to understand this.
- To help clients understand changing relationships in cats, ask to see their photo albums before and after the addition of a new cat. Social rearrangements will make any conflict clear.
- If clients are encouraged to videotape their cats' favorite resting and sleeping places, litterboxes, food

dishes, and places they spend their time, they will video the important differences in interaction between the cats that will help guide vets to help them. Have everyone make a video.

- At every visit, let people know that new cats should be introduced in a way to mitigate any conflict. This gives you a chance to encourage people to ask about adding new animals and to pick ones that may fit seamlessly into the household.
- Venn diagrams are not something that veterinarians use every day, but there is no better way to diagram the social relationships in feline households. If clients can diagram who can spend time with whom in mutual grooming and who can sleep in whose presence, they will have effectively provided a key for how to divide living space should aggression occur. Clients have to be taught how to use these diagrams of overlapping circles, but diagramming multi-cat households yearly may focus clients on their cats' behavioral health like nothing else does. Remind them to include litterboxes, food and water dishes, beds, perches, and spots where humans spend a lot of time.

PATHOLOGIES NOT RELATED TO AGGRESSION

Fear/Fearful Behavior
Diagnostic Criteria and Description
- True fear involves responses to stimuli (social or physical) that are characterized by withdrawal and passive and active *avoidance behaviors* associated with the sympathetic branch of the autonomic nervous system and in the absence of any aggressive behavior.
- Fear and anxiety have signs that overlap. Some non-specific signs, such as lowering of the back, shaking, and trembling, can be characteristic of both fear and anxiety.
- Truly fearful cats disappear. Those who can be seen withdraw and fold their limbs into themselves to the extent possible. The normal feline behavioral response to fearful stimuli is hiding.
  - Cats who are allowed to hide as a choice when faced with a scary situation and/or have more complex environments have decreased serum and urinary cortisol levels (Carlstead et al., 1992, 1993; McCobb et al., 2005).
  - Table 9-4 contains a scale by which cats' withdrawal responses can be measured.
- The physiological signs of fear and anxiety probably differ at some very refined level, and the neurochemistries of each are probably very different in a way that is not addressed by the *relatively* non-specific medications we commonly use (see Table 10-4 for a discussion of the complexity of the distribution of subtypes of serotonin receptors).

- Refinements in qualification and quantification of the observable behaviors will hopefully parallel these differences.
- True fear always involves avoidance, with an apparent intent to decrease the probability of social interaction. This is in contrast to anxiety, where avoidance is not the first choice.

Common Non-Specific Signs
- Specific behavioral responses may include:
  - tucking of neck, head, tail, and all limbs,
  - hunched backs,
  - ears down and folded over the side of the head,
  - becoming as small as possible,
  - pupils dilated and round,
  - hiding (even if the only hiding possible is by curling into oneself), and
  - increased respiratory rates may be possible to observe by watching the cat's chest.
- Very distressed cats may pant and/or open mouth breathe with their tongue rolled.

Rule Outs
- Endocrinopathies, including hyperthyroidism, can result in many of the same signs, but the pattern is usually different.
- Cardiomyopathy and other serious cardiac illness can cause cats to exhibit many of the same signs, and they may, in fact, be fearful about how they feel.
- Because of their propensity to withdraw, very ill cats can look like very fearful cats. Fearful cats are watchful and can react, whereas many very ill cats are not watchful and may be less reactive.

Etiology, Epidemiology, and Risk Groups
- We know that there are "genetically" fearful/shy/timid cats and that there are cats who would have been more outgoing had they been handled between 2 and 9 weeks of age.
  - Early handling may have a limited to no effect if the cat has a heritable propensity for fear.
  - During any part of the sensitive period, if cats lack exposure to humans, other animals, or novel stimuli (e.g., car travel) and environments (e.g., the vet's office), the risk that the cat will experience pathological fear of these stimuli is great.
- Cats can also develop profound fear if exposed to a truly horrific circumstance. How often this happens is unknown, and it is seldom reported, but it likely occurs. The extent to which cats mitigate their own neurochemical response by hiding and shutting down neurochemical reactions may protect them from the types of phobias and post-traumatic stress disorder events to which dogs may be more prone.
- If the cat does not have a genetic predisposition to be behaviorally inflexible, exposure to cats, bicycles, dogs, kids, animal hospitals, physical exam needs, claw trimming, teeth brushing, venipuncture, vacuums, et cetera, within the first 12 weeks of life

(and the earlier the better) through 6 months of age can help the cat to accept these stimuli as part of the "normal" world.

- Cats do not have the expanded sensitive periods that dogs do, likely because they did not undergo the same domestication or evolutionary history.
  - Left to themselves, cats would explore many environments on their own but would not put themselves in the situations with humans and most other animals to which "pet ownership" constrains them.

Common Myths That Can Get in the Way of Treatment or Diagnosis
- He's just "shy."
  - Being "shy" is fine if the cat is also not actively unhappy or suffering a decrement in his QoL, but these concerns need to be assessed. However, being "shy" could be a major impediment to getting needed and excellent veterinary care, so clients should discuss medication and other interventions that may make trips to the vet less distressing (Rodan et al., 2011).
- Cats are not supposed to be outgoing—fear is normal for them.
  - This is not true at all. Although there are a range of behaviors from less outgoing to being effusively social that characterize cats, no pathology, including pathological fear, should ever be considered "normal."
- Don't worry—she will "grow out of it."
  - These fearful cats do not "grow out of it." Instead they learn that everything is a threat, and they hone their avoidance and withdrawal skills in the absence of medication and behavior modification specifically designed to address the concern.

Commonly Asked Client Questions
- Will he/she ever be normal?
  - Not completely, but with some protection and good treatment, these cats can have a good QoL. Some of them may even improve dramatically, but this outcome depends entirely on genetics and early exposure. If the cat is fearful only situationally, such as when going into carriers, into cars, to the vet's, et cetera, medication, behavior modification, clicker training, and other reward-based approaches can help these cats not to be distressed. Veterinarians do not place a high enough emphasis on the importance of avoiding stress and distress in the life of cats, yet they are almost model organisms for the adverse effects of stress on infectious disease.
- Are drugs needed for the rest of his life?
  - If medication is helping, and if the medication is causing no untoward side effects, treatment may be for life because this may be what the cat needs. Emphasis must be on QoL, and if the cat has learned to fear a housemate who is still living in

the house, part of the integrated treatment plan may be lifelong medication for both cats—as long as it is helping.
  - If the cat requires medication for something specific, such as veterinary visits, an interesting pattern emerges. The less distressed the cat is for each visit, the more he learns that they do not have to be painful. If clients make the effort to take the cat to the clinic frequently and reward non-fearful responses (even if they do so with a click for cats who will not or cannot take treats), the cat may not need medication after the fifth or sixth visit. Cats can learn that they do not have to fear something, but they have to have it demonstrated to them that not fearing the circumstance is a sane and safe approach.
- Could we have prevented this fear?
  - We do not know because although we know some forms of fear appear to be heritable, we do not know at what level or mechanism the pathology resides.
  - If the cat lacked early exposure, unless the cat was genetically predisposed to withdraw, such exposure would have helped. Unfortunately, most people do not have the cats at the time when exposure would make the biggest difference (2 to 9 weeks). *Breeders need to work with kittens to accustom them to as many environments, stimuli, and social situations as is humanly possible.*
- The cat was sitting at the back of the cage at the shelter—should we have known this would happen?
  - It's hard to know whether that cat was rationally or irrationally fearful. Most shelters now know that cats who are sitting at the backs of cages are seen as less adoptable, and they are now working to reduce shelter-related fear. Prospective adopters need to see the cat over a period of time, preferably in a few environments. If the cat has a relative who also needs adoption, adopting the core social unit may mitigate some of the cat's withdrawal.

Treatment
- Management:
  - Part of the management of this condition involves screening for it at every single veterinary visit.
    - Veterinarians see cats at a very young age. They should observe cats and ask about interactions with people and other animals at every visit.
    - No cat should ever be dumped or pulled from a cat carrier for examination or to remove them from the carrier once home.
      - The cat should be allowed to emerge on his own at home (and the amount of time this takes may give the clients an idea of how stressful an event it was).
      - If the cat will not emerge from the carrier at the veterinary hospital, the client should

invest in a carrier where the top can be removed, and a blanket or towel should be used to cover all of the cat except the part being examined at that second. Cats may be incredibly amenable to veterinary manipulation if they can be handled while hiding (Anseeuw et al., 2006; Rodan et al., 2011).

- Even the most pathologically fearful cat may adapt to some level of human interaction. Part of treating—or at least managing the fear so as not to trigger a fearful event—involves being predictable by using behaviors with which the cat is maximally comfortable and protecting the cat from circumstances that the cat cannot manage.
- Behavior modification:
  - Behavior modification may help more than people realize. Fearful cats are the ideal subjects for clicker training (www.clickertraining.com/cattraining).
    - Clicker training does not require that anyone approach, handle, or reach for cats. Cats can learn quickly that a favorite treat appears on the floor when they hear a click.
    - Once the cat understands the basic principles, more outgoing behaviors can be shaped, as can behaviors that will make veterinary examination less stressful.
    - Cats can be taught to "go to their mat" just like dogs and can learn that when there they are unmolested by others in the household. Simple skills such as this can prevent swatting and hissing that is common in some milder fears.
  - Clients may need help implementing such programs and could benefit from help from certified pet dog trainers, applied animal behaviorists, or others trained in these techniques. Many dog trainers also work with cats or horses, so clients should check with all individuals in their area.
- Medication/dietary intervention:
  - Supplements containing omega-3 fatty acids and other PUFAs may have a beneficial effect on fearful behaviors by preventing damage to neurons that could inhibit the ability to recover from a fearful event.
  - The available nutriceuticals (Zylkene (Beata et al., 2007b), Anxitane, Calmex and Harmonease) may benefit fearful cats because they all have some effect on GABA and promote calmer behaviors through inhibition. Some of these may also have neuroprotectant effects (see Chapter 10).
  - In all but the mildest circumstances, medication may be warranted because QoL matters. Medication is the recommended course for cats who are fearful because they are the victims of inter-cat aggression.
  - Medications that may help come from the following classes of drugs:

- TCAs (amitriptyline, nortriptyline, clomipramine) may help cats to be less anxious and more outgoing as they modulate neurochemical activity. Broad-spectrum TCAs affect many norepinephrinergic/noradrenalinergic and 5-HT receptors and so may address a variety of neurochemical variants of fear. If the fearful response involves any ritualistic components, clomipramine may be the first drug of choice.
  - SSRIs (fluoxetine, sertraline) have been shown to be helpful in some forms of panic, fear, and profound anxiety. Because they target specific 5-HT_{1A} subtype receptors, they mostly affect regions of the brain involved in learning and so may cause their greatest effect in combination with behavior modification designed to teach patients more successful and less distressing behaviors.
  - BZDs (alprazolam, clonazepam) and related compounds (gabapentin) may be essential for alleviating fear and can be given daily or as needed.
  - SARIs (trazodone) affect 5-HT_{2A} receptors and given the distribution of these may modulate some activity/motion associated with fear. However, in profound, non-situational fear, treatment with trazodone alone is unlikely to be helpful.
- Cats should always have a complete physical exam and cardiac evaluation before treatment with behavioral medications. Cats treated with a BZD can undergo paradoxical excitement or sedation, as can dogs. There have been a series of cases reported during a limited period of time involving hepatotoxicity and BZD treatment. This experience appears to have been exceptional but is discussed in detail in Chapter 10.
- Miscellaneous interventions:
  - Protection is under-valued as a treatment strategy, although people recognize its value as a coping strategy. Risk assessment is essential here. When nothing good is likely to come from the interaction and it's not necessary (e.g., the cat does not have a broken leg) avoiding the fearful situation will protect the cat from making molecular changes that will reinforce the memory of situation-associated fear.

Helpful Handouts

- "Protocol for Deference"
- "Protocol for Teaching Cats and Dogs to 'Sit,' 'Stay,' and 'Come'"
- "Tier 2: Protocol for Desensitizing and Counter-Conditioning a Dog or Cat from Approaches from Unfamiliar Animals, including Humans"
- "Protocol for Understanding and Treating Dogs with Fear/Fearful Aggression"
- "Protocol for Treating Fearful Behavior in Cats and Dogs"
- "Protocol for Using Behavioral Medication Successfully"

Last Words

- None of us are perfect, and no cat needs to be perfect. Clients who can adequately protect cats from the objects of their fear may choose protection as a strategy, but they need to ensure that they can continuously implement the protection over a decade or more. Few clients have stable enough lives to guarantee this approach.
- Cats who are fearful may be difficult to assess medically, especially for pain. The sympathetic response to fear will mask a number of non-specific signs of physical ailments and may ultimately worsen pain (Hellyer et al., 2007). Medication and rehabilitative therapy to alleviate the pain should be considered, especially because nociceptive perception and anxiety become neurochemically associated centrally.

Separation Anxiety

Diagnostic Criteria and Description

- Physical, physiological, and/or behavioral signs of distress exhibited by the animal *only* in the absence of, or lack of access to, the client.
- The diagnosis is confirmed if there is consistent, intensive destruction, elimination, vocalization, or salivation exhibited *only* in the virtual *and/or* actual absence of the client. In virtual absences, the client is present, but the cat does not have access to the client (e.g., a door is closed).
- Signs of distress should be evaluated in currency and terminology that are meaningful to the cat.
  - The most commonly reported behaviors include inappropriate elimination, excessive vocalization, destructiveness, and over-grooming/self-mutilation (Schwartz, 2002). These are the signs that the client can recognize.
    - Cats may exhibit other signs of distress (e.g., withdrawal, vigilance and scanning, remaining awake and tense, anorexia, et cetera) when left that clients may not appreciate. If clients are unsure whether their cat is distressed when left, a video of the cat will be informative.
      - Streaming video is an increasingly popular option for understanding the lives of cats.

Common Non-Specific Signs

- Specific behavioral signs may include (Beata et al., 2007b; Schwartz, 2002; Seksel and Lindeman, 1998):
  - inappropriate urination,
  - inappropriate defecation,
  - vocalization,
  - destructiveness, and
  - self-mutilation/over-grooming.
- Other non-specific signs may occur in separation anxiety. If the criterion "distress only in the absence of the client(s) or access to the client(s)" is met, it doesn't matter whether the behavior is in the above list. We know very little about these types of anxieties in cats.

- Much of the study of separation anxiety in dogs has focused on "attachment" and "attachment" behaviors. Given the different "domestication" and evolutionary histories of dogs and cats, we might expect some different manifestations of separation anxiety, yet the top complaints are the same as those for dogs.
  - It's possible that cats who experience and show separation anxiety may have different social relationships with humans than those who do not.
  - We cannot rule out that most people would miss signs of separation anxiety in cats because they don't think it can happen to cats or that cats are not sufficiently "social" to allow the development of separation anxiety.

Rule Outs

- The most common medical rule out is thyroidal illness. Hyperthyroid cats can exhibit all of the behaviors exhibited by cats with separation anxiety.

Etiology, Epidemiology, and Risk Groups

- Separation anxiety has been postulated to be an outgrowth of a distress response from separation associated with a highly social state. Physiological signs such as anorexia, depression, diarrhea, vomiting, and excessive licking represent non-specific neuroendocrine correlates of anxiety.
  - The very narrow sensitive periods in cats may provide some understanding about the extent to which social anxieties are associated with degree of exposure. To date, no such studies exist.
  - Numerous studies on "attachment" to humans have shown that dogs demonstrate true attachment (Palestrini et al., 2005), but the extent to which alterations in attachment behaviors affects re-homed or abandoned/relinquished dogs remains unclear. We have even fewer data for cats.

Common Myths That Can Get in the Way of Treatment or Diagnosis

- The cat is urinating, destroying, defecating, et cetera, because he is "angry" or "spiteful."
  - If the behaviors of concern occur in the contexts defined, they have nothing to do with "anger" or "spite." Concerns about anger and spite suggest that the client is seeing the situation only from his or her perspective. Seen from the cat's perspective, these behaviors are about distress. A video will convince even the most narcissistic client.
- The cat is "punishing" the client for his or her behavior/schedule/choice in boyfriends/girlfriends.
  - See the previous comment. The cat may not like the new friend, but self-injury is an extreme way to punish another individual.
- The cat is exhibiting the problem behaviors because he loves me too much not to be with me.
  - The cat may adore the client, but, again, these behaviors are about distress. Love should not be pathological.

- The cat develops separation anxiety because the clients "spoil" the cat by allowing the cat to sleep in their bed, lie on the sofa, et cetera.
  - No study has been able to demonstrate that separation anxiety is more common in dogs who are treated well and deeply loved, and it would be unlikely that any study would demonstrate a causal link for cats treated the same way.

Commonly Asked Client Questions

- Can this condition be cured?
  - No, because treatment does not change the cat's response surface. At the heart of this condition, similar to all other behavioral conditions, is an abnormal perception, abnormal information processing, and/or an abnormal response to information perceived and processed. *The extent to which the cat can learn calm behaviors is key, and this ability is usually aided by medication.*
- If medication is used, is it for life?
  - Maybe. The probability that long-term medication use is needed may be related to the duration of the condition and the severity of the signs. This is why screening for behavioral problems at each visit is so important. Annual laboratory and physical examination can identify risks that may warrant changing medications or dose reduction.
- Is this condition heritable, or are there liability genes?
  - We do not know the answer to this question. Most behavioral conditions are complex. Behavioral studies in cats are distinctly lacking.
- Would this cat do better in another home?
  - *The best outcomes occur in families where the primary interest of the humans is to meet the cat's needs humanely and provide the best QoL.* Unless the clients know that they cannot meet the cat's needs *and* know of a home that can meet these needs that also wants the cat *and* the home is familiar to the cat *and* the cat is happy to go—all of which is exceedingly unlikely—they will do more harm than good in re-homing this cat.

Treatment

- Management:
  - *Questions about the presence and patterns of behaviors associated with separation anxiety should be included in all histories for all visits because the problem is among the most common canine problems and yet is so often missed in its early stages. The diagnosis may be missed even more frequently in cats because people do not expect it. The long and short screening questionnaires in this text have sections that assess these complaints. Early intervention is important.*
  - Clients should be encouraged to keep a log of the cat's behaviors using the non-specific signs exhibited by the cat on the video (Table 9-5; a client version of this log is included with the handout, "Daily/Weekly Schedule/Log for Cats with Separation Anxiety"). Monitoring the non-specific signs allows the client and the veterinarian to recognize patient progress or lack thereof. The pattern of the signs can also be essential in helping the clinician decide if the patient meets the criteria for diagnosis, in cases where multiple behavioral conditions may be ongoing.
    - If the client learns that the cat can be left for 4 hours without elimination, but not 6 hours, the client knows that—for now—he needs to avoid longer absences. Avoidance is key in the treatment of all behavioral problems because every time the behavior—no matter how undesirable or abnormal—is repeated, the cat will be reinforced for the behavior. Practice reinforces learning at the molecular level. Logs are best used in combination with video surveillance because some signs are much easier for clients to note than others.
  - Petsitters are great options for these cats if the cat is social with non-family members.
  - Food toys *may be good indicators of when cats start to improve* enough to eat, but *they are not a treatment* for separation anxiety. Cats who are profoundly distressed cannot eat. If a fresh food toy with something really special is left for the cat daily, the day he starts to use it flags the first time his distress lessened enough to take food. The food also acts as a reward for the calmer behavior.
- Behavior modification:
  - Clients inadvertently reward anxious behaviors for two common reasons:
    - They think the cat is just seeking their attention and they don't distinguish between *cats who want attention* and *cats who need it,* so the latter group of cats is inadvertently rewarded for anxious, pesky behaviors.
    - They recognize that the cat is distressed, and they are seeking to reassure the cat. Unless the cat is rewarded only when calm, anxious behaviors are also being reinforced, resulting in a miscommunication.
  - If clients use the "Protocol for Deference" for all interactions with their cats—no matter how brief or benign—the cat will learn that he is rewarded for sitting calmly and looking at the client, and the client will be able to reinforce calm behaviors.
    - Clicker training will really help here because it helps the cat to focus on the client and take all cues from them while being calm (www.clickertraining.com/cattraining).
- Medication/dietary intervention:
  - Diets such as the CALM Diet formulated by Royal Canin, which contains alpha-casozepine and an anti-oxidant complex of vitamin E, vitamin C, taurine, and lutein, is intended to be fed before

TABLE 9-5

Daily/Weekly Schedule for Cats with Separation Anxiety

Day/Date: _____

Absence No./Time Left	Maintenance Style	Amount of Time Left	Signs Noted
Absence 1 Time: ___	Left free Confined in room Left outside—fenced Outside—free/unrestrained Other—please note: ___	<5 minutes 5-10 minutes 10-20 minutes 20-30 minutes 30 minutes to 1 hour 1-2 hours 2-4 hours 4-6 hours 6-8 hours >8 hours	None Urination Defecation Destruction Vocalization Self-mutilation/over-grooming Other—please note: ___
Absence 2 Time: ___	Left free Confined in room Left outside—fenced Outside—free/unrestrained Other—please note: ___	<5 minutes 5-10 minutes 10-20 minutes 20-30 minutes 30 minutes to 1 hour 1-2 hours 2-4 hours 4-6 hours 6-8 hours >8 hours	None Urination Defecation Destruction Vocalization Self-mutilation/over-grooming Other—please note: ___
Absence 3 Time: ___	Left free Confined in room Left outside—fenced Outside—free/unrestrained Other—please note: ___	<5 minutes 5-10 minutes 10-20 minutes 20-30 minutes 30 minutes to 1 hour 1-2 hours 2-4 hours 4-6 hours 6-8 hours >8 hours	None Urination Defecation Destruction Vocalization Self-mutilation/over-grooming Other—please note: ___

and during stressful events. There are no specific, controlled data for the treatment of cats with separation anxiety, and in the published literature the effects are mild.

- Nutraceuticals such as Zylkene, Anxitane, Calmex, and Harmonease have been reported to help distressed and anxious animals, but there are no specific, controlled data for separation anxiety.
- Because the act of being distressed, anxious, and panicky can itself contribute to the production of ROS and other neurochemical stressors, nonspecific treatment with anti-oxidants and omega-3 fatty acids (Nordic Naturals) may provide an ancillary benefit for patients with many behavioral conditions, including separation anxiety.
- Medication is almost always an essential part of treatment of clinical separation anxiety. In the United States, two medications have veterinary labels and are licensed for use in dogs with separation anxiety and can also be helpful for cats (Landsberg and Wilson, 2005; Pryor et al., 2001; Seksel and Lindeman, 1998): fluoxetine (Reconcile) and clomipramine (Clomicalm).

- Medications to which these cats may best respond include/may include:
  - TCAs (clomipramine, amitriptyline if in combination with a SSRI)—*if the separation anxiety is primarily characterized by ritualistic components, clomipramine may be the drug of choice.*
  - SSRIs (fluoxetine, sertraline, luvoxamine)—*if the separation anxiety is primarily characterized by explosive components, fluoxetine may be the drug of choice.*
  - SARIs (trazodone)—*trazodone affects regions of the brain associated with motor activity and so may be a suitable ancillary medication for some affected cats.*
  - Gabapentin, alone or in combination with TCAs and/or SSRIs, may be useful if reactivity is the primary concern. The side-effect profile of this medication is favorable, so clients may feel more

confident when using it in combination with other medications. Because it affects BZD receptors, it may also augment BZDs without some of the more systemic potential side effects of BZDs (e.g., concerns about hepatic metabolic pathways).

- Not all signs are equally controlled by all medications; this concern may be addressed with polypharmacy.
- Miscellaneous interventions:
  - Synthetic analogue products of feline pheromones have been frequently suggested as an aid in the treatment of separation anxiety. There are no sufficiently controlled or reported studies that suggest a helpful effect (Frank et al., 2010). Some BZDs appear to affect both the olfactory epithelia involved in pheromone detection and the limbic regions to which ultimate connections project. By regulating Fos expression in these regions, the BZDs may affect some regions involved in defensive behavior (e.g., the prelimbic cortex and the medial amygdala) but not affect defensive behavior and defensive aggression in the ventromedial hypothalamic nuclei. It's possible that the reported weak and variable pheromonal responses are due to effects on these and related pathways. If true, this could provide a putative mechanism that could be tested.

Helpful Handouts
- "Protocol for Deference"
- "Protocol for Using Behavioral Medication Successfully"

Last Words
- Separation anxiety is a condition that is often *a problem for the client,* so it gets a lot of attention, but most of the attention goes to dogs. Only lucky cats have people who seek help.
- Veterinarians can use the increasing awareness of separation anxiety to educate clients about the extent to which separation anxiety and other behavioral conditions are *problems for the cat and his QoL.* If clients understand that early intervention may prevent co-morbidity of behavioral problems and they understand which behaviors indicate problems, there is an increased chance that they will be better participants in the cat's behavioral and overall veterinary care.
- *All cats should be screened for all behavioral conditions at all appointments.* The short history form in this text can help any veterinarian do this. Cats, similar to dogs with separation anxiety, worsen the longer they are untreated.

Cognitive Dysfunction/Cognitive Dysfunction Syndrome
Diagnostic Criteria and Description
- CD is defined by changes in interactive, elimination, sleep-cycle, navigational behaviors, and/or related cognitive behaviors, attendant with aging, which are explicitly *not* due to primary failure of any organ system.
- The changes must be ongoing (this diagnosis cannot be made on the basis of a one-time event) and progressive.
- CD is a potential animal model for the age-dependent cognitive changes that occur in humans. The affiliated behaviors may be associated with Alzheimer's-like (senile dementia of the Alzheimer type) lesions (Gunn-Moore et al., 2007).
- It is unclear if this condition in dogs or cats is associated with age-dependent changes in dopaminergic (suggested because selegiline, a MAO inhibitor with large effects on dopamine, is used to treat CD) or other neurotransmitter function, micro-embolic events.
- The main methods for evaluating CD in humans are not applicable to cats and dogs because they primarily rely on written and verbal responses for assessment. Refinements in cognitive tests based on learning, memory, problem solving, olfactory function (Overall and Arnold, 2007), and navigational skills (Sherman et al., 2013) should enhance our understanding of this condition, especially when combined with imaging and serum, plasma, urine, and cerebrospinal fluid biomarkers.
- Not all dementias are the same in humans, and this is also likely to be true in animals. *Neither dogs nor cats make neurofibrillary tangles, but they make β-amyloid plaques. Whether the burden of plaque correlates with the burden of the CD is an open question in all species.* Even when we make the relevant and necessary mechanistic refinements (e.g., characterization and tracking of amyloid load correlations with age and performance), we will likely have some populations with relatively large amyloid burdens but little impairment.
- Although we know that some genotypes of humans may render them more susceptible to certain types of or onset times for Alzheimer's disease, these data do not currently exist for cats across or within breeds.
- There are three main contributors to problematic, age-related brain aging changes, all of which interact to compromise brain function:
  - Oxidative changes associated with processes such as free radical formation, formation of lesions including those composed of amyloid, and shifts in oxygen and energy availability.
- Aging is associated with increased expression of *genes associated with stress and inflammation,* especially in the brain region primarily involved in associational learning, the hippocampus.

Common Non-Specific Signs
- In this condition, the signs are extremely variable and non-specific and may include:
  - Nocturnal vocalization—this may be the most frequently noticed sign in cats, but it can also be a common non-specific sign of hyperthyroidism.

- Disorientation, including getting stuck in corners or going to the wrong side of a door
- Alterations in social/interactive behaviors; early in the condition, this may appear as a form of increased "neediness"; late in the condition, this appears as a truly disengaged cat.
- Changes in locomotor behavior
- Changes in sleep cycle—this pattern is tricky in cats because their sleep schedules so depend on stimulation that many clients will have difficulty accurately assessing change, but sleep cycles are profoundly affected by changes in hypocretin neuron density and function.
- "Loss of housetraining"—cats either miss or do not even seem to go to the litterbox.
- Increased anxiety in situations in which the cat was formerly comfortable

Rule Outs

- This is one condition where our ability to assess the cognitive component is confounded by age-associated changes and debility. By monitoring both abilities of cats over time and clients' perceptions of them, we may be able to note problems as they occur. An example of a tick sheet that could be used at each visit to assess age-related physical and behavior change is part of the accompanying questionnaire.
- Cats who are arthritic may appear to interact less but may choose to move less because of pain.
- Cats who are arthritic may have more elimination accidents because they cannot navigate as fluidly as is needed to get outside and, once outside, they may be sufficiently painful that they interrupt urination or defecation.
- With pain, arthritis, and other degenerative physical changes, a cat's ability to digest food may change, necessitating a change in their elimination schedules and/or diet. If clients are unaware of these potential needs, they will not meet them, and it could look like the elimination indoors is associated with cognitive change when it is associated with physical change and unmet needs.
  - Cats with dental disease or dental pain may also chew differently and/or be impeded in their ability to smell food. Both of these factors could mimic behaviors associated with cognitive change.
- Cats who are experiencing decrements in visual and auditory capability may change the manner in which they interact because they are lacking social cues. These cats may startle more frequently, which could appear as a social and interactive change to their people, especially if the cat protects herself from startle by hiding.
- Activity level can be directly affected by whether the cat can see and hear. If cats perceive that they are at risk, they will hide. This outcome can translate to sleep cycle changes.

- Old cats, similar to old people, are often taking a variety of medications. These medications can have adverse interactions including sedation and ataxia, which, especially when combined with arthritides, can *make a cat appear as if she has CD/cognitive dysfunction syndrome (CDS) when she does not.*
- A good *medical* history is required to diagnose this condition because non-specific signs of renal, hepatic, or gastrointestinal illness; endocrinopathies; many infectious diseases; and central nervous system lesions (Gunn-Moore et al., 2007) all could be compatible with the non-specific signs that correlate with CD/CDS.
- Figure 9-21 is a behavior screen for age-associated changes that can be used at each visit to monitor physical and behavioral patterns that could be associated with cognitive dysfunction.

Etiology, Epidemiology, and Risk Groups

- Estimates from numerous studies suggest that at least 25% of cats 11 to 14 years old have at least one geriatric-onset behavior problem, and at least 50% of cats older than 15 years are affected.
  - Caution is urged in uncritical acceptance of these estimates. The data are taken primarily from phone surveys and client questionnaires that focus on presence/absence of certain predetermined categories and not on the reasons for the patterns noted.
  - The best data come from a combined approach using client reporting and direct physical and behavioral examination. This approach is almost never taken.
- One study on research colony cats aged 1 to 3, 5 to 9, and 11 to 16 years assessed locomotor activity, plank walking, reactivity, and spatial reversal learning (Levine et al., 1987). It should be noted that all of the cats tested came from breeding colonies and so may have had *more complex cognitive and experiential lives than most people's pet cats do, if the cats are indoor cats with little social or physical stimulation.*
  - Cats in the oldest group were relatively insensitive to habituation in locomotor sessions, but younger cats habituated quickly.
  - *Older cats made fewer mistakes in walking planks* than the youngest cats and showed no differences in any neurobiological assessment compared with the other two age groups.
  - *Older cats were more reactive to auditory stimuli* than younger cats, and they sustained their reactive responses longer. No data exist on auditory acuity, but heightened auditory reactivity is common as decrements in hearing begin to appear.
  - The *oldest cats (11 to 16 years old) actually performed better on a spatial reversal learning task than the younger cats.* They made fewer errors and learned to reverse faster, although they *did not appear to maintain learning between tasks.*

Behavior screen for age-associated changes that can be used at each visit to monitor physical and behavioral patterns that could be associated with cognitive dysfunction

1. Locomotory/ambulatory assessment (tick **only** 1)
   - ☐ a. No alterations or debilities noted
   - ☐ b. Modest slowness associated with change from youth to adult
   - ☐ c. Moderate slowness associated with geriatric aging
   - ☐ d. Moderate slowness associated with geriatric aging plus alteration or debility in gait
   - ☐ e. Moderate slowness associated with geriatric aging plus some loss of function (e.g., cannot climb stairs)
   - ☐ f. Severe slowness associated with extreme loss of function, particularly on slick surfaces (may need to be carried)
   - ☐ g. Severe slowness, extreme loss of function, and decreased willingness or interest in locomoting (spends most of time in bed)
   - ☐ h. Paralysed or refuses to move

2. Appetite assessment (may tick **more** than 1)
   - ☐ a. No alterations in appetite
   - ☐ b. Change in ability to physically handle food
   - ☐ c. Change in ability to retain food (vomits or regurgitates)
   - ☐ d. Change in ability to find food
   - ☐ e. Change in interest in food (may be olfactory, having to do with the ability to smell)
   - ☐ f. Change in rate of eating
   - ☐ g. Change in completion of eating
   - ☐ h. Change in timing of eating
   - ☐ i. Change in preferred textures

3. Assessment of elimination function (tick **only** 1 in **each** category)

   a. Changes in frequencies and "accidents"
   - ☐ 1. No change in frequency and no "accidents"
   - ☐ 2. Increased frequency, no "accidents"
   - ☐ 3. Decreased frequency, no "accidents"
   - ☐ 4. Increased frequency with "accidents"
   - ☐ 5. Decreased frequency with "accidents"
   - ☐ 6. No change in frequency, but "accidents"

   b. Bladder control
   - ☐ 1. Leaks urine when asleep, only
   - ☐ 2. Leaks urine when awake, only
   - ☐ 3. Leaks urine when awake or asleep
   - ☐ 4. Full-stream, uncontrolled urination when asleep, only
   - ☐ 5. Full-stream, uncontrolled urination when awake, only
   - ☐ 6. Full-stream, uncontrolled urination when awake or asleep
   - ☐ 7. No leakage or uncontrolled urination, all urination controlled, but in inappropriate or undesirable location
   - ☐ 8. No change in urination control or behavior

   c. Bowel control (Circle appropriate answer, if this occurs, please)
   - ☐ 1. Defecates when asleep
     - Formed stool   Diarrhea   Mixed
   - ☐ 2. Defecates without apparent awareness
     - Formed stool   Diarrhea   Mixed
   - ☐ 3. Defecates when awake and aware of action, but in inappropriate or undesirable locations
     - Formed stool   Diarrhea   Mixed
   - ☐ 4. No changes in bowel control

Fig. 9-21 Behavior screen for age-associated changes.

4. Visual acuity–how well does the client think the cat sees? (tick **only** 1)
   - ☐ a. No change in visual acuity detected by behavior - appears to see as well as ever
   - ☐ b. Some change in acuity **not** dependent on ambient light conditions
   - ☐ c. Some change in acuity dependent on ambient light conditions
   - ☐ d. Extreme change in acuity **not** dependent on ambient light conditions
   - ☐ e. Extreme change in acuity dependent on ambient light conditions
   - ☐ f. Blind

5. Auditory acuity–how well does the client think the cat hears (tick **only** 1)
   - ☐ a. No apparent change in auditory acuity
   - ☐ b. Some decrement in hearing–not responding to sounds to which the cat used to respond
   - ☐ c. Extreme decrement in hearing–have to make sure the cat is paying attention or repeat signals or go get the cat when called
   - ☐ d. Deaf–no response to sounds of any kind

6. Play interactions–if the cat plays with **toys** (other pets are addressed later), which situation best describes that play? (tick **only** 1)
   - ☐ a. No change in play with toys
   - ☐ b. Slightly decreased interest in toys, only
   - ☐ c. Slightly decreased ability to play with toys, only
   - ☐ d. Slightly decreased interest and ability to play with toys
   - ☐ e. Extreme decreased interest in toys, only
   - ☐ f. Extreme decreased ability to play with toys, only
   - ☐ g. Extreme decreased interest and ability to play with toys

7. Interactions with humans–which situation best describes that interaction? (tick **only** 1)
   - ☐ a. No change in interaction with people
   - ☐ b. Recognizes people but slightly decreased frequency of interaction
   - ☐ c. Recognizes people but greatly decreased frequency of interaction
   - ☐ d. Withdrawal but recognizes people
   - ☐ e. Does not recognize people

8. Interactions with other pets–which situation best describes that interaction? (tick **only** 1)
   - ☐ a. No change in interaction with other pets
   - ☐ b. Recognizes other pets but slightly decreased frequency of interaction
   - ☐ c. Recognizes other pets but greatly decreased frequency of interaction
   - ☐ d. Withdrawal but recognizes other pets
   - ☐ e. Does not recognize other pets
   - ☐ f. No other pets or animal companions in house or social environment

9. Changes in sleep/wake cycle (tick **only** 1)
   - ☐ a. No changes in sleep patterns
   - ☐ b. Sleeps more in day, only
   - ☐ c. Some change–awakens at night and sleeps more in day
   - ☐ d. Much change–profoundly erratic nocturnal pattern and irregular daytime pattern
   - ☐ e. Sleeps virtually all day, awake occasionally at night
   - ☐ f. Sleeps almost around the clock

10. Is there anything else you think we should know?

Fig. 9-21, cont'd

- The *oldest cats appeared to have some short-term memory deficits* compared with the younger cats but appeared to view each trial of the specific task used as a new learning experience, as determined by a test for randomness in their first few sets of responses (the cats in the two younger groups did not show this randomness in response), and the older cats learned from their incorrect responses.
- A more recent study with a slightly different design (McCune et al., 2008) also showed a lack of evidence for age-related cognitive decline in spatial learning, again suggesting that brain aging in cats and dogs differs.
- Studies of the brains of old cats compared with the brains of young cats have shown decreased neuronal density in each layer of the cerebellar cortex, denser astrocytes, and fewer neurofilamentary immunoreactive neurons (suggesting loss of dendrites) (Zhang et al., 2006). Together, these changes support that neurons and affiliated function are lost with age.
- This loss of neurons is associated with decreased expression of genes that are involved in the ability of neurons to send and receive signals.
  - Brain-derived neurotrophic factor (BDNF) is essential for the processes of making and repairing all components of neurons.
  - BDNF, which stimulates cytosolic response element binding protein, has three main functions:
    - Enhances growth of serotoninergic (5-HT) and norepinhrinergic neurons
    - Protects these neurons from neurotoxic damage
    - Helps in remodeling neuronal receptors, altering function by enhancing messenger RNA transcriptional changes in translated protein products (i.e., receptors)
- When amyloid deposition is sufficiently extensive, it physically disrupts communication between neurons worsening the processes discussed previously. β-Amyloid in cats is deposited in extremely diffuse plaques, but it still appears to be involved in age-related feline behavioral changes, as does the deposition of tau proteins (Head et al., 2005). β-Amyloid deposition within and/or closely associated with neurons and/or blood vessels appears to be age-dependent in cats, regardless of any effect on behavior (Gunn-Moore et al., 2006).
- P300 potentials are scalp potentials that are task related and so are useful as a measure of stimulus discrimination, sequential information processing, and short-term memory. These potentials can be affected by brain disease. P300 potentials in young cats (1 to 3 years old) are larger in response to rare stimuli compared with frequent stimuli, but in older cats (>10 years old), P300 potentials do not differ between rare and frequent stimuli (Harrison and

Buchwald, 1985). Old cats, similar to old humans, appear to show no consistent response.
- *Old cats experience decreases in the function/density of hypocretin (orexin) neurons* compared with adult controls (Zhang et al., 2002). Because hypothalamic hypocretin-containing neurons project to brainstem nuclei that control sleep and wakefulness, *this could be one mechanism for changes in nocturnal motor activity and vocalization about which clients so often comment in old cats.* In old cats, the locus ceruleus appears to be particularly affected.
- As is true for dogs, because *the feline behaviors we evaluate to make the diagnosis of CD are so general,* we must remember that these behaviors could be natural sequelae to a variety of organ system changes. *If so, the diagnostic criteria will lead to many false-positive diagnoses.*

Common Myths That Can Get in the Way of Treatment or Diagnosis

- Behavioral changes that occur with age are "normal," and there is nothing you can do about this.
  - There is a lot of variation in how well animals within any species age, and there is a lot of variation in how "successful aging" (i.e., aging without cognitive impairment) occurs.
  - There are a number of animals who are ancient and yet have few demonstrable cognitive changes.
  - Patient needs may change (e.g., the cat needs to have a litterbox on each floor), but if met, old cats can do well.
  - Increased aerobic exercise of any kind is helpful because of its effects on ROS and vascular health, and alterations in diet/supplements and enhanced cognitive stimulation can help slow or derail behavioral changes associated with aging.
- Old cats have had their time, there is no sense trying to treat them, things will just continue to go wrong, so the treatment of choice is euthanasia, and there are a lot of young cats in shelters who need homes.
  - It is true that there are many cats in shelters who need homes, and anyone who can give a quality home to a homeless animal of any kind should be encouraged to do so.
  - Prevention and early intervention through diet, exercise, and cognitive stimulation matter for both behavioral and physical conditions. Aging *per se* is not a death sentence.
  - We cannot make cats young again, but we can provide them a better QoL with such intervention.
  - Euthanasia is not a treatment.
    - Although it was commonly believed that old cats should just be "put out of their misery," we have more options now, and people should visit their vets to avoid euthanasia in older cats. Euthanasia should be a decision of last, not first resort. Many clients with old animals

would be content with natural deaths for their companions if they have done everything they could; the cat's dignity was respected; and there was no pain, discomfort, or suffering left unaddressed.

- Veterinarians should know that clients avoid or delay seeking treatment if they are afraid that the vet will recommend euthanasia. This pattern is ironic in that it increases the likelihood of serious pathology that could *render euthanasia more likely.*

Commonly Asked Client Questions
- Can this condition be fixed?
  - We cannot reverse the cat's age, and we cannot rid them of any amyloid lesions. However, we can address the pathologies associated with these by addressing functional change using diet/supplements, exercise, medication, and cognitive stimulation. There are promising experimental studies in rodents suggesting that amyloid burdens can be altered (Cramer et al., 2012), but these interventions are not yet clinically applied.
- How long will the cat have left if he or she is treated?
  - We cannot know the answer to this question, but the earlier intervention is attempted, the greater the likelihood of a longer and happier life. Overall, the amount of life left will increase, but the QoL will increase even more.

Treatment
- Management:
  - Helpful management changes include the following:
    - Ensure that the cat has easy access to simple cat doors and/or has multiple litterboxes within easy walking distance of where she spends most of her time and that the box is easy for her to enter and exit.
    - If the cat is not getting a lot of exercise, stimulate his muscles with a range-of-motion exercises and/or massage daily.
    - Cats can learn to use swimming pools, heated baths, and underwater treadmills to help ameliorate alterations in mobility, but most people are reluctant to try such interventions if cats did not engage in such activities when young.
    - Food toys that move a bit but are still relatively easy for arthritic cats to use or toys that allow the cat to problem solve without having to be so physically robust (Fig. 9-22) may stimulate activity.
  - Ensure that the medications the cat is taking are the medications he or she needs, and review all potential and present side effects every 3 months or earlier, if needed.
  - Teach the client to signal clearly to the cat to address any deficits in vision or hearing common to aging cats. This can be done by touching or

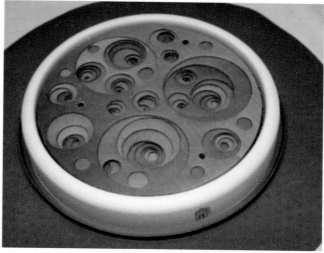

Fig. 9-22 A Catit food toy made of layered cardboard cutouts that allow different sizes and textures of dry food to be "hunted" by cats. This toy comes with a rubber collar so that it does not slip on the floor, which can be helpful for older cats.

tapping the cat, and if the client does so frequently, the cat will be less isolated because of such changes.
  - Providing surfaces that have traction by using rubber mats or rugs can help cats get more exercise and have fewer elimination accidents.
- Behavior modification:
  - Unless clients worked with some training or behavior modification when the cat was young, they are unlikely to do so with older cats, but they should still be encouraged to engage in reward-based programs.
    - Old cats can be clicker trained to stretch body parts and move in certain directions.
    - Scent work is common for dogs, but cats also have an excellent sense of smell and may benefit from puzzles or feeding designs that encourage them to use their nose and "hunt."
    - Bird feeders may encourage cats to attend and respond to movement.
- Medication/dietary intervention:
  - This is the area where most work is being done and where we currently have so much help and hope. The best time to implement dietary or supplement intervention is before the cat is showing any signs of brain aging. This means that dietary/supplement changes should be made once the cat has reached about 7 years of age, as they are entering middle age.
    - PUFAs, especially arachidonic acid (ARA), DHA, and EHA, play roles in maintaining neuronal integrity and enhancing energy use by neurons.

- All of these PUFAs are essential for early brain development.
- ARA is thought especially to maintain hippocampal cell membrane fluidity and protect cells in the hippocampus from oxidative stress.
- DHA may encourage development stage–specific associational learning, although the data are mixed.
- Supplementation with DHA and EPA affect concentration of these substances in rat brains, and their distribution is not uniform (see www.nordicnaturals.com for compounds specially formulated for dogs and cats, and note that cat and dog dosages and formulations differ).
- Diets deficient in α-linoleic acid (an essential fatty acid for cats) especially cause decreases of DHA in the frontal cortex—the part of the brain responsible for complex learning and integration of information and executive function.
- We currently lack detailed data on effects of omega-3 fatty acids and medium-chain triglycerides on brain function for cats, but this is an active area of research.
- Diets for cats older than 7 years focus on roles for anti-oxidants (Nestlé Purina Pro Plan Age 7+, Hills Science Plan Feline Mature Adult 7+). One study of life expectancy in cats 7 to 17 years old in three dietary treatment groups showed that, regardless of age, cats fed diets high in linoleic acid (an essential n-6 fatty acid in cats) and the anti-oxidants vitamin E and beta carotene lived longer (Cupp et al., 2006).
  - Supplements:
    - Senelife (Ceva Santé Animale) uses anti-oxidants (reservatrol), structural enhancers of neuronal membranes (phosphatidylserine), and a co-enzyme of neurotransmitter function (pyroxidine) to address three factors that can affect brain aging.
    - Aktivait (Vet Plus, UK; available online only in the United States at this writing) also addresses structural concerns by providing DHA, EPA, and phosphatidylserine, plus the antioxidants vitamins C and E, selenium, and acetylcysteine. An α-lipoic acid–free version has been introduced more recently for cats.
  - NOVIFIT (NoviSAMe; Virbac) is S-adenosylmethionine, an anti-oxidant frequently used in cats that may help brain function.
  - Medications:
    - No medications are licensed for use for the treatment of CD/CDS in cats in the United States at this writing.
    - Selegiline (Anipryl; Pfizer, Ceva Santé Animale) is a MAO B inhibitor licensed to treat CD/CDS

in dogs that has been used *extra-label in cats*. It works by inhibiting the degradation and recycling of the monoamine neurochemicals (i.e., norepinephrine, serotonin, dopamine), with its largest effect on dopamine. By providing increased neurochemical stimulation to neurons, their synapses are maintained, and the effects of BDNF are able to occur. This medication works best as a preventive and treatment if given when the first signs of CD begin. The most dramatic effect is noticed by clients if the cats are moderately affected, but that's because the decline was so apparent. Treatment of CD with medication is another example of a situation when treating early and often is preferred.
- Propentofylline—xanthine derivative with neuroprotectant effects and helps to improve blood flow
- Nicergoline—ergot derivative that is a potent vasodilator that putatively works by improving blood flow
- For some cats who exhibit non-specific signs of anxiety as their first behavioral changes with age, treatment with TCAs or SSRIs may help. The effects that the clients see are the ones on anxiety, but because these medications also cause their effects by increasing signal transduction efficiency, they help to keep neurons and their second messenger systems healthy and able to make useful connections with other neurons. As a result, TCAs and SSRIs may have protective and treatment roles for CD.
- Cats who are experiencing some sleep cycle changes may also benefit from treatment with a BZD because of the calming effects on the reticular activating system. Avoiding BZDs with sedative intermediate metabolites that could pose a risk for older cats (e.g., diazepam) may be helpful. Shorter acting BZDs such as alprazolam, oxazepam, and lorazepam may be helpful.
- Miscellaneous interventions:
  - The most commonly omitted intervention is the cognitive one.
    - Food toys and puzzles are commercially available, but they can also be homemade (Fig. 9-23).
    - We know from the human literature that all conditions involving cognitive impairment also involve decrements in olfactory ability. Cats can be encouraged to use their noses by putting different food items under an array of paper cups, by placing small amounts of food in tiny dishes in multiple locations/at multiple levels, et cetera.
    - This association between decrements in cognition and olfactory function may also suggest that we need to pay attention to the

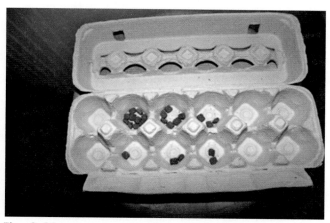

Fig. 9-23 An extremely cheap and easy-to-make feline food toy that stimulates olfaction, cognition, and physical movement.

volatile olfactory component of our cat's dinners. Warming food and providing warm broth allows odorant molecules to volatilize, stimulating the cat's brain and encouraging eating.

- Smelling the air and all the information that it carries to cats can be a huge benefit to a cat whose ambulatory skills are compromised. Cats who enjoy rides in cars and are bold may like to go for a walk in an animal stroller.
- Social interaction and exposure to new stimuli are essential for keeping cognitive skills sharp. Older cats may benefit from interaction with and the stimulation of younger animals.

Helpful Handouts
- "Protocol for Understanding and Helping Geriatric Animals"
- "Protocol for Preventing and Treating Attention-Seeking Behavior"

Last Words
- People who have sought veterinary practices that are behavior centered and who have fed, exercised, and cared for their cats well do not wish to hear that their cats are "just getting old." Fortunately, clients no longer need to hear that their cat is "just old." Veterinarians should prepare patients and clients for age-based and stage-based care and evaluate whether supplements and dietary change are warranted as cats move into middle age.

Depression
Diagnostic Criteria and Description
- There is debate about whether the term "depression" should be used for non-human animals. We lack the data that exist in human medicine for population-wide descriptions and determinations of animals affected with depression.

- A reasonable set of diagnostic criteria could include a prolonged (>1 to 2 weeks) endogenous or reactive pattern of behavior that may include withdrawal from social stimuli, withdrawal from activities that were previously engaging and enjoyable, alterations in appetite, and/or alterations in sleep-wake cycles that are not incidental.
- The condition is likely confirmed if the patient also exhibits decreased locomotor/motor activity and actual physical removal from normal social and environmental stimuli in the absence of any neurological or physiological condition.
  - The problem with using this criterion in cats is that these signs are also non-specific signs of anxiety, stress, and pain, so *the context in which the withdrawal occurs becomes essential.*
- The reactive form of depression will be easiest to recognize and acknowledge in cats.
  - Some forms of reactive depression in dogs may be comparable to "adjustment disorder" in humans.
  - In an "adjustment disorder" type of depression, the behaviors are shared with those enumerated here but are a *response* to a drastically altered environment over which the patient had no control (e.g., relinquishment, abandonment, re-homing, death of a close human or another pet). *Bereavement and grief can be the essential targets for this type of depression.*

Common Non-Specific Signs
- Some of the signs seen in human depression may be applicable to cats, but they are non-specific and must be interpreted in the context required by the definition for feline depression.
  - The definition used here allows individuals sensitized to watching for the signs to recognize the following in a context that should be meaningful to the cat:
    - loss of appetite,
    - disruptions in sleep cycles,
    - poor to no grooming (clients may notice spiky coat, mats, dry skin, et cetera),
    - sleeping a lot when normally awake,
    - weight loss (weight gain and hyperphagia occur in this context only rarely in cats); cats who have lost a companion of any species should be weighed multiple times a week to monitor this key aspect of grief and depression, and small cats are especially at risk,
    - loss of range of behavioral and emotional expression, loss of interest in formerly enjoyable activities (playing with the feather toy, watching the birds at the feeder),
    - decrease in energy and activity levels,
    - social withdrawal,
    - unexplained, non-specific, and transient pain and stiffness, and
    - gastrointestinal distress (sporadic diarrhea, tenesmus, mucousy feces).

- These behaviors are recognizable and could be noted on a daily log that allows clients to record time of day, circumstance, and response. If clients make a schedule of how the cat formerly spent her day, they will likely recognize deviations from this.
- Clients can be provided with tick sheets to note the occurrence and frequency of certain behaviors.
  - The behaviors assessed would have to be relevant to the patient and the household of which he or she is a member.
  - For example, if the cat usually greets the kids when they return from school and ceases to do this, this change is a concern.
- If the cat used to lie in someone's lap each night for petting and grooming and no longer seeks out such attention, this is a concern.
- Any assessment measure used must matter *to the cat and specifically to that cat.*

Rule Outs

- The non-specific signs of depression are common ones that can be associated with "malaise" resulting from almost any illness.
- Conditions that are sufficiently common that they should be ruled out include:
  - infectious diseases,
  - endocrine conditions,
  - early cardiac, renal, or hepatic failure, and
  - neoplasia.

Etiology, Epidemiology, and Risk Groups

- We do not know which cats are at risk for this condition, but profound life changes resulting in loss (e.g., the loss of a human, companion animal, home) can put cats at risk for the reactive form of depression.
  - Cats who are relinquished to shelters, regardless of vaccination history, are at high risk for infectious respiratory disease because their immune system is stressed by the relinquishment and relocation. These signs are compatible with depression.

Common Myths That Can Get in the Way of Treatment or Diagnosis

- There is a common belief that cats accept and survive tragedy much better than humans do and that they will—and should—just "snap out of it."
  - This myth may have developed because humans realize that the number of cats abandoned and/or in shelters is truly appalling. By believing that cats are good survivors and can handle such abandonment better than we can, we relieve ourselves of guilt.
  - *No one—regardless of species—just "snaps out of it."*

Commonly Asked Client Questions

- Is it possible that my cat is depressed?
  - Clients have been told cats don't get depressed. If you query them, they will tell you that something may have happened that seemed to cause the cat to lose all joy. Such a description meets the criteria for depression.
- Can the depression my cat is experiencing be treated?
  - Yes. Use of anti-anxiety medications and structured attention to ensure that the cat is included in activities and monitored for physical side effects can help.

Treatment

- Management:
  - Cats should be encouraged, not forced, to engage in behaviors that they previously found pleasurable.
  - Cats should be protected from interactions that clearly distress or frighten them.
  - As long as the cat is maintaining his weight, dietary intervention isn't necessary, but if the cat stops eating his normal diet, hepatic lipidosis is a serious concern.
    - Tempting cats with favored foods that are warmed to ensure maximal olfactory stimulation may help them to eat and stimulate the olfactory-cognition link.
  - Supplements, particularly those rich in antioxidants to protect cats' brains from the toxic effects of ROS, may help and may help many diets to appear more palatable (e.g., adding salmon or cod liver oil may have two effects).
  - Try to keep the cat on a regular schedule.
- Behavior modification:
  - Behavior modification with these cats is tough, but if the cat can be convinced to crave any food, work with clickers or simply rewards for walking with the person and/or presenting body parts for grooming may help.
- Medication/dietary intervention:
  - PUFA supplements, including omega-3 fatty acids, may help prevent the cat from worsening by helping to combat inflammation and oxidative stress.
  - Medication is key to helping these cats regain joy in their lives.
    - Most cats will need a SSRI or one of the newer derivatives. Fluoxetine, sertraline, and paroxetine all have been used in these conditions.
    - Selegiline, a MAO inhibitor, has been used in Europe for similar conditions but is not widely used in the United States except for CD. The primary effect of selegiline is as a MAO inhibitor whose main target is dopamine, although all other monoamines (e.g., serotonin, norepinephrine, phenylethylamine) are affected to some extent. The effects of the medication will be determined, in part, by the distribution of central dopaminergic neurons.
    - Alpha-casozepine (Zylkene) may be helpful for non-specific anxiety and withdrawal in cats.
    - BZDs may help because they stimulate appetite as a fortuitous side effect and so may facilitate appetite and any behavior modification using

food treats. BZDs have been postulated to disinhibit inhibited behaviors, so some recovery of appetite may be attributable to this effect on the hypothalamus.

Miscellaneous Interventions

- Massage, grooming, sitting with the cat in the sun, spending time with another pet, and any other actions that may make the cat happy may help.
- In this condition, time matters. If tincture of time and behavior modification has not helped in a week or so, do not delay treatment with medication further. This is especially true if the cat is tiny and is losing weight.
- For cats who are very close to specific people or other animals and/or who rely on them, death of the companion/friend can be devastating.
  - Dogs and cats should be given the chance to visit with their dying human companions and to see them after death.
  - They should also be able to visit with their ill and dying canine and feline companions and to spend time with them after death.
    - This last recommendation is especially important for dogs and cats who are rescues.
    - Dogs and cats can understand death but may not understand absence.
    - Given their own relinquishment history, uncertainty could contribute to anxiety and depression in rescued patients.
    - If end of life involves euthanasia, the other dogs and cats should be given the opportunity to be present. As we move more toward humane home hospice care for terminally ill animals, it will be easier for the other dogs and cats in the family to be present, which may greatly comfort the dying animal if the dogs/cats were close.
    - If signs of unremitting depression appear at any stage of the hospice care for or after the death of the companion, treatment as soon as possible may shorten the treatment course.

Helpful Handouts

- "Protocol for Using Behavioral Medication Successfully"
- "Protocol for Teaching Cats and Dogs to 'Sit,' 'Stay,' and 'Come'"

Last Words

- The definition of depression in humans does not adapt easily to cats or other animals. Because of the variable relationships we share with animals, *it is important that any definition of depression be relevant from the animal's viewpoint and that assessment takes into account the evolutionary history of the animal, roles played, and the context in which the diagnosis is being made.*
- In humans, depression can be defined as "an illness that involves the body, mood, and thoughts, that affects the way a person eats and sleeps, the way one feels about oneself, and the way one thinks about things" (www.medterms.com/script/main/art.asp?articlekey=2947). It has also been termed "a clinical mood disorder associated with low mood or loss of interest and other symptoms that prevents a person from leading a normal life" (www.webmd.com/depression/depression-glossary?page=2). Depression has been termed by the World Health Organization as a "common mental disorder that presents with depressed mood, loss of interest or pleasure, feelings of guilt or low self-worth, disturbed sleep or appetite, low energy, and poor concentration" (www.who.int/mental_health/management/depression/definition/en).
- A diagnosis of depression in humans is made on the basis of meeting the definitional criteria and on the types, duration, and frequency of the signs. We must remember that most human conditions that use such information pertaining to signs are able to do so because of large prospective or retrospective studies seldom possible or available in veterinary medicine.
- *No matter what the species, depression is a serious QoL condition, and very few individuals "spontaneously" recover.*

Obsessive-Compulsive Disorder/Compulsive Disorder with Special Emphasis on Feline Hyperesthesia

Diagnostic Criteria and Description

- Repetitive, stereotypic motor, locomotory, grooming, ingestive, or hallucinogenic behaviors that occur out of context to their "normal" occurrence or in a frequency or duration that is *in excess of that required to accomplish the ostensible goal.*
- As this condition progresses, the behaviors are manifest in a manner that interferes with the animal's ability to function otherwise in his or her social environment.
- When fully manifest, the cat is unresponsive to human or animal intervention and to pain.
- This diagnosis is sometimes called only compulsive disorder in the veterinary literature because we cannot directly assess the obsessive component in dogs and cats.
  - In humans, the behaviors are abnormal ones that have as characteristics recurrent, frequent thoughts or actions that are out of context to the situations in which they occur.
  - These behaviors in humans can involve cognitive or physical rituals and are deemed excessive (given the context) in duration, frequency, and intensity of the behavior.
  - *It would be a mistake to believe that this condition does not have cognitive components or forms in animals.* In fact, one could argue that the compulsive behaviors are the result of obsessive "thoughts."

- There is now ample evidence that dogs and cats are cognitive and that they mirror assays of human performance when adapted to a species that is non-verbal.
- The ways we assess whether humans "obsess" involves asking about obsessions and observing patterns of speech and behavior. Independent assays of obsession (e.g., imaging) are seldom done.
- For dogs and cats, *direct observation, especially under a variety of conditions, can confirm that this condition has cognitive aspects involving intense, unremitting focus (e.g., obsession).*
- Separate from the obsession issue is the one of relative intensity: whether a behavior is excessive or a manifestation of OCD may be a determination of degree. *Careful description and recording of behaviors and their durations could provide data that would permit evaluation of the extent to which such behaviors may lie on a continuum.*
- Good histories and observation are important because in some peculiar forms some OCD—especially odd, episodic grooming and mutilation behaviors in cats—could resemble seizure-like activity. However, we should remember that "seizure-like" activity is more poorly defined than are most behavioral conditions. By definition, some epileptic or seizure-like activity is stereotypic, which is one reason why this very explicit and specific diagnosis category is preferable to that of stereotypy.
  - The issue of arousal cannot be overestimated in cats. Because of the unique neuromodulatory patterns of feline arousal and reactivity, behaviors such as over-grooming, self-mutilation, and hyperesthesia can be fierce and episodic. These behaviors still meet the requirements for OCD, but the intensity is shaped by the evolutionary history of cats that has affected their neuromodulatory patterns.
- A hallmark of OCD that distinguishes it from neurological conditions involving motor tics, et cetera,

is that OCD behaviors follow *a set of rules created by the patient.* This condition is likely to be mechanistically heterogeneous (e.g., multifactorial). *Regardless of the type of behavior in which the cat engages, it must be sufficiently pronounced to interfere with normal functioning to make this diagnosis.*

- OCD can be primary (truly endogenous) or secondary and likely associated with thresholds for stimulation (Fig. 9-24).

Common Non-Specific Signs

- Depending on the form the OCD takes, the cat will exhibit the repeated behavior in a manner consistent with some internal and unforgiving rule structure. For example, cats who suck and/or chew on fabrics (and these are likely different at some mechanistic level) will have a rule for a subset of fabrics they prefer, and a rule for how they acquire them, and a rule for how they handle them (e.g., do they "shake" the fabric first or do they knead and suck on it?).
- Cats may seek out opportunities to engage in the OCD behavior, especially if they have been reprimanded or disciplined for engaging in them. As a result, clients can ensure that the cat hides the behavior from them. However, most cats engage in these behaviors where people can see them.
- The demography and epidemiology of OCD in cats is poorly described, but the most commonly noted behaviors include (Fig. 9-25):
  - chewing, sucking, or ingesting fabrics (pica),
  - chewing cords or linear objects (pica), and
  - over-grooming, possibly with true self-mutilation (Fig. 9-26).
    - Feline hyperesthesia may be a variant OCD that can be combined with over-grooming if the cats actually bite at themselves. Otherwise, the skin rippling, arousal, and attentive responses to rippling and escape behaviors may characterize yet another form of feline OCD.
- Most forms of feline OCD that have been reported have noted that cats begin to express the OCD only after physical trauma or a change in feline or human

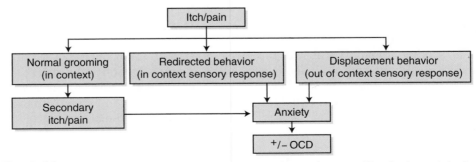

Fig. 9-24 Schematic for how OCD can develop as a secondary condition to dermatological concerns involving pruritus and/or pain.

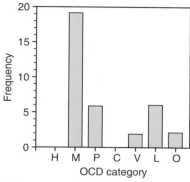

Fig. 9-25 Relative frequencies of types of OCD behaviors for patients the study by in Overall and Dunham (2002). *H,* Hallucination; *M,* self-mutilation; *P,* pica; *C,* coprophagia; *V,* vocalization; *L,* locomotor behavior; *O,* other. (Data from Overall and Dunham, 2002.)

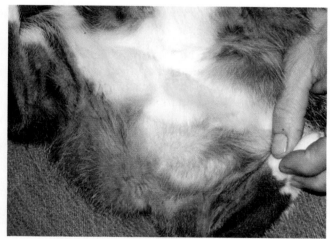

Fig. 9-26 Sparse hair in the inguinal region of a cat who licks and plucks; note that the hair loss is not symmetrical and is not over the bladder region—the hair loss is in the hind limb and inguinal region. (Photo courtesy of Anne Marie Dossche.)

social circumstances that affected the cats (Overall and Dunham, 2002).

Rule Outs

- Depending on the form the OCD takes, medical rule outs can be numerous.
- The most common conditions to rule out are:
  - endocrine conditions,
  - treatment with progestins,
  - atopy/allergy,
  - FLUTD/UTI/FIC—cats with painful bladders may pluck the hair on their abdomen over the bladder region,
  - primary neurological disease (especially if the cat engages in motor or locomotor activity),
  - toxicity (including heavy metals like lead),
  - gastrointestinal parasites (because of some of the odd and possibly high-fiber objects consumed),
  - dental disease,
  - infectious diseases,
  - undiagnosed or untreated pain secondary to another condition, and
  - other behavioral conditions, including attention-seeking behavior.
- Diagnosis may be difficult to confirm, but most of the rule outs listed can be dismissed on the basis of radiology, imaging, laboratory evaluation (which may include a cerebrospinal fluid analysis), and some toxicology panels.
- Video is essential in correct diagnosis: the pattern of the behaviors involved in OCD tend to separate this diagnosis from other conditions that cause related and possibly confusing behavioral shifts.

Etiology, Epidemiology, and Risk Groups

- When the families are known, the condition runs in family lines. Careful questioning reveals no generations are skipped (Overall and Dunham, 2002).
- Oriental breeds appear to be over-represented, especially for ingestion of fabrics, but recently created breeds (e.g., Bengal cats) appear to be at risk for OCD involving grooming unless they have a large amount of space and stimulation. These are not good cats for tiny apartments where humans are seldom home.
- The extent to which an OCD may be expressed can depend on the physical and social environment. It's likely that in cats, the underlying genetic sensitivity is less latent in some physical and social environments than others. When examined, changes or stressors always seem to precede the development of the condition in cats (Overall and Dunham, 2002).
  - Cats who chew on fabrics or other substances in the environment, may do so because of effects on cholecystokinin B receptors (Singh et al., 1991).
  - *If the cat is presenting multiple times for foreign body obstruction or possible foreign bodies, OCD should always be considered as a causal condition.*
- Cats, similar to dogs, appear to begin to express the condition during social maturity (median age of onset, 12 months; mean age of onset, 28.2 months) (Overall and Dunham, 2002), suggesting that the neuronal remodeling associated with social maturity is involved in the pathology.
- There is variation in response surfaces in cats from different lines; some cats require extreme stress to develop OCD, whereas others may display signs consistent with OCD under less stressful conditions.
- In cats, in contrast to in dogs, forms do not seem to vary among relatives, but the data are few.
- An inability to inhibit behavior has been proposed as an endophenotype in human OCD (Chamberlain, 2005).
  - This type of criterion might allow us to understand variation in arousal in cats.

- OCD spectrum conditions in humans are thought to include attention-deficit/hyperactivity disorder, Tourette's syndrome, and trichotillomania (compulsive hair pulling) (Chamberlain, 2005). We lack the data to use such an approach in veterinary behavioral medicine, but it could doubtless identify diagnostic subgroups that are important.
- Treatment of OCD generally requires lifetime medication once diagnosed. Cats removed from medication usually relapse (Overall and Dunham, 2002).
- *Especially when dermatological conditions are co-morbid, all aspects of roles for anxiety, pain and pruritus must be addressed because we now know that pain, anxiety, and pruritus are related at both the central level and the level of the dorsal horn of the spinal ganglion (Fig. 9-27).*

Common Myths That Can Get in the Way of Treatment or Diagnosis

- The most common myth pertaining to OCD is that it is a variant of normal behavior. Pathologies may have been deliberately or accidentally selected for in the breed, but they are hardly "normal."
  - By accepting/asserting a pathological behavior as normal, we do the following things:
    - We fail to address that the cat may be suffering and that the behavior is a non-specific sign of stress or pathology.
    - We relinquish the chance to intervene early when intervention will be most simple and helpful.
    - We tacitly approve breeding for the pathology.
    - We fail to acknowledge that something associated with this concern must have been desirable at some point if a large proportion of any line or breed is affected. If we fail to acknowledge this pattern, we will be unable to understand the genetic variance-covariance matrix that is operating and so cannot know if it is possible to select for desirable traits without carrying along traits that are injurious.
    - We pass on the misery to the next generation.

Commonly Asked Client Questions

- Can this cat improve and become normal?
  - These are not the same questions.
    - All affected cats can improve—we are discussing the matter of the degree to which they can improve. Some cats will need medication for an extended period just to break through their distress long enough to render them susceptible to learning an alternative way to live.
    - Some cats will become so happy and so free of their non-specific signs that people will think that they are "cured" or "normal." This is the second question. Unfortunately, these cats never become "normal." If we think about treatment in terms of the response surface for the individual cat, behavioral, environmental, and genetic factors all contribute to the outcome.
    - Some cats exhibit less profoundly affected behaviors, some have greater space for environmental intervention, and some have a greater degree of genetically based plasticity for learning new ways to cope and make their lives more predictable. This trifecta will help the cat look "normal." He will never be normal, and the clients must understand what this means.
    - Stressors could have profound effects on these cats, so if there is a social or physical disruption, the clients should expect to see some backsliding. Resiliency likely has genetic components, but using behavior modification we can teach

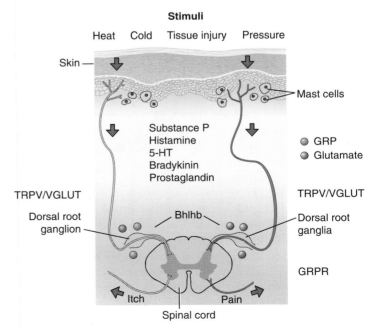

Fig. 9-27 Pain, anxiety, and pruritus are related at both the central level and the level of the dorsal horn of the spinal ganglion. *DRG,* Dorsal root ganglia; *Glu,* glutamate; *Vglut,* vesicular glutamate transporter; *GRP,* gastrin-releasing peptide; *GRPR,* gastrin-releasing peptide receptor; *TRPV1,* vanilloid receptor; *Bhlhb,* a transcription factor. (Adapted from Patel and Dong, 2010, and Rang et al., 2012.)

resiliency by rewarding a range of acceptable alternative responses.

- Will medication be lifelong?
  - Yes, unless the problem just started and responded almost instantly to treatment, it is far safer to treat the cat for life. Once established, the story of OCD is one of staying the course and managing minor slips from grace. In almost all cases, continuous medication makes this possible.

Treatment

- Management:
  - Recognizing, understanding, planning for, and managing stimuli that provoke an OCD burst in the cat are essential steps in recovery. This is especially true because for OCD involving any aspect of grooming, including hyperesthesia, the extent to which the cat is aroused could pose a risk for human intervention.
    - Re-directed aggression has been seen when some clients try to stop the cat from licking, chewing, or biting/swatting at herself.
    - More commonly, the re-directed behavior is manifest as flight, but this is still a concern for clients.
  - This is a condition that is about patterns. The cats are using a failed rule structure to—ostensibly—help them cope with situations that, regardless of the level of the pathology, the cat finds distressing. We help the cat by substituting rules associated with relaxation and non-reactivity for rules that cause them to react and become distressed. The clients should be able to recognize the patterns that appear in the cat's behaviors when the rules begin to slip and re-direct the cat as early in the sequence as possible.
- Behavior modification:
  - In extreme cases where the behaviors are unremitting, it may be exceedingly difficult to engage in any behavior modification until the cat has experienced some relief from medication. This may mean that clients cannot begin to engage in active behavior modification for 3 to 5 weeks.
    - In such cases, clients should not think that they can do nothing. Instead, they should focus intensely on any possible form of passive behavior modification.
    - Having the cat learn to sit on cue or clicker training the cat to engage in a behavior that is incompatible with the particular OCD may help.
    - Rewarding the cat when her arousal level is below that which is usually involved in the commission of the OCD may help teach the cat the association of being calmer and being happier.
    - Regardless, we want to teach the cat a behavior that competes with the OCD in a manner that not only inhibits the performance of the OCD but that also helps the cat to relax and learn that

he has some control over his behavior. Clients should be reminded that this type of intervention may not be possible until the medication has begun to take effect.

- Medication/dietary intervention:
  - Medications that can be helpful in controlling the anxiety that drives OCD may include (Overall and Dunham, 2002; Seksel and Lindeman, 1998):
    - TCAs—most TCAs have some anti-pruritic effects and may help to alleviate pain.
      - Amitriptyline
      - Clomipramine was developed for the treatment of OCD and may be the medication of choice if the manifestation of the condition can be characterized by ritualistic activity.
      - Doxepin is an H_1 antagonist—especially useful if there are dermatologic manifestations of the OCD; can be used in combination with other medications with care and reduced dosages. It is heavily sedative in cats and getting the right, low dosage may be very tricky. In extreme cases, it can be considered for use as a later resort.
      - Nortriptyline
    - SSRIs:
      - Fluoxetine is generally preferred if the OCD has explosive components or an explosive start to the bout. If the entire form of the OCD can be characterized by its impulsivity, fluoxetine may be a more efficacious medication.
      - Fluvoxamine
      - Paroxetine
      - Sertraline
    - SARIs:
      - Trazodone may be best used as an adjuvant medication with others that are more specific for other receptor classes. Its associated effect on movement affected by $5\text{-}HT_{2A}$ receptors suggests that its addition may be helpful in some situations.
    - Other:
      - Gabapentin may be especially useful if any neuropathic pain is involved but may be extremely helpful as a second or third medication to help address arousal and more global anxieties.
      - Memantine (a NMDA antagonist) has been efficacious as an adjuvant in OCD that resolves incompletely, suggesting that regulation of signal transduction pathways on more general levels may be useful.
    - Some cats with OCD, especially if there is a self-mutilation component, do themselves considerable damage. Under no circumstances, unless used as a last resort to spare the remaining limb, should digits or limbs be amputated

as a "treatment" for OCD. The pathology that is in the cat's head will not be addressed by the removal of a limb or tail, and affected patients with true OCD will continue to mutilate more proximal body areas. Instead, these cats should be treated with medications that will treat pain and pruritus, and possibly long-term antibiotics to control any residual infection. If needed, butorphanol injections may help.

- Miscellaneous interventions:
  - Re-directing the cat to a more suitable outlet for the particular behaviors may help (e.g., encourage the cat to chew on the freshly cooked beef bone, not herself), but these are stop-gaps. The ease with which such re-direction is accomplished can serve as an index of improvement.
  - Massage may help because it is incompatible with virtually all OCDs and may be able to be worked into the behavior modification plan as a way of teaching the cat that he can have some control over his own behaviors. Caution is urged for attempting this when the cat is at all aroused.
  - Aerobic exercise that achieves true aerobic scope may help modulate the intensity and frequency of the behaviors and so act as part of an integrated treatment plan.
  - Elizabethan collars are likely just to distress these cats more because of the difficulty they can cause for navigation.
  - For cats who self-injure, bandages and wraps should be avoided when possible because they may serve as foci for more licking and chewing. If a wrap sufficiently changes the stimulus so that it is less noticeable, it may help, so some cast or splint designs may help lesions to heal. Such interventions are not often used but may be most successful in combination with topical anesthetics.
  - Cats who self-injure may have a particular sensitivity to sutures, and so if they recover from their OCD and require any surgery this concern should be noted and factor into decisions made. Knowing that some intervention may be problematic for the cat causes the humans charged with his care to watch that cat differently and so makes early intervention possible. This is a form of anticipatory guidance.
  - If cats chew on/ingest certain classes of items, exposure to these must be minimized both so that the cat does not practice her particular form of OCD and so that the risk of a foreign body is minimized. *If restricted exposure causes the cat to become more anxious, the client has just confirmed the diagnosis.*

Helpful Handouts
- "Protocol for Understanding and Treating Obsessive-Compulsive Disorder (OCD)"
- "Protocol for Preventing and Treating Attention-Seeking Behavior"

- "Protocol for Using Behavioral Medication Successfully"
- "Protocol for Teaching Cats and Dogs to 'Sit,' 'Stay,' and 'Come'"

Last Words
- Co-morbidity is the rule with OCD. Screen all cats for other anxiety-related conditions, and treat all of them.
- Other conditions that may be neurodevelopmental (e.g., blindness, deafness, epilepsy, "seizure" activity) often co-occur in families where OCD (and other anxiety-related conditions, such as noise phobia) has been identified. Although the behavioral condition always appears to be inherited separately from the other conditions, including when these may be due to inborn errors of metabolism (Uchida et al., 1997), it is possible that in polygenic conditions there may be shared liability genes that could affect how profoundly ill the patient can become. Anyone interested in understanding the molecular genetics and neurobiology of these conditions may wish to consider these associations.
- We don't know what the early stages of OCD look like. Encourage all clients, especially those with breeds or breed groups in which OCD is either relatively common or may have been directly or indirectly selected for, to monitor kittens for odd, ritualistic behaviors and to interrupt them. Ease of interruption is a good indicator of how severe the problem may be.

Feline Hyperesthesia—Likely a Special Case of Obsessive-Compulsive Disorder
Diagnostic Criteria and Description
- One example of the complexity of OCD conditions is found in feline hyperesthesia. Hyperesthesia syndrome has been variously called "rolling skin syndrome," "neuritis," "twitchy cat disease," and "atypical neurodermatitis" (Shell, 1994).
  - Our lack of knowledge has encouraged the word "syndrome" to be attached to the descriptor because syndromes are collections of related non-specific signs that may co-occur but may have variable underlying etiologies and may not represent a singular diagnosis. It would be a mistake, however, to view these behaviors as randomly associated collections. They are not. All of the non-specific signs associated with hyperesthesia are linked in their presentation by the effects that arousal and reactivity have on them.
  - The behaviors demonstrated in feline hyperesthesia occur in many conditions and can include:
    - those mimicking estrus (e.g., rolling),
    - biting at the tail, flank, anal, or lumbar areas, generally with barbering and/or self-mutilation, and

- skin rippling and muscle spasms or twitching (usually dorsally) often accompanied by vocalization, running/jumping (possibly escape behaviors), hallucinations, and self-directed aggression (ritualistic motor behavior).

Common Non-Specific Signs

- The presenting signs in hyperesthesia are related or subsequent to skin rippling on the dorsal neck and spine. This rippling can occur spontaneously or in response to any tactile stimulus (e.g., touch by a human or another animal, self-licking, brushing against a solid surface).
- Specific primary behaviors that are seen in many other conditions may include:
  - tail twitching,
  - dorsal skin rippling,
  - piloerection on dorsal spine,
  - muscle spasms on dorsum and flank, and
  - mydriasis often accompanies increased arousal.
- Secondary behaviors that may follow the primary behaviors (and, in some cases, may induce them) include:
  - vocalization (hissing, growling, meowing)—owners often report that the cat appears distressed, as if seeking something,
  - running/jumping (escape behaviors),
  - barbering,
  - rolling in a manner that may resemble estrus behaviors,
  - overt aggression in response to touch, re-directed aggression to self or others nearby, and
  - self-directed aggression (ritualistic motor behavior including licking, sucking, chewing, barbering, self-mutilation, and biting). It is this suite of behaviors that most likely meets the criteria for a diagnosis of OCD (Overall and Dunham, 2002).
- Clinical physical signs can include dermatological lesions (e.g., crusts, scales, scabs, pustules), barbered hair, sucked skin that may have hair loss and become erythematous, saliva staining, and regions where plucking or scratching are apparent.
- Clients should provide a history that includes age of onset of first event; behaviors involved; pattern of development of the condition including number, order, and extent of body regions involved; any correlating factors that trigger, worsen, or ameliorate the condition; and any interventions that disrupt the behavior, once initiated. Clinicians should be encouraged to use a standardized questionnaire or assessment tool to ensure that they are exploring all relevant aspects of the behavioral history in a manner that allows them to compare patients.

Rule Outs

- Trauma—current or historical
- At the broadest level, rule outs should include normal behaviors (e.g., estrus), dermatological (atopy/pruritus) conditions, and neurological conditions.

- Attention-seeking behavior and inappropriate play behavior may be concerns, especially if a description is provided by a novice cat client and the behaviors are not seen by the veterinarian.
- These behaviors could be a non-specific response to anxiety.

Etiology, Epidemiology, and Risk Groups

- Some genetic liability is likely present.
- Social and environmental stressors (e.g., new additions to household, alterations in schedules, moving house) may provoke the behaviors or more frequent incidence of them.
- Anxiety-related conditions are notoriously heterogeneous and vary depending on duration of condition (which likely alters neurochemical pathology) and brain regions recruited. Progress is being made in the rodent and human literature through investigations into effects of sensory stimulation.
- Processing and extent of sensory stimulation and/or its perception is key.
  - Arousal is associated with a cutaneous response generated by types 1 and 2 slow-adapting epidermal units.
  - Rate of discharge that is proportional to the amount of displacement of the hair or the indentation of the skin in cats.
  - Interactions of slow-adapting units with rapid-adapting units in the vibrissae around the face, lips, mouth, and guard hairs to generate the classic biting response that follows vibrissae stimulation in predatory situations.
  - Feline body and head posture affect mediation of responses through descending spinal tracts and may augment the duration and intensity of extensor activity.
  - Cutaneous and proprioceptive feedback interact to program the relative timing of flexor and extensor activity. In the fulminant form, these bouts resemble the classic chewing/aggression mediated by the ventromedial hypothalamus/amygdala.
  - Cholecystokinin B (central brain) receptors are involved in the firing of feline jaw musculature and so may affect the form of some of these behaviors that involve licking or biting (Singh et al., 1991).
  - Anxiety, pain, and pruritus are related at both the central level and the level of the dorsal horn of the spinal ganglion (see Fig. 9-27).
- Etiology is complex but doubtless involves numerous serotonin receptors.
  - There is now considerable evidence that nociception and anxiety affect the same serotonin receptors, especially the 5-HT_{1A} and 5-HT_{2A}, which is particularly important for peripheral nociception (Lanfumey et al., 2008).
  - Itch and pain also share peripheral and central pathways (Patel and Dong, 2010).

- Sensitization of a stimulus response to pain or itch is possible at both the peripheral and the central level and may involve endorphins, cytokines, histamine, nerve growth factor, and other receptors/neurotransmitters already discussed.
- There is virtually no research on feline hyperesthesia, so the extent to which social and environmental change and associated anxiety versus endogenous factors contribute to anxiety is unknown.
- In its full-blown form, feline hyperesthesia meets the diagnostic criteria for OCD/compulsive disorder (repetitive, stereotypic motor, locomotory, grooming, ingestive, or hallucinogenic behaviors that occur out of context to their "normal" occurrence or in a frequency or duration that is in excess of that required to accomplish the ostensible goal).
  - When this occurs, clients report that their cat is extremely focused in his response to the rippling and that it can be impossible to distract him from it. The behavior may cease only when the cat is exhausted, physically prevented from responding (e.g., wrapped in a blanket), or disrupted by a profound (and often startling) sensory change (e.g., being scooped up and put outside).
- Cats have an atypical response to arousal in general when their hypothalamus is stimulated.
  - Cats isolated from other cats for most of the first year of life exhibit a response characterized by galvanic skin responses and disruption of regular sleep rhythms.
  - Excitation of the VMH and amygdala leads to a defensive response in cats.
  - Stimulation of the lateral amygdala facilitates predatory attack and defensiveness in cats, but stimulation of the lateral amygdala using high intensity also recruits the ventral hippocampus in these behaviors, providing a partial explanation for why repetition is so problematic. The hippocampus plays a major role in associational learning.

Common Myths That Can Get in the Way of Treatment or Diagnosis

- Cats do weird things—that's the way they are.
  - Yes, cats are interesting animals. However, any time they engage in behaviors that cause them distress, potentially could injure themselves or others, or that result in a decreased QoL, we should question whether they need help. Every behavior that people consider odd and cat-like may not be normal.

Commonly Asked Client Questions

- Can this cat improve and become normal?
  - These are not the same questions.
    - All affected cats can improve—we are discussing the matter of the degree to which they can improve. Some cats will need medication for an extended period just to break through their

distress long enough to render them susceptible to learning an alternative way to live.
    - Some cats will become so happy and so free of their non-specific signs that people will think that they are "cured" or "normal." This is the second question. Unfortunately, these cats never become "normal." If we think about treatment in terms of the response surface for the individual cat, behavioral, environmental, and genetic factors all contribute to the outcome.
    - Some cats exhibit less profoundly affected behaviors, some have greater space for environmental intervention, and some have a greater degree of genetically based plasticity for learning new ways to cope and make their lives more predictable. This trifecta will help the cat look "normal." He will never be normal, and the clients must understand what this means.
    - Stressors could have profound effects on these cats, so if there is a social or physical disruption, the clients should expect to see some backsliding. Resiliency likely has genetic components, but using behavior modification we can teach resiliency by rewarding a range of alternative, acceptable responses.
- Will medication be lifelong?
  - Possibly.

Treatment

- Management:
  - *Recognizing, understanding, planning for, and managing stimuli that provoke hyperesthesia in the cat are essential steps in recovery.* This is especially true here because the extent to which the cat is aroused could pose a risk for human intervention.
    - Re-directed aggression has been seen when some clients try to stop the cat from licking, chewing, or biting/swatting at herself.
    - More commonly, the re-directed behavior is manifest as flight, but this is still a concern for clients.
  - This is a condition that is about patterns. The cats are using a failed rule structure to—ostensibly—help them cope with situations that, regardless of the level of the pathology, the cat finds distressing. We help the cat by substituting rules associated with relaxation and non-reactivity for rules that cause them to react and become distressed.
- Behavior modification:
  - In extreme cases where the behaviors are unremitting, it may be exceedingly difficult to engage in any behavior modification until the cat has experienced some relief from medication. This may mean that clients cannot begin to engage in active behavior modification for 3 to 5 weeks.
  - In such cases, clients should not think that they can do nothing. Instead, they should focus

intensely on any possible form of passive behavior modification.

- Having the cat learn to sit on cue or clicker training the cat to engage in a behavior that is incompatible with the hyperesthesia may help.
- Rewarding the cat when her arousal level is below that which triggers the hyperesthesia may be the most important part of treatment, but clients must be good observers with good timing.
- If possible, we want to teach the cat a behavior that competes with the hyperesthesia. Clients should be reminded that this type of intervention may not be possible until the medication has begun to take effect.
- Teach the cat some relaxed and distracting behaviors with conditioned responses. For example, the cat could be taught to lie on his side and then rear up in response to movement when he sees a feather on a pole.
- Early in the condition, clients may help cats to relax and take deep breaths by rewarding this behavior in response to long, slow, deep dorsal petting. Clients should be cautioned that such petting may act as a focus for aggression as the condition progresses.

- Medication/dietary intervention:
  - Medications that can be helpful in controlling the anxiety that drives OCD may include:
    - BZDs:
      - Alprazolam (especially useful if there are explosive components to the OCD and/or ones that are provoked by known triggers)
      - Clonazepam
      - Lorazepam (start low; be aware that with long half-life repeat dosages will be additive)
    - TCAs:
      - Most TCAs have some anti-pruritic effects and may help to alleviate pain.
      - Amitriptyline
      - Clomipramine (Overall and Dunham, 2002; Seksel and Lindemann, 1998)
      - Doxepin (H_1 antagonist—especially useful with dermatological manifestations; can be used in combination with other medications with care and reduced dosages) (start low—this is highly sedative in cats)
      - Nortriptyline
    - SSRIs:
      - Fluoxetine
      - Fluvoxamine
      - Paroxetine
      - Sertraline
    - SARIs (best use may be as an adjuvant medication with others that are more specific for other receptor classes)
      - Trazodone—dosage not established in cats but because the elimination half-life is three times that of dogs, cats may be effectively dosed every 3 days. Because trazodone affects the 5-HT 2A receptor it has particular resonance for noiception x anxiety conditions.
    - Other:
      - Gabapentin (especially useful if any neuropathic pain is involved but may be extremely helpful as a second or third medication to help address arousal and more global anxieties)
      - Memantine (a NMDA antagonist) has been efficacious as an adjuvant in OCD that resolves incompletely, suggesting that regulation of signal transduction pathways on more general levels may be useful.
- Miscellaneous interventions:
  - Re-directing the cat to a more suitable outlet for the particular behaviors may help (e.g., encourage the cat to chase a feather, not her back), but these are stop-gaps. The ease with which such re-direction is accomplished can serve as an index of improvement.
  - Massage may help because it is incompatible with virtually all OCDs and may be able to be worked into the behavior modification plan as a way of teaching the cat that he can have some control over his own behaviors. *Caution is urged for attempting this when the cat is at all aroused. Cat bites and scratches could result. Cat bites and scratches can be serious injuries.*

Helpful Handouts

- "Protocol for Understanding and Treating Obsessive-Compulsive Disorder (OCD)"
- "Protocol for Preventing and Treating Attention-Seeking Behavior"
- "Protocol for Using Behavioral Medication Successfully"
- "Protocol for Teaching Cats and Dogs to 'Sit,' 'Stay,' and 'Come'"

Last Words

- Clients should obtain videos of as many of the episodes as possible, including in the videos behaviors that precede and follow the events, if possible.
- A good physical examination is essential for all behavioral concerns. Depending on the dermatological/neurological findings, scrapings, radiographs, nerve conduction studies, et cetera, may be warranted.
  - *If self-mutilation and anxiety are involved, caution is urged for biopsy, unless there is a strong suspicion that it will be informative in a manner that alters treatment. Healing wounds often act as a focus for self-mutilation in these cats, which could worsen the condition.*

BEHAVIORAL CONCERNS THAT DO NOT RISE TO THE LEVEL OF A DIAGNOSIS BUT THAT STILL WORRY CLIENTS

As noted, clients do not intuitively understand cats. Many cat behaviors that have been unchanged as a result of their quasi-domesticated relationship with humans are puzzling to and scary for clients. The most common of these normal but annoying and/or scary behaviors are discussed in this section. There is an accompanying client handout that presents the same information in plain language for clients who love but are confused by their companions ("Protocol for Understanding Odd, Curious, and Annoying Feline Behaviors").

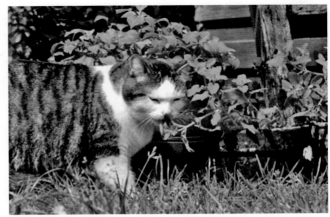

Fig. 9-28 Cat eating a mint grown especially for cats. (Photo courtesy of Anne Marie Dossche.)

Eating Plants

Most cats will eat plants if they have access. Cats appear to enjoy fresh grass. Whether this is due to a taste preference or whether the cats want or need the roughage is unknown. We know that roughage can be important and may help cats who become constipated. Adding fiber to a diet may help regulate some feline diabetics. Clients need to be reassured that eating plants is normal for cats, but they may need some direction about how to ensure cats eat safe plants.

The needs of cats who like and seek out plants to ingest can be met safely. Commercially available "grass gardens" can be grown indoors for cats. Certain herbs and mints will also grow indoors and are favored by many cats. Some aromatic plants may also act as anti-parasite agents, so their choice may be a healthy one.

Concerns about eating plants focus primarily on toxic issues. *Many houseplants (e.g., all lilies) are far more toxic to cats than they would be to dogs.* (Go to www.aspca.org/Pet-care/poison-control/plant-list-cats.aspx for more information.) Pesticides, chemicals used in lawn treatments, and fertilizers can also be toxic for cats, so if the clients are happy to have their cat eat plants, it may be best to grow plants especially for the cat (Fig. 9-28). If clients do not wish for their cats to experience the arousal effects of catnip, they may wish to grow other mints instead. Clients should be informed that the ability to respond to catnip is genetically determined. *If there are any social aggressions within the household, having a cat who responds to catnip with aroused behaviors may be problematic.*

Scratching Behavior

Cats scratch objects for two main reasons: (1) to remove the layered sheaths that comprise their claws and (2) to leave visual and olfactory marks. Similar to spraying, the act of scratching is also a behavior that is very obvious and can be seen by any watching cats. The scratches left by the behavior act a mark to inform other

cats who was there and when the tree was last scratched (Fig. 9-29).

The conventional wisdom regarding onychectomy is changing. In Canada, Australia, and most European nations, declaw is not considered a valid or legal veterinary procedure unless injury is involved (i.e., the procedure is done only when medically warranted). Most declaws in the United States are elective, meaning that there is not a medical reason for the procedure. Attitudes are changing in the United States, and more veterinarians, welfare groups, and veterinary groups now feel that declaw should be a last resort, not a first choice. *Were cats given their choice, they would never have their claws and the end segment of their toes surgically removed:* they would scratch in materials like tree trunks, lawns, fabric-like surfaces of peeled bark, et cetera. Removing the claws and a section of their toes doesn't alter the glandular secretions that are produced when cats scratch, so declawed cats can still leave the odorants associated with these glands and, in some cases, a visual residue.

Tenectomy prohibits flexion of the claw and so can modulate destructive scratching. Claws continue to grow and must be routinely trimmed, but the cat cannot extend the claws to scratch on furniture or other living things.

Pain can be involved with both of these procedures, but according to published reports tenectomy appears to have faster recovery and fewer long-term side effects (Jankowski et al., 1998; Cambridge et al., 2000; Romans et al., 2004). Long-term pain and discomfort is the exception, but only one good *behavioral* study has been done that compared cats' personal behaviors, activity, and interactions before and after declaw (Cloutier et al., 2005). Cloutier et al. suggest that tenectomy is not less painful than onychectomy, based on behavioral assays. As Jankowski et al. (1998) note, complications are common sequelae to both of these techniques. These studies strongly suggest that meeting the cat's needs is

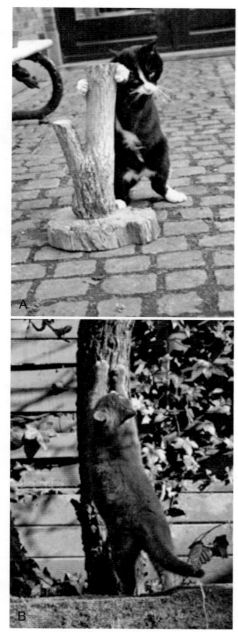

Fig. 9-29 The cat in **A** is using a "homemade" scratching post crafted from tree branches. The cat in **B** is using a real tree in the yard (**B**). (Photos courtesy of Anne Marie Dossche.)

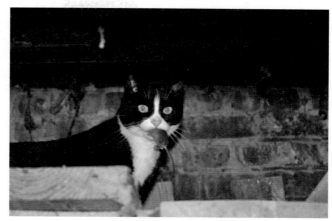

Fig. 9-30 A well-fed indoor/outdoor cat with a rodent he caught. (Photo courtesy of Anne Marie Dossche.)

a strategy that should come early in the decision-making process. Were this to be the case, surgical interventions could be exceptional.

Scratching on furniture can be done for either of the reasons cats commonly scratch, but it usually occurs because the fabric resembles the natural surfaces that the cat would otherwise seek out and/or the furniture is placed in a socially meaningful spot. Clients should be encouraged to provide all cats with appropriate scratching surfaces when they enter the household and encourage the cats to use them. Scratching is self-rewarding, but clients can further reward attentive behavior to the scratching post using food treats.

Hunting and Caching

Indoor/outdoor cats or outdoor cats may hunt (Fig. 9-30). Cats have to learn to hunt, and they are generally taught to do so by their mother. Starved cats can learn to hunt. Even well-fed cats will hunt if they are "hunters." They may or may not eat their prey. Cats often cache prey for later use. Were the cats free-ranging, this would be an adaptive behavior.

Hunting is an intellectual endeavor. The more clients are able to stimulate their cats using problem-solving activities, the less likely they are to hunt and provide clients with partial or complete corpses.

Clients should understand that cats eat one small meal multiple times per day, so rodents are the feline version of a boxed or "take-out" meal. The mental stimulation involved in this activity is not trivial. When we "meal feed" cats, they not only don't get to hunt, but also they get all their calories in one sitting. After they empty their dish, they have 23 hours and 55 minutes of their day to fill.

Cats fed dry food can be encouraged to mimic hunting behaviors by having all their food placed in treat balls: as the cats bat these, one or two pieces of kibble come out. Filling these with a tiny amount of food three to five times a day can mimic the native hunting behavior. If clients feed moist food, they can still create food puzzles by putting small amounts of food into holes in peg boards or into small Kongs and other washable food toys (Figs. 9-31 and 9-32). A cafeteria tray can be outfitted with small flower pots covering food or rocks and large pebbles that hide food. Clients should be encouraged to remember that although it is not bad that they find the toy esthetically appealing for design reasons, the cat must find it appealing for his or

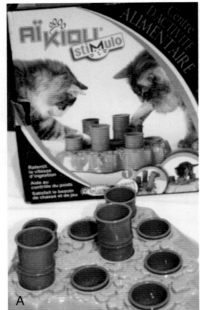

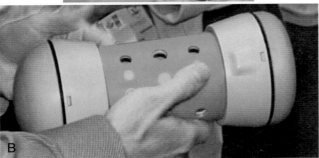

Fig. 9-31 Aïkiou toys for cats can be made simpler or harder by changing the feeding cup depth for the Stimulo (**A**) or the size of the holes for the Pipolino (**B**). The Pipolino is best for dry food, but the Stimulo can work for moist or dry food.

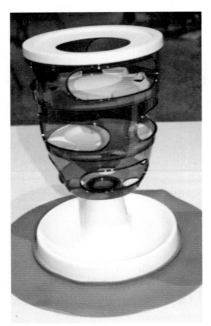

Fig. 9-32 A Catit food toy where access requires dexterity, and dry food can change position.

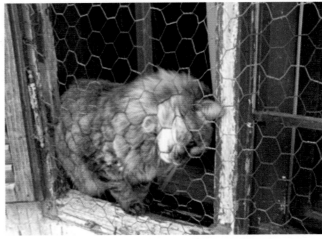

Fig. 9-33 A cat rubbing her cheeks and whiskers across a metal screen, which leaves behind some waxy secretions and odor.

her own reasons. If clients watch their cats, they will know which kinds of toys best stimulate them.

Clients should be aware that *hunting has wildlife conservation implications*. In many parts of the world, cats have been responsible for the extinction of native species. Many island species are particularly victimized, and large extermination programs are necessary to control the cat population if we are to have any wildlife left in these areas. More countries, provinces, states, and townships are legislating the extent to which cats are allowed to roam.

Rubbing

Cats rub people, cats, other animals, walls, and inanimate objects. Rubbing is a normal behavior that has tactile, social, and olfactory components. Cats rub when they are exhibiting "affiliative" behavior—these are behaviors associated with being close, with being in relaxed and friendly social circumstances.

Cats have large numbers of glands that secrete a volatile, waxy substance that is deposited by rubbing. These compounds likely differ depending on the region of the body, which may explain why certain patterns of rubbing seem to occur more frequently in some environments than others.

When cats rub against humans, they may rub with only their tail and their hind end, or they may "bunt." Bunting is the behavior where the cat pushes his head up into someone and rubs the area just in front of the ears across the individual being rubbed.

Cats will also rub the sides of their checks (Fig. 9-33), the area in front of the ears, and their chin on corners of walls or furniture. You can learn if your cat has been doing this by looking at hallways, entrances, et cetera, at cat height—you'll see the slightly waxy deposit. This behavior has created a market for "corner combs," devices that can be attached to edges of walls where cats can rub and groom their facial hair at the same time.

Cats will also move back and forth along edges while pressing the base of their tail and their rump against them. These are normal behaviors. When patterns of these marking behaviors begin to change, the change may indicate difficulties in the feline social environment. *Clients are unable to recognize when something changes without knowing what normal is. If veterinarians discuss watching their cats with them and have videos available to watch with clients, clients will be more compliant and helpful.*

Nocturnal Activity

Cats hunt alone and focus on animals that are awake at night (e.g., mice, voles, et cetera). Cats are innately much more nocturnal than we or dogs are. Cats do not have to swing from chandeliers at 2 AM, but if they are young, left alone all the time, and get little attention, clients will learn that the cats will be awake at night because it is the only time that they will get any attentions. Clients will benefit from getting detailed information from their veterinarian about how they can best meet their cat's age-specific needs. Such suggestions might include:

- playing games with the cat before the client goes to bed,
- getting another cat with the same playful temperament,
- having the cat play with a dog who likes cats,
- feeding the cat 1 to 2 hours or so before bed because cats often nap after eating,
- leash-walking cats,
- taking cats out in strollers, and
- clicker training cats to do specific tasks.

Roaming and Cat Enclosures

Roaming cats who defecate in neighbors' gardens are nuisances. The esthetic aspect is one problem; the public health aspect is more severe. Illness is a concern in areas where humans garden in soil in which cats have defecated or where children play in sandboxes used by cats. The soil or sand may harbor fecal parasites that can make humans ill, and toxocariasis is a serious concern in many urban and rural communities. This public health issue requires people who have cats to take responsibility for the actions of their pets (www.petsandparasites.org./cat-owners;www.cdc.gov /parasites/toxoplasmosis/gen_info/pregnant.html).

Veterinarians should remind the clients with cats that:

- Neutering cats renders them more likely to stay close to home and less likely to roam.

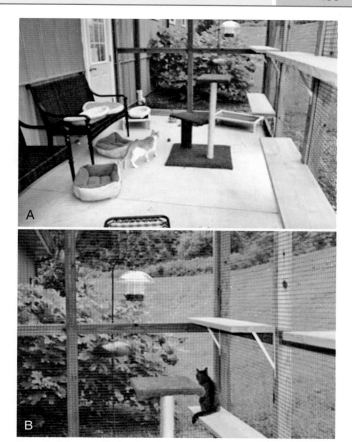

Fig. 9-34 A cat enclosure that humans can share. The cat pen is made from enclosing a concrete slab porch (**A**). This is a safe way for the cats to be outdoors and experience mental stimulation (**B**).

- Having an entertaining and stimulating environment at home will keep cats closer to home.
- Providing cats with physical exercise and mental stimulation will keep the cats closer to home.
- Keeping cats indoors can keep them safe, and they will live longer than outdoor cats.

If clients wish their cats to have outdoor exercise, cat enclosures (Fig. 9-34) may be the perfect solution for meeting the cat's needs. Custom-made enclosures are more commonly seen in Europe than in the United States, and they can be wonderful. These enclosures are made from various kinds of fencing and mesh, can be built into a window or a cat door, and can even be designed to include most of a tree so that the cats can see the birds but not snack on them (www.catsondeck.com, http://habitathaven.com, http://catnet.stanford.edu). Fencing additions can also restrict cats to their own yards safely and humanely (www.kittyfence.com, www.catfence.com, www.purrfectfence.com). These are two ways to bring the rich stimulation of the outside world to the indoor cat and make everyone happy while meeting the cat's needs.

Inappropriate Play Behavior

Although play aggression is a truly problematic and possibly pathological condition, inappropriate play behavior is a management-related problem. This concern is discussed in depth for clients in the handout "Protocol for Teaching Kids—and Adults—to Play with Dogs and Cats," but a short discussion may be helpful here.

Puppies and kittens, similar to young children, are energetic, can quickly progress to out-of-control and exhausted play, and make mistakes in both the objects and the intensity of their play behaviors. Kittens box and rear and pounce on each other as part of play, and because they lack opposable thumbs, they may grab people. If the kitten's tooth or claw is caught in the human's clothing, the cat may learn that fierce struggle frees them. If the clients think it is cute when a kitten acts fierce, the client may unintentionally reinforce inappropriate play behaviors. Some guidance from the veterinary staff can be useful.

Tackling, pawing, mounting, et cetera, by young animals *can be* acceptable *if* the client can (1) always stop the behavior by saying "no" or by withdrawing, (2) re-direct the behavior to another focus such as a toy, and (3) gently change the behavior so that it decreases in the future should the behavior be too rough.

If the animal's response to a gentle "correction" of standing up or withdrawal of your leg is to attack more forcefully, *a serious problem already exists, and we may be dealing with the first signs of play aggression.* It's possible that this behavior is a response to overly forceful behaviors on the part of the human. Clients should understand that appropriate correction for forceful tackles or pouncing includes stopping, saying "no," re-directing the animal's attention to a toy, and asking the cat to exhibit a more appropriate behavior. Preferred behaviors include sitting and waiting for a toy or being re-directed to pounce on a preferred object (Figs. 9-35 through 9-38). In each of the examples illustrated in

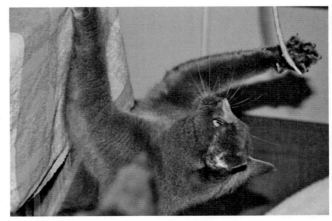

Fig. 9-36 A cat re-directed to chasing a shoelace, rather than the human who owns the laces (note that the cat has claws and they are fully extended). (Photo courtesy of Anne Marie Dossche.)

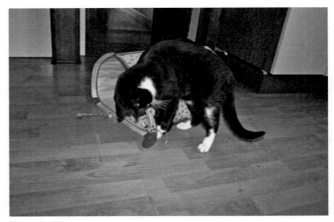

Fig. 9-37 A cat who captured his tossed catnip mouse. (Photo courtesy of Anne Marie Dossche.)

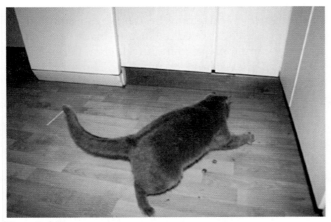

Fig. 9-35 A cat chasing hazelnuts that have been tossed across the floor to re-focus his attention. (Photo courtesy of Anne Marie Dossche.)

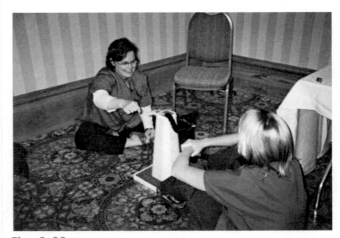

Fig. 9-38 Play with a rescue kitten using a toy and a hemp scratching post. Notice that this cat is very physical in the use of his paws and claws and that this mode of play keeps everyone safe, while encouraging the kitten to use his claws on the scratching post.

Figures 9-35 through 9-38, the cats are getting intellectual and physical exercise and humans are no longer at risk.

Clients must be told not to "correct" animals by swatting them in the face or thumping them on the rump. These human behaviors encourage cats to play more roughly or to be frightened. Clients should refrain from using "correctional" behaviors, including hanging a kitten by its scruff; rolling a dog over forcefully and lying on it while growling in its face; shaking a dog by the jowls, scruff, or neck; swatting a dog across the ears; slapping a dog under the chin, et cetera. If clients persist, examine the human household: rough treatment of animals is linked to rough treatment of humans. Ask yourself whether you need to have as a consultant in your practice a psychiatrist, psychologist, or social worker. The American Humane Association (AHA), the Humane Society of the United States (HSUS), and the Latham Foundation all have demonstrated that *child abuse and pet abuse are linked.* People who are abused as children will hone their abuse skills on their pets before continuing the cycle by abusing their own children. Pets that are abused may act as a red flag for child abuse.

The concepts of abuse and discipline are changing as we learn more about ourselves and our pets. Harsh punishment of pets may act as guides to other problems that we have not previously understood. More recent research shows that people who are best able to play and signal as dogs and cats would have the best relationship with their pets and report few behavioral complaints.

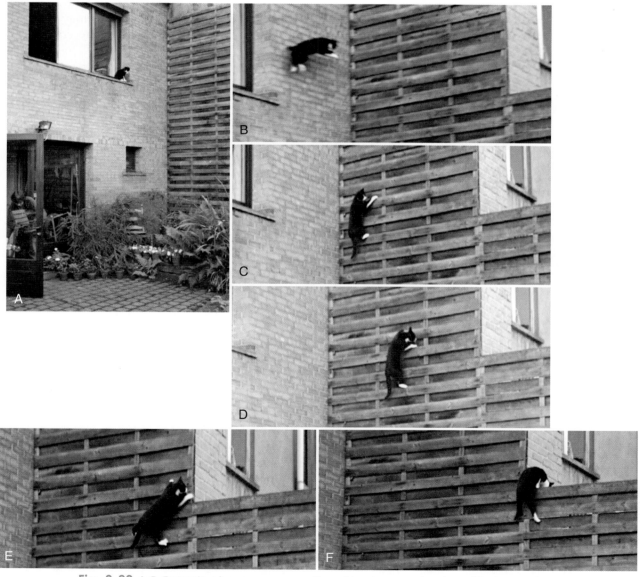

Fig. 9-39 **A-F,** Example of a young, energetic cat having an adventure. (Photos courtesy of Anne Marie Dossche.)

Overactivity

Clients, especially clients with young kittens, complain about overactivity. They may also complain about nocturnal activity, but these two sets of complaints are separated here to distinguish the clients with cats who stalk them, get in their way, crawl up curtains, swat at any paper that is being read, et cetera. Overactivity is best defined as motor activity that is in excess of that exhibited when the animal experiences a regular exercise and interaction schedule and that occurs in the absence of any signs of organic disease or true hyperactivity. *Overactivity resolves with increased aerobic activity and interaction.* Overactivity is a management-related "diagnosis" that is contingent on contexts that include the age of the cat, the age of the client, and the cat's social and physical environment. Overactivity in cats must be distinguished from attention-seeking behavior, inappropriate play behavior, and hyperactivity associated with disease (usually hyperthyroidism) in cats.

The perception of overactivity by a client may be the result of not understanding the cat's needs at all, which differs from the canine situation, where those needs are simply not met. If clients understood the extent to which cats are curious and active, they might have a better sense of why their cat was engaging in his chosen activities. Figure 9-39 shows a normal, healthy, young cat, who is bold and outgoing, having an adventure. If clients can learn to appreciate that these adventures are "normal" behaviors, they may be better mentally equipped to meet their cat's needs. Could someone living in an apartment recreate an environment such as the one shown in Figure 9-39, *A-F?* Yes. One wall of a garage or a study could be covered with burlap. The burlap could have ropes hanging from it and built-in platforms where plants could be anchored. Food could be hidden in pockets in wall. Interactive cat toys could be attached to the wall. The process of working through these concepts with clients may not result in any change in the behavior of the clients, but it might result in a greater understanding of cats and more curiosity on the part of the clients. Such discussions may lead to behaviorally healthier cats whose welfare and QoL needs are met.

Behavioral Supplements and Medications

CHAPTER 10

Pharmacological Approaches to Changing Behavior and Neurochemistry: Roles for Diet, Supplements, Nutraceuticals, and Medication

As diets and supplements become more sophisticated, the lines between "treating" a dog or cat and "supplementing" that same dog or cat are going to become more blurred. Because some of the supplements, nutraceuticals, and dietary ingredients have the potential to interact with medication, a modern, holistic approach to getting substances that may affect their behavior into patients is taken here. This chapter first addresses common questions and issues in the diet/supplement fields, with detailed discussions provided of more recent findings and new research foci (e.g., new energy source use that may help aging brains). The second part of the chapter focuses on medication.

After reviewing which medications are used and which neurochemical systems are involved, the focus here is on how specific medications work, with an emphasis that will allow the clinician to decide which drug is suitable for which patient based on risk of undesirable effects (usually called side effects) and hoped-for outcomes. Earlier chapters in this text focused on specific behavioral diagnoses and made medication recommendations based on data and suitability. Combined with the information in this chapter, the clinician should gain confidence in and understanding about the use of behavioral medications.

OVERVIEW OF DIET AND BEHAVIOR

Dietary composition has long been a focus for improving performance in working dogs, such as sled dogs, where fats have been used to provide sources of both calories and water. Diet continues to play a large role in the treatment of many medical conditions, including diabetes, cardiac disease, and renal disease, by helping to control substances that may exacerbate disease. For behavioral concerns, commercial dietary and dietary supplement strategies have largely focused on the role that anti-oxidants and related compounds can have for behavioral changes that occur with age. Substances that have been used as either supplements or additives

include, but may not be restricted to, the substances listed alphabetically in Table 10-1.

POTENTIAL ROLES FOR THE MOST COMMON DIETARY COMPOUNDS AND SUPPLEMENTS

The most common roles for compounds found in, or added to, diets fall into a few classes:
1. neuroprotective agents,
2. anti-oxidants, most of which should be neuroprotective,
3. reactive oxygen species (ROS)/free radical scavengers, most of which should be neuroprotective,
4. precursor neurochemicals, which are postulated to affect the behaviors associated with the neurochemical of interest with the intent to enhance cognition or decrease reactivity,
5. enzymes, co-enzymes, or co-factors for some aspect of Kreb's cycle function or neurochemical production, and
6. sources of energy for brain metabolism for enhanced cognition and neuroprotection.

These compounds are united by their contributions to the maintenance of cellular metabolism and to efficient neuron-to-neuron communication, processes essential to keeping brain neurons plump, healthy, and functional.

PRECURSOR NEUROCHEMICALS THAT POSSIBLY AFFECT BEHAVIORS ASSOCIATED WITH SPECIFIC NEUROCHEMICALS

Tryptophan

Our understanding of dietary effects on behavior is nascent. One of the most controversial dietary supplements is tryptophan, which is a precursor to serotonin (tryptophan → 5-hydroxy-L-tryptophan [5-HTP] → serotonin/5-hydroxytryptamine [5-HT]) and an

458

TABLE 10-1

Putative Dietary Substances with Behavioral Effects and Presumptive Effects

Substance	Presumptive Effect
Acetate	Brain energy source
Alpha-lipoic acid	Free radical scavenger and co-factor for mitochondrial respiratory chain enzymes (redox reactions that would recycle other anti-oxidants and increase glutathione)
Arachidonic acid	Essential fatty acid; maintains hippocampal cell membrane fluidity and protects from oxidative stress
Carotenoids (alpha-, beta-, and cys-beta-carotene, lutein, zeaxanthine, alpha-cryptoxanthine, lycopene, cis-lycopene)	Anti-oxidant and generalized neuroprotective agents
Chondroitin sulfate	Chondroprotective agents
Cod liver oil	Anti-oxidant and neuroprotective agent
Co-enzyme Q/co-enzyme Q10	Provides cellular energy by generating it on the inner mitochondrial membrane
D-Alpha-tocopherol (vitamin E)	Anti-oxidant and neuroprotective agent ("natural" form)
Docosahexaenoic acid	Long-chain polyunsaturated fatty acid integral to brain membrane development and integrity and to neurodevelopment; may have direct effect on learning ability, especially during development; essential for the development of the brain and retina in dogs
Eicosapentaenoic acid	Long-chain polyunsaturated fatty acid integral to brain membrane development and integrity and to neurodevelopment
Essential fatty acids	Examples: docosahexaenoic acid, eicosapentaenoic acid, arachidonic acid
Ginkgo biloba	Anti-oxidant with postulated cerebrovascular metabolism effects
Glutamate	Brain energy source and excitatory amino acid that is responsible for much neuron-neuron communication
Insulin-like growth factor-I	Control of brain energy expenditure and neuronal plasticity with concomitant neuroprotective effects
L-Carnitine	Precursor to acetyl-L-carnitine involved in mitochondrial function
L-Theanine (5-N-ethyl-L-glutamine)	Psychoactive agent that appears to affect GABA synthesis; may affect other neurochemicals
Long-chain polyunsaturated fatty acids	Anti-oxidant and neuroprotective agents
N-acetyl cysteine—precursor to glutathione	Free radical/reactive oxygen species scavenger
Phosphatidylserine	Constituent of neuronal membranes that affects plasma membrane functionality
Pyroxidine (vitamin B_6)	Co-enzyme for neurotransmitters including serotonin
Resveratrol (polyphenolic compound from grape skins)	Free radical scavenger
Salmon oil	Omega fatty acids
Selenium	Trace element with neuroprotective properties
Tryptophan	Precursor neurochemical
Vitamin C	Free radical scavenger and required for maintaining oxidative protection in soluble cell phases

essential amino acid (AA) in humans. Of the essential AAs—arginine, histidine, methionine, threonine, valine, isoleucine, phenylalanine, tryptophan, leucine, and lysine—arginine and histidine have also received a lot of attention because they are thought to be essential during growth, a period of high anabolic activity (Bosch et al., 2007).

Studies in rodents, humans, and pigs suggest tryptophan may affect behavior but not always in the desired direction. Pigs fed diets supplemented with tryptophan have been reported to experience better recovery from stressful situations (Koopmans et al., 2005). Horses fed diets supplemented with tryptophan and then isolated showed increases in motor activity and heart rates compared with horses not receiving supplements (Bagshaw et al., 1994). Rats fed diets high in tryptophan have been reported to decrease killing of mice (Chamberlain et al., 1987) and to recover better from stressors (Dunn, 1988), but increased tryptophan has been associated with increased aggression in male mice who are territorial (Lasley and Thurmond, 1985). The finding that humans who are depressed have lower tryptophan concentrations compared with humans who are not depressed led to the hypothesis that because stressors initially decrease serotonin turnover, precursor AA may be depleted, which could contribute further to decreases in serotonin (Branchey et al., 1984). Were this true, supplementation with tryptophan may be beneficial.

As a result, tryptophan has been suggested as a nonspecific treatment or preventive for "aggressive" behavior based on its potential neuromodulatory effects on serotonin. The results from the literature are not as clear as one would hope. Numerous factors affect whether there is a detectable effect of tryptophan in laboratory and clinical studies, and the first and possibly most important of these is the innate metabolism of tryptophan.

Tryptophan is one of three members of a group of aromatic AAs—tryptophan, tyrosine, and phenylalanine—that are precursors in the biosynthetic pathway for the neurotransmitters serotonin, dopamine, and norepinephrine (NE) (Table 10-2). The amount and timing of food intake, composition of diet, and overall digestibility of the diet all affect availability of these AAs (Bosch et al., 2007). Aromatic AAs are postulated to affect brain function, which requires that the food ingested alters the level of these AAs in the brain, but not all tryptophan is equally available.

Only very small molecules cross the blood-brain barrier (BBB), and for any AA to have an effect on behavior it must cross the BBB. Tryptophan is a relatively small molecule, but whether it crosses the BBB depends on the relative availability, the availability of the appropriate carrier, and the extent to which the tryptophan remains protein bound in the serum. To make matters more complex, factors pertaining to the

TABLE 10-2

Precursor Amino Acids and Neurotransmitter Pathways That They Affect

Precursor Amino Acids	Neurotransmitter Pathway Effects
Tryptophan	tryptophan → 5-HTP → serotonin → melatonin
	tryptophan →5-HTP→serotonin→5-HIAA
	tryptophan → N'-formylkynurenine → kynurenine → 2-amino-3-(3-oxoprop-1-enyl)-fumaric acid → quinolinate → niacin (vitamin B_3)
Tyrosine	phenylalanine → tyrosine → DOPA → dopamine → norepinephrine → epinephrine
Phenylalanine	phenylalanine → tyrosine → DOPA → dopamine → norepinephrine → epinephrine

DOPA, Dihydroxyphenylalanine; 5-HIAA, 5-hydroxyindoleacetic acid; 5-HTP, 5-hydroxy-L-tryptophan.

patient including, but likely not restricted to, breed, sex, age, activity level, social status, and arousal level all affect metabolism and transport of tryptophan across the BBB, whereas composition of the diet is responsible for availability of dietary tryptophan (Bosch et al., 2007).

Relative Availability of Tryptophan
As noted, the extent to which tryptophan is available depends on the diet. Tryptophan is found in most protein-containing foods, but its *relative availability* depends on the other AAs present. Large neutral AAs that may affect accessibility of tryptophan include phenylalanine (an AA and neurotransmitter thought to affect affiliative social behavior), leucine, isoleucine, valine, and tyrosine (a precursor in the synthesis of dopamine and NE [tyrosine → dihydroxyphenylalanine → dopamine → NE]). High-protein meals generally increase tyrosine concentrations in the brain but decrease concentrations of tryptophan (Bosch et al., 2007; Leathwood, 1987).

Availability of an Appropriate Carrier
Gaining access to the brain across the BBB requires a *carrier*, and all large neutral AAs share the same carrier. Because tryptophan is usually present in small concentrations in most dietary proteins, increasing dietary protein may actually decrease the ratio of tryptophan to other large neutral AAs because other large neutral AAs are preferentially transported by the carrier.

Extent of Protein Binding in Serum
Tryptophan is also *highly bound* to albumin (80% to 90% of all blood tryptophan is bound to serum albumin), so

any process that affects either bound or unbound tryptophan can affect tryptophan availability for neurons in the brain. Both bound and unbound tryptophan can be available to brain neurons, but *none of the transmission processes appear to be strictly linear with diet*. One concern is uptake into peripheral tissues. For example, elevations in insulin owing to carbohydrate ingestion facilitate the uptake of large neutral AAs into skeletal muscle but not of tryptophan that is bound to albumin, and so the *relative* amount of tryptophan available to be transported increases because the ratio of tryptophan to large neutral AAs increases. However, very small increases in overall protein in a meal (2% to 4% by weight) can prevent availability of this tryptophan to central nervous system neurons.

Whether increased protein—or supplementation using tryptophan itself—has an effect on the amount of serotonin produced in the neurons depends on how efficient the regulation of the synthesis and recycling components of central nervous system neurons is. Studies show that in normal/unstressed animals, tryptophan supplementation appears not to make a difference in behavior. Even in some forms of stress-related behavior, no effect of supplementation has been seen (Bosch et al., 2007).

When some effects of tryptophan supplementation are found, they tend to be non-specific (e.g., less exploratory behavior). If exploratory behavior decreases, but activity does not (as has been the case in many studies), there may have been a change in the *form* of anxiety measured, without affecting the *amount* of anxiety measured (Janczak et al., 2003). Clients attempting supplementation should be aware of this finding because a change in the way the anxiety is shown or conveyed may not be an improvement from the dog's or cat's perspective.

In the published studies focusing on combined tryptophan and protein supplementation in dogs, the effects noted may be non-specific effects of changes in locomotor behavior and not qualitative shifts in the behaviors about which people are usually concerned (DeNapoli et al., 2000; Dodman et al., 1996). For example, if an aggressive dog moves around more on one diet than another, we may have altered the probability that he will encounter a stimulus that will encourage his aggression, rather than altering the aggressive response itself. Clients should be aware that *although altering the probability of encountering provocative situations may be helpful, supplementation does not seem to affect the actual behaviors once the dog reacts.*

One rigorous study that demonstrated an increase in plasma tryptophan by 2.6 times with supplementation failed to show behavioral changes attributable to this treatment in privately owned, mildly anxious pet dogs over the 8 weeks of the study (Bosch et al., 2009). In this study, plasma tryptophan levels were increased by 37.4%, and the tryptophan ratio with large neutral AAs was increased by 32.2%, levels theoretically sufficient to engender a possible effect.

The best evidence for the effect of tryptophan for modulating non-specific aggressive responses via serotonin metabolism may come from experimentally induced tryptophan depletion. In studies where tryptophan is "depleted" (an artificial and incredibly difficult situation to produce), rodents and humans become "aggressive" in situations in which they otherwise would have been non-reactive (Bell et al., 2011). This extreme laboratory result may have limited application to the real world.

Tryptophan has been used as an ancillary, potentiating treatment in human patients taking monoamine oxidase (MAO) inhibitors for the treatment of depression. The effects of clomipramine (a tricyclic antidepressant [TCA]) and paroxetine (a selective serotonin reuptake inhibitor [SSRI]) are altered with reduced tryptophan levels, but medications primarily affecting the reuptake of NE are not. For this reason, tryptophan has sometimes been added to some psychotropic medications in humans in the hope of converting a non-responder to a responder. Outcomes have not been dramatic. There is an absence of rigorous, peer-reviewed literature on this subject in dogs or cats.

Metabolism of tryptophan is also informative when considering supplementation. Indoleamine 2,3-dioxygenase (IDO) and tryptophan 2,3-dioxygenase (TDO) degrade tryptophan. IDO is responsible for converting tryptophan into kynurenine. TDO is specific to the liver and regulates circulating levels of tryptophan (Turner et al., 2006).

Both IDO and TDO are stimulated by pro-inflammatory cytokines, which make less tryptophan available for conversion into 5-HTP and serotonin. Corticoids also induce TDO (Salter and Pogson, 1985), lowering tryptophan levels, which is one possible mechanism for the adverse changes in behavior (e.g., greater reactivity) that can occur when some patients are treated with corticosteroids (Notari and Mills, 2011). Depressed human patients often can have increased cortisol levels (Porter et al., 2004) and so may have lowered serotonin levels as a result of the effect cortisol has on increasing TDO, which then lowers tryptophan, 5-HTP, and serotonin. Finally, at concentrations in excess of those found in normal physiology, tryptophan itself induces TDO and/or IDO, so increased dietary intake may not cause increases in either tryptophan or its derivative neurochemicals (Turner et al., 2006).

Administration of exogenous tryptophan is not risk-free. Side effects can include eosinophilia and myalgia, followed by progressive myopathy and neuropathy. Tryptophan supplementation has been associated with conditions involving fibrosis. Pancreatic atrophy has also been reported in patients given tryptophan supplementation. Tryptophan is the most potent AA in stimulating pancreatic synthesis in dogs.

Roles for Other Amino Acids in Neurotransmission

Glutamate and aspartate are acidic AAs that act as neurotransmitters, but they are not readily available to the brain through diet even though they are almost ubiquitous in proteinaceous foods. The same is *not* true for additives such as monosodium glutamate and aspartame (which contains the AA aspartate), which have been noted to affect brain neurochemical function.

STRUCTURE OF NEURONAL MEMBRANES AND POTENTIAL ROLES FOR SUPPLEMENTS AND DIET

Arachidonic acid (ARA), docosahexaenoic acid (DHA), and eicosahexaenoic acid (EHA) are long-chain polyunsaturated fatty acids (PUFAs) that are essential for developing and maintaining the integrity of cells of the brain's membranes. These PUFAs are related by their synthetic sequence: linoleic acid (18:2n-6) < ARA (20:4n-6) < docosapentaenoic acid (22:5n-6). Elongation of alpha-linoleic acid produces eicosapentaenoic acid (EPA) (20:5n-3) < DHA (22:6n-3) (Bosch et al., 2007).

All of these PUFAs are essential for early brain development. ARA is thought especially to maintain hippocampal cell membrane fluidity and protect cells in the hippocampus from oxidative stress. The hippocampus is one of the main areas involved in long-term potentiation (LTP), a form of molecular learning, and is one of the main regions where associational learning takes place.

DHA may encourage development stage–specific associational learning, although the data are mixed (Fahey et al., 2008). Supplementation with DHA and EPA affects concentration of these substances in rat brains, and their distribution is not uniform. Diets deficient in alpha-linoleic acid especially cause decreases of DHA in the frontal cortex—the part of the brain responsible for complex learning and integration of information and executive function. In dogs, low concentrations of DHA during gestation and/or lactation depress the retinal sensitivity of puppies, which can have profound and complex behavioral outcomes. *The current data support the need for DHA for optimal neurological development in puppies, and there are hints that it may improve both early and long-term cognitive abilities, but the data are scant.*

It has been suggested that PUFAs are also important in some canine behavioral conditions. In one study of German shepherd dogs with a history of aggressive behavior, aggressive dogs showed a significantly lower concentration of DHA (22:6n-3) and a higher omega-6/omega-3 ratio compared with unaffected dogs (Re et al., 2008). Plasma concentrations of ARA (20:4 n-6) and EPA (20:5 n-3) did not differ. These same animals showed reduced levels of cholesterol compared with control dogs. Similar, non-specific findings regarding cholesterol have been reported for aggressive dogs (Sentürk and Yalçin, 2003). It is important to realize that the characterization of "aggression" in these studies is variable and that such correlations say nothing about cause. Such findings could be the outcome of aberrant neurochemical function. However, one of the main roles for PUFAs appears to be maintenance of membrane fluidity and protection from oxidative stress, especially in the part of the brain essential to associational learning, the hippocampus.

Finally, in humans, the brain contains 600 g lipid/kg, with approximately equal amounts of ARA and DHA. It's been postulated that a dietary intake of Rift Valley lake fish and shellfish comprising 6% to 12% protein provided sufficient DHA and ARA that allowed the early hominoid cerebral cortex to grow disproportionately larger without requiring an increase in body mass (Broadhurst et al., 1998). Any putative effects of these PUFAs on cognitive abilities are likely routed in this evolutionary history. PUFA levels in brains of young versus geriatric dogs, when measured, have not been shown to be different (Swanson et al., 2009), but effects of varying amounts in different regions of the brain (e.g., the hippocampus, which is key to learning, and the frontal cortex, which is involved in learning and is essential for executive function or application of that learning) in older animals have not been studied, the beneficial effects of ARA on membrane fluidity in the hippocampus notwithstanding.

NEUROPROTECTIVE AGENTS

As the canine population has aged, thanks to much improved and regular, lifelong veterinary care, changes in brain function have become apparent as part of what is often called "cognitive dysfunction syndrome." Not all dementias in humans are due to Alzheimer's disease or even to tauopathies (of which Alzheimer's disease is but one form), so we should be mindful that not all cognitive dysfunction syndrome will be due to the same underlying pathology. Some cognitive dysfunction syndrome may be due to vascular and blood flow changes. There has been a small explosion in studies investigating the value of free radical scavengers, neuroprotective agents, and anti-oxidants and, more recently, studies investigating sources of brain energy that could be compromised because of vascular deficits.

Regardless of the mechanism involved, all degenerative brain changes result in smaller neurons and ones less likely to undergo communication with each other with resultant second messenger system–dependent neurotrophic changes. Treatments augmenting brain energy and treatments using neuroprotectants both seek to keep cells lush and vibrant and to keep intracellular signaling systems intact and efficient. If this can be done, receptors will continue to talk to each other, cells will fire, and memory and cognition have a greater chance of remaining intact.

NUTRITIONAL REDRESS OF OXIDATIVE STRESS

One of the major foci of age-related and illness-related changes is the effect of a cumulative burden of oxidative stress over time. Increased oxidative stress is one of the most common topics examined in brain aging, and it appears to affect all major classes of molecules involved in neurotransmission. Development of oxidative stress may not be independent of energy source or use (see section on energy sources, p. 464).

Intermittent fasting has been reported to induce the production of brain-derived neurotrophic factor (BDNF), which is associated with neurogenesis and molecular learning and memory, particularly in the hippocampus. Increases in BDNF affect numerous signaling pathways involving tyrosine kinase B (trkB), which may directly or indirectly affect regional brain metabolism and function. Production of BDNF may also be encouraged by various anti-oxidants and free radical scavengers that are now found in may prescription diets for old animals (e.g., Hill's B/D) and in many of the supplements currently available (e.g., Aktivait, Senelife).

Effects for enhancement are pronounced in the regions of the brain associated with making and consolidating associational memories—the hippocampus and the cerebral cortex. Anti-oxidants improve cognitive performance on memory tests for old dogs, but not young dogs (Cotman et al., 2002; Siwak et al., 2005). Data from the brains of both old dogs and old rodents show that dietary enhancements using anti-oxidants appear to work best when they are accompanied by cognitive enhancement that is an intensive part of the daily routine (Milgram et al., 2002, 2004; Nippak et al., 2007; Opii et al., 2008; Roudebush et al., 2005; Siwak et al., 2005; Wedekind et al., 2002). For young dogs, such enhancement may be ongoing because of their activity levels. As activity levels wane, old dogs may be more at risk for cognitive degeneration associated with a lack of stimulation of complex social tasks and problem solving. We overlook such effects all the time in patients, and part of routine exams should be to assess the cognitive stimulation and exercise available to the patient.

Astrocytes are responsible for *de novo* synthesis of two neurotransmitters: glutamate and D-serine (Dienel and Cruz, 2006). Glutamate, the excitatory neurotransmitter that is responsible for an estimated 85% of synaptic activity, appears also to be essential in metabolic activity of the brain. Glutamate may be responsible for energy regulation by affecting neurovascular exchange (Magistretti, 2009). Glutamate has as its signaling targets the synapse, astrocytes, and intra-parenchymal capillaries.

In normal brain function, glutamate effects its signaling by altering flow of calcium and sodium ions. Postsynaptically, it modifies the permeability of N-methyl-D-aspartic acid (NMDA) receptors to sodium and calcium and the alpha-amino-5-hydroxy-3-methyl-4-isoxazole propionic acid (AMPA) receptors to sodium; presynaptically, it affects NMDA receptors and metabotropic receptors via calcium. This interaction is what causes an excitatory postsynaptic potential. Glutamate activity is also thought to be involved in pathological conditions in which excitatory sensitivity has been implicated (e.g., strokes, impulsively aggressive states, cortical and hippocampal epileptogenic activity). In both normal and pathological conditions, the main effect of glutamate is on excitability and synaptic plasticity.

Glutamate also affects astrocytes, which are non-neuronal cells (Magistretti, 2009). Glutamate transporters appear to use the sodium gradient to facilitate glutamate uptake by astrocytes. More recent anatomical studies show that astrocytic processes ensheath intra-parenchymal capillaries and synapses and that many of these processes have receptors and reuptake sites for neurotransmitters. It is these findings that allow glutamate to act as a metabolic intermediary. In short, glutamate stimulates the conversion of glucose into lactate in astrocytes.

Many pathways that affect glycolysis for brain energy are also adversely affected at some point by oxidative change. Many of these effects may be modulated by anti-oxidant or co-factor treatment, coupled with active behavioral interventions/enrichment. Alpha-enolase inter-converts 2-phosphoglycerate and phosphoenolpyruvate. Alpha-enolase has been shown to be altered in canine models of neurodegenerative disorders and responds to treatment with anti-oxidants, mitochondrial co-factors (lipoic acid), and behavioral/social/cognitive enrichment (Opii et al., 2008). Decreased oxidation of alpha-enolase and glyceraldehyde-3-phosphate dehydrogenase could improve glycolytic function, with a resultant increase in adenosine triphosphate (ATP) production. Together, these alterations appear to lead to neuronal recovery and improved cognitive function in the canine model of human brain aging (Opii et al., 2008).

In a study of gene expression in brains of old dogs, the expression of genes involved in neurochemical signaling and synaptic transmission was decreased (Swanson et al., 2009). Particularly affected were levels of growth and transmission factors already discussed, including BDNF and trkB. These factors did not respond to anti-oxidant diet supplementation. In the same study, compounds such as glutathione S-transferase—responders to oxidative stress—were also decreased in geriatric dogs. Such findings show the ultimate inter-relatedness of available brain energy, neurotransmission, and neuroregulator function and structural changes in aging dogs.

EMERGING ROLE FOR BRAIN ENERGY IN COGNITIVE FUNCTION IN DOGS

Diet can affect behavior through chemical interactions between AAs and by altering brain energy sources, allowing alterations in use of resources. Energy sources for the brain can be variable, and lactate, acetate, and pyruvic acid are now considered viable energy sources, in addition to what has traditionally been considered the main energy source, glucose.

Glucose is considered the common brain energy currency, but it is not stored. The stored form of glucose is glycogen. Glycogen is found mainly in astrocytes, and the amount of glycogen available is affected by glucose concentration and neurotransmitter presence and function (Brown and Ransom, 2007; Pellerin et al., 2007). During hypoglycemia, glycogen is converted to lactate via pyruvate (glucose → pyruvate → lactate). The lactate is transferred to adjacent neurons. This conversion and transfer allow the neurons to use a source of aerobic fuel.

Glycolysis can also be anaerobic and is faster at producing energy than oxidative phosphorylation (Raichle and Minton, 2006). In fact, glycolysis makes pyruvate faster than it can be oxidized: by converting glucose to lactate, ATP is made twice as fast than would be the case were glucose oxidized completely.

Lactate

The use of lactate in hypoglycemic events can extend axon functions for 20 minutes or longer (Pellerin et al., 2007). This conversion of astrocyte glycogen to lactate also occurs during periods of intense neural activity, demonstrating the role of astrocytes as bankers of energy-conversion compounds.

After glucose, lactate is the preferred energy source for the human brain (van Hall et al., 2009), and there is no reason to assume that this may not also be an important pattern in dogs. Most lactate used as an energy source is thought to come from glycogenic processes because most lactate is too large a molecule to pass through the BBB. However, blood lactate has been measured in oxidized form and may be a source of some energy for brain tissue. Some astrocytes appear to "prefer" to process glucose glycolytically into lactate (Magistretti, 2009). Lactate can then be converted into pyruvate and enter the tricarboxylic acid cycle, providing energy in the form of ATP.

Medium-Chain Triglycerides

Ketone bodies and fatty acids have been proposed as alternative energy sources because of their modulating effects on hypoglycemia. 8-Hydroxybutyrate (8-OHB), in particular, may be useful for protecting hippocampal neurons from toxicity (Reger et al., 2004). A placebo-controlled, double-blind study found that patients with Alzheimer disease with mild impairment who were supplemented with medium-chain triglycerides (MCT) showed improvement in a number of pre-treatment versus post-treatment cognitive test measures and that such improvement correlated with 8-OHB increases. It should be noted that this result depended on the apo-lipoprotein E (APOE) genotype: only patients without an APOE-epsilon4 allele responded to acute elevation of 8-OHB. Assessment of genetic risk factors has not been pursued in dogs, which, because of the presence of breeds, may be rich sources for such information.

Fatty acid oxidation in the brain has been studied in rats using nuclear magnetic resonance spectroscopy (NMRS). One of the MCTs, octanoate, is thought to constitute up to 13% of the free fatty acid pool in humans. Because it readily crosses the BBB, it has been studied in a variety of clinical and experimental settings. In a labeling study in rats subjected to NMRS, octanoate could contribute 20% of brain energy in an intact, physiological system (Ebert et al., 2003). The mechanism for this change in brain energy balance was likely incorporation into both glucose and ketones and secondary effects on the metabolism of the excitatory neurotransmitter, glutamate.

In a study of eight beagles (four in a control group and four in a treatment group) 9 to 11 years of age, supplementation with MCT at a dosage of 2 g/kg/day resulted in improved mitochondrial function, which was most pronounced in the parietal lobe (Studzinski et al., 2008). Steady-state levels of amyloid precursor protein also decreased in the parietal lobe after short-term supplementation leading the authors to conclude that short-term MCT supplementation can improve brain energy metabolism and decrease amyloid precursor protein levels in old dogs.

Age-related cognitive decline in dogs may be associated with decreases in omega-3 PUFAs in the brain. Because MCTs increase fatty acid oxidation, they may increase omega-3 PUFAs in the brain via metabolism of adipose tissue. In a 2-month study of eight beagles (four in a control group and four in a treatment group) fed an MCT-enriched diet (EN Purina Veterinary Diet), enrichment was shown to result in increases in brain phospholipid and total lipid concentrations.

SUPPLEMENTS

Aktivait

The nutritional supplement Aktivait (VetPlus Ltd; available online but not in the United States) contains a number of anti-oxidants and free radical scavengers. The listed components are *N*-acetyl cysteine, alpha-lipoic acid, vitamins C and E, L-carnitine, co-enzyme Q10, phosphatidylserine, selenium, DHA, and EPA. The supplement Senilife (CEVA/Sanofe) contains phosphatidylserine and *Ginkgo biloba*. Phosphatidylserine appears to be important for neuronal membrane stability and function (Osella et al., 2008) and has been shown to improve learning and memory test outcomes in rodents in a dose-dependent manner (Suzuki et al., 2001) and in aged beagles (Araujo et al., 2008).

In one trial of Aktivait involving 24 control dogs and 20 dogs who met the inclusion criteria for cognitive dysfunction syndrome (the dogs had to be >8 years of age and show some signs of disorientation associated with signs of either alterations in social interaction or changes in sleep/wake cycle or alterations in house soiling incidents), there was a significant difference between placebo and treatment groups. The largest effects were found for improvement in disorientation, interaction, and house soiling scores (Heath et al., 2007).

Trials of individual components must be interpreted cautiously. In one study that supplemented acetyl-L-carnitine and alpha-lipoic acid, a decrease in the number of errors for learning a new task was noted, but there was no effect for variable delay versions of standard spatial memory tasks in laboratory dogs (Milgram et al., 2005). Tests of single or paired components of supplements for spatial learning have been disappointing (Christie et al., 2010), so the mechanism by which supplements may work is still unclear.

What is clear is that the best effects of anti-oxidant diets and supplements is found when they are given to patients who also have increased physical and cognitive exercise (Cotman et al., 2007; Fahnestock et al., 2012; Head et al., 2009; Siwak-Tapp et al., 2008) suggesting that inflammation and components in the inflammatory cascade may also be involved in brain aging (Cotman et al., 2007). Similar to humans and rodents, old dogs show increased expression of genes associated with inflammation and stress response and decreased expression of genes associated with neuropeptide signaling and synaptic transmission (Swanson et al., 2009). We should expect dietary interventions and supplements to address and test relevant interventions that could affect inflammation and expression of genes involved in inflammatory/stress responses in a preventive manner.

Novifit

NOVIFIT (NoviSAMe, Virbac) is *S*-adenosyl-L-methionine (SAMe). One study showed improvements in social interactions, disorientation, and changes in sleep-wake cycles in dogs with mild to moderate cognitive dysfunction syndrome (Remé et al., 2008). The side effects of these supplements appear minimal, suggesting that there will be future market expansion both as independent supplements and as constituents of specially targeted diets. The unexplored role for such supplements is as protectants for the neurochemical stress experienced by patients with behavioral problems and preventive agents for age-associated neurophysiological assaults.

Melatonin

Melatonin is often offered as a "safe," over-the-counter alternative to behavioral medications. Melatonin (*N*-acetyl-5-methoxytryptamine) is synthesized from serotonin in the pineal gland, which is largely responsible for diurnal hormonal and physiological responses associated with sleep-wake cycles. Melatonin has been shown to inhibit TDO competitively (Turner et al., 2006) and, independent of its effects on TDO, may stimulate pro-inflammatory cytokines. Both of these effects of melatonin ultimately lead to a decrease in the biosynthesis of 5-HTP and serotonin. Melatonin is also an anti-oxidant that easily crosses the BBB, and it may act as a ROS scavenger. It also appears to prohibit the organization of β-amyloid into neurofibrillary tangles, but clinical data are lacking.

5-Hydroxy-L-tryptophan

5-HTP is an over-the-counter supplement that readily crosses the BBB and is converted to serotonin. It has a relatively short half-life (approximately 4 hours) and an even shorter time to maximum concentration (1 to 2 hours) in humans, times that are likely to be similar or less in dogs. Because 5-HTP is so readily available to be converted to serotonin, serotonin syndrome is a risk, and serotonin syndrome has been reported in rodents at dosages of 5-HTP of 100 to 200 mg/kg (Turner et al., 2006). The signs seen in rodents were potentiated by concomitant administration of SSRIs.

Gastrointestinal and neurological signs consistent with serotonin syndrome in dogs have been reported for dosages of 5-HTP ranging from 2.5 to 573 mg/kg. The minimum toxic dose in one study was 23.6 mg/kg (Gwaltney-Brant et al., 2000). The most common signs of toxicosis in dogs were vomiting or diarrhea, abdominal pain, and hypersalivation for gastrointestinal signs and seizures, depression, tremors, hyperesthesia, and ataxia for neurological signs. Death is a possible sequela. The minimum lethal dose reported was 128 mg/kg. Onset of signs can occur within 10 minutes, and signs can last 36 hours.

5-HTP has not been shown to lead to serotonin syndrome in humans, even when combined with TCAs and SSRIs in reasonable dosages, and it has been hypothesized to be efficacious alone or in combination with other medications in the treatment of human depression (Turner et al., 2006).

NUTRACEUTICALS

A "nutraceutical" is generally defined as a food product that provides health and medical benefits by affecting physiology and that is available in forms not packaged or marketed as food. Nutraceuticals can be herbals, can be isolated from nutrients, can be derivatives of food products, or can be manufactured as dietary supplements. The nutraceuticals that have been investigated for effects in veterinary behavioral medicine are:

- alpha-casozepine (Zylkene),
- L-theanine (Anxitane),
- Harmonease, and
- Calmex (VetPlus), which contains a combination of L-theanine, L-tryptophan, an array of B vitamins, and *Piper methysticum.*

Alpha-casozepine, an alpha casein derivative, has been used to treat non-specific anxiety in cats and dogs (Beata et al., 2007a, 2007b). Alpha-casozepine is similar in structure to gamma-aminobutyric acid (GABA) and has an affinity for GABA-A receptors (Beata et al., 2007a). In a blinded, controlled study, dogs with a variety of anxiety-related conditions improved when treated with alpha-casozepine to the same extent as dogs treated with selegiline using a standardized, scored assessment (the Emotional Disorders Evaluation in Dogs [EDED] scale) (Beata et al., 2007b). However, the conditions varied considerably, and outcomes were based on client scores, so it is likely that this study could be replicated or that a placebo effect of simply participating in a study could be ruled out.

Palestrini et al. (2010) conducted a placebo-controlled, double-blind study on the effects of a diet containing caseinate hydrolysate using both behavioral and physiological assays in anxious and non-anxious laboratory beagles. Anxiety scores were not affected by diet, and behavioral scores were only mildly affected. A large and statistically significant effect was found for decreased cortisol for anxious dogs fed the diet with caseinate hydrolysate, suggesting that such diets may play some role in alleviating some aspects of distress.

Alpha-casozepine is also one of the main ingredients in the CALM Diet (Royal Canin). This diet, which also contains an anti-oxidant complex of vitamin E, vitamin C, taurine, and lutein, is intended to be fed to a dog 10 days before an expected stressful procedure and then for an additional 2 to 3 months. Kato et al. (2012) examined the effect of the CALM Diet compared with a control diet (both with approximately 25% protein) on behavior and urinary cortisol creatinine ratios (UCCR) in anxious pet dogs. They found a small but statistically significant effect on UCCR for the dogs eating the CALM Diet. UCCR increased less in response to a stressor in the dogs fed the CALM Diet than in dogs fed a control diet, but this effect could have been confounded by the casozepine or slightly higher fat and protein (in g/kg) in the CALM Diet. Also, the study design used did not control for effects of habituation, a common design concern in many behavioral studies. An additional confounding factor in determining effects of such therapeutic diets is that of determining

the effect of dosage. Animals vary in size and intake and if fed other foods may experience effects such as those of large neutral AAs on tryptophan.

Harmonease (Veterinary Products Laboratories) is a "natural proprietary blend of a patented extract of *Magnolia officinalis* and a proprietary extract of *Phellodendron amurense*" (www.vpl.com/literature/pdfs/Harmonease_NewProductVet_DM_300503660_08-2057.pdf; last accessed October 8, 2011). These compounds have been reported to decrease mild, transient stress (Kalman et al., 2008), and the derivatives honokiol and magnolol from *Magnolia* have been shown to have *in vitro* GABA$_A$ modulation capability (Kuribara et al., 1998, 1999). In one cross-over study of laboratory beagles who were mildly reactive to recordings of storms but who did not show clinical signs of noise phobia, there was a mild but significant effect of Harmonease on activity level (De Porter et al., 2012).

L-Theanine (Anxitane; Virbac Animal Health) is the levorotatory isomer of theanine. It is naturally occurring in the tea plant and thought to lessen some stress conditions and mild anxiety-related problems in pets (Araujo et al., 2010; Kimura et al., 2007). L-Theanine is an analogue of glutamic acid. As such, it may inhibit reuptake of glutamate by the glutamate transporter (Sadzuka et al., 2001) and so increase GABA concentrations. Because high glutamate levels have been associated with neurocytotoxicity, L-theanine may also have a neuroprotectant effect and may modulate any neurotransmitters that interact with glutamate receptor subtypes (e.g., serotonin, dopamine). As with most nutraceuticals, side effects are inapparent even at dosages in excess of the recommended dose (www.virbacvet.com/images/resources/other/anxitane; last accessed October 8, 2011).

The supplements discussed and some prescription diets (e.g., Hill's B/D) contain bioactive compounds that may act as precursors or enhancers for some neurochemicals. Although side effects are rare, attention should be paid when also treating these patients with medication. No dosage adjustments will be necessary in most cases but we should be mindful of what we do not know. The recommended amounts of supplements/nutraceuticals for cats and dogs are presented in Table 10-3.

SUMMARY OF EFFECTS OF SUPPLEMENTS AND DIET ON BEHAVIOR

Use of supplemental AAs that are specific neurochemical precursors (e.g., tryptophan) for treatment of behavioral conditions has been disappointing (Janczak et al., 2001). Utility of any AA supplement will be affected by relative availability, overall amount of protein available, composition of protein available with respect to other AAs that might compete for transporters, availability of transporters, and the extent to which the AAs are protein bound and present but inaccessible (Bosch

TABLE 10-3

Recommended Amounts of Supplements/Nutraceuticals to Administer Based on Manufacturer Information

Supplement/Nutraceutical	Dosage/Recommended Capsule Size/Frequency
Aktivait	Cats: 1 tablet daily (DHA/EPA 35 mg; no alpha-lipoic acid) Small dog breeds (<10 kg), 1 tablet daily (DHA/EPA 35 mg) Large dog breeds: <20 kg, 1 tablet daily; >20 kg, 2 tablets daily (DHA/EPA 35 mg)
Senilife	Regular: Cats and dogs up to 30 lb, 1 capsule; 31-50 lb, 2 capsules Senilife XL: Dogs >50 lb, 51-99 lb, 1 capsule; ≥100 lb, 2 capsules
NOVIFIT	S—for dogs ≤22 lb and cats M—for dogs 22.1-44 lb L—for dogs 44.1-88 lb
Zylkene	Cats and small dogs: 75 mg once daily Medium-sized dogs: 10-20 kg, 225 mg once daily Large dogs: 20-40 kg, 450 mg once daily; >40 kg, twice daily
Anxitane	50-mg tablets (S) for dogs and cats ≤22 lb 100-mg tablets (M and L) for dogs >22 lb
Harmonease	500-mg tablets of extracts of *M. officinalis* and *P. amurense*: for dogs ≤50 lb, ½ tablet daily; for dogs >50 lb, 1 tablet daily

DHA/EPA, Docosahexaenoic acid/eicosahexaenoic acid.

et al., 2007). It's unwise to recommend supplementation with AAs for the treatment of specific behavioral concerns at this time.

Protein levels themselves affect availability of AA. Low protein levels may have relatively minor effects on non-specific signs of behavioral problems such as activity levels, and there may be an indirect role for AA levels in activity levels. Recommendations about protein levels should be made in the context of the overall health and activity level of the cat or dog. For dogs, recommendations should also take into account whether they work (e.g., police dogs, detection dogs, guide dogs). Qualified suggestions about the effects of increased energy levels or decreased overall protein levels on the effects of behaviors that have an activity component may be cautiously made.

DHA and EPA appear to play major roles in the development and maintenance of cognition through various mechanisms, and we should expect to see widespread inclusion of them in a variety of dietary/nutraceutical/supplemental products.

Neuroprotection appears to be both important and possible to address. Diets such as Hill's B/D and supplements such as Aktivait have opened the door to exploration of the manipulation of large combinations of precursor neurochemicals, membrane constituent chemicals, and agents that thwart ROS. The easiest conditions in which to explore such efficacy are those associated with learning and memory: cognitive dysfunction syndrome and early puppyhood/kittenhood developmental impairment associated with under-nutrition or malnutrition and lack of appropriate social exposure (puppy and kitten farms/mills). Because behavioral conditions may cause so much neuronal damage by

excessively stimulating some excitatory AAs such as glutamate, these interventions may have much broader applications.

Altering brain energy and effects of compounds that affect it is a novel and promising strategy that should have applications across behavioral and primary physiological conditions. Such interventions also have implications for longevity, and we should expect to see some creative applications.

EFFECT OF ENDOGENOUS HORMONES ON BEHAVIOR

Much attention has been given to the role of sex hormones and behavioral concerns in cats and dogs, but the data are scant (Hart, 1974b). It may be appropriate to view testosterone as a behavioral modulator that may facilitate the attainment and escalation of the aggressive state. An intact dog may react more easily, escalate any response more quickly, plateau at a higher level of reactivity, return to baseline at a slower rate, and possibly alter his baseline to a higher level than a neutered dog.

Both neutered and intact dogs may have behavioral concerns, and only some of these concerns are affected by sexual dimorphism. Dimorphic behaviors associated with the presence of testosterone include urine marking with lifted leg, roaming, and some types of mounting. Mounting is an unclear issue because it is a challenge and control behavior as well as a sexual one; little work has been done to determine whether the nuances of the mounting behavior are identical in both situations. Castration results in a decrease in androgen within 6 hours of the procedure; most of the hormonal decrease is complete in 72 hours (Hopkins et al., 1976). In one study (never replicated or expanded) roaming decreased by approximately 90%, male-male aggression by approximately 75%, urine marking by approximately 60%, and mounting by 80% in dogs who were neutered/castrated. However, marking, mounting, and fighting are complex behaviors not wholly controlled by hormones. There is a significant learning component in these behaviors that will not be redressed by castration. Most situations in which these concerns are problematic involve anxiety disorders, and so medication may be an essential part of treatment.

Less attention has been paid to the role of female sex hormones and aggressive behavior, but work suggests a potential, if restricted, role for them (O'Farrell and Peachey, 1990). Female puppies *who were already showing signs of "dominance aggression" (now impulse control/ conflict aggression) only became worse after spaying.* Spaying did not have an effect on any other age and behavior group combinations (Overall, 1995c). It is possible that for these young, aggressive bitches, sex hormones may play a helpful role in modulating their reactivity. If these dogs are in a responsible household where breeding is prohibited, allowing them to have a heat cycle may be beneficial in terms of ameliorating their aggression, but there are few to no prospective data.

Neutering/desexing (castration or ovariohysterectomy [OHE]) is usually recommended for aggressive dogs and cats because if there is a heritable component to the behaviors, neutering affected animals prevents them from passing on the condition. If heritability is complex and/or has a large environmental component to expression, neutering dogs known to be aggressive may not substantially decrease genetic risk *within the population of breeding dogs.*

Reasons for neutering owned dogs may vary by sex. Common reasons for neutering male dogs include the dog marks with urine, the dog has an enlarged prostate or prostatic or testicular neoplasia, or the dog is not focusing on his job if a working dog but on odors of other dogs. Common reasons for neutering females include a desire to decrease the risks of mammary neoplasia, the client cannot or will not or does not wish to monitor for pyometra, the client doesn't want to deal with the behavioral and physical consequences of heat cycles, and there are behavioral issues pertaining to heat or being intact that are problematic for the dog and/or household.

The most common reason for OHE is to spare dogs the risk of mammary neoplasia, which is extremely common in dogs, although malignant only about half the time (Brodey et al., 1983). In countries where dogs are not routinely spayed, the risk for mammary neoplasia may be as high as 53.3% (Moe, 2001). Neutering female dogs before their first heat decreases the risk of mammary neoplasia to 0.5%. If clients wait until the second heat, the risk is 8%, and after the second heat

the risk increases to 26% (Overly et al., 2005; Schneider et al., 1969). Although spaying after the second heat does not substantially reduce risk, spaying at the time that the mammary tumors are removed appears to have a beneficial effect on survival (Overly et al., 2005; Sorenmo et al., 2000). The patterns for OHE and mammary neoplasia are similar in cats, but 85% to 90% of feline mammary tumors are malignant (Brodey et al., 1983; Lana et al., 2007).

Repeated heat cycles increase the risk of pyometra (Johnston et al., 2001). In one Swedish study, 25% of the females studied developed pyometra by 10 years of age. There are strong breed effects that may increase or decrease this risk (Egenvall et al., 2001, 2005). Spaying eliminates the risks of pyometra.

The risk of prostatic disease in male dogs increases with age, and benign hypertrophy may affect 60% or more of dogs older than 7 years (Berry et al., 1986). Castration both prevents and treats benign prostatic hyperplasia. Testicular tumors are rare, but all are prevented or treated by castration.

Concerns have been raised about adverse effects of neutering on other health issues. Castration may increase the risk of bladder transitional cell carcinoma (Bryan et al., 2007) and prostate carcinoma (Bryan et al., 2007; Sorenmo et al., 2003), an effect augmented by breed. At least one study suggests that neutering may facilitate tumor growth, while having no effect on initiation of the development of the cancer (Teske et al., 2002). Neutered dogs have been reported to have a higher risk for osteosarcoma than intact dogs (Cooley et al., 2002; Ru et al., 1998), but the studies are complicated, and the neutered dogs in the studies lived longer than the intact dogs.

Spayed females have been reported to have an increased risk of hemangiosarcoma compared with intact females (Prymack et al., 1988; Ware et al., 1999), a finding that may be heavily influenced by breed. Transitional cell carcinoma may affect more neutered than intact females, but it is very rare, although more common in females (Norris et al., 1992).

Early neutering, as practiced by shelters to reduce the number of unwanted dogs and cats, may have different effects on health than neutering later in life. Early neutering increases long bone growth, which may pose risks for later skeletal conformations that could affect hip dysplasia (Salman et al., 1998, 2000; Salmeri et al., 1991; Spain et al., 2004), but these findings are not supported by all studies (Howe et al., 2001), and even when present the effect may be relatively weak (Spain et al., 2004). If OHE for female shelter puppies can be delayed until 3 months of age, risks for temporal related cystitis and later urinary incontinence may be decreased (Spain et al., 2004), but the effect may matter less than anticipated (Howe et al., 2001), and if the risk is that the pup would not otherwise be neutered, neutering of shelter dogs is always preferred.

Chemical castration with implantable deslorelin, a gonadotropin-releasing hormone agonist is occasionally used because it renders animals treated with it functionally sterile, a condition that is reversible with removal of the implant (Junaidi et al., 2003). Deslorelin decreases testosterone and luteinizing hormones to undetectable levels in dogs and so may affect testosterone-modulated behaviors. When alpha agonists fail, deslorelin may successfully treat estrogen-dependent urinary incontinence in female dogs (Reichler et al., 2003). Ferrets treated with deslorelin showed decreased fighting between males in association with sexual behavior and increased play behavior compared with ferrets who had been surgically castrated (Schipper et al., 2008). One study that examined play, fear, and aggressive behaviors in dogs treated with deslorelin compared with surgically castrated dogs found no differences between groups in these behaviors (Steur, 2011). When given to cats, deslorelin rendered them infertile and caused decreases in testicular volume and disappearance of penile spines (Goericke-Pesch et al., 2011). Cats who were given implants experienced decreased libido, decreases in mounting and mating behaviors, and decreased spraying, but food intake increased, a potential concern given the obesity epidemic in cats in the United States.

Farhoody and Zink (2010) in an unpublished, non–peer-reviewed, online summary of a Masters thesis suggested that neutered dogs are more fearful, excitable, and aggressive and less trainable than intact dogs. However, this study is fatally flawed in that it does not follow dogs through time and instead relies on unmatched cohorts. We do not know whether these dogs were evaluated at the same age (control for ontogeny) or at a pre-determined time after neutering (control for postoperative effects). Without these controls, most correlations—especially using scored and ranked data, as is the case here—are likely to be spurious. There are other major methodological issues that preclude accepting these conclusions as valid, and they are common enough mistakes in studies that they warrant an outline here.

1. The data are scored *client* assessments of their own dog's behaviors using a scale that was not validated to ensure that it represented reliable, repeatable behaviors (e.g., whether the dog was actually "aggressive" if she barked).
2. No inter-rater reliability data are provided. In other words, we have no idea how variable clients' interpretations of the dogs' behaviors were or how variable their interpretation of the terms and scales used were.
3. Scaled data are difficult to interpret because they are so subjective and without inter-rater and intra-rater reliabilities that it is impossible to know, for example, if person A's 4.5 is equivalent to person B's 4.5. This is one reason why such scales should be avoided in population studies, unless they are defined, validated, and tested for inter-rater agreement (e.g., kappa scores).
4. The data are presented graphically, and the axes are not the same. As a result, differences appear larger than they truly are. When plotted on the same scale, differences are modest, especially given that very small changes in scores obtained from scaled responses are calculated for a very large number of responses.
5. The sample size is huge because this is a survey study, and with a sample size so large it would be odd if some findings were not significant by chance alone. This effect is magnified when scores are calculated from scales. Even for those relationships that are *statistically* different, we have no idea if the differences noted are *biologically meaningful.*
6. Analysis of ratios (here, bone length) is complex and requires certain assumptions that we cannot know were met here.

In short, any causal attribution for neutering and problematic behavior is premature (Kim et al., 2006 [see discussion on p. 176]; Overall, 2007). When one considers the difficulty of identifying physical pathologies that may be affected by neutering, as discussed earlier, one should take special care with behavioral evaluations, which are much more difficult to evaluate in an unbiased, valid, and repeatable manner.

There is no one recommendation that will fit each client and each dog. Issues pertaining to neutering and associations with neoplasia are complex, and issues associated with a putative causal relationship appear to be more so. Clients making decisions about their pets should be apprised of this complexity, should understand relative risk as it affects breed, and should be informed about what we do not know. Regardless of the possible effects of hormones on later health, *we rank risks differently when dealing with unwanted animals or patients with known behavioral concerns than is the case when theoretically addressing dogs in general.* Because there is a non-trivial risk that shelter dogs, if adopted intact, will not be neutered and will reproduce, thus contributing to perpetuation of the shelter euthanasia cycle, animals in shelters should be neutered prior to adoption. In terms of costs and surgical time, early neutering is an excellent strategy for shelter puppies and kittens.

MEDICATION OVERVIEW

The use of medication is essential for the treatment of many behavioral problems. Although medication is most commonly recommended for ongoing or severe behavioral problems, it may be used even more effectively *early* in the course of the condition.

The one outstanding finding from placebo-controlled, double-blind studies is that the addition of psychotherapeutic agents to behavioral and environmental modification leads to faster and better treatment outcomes (King et al., 2000a, 2000b, 2004b; Landsberg et al., 2008; Simpson et al., 2007). The reason for the enhanced efficacy of treatment approaches that combine medication with behavioral work and environmental change lies in the effects of these medications on neurons: both learning and behavioral medications rely on the same molecular changes, and serotoninergic neurons, which are affected by many of the medications routinely used, are most dense in the frontal cortex and hippocampus, the parts of the brain primarily involved in learning.

Treatment of non-specific behavioral complaints and signs—without addressing the contextual framework provided by a diagnosis—is unacceptable. Instead, treating specific diagnoses whose diagnostic criteria are met offers the clinician the chance to choose treatment that addresses the putative, underlying neurochemical mechanisms (Overall, 1997, 2005). This approach leads to the best treatment outcomes.

Supplements, diet, and nutraceuticals are now sufficiently sophisticated that many of them are being designed with a focus on specific neurochemical or behavioral effects. Clinicians will want to know whether their clients are using any of these avenues of treatment because some of them may interfere with or augment the effects of traditional pharmacological intervention. Additionally, clinicians may wish to employ some of these interventions in their own treatment plans for distressed and troubled patients.

Clients must appreciate that neither drugs nor diets are a "quick fix." Behavioral medication, especially, is not intended to blunt, mask, or disguise problematic behaviors or to sedate or drug the dog or cat. In fact, if any of these outcomes occur, they should be viewed as side effects. However, knowing that behavioral medication can facilitate the learning involved in behavior modification can help clients to comply with such programs and make their implementation easier.

The client handout, "Protocol for Using Behavioral Medication Successfully," covers the questions most often of concern to clients, which are also addressed in more detail in this chapter:

- What medications are used?
- How do these work?
- What are the potential side effects?
- How should the client monitor for side effects?
- Can these medications interact with other medications (e.g., thyroxine, antiinflammatories, tramadol), and, if so, how?
- What effects can be seen and when?
- How long must the patient take the medication?
- How do we wean or remove the patient from the medication?
- What does the client do if he or she is scared or worried about changes in the pet's behaviors?

Because all of the medications we use in veterinary behavioral medicine are also human medications, clients may have at least some passing familiarity with the medication. Such knowledge may render them less or more worried about giving the medication to their pet. Having someone on the staff who is comfortable

explaining the principles of behavioral drug use review the handout with the client can assuage fears, help with compliance, and encourage a better treatment outcome.

At every step of the decisions made in treating patients with behavioral complaints, *veterinarians should remember that medication can play an essential role in saving lives and improving the quality of life (QoL) of their patients and the people who love them. Behavioral complaints and problems remain the single most common cause of euthanasia and/or relinquishment of pet dogs and cats, and clients should be told this.*

ROLE FOR ACCURATE DIAGNOSIS

The issues pertaining to accurate diagnosis and the terminology used in veterinary behavioral medicine have been discussed in depth in Chapter 2. It is important to understand these issues because our thinking affects what treatment plans we select, how we explain our choices and plans to clients, and how we use the patients' behavioral responses to modify treatment plans and inform our thinking about their conditions.

Most behavioral conditions are best represented by non-linear models (i.e., models that represent multifactorial, heterogeneous disorders). For example, there is no one drug to treat feline spraying: spraying can be a behavioral description *or* a species-typical normal behavior, *or* a nonspecific sign, *or* a phenotypic diagnosis. The behavior of spraying is caused by a variety of social circumstances and may be the result of various, interacting neurochemical systems, even when everyone agrees that it is a non-specific sign of anxiety.

If diagnoses are made using rigorous, repeatable criteria, and if the patient population is sufficiently large, failure of some significant portion of the population to respond to one medication when another significant portion responds well suggests that there is neurochemical and/or molecular variability within the diagnosis. This means that not all patients exhibiting the same diagnosis are affected for the same reasons. In human psychiatry, large, multicenter treatment trials are common and serve to identify subpopulations of patients who share a phenotypic diagnosis but who vary in their neurochemical mechanism for that diagnosis. There are no large-scale studies in veterinary behavioral medicine that would permit the use of the type of empiricism that is possible in human psychiatry.

Understanding that such variation exists is essential for rational use of behavioral medications. It is important that clients know what we do not know and that we may need to try a series of diets, medications, or combinations before we find the best choice for their dog or cat. Clients can understand that all SSRIs vary in structure, and all of these vary to some extent in structure and effect compared with TCAs and other groups of useful medications. If a patient does not respond to the first medication of choice, he or she may

Benefits of Early Treatment

- Fewer medications and/or a lower dose may be needed
- A quicker resolution may occur
- Shorter treatment course may be needed
- Because behaviors that are practiced and repeated become learned, the role of practice and learning is shortened
- The patient may be more flexible in his or her overall behavioral profile and may acquire new behaviors (via behavior modification) more quickly and easily
- The patient may develop a less severe version of the condition and so may have fewer signs that are easier for the clinician and client to recognize and monitor for intervention
- Stress and distress for both the patient and the client are reduced, with concomitant lowering of any risk for anger, abuse, relinquishment, or death

respond to another simply because this patient's neurochemical profile is not the same as another patient's, although they have been diagnosed with the same behavioral condition. If we explain these facts to clients as soon as we or they notice any behavioral concerns, they will have an accurate impression of what is involved in treating a behavioral condition, may elect to treat it earlier, and can become true partners in treatment. The benefits of earlier treatment that can be explained to clients are listed in Box 10-1.

WILL MEDICATION WORK?

Although medication alone may render the patient globally less anxious, if the patient is still being provoked by social or physical environmental stimuli, the benefit of treatment with medication will be minimized. Without an adequate history to ensure that no provocation is still ongoing, many clients and veterinarians will falsely believe that medication does not work. The newer serotonin-affecting medications, protective nutraceuticals, and enhanced dietary regimens have a huge potential to improve life for troubled pets and their distressed people, and rational drug use should now be considered part of basic humane treatment of our patients.

MEDICATIONS USED MOST FREQUENTLY TO TREAT BEHAVIORAL CONDITIONS

Medications commonly used to treat behavioral conditions in dogs and cats are usually antidepressants, antianxiety agents, and anxiolytics that fall into three main classes (Overall, 2001; Simpson and Papich, 2003):

- benzodiazepines (BZDs) (e.g., alprazolam, clorazepate, diazepam, midazolam, oxazepam, clonazepam, lorazepam, temazepam),
- TCAs (e.g., amitriptyline, nortriptyline, clomipramine, imipramine, doxepin), and
- SSRIs (e.g., fluoxetine, paroxetine, sertraline, fluvoxamine, citalopram, escitalopram).
Increasingly, we see patients treated with:
- *noradrenergic reuptake inhibitors (NRIs) (e.g., reboxetine),*
- dual serotonin NE reuptake inhibitors (SNRIs) (e.g., venlafaxine, duloxetine),
- dual serotonin 2A agonist/serotonin reuptake inhibitors (SARIs) (e.g., trazodone, nefazodone), and
- noradrenergic and specific serotoninergic antidepressants (NaSSAs) (e.g., mirtazapine).

Less commonly used medications, or medications with more restrictive populations likely to benefit, include:
- MAO inhibitors (e.g., selegiline),
- azaspirones (e.g., buspirone),
- centrally acting alpha agonists, which may act as hypotensives decreasing cardiac output and peripheral vascular resistance (e.g., clonidine, guanfacine, medetomidine, and dexmedetomidine [all centrally acting alpha-2A-adrenergic receptor agonists; dexmedetomidine also affects alpha-1A-receptors]),
- NMDA antagonists (e.g., memantine),
- sympathomimetics (e.g., dextroamphetamine, methylphenidate), and
- hormonal agents.

All of these medications cause their effects through modulation of the neurotransmitters serotonin (5-HT), dopamine, noradrenaline/NE (NA/NE), and/or GABA and their related metabolites (e.g., the excitatory AA glutamate, which becomes GABA). Accordingly, any medication, supplement, or dietary constituent that shares a metabolic or synthetic pathway with any of these neurotransmitters or medications can affect the amount of any medications available and their utility.

Most medication use in veterinary behavioral medicine is "extra-label"; this means that there is no veterinary product that is equivalent to the human product chosen. Such use is legal in the United States, although it should be explained to the client. Published data for medications used "extra-label" may or may not exist, but all licensed relevant medications were required to undergo toxicology studies in dogs in the United States and so may have these data available, even though no therapeutic data may be published. As of this writing, clomipramine (Clomicalm; Novartis), fluoxetine (Reconcile; Lilly), and selegiline (Anipryl; Pfizer) are available in veterinary formulations. The availability of these formulations in the United States does not preclude the use of the human formulation or re-compounding.

Clients should understand that although we may know a lot about toxicity of these medications for laboratory dogs, most of the medications have not been formulated or tested at clinically therapeutic levels in clinical settings for dogs or cats. Accordingly, there is much we do not know. Our use of these medications is shaped by strong inference, and clients need to be a part of the treatment team and monitor their pet's reaction to the medication.

ADVERSE EFFECTS

Clients worry about undesirable effects or side effects, so it is essential that the veterinary team has an accurate understanding of relevant risk. Common adverse effects of psychotherapeutic drugs are usually caused by a blockage of the muscarinic acetylcholine receptors, which have diffuse connections throughout the brain. These "common" side effects are actually not very common and generally manifest as *transient* changes. The most common complaints are related to gastrointestinal function, appetite change, sedation, or alterations (usually increases) in heart rate. For most patients, any side effects will truly be transient, occurring within the first week; however, if any side effect is *not* transient, clients need to understand that their pet may be experiencing a serious problem. For this reason, it is important to encourage clients to help monitor both their animal's response to the medication and any side effects that their pet may experience.

Although many BZDs can be sedative, the BZDs now used most commonly (e.g., alprazolam, oxazepam, clonazepam) are less sedative than diazepam and clorazepate. Because dogs and cats, similar to humans, can experience a huge range of effects when given a BZD, clients should be encouraged to give any BZD when they can monitor the patient. This means that the first one or two doses should be given when the client is home and can watch the dog. The client handout, "Generalized Guidelines for Using Alprazolam for Noise and Storm Phobias, Panic, and Severe Distress," details how clients can test and monitor for side effects and how they can learn if a BZD is effective for their pet.

Because the most severe side effects of TCAs, SSRIs, and the more recently popular SARIs can involve cardiac affects, *clients should and can easily learn to take pulse rates, which may be the first sign of developing serotonin syndrome.* Slight increases in pulse rate are not worrisome. Huge, sustained increases in heart rate *are* problematic. If clients know that their dog's resting heart rate is 65 beats/min and with medication this changes to 150 beats/min, they can immediately bring this change to the veterinarian's attention. Likewise, if the increase is minor (65 to 75 beats/min), the client can take notes and not worry. *For this reason, baseline electrocardiograms (ECGs) are recommended for any patient who has had a history of any arrhythmia, heart disease, or prior drug reactions; who is on more than one medication; and who may be undergoing anesthesia or sedation* (Reich et al.,

2000). Cats may be more sensitive to cardiac side effects than dogs, and, at a minimum, a lead II ECG evaluation for any arrhythmias should be done before treating cats with agents that may affect serotonin (Lainesse et al., 2007b; Martin, 2010).

Most behavioral drugs are metabolized through renal and hepatic pathways, so knowledge of baseline, pre-medication values is essential. Liver dyscrasias and cardiac arrhythmias may not rule out the use of a drug, but knowing that they exist can serve as a guide to dosage and anticipated side effects. Annual laboratory evaluation can help monitor changes in renal or hepatic function that may affect metabolism of behavioral medications. Should changes occur, their magnitude can guide alterations (usually decreases) in the dosages of behavioral medication.

Atypical reactions can occur, and laboratory evaluation is essential for any unexplained or sudden illness. If any rare but profound alteration in hepatic function occurs, immediate withdrawal from behavioral medicine is an option while the patient receives supportive care. Although dogs have been known to die of toxic overdose of their owners' medication, there have been few confirmed cases of death resulting from behavioral medication prescribed for the dog at therapeutic canine dosages.

Educated clients will monitor their pets better, will be more willing to use medications and behavior modification appropriately, and will be more enjoyable clients for their veterinarian. Clients should receive a complete list of all potential adverse responses and should be encouraged to communicate with the veterinarian at the first sign of any problem. Clients are often very distressed after a behavioral consultation and need a written reminder of situations for which they should be alert. The handout, "Protocol for Using Behavioral Medication Successfully," lists such concerns, and if the veterinary team reviews and highlights the concerns for the clients, compliance will improve.

This practice of encouraging clients to be active participants in care and monitoring of their pet is extremely helpful in ensuring that we recognize animals with atypical or serious sedative responses so that we can find more appropriate medications with which to treat them.

ANCILLARY CONCERNS

All psychotropic medications can interact with other medications. For example, use of TCAs, SSRIs, and related drug classes will cause thyroidal values—whether or not supplementation is involved—to read falsely low (Martin, 2010). It is essential to know about this interaction when evaluating an animal's true thyroid status. This issue is especially germane for dogs, for whom there has been a cyclic vogue for non-specifically treating dogs with behavioral concerns and borderline thyroid values with thyroxine. There is now good evidence showing that most behavioral concerns are not directly associated with any thyroid dysfunction, although such dysfunction may affect behavior.

Many serotoninergic agents are thought to lower seizure thresholds and are recommended with caution in patients treated with a history of seizures. The story is considerably more complex than this. For both humans and dogs, anxiety itself may lower seizure thresholds and so *treatment of the anxiety may actually raise the seizure threshold* and allow the patient to decrease successfully the amount of seizure medication needed.

Finally, the client household must be considered when the decision to use behavioral drugs is made. Substance abuse is rampant in humans, and some medications used to treat canine and feline behavioral conditions have a high human abuse potential.

EFFICACY AND MECHANISM OF ACTION

It's important for clients to understand that newer, more specific, and more efficacious drugs have a relatively long lag time between initiation of treatment and apparent changes in the patient's behavior. This delay is due to the mechanism of action of TCAs and SSRIs, which involves altered transcription of new proteins, including proteins involved in creating new receptors.

A review of the neurochemical functions and characteristics will lead to a logical understanding of what medications are available to treat different conditions.

Serotonin

Serotonin (5-HT) receptors are all G protein–coupled receptors. There are 14 identified classes of serotonin receptors. The 5-HT$_1$ receptors are linked to the inhibition of adenylate cyclase and are the primary receptors thought to affect mood and behavior.
- Presynaptic 5-HT$_{1A}$ receptors predominate in dorsal and median raphe nuclei.
- Postsynaptic 5-HT$_{1A}$ receptors predominant in limbic regions (hippocampus and septum) and some cortical layers. It's helpful to remember that the hippocampus is the part of the brain where associational learning takes place, so it should be transparent how anxiety can adversely affect learning.

Distribution of serotonin receptors within the brain can help guide choice of medications based on expected regional effects (Table 10-4). The extent to which individuals vary in regional density of specific receptors is currently unknown but could become an important area of study as we attempt to tailor choice and effect of medications better.

TABLE 10-4

Serotonin Receptor Subtype for Region of the Brain Where Receptors or Messenger RNA Activity Has Been Identified

Receptor Subtype	Region of Brain with Messenger RNA Activity
5-HT$_{1A}$	Hippocampus (dentate gyrus, CA1, CA3), lateral septum, raphe nuclei, entorhinal cortex, central amygdala
5-HT$_{1B}$	Globus pallidus, substantia nigra (pars reticula), olivary pretectal nuclei, dorsal subiculum, superior colliculi (superficial layer)
5-HT$_{1D}$	Globus pallidus, substantia nigra, caudate, putamen, accumbens nuclei, frontal cortex
5-HT$_{2A}$	Claustrum, olfactory tubercle, frontal cortex, neocortex (layer IV), raphe nuclei
5-HT$_{2B}$	Cortex, amygdala, caudate, hypothalamus
5-HT$_{2C}$	Choroid plexus, substantia nigra, globus pallidus, neocortex (layer III), hippocampus (CA1, CA3), raphe nuclei
5-HT$_3$	Amygdala (basolateral nuclei), entorhinal cortex, hippocampus
5-HT$_{3A/3B}$	Amygdala, hippocampus
5-HT$_4$	Hippocampus (CA1), caudate, amygdala, colliculi (superior layer)
5-HT$_5$	Hippocampus, habenula
5-HT$_{5B}$	Habenula, hippocampus (CA1), raphe nuclei
5-HT$_6$	Piriform and prefrontal cortex, striatum, hippocampus (CA1-CA3, dentate gyrus), amygdala
5-HT$_{7A}$	Hippocampus, amygdala, cortex, raphe nuclei
5-HTP	Hippocampus

From Meneses, 1999; see paper for references for regional attributions.

Urinary excretion of 5-hydroxyindoleacetic acid (5-HIAA) is a measure of 5-HT turnover and has been used to assess neurochemical abnormalities in human psychiatric patients and is beginning to show potential in this regard for veterinary behavioral medicine, especially for patients with anxiety-based aggression diagnoses (Riva et al., 2010, 2012). The medications that most affect serotonin receptors are TCAs, SSRIs, SNRIs, and SARIs, all of which act to inhibit reuptake of serotonin in the presynaptic neuron, and partial agonists, such as the azaspirone, buspirone, which selectively stimulates the presynaptic 5-HT_{1A} subtype receptor.

Nutraceuticals designed to augment 5-HT and 5-HT supplements may not engender the same response as pharmacologic agents because, as is true for tryptophan, 5-HT does not pass easily through the BBB and instead requires the help of a transport protein. This transport protein is also used to move other AAs across the BBB, and so even if 5-HT-containing substances are absorbed unchanged from the gastrointestinal tract, they may be excreted depending on the pharmacodynamics of the other AAs present (Grimmett and Sillence, 2005).

Noradrenaline/Norepinephrine

The most prominent collection of noradrenergic neurons is found in the locus coeruleus of the gray matter of the pons and in the lateral tegmental nuclei. There is also a cluster in the medulla.

NE has been postulated to affect:

1. mood,
2. functional reward systems, and
3. arousal.

NE has been shown to be decreased in depression and increased in manic states. Centrally acting alpha agonists (e.g., clonidine) and, to a lesser extent, TCAs and SNRIs (e.g., venlafaxine) exert their affects through NE. SSRIs have quite small but variable effects on NE.

Dopamine

The distribution of dopamine in the brain is nonuniform but is more restrictive than the distribution of NE. Dopaminergic nuclei are found primarily in:

1. the substantia nigra pars compacta, which projects to the striatum and is largely concerned with coordinated movement,
2. the ventral tegmental area, which projects to the frontal and cingulate cortex, nucleus accumbens, and other limbic structures, and
3. the arcuate nucleus of the hypothalamus, which projects to the pituitary.

A large proportion of the brain's dopamine is found in the corpus striatum, the part of the extrapyramidal system concerned with coordinated movement. Dopamine is metabolized by MAO and catechol *O*-methyl transferase (COMT) into dihydrophenylacetic acid (DOPAC) and homovanillic acid (HVA). HVA acid is used as a peripheral index of central dopamine turnover in humans, but this use has not been explored extensively in veterinary medicine.

All dopaminergic receptors are G protein–coupled transmembrane receptors.

- D_1 receptors exhibit their postsynaptic inhibition in the limbic system and are affected in mood disorders and stereotypies.
- D_2, D_3, and D_4 receptors all are affected in mood disorders and stereotypies.

The distribution of dopaminergic neurons means that excess dopamine, as produced by dopamine-releasing agents (amphetamines and dopamine agonists, such as apomorphine) is associated with the development of stereotypies.

Acepromazine, a phenothiazine, neuroleptic tranquilizer, is a dopamine antagonist that binds dopamine receptors without activating them, decreasing the amount of dopamine available. The tranquilization function acts to scramble memory but does not prevent or treat anxiety. *Acepromazine should never be used as a behavioral medication or as a treatment for storm or noise phobias, unless the intent is to sedate the dog completely because if the dog is less able to process rationally information pertaining to stimuli he or she perceives, the dog is more, not less, anxious.*

Additionally, animals already sensitized to noise experience profound reactivity and distress when given acepromazine and then exposed to noise in the environment (Clough, 1982). Because of this sensitization, the *continued use* of acepromazine may make the dog *more reactive to noise* but less able to do anything about it and so render the animal considerably more anxious with time. Dogs and cats who are fearful, panicky, or distressed when left alone should not be treated with phenothiazines, for similar reasons.

Acepromazine, especially in combination with medications such as butorphanol, *can* help to control perioperative pain (Grint et al., 2010; Hofmeister et al., 2010) and possibly some of the anxiety attendant with this and other pain, but its use should not be indiscriminate and may be problematic for patients who react to noise. Low dosage of acepromazine in combination with anti-anxiety medication, especially if some pain is involved, may be helpful for some patients whose complaints do not involve noise reactivity/phobia.

Phenothiazines can have effects on multiple systems that may affect behavior.

- Phenothiazines can depress the reticular activating system affecting body temperature control, basal metabolic rates, vasomotor tone, alertness, emesis, and hormonal balance.
- Phenothiazines can also have—and may be used for—anti-cholinergic, anti-histaminic, anti-

spasmodic, and alpha-adrenergic–blocking effects. The alpha-adrenergic antagonist effect is relevant if clonidine, TCAs, SSRIs, SARIs, or SNRIs are concomitantly used.

- More recent research indicates that acepromazine does not increase the risk of seizure activity, as previously thought, within therapeutic ranges (Tobias et al., 2006; McConnell et al., 2007).

Animals who are profoundly fearful or anxious for any reason and who experience the reticular activating system and alpha-adrenergic–blocking effects of phenothiazines will become worse quickly because they are experiencing profoundly scary and unpredictable stimuli that they cannot understand *and so will worsen with such treatment.* Over time, long-term use of acepromazine necessitates higher dosages because treatment re-regulates the dopaminergic system and is often associated with extrapyramidal motor signs. These signs also worsen any anxious, fearful, or panicky responses.

Acepromazine is not a behavioral medication and should be used with caution in any patient with any behavioral concern and avoided, if possible, in patients with heightened sensitivity or reactivity to noise.

Gamma-Aminobutyric Acid

GABA, the inhibitory neurotransmitter found in short interneurons, is produced in large amounts only in the brain and serves as a neurotransmitter in approximately 30% of the synapses in the human central nervous system. GABA is formed from the excitatory AA glutamate via glutamic acid decarboxylase (GAD), catalyzed by GABA-transaminase (GABA-T) and destroyed by transamination (Fig. 10-1). Glutamine can readily cross the BBB; glutamate cannot.

There are two main groupings of GABA receptors— $GABA_A$ and $GABA_B$.

- $GABA_A$ receptors:
  - are transmembrane receptors affected by many compounds,
  - are ligand-gated ion channels,
  - mediate postsynaptic inhibition by increasing Cl^- influx, and
  - increase mean channel opening time when potentiated by barbiturates but increase the probability of the Cl^- channel opening when potentiated by BZDs.
- $GABA_B$ receptors:
  - are G protein–coupled, seven-domain transmembrane receptors,

- are involved in the fine-tuning of inhibitory synaptic transmission,
- inhibit neurotransmitter release via high-voltage activated Ca^{2+} channels when the $GABA_B$ receptor is presynaptic, and
- decrease neuronal excitability by activating inwardly rectifying K^+ conductance underlying the late inhibitory postsynaptic potential when the $GABA_B$ receptors are postsynaptic (Lauder et al., 1998).

GABA also has various tropic effects on developing brain cells (Melzer et al., 2012; Waagepetersen et al., 1999). During ontogeny, GABAergic axons move through areas where other neurotransmitter phenotypes are being produced and so may be related to later monoaminergic imbalances. The extent to which such ontogenic effects are relevant for behavioral conditions is currently unknown but bears investigating.

Excitatory Amino Acids (Glutamate, Aspartate, and Possibly Homocysteate)

Excitatory AAs have a role as central neurotransmitters and are produced in abnormal levels in aggressive, impulsive, and schizophrenic disorders. The main fast excitatory transmitters in the central nervous system are excitatory AAs. Glutamate, widely and uniformly distributed in the central nervous system, is involved in carbohydrate and nitrogen metabolism. Glutamate is stored in synaptic vesicles and released by Ca^{2+}-dependent exocytosis, so calcium channel blockers may affect conditions associated with increased glutamate.

Both barbiturates and progesterone suppress excitatory responses to glutamate, as does the newer NMDA receptor antagonist, memantine (Namenda), which has been approved for treatment of humans with Alzheimer's disease. Barbiturates inhibit calcium uptake presynaptically and decrease synaptosomal release of neurotransmitters, including GABA and glutamate.

Other Chemical Mediators

Nitric oxide and arachidonic acid metabolites (e.g., prostaglandins) can mediate neurotransmitter release. These are synthesized on demand and released by diffusion, requiring no specialized vesicles or receptors. These mediators are extruded through exocytosis after binding with the synaptic membrane. These chemical mediators are activated by an increase in calcium and so may be affected by calcium channel blockers.

MOST USEFUL MEDICATION CLASSES FOR VETERINARY BEHAVIORAL MEDICINE

Anti-histamines, anti-convulsants, progestins/estrogens, sympathomimetics/stimulants, tranquilizers,

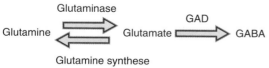

Fig. 10-1 Main synthetic pathways for glutamate and GABA. *GAD,* Glutamic acid decarboxylase.

and narcotic agonists/antagonists have *extremely limited use* in modern behavioral medicine.

Tranquilizers

Tranquilizers are the least useful of most modern medication classes. Tranquilizers decrease spontaneous activity, resulting in decreased response to external or social stimuli, and so they interfere profoundly with any behavioral modification.

- Neuroleptic butyrophenones such as haloperidol decrease both appropriate and inappropriate activity, and because of side effects associated with the most effective mode of delivery (i.e., intravenous), they have limited use.
- Use of phenothiazines (e.g., chlorpromazine, promazine, acetylpromazine, and thioridazine), which target the dopamine receptor, is outdated, as discussed earlier. All phenothiazines have side effects from long-standing use (e.g., cardiovascular disturbance, extrapyramidal signs). As noted, acepromazine makes animals more reactive to noises and startle and so is wholly inappropriate for use in patients with noise phobia.

Benzodiazepines

Compared with barbiturates, cortical function is relatively unimpaired by BZDs. All BZDs potentiate the effects of GABA by increasing binding affinity of the GABA receptor for GABA and by increasing the flow of chloride ions into the neuron, primarily affecting the $GABA_A$ receptors. $GABA_A$ receptors are ionotropic, transmembrane receptors. Barbiturates also affect the $GABA_A$ receptor BZD receptor–chloride ion channel complex using a slightly different mechanism than BZDs, but because of detrimental effects on cognition, barbiturates have been superseded by BZDs and TCAs in the treatment of anxiety and aggression.

BZD effects are dose dependent.

- At low dosages, BZDs act as calming agents or mild sedatives, facilitating calmer activity by tempering excitement and engendering muscle relaxation.
- At moderate dosages, they act as anti-anxiety agents, facilitating social interaction in a more proactive manner.
- At high dosages, they act as hypnotics, facilitating sleep.
- Ataxia and profound sedation usually only occur at dosages beyond those needed for anxiolytic effects.

BZDs easily cross the BBB and are lipophilic. The rate at which they diffuse through the brain depends on the individual BZD and is largely controlled by its lipophilicity. The faster the diffusion rate, the quicker the onset of action. Distribution half-lives of intravenously administered BZDs can be on the order of minutes. Orally administered BZDs reach their maximum concentrations in 30 minutes to a few hours in humans (Riss et al., 2008).

BZDs can be classified as low-, moderate-, or high-potency compounds based on their *in vivo* affinity and that of their metabolite for the receptor. Clonazepam and lorazepam are considered high-potency BZDs with concomitantly long half-lives, whereas clorazepate and diazepam are considered moderate-potency BZDs (Riss et al., 2008).

BZDs decrease muscle tone by a central action that is independent of the sedative effect but may function as a non-specific anxiolytic effect because many distressed animals tense their muscles. Some newer BZDs such as clonazepam have muscle relaxation effects at smaller dosages than those needed for behavioral effects.

BZDs are essential for treatment of sporadic events involving profound anxiety or panic (e.g., storms (Crowell-Davis et al., 2003), fireworks, panic associated with departures of humans signaled by an outside indicator such as an alarm clock).

- For these drugs to be efficacious, based on patterns of suspected maximal concentrations, they should be given to the patient *at least 1 hour before the anticipated stimulus and preferably before the patient exhibits any anticipatory signs of distress.*
- BZDs can also be used as interventional drugs. Advance thought allows repeat dosing that makes use of the half-life of parent compounds and intermediate metabolites and permits concomitant use with daily TCA or SSRI treatment.

The preferred paradigm for the use of the panicolytic BZD, alprazolam, adapted from the client handout, "Generalized Guidelines for Using Alprazolam for Noise and Storm Phobias, Panic, and Severe Distress," is presented in Box 10-2.

Many of the long-term effects and side effects of BZDs are the result of intermediate metabolite function. *N*-desmethyldiazepam is heavily sedative and in high dosages can lead to confusion, ataxia, and apparent amnesia. These conditions are noted in humans and appear to be riskier for elderly adults. We have only poor data on effects for elderly cats and dogs. Amnestic effects can be seen for most BZDs even at clinically relevant levels, and sometimes this is a desired effect, but if BZDs are to be used as part of a treatment plan that requires active learning, some assessment of whether the patient is learning is helpful. Clients can become quite good at noting when their dogs or cats are able to acquire and use new information versus situations where they seem sedated or unable to learn.

Clients often ask about the potential side effects of continued BZD use, *tolerance* and *dependence.*

- In human medicine, "dependence" refers to the desire/compulsion to take the medication to a certain desired effect or to avoid the effects of

BOX 10-2

Generalized Paradigm for Using Alprazolam for Panic and Severe Distress

Alprazolam: The preferred dosage range for dogs is 0.02 to 0.04 mg/kg. With a medium-sized dog as used in this example, the dosage may be 0.25 to 0.5 mg every 12 hours or every 4 to 6 hours as needed.

Alprazolam is the "panicolytic" medication used in dogs and humans, and used well, it can be very effective. There are three ways to use alprazolam: as a preventive, as an interventional medication, and in a truly panicolytic context. Many patients will benefit from all three modes of use.

Preventive: To use as a true preventive, the client must be able to anticipate when there will be a provocative stimulus: a guest, the last walk of the day when there is traffic, an approaching storm.

Give a 0.25-mg tablet 2 hours before anticipated event (either an expected storm—expected means ≥50% chance—or a planned trip) and repeat a full or half dose 30 minutes before event. Repeat every 4 to 6 hours as needed using either the low or the high dose. Start with the low dose because this dosing is cumulative.

Interventional: If the dog has a history of reacting to some stimulus (e.g., the dog becomes distressed outside on a walk, where the distress may have been triggered by a noise, or an unexpected storm, precluding a preventive strategy, and not yet full-blown), clients can continue or discontinue the walk depending on the dog's response, but it's really important that the dog *not* make a molecular memory of the fear and his or her own response to it, which means that clients may wish to give the dog a half or a whole 0.25-mg tablet. Clients learn to walk the fine line between learning whether the dog really needs the medication and

not intervening early enough to avoid the distress that will make a molecular memory. No one is perfect at this, so being attentive to the issues is important. This strategy requires that clients have alprazolam with them at all times.

On distressing days, a combination of the above-described strategies is the best choice. For example, clients can give a dose as soon as the dog awakens, repeat the dose in 2 hours and then again at 30 minutes before the anticipated upsetting event, and continue to give ½ to 1 tablet as needed depending on how upset the dog is. Clients may wish to expand this strategy in dogs who respond beneficially to alprazolam to repeated use daily for a few days preceding an event that may be distressing. If clients are able to medicate the dog before he or she becomes distressed, the dog will always need less medication.

Panicolytic: If something happens that is truly frightening (e.g., the dog has a panic attack at the veterinary hospital, the dog is jumped by another dog in the park, a surprise thunderstorm erupts, there is a huge fire with attendant fire trucks next door) and the dog has a full-blown panic attack, give the full dose immediately. If the dog is still distressed in 30 minutes, give another half or full dose. The pill can be dissolved in a tiny amount of liquid or will dissolve in the dog's cheeks.

Similar patterns for alprazolam use—albeit at much lower dosages—also benefit distressed cats. The most important uses of alprazolam for cats may be before visiting the veterinarian, after visiting the veterinarian if the visit caused distress, and for any travel. Concerns about use of BZDs in cats and feline hepatic metabolism are discussed later.

---

not taking the medication (*sensu* Riss et al., 2008). As such, the ability to become dependent relies on the presence of opposable thumbs and access to the medication at will. Canine and feline patients do not have such access. Because of this concern, certain human households should not have access to BZDs.

- Physiological tolerance occurs with BZDs. Cross-tolerance is possible with BZDs and may be specific to the compound used. In humans, the tendency to develop physiological tolerance does not depend on the chemistry or pharmacokinetics of the involved compound but may depend on the individual BZD and the patient's reaction to it. This suggests that changes in receptor function, as are thought to occur when TCAs or SSRIs have been discontinued and then re-started, are responsible. Although dependence is associated in humans with high dosages of BZDs, high potency, short duration of action, and

long duration of treatment, these factors appear to be only partially involved in physiological tolerance.

- Rebound and withdrawal phenomena/syndromes are well known for BZDs but also occur with TCAs, SSRIs, NaSRIs, et cetera. With rebound syndrome, the patient's original signs reappear when medication is discontinued. With withdrawal syndrome, new and distress signs appear when medication is discontinued. Gradual weaning (over a period of weeks) to the lowest effective level of medication usually minimizes the chance of occurrence for both of these phenomena. Abrupt withdrawal, especially with shorter acting compounds, may place patients more at risk for these phenomena.

  - If the medication is given twice a day, weaning may involve halving the amount given—if this is possible—twice a day for 7 to 10 days, then giving the medication once a day for 7 to 10 days, then giving it every other day for 7 to 10 days.

TABLE 10-5

Half-Lives of Parent Compounds and Intermediate Metabolites of Target Benzodiazepines in Humans

Parent Compound	Half-Life Parent Compound	Half-Life Intermediate Metabolite	Overall Duration of Action
Triazolam	2-4 hr	2 hr	Ultra-short: 6 hr
Oxazepam	8-12 hr		Short: 12-18 hr
Alprazolam	6-12 hr	6 hr	Medium: 24 hr
Diazepam	24-40 hr	60 hr	Long: 24-48 hr
Clonazepam	50 hr (19-60 hr*)		Long: 24-48 hr

*Riss et al., 2008.
Adapted from Greenblatt et al., 1981, 1983.

- Clients who can halve an individual dose may be more comfortable if they halve the evening dose for 7 to 10 days, then the morning dose for another 7 to 10 days, then give only one dose for 7 to 10 days, then move to an every-other-day dose. This longer weaning period is fine and may provide a needed added comfort level.
- By the time dosing gets to every other day, it's usually safe to stop after 7 to 10 days of this, but if clients worry or the animal becomes reactive, giving the medication every third day for 2 weeks and then titrating it even more slowly are options.

Parent compound and intermediate metabolite half-lives are listed in Table 10-5 for humans and in Table 10-6 for domestic species (Greenblatt et al., 1981, 1983; Schwartz et al., 1965).

Patients who react adversely or not at all to one BZD may do well with another. Routes of metabolism and cytochrome P-450 (CYP) enzymes involved in metabolism may affect outcome. Some inhibitors and inducers of BZD activity are listed in Table 10-7.

The BZDs currently and commonly used in dogs and cats are listed in Table 10-8, along with their major properties, extrapolated from the human and rodent literature. A schematic of the metabolic paths of commonly used BZDs is found in Figure 10-2. There are a number of BZDs that are not or seldom used in dogs that may have treatment benefits.

All BZD end products are glucuronidated and excreted, and these usually appear with parent compounds in the urine.

Occasionally, a dog or cat will not respond to one BZD but may respond to another. Some animals respond to none, which likely is the result of a genetic variant in hepatic CYP systems.

Other Agents That Affect Gamma-Aminobutyric Acid

Rarely, a dog or cat experiences excitement when given a BZD. This excitement will resolve in a few hours, during which the animal should be protected, but can also be aborted by *flumazenil*, a specific BZD antagonist

TABLE 10-6

Duration of Action of Parent Compound, Diazepam, and Its Intermediate Metabolite, Nordiazepam (N-Desmethyldiazepam) in Selected Domestic Animals

Species	Diazepam	N-Desmethyldiazepam
Horse	24-48 hr	51-120 hr
Cat	5.5 hr	21 hr
Dog	3.2 hr	3-6 hr

Adapted from Schwartz et al., 1965.

(0.01 to 0.02 mg/kg intravenously). Patients with extreme excitement to more than one BZD may not be good candidates for BZD treatment.

Gabapentin is considered a GABA analogue—it structurally looks like GABA to the receptors—but it is not active and is not physiologically regulated. Gabapentin was originally developed with the intent to have benzodiazepine-like activity by acting as a $GABA_A$ receptor agonist. While we now know that it does not act as a GABA precursor, agonist, or antagonist it does have an effect on the AA active transporter at the BBB. This transporter interaction increases the amount of brain and intracellular GABA. It also appears to affect numerous enzymatic regulatory mechanisms and may increase GAD.

In addition to its direct effects on GABA, gabapentin:
- increases non-synaptic GABA release from glia,
- modulates glutamate metabolism—possibly very important for conditions involving impulsivity, and
- modulates sodium and calcium channels.

As a by-product of all of this, gabapentin also increases whole blood serotonin levels.

Common uses for gabapentin include:
- myogenic and neurogenic pain,
- anxiety disorders including panic,
- generalized anxiety disorder and social phobias, and
- as an adjuvant to other treatments for obsessive-compulsive disorder (OCD) and some seizure disorders.

TABLE 10-7

Inhibitors and Inducers of Cytochrome P-450 Enzymes for Various Benzodiazepine Substrates

CYP Enzyme	BZD Substrate	Inhibitor	Inducer
CYP2C19	Diazepam	Fluvoxamine Omeprazole Oxcarbazepine	Dexamethasone Phenobarbital Phenytoin St. John's wort
CYP3A4	Clonazepam Diazepam Midazolam	Azole anti-fungals (e.g., ketoconazole) Cimetidine Clarithromycin Diltiazem Erythromycin Fluoxetine Nefazodone Sertraline	Carbamazepine Phenobarbital Phenytoin St. John's wort
UGT	Lorazepam Oxazepam	Valproate	Carbamazepine Phenobarbital Phenytoin

BZD, Benzodiazepine; CYP, cytochrome P-450.
Adapted from Riss et al., 2008.

TABLE 10-8

Characterization by Activity of, Interaction of, and Potential Uses for Select Benzodiazepines Currently and Commonly Used in Dogs and Cats

BZD Compound	Characterization	Potential Uses
Alprazolam	• Intermediate-acting • Extended release form available • Absorption delayed by food • Substrate of CYP enzyme 3A4 • No interactions between alprazolam and sertraline or paroxetine • Fluoxetine prolongs $t_{1/2}$ and increases AUC of alprazolam • Fluvoxamine increases alprazolam concentrations (up to 100%) • Venlafaxine lowers the AUC by ~30%	• Panic and panic disorder • Short-term treatment of acute and severe anxiety
Clonazepam	• Long-acting • Completely absorbed with high (90%) bioavailability • Biotransformation possibly involving CYP3A • Undergoes extensive metabolism, but no active intermediate metabolites are formed	• Anti-convulsant • Muscle relaxant • Anxiety
Clorazepate	• Undergoes complete conversion to N-desmethyldiazepam in gastrointestinal tract, and its effects are almost wholly due to the level attained of this intermediate metabolite	• Panic • Profound anxiety • Seizures
Diazepam	• Action is primarily due to N-desmethyldiazepam, especially with repeat dosing • Temazepam and oxazepam are relatively minor metabolites	• Seizures • IV for status epilepticus • Anxiety • Preoperative anesthesia

Continued

TABLE 10-8

Characterization by Activity of, Interaction of, and Potential Uses for Select Benzodiazepines Currently and Commonly Used in Dogs and Cats—cont'd

BZD Compound	Characterization	Potential Uses
	• Demethylation of diazepam is catalyzed by CYP2B6 exclusively and preferentially by CYP2C8, CYP2C9, and CYP2C9R144C • CYP3A4 and CYP3A5 catalyze 3-hydroxylation • A genetic polymorphism of CYP2C19 affects influence • Diazepam and nordiazepam (*N*-desmethyldiazepam) pharmacokinetics in humans, but the effect is only 2-fold • Characterized by long $t_{1/2}$ of parent compound (diazepam $t_{1/2}$ 20-50 hr) and main metabolite (nordiazepam $t_{1/2}$ up to 200 hr) • Phenobarbital is a powerful inducer of CYP and so decreases AUC, bioavailability, et cetera, increasing T_{max} • Omeprazole inhibits the formation of nordiazepam, temazepam, 4'-hydroxydiazepam • Readily absorbed orally, rectally, and nasally	
Lorazepam	• Premedication for general anesthesia • Poorly water and fat soluble • Metabolism impaired by fluconazole, miconazole, and ketoconazole because of competitive inhibition of CYP enzyme	• Anxiolytic • Sedative • Amnestic agent (possible use for panic associated with awful experience) • Insomnia (primarily in humans) • IV for status epilepticus
Midazolam	• Short-acting • Effects dose-dependent and even with CYP3A induction $t_{1/2}$ increases with high dosages because of a concomitant increase in volume of distribution • Can be given orally, sublingually, or IV with high bioavailability	• Sedative • Premedication for anxiety and before anesthesia induction • Sedation for serious in-hospital cases • Status epilepticus
Oxazepam	• Intermediate-acting • Less likely to accumulate than other BZDs with hepatic impairment	• Anxiety • Anorexia in cats
Triazolam	• Short-acting • Historically associated with side effect of aggressiveness but considered safe in United States at low dosages; banned in United Kingdom	• Insomnia (primarily in humans)

AUC, Area under the curve; BZD, benzodiazepine; CYP, cytochrome P-450; IV, intravenously; T_{max}, maximum threshold; $t_{1/2}$, half-life. Adapted from Mandrioli et al., 2008.

The starting dose in dogs is generally 200 mg (100 mg for small dogs) one to three times per day, depending on the other medications the dog is taking, with a recommended starting dosage of 10 to 20 mg/kg orally every 12 hours. In cats, the starting dosage is 3 to 5 mg/kg orally every 12 to 24 hours. In humans, 3600 mg/day have been given with a good therapeutic outcome.

Because gabapentin has no active metabolites, no plasma binding, and no CYP auto-inductions, it is a relatively "safe" medication to use, especially in animals with renal and hepatic compromise. Side effects in

humans include "psychosis," so clients should be asked to watch for "personality changes," but the most often reported side effect is sedation.

Monoamine Oxidase Inhibitors

MAO inhibitors act by blocking oxidative deamination of brain amines (dopamine, NE, epinephrine, 5-HT), increasing these substances and elevating mood. The MAO inhibitor for the subtype B receptor, selegiline (Anipryl), is used for the treatment of cognitive dysfunction in cats and dogs. It affects reuptake and

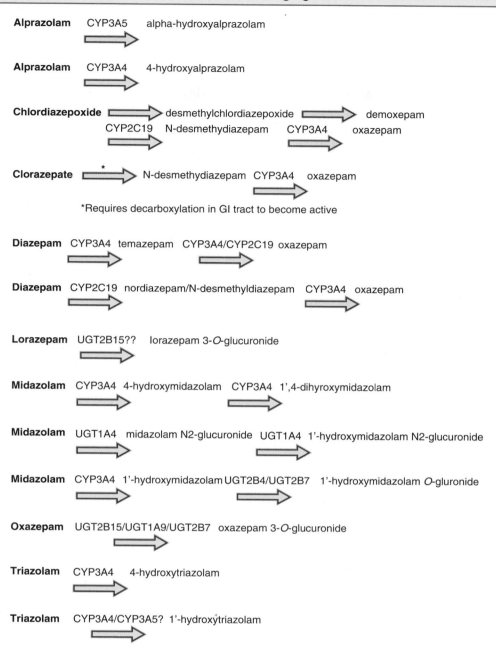

Fig. 10-2 Metabolic pathways of some common benzodiazepines, with the cytochrome P-450 enzymes involved in the specific metabolic steps. *UGT,* Uridine diphosphate–glucuronosyltransferase, an enzyme that leads to glucuronidation. (Adapted from Mandrioli et al., 2008.)

recycling of dopamine, in a manner similar to TCAs and SSRIs and other neurotransmitters. Selegiline is fairly specific for dopamine and as an antagonist slows destruction of synaptic knobs of presynaptic neurons (Milgram et al., 1993). As a result, neuronal transmission and use of dopamine may become more efficient, leading to neurotrophic effects that may aid decreasing cognitive abilities. Selegiline is metabolized into a relatively small amount of amphetamine, which may account for some small proportion of its effects (Milgram et al., 1993).

Because of the life stage of the cat or dog when selegiline is likely to be recommended, treatment, if helpful, should be considered lifelong, barring serious side effects. Animals without cognitive impairment will not benefit from selegiline and may become agitated because it is metabolized into amphetamine-like compounds, a potential benefit for aged patients.

Tricyclic Antidepressants

TCAs are structurally related to the phenothiazine anti-psychotics and are used in humans to treat endogenous depression, panic attacks, phobic and obsessive states, neuropathic pain states, and pediatric enuresis. There are three major effects of TCAs that vary in degree depending on the individual drug:

1. sedation,
2. peripheral and central anti-cholinergic action, and
3. potentiation of central nervous system biogenic amines by blocking their reuptake presynaptically.

In treatment of behavioral conditions we aim for this last effect.

The ability of TCAs to inhibit presynaptic reuptake of NE and 5-HT is largely responsible for their antidepressant effect. With long-term use, TCAs may cause a decrease in the number of beta-adrenergic and $5-HT_2$ receptors. Many TCAs also have potent muscarinic, alpha-1-adrenergic, and H_1 and H_2 blocking activity, which can account for common side effects reported in humans (e.g., dry mouth, sedation, hypotension). The H_1 and H_2 side effects may be useful in treating pruritic conditions in veterinary medicine, and this is the primary use of the TCA, doxepin, which has 600 to 800 times the H_1 antagonist properties of diphenhydramine (Benadryl).

Most dogs treated with clomipramine (Clomicalm) reach steady-state levels in 3 to 5 days, attain peak plasma concentrations in approximately 1 to 3 hours, and experience a half-life of 1 to 16 hours of the parent compound and 1 to 2 hours of the active intermediate metabolites (Hewson et al., 1998; King et al., 2000a, 2000b), suggesting that dogs may require higher dosages or more frequent dosing than humans. Cats differ in their pharmacokinetics and reach peak plasma levels of the parent compound in 3 hours and within 7 hours for desmethylclomipramine, the main intermediate metabolite (Lainesse et al., 2006, 2007a, 2007b). Cats also may have a lower capacity to hydroxylate metabolites of clomipramine compared with dogs and humans (King et al., 2004; Lainesse et al., 2007b).

Knowledge of intermediate metabolites can be important; animals experiencing sedation or other side effects with the parent compound may do quite well when treated with the intermediate metabolite alone. For example, cats that become sedated or nauseous when treated with amitriptyline, may respond well when treated with nortriptyline at the same dose. Table 10-9 lists parent compounds, intermediate metabolites, and their relative effects on NE and 5-HT.

Side effects of TCAs in humans can include a dry mouth, constipation, urinary retention, tachycardias and other arrhythmias, syncope associated with orthostatic hypotension and alpha-adrenergic blockade, ataxia, disorientation, and generalized depression and inappetence. Side effects appear to be more rare and less diverse in dogs and may include gastrointestinal distress, changes in appetite, occasional serious sedation, and discomfort associated with unremitting tachycardia that resolves when drugs are withdrawn.

Use of TCAs is contraindicated in animals with a history of urinary retention, glaucoma, and uncontrolled cardiac arrhythmias (Reich et al., 2000). The common side effects of TCAs as manifest on ECG include:

- flattened T waves,
- prolonged Q-T intervals, and
- depressed S-T segments.

In high doses, TCAs have been implicated in sick euthyroid syndrome. If laboratory evaluation occurs while the patient is undergoing treatment with TCAs, thyroid levels should be interpreted with caution

TABLE 10-9

Relative Effects of Tricyclic Antidepressant Parent Compounds and Intermediate Metabolites on Norepinephrine and 5-Hydroxytryptamine Reuptake

Parent Compound	Intermediate Metabolite	NE	5-HT	Potential for Sedation*	Potential for Anti-Cholinergic Effects
Desipramine		++	+	Low	Low
Imipramine	Desipramine	+++	++	Moderate	Moderate
Amitriptyline	Nortriptyline	++	++	High	High
Nortriptyline		+	+	Moderate	Moderate
Clomipramine	N-Desmethyl clomipramine + clomipramine[†]	++	+++	High	High

5-HT, 5-Hydroxytryptamine; NE, norepinephrine; +, mild effect; ++, moderate effect; +++, large effect.
*At therapeutic levels in dogs and cats, any true sedative effect should be transient. Dogs and cats may sleep more deeply and soundly but should awaken refreshed and not groggy. If the patient is groggy or sedated after 3 to 4 days, this should be considered a true side effect resulting in changes of medication and/or dose.
[†]Does not include the specific effect of the intermediate metabolite as a selective serotonin reuptake inhibitor.

because TCAs (and SSRIs) can artificially lower laboratory thyroid values.

In older or compromised animals, complete laboratory evaluations are urged because high doses of TCAs are known to alter liver enzyme levels. Extremely high doses are associated with convulsions, cardiac abnormalities, and hepatotoxicity. Cats are likely to be more sensitive to all TCAs than dogs because TCAs are metabolized through glucuronidation, a pathway for which cats have decreased facility compared with dogs.

These medications have been extremely successful in treating many canine and feline conditions, including separation anxiety, generalized anxiety that may be a precursor to some elimination and aggressive behaviors, pruritic conditions that may be involved in or precursors to conditions involving self-mutilation, acral lick dermatitis, compulsive grooming, and some narcoleptic disorders.

Amitriptyline, an older TCA, can be very successful in treating separation anxiety and generalized anxiety. Imipramine has been useful in treating mild attention-deficit disorders in people and may be useful in dogs because it has been used to treat mild narcolepsy. A TCA derivative, carbamazepine, has been used successfully to control aberrant activity in psychomotor seizures in dogs (Holland, 1988). Clomipramine has been successful in the treatment of human and canine OCD (Overall and Dunham, 2002). Clomipramine has one active, intermediate metabolite, clomipramine, which acts as a serotonin reuptake inhibitor.

Tricyclic Antidepressant Derivatives

Carbamazepine (Tegretol) is an iminodiabenzyl derivative of imipramine (Barratt, 1993). Carbamazepine has been used in humans to treat temporal lobe epilepsy, trigeminal neuralgia, acute mania, and explosive aggression (Barratt, 1993). It has also been used, with some success, prophylactically in the treatment of bipolar disorder in humans. The efficacy of carbamazepine in such cases has been postulated to be the result of its effects on sodium ion channels and potential effects on peripheral BZD receptors in the brain. It also may potentiate alpha-adrenergic receptors. Carbamazepine is slowly and erratically absorbed from the gastrointestinal tract and is better absorbed if ingested with food. In humans, it reaches peak plasma levels within 2 to 8 hours, has a half-life of 12 to 17 hours, and has an active intermediate metabolite that also has anticonvulsant properties. Canine dosages overlap dosages in humans (400 to 1600 mg/day in divided doses) (Holland, 1988), and, as with humans, the therapeutic concentration necessary to obtain anti-epileptic effects (6 to 10 μg/mL) is lower than that necessary to obtain psychiatric or behavioral effects (8 to 12 μg/mL); however, serum levels were not a useful guide for response. Carbamazepine can have profound side effects that include agranulocytosis, aplastic anemia

(these occur in 1:20,000 human patients), and decreases in triiodothyronine (T_3), thyroxine (T_4), and the free T_4 index. Carbamazepine, similar to some TCAs and SSRIs, may increase the activity of the enzyme that converts T_4 to T_3 (5′-iodinase) in rodents, but the effect is not independent of diurnal rhythm, brain region, or extent of sleep deprivation (Baumgartner et al., 1997). Free T_4 concentrations have repeatedly been reported to be decreased by carbamazepine in humans without concomitant endocrine illness (Simko and Horacek, 2007), but these rebound on discontinuation of medication, even if carbamazepine treatment had been long-term (Lossius et al., 2009).

Partial Serotonin Agonists

Partial 5-$HT_{1A/B}$ agonists (e.g., buspirone) have few side effects; do not negatively affect cognition; allow rehabilitation by influencing cognition, attention, arousal, and mood regulation; and may aid in treating aggression associated with impaired social interaction. Buspirone—the primary partial serotonin agonist used in veterinary behavioral medicine—has been used with varying but unimpressive success in the treatment of canine aggression, canine and feline ritualistic or stereotypic behaviors, self-mutilation, possible OCD, thunderstorm phobias, and feline spraying. It may be best used in combination with other compounds. However, buspirone may be useful as a solitary agent in the treatment of the victim in true inter-cat aggression. TCAs and the BZDs, alprazolam and lorazepam, can also be considered in the treatment of inter-cat aggression (see Chapter 9).

When buspirone is used for cats who are victims of inter-cat aggression, clients should understand that buspirone acts by making the cat less anxious and more interactive/assertive, which could lead to confrontations. The anecdotal reports that buspirone renders animals more "aggressive" are misleading and an outgrowth of unclear labels. Cats treated with buspirone tend to become more outgoing and less anxious but are still living within a social environment where they are treated as victims by the other cat. Treatment with buspirone may alter their former response, which could lead to an agonistic encounter. This example highlights how pharmacological changes do not occur in a vacuum, and behavioral and environmental changes—including those in the social environment—are important to monitor.

Selective Serotonin Reuptake Inhibitors

The SSRIs (fluoxetine, paroxetine, sertraline, and fluvoxamine) are derivatives of TCAs. These compounds often have a long half-life, and after 2 to 3 weeks plasma levels peak within 4 to 8 hours. As for the TCA, clomipramine, which is converted into an SSRI, treatment must continue for a minimum of 6 to 8 weeks before a determination about efficacy can be made. These medications induce receptor conformation changes through the production of new protein—an action that can take 3 to 5 weeks to be consistent, so a minimum treatment period of 8 weeks is required before a treatment "failure" can be pronounced.

Fluoxetine is efficacious in the treatment of profound aggressions, separation anxiety (Landsberg et al., 2008; Simpson et al., 2007), panic disorder, and OCD. Paroxetine is efficacious in the treatment of depression, social anxiety, and agitation associated with depression. Sertraline is thought to be useful particularly for generalized anxiety and panic disorder.

Most SSRI effects are due to highly selective blockade of the reuptake of 5-HT_{1A} into presynaptic neurons *without* major effects on NE, dopamine, acetylcholine, histaminic, and alpha-adrenergic receptors.

SSRIs should not be used with MAO inhibitors because of risks of serotonin syndrome (Brown et al., 1996; Lane and Baldwin, 1997). Although many MAO inhibitors have few to no effects on serotonin directly, dopamine is converted to NE, so co-administration may cause a stimulatory synergy with far-reaching effects. Serotonin syndrome is covered in more depth later in this chapter.

Co-administration of buspirone with SSRIs may decrease the efficacy of buspirone and potentiate extrapyramidal symptoms, but there have also been reports of synergistic effects. Concomitant use of TCAs or BZDs increases the plasma levels of both of these and may prolong the excretion of fluoxetine.

Polypharmacy can be safe, rational, and cheap and can save animals' lives, but an understanding of how the medications act is required. The effects of the CYP system on metabolism of related compounds are discussed later in the chapter. Examples of potentially efficacious combinations of these medications are presented in Box 10-3.

Table 10-10 summarizes the "gestalt" of TCA and SSRI use. This algorithm is extrapolated from the human literature based on the similarity of dogs and humans with respect to pharmacokinetics and pharmacodynamics when treated with TCAs or SSRIs (Hewson et al., 1998; King et al., 2000b; Yokota et al., 1987). This algorithm is intended to provide a model for thinking about how to choose and change medications based on what is known and learned about the manifestation of the patient's condition, but it should be remembered that although dogs and humans may be similar, their metabolisms still vary, and cat responses can be very different from responses of humans and dogs.

Serotonin Norepinephrine Reuptake Inhibitors

There are few to no data on the use of SNRIs in veterinary patients, but these agents have anecdotally been

---

BOX 10-3

Sample Combinations of Medications That May Allow the Dosage of Each to Be Lowered with Enhanced Efficacy

Amitriptyline (TCA) (anxiety-related diagnosis) + fluoxetine (SSRI) (anxiety-related diagnosis)

Amitriptyline (TCA) (anxiety-related diagnosis) + fluoxetine (SSRI) (anxiety-related diagnosis) + alprazolam (BZD) (panic/phobia/severe distress with known trigger)

Amitriptyline (TCA) (anxiety-related diagnosis) + alprazolam (BZD) (panic/phobia)

Fluoxetine (SSRI) (anxiety-related diagnosis) + alprazolam (BZD) (panic/phobia)

Clomipramine (TCA—relatively specific) (anxiety-related diagnosis) + alprazolam (BZD) (panic/phobia)

Clomipramine (TCA—relatively specific) (anxiety-related diagnosis) + diazepam (BZD) (panic/phobias)—could be fairly sedating

Amitriptyline (TCA) (anxiety-related diagnosis) + diazepam (BZD) (panic/phobia)—could be fairly sedating

Selegiline (MAO inhibitor) (cognitive dysfunction) + diazepam (BZD) (panic/phobias)

Selegiline (MAO inhibitor) (cognitive dysfunction) + alprazolam (BZD) (panic/phobia)

Paroxetine (SSRI) (social anxiety) + alprazolam (BZD) (panic/appetite stimulation in cats)

TABLE 10-10

"Gestalt" of Tricyclic Antidepressant and Selective Serotonin Reuptake Inhibitor Use Based on Half-Life of Parent Compounds and Active Intermediate Metabolites, Relative Effects on Norepinephrine and 5-Hydroxytryptamine, and Extrapolations from Multicenter Human Studies

Diagnosis/Type of Condition	First Drug of Choice
Narcolepsy	Imipramine
Milder, relatively non-specific anxieties	Amitriptyline
Milder, relatively non-specific anxieties with avoidance of sedation	Nortriptyline
Social phobias/anxieties concerning social interaction	Paroxetine
Panic/generalized anxiety	Sertraline
Outburst aggression/related anxieties; explosive forms of OCD or separation anxiety	Fluoxetine
Ritualistic behavior associated with anxiety, including OCD and separation anxiety	Clomipramine

OCD, Obsessive-compulsive disorder.

used extensively. These medications may be viable choices for patients who are experiencing an incomplete response to SSRIs and for whom administration of both a TCA and a SSRI is undesirable.

Venlafaxine has a half-life of 2 to 4 hours in dogs (Curtis, 2008; Howell et al., 1994), which may render it less practical for canine use than treatment with a combination of medications chosen for their efficacy of action, potential beneficial interactions, and half-lives.

Serotonin 2A Antagonist/ Reuptake Inhibitors

More recent attention has been given to the SARI, trazodone, which may be useful for panic and phobias as an adjuvant to BZD, TCA, and/or SSRI treatment. The primary action of SARIs is to antagonize 5-HT_{2A} receptors and to inhibit 5-HT reuptake, although there are also effects of its metabolite on 5-HT_1 receptors.

Trazodone acts as a 5HT_{1A} agonist at relatively low dosages (0.05 to 1 mg/kg), very similar to buspirone, and can act as an antagonist at high dosages (6 to 9 mg/kg) (American Hospital Formulary Service, 1999). There is no established dosage, but ranges of 1.7 to 9.5 mg/kg/day have been reported for trazodone use in dogs (Gruen and Sherman, 2008).

Although G protein–coupled systems such as those involved in the effects of TCAs, SSRIs, SARIs, and SNRIs can respond almost instantly, the effects of these over time on molecular transcription and translation are thought to underlie the mechanism of these medications (Duman, 1998). If this is true, it is unlikely that as-needed usage of these compounds will be effective, unless the patient is already taking a medicine in this class. Assays of efficacy are best done in placebo-controlled, double-blind studies (Overall and Dunham, 2009) so that the effects of the non-medication intervention can also be assessed.

Other Adjunctive Agents

Medications Affecting Blood Pressure
Beta-Adrenergic Receptor Antagonists
Beta-adrenergic receptor antagonists (beta blockers) are used in humans to treat self-injurious behavior, intermittent explosive disorder, conduct disorders, dementia, brain disease/injury, autism, and schizophrenia.

- Older beta blockers, such as propranolol (a beta-1 and beta-2 blocker), have not been as successful as hoped in treating canine or feline aggression but have been used with mixed success in combination with TCAs or SSRIs to treat some anxieties and noise phobias. Dogs do not respond the way humans do to beta-adrenoreceptor blocking drugs because, at rest, dogs appear to lack tonic adrenergic tone, which these medications would suppress (Kantelip et al., 1982).

- Pindolol, a beta-adrenoreceptor antagonist/blocker, has been used successfully to potentiate the action of TCAs and SSRIs by blocking the presynaptic autoreceptor—the "thermostat"—aborting the initial "down-regulation" phase of monoamine release: the relevant monoamine continues to be produced despite accumulation in the synaptic cleft owing to presynaptic reuptake inhibition (Duman, 1998).

Alpha-Adrenergic Agonists
- Clonidine, a centrally acting, alpha-adrenergic agonist, which lowers heart rate and blood pressure, has been used in the treatment of noise reactivity and panic/panic disorder in dogs (Ogata and Dodman, 2010). Dogs appear to be less sensitive to the hypotensive effects than many other species (Murrell and Hellebreker, 2005).

- Clonidine and guanfacine (Tenex), both potent centrally acting $alpha_{2A}$-adrenergic receptor agonists, decrease cardiac output and peripheral vascular resistance by extremely efficient binding of alpha-adrenergic receptors in the vasomotor center, the locus coeruleus, in the brainstem. This binding decreases presynaptic calcium release, and so adrenergic receptors do not fire, which subsequently inhibits adrenal release of NA/NE. Consequently, one undesirable side effect is sedation, but decreased arousal below the level of sedation is considered a desired effect.

- Adenyl cyclase is also inhibited by alpha agonists, altering cellular function by decreasing levels of cyclic adenosine monophosphate (cAMP) and subsequently decreasing the reactivity of central nervous system neurons.

- The sedative effect of $alpha_{2A}$ agonists appears to be largely due to action on the locus coeruleus.

- $Alpha_2$ receptors are also found in high densities in the vagus nerve, primary sensory nerves, and the dorsal horn of the spinal cord. The receptors in the dorsal horn are largely $alpha_{2A}$ subtype receptors, whereas receptors in sensory neurons are mixed $alpha_{2A}$ and $alpha_{2C}$ subtype receptors (Murrell and Hellebrekers, 2005).

- Because neurons from the locus coeruleus project to limbic structures (e.g., amygdala) and to the forebrain, general applications for the treatment of anxiety-related conditions are clear.
  - Clonidine may also increase $GABA_A$ activity (Lipman, 1996).
  - Clonidine has been used to treat autonomic hyperarousal in human post-traumatic stress disorder and may be useful in conditions in dogs involving hyperarousal and hyper-reactivity.
  - Guanfacine appears not to be as sedating as clonidine, although it has a longer duration of action (Scahill et al., 2001). Guanfacine also improves pre-cortical function in non-human primates (Casey et al., 1997) and so may be promising for

use in dogs when anxiety affects cognitive performance. Guanfacine is not widely used in dogs, but it may be a consideration for reactive dogs when other medications do not seem to help. Dosages for children range from 0.5 to 4 mg/day, with dosage intervals of one to four times per day.

- Neither clonidine nor guanfacine should be used incautiously with TCAs because TCAs block alpha$_1$-adrenergic receptors. Clonidine has weaker but measurable effects on alpha$_1$-adrenergic receptors, possibly permitting informed use, but the effects of TCAs and alpha-agonists may be generally antagonistic. Hypertensive crises have been reported in humans given both medications.

Medications Affecting N-Methyl-D-Aspartate Receptors

Memantine (Schneider et al., 2009) has been used for the treatment of OCD, both alone and as an adjuvant. Memantine blocks NMDA glutamate receptors and so lessens the effect of glutamate. It is thought to have a positive effect on cognition, mood, and behavior by modulating the neurocytotoxic and synaptic sensitization effects known to occur with unregulated or excess glutamate. Memantine acts as an agonist at the D$_2$ receptor, acts as a non-competitive antagonist at the 5-HT$_3$ receptor, and may contribute to some signs of cholinergic effects. Because of its effects on the NMDA glutamate receptors, memantine may have a role in treating impulsive conditions beyond those involving OCD.

Narcotic Agonists/Antagonists

Narcotic agonists/antagonists have been useful in human OCD (Herman et al., 1989; Pickar et al., 1982) and in domestic animal self-mutilation and ritualistic disorders (Dodman et al., 1987, 1988a, 1988b). These include naloxone and naltrexone (pure antagonists) and nalorphine and pentazocine (mixed agonist-antagonists). Pure antagonists appear to block delta, mu, and kappa receptors equally. Naloxone reverses opioid-induced analgesia and may be a useful diagnostic tool for practitioners attempting to determine whether stereotypic behavior is associated with endogenous, self-stimulation of opioid receptors (Brown et al., 1987). Naloxone suppresses food intake in most domestic animals (Foster et al., 1981). Hydrocodone (Hycodan) can be useful in long-term treatment of canine acral lick granulomas and in self-mutilation by cats. The common human side effect of constipation does not appear to be a problem, but the drug is abusable by humans. Morphine opiates can be physiologically addictive in dogs (Martin et al., 1974; Segall, 1964).

Progestins/Estrogens

The use of progestins and estrogens has largely been superseded by the newer classes of medications discussed in this chapter. The progestins (medroxyprogesterone acetate [Depo-Provera], megestrol acetate [Ovaban, Megace], and diethylstilbestrol [DES]) have historically been used in behavioral medicine because of their putative "calming effects" on canine aggression (Beaver, 1982; Hart, 1974a, 1979c, 1980; Knol and Egberink-Alink, 1989a, 1989b) and possibly because of their ability to suppress the excitatory effects of glutamate (Sohn and Ferrendelli, 1976) and their suppressant effects on male stereotypic behaviors. In rodents, progestins have been noted to decrease aggression without a decrease in general locomotor behavior (Fraile et al., 1988).

In humans, cyclicity of epileptic seizures (decreases in seizure susceptibility) has been associated with increases in estrogen and progesterone. Progesterone has been reported to have anti-convulsant effects. Progesterone metabolites have been reported to be 10 to 50 times more potent than barbiturates in potentiating GABA receptor–coupled Cl$^-$ conductance in cultured embryonic rat hippocampal neurons (Taubøll and Gjerstad, 1993).

Progestins are no longer recommended for use because of their systemic side effects, which may include diabetes, increased insulin levels, increased growth hormone, acromegaly, polyphagia, polyuria, decreased packed cell volume, decreased exercise tolerance, jaundice associated with thickening of the gallbladder walls, gynecomastia, mammary gland hyperplasia, adenocarcinoma, endometrial hyperplasia/pyometra, adrenocortical suppression, and bone marrow suppression (Eigenmann and Eigenmann, 1981a, 1981b; Peterson, 1987). There are safer agents than progestins, such as DES, to use to treat resting urinary incontinence. Bethanechol is particularly effective if the bladder is enlarged. Phenylpropanolamine is a sympathetic agonist whose side effect is increased bladder tone, which means that it is contraindicated in cases of urinary retention.

Sympathomimetics/Stimulants

There are few treatment and diagnostic situations that have been more misunderstood than those involving stimulants and "hyperactivity." The original literature on "hyperkinesis/hyperactivity" in dogs actually focused on laboratory dogs as a potential animal model for a very restrictive variant of hyperactivity in humans ("hyperkinesis") (Corson et al., 1971). Truly hyperkinetic human patients were defined as displaying physiological signs of hyperactivity (heart rate, respiratory rate increases) in addition to congruent behavioral signs. Stimulants such as dextroamphetamine

(Dexedrine), methylphenidate (Ritalin), and pemoline (Cylert) were expected to have paradoxical effects in truly "hyperkinetic/hyperactive" animals, including humans. These medications were thought to produce excitement in "normal" individuals and paradoxical calm in "hyperkinetic/hyperactive" individuals. Dogs were defined by Corson as being "hyperkinetic/ hyperactive" *only* if they responded to treatment with 0.2 to 1.0 mg/kg methylphenidate with a 15% decrease in heart rate and respiratory rate 75 to 90 minutes after treatment (Corson and Corson, 1976; Corson et al., 1971, 1980). Were the dogs to become more aroused when given the medication, they were considered not to meet the criteria for "hyperkinesis/hyperactivity." *Truly hyperactive states that meet these conditions are rare in canine and feline patients* (Marder, 1991) and may not be common in humans.

In the past 20 years, the focus in humans has shifted to attention deficits, inattentiveness, and related high activity levels (attention-deficit/hyperactivity disorder [ADHD]), with stimulants, TCAs, SSRIs, and many other medication groups being prescribed as treatments. Methylphenidate and other related compounds became commonly used in humans to decrease inattention and to increase self-control (Gadow et al., 1990) as well as to increase motivation for and compliance with attendant behavior modification (Arnold et al., 1973). The number of indications and conditions for which sympathomimetic amines are now used has grown, not because more humans and dogs are recognized as truly "hyperkinetic/hyperactive" using the original criteria but because we now recognize that these compounds also affect neurotransmitters and receptors that affect anxiety, attentiveness, and memory.

Dogs who are treated with sympathomimetic amines should not be considered truly hyperkinetic or hyperactive or to have a canine version of ADHD. It is difficult to find diagnostic criteria for dogs for any of these conditions except for the original derivative definition from Corson (Marder, 1991; Overall, 1997). Assessment of attention is seldom done in dogs, and we may wish to consider whether the dogs who might be good candidates for the attentional benefits of these medications are *hyper-reactive*, rather than truly hyperactive. This approach more clearly defines the clients' concerns and behaviors that we can actually assess, while avoiding the historical confusion that arose as a result of a search for a laboratory dog model for a human condition. Some hyper-reactive dogs may benefit from sympathomimetic amines, in combination with or instead of SSRIs, TCAs, BZDs, and related medications such as gabapentin, all of which are now also used to enhance learning and decrease anxiety and reactivity.

All sympathomimetic amines have central nervous system stimulant activity. The predominant responses for amphetamine are increased extracellular concentrations of dopamine and 5-HT in the caudate nuclei and increased extracellular concentrations of NE in the hippocampus (Kuczenski et al., 1995). These actions are thought to increase focus and facilitate learning. Dextroamphetamine also increases dopamine in the prefrontal cortex where activation of the dopamine D_2 receptor inhibits glutamate release and activation of the dopamine D_1 receptor increases glutamate in the nucleus accumbens. Humans with ADHD may have low levels of glutamate in prefrontal cortex regions (and so respond to amphetamines, which would increase it), whereas glutamate appears to be high in these regions of humans with OCD (Carlsson, 2000). This responsivity of the prefrontal cortex to amphetamine with respect to glutamate may affect addiction in humans (Shoblock et al., 2003) and, possibly, how animals learn and are rewarded for learning some behavioral patterns.

Somatic effects of stimulants can include increased heart and respiratory rates, possible anorexia, and tremors with possible hyperthermia. Stimulants are contraindicated for patients with cardiovascular disease, glaucoma, concurrent MAO inhibitor therapy, and hyperthyroidism. The half-life of dextroamphetamine is 8 to 12 hours, and the half-life of methylphenidate is 3 to 4 hours. Both of these are administered two to three times per day and reach peak levels in 1 to 2 hours. Pemoline has a very long half-life, allowing for dosing once every 24 hours.

Newer Ideas

Nasal oxytocin has been used to treat post-traumatic stress disorder and social phobias in humans (Maes et al., 1999). Oxytocin is an affiliative neurochemical and may facilitate social bonding and interaction (Mitsui et al., 2011; Panksepp, 1993). Dogs and cats can learn to accept nasal vaccines, but this route is seldom considered for other medications. Nasal administration of medication may be extremely beneficial in cats and dogs. Because intranasal administration delivers medication to the rich nasal vasculature, it is quickly absorbed, bypasses the bloodstream, and can appear in the cerebrospinal fluid within 30 minutes, while minimizing systemic side effects (Born et al., 2002). Nasal oxytocin may have promise for distressed and panicked dogs, dogs with true fear or generalized anxiety disorder, and dogs with canine post-traumatic stress disorder. Intranasal use of BZDs has been shown to be effective in dogs (Platt et al., 2000).

Exaggerated amygdala reactivity has been associated with facial social cues that are aversive and threatening for humans with generalized and social anxiety (Phan et al., 2006). In a placebo-controlled functional magnetic resonance imaging study, administration of 24 IU of oxytocin before scanning attenuated responses to facial signals that the patients perceived as scary (Labuschagne et al., 2010). Oxytocin may enhance the

TABLE 10-11

Half-Lives (for Humans) and Kinetics of the Most Commonly Used Medications in Veterinary
Behavioral Medicine

Medication	Class	Half-Life (Humans) (hr)	Kinetics
Amitriptyline	TCA	24	Linear
Carbamazepine	Anti-convulsant	10-25	Non-linear
Citalopram	SSRI	75	Linear
Clomipramine	TCA	24	Linear
Duloxetine	SNRI	12.5	Linear
Fluoxetine	SSRI	90	Non-linear
Fluvoxamine	SSRI	15	Non-linear
Gabapentin	Anti-convulsant	5-7	Non-linear
Imipramine	TCA	22	Linear
Mirtazapine	NaSSA	35	Linear
Nefazodone	SARI	4	Linear
Nortriptyline	TCA	26	Linear
Paroxetine	SSRI	24	Non-linear
Sertraline	SSRI	24	Linear
Trazodone	SARI	8	Linear

Note: For most medications investigated, the half-life for the listed compounds is shorter in dogs than in humans; however, the profiles are often similar, so if there is a beneficial effect but also some undesirable effects (e.g., sedation), switching the patient to a compound that is a metabolite of the one originally chosen or one within the same or related class with a shorter half-life may help. NaSSA, Noradrenergic and specific serotoninergic antidepressant; SARI, serotonin 2A agonist/serotonin reuptake inhibitor; SNRI, serotonin norepinephrine reuptake inhibitor; SSRI, selective serotonin reuptake inhibitor; TCA, tricyclic antidepressant. Adapted from Rang et al., 2012.

ability to interact socially, where it is impaired, and help patients to improve their control over their stress and anxiety responses in social situations (Kirsch et al., 2005). Dosages of intranasal oxytocin for adult humans range from 18 to 54 IU 30 to 60 minutes before testing or expected stimuli, or up to 40 IU every 12 hours (Kirsch et al., 2005; Labuschagne et al., 2010; MacDonald and MacDonald, 2010; Savaskan et al., 2008). A similar regimen could benefit anxious dogs.

The half-lives for humans for medications commonly or increasingly used to treat dogs and cats are shown in Table 10-11. A list of the medications discussed and relevant dosages can be found in Tables 10-18 and 10-19 at the end of the chapter.

WHAT MAKES TRICYCLIC ANTIDEPRESSANTS AND SELECTIVE SEROTONIN REUPTAKE INHIBITORS SPECIAL, AND WHY ARE THEY SO USEFUL FOR TREATMENT OF ANXIETY DISORDERS?

The short answer to these questions is that these medications facilitate learning and acquisition of changes in behavior through behavior modification because they use the same second-messenger systems and transcription pathways used in cellular/molecular "learning"

(e.g., LTP). This pathway involves cAMP, cytosolic response element binding protein (CREB), BDNF, NMDA receptors, and protein tyrosine kinases (PTK), particularly Src, which regulate activity of NMDA receptors and other ion channels and mediate the induction of LTP, which is a special case of synaptic plasticity (Fig. 10-3).

These actions are particularly prominent in the CA1 region of the hippocampus—the part of the brain so important for associational learning (e.g., sitting for a signal ["sit"] and receiving a treat for doing so). Chronic treatment with TCAs, SSRIs, SARIs, SNRIs, et cetera appears to stimulate neurogenesis in the hippocampus (Santarelli et al, 2003; Sapolsky, 2011). Behaviors are reinforced or learned best if every time they occur they are rewarded. At the cellular level, repeated reinforcement ensures better, more numerous, and more efficient connections between neurons (Carter et al., 2002; Wittenberg and Tsien, 2002). This stimulation of neurons with repeated reinforcement leading to more efficient connections between neurons is the goal of treatment with most newer behavioral medications and of many dietary interventions.

Stimulation is induced when a neurochemical in a synapse triggers a receptor to engage it. This stimulation of the receptor engages second-messenger systems

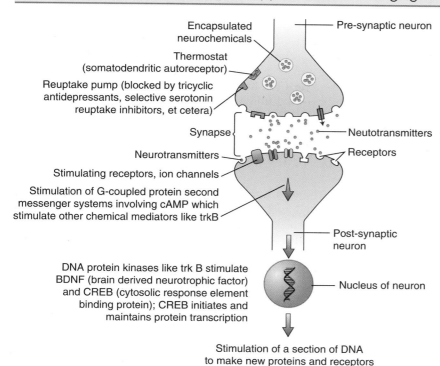

Stimulation of a section of DNA
to make new proteins and receptors

Fig. 10-3 Effect of TCAs and SSRIs on the molecular basis of learning. Both the anti-anxiety effects and the molecular basis of learning, which involves making new protein, require activation of second-messenger system pathways that stimulate BDNF and CREB in the nucleus. The effect on protein transcription is not immediate and involves G-gated protein reception, ion receptors and NMDA receptor activation, and ongoing stimulation. This may be one reason why the most profound effects are not apparent for 3 to 5 weeks after beginning treatment for more specific TCAs, SSRIs, and derivatives. (From Overall, 2001.)

in the postsynaptic cell, usually cAMP. The result is cellular memory or LTP. By itself, initial cAMP-stimulated LTP represents "early phase LTP" (E-LTP) and short-term memory. The process is short-lasting and independent of RNA and protein synthesis, and the result does not persist or become self-potentiating, unless the stimulus is consolidated into "late phase LTP" (L-LTP), which is a more permanent form (Schafe et al., 2001). E-LTP can be induced by a single train of stimuli in either the hippocampus or the lateral amygdala.

In contrast, L-LTP and LTM requires repeated stimulation of cAMP and induction of CREB (a nuclear transcription factor) and is long-lasting, protein synthesis dependent, and RNA transcription dependent (Schafe et al., 2001). When stimulation continues, BDNF enhances neurotransmission and potentiates what is called "activity-dependent plasticity" at synapses (e.g., learning), particularly in the region of the brain most involved in learning, the hippocampus. This effect can also occur in the lateral amygdala and is one modality postulated to be involved in learned or conditioned contextual fear (Schafe et al., 2001).

The range of optimal levels of CREB is dependent on the range of optimal levels of BDNF (Peters et al., 2004). These levels are dependent on levels of cortisol. If cortisol is low, arousal is sufficiently low that learning does not occur. If arousal is high, cortisol is high. High levels of cortisol may interfere with the production of cellular/molecular memory because cortisol at these levels acts as a hormone response element that inhibits the action

of CREB to transcribe nuclear protein. Without this transcription, no translation of protein is possible, and learning is inhibited (see Fig. 10-3) (Truss and Beato, 1993; Yau et al., 2002). The role of steroid transcription regulation by steroid hormones may have complex, but widespread application for behavioral concerns (Beato et al., 1996).

There are two phases of TCA and SSRI treatment: short-term effects and long-term effects. Short-term effects result in a synaptic increase of the relevant monoamine associated with reuptake inhibition. The somatodendritic autoreceptor of the presynaptic neuron decreases the firing rate of that cell as a thermostatic response. There is increased saturation of the postsynaptic receptors resulting in stimulation of the beta-adrenergic coupled cAMP system. cAMP activation increases PTK as the first step in the long-term effects. PTK translocates into the nucleus of the postsynaptic cell, where it increases CREB, which has been postulated to be the postreceptor target for these drugs. Increases in CREB lead to increases in BDNF and tyrosine kinases (e.g., trkB), which stimulate messenger RNA transcription of new receptor proteins. The altered conformation of the postsynaptic receptors renders serotonin stimulation and signal transduction more efficient (Duman, 1998). Knowledge of the molecular basis for the action of these drugs can aid in treatment. For example, the presynaptic somatodendritic autoreceptor is blocked by pindolol, so augmentation of TCA and SSRI treatment with pindolol can accelerate treatment onset.

Long-term treatment, particularly with the more specific TCAs (e.g., clomipramine) and SSRIs, employs the same pathway used in LTP to alter reception function and structure through transcriptional and translational alterations in receptor protein. This can be thought of as a form of *in vivo* "gene therapy" that works to augment neurotransmitter levels and production, making the neuron and the interactions between neurons more coordinated and efficient.

In some patients, short-term treatment appears to be sufficient to produce continued "normal" functioning of the neurotransmitter system. The fact that there are some patients who require lifelong treatment suggests that the effect of the drugs is reversible in some patients, further illustrating the underlying heterogeneity of the patient population considered to have the same diagnosis.

PATIENT MONITORING

Patient monitoring by clients and veterinarians is essential. Annual physical and laboratory evaluation should be done for all patients; the frequency should be increased for older patients. Age-related changes in hepatic mass, function, blood flow, plasma drug binding, et cetera, cause a decrease in clearance of some TCAs. Adjustment in drug dosages may be necessary with age. BZDs may impair memory more in older patients than in younger ones, so attention should be paid to mentation status and ability to acquire and act on new behaviors. If any patient becomes ill for any reason or shows signs of side effects, re-assessment is essential.

The minimum pre-medication and follow-up database should include a complete blood count, serum biochemistry profile, and urinalysis with or without culture as indicated. Additional tests that may be recommended depending on clinical signs include fecal analysis/culture, tic titers, toxicity panels (especially for lead), thyroid profiles (the concern is a hyperthyroid component to the behavior of concern in cats and a hypothyroid component in dogs) using the dialysis method, and ECGs. Because of the small but real risk for conduction disturbances in cats being treated with TCAs, SSRIs, et cetera, a pre-medication lead II ECG is a good idea. For any animal with obvious or postulated conduction anomalies, a complete cardiac evaluation is warranted.

Older medications are traditionally thought to have more side effects than newer ones, but this pattern has not been investigated for dogs and cats and may not be relevant for species who are not susceptible to litanies of verbal complaints and marketing folklore. Most TCAs and SSRIs have shorter half-lives in dogs than in humans, and so some of the ultra-short-acting newer SSRIs, SNRIs, and SARIs may have sufficiently short half-lives in dogs that rebound syndrome may pose a risk (see the earlier discussion on rebound and withdrawal syndromes pertaining to BZDs). For these newer medications, the dosage interval is critical: every

24 hours means once every 24 hours, not once a day, where a "day" is defined by the date, not a clock. Fluoxetine, a commonly prescribed SSRI for dogs (Reconcile), has numerous active intermediate metabolites and a long half-life in dogs and humans. This profile carries with it a different set of risks of side effects but means that if someone forgets to give the patient the medication for a few days, the dog will likely be okay.

It is preferable to withdraw most patients from one class of drug before starting another.

- For changing between SSRIs and MAO inhibitors, the recommended drug-free time in humans and dogs is 2 weeks (2 + half-lives—the general rule of thumb for withdrawal of any drug).
- SSRIs can be added to TCAs and may exhibit a faster onset of action than when they are given alone. This is due to the shared molecular effects on second-messenger systems of both TCAs and SSRIs. Combination treatment allows the veterinarian to use the lower end of the dosage for both compounds, which minimizes side effects while maximizing efficacy.
- BZDs can be used to blunt or prevent acute anxiety-related outbursts on an as-needed basis in patients for whom daily treatment with a TCA or SSRI is ongoing. Together, the combination of BZDs and TCAs/SSRIs may hasten improvement and prevent acute anxiety-provoking stimuli from interfering with treatment of more regularly occurring anxieties.

When stopping a behavioral medication, weaning is preferred to stopping abruptly. If patients are withdrawn suddenly, rather than weaned from medication, they may not have the same response to the medication that they had originally if they re-start the medication at a later date. Weaning minimizes potential central withdrawal signs, including those associated with serotonin discontinuation syndrome (Rosenbaum et al., 1998; Zajeka et al., 1998) and allows determination of the lowest dosage that is still effective (Overall, 1997). Patients with rebound/discontinuation/cessation syndrome become moody and lethargic, but these effects usually pass within a week. Extreme effects, including psychosis, have been noted for humans discontinuing medications with very short half-lives. If these signs do not remit, re-assessment of the wisdom of stopping medication is warranted. Medications that have the longest half-life of intermediate metabolites (e.g., fluoxetine) are less likely to cause problems when withdrawn quickly than are medications with short half-lives or no functional intermediate metabolites (e.g., paroxetine). However, SSRIs that have the greatest *in vivo* reuptake capabilities (e.g., paroxetine) may be more at risk for involvement in serotonin syndrome (Box 10-4). Long-term treatment may be the rule with many of these medications and conditions, but maintenance may be at a considerably lower level of drug than was prescribed at the outset. The only way the veterinarian will discover this is to withdraw the medication slowly.

Algorithm for Treatment Length and Weaning Schedule*

1. Treat for as long as it takes to begin to assess effects:
   - 7 to 10 days for relatively non-specific TCAs
   - 3 to 5 weeks **minimum** for SSRIs and more specific TCAs

Plus

2. Treat until "well" with either no signs associated with diagnosis or some low, consistent level of signs:
   minimum of another 1 to 2 months

Plus

3. Treat for the amount of time it took to attain the level in (2) so that reliability of assessment is reasonably assured:
   minimum of another 1 to 2 months

Plus

4. Wean over the amount of time it took to get to (1) or more slowly. Remember, if receptor conformation reverts, it may take 1 or more months to notice the signs of this. Although there are no acute side effects associated with sudden cessation of medication, a recidivistic event is a profound "side effect." Full-blown recidivistic events may not be responsive to re-initiated treatment with the same drug and/or same dose:
   - 7 to 10 days for relatively non-specific TCAs
   - 3 to 5 weeks minimum for SSRIs and more specific TCAs

Total: Treat for a minimum of 4 to 6 months

Remember, you cannot pronounce a treatment failure with more specific medications until the patient has been treated for 8 weeks.

Because of these patterns, it is best *not* to withdraw animals from medication before anesthesia but instead to adjust the pre-medication sedation so that fewer interactions—particularly of the adrenergic variety—can be expected. Finally, many animals appear to stop responding to medication. Staying the course may be the best decision in some of these cases because the CYP system is an inducible one, and multiple medication changes may make the animal more—not less—refractory. Additionally, there is a huge range of genetic polymorphisms that determine how this system acts. These are poorly understood in dogs and cats because there has been so little investigation.

ANCILLARY CONCERNS

Roles for Food

The absorption of behavioral medications occurs passively in the small intestine, and the efficiency of absorption is affected by the physiology/metabolism of the patients, whether food is present, and how the medication itself is compounded.

Most behavioral medications used are best absorbed on an empty stomach. Food decreases the rate of absorption, which may be part of the desired effect, but if a quick peak effect is desired (e.g., as is true for treating panic), full stomachs may alter the rate at which medication is absorbed (but not usually peak levels). For animals being treated for conditions that may require the presence of food (e.g., diabetes) or adherence to strict feeding schedules (e.g., hyperthyroidism in cats), knowing about half-lives, absorption rates, and any effects on peak levels may be important.

It is also important to consider that the overall physical state of the animal (e.g., fat or thin) may affect how medications act. For example, all BZDs are lipophilic, meaning that the BZD may be quickly re-distributed into the fat away from its target, but the fat then acts as sink or storehouse for the BZD, slowly releasing it.

Finally, BZDs have the side effect of increasing hunger. For animals who are anorectic, especially because of grief or situational stress, short-term treatment with a non-sedating BZD (e.g., oxazepam) may help.

Thyroidal Illness and Assessment

The use of TCAs, SSRIs, and related compounds artificially lowers measurements of T_3 and T_4 levels in standard thyroid panels. It is essential to know about this interaction when evaluating an animal's true thyroid status. This issue is especially germane for dogs, for whom there has been a cyclic vogue for non-specifically treating dogs with behavioral concerns and borderline thyroid values with thyroxine. There is now good evidence showing that most behavioral concerns in dogs are not directly associated with any thyroid dysfunction, although such dysfunction may affect behavior, and behavioral complaints may be the first sign of hyperthyroidism for cats (Dodds, 2011; Kemppainen and Birchfield, 2006; Peterson et al., 1997, 2001). See the discussion on page 217 for a justification for avoiding facile treatment of behavioral conditions using thyroxin.

In high doses, TCAs have been implicated in sick euthyroid syndrome, now more commonly called non-thyroidal illness syndrome (NTIS). In NTIS, thyrotropin (thyroid-stimulating hormone) levels are low. NTIS has been postulated possibly to be an adaptive response to illness, and with recovery thyrotropin has been reported to increase to normal levels (Koenig, 2008; Peterson and Gamble, 1988; Warner and Beckett, 2010). Diminished calorie intake appears to decrease thyrotropin-releasing hormone (TRH) from the paraventricular nucleus, and neuropeptide Y and other proteins that are increased in fasting suppress TRH gene expression, as do sepsis and trauma. Almost half of cats with NTIS have serum T_4 concentrations below the normal range. Patients who do poorly with NTIS lose TRH gene expression (Graves, 2011), and so understanding pre-medication thyroidal status may be important.

Seizure Activity and Medications

Many serotoninergic agents are thought to lower seizure thresholds and so are recommended with caution in patients with seizures. There is now evidence in both the human and the canine literature that anxiety itself may lower seizure thresholds, and *so treatment of the anxiety may raise the seizure threshold and allow the patient to decrease successfully the amount of seizure medication needed.*

There is some evidence that omega-3 fatty acids may aid in the treatment of some forms of epilepsy in dogs (Scorza et al., 2009), suggesting that anti-oxidants and inflammation may play broad roles in aging, brain diseases such as epilepsy, and anxiety (Lakhan and Vieira, 2008). Carbamazepine is used to treat seizure activity and some behavioral conditions, and medications used to treat seizure activity and behavioral conditions can interact. Mechanisms of interaction are shown in Table 10-12.

First-Pass Effects

Similar to other orally ingested medications, behavioral medications are subject to a first-pass effect (e.g., hepatic metabolism and biotransformation/elimination). Medications given intravenously, intramuscularly, subcutaneously, or intranasally are not subject to first-pass effects.

First-pass effects mean that less of the parent compound actually is, or more of the metabolites (which may be the desired compounds) are, available in the circulation or to reach the target. First-pass metabolism is often important for behavioral and other medications and is a source of inter-individual variation in effect because it is the result of CYP enzymatic action in the intestinal luminal cells and in the liver.

When a second dose is added, timing becomes important. The second-dosing effect describes the phenomenon in which if a second drug dose taken immediately after the effect of the first dose stops, the duration of that dose is longer, and the intensity of its effect is greater. If repeated dosing occurs before the first dose is completely eliminated, there is a greater effect of subsequent doses, although the intensity of the effect may level off.

Atypical Benzodiazepine Responses

Special Case of Atypical Benzodiazepine Reactions and Whether to Use Them in Cats

Many of the long-term effects and side effects of BZDs are the result of intermediate metabolite function. Parent compound and intermediate metabolite half-lives must be considered. The active intermediate metabolite in diazepam (and any compound that shares its metabolic pathway) is nordiazepam or *N*-desmethyldiazepam, which is extremely sedative and has a very long half-life in all species examined (Fig. 10-4 and see Table 10-6). This is a first-pass effect. One of the reasons use of diazepam may be a concern in cats involves the half-life of this compound. In dogs, diazepam has a half-life of 3.2 hours,

TABLE 10-12

Mechanism of Action for Medications Commonly Used to Treat Seizures in Dogs and Cats

Medication	Acts via Potentiation of GABA	Acts via Inhibiting Glutamate Neurotransmission	Acts by Blocking Na⁺ and/or Ca⁺⁺ Channels
Clorazepate*	+	–	–
Diazepam*	+	–	–
Clonazepam*	+	–	–
Carbamazepine*	+/–	+/– (NMDA)	+/– (Na⁺/Ca⁺⁺)
Felbamate	+	+ (NMDA)	+ (Na⁺/Ca⁺⁺)
Gabapentin*	+/–	–	+ (Ca⁺⁺)
Levetiracetam	+/–	+/–	+ (Ca⁺⁺)
Pregabalin	–	–	+ (Ca⁺⁺)
Phenobarbital†	+	–	+/– (Ca⁺⁺)
Phenytoin	–	+/–	+ (Na⁺)
Topiramate	+	+ (AMPA)	+ (Na⁺/Ca⁺⁺)
Zonisamide	+/–	–	+ (Na⁺/Ca⁺⁺)

AMPA, Alpha-amino-3-hydroxy-5-methylisoxazole-4-propionic acid; GABA, gamma-aminobutyric acid, NMDA, N-methyl-D-aspartate.
*Also used to treat non–epilepsy-related behavioral conditions.
†Primidone is converted into phenobarbital.
Adapted from Mula, 2008.

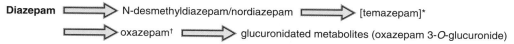

Fig. 10-4 When cats ingest diazepam, they are actually being given three or four active compounds, depending on which CYP enzymes are involved; two or three of these are themselves parent compounds, and all must be glucuronidated. It's no surprise that some cats may experience profound side effects when given diazepam. *If use the CYP34A pathway. †If use CYP2C19 and CYP3A4 pathway.

whereas nordiazepam has a half-life of 3 to 6 hours. For cats, these half-lives are 5.5 hours and 21 hours, respectively. This means that an extremely sedative intermediate metabolite, plus a parent compound, now must be metabolized through a glucuronidation pathway in a species—the cat—for which glucuronidation is not very efficient (see Fig 10-4). Sedation can be a real concern in cats.

All BZDs are lipophilic, so all BZDs in any metabolic pathway will pool in the fat, creating an almost continuous infusion source in some cats. Use of BZDs that avoid the nordiazepam intermediate metabolite and are less affected by glucuronidation (e.g., oxazepam, alprazolam) may be highly desirable in cats.

Cats have been reported to experience an atypical hepatonecrosis associated with diazepam administration (Center et al., 1996; Hughes et al., 1996). After the initial publications using the same pathological samples, reports of hepatotoxicity in cats treated with BZDs became almost non-existent. No country other than the United States ever reported any concerns. It's most likely that although BZDs were involved in the hepatic failure in these cats, the issue was more complex and that something else made these particular cats extraordinarily susceptible, even given the concerns about metabolism of BZD in cats. Regardless, the cited studies on this issue serve as an important reminder of several issues.

- Treat a diagnosis, not a non-specific complaint.
- The units of mass for accurate dosing are "grams" or "kg," not "cats"; most cats in these studies received one size of medication regardless of *their* size.
- BZDs are lipophilic; this means that fat cats have a pool of stored BZDs that may increase with every dose.
- Diazepam and other BZDs that have *N*-desmethyldiazepam as an intermediate metabolite are more sedative than BZDs that do not use this pathway. Our goal is not to sedate patients and suppress normal behaviors. Our goal is to redress anxiety so that normal behaviors can be expressed and help the patient better negotiate the world. By choosing other BZDs (e.g., oxazepam, alprazolam), we can achieve this goal while minimizing risk.

Other Concerns about Extreme Responses to Benzodiazepines in Cats and Dogs

Excitement
Occasionally, a dog or cat will not respond to one BZD but may respond to another. Some animals respond to

none, which likely is the result of a genetic variant in hepatic CYP systems. Rarely, a dog or cat experiences excitement when given a BZD. This excitement will resolve in a few hours, during which the animal should be protected, but can also be aborted by flumazenil, a specific BZD antagonist (0.01 to 0.02 mg/kg intravenously). If dogs or cats experience this side effect with more than one BZD, these patients are not good candidates for BZD treatment.

Disinhibition
Use of BZDs is often restricted in animals because of the concern that their behaviors will become "disinhibited." The particular concern is for disinhibition of aggression in animals being treated for problem aggressions.

Data from the literature on human responses to BZDs suggest that concerns about disinhibition are overblown and that there is no direct evidence for BZDs engendering disinhibition. Many of the behaviors attributed to this action may actually be due to the side effect of sedation as it affects memory and cognition. Adverse effects on cognition appear to co-vary with the sedative properties of the BZD chosen, again suggesting that BZDs that go through the *N*-desmethyldiazepam pathway may be implicated (Riss et al., 2008).

In a study of one population where one could expect to see disinhibition effects, were they to occur, Rothschild et al. (2000) found no evidence for disinhibition in terms of acts of self-injury, assaults on staff or other patients, need for seclusion or restraints, increased need for observation while hospitalized, or decreases in patient privileges (which would result from behavioral disinhibition) for patients treated with alprazolam or diazepam compared with patients not treated with a BZD. The findings of this study are consistent with other reviews and meta-analyses when these use controlled, blinded studies (Jonas and Hearron, 1996; Rothschild, 1992).

One might expect that if these BZDs were used at anti-anxiety levels, some behaviors that patients were suppressing because of their anxiety may appear, a scenario relevant for veterinary behavioral medicine. Although only truly inhibited aggressions might be postulated to be at risk for appearance with treatment using BZDs, the risks are likely offset by the improvement in pathology that would make expression of aggression less likely.

Reports of disinhibition have been anecdotal in veterinary behavioral medicine, and their interpretation is confounded by the sedative effects of intermediate metabolites, already discussed. For this reason, when possible, choosing BZDs that have lower risks for sedation is preferable. If the veterinarian has a concern about the effects/side effects of one BZD, he or she can change the BZD and may find that the patient responds better.

POLYPHARMACY

Combination Treatment/Polypharmacy and Undesirable Drug Interactions

The combination of medications from the same or a related class (e.g., TCAs, SSRIs) may increase the risk of side effects, unless dosages of each are adjusted (usually downward). Combinations may also be subject to the changes in metabolism discussed previously. Combining medications from different classes may also lead to enhanced side effects if the medications share side effects (e.g., sedation associated with combining barbiturates and BZDs).

- Combinations of TCAs or SSRIs and MAO inhibitors are not recommended because of the risk of serotonin syndrome. In serotonin syndrome, the patient experiences tachycardia, tachypnea, agitation, anorexia, hyperpyrexia, irritability, hypertension, diarrhea, and ultimately seizures.
- MAO inhibitors also should not be combined with narcotics, especially meperidine, which has been associated with a potentially fatal reaction.
- Serotonin syndrome can be a rare concern for patients receiving TCAs/SSRIs and tramadol, a mu opioid analogue that also affects adrenergic and serotonin receptors (KuKanich and Papich, 2004). It may help to note that the opioid effect is small in dogs (Giorgi et al., 2009a, 2009b; KuKanich and Papich, 2004). While tramadol and its active intermediate metabolite O-desmethyltramadol (which is partly responsible for the opioid effect) (Pypendop and Ilkiw, 2008), affect circulating and platelet serotonin levels, but the risk of serotonin syndrome has been found to be extremely low (Lange-Asschenfeldt et al., 2002; Wedge, 2009), is dose-dependent, and apparent only at dosages of tramadol or TCAs/SSRIs that *exceed the normal treatment range* (Gillman, 2010).
- Combining TCAs/SSRIs with tryptophan may be more likely to be associated with the signs of serotonin syndrome but *only* if catecholamine release is enhanced (Gillman, 2006, 2010).

It has become clear that a small, acidic protein, p11, is responsible for facilitating the movement and attachment of serotonin receptors at the cell surface, enhancing the excitability of neurons (Svenningsson et al., 2006). The primary effect of p11 appears to be on 5-HT_{1B} receptors, but TCAs and SSRIs that primarily affect other receptors appear to interact with p11 (Warner-Schmidt et al., 2011). In rodents, both TCAs and SSRIs (and electroconvulsive therapy) increase levels of p11 in the cerebral cortex and hippocampus, which is apparently mediated by an increase in the cytokines tumor necrosis factor α and interferon-γ (Fig. 10-5). Tumor necrosis factor α increases production of nerve growth factor, BDNF, and glial cell–derived neurotrophic factor (GDNF) in the astrocytes and BDNF in endothelial cells in the human cerebrum. BDNF increases p11 in the murine cerebral cortex, and many of its neurotrophic effects, including effects involved in its antidepressant action, appear to require p11. Interferon-γ also appears to require p11 for its antidepressant effects, among which are neuritic growth and differentiation (Warner-Schmidt et al., 2011).

The reason this aspect of molecular biology is discussed here is that non-steroidal anti-inflammatory drugs (NSAIDs) appear to inhibit antidepressant-induced increases in p11 and may interfere with medications that act solely or primarily by affecting serotoninergic receptors (SSRIs) (Warner-Schmidt et al., 2011) in human patients treated with these medications. This effect is not seen with TCAs, which primarily affect NA/NE. Such effects could cause recidivistic events in patients being successfully treated for behavioral conditions or may cause some patients to be non-responders to SSRIs. There are few clinical data on dosage effects, half-lives, peripheral versus central effects, et cetera, but the data that exist suggest co-administration of such medications may affect behavioral outcomes and that careful monitoring should ensue if NSAIDs are given with SSRIs.

Cytochrome P-450 System

The CYP system relies on a series of enzymes that are either inhibited or induced by various medications. Enzymes affected by behavioral/psychotropic medications include 1A2, 2A6, 2B6, 2C9, 2C19, 2D6, 2E1, and 3A4. Many of these medications also act as substrates for this enzyme system, with an especially large number being substrates for the 3A4 enzyme (e.g., alprazolam, amitriptyline, carbamazepine, diazepam, fluoxetine, imipramine, nefazodone, sertraline,

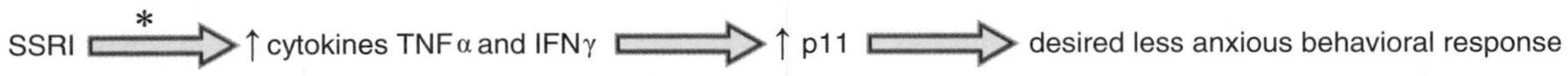

SSRI $\xrightarrow{\quad * \quad}$ ↑ cytokines TNFα and IFNγ $\Longrightarrow$ ↑ p11 $\Longrightarrow$ desired less anxious behavioral response

Fig. 10-5 Schematic of action of SSRIs on cytokine and p11 levels. NSAIDs block the step marked by the *asterisk*. *TNFα,* Tumor necrosis factor α; *IFNγ,* interferon-γ. (Adapted from Warner-Schmidt et al., 2011.)

trazodone, triazolam, venlafaxine). Behavioral medications that are inducers of the above-mentioned systems are listed in Table 10-13. Other medications that are commonly prescribed and are inhibitors or inducers of these enzymes are listed in Table 10-14. Because such interactions can slow (inducers) or enhance (inhibitors) the rate at which medication is available and the amount available, knowing which medications use the same enzyme systems can be helpful. For more information, see the text from which the information in these tables was adapted (Schatzberg and Nemeroff, 2004, 2009).

Genetically Determined Variation of Cytochrome P-450 Enzyme Systems

In humans, we know that there are genetic variants of the CYP system enzymes and that these can have clinical consequences for patients. The percentage of variants noted depends on race. In dogs and cats, where breeds act to canalize genetic variation, it would be surprising if CYP system enzyme variants did not exist, but almost no work has been done on this topic (Lesch and Mössner, 1998; Lucki et al., 2001). However, knowing about some of the patterns in humans may provide insight into why this is important.

- Variants of the 2D6 enzyme may result in high drug concentrations of desipramine and nortriptyline, possibly resulting in toxicity.
- Variants of the 2C9 enzyme cause reduced substrate clearance for substrates such as phenytoin.
- Variants of the 2C19 enzyme result in high drug concentrations, increased sedation, and possible toxicity for diazepam.

Because of the CYP enzyme interactions, some generalizations can be made about effects of other

TABLE 10-13

Behavioral Medications That Are Inhibitors or Inducers of Listed Cytochrome P-450 Enzymes

CYP Enzyme	Substrate	Inhibitor	Inducer
CYP1A2	TCAs Fluvoxamine Mirtazapine Duloxetine	Fluvoxamine Fluoxetine Paroxetines Sertraline Some TCAs	Phenobarbital Carbamazepine Phenytoin
CYP2A6			
CYP2B6			
2CYPC9/CYP2C9/10	Sertraline Fluoxetine Amitriptyline	Fluvoxamine Fluoxetine Sertraline	Carbamazepine
2C19/CYP2C19	Citalopram Sertraline Clomipramine Imipramine	Fluvoxamine Fluoxetine Sertraline	Carbamazepine
CYP2D6	Fluoxetine Fluvoxamine Citalopram Duloxetine Paroxetine Venlafaxine Trazodone Nefazodone TCAs	Duloxetine Fluoxetine Paroxetine Norfluoxetine Citalopram Sertraline Some TCAs	
CYP2E1			
CYP3A4	Nefazodone Sertraline Venlafaxine Trazodone TCAs	Fluvoxamine Norfluoxetine TCAs nefazodone	Carbamazepine

Note: Inducers slow the rate at which the substrate medication is available and reduce the amount available. Inhibitors increase the rate at which the substrate medication is available and increase the amount available.
CYP, Cytochrome P-450; TCA, tricyclic antidepressant.

TABLE 10-14

Commonly Used Medications That Could Be Given Concomitantly with Behavioral Medication and That Are Inducers or Inhibitors of Listed Cytochrome P-450 Enzymes

CYP Enzyme	Inhibitor	Inducer
CYP1A2	Fluoroquinolones	Charcoal-broiled beef Cruciferous vegetables Marijuana smoke Omeprazole Phenobarbital Phenytoin
CYP2A6	Tranylcypromine	Barbiturates
CYP2B6		Phenobarbital
CYP2C9/CYP2C9/10	Propoxyphene Disulfiram Fluconazole Sulfaphenazole	Rifampin Phenobarbital Phenytoin
CYP2C19	Omeprazole	Rifampin Phenytoin
CYP2D6		
CYP2E1	Disulfiram	Ethanol
CYP3A4	Fluconazole Ketoconazole Cimetidine Clarithromycin, erythromycin (macrolides in general) Propofol	Barbiturates Dexamethasone/long-term glucocorticoids Phenytoin St. John's wort* Flucloxacillin

Note: Inducers slow the rate at which the substrate medication is available and reduce the amount available. Inhibitors increase the rate at which the substrate medication is available and increase the amount available.
CYP, Cytochrome P-450.
*Hyperforin is the compound that is the inducer.

medications on the level of behavioral medications in the plasma (Mula, 2008).

- Phenobarbital lowers plasma levels of:
  - all TCAs,
  - most SSRIs (except fluoxetine),
  - the NDRI bupropion,
  - the SNRI duloxetine, and
  - the NaSSA mirtazapine.
- Carbamazepine lowers plasma levels of:
  - all TCAs,
  - most SSRIs (except fluoxetine),
  - the NDRI bupropion,
  - the SNRI venlafaxine,
  - the NaSSA mirtazapine, and
  - the SARI nefazodone.
- Gabapentin appears to leave plasma levels of these compounds unchanged.

Serotonin Syndrome

Serotonin syndrome—which may better be described as serotonin toxicity—is the most severe side effect that can occur with any medication affecting serotonin, and

it can be fatal if untreated. Although serotonin syndrome is rare, when it does occur, it occurs most commonly within the first week or so of treatment and/or when switching or addition of other medications affecting serotonin (Hegerl et al., 1998). Serotonin must be elevated 10 to 50 times above the baseline level for a toxic effect to be experienced (Gillman, 2006, 2010). The non-specific signs for serotonin syndrome can be grouped by system: cognitive alterations (disorientation, confusion), behavior (agitation, restlessness), autonomic nervous system (fever, shivering, diaphoresis, diarrhea), and neuromuscular activity (ataxia, hyperreflexia, myoclonus) (Lane and Baldwin, 1997). It has been suggested that a diagnosis of serotonin syndrome can be made *only* when three of the following signs occur, coincident with the addition or increased dosage of a known serotoninergic agent and only in the absence of another etiologic agent and when the signs do not pre-date when the medication was started/increased: *agitation, mental system changes (confusion, hypomania), myoclonus, hyperreflexia, diaphoresis, shivering, tremor, diarrhea, incoordination, and fever.* Canine—and one would assume feline—patients experiencing serotonin syndrome become anxious, agitated, anorectic, and unfocused and are often tachycardic and tachypneic. They may not sleep, cannot calm, may have a seizure, and can become hyperthermic whether or not they have a seizure. It is the hyperthermia that poses the largest risk, including that of seizure.

Serotonin syndrome, although rare, can occur when a patient is given one medication affecting serotonin or a combination of them. When using polypharmacy, decreasing the dose of the medications involved—especially if they are affected by or affect the same CYP systems—is essential.

Clients should and can easily learn to take pulse rates, which may be the first sign of developing serotonin syndrome in dogs. Slight increases in pulse rate are not worrisome. Huge, sustained increases in heart rate *are* problematic. If clients know that their dog's resting heart rate is 65 beats/min and with medication this changes to 150 beats/min, they can immediately bring this change to their veterinarian's attention. Likewise, if the increase is minor (65 to 75 beats/min), the client can take notes and not worry. For this reason, baseline ECGs are recommended for any patient who has had a history of any arrhythmia, heart disease, or prior drug reactions; who is on more than one medication; and who may be undergoing anesthesia or sedation. Cats, especially, may benefit from a pre-medication lead II ECG to rule out risks from conduction disturbances that may be triggered by medications affecting serotonin.

One concern about serotonin syndrome involves the concomitant use of tramadol, the synthetic mu opioid inhibitor that is a commonly used pain medication. In experiments with synaptosomes in rodent brains, tramadol acts as a 5-HT uptake blocker (Gobbi and Mennini, 1999). Studies in human liver microsomes have shown that inhibitors of CYP2D6 (fluoxetine, amitriptyline, and quinidine) also may inhibit the metabolism of tramadol. In dogs, CYP 2B and 3A appear to metabolize tramadol to large amounts of two metabolites that do not affect mu opioid receptors and to low levels of the metabolite that does (Giorgi et al., 2009b; Kongara et al., 2009), suggesting that not only are the pharmacokinetics different than in humans, but that pain relief may be due to tramadol's effects on serotonin and adrenergic receptors. Accordingly, we should remember that giving tramadol and SSRIs, TCAs, SARIs, or SNRIs may result in increases in tramadol concentrations. We also know that tramadol is metabolized by CYP3A4, so CYP3A4 inhibitors, such as ketoconazole and erythromycin, or inducers, such as St. John's wort, may affect tramadol metabolism and enhance exposure to it.

- This *does not mean* that tramadol cannot be used to mitigate pain in patients taking SSRIs, TCAs, SARIs, or SNRIs.
- Instead, when tramadol *is* used with these medications, lower dosages of each may be necessary, and

clients should be instructed to monitor the patient for early signs of serotonin syndrome which, they should be reminded, usually occurs early in the dosing.

- QoL matters, and pain takes a toll on QoL. Tramadol in the immediate release (not sustained release) form has been shown to increase nociceptive thresholds in dogs (Kongara et al., 2009; KuKanich and Papich, 2011) and so has a place in QoL decisions. Peak effects are seen about 6 hours after oral treatment at 9.9 mg/kg (KuKanich and Papich, 2011). Balancing the patient's needs with risks from helpful medication can be done with educated clients, careful dosing, and calm monitoring by all parties. Anxiety and pain have positive feedback on each other. Rational treatment strategies mandate that we address both and understand that by decreasing pain we may also be decreasing anxiety, especially when using agents that affect serotonin.

Cyproheptadine is a non-specific serotonin antagonist that can be used at a dosage of 1.1 mg/kg orally as an aid in combating serotonin syndrome (Wismer, 2000). Cyproheptadine is anti-serotoninergic, antihistaminic, and anti-cholinergic and a 5-HT$_2$ antagonist. It is most commonly used to stimulate appetite in cats and dogs and to control incompletely controlled asthma in cats. In some cases, cyproheptadine has been helpful in treating otherwise non-responsive urinary spraying in cats.

In human medicine, methysergide, another non-specific serotonin antagonist (5-HT$_{1A}$ and 5-HT$_{2B,D}$ receptors) is also used to treat serotonin syndrome. A number of phenothiazine derivatives are potent and specific antagonists for the 5-HT$_2$ receptor, but the concern has been further lowering of seizure thresholds. Because this concern has been shown to be over-rated for acepromazine in dogs, acepromazine may be helpful in treating some cases of serotonin syndrome. However, the antagonism of the 5-HT$_2$ receptor again highlights why one reason *acepromazine may render storm/noise phobic/reactive patients worse.* Acepromazine also impairs ability to process information, so these combined effects will put storm/noise phobic/reactive patients at risk for more profound suffering.

Occasionally, human patients diagnosed with serotonin syndrome have benefited from treatment with propranolol, a beta blocker that also blocks the 5-HT$_{1A}$ subtype receptor, but the data do not support widespread efficacy of this approach (Gillman, 2010). Care for serotonin syndrome is supportive and symptomatic.

Because the non-specific signs/diagnostic criteria for serotonin syndrome are overly broad, it is possible that all undesirable effects of any medications affecting serotonin are lumped as "serotonin syndrome" or as precursors to serotonin syndrome, leading many researchers to question the legitimacy of the diagnosis. This is one reason why the monitoring discussed previously is recommended. *If clients can rationally monitor side effects, they are more likely to treat the dog or cat long enough to assess and experience any beneficial effects and can do so without undue concern.* Such rational thought is particularly important if Gillman (2010) is correct, and he likely is, that activation of the 5-HT$_{2A}$ receptor, not the 5-HT$_{1A}$ receptor, is required for serotonin syndrome, as indicated by the dose-related action of serotonin or serotonin agonists on this receptor and the response to cyproheptadine, a 5-HT$_{2A}$ antagonist.

Accidental Overdose

Although truly adverse side effects are rare for most patients treated with behavioral medications, accidental ingestion of either the patient's own medication or client prescriptions of the same medication is a true emergency. Poison control centers report that the most common reason for accidental overdose of psychotropic medication is ingestion of the *client's medication* by the dog.

Toxic effects from overdose can be noted within the first 1 or 2 hours of ingestion, or they may not be seen for 8 to 10 hours after ingestion, depending on the medication. Treatment is supportive. The safest intervention, which is recommended by American Society for the Prevention of Cruelty to Animals Poison Control Center, involves emesis, gastric lavage, and activated charcoal every 6 hours. Emesis should be considered only if the patient is asymptomatic. Otherwise, supportive and symptomatic care designed to protect the patient and to regulate body temperature, if needed, is usually sufficient. Fluids will help with temperature regulation, blood pressure maintenance, and support of renal function, but almost all behavioral medication is highly protein bound, and so diuresis will not aid excretion.

Concerns for Patients Undergoing Sedation or Anesthesia

Patients who are taking behavioral medications should not have them withdrawn before anesthesia or surgery, unless the medications will cause an adverse outcome in an emergency situation and/or the patient is already experiencing profound side effects that will potentially affect the outcome of the procedure warranting sedation/anesthesia. These situations are rare.

Removing patients from their behavior medication, especially if the medication is helping, is not a good idea for three reasons:

1. The patients could become more anxious, which would compound the anxiety of the procedure itself. Increased anxiety is accompanied by high levels of sympathetic tone, a risk itself.

2. The patient could become neurochemically less stable because of discontinuation/rebound syndrome. In patients taking long-term BZDs, withdrawal syndrome is also a concern.

3. The patient who was doing well on medication may not respond in the same manner when re-introduced to the medication. Although widely recognized, this phenomenon is poorly understood, but it appears to be due to receptor desensitization. Alteration in subunit configuration and composition may result in the receptors no longer recognizing the medication in the manner that had been previously helpful. These alterations would be postulated to affect gene transcription and its coding. For this reason, weaning from or discontinuation of successful long-term treatment is not a decision to be undertaken lightly.

Instead, using the available data on interaction of side effects, interaction at the level of CYP enzymes, and data available on shared effects (see Box 10-4), premedication, sedative and anesthesia cocktails should be adjusted with presumed interactions and their effects on the respiratory and cardiovascular systems in mind. Some basic rules should be clear.

- Avoid acepromazine in noise-sensitive or phobic dogs.
- Use BZDs, particularly alprazolam, if the patient is responsive, at home to lessen any anxiety associated with the procedure because such anxiety enhances cardiovascular risks because of sympathetic effects on cardiac function.
- Many pre-anesthetic medication cocktails contain a BZD. If the patient is also taking a BZD for anxiety or panic, these may interact, enhancing and/or prolonging the plane of anesthesia and perhaps acting as a respiratory suppressant.
- If dexmedetomidine (Dexdomitor) is used, understand that clonidine has the same mechanism of function as a central alpha-adrenergic agonist, and effects will be cumulative. If clonidine is used as an anti-anxiety or panicolytic medication for veterinary evaluation, adjust dosages (lower them) accordingly.
- Any medication that affects NE (TCAs, SARIs, NaSSAs, NRIs, and some SSRIs) can alter cardiovascular tone, so it may be helpful to avoid pre-anesthetic and anesthetic agents that could affect an additional increase in cardiovascular tone.
- Many patients who are taking a TCA or SSRI may also be taking alprazolam because of the co-morbidity of panic and other anxiety-related diagnoses. The pharmacodynamics of these medications vary as shown in Tables 10-7 and 10-12 and Figure 10-2 depending on medications chosen. Knowing how these medications affect each other can help in determining which pre-anesthetic medications to use.

- Propofol, a commonly used induction agent, is a potent CYP3A4 inhibitor, as are the behavioral medications fluvoxamine, norfluoxetine (one of the active metabolites of fluoxetine), TCAs, and nefazodone. These medications will potentiate each other, so less propofol might be needed for anesthetic induction.
- Propofol and BZDs may act synergistically by potentiating the $GABA_A$ receptor (Reynolds and Maitra, 1996). Respiratory depression could be a problem.
- Any patient who is taking any behavioral medication should be fully monitored during anesthesia and surgery, and any alterations in respiratory or cardiovascular function should be attended to immediately. Continuous ECG monitoring will ensure that even subtle changes in conduction are noted before they become problems.

Studies That Support Use and Dosing

Controlled studies, especially studies that involve a placebo and are double-blind, are quite rare in veterinary behavioral medicine. Studies that meet this requirement (King et al., 2000a, 2000b, 2003; Landsberg et al., 2008; Simpson et al., 2007) have been funded by pharmaceutical companies as part of licensing requirements to obtain a canine (or feline) label. Laws vary among countries, as do some of the rules for the types of studies needed. Doing such studies is expensive, and so it is extremely unlikely that anyone will fund what is really needed: good, comparative studies across different medications used to treat the same condition. In other words, *for most medications and indications, we have not met the requirements of evidence-based medicine, let alone hypothesis testing about mechanisms of action and outcomes. This means that we may not understand all the effects or the side effects of any medication.* Most studies are small sample, open-label trials or incompletely controlled trials. That human medicine finds itself in much the same position is small comfort. In human medicine, in contrast to in veterinary medicine, studies are at least large, so we can hope to use humans as a partial model for effects and side effects of these medications in at least dogs, who are so often used as toxicology models for humans (Mahmood et al., 2003). Post-surveillance monitoring for atypical effects is done in the United States by the Food and Drug Administration Center for Veterinary Medicine (www.fda.gov/AboutFDA/CentersOffices/CVM/default.htm), but the effort depends on voluntary reports. We need to strive to begin to collect data in collaborative, systematic ways if we are to overcome the power of anecdote. Such efforts could be organized online and would be publishable.

One preliminary study (Overall and Dunham, unpublished) examined the effects of treatment with TCAs and/or SSRIs for 46 dogs (29 males, 17 females) and 8 (3 males, 5 females) cats on laboratory evaluation of renal and hepatic function. The age range for the dogs at first treatment was 6 to 124 months (mean, 46.2 months). The age range of the cats at first treatment was 12 to 135 months (mean, 80.5 months). The length of treatment for dogs varied from 1 to 73.25 months (mean, 26.2 months), and for cats, treatment ranged from 1 to 72 months (mean, 21.8 months). Duration of treatment, age, and frequency of laboratory evaluation were *not independent.* Table 10-15 shows changes in laboratory values as a function of evaluation number. It's clear that in this small, preliminary study, treatment with TCAs and SSRIs relatively rarely affected laboratory measures of renal and hepatic function. For only three of the measurements noted were the increased values actually outside of the reference range, and none of the patients evaluated showed any clinical signs that could be associated with their solitary evaluations. These data suggest that long-term treatment with these medications, especially if rationally monitored, is relatively low risk.

Which Client?

Finally, the client household must be considered when the decision to use behavioral drugs is made. Substance abuse is rampant in humans, and some medications (e.g., BZDs) used to treat canine and feline behavioral conditions have a high human abuse potential. Relevant Drug Enforcement Administration schedule information for the United States is provided in Table 10-16.

All clients should be provided with informed consent statements (see handouts/protocols at the end of the text and on the DVD) for medications that are "extra-label" (not yet approved for use) for cats and dogs. If the clients are given written discharges, which they sign, plus the "Protocol for Using Behavioral Medication Successfully," which should be referenced in the discharges, these can act as an equivalent notice of informed consent. The client handout, "Protocol for Using Behavioral Medication Successfully," can help clients make rational decisions.

Getting Medications into the Patient

The easiest time to teach veterinary patients how to take medication is before they need it. All puppies and kittens should learn to take pills, preferably in some food, at a very young age. In fact, giving them "blanks" on a regular or even daily basis can facilitate giving them medication when they need it (see the handout, "Protocol for Activities for Clients to Practice with Puppies and Kittens"). If one animal in the household is taking medication, all of them can have "blanks," which may mitigate the distress that the animal

TABLE 10-15

Number of Renal and Hepatic Measures That *Significantly* Increased (1-fold Increase) or Decreased and Elevated Pre-existing Values That Did Not Change with Treatment with Selective Serotonin Reuptake Inhibitors and/or Tricyclic Antidepressants

	Second Evaluation	Third Evaluation	Fourth or Subsequent Evaluation
Cats (n)	4	3	1
No. values significantly increased (+ 2 SD) with treatment	ALT—2	ALT—1	
	Albumin—1	Albumin—1	
No. pre-existing significantly high values that did not change with treatment	Albumin—1		
No. significantly high values that decreased with treatment	ALT—2		
Dogs (n)	24	13	9
No. values significantly increased (+ 2 SD) with treatment	Creatinine—2	ALT—2	ALT—1[†]
	ALT—2	SAP/ALP—2*	
	AST—1[‡]		
	SAP/ALP—1		
	GGT—1[†,‡]		
No. pre-existing significantly high values that did not change with treatment			SAP—3
No. significantly high values that decreased with treatment	ALT—1	ALT—1	ALT—3
	SAP/ALP—5	AST—1	Total bilirubin—1
		SAP/ALP—2	
		GGT—1	

Note: The number of the laboratory evaluation reflects that subsequent to the baseline, premedication evaluation against which the results were compared; only three values were outside the reference range.
ALT, Alanine aminotransferase; AST, aspartate aminotransferase; GGT, gamma-glutamyltransferase/transpeptidase; SAP/ALP, serum alkaline phosphatase.
* One elevated SAP/ALP value was outside the reference range.
[†]Single values outside the reference range.
[‡]Decreased to original value on third evaluation.

requiring the pill feels, while taking advantage of social facilitation.

Cats are unique creatures and can become unduly attached or averse to textures at young ages unless they are chronically exposed to them. This generalization extends to textures and tastes of ingested items. Because cats do not taste "sweet" in the way dogs do, foods for providing treats and medication can be more difficult to identify, but many cats like yeasty, salty spreads (Marmite, Vegemite) and can have small amounts of these on a special but regular basis. Cats who like fishy oils have another compounding option for when they require medication. It cannot be emphasized enough to clients that they need to encourage cats to eat and like special foods (chicken liver, shrimp, sardines) or treats (including the yeast spreads of Marmite, Vegemite) that will facilitate medication ingestion when the time comes.

Virtually all behavioral medications are extremely bitter. For some patients, the palatable veterinary versions of the medication (Reconcile, Clomicalm) may be acceptable. If the client must pill the dog or cat, this will be relatively simple if they can find a food that the patient will swallow greedily. It also helps to remember that most, but not all, BZDs are very water-soluble and can be easily made into a tiny amount of paste the cat or dog can lick from their nose or lips. In a worst-case scenario, a paste of the tablet can be smeared on their inner lips and will be ingested the next time they swallow.

The difficulty in delivering medication to canine and feline patients has encouraged investigation of transdermal (Ciribassi et al., 2003) and intranasal (Platt et al., 2000) medication routes. However, for transdermal fluoxetine to provide equivalent blood levels to those obtained orally, the concentration of the

TABLE 10-16

Relevant Drug Enforcement Administration Schedule Information

Schedule Level	Concerns and Requirements	Relevant Medications
DEA schedule II	High abuse potential Severe physical dependency Psychological dependency (humans) No refills No phone prescriptions	Amphetamine Codeine Fentanyl Hydromorphone Meperidine Methylphenidate Pentobarbital
DEA schedule III	Abuse potential less than schedule I and II Moderate, low physical dependency High psychological dependence (people) New prescription after 6 months or five refills	Buprenorphine Compounds with codeine (≤90 mg) Hydrocodone Ketamine (Naltrexone) Anabolic steroids
DEA schedule IV	Low abuse potential Limited physical dependence Limited psychological dependence Prescription after 6 months or five refills	Benzodiazepines (treated as a schedule II drug in New York state) including alprazolam, clonazepam, clorazepate, diazepam, lorazepam, midazolam, temazepam, and triazolam Meprobamate Phenobarbital

DEA, Drug Enforcement Administration.

medication has to be 10 times that of the oral medication, which creates a toxicity hazard should the cat ingest the patch or compound (Ciribassi et al., 2003). No one should assume that compounding an oral medication into a transdermal form maintains the medication's bioequivalence or efficacy. Many oral medications require action in the stomach, intestines, and/or liver (e.g., biotransformation through first-pass metabolism) to deliver the desired compound, and dosages obtained transdermally may not be equivalent to dosages obtained orally.

Intranasal medication delivery is being closely examined because of ease of administration and the potential to lower the dosage of some medications that effectively cross into the systemic circulation. Additionally, intranasal delivery allows some medications to pass into the cerebrospinal fluid quickly and at concentrations that otherwise may be difficult to achieve. Intranasal administration of oxytocin appears reasonable and successful.

In summary, teaching cats and dogs to take medication really is a priceless skill.

PHEROMONES

True pheromones are chemicals excreted or secreted by a member of a species that trigger a *specific social response in other members of the same species.* Classic responses include behavioral and/or physiological changes that affect reproduction, social status, prey identification, et cetera (Dorries et al., 1997; Liman, 2001). By definition, pheromonal responses must be *biochemically specific* and *not* occur in the absence of the compound. Pheromonal responses are mediated through receptors in the vomeronasal organ (VNO) and the main olfactory epithelium (OE). The cells in these sensory epithelia are heterogeneous in the receptors that they express and in the odorants or ligands that the receptors bind. In mice, specific pheromones appear to be detected by nonoverlapping populations of cells (Liman, 2001). A small fraction of any set of VNO cells responds to bioactive chemicals (Holy, 2003). The cells of the VNO appear fine-tuned to specific pheromones, whereas neurons in the OE appear to be more broadly tuned to general odorants. Given the function of VNO in ensuring behavioral responses tied to species survival, this may not be surprising.

Processing of information from the VNO and OE differs, but there is more functional overlap than often thought.

- Axons from neurons in the VNO project to the accessory olfactory bulb. Neurons of the accessory olfactory bulb appear to respond only after direct contact, which has suggested that these neurons are not stimulated from a distance by volatile compounds in the air (Holy, 2003), and these neurons are very selective in their response with respect to aspects such as sex of the individual and, in mice, strain of the mice studied (Dulac, 2000; Luo et al., 2003). Neurons from the accessory olfactory bulb then project to the amygdala (Dulac and Axel, 1995; Lin et al., 2005). From the amygdala, neurons project to the hypothalamus, with subsequent responses dependent on region and type of hypothalamic stimulation.

• Neurons from the OE terminate in the olfactory bulb, where they synapse on neurons that project directly to the olfactory cortex.

Because of these differences, it has been thought that much of the response to an odorant is cognitive, but responses from the VNO were not. Immunohistochemistry studies have made it clear that VNO neurons can detect both odorants and pheromones (Sam et al., 2001). There is overlap between VNO and OE odorant recognition, and both the VNO and OE are neurogenic (Dennis et al., 2003). Beyond this, there is also considerable integrated function and processing that is facilitated by oxytocin and vasopressin (Bielsky and Young, 2004). Bielsky and Young (2004) have proposed that such integration may be necessary for social discrimination.

Since the 1990s, pheromonal analogue products (e.g., Feliway, DAP, Adaptil, Felifriend, depending on country) have been available and marketed for the treatment of behavioral concerns. Pheromonal analogue products are not true pheromones, and purported active ingredients and complete chemical structures have not been reported in the peer-reviewed literature. These products have been asserted to work like pheromones, a claim that has been inadequately substantiated. Few controlled studies have been published in the peer-reviewed literature, and most studies that assess the effects of these products have used inadequate designs and controls and insufficient sample sizes (Frank et al., 2010). There is *very limited evidence that these products produce any consistent behavioral effects* (Frank et al., 2010), even when sufficient data and experimental controls exist to evaluate outcome scientifically. The results for which there *may* be adequate data for an effect tend to involve non-specific responses associated with mild changes in activity levels (sitting vs. lying down, moving a lot vs. being more still (Denenberg and Landsberg, 2008; Griffith et al., 2000; Mills et al., 2006). *The methodology in these studies is flawed, and effects attributed to the product may be coincident.* Because these products lack testing for specific mechanism of action, and because any outcomes that affect the VNO and OE are complex, clinical trials of such products need to be controlled and double-blinded, to focus on well-defined, repeatable clinical entities that are sufficiently narrow to be assessed with the numbers proposed, and to use assessment criteria that are biologically meaningful (a comment on statistical concerns and relevance is found in Box 10-5) and

valid. Such studies should meet or exceed the level required for pharmaceuticals, where mechanisms of action of strongly supported or identified. To date, such studies are lacking.

Clients anecdotally report a range of responses to these products, including behaviors associated with *both increased and decreased arousal.* Based on the heterogeneity of the response of VNO, discussed previously, it's possible that the compounds in these products may stimulate the VNO and/or OE in highly variable ways, which may not be independent of the genetic background of the individual affected.

No data on specific and/or variable responses of individuals who may represent different subpopulations are available. The indication for these products is over-broad and non-specific (e.g., "stress"), complicating any potential identification of putative population-specific effects. These products are recommended for use *in conjunction with environmental and behavior modification,* so any attribution of effect becomes complex. This is why rigorous, specific, quantitative, placebo-controlled studies are required, and the less specific the effect, the more rigorous the study must be. *Placebos* are often mistakenly viewed as the effect of doing nothing, when they actually *measure the effect of participating in the study, which includes the effects of:*

• Communication between study participants and veterinarians
• Behavioral and environmental modification
• Watching the animal differently because of participation in the study
• Altering impressions of the pet's behavior and/or the client's own tolerance of the behavior because of new knowledge
• Any direct effect of the compound studied

These factors may also interact. In well-designed studies, the above-listed effects are identifiable and measurable. In all of the placebo-controlled studies used in licensing clomipramine and fluoxetine use for specific diagnostic indications in dogs, when compared with the placebo group, dogs treated with medication increased the rate at which they acquired changes associated with behavior modification (King et al., 2000a, 2000b; Landsberg et al., 2008; Simpson et al., 2007). No comparable data published in the peer-reviewed literature currently exist for the pheromonal analogue products.

It may be best to recommend that veterinarians wishing to use such products should consider the financial cost of the product to the client in the context of the potential benefits and fully disclose the state of the extant data in any discussion of use and cost. Both cost and outcomes may reflect on clients' opinions of veterinarians, so full disclosure about what we do not know and about the lack of strong, definitive studies is always a good idea.

BOX 10-5

What It Means to Have a *Statistically* Significant Finding and a *Biologically* Meaningful Finding

- A comment on statistical significance and its limitations may be helpful.
- Assessment of changes in behavior can be difficult and requires good definitions of behaviors, validation of those behaviors as assays of the condition in question, and quantitative ways to measure change. These requirements are usually incompletely met.
- In *a priori* statistical tests, a significance level is set in advance of the analysis of the data.
  - This level is generally 0.05, meaning that 5 times out of 100, the finding is due to random factors, and 95 times out of 100, the finding is due to the tested association or pattern.
  - In other words, in a laboratory panel that measures 20 compounds, the finding that one of the measures is beyond the limits of the reference range could be random.
  - The interpretation of the laboratory finding that is beyond its reference range will depend on the actual numbers and the clinical signs of the patient.
    - For example, if the reference range in the laboratory used for alkaline phosphatase is 10 to 150 U/L and the reading for patient A is 160 U/L, in the absence of clinical signs or any other elevated liver enzyme level, a less than 10% increase in the upper end of the reference range is unlikely to be biologically meaningful.
    - A small change such as this is not informative about the patient.
    - In a lengthy panel, this finding could also be legitimately due to chance. True accuracy—a separate concern—is also an issue in interpretation.
    - Consider a patient with cancer who is given a new treatment that significantly decreases one cell class that is increased in that cancer. Even a statistically significant decrease in cell number will not bring a new medication to market in the absence of an accompanying clinical effect, a change in outcome (longevity or QoL), or a link between the finding and a specific mechanism that affects disease course.
- In behavioral medicine, it is difficult to meet the above-listed criteria because few behavioral assays are validated. However, changes in clinical signs can be used.
  - In our example, we will consider a canine patient who has a noise phobia, as defined in this text.
  - This patient pants, paces, dilates her pupils, trembles, and cannot eat when distressed.

- This patient is treated with compound X.
- The number of breaths per minute decreases to a level that achieves significance at the 0.05 level.
- No other behavioral measures used change significantly. In this example, we have a statistically measurable finding for which the intervention may be responsible, but this finding is of limited to no biological value because although the patient decreased her rate of panting, no one would doubt that given the other signs present, she is still suffering.
- Interventions are often assessed by asking clients whether they perceive a change and in which direction they perceive a change.
  - Such subjective measures are tricky because a "good" improvement for one client may be only a "marginal" improvement for another.
  - Without measuring the behaviors and knowing the goals of the client, we cannot tell whether the difference in opinion is due to a difference in client goals and expectations or a real, quantitative change in meaningful behaviors.
  - For marketing purposes, any positive change that clients can identify is considered excellent and touted, but enduring results depend on real, measured change using valid assessments and accurate measures. Without these, we are actually treating dogs based on client opinion rather than patient needs and signs.
- Finally, authors often are distressed when their data achieve a significance level of, for example, 0.058, and their goal was 0.050.
  - Even with this small difference, authors should not report that "findings approached significance." Regardless, their findings were not significant.
  - However, authors may wish to measure the power of the test, which could tell them whether, given the pattern of responses, they had a sufficient sample size to detect an effect.
    - The bigger the effect, the lower the sample size can be.
    - The smaller the effect, the larger a sample size needed to detect it.
  - Regardless of this discussion of significance level, the issue of whether the finding is biologically meaningful must still be considered.
- In short, establishing effects of interventions in veterinary behavioral medicine can be a hornet's nest, but with care and due consideration, it can be done.

HOMEOPATHY

No study has shown any statistically significant, beneficial effect for behavioral change for any homeopathic compound studied (Cracknell and Mills, 2008, 2011; Overall and Dunham, 2009). "Homeopathy" refers to high-dilution homeopathic preparations in which not a single molecule of the original substance can be shown to exist (Cracknell and Mills, 2008). No homeopathic preparation has demonstrated a scientifically plausible, biochemical mechanism of action beyond that of the placebo effect. Hypothesis testing and falsification are at the very core of the scientific approach, and so homeopathy must be shown to be valid using methods that science uses to evaluate all treatment modalities, including those discussed in this chapter. No field or treatment can claim a special exemption and be considered to be scientific or a best practice. Finally, what so many engaging in such studies fail to understand is that one of the most valued attributes of study designs that test for potential effects of intervention and use placebos is that the effect of the placebo is *not* the effect of doing nothing: it is the effect of doing the study, as discussed.

SUMMARY: USING DIETS, SUPPLEMENTS, NUTRACEUTICALS, AND MEDICATION TO ADDRESS BEHAVIORAL CONCERNS IN DOGS AND CATS

Diet, Nutraceuticals, and Supplements

- The appeal for using diets, nutraceuticals, and supplements, rather than medication, is in ease of administration and because these interventions are seen to affect behavior in a more "natural" manner. For clients who are averse to and concerned about side effects, these types of interventions are relatively free of side effects, although gastrointestinal distress can occur for any oily/fatty diet/supplement.
- Diets/nutraceuticals/supplements offer tremendous promise for favorably manipulating behaviors at the molecular and neurochemical level in a way that may have fewer side effects if processes can be beneficially affected early in their pathways.
- Just because a supplement does not have to go through FDA approval, this does not mean it is safe or efficacious. 5-HTP has been demonstrated to cause signs associated with serotonin syndrome in dogs at dosages that do not affect humans. St. John's wort contains a compound that is a potent CYP3A4 inducer.
- The strongest evidence for the beneficial use of diets/nutraceuticals/supplements is found for the neuroprotectant/anti-oxidant effects on neurodegenerative changes associated with aging. Whether delivered by diet or supplement, the effects of neuroprotectants have been found at the behavioral, cognitive, and molecular levels. Neuroprotection is a growing field.
- The best results from any of the dietary/supplementation studies on aging brains are obtained by a combination of diet/supplement and cognitive stimulation.
- Cognitive stimulation benefits from aerobic exercise.
- Newer approaches to cognition use novel sources of energy to enhance neuronal function and to facilitate neuroprotection.
- Most studies showing positive results have been for laboratory dogs, who are not representative of the pet dog population. Results may be different in pet dogs who do not live in an environment where cognitive stimulation and exercise are restricted. Regardless, the neurochemical mechanisms are the same and should be emphasized.
- Intervention with diets/nutraceuticals/supplements (plus exercise and cognitive stimulation) likely will be most effective when it is lifelong, but special attention should be paid no later than when cats (8 to 10 years) and dogs (5 to 8 years) enter early middle age.
- Many new developments are likely in these fields.

Medication

- Behavioral problems should always be viewed as QoL issues. Regardless of severity, behavioral problems are often life-threatening. Behavioral medication, when competently prescribed and monitored, is the humane choice for all patients who are at risk of being relinquished, abandoned, or euthanized and for most patients for whom a diagnosis can be determined.
- No matter how helpful medications can be, they are not the right choice for some *clients*. Chemical abuse issues aside, any client who is going to worry about medication to the point that they hang over the dog's or cat's every move will worsen the dog's or cat's behavior by making them more anxious. Conversely, if the client cannot or will not monitor the patient for side effects, they have increased the risk of medication for their pet.
- Given early, behavioral medication prevents the worsening of the behavioral condition and, similar to dietary intervention, acts in a neuroprotectant manner because the medication addresses the neurocytotoxic stress associated with increased distress and behavioral reactivity. Consider the possible effect of ongoing stress and anxiety as it relates to the neuroendocrine response and its detrimental effect on lifelong physical health.
- Behavioral medications can safely be given as lifelong treatment, but the earlier in the course of the condition that the medications are given, the less likely lifelong treatment is in most situations.

- Behavioral medications can have side effects, but they are usually mild and transient. If side effects are not transient, adjustments must be made.
- Clients can be schooled to monitor for more severe side effects, but they must understand what to monitor (e.g., heart rate). Because most behavioral medications for dogs and cats are "extra-label," informed consent statements can be useful to ensure that clients understand what is unknown, what is expected, why they must monitor their pet's response, and when to call for help. Having the clients sign that they have reviewed with you and understood the "Protocol for Using Behavioral Medication Successfully" can act as an informed consent statement.
- Behavioral medications speed the rate at which behavior modification is acquired, a finding supported by all published placebo-controlled, double-blind studies.
- Many of the medications used are metabolized by enzymes that affect other medications, and knowing how medications can interact is important both for the patient's safety and for obtaining the desired, favorable effects of the medications. It's important to remember that although outcome may not scale with dosage and blood level for many of the medications used in veterinary behavioral medicine, side effects can and do. Any time multiple medications are given, the risk of side effects can increase. Such risk is minimized by understanding how these medications work and how they are metabolized. These properties should be reviewed when treating any animal with any medication.
- Routine monitoring (e.g., physical exam, complete blood count, chemistry panel, urinalysis) once or twice a year can ensure that there are no adverse effects of long-term treatment. Pre-medication laboratory evaluation can minimize side effects by alerting the clinician to any underlying concerns and will allow the clinician to attribute any side effects to the medication, rather than an underlying condition that may not be apparent, in patients that are otherwise healthy. Without pre-medication laboratory evaluation, the trend will be for the client to blame any and all physical changes or concerns on the medication, an attribution that may be meritless.
- Long-term treatment is preferable to abrupt cessation of treatment. If the client wishes to see if the dog or cat still "needs" the medication, the client should wean as slowly as possible. However, clients should understand that some patients, once removed from the behavioral medication, become refractory to it. This means that they do not respond to it when treated with it again, although they responded well when first treated. This phenomenon is poorly understood but appears to be due to receptor desensitization. Alteration in subunit configuration and composition may result in the receptors no longer recognizing the medication in the manner that had been previously helpful. These alterations would be postulated to affect gene transcription and its coding. For this reason, weaning from or discontinuation of successful long-term treatment is not a decision to be undertaken lightly.
- Medications should be given as part of an integrated treatment program involving environmental, social, and behavioral modification. Many certified pet dog trainers are now familiar with the numerous behavior modification programs available and can help clients to develop the skills necessary to help the dog.
- Many patients treated with behavioral medication may never be "normal," but they can be happy and have a good QoL, and their people can be safe and happy as well.

FINAL ADVICE

In the industrial world, behavioral problems in pets are responsible for more relinquishment and death than are infectious disease, neoplasia, and cardiac disease combined. *Rational use of behavioral medication represents a real and ongoing chance for veterinarians to treat their patients more humanely and to provide guidance to clients about more humane guardianship.* Investing in the time and knowledge needed to help these troubled patients and their distressed humans can be one of the most rewarding aspects of any veterinarian's career and, as such, can change us and the future of veterinary medicine for the better.

Drugs alone cannot accomplish these goals, but they can be part of effective, humane, state-of-the-art treatment. The standard of care is evolving to include the effective use of psychotropic medication. It is essential to incorporate all new modalities of treatment that can aid clients in helping their troubled pets better, and that can help protect these troubled pets from circumstances that upset them. *No discussion of the use of behavioral medication should happen without a discussion of "true" behavioral modification that effects cognitive change to help the troubled cat and dog to alter their behaviors* (see accompanying client handouts, "Protocol for Teaching Your Dog to Take a Deep Breath and Use Other Biofeedback Methods as Part of Relaxation" and "Protocol for Generalized Discharge Instructions for Dogs with Behavioral Concerns").

Acquisition of the changes associated with behavior modification can occur more quickly with the use of medication, and both of these treatments should include in their discussion the following:

1. use of canine head collars and harnesses,
2. cognitive needs of "captive" cats and dogs,
3. role of appropriate and repeated exercise, and
4. need for and rational use of pain medications and dietary supplements and treatments that can aid in passage through each life stage.

Text continued on p. 512

TABLE 10-17

Client Questions about Medications and Their Answers

Client Question	Quick Answer
What medications are used?	We use most of the same medications or classes of medication that are used for the same conditions in humans. Most commonly used medications come from the BZD, TCA, and SSRI classes of drugs.
How do these work?	All of these medications affect how brain neurons communicate with each other and the neurochemistry that appears impaired in anxiety.
What are potential side effects?	Side effects (medication effects that clients, clinicians and/or patients find undesirable) are usually rare and transient but can include gastrointestinal distress including diarrhea and/or regurgitation/vomiting, changes in appetite including anorexia, sedation, changes in energy level, atypical reactivity, and increased heart and respiratory rates. If any of these side effects are profound or last longer than a few days, the patient should be re-evaluated. Anorexia is a rare but profound problem for some patients given SSRIs. Serotonin syndrome is a concern for any patient taking any medication that affects serotonin and who is experiencing profound increases in heart rate, body temperature, and/or agitation.
How should the client monitor for side effects?	Clients should keep a log of worrisome behaviors, and compare them with normal behaviors. To do this, they need to know if the dog or cat occasionally has diarrhea and what their behaviors were before starting medications. Clients can learn to take patients' heart rates and report any significant increases or decreases immediately to the veterinarian. Clients can also comply with the recommendation for annual physical and laboratory evaluation for younger animals and biannual evaluation for older animals. Evaluation should also occur if the dog or cat becomes ill.
Can these medications interact with other medications (e.g., thyroxine, anti-inflammatories, pain medications such as tramadol), and, if so, how?	Yes, any medications that use the same enzyme system in the liver can have their effect exaggerated or decreased, depending on the enzyme function, and those medications can have the same effect on the behavioral drugs. This is why it is so important for clients to ensure that they tell their veterinarian every single medication and supplement that their dog or cat is being given. Clients need to understand that this list includes "homeopathic," "herbal," and "natural" products. For example, St. John's wort is a potent CYP3A4 inducer. For medications such as thyroxine, there may be effects on measured blood levels of the medication or on the compounds it is intended to affect. Pain medications (e.g., tramadol), antibiotics, and anti-inflammatories can be given with behavioral medications if they are needed, the dosages are appropriately adjusted, and the patient is monitored, which is easy to do. *Anti-inflammatories may block some effects of SSRIs, but there are no data yet for dogs and cats.*
What effects can be seen and when?	Dogs and cats treated with medications affecting anxiety should become calmer and less anxious. This may mean a decrease in activity, which can appear as weight gain. Patients may eat more and may finish their food treats/food toys when the clients are not with them. Contrast this with anxious patients who cannot eat when distressed and who will not eat or finish treats/food toys when alone. Patients who are less anxious may react less quickly to a stimulus. Patients who are less anxious may react to a certain stimulus using a lower level of reactivity than was previously possible. Patients who are less anxious may raise their threshold for reacting and so not react as readily as they had previously. It takes more of a stimulus to make them react. Patients who are improving may show a decreased amount of time between hearing the request to lie down or sit down and compliance with the request. They are less worried and so can comply more readily. Patients who are deriving beneficial effects from medication may pause before reacting or become more thoughtful and less concerned in general. They may be able to attend more to cues in the environment and assess whether they need to react before reacting. Patients may sleep longer and more soundly (more restorative sleep) as their anxiety resolves. Patients may be more receptive to learning to change their behavior through behavior modification.

TABLE 10-17

Client Questions about Medications and Their Answers—cont'd

Client Question	Quick Answer
	Patients may become more attentive to the helpful cues they are given, and they may solicit cues more often.
	Dogs who are improving may take treats more gently rather than grabbing forcefully at them as concerned dogs often do. It is important here to separate poor delivery technique from patient anxiety.
	Cats who are improving may become more interested in behavioral modification using food treats and be willing to remain with the client to learn about these.
	Clients may be best able to appreciate these effects by taking before and after treatment videos in the same situations and comparing them. If the clients are uncertain of any behavior on video, they should watch the video with their vet—a new set of eyes may help clarify a situation or spot improvement.
How long must the patient take the medication?	Patients affected for a long time may require or benefit from long-term treatment. Patients with relatively uncomplicated, recent concerns may require medication for only a few months. Length of treatment is determined by the patient's history, the patient's treatment response, the client's concerns, and the patient's stimulatory environment.
How do we wean or remove the patient from the medication?	If there is an emergency, patients can be abruptly taken from the medication, but weaning is preferred in planned cessations. Weaning permits the avoidance of rebound syndrome and allows clients to learn if their pet would benefit from a lower dose of the medication. Some patients who are removed from a medication will not respond to it when exposed again, no matter how well they did when treated with it the first time.
What should the client do if he or she is scared?	The client should call the vet immediately and relate the details of the concern to a member of the treatment team. If the concern is after hours and no one returns a phone call quickly, the client should take the dog or cat to any emergency service to err on the safe side and to prevent the possibility of feeling guilt.

Note: A client-friendly version of these questions and answers can be found in the handout, "Protocol for Using Behavioral Medication Successfully."
BZD, Benzodiazepine; SSRI, selective serotonin reuptake inhibitor; TCA, tricyclic antidepressant.

TABLE 10-18

Psychopharmacological Agents That May Be Useful in the Treatment of Feline Behavioral Diagnoses

Psychopharmacological Agent	Dosage Information
Alprazolam (tablets: 0.25, 0.5, 1, 2 mg; 1- and 2-mg tablets scored)	0.0125-0.025 mg/kg PO q12h **to start** (this means that the smallest tablets may have to be quartered for small cats; smaller cats may take the relatively high end of the dose and larger cats may take the relatively smaller end of the dose because of differences in mass-dependent metabolism; a 3-kg cat may take 3×0.025 mg = 0.075 mg, which is ¼ of a 0.25 mg tablet); *some cats may do well with dosages starting at 0.05 mg to 0.1 mg/kg, but start low*; dosages should be gradually increased to see if a desired effect can be achieved
	Notes: All BZDs can cause rare paradoxical (excitement) reactions in dogs, cats, and primates. Undesirable reaction (profound sedation or excitement) to one BZD does not mean that you will have a reaction to another. All BZDs are lipophilic. This means that fat cats may store drug, which suggests starting at a lower dose.
Amitriptyline (tablets: 10, 25, 50, 75, 100, 150 mg)	0.5-2.0 mg/kg PO q12-24h; start at 0.5 mg/kg PO q12h
Buspirone (tablets: 5, 10, 15 mg)	0.5-1 mg/kg PO q8-12-24h (2.5-5 mg/**cat**)

Continued

TABLE 10-18

Psychopharmacological Agents That May Be Useful in the Treatment of Feline Behavioral Diagnoses—cont'd

Psychopharmacological Agent	Dosage Information
Chlorpheniramine (tablets: 4 mg)	1-2 mg/**cat** (low dose) to 2-4 mg/**cat** (high dose) PO q12-24h
Clomipramine (capsules: 25, 50, 75 mg in human formulation [Anafranil]; 20, 40, 80 mg scored tablets in veterinary formulation [Clomicalm]; 5-mg scored tablets available in Australia and Europe)*	0.25-0.5 mg/kg PO q24h
Clonazepam (tablets: 0.125, 0.25, 0.5, 1.0, 2.0 mg)	0.05-0.1-0.2 mg/kg PO q12-24h (note range of dosages and start low; low dose can be used q8h)
Clorazepate (tablets: 3.75, 7.5, 11.25, 15, 22.5; capsules: 3.75, 7.5, 15 mg)	0.5-2.2 mg/kg PO as needed for profound distress; 0.2-0.4 mg/kg q12-24h
Cyproheptadine (tablets: 4 mg; solution: 4 mg/mL)	1-4 mg/**cat** PO q8-12h; 1.1 mg/kg to combat serotonin syndrome
Diazepam (tablets: 1, 2, 5, 10 mg; solution: 5 mg/mL)	0.2-0.4 mg/kg PO q12-24h (start at 0.2 mg/kg PO q12h)
Doxepin (capsules: 10, 25, 50, 75, 100, 150 mg; solution: 10 mg/mL)	0.5-1.0 mg/kg PO q12-24h (start low) and monitor—very sedative
Flumazenil (intravenous solution: 0.1 mg/mL)	0.01-0.02 mg/kg IV for antagonism of profound, adverse BZD effects
Fluoxetine (capsules: 10, 20 mg; solution: 5 mg/mL)	0.5-1.0 mg/kg PO q24h
Flurazepam (capsules: 15, 30 mg)	0.1-0.2 mg/kg PO q12-24h as appetite stimulant
Fluvoxamine (capsules: 10, 20 mg)	0.25-0.5 mg/kg PO q24h
Gabapentin (capsules: 100, 300, 400 mg; solution: 250 mg/5 mL)	3-5 mg/kg PO q12-24h (note that this is lower than the 5-10 mg/kg PO q8h dosage for pain)
Hydrocodone (tablets: 5 mg; solution: 1 mg/mL)	0.25-1.0 mg/kg PO q12-24h; may be given up to q8h if effective
Imipramine (tablets: 10, 25, 50 mg; capsules 75, 100, 125, 150 mg)	0.5-1.0 mg/kg PO q12-24h (start at 0.5 mg/kg PO q12h)
Lorazepam (tablets: 0.5, 1.0, 2.0 mg)	0.05 mg/kg (range: 0.03-0.08) PO q12-24h up to 0.125-0.25 mg/**cat** (start low; with longer half-life, repeat doses will be additive)
Midazolam (solution 1 mg/mL, 5 mg/mL)	0.05-0.3 mg/kg IV, IM, SC; start low to medium dose
Naltrexone (tablets: 50 mg)	5-10 mg/kg PO q24h; 25-50 mg/**cat** PO q24h
Nicergoline (tablets: 5, 10, 30 mg)	0.25-0.5 mg/kg PO q24h
Nortriptyline (capsules: 10, 25, 50, 75 mg)	0.5-2.0 mg/kg PO q12-24h
Oxazepam (tablets: 15 mg; capsules: 10, 15, 30 mg)	0.2-0.5 mg/kg PO q12-24h; high dose:1.0-2.5 mg/kg PO q12-24h; 3 mg/kg PO as a bolus for appetite stimulation
Paroxetine (tablets: 10, 20, 30, 40 mg; suspension: 10 mg/5 mL)	0.5 mg/kg PO q24h × 6-8 wk to start; may increase to 1.0 mg/kg PO q24h but monitor heart rate and function
Phenobarbital (tablets: 8, 16, 32, 65, 100 mg; solution: 5, 10, 15, 20 mg/mL)	2-3 mg/kg PO as needed for mild sedation (e.g., car travel)
Propentofylline (tablets: 50, 100 mg)	12.5 mg/cat PO q24h
Protriptyline (tablets: 5, 10 mg)	0.5-1.0 mg/kg PO q12-24h (start at 0.5 mg/kg PO q12h)
Selegiline (Anipryl; Selgian) (tablets: 5, 10, 15, 30 mg*)	0.25-0.5 mg/kg PO q12-24h; up to 1 mg/kg PO q24h; start low
Sertraline (tablets: 25, 50, 100 mg)	0.5 mg/kg PO q24h × 6-8 wk to start; may go to 1 mg/kg but must monitor for undesirable effects
Triazolam (tablets: 0.125, 0.25 mg)	0.5 mg/kg (2.5-5 mg/**cat**) PO q8h

BZD, Benzodiazepine; IM, intramuscularly; IV, intravenously; PO, orally (per os); SC, subcutaneously.
*Veterinary label for some canine and feline conditions; label depends on country and species. Please note the range of the dosages listed for TCA, SSRIs, et cetera may be lower than commonly cited. Above these dosages, serotonin augmenting medications may cause increased arousal and agitation, usually associated with increased heart rate (which clients can monitor). Should these signs be seen with increasing dose, it is wise to decrease the dose to the level where the arousal does not occur, and if additional treatment effects are needed, consider possible polypharmacy.

TABLE 10-19

Psychopharmacological Agents That May Be Useful in the Treatment of Canine Behavioral Diagnoses

Psychopharmacological Agent	Dosage Information
Alprazolam (tablets: 0.25, 0.5, 1, 2 mg; 1- and 2-mg tablets scored)	0.01-0.1 mg/kg PO as needed for phobic or panic attacks; common efficacious starting range is 0.02-0.04 mg/kg; profound lethargy and incoordination may result at high dosages (0.75-4.0 mg/**dog**/day; may increase slowly over 4.0 mg/**dog**/day if obtaining some effect at a lower dose); start with 1 mg maximum for a 25-kg **dog**; alternatively can start at 0.25 mg (0.02-0.04 mg/kg range) and repeat q2-4h to effect—that then becomes new starting dose; if you are in the 4-mg range and there is no effect, this is not likely to be a useful drug for that dog
Amitriptyline (tablets: 10, 25, 50, 75, 100, 150 mg)	1-2 mg/kg PO q12h to start
Buspirone (tablets: 5, 10 mg)	1 mg/kg PO q8-24h (mild anxiety) to start (range is 0.5-2 mg/kg PO q8-24h); 2.5-10 mg/**dog** q8-24h (mild anxiety); 10-15 mg/**dog** PO q8-12h (more severe anxiety; use high dose for thunderstorm phobia)
Carbamazepine (tablets: 200 mg [scored]; chewable tablets: 100 mg [scored])	4-8 mg/kg PO q12h; 0.5-1.25 mg/kg PO q8h; 4-10 mg/kg/day divided q8h
Chlordiazepoxide (tablets: 5, 10, 25 mg; also available as a powder for injection)	2.2-6.6 mg/kg PO as needed (start low—very sedating)
Citalopram (tablets: 20, 40 mg)	0.5-1 mg/kg PO q24h to start; up to 2 mg/kg PO q24h; equivalent human dose is 20 mg/day; dogs experience profound toxicity and can die at 8 mg/kg/24 hr
Clomipramine (capsules: 25, 50, 75 mg in human formulation [Anafranil]; 20, 40, 80 mg scored tablets in veterinary formulation [Clomicalm]; 5-mg scored tablets available in Australia and Europe)*	1 mg/kg PO q12h × 2 wk, then 2 mg/kg PO q12h × 2 wk, then 3 mg/kg PO q12h × 4 wk and then as maintenance dose; or 2 mg/kg PO q12h × 8 wk to start; may need higher maintenance dose; constant dosage associated with slight increase in gastrointestinal side effects. *Note:* Dosing q24h is insufficient for most animals, particularly animals with multiple signs, early age onset, or long-standing complaint.
Clonazepam (tablets: 0.125, 0.25, 0.5, 1.0, 2.0 mg)	0.125-1.0 mg/kg PO q8-12h; range, 0.01-0.1 mg/kg PO as needed q4-8h for phobic or panic attacks; profound lethargy and incoordination may result at dosages >4.0 mg/day, but higher dosages may be used incrementally if there has been some effect at a lower dose; start with 1-2 mg for a 25-kg dog
Clonidine (tablets: 0.1, 0.2, 0.3 mg)	0.01-0.05 mg/kg PO as needed q12h; maximum dose = 0.9 mg total for medium dog range
Clorazepate (tablets: 3.75, 7.5, 11.25, 15, 22.5; capsules: 3.75, 7.5, 15 mg)	0.5-2.2 mg/kg PO at least 1 hr before provocative stimulus (departure) or anticipated noise (storm, fireworks); repeat q4-6h as needed; 11.25-22.5 mg/**dog** PO q24h (~22.5 mg/large dogs; ~11.25 mg/medium **dogs**; ~ 5.6 mg/small **dogs**)
Cyproheptadine (tablets: 4 mg; solution: 4 mg/mL)	1 mg/kg PO q8-12h; 1.1 mg/kg to combat serotonin syndrome
Dextroamphetamine (tablets: 5, 10 mg; extended-release capsules: 5, 10, 15, 20, 25, 30 mg)	0.2-1.3 mg/kg PO as needed; 5-10 mg/dog PO q8h for narcolepsy
Diazepam (tablets: 1, 2, 5, 10 mg; solution 5 mg/mL)	0.5-2.2 mg/kg PO at least 1 hr before provocative stimulus (departure) or anticipated noise (storm, fireworks); repeat q4-6h as needed; intranasal administration at 0.5-2 mg/kg is superior to rectal administration in terms of mean systemic availability and time to onset (only intravenous administration is faster)
Diphenhydramine (tablets: 25, 50 mg; capsules: 50 mg; solution: 12.5 mg/5 mL)	2.2 mg/kg PO q8h
Doxepin (capsules: 10, 25, 50, 75, 100, 150 mg; solution: 10 mg/mL)	3-5 mg/kg PO q8-12h
Flumazenil (intravenous solution: 0.1 mg/mL)	0.01-0.02 mg/kg IV for antagonism of profound, adverse BZD effects

Continued

TABLE 10-19

Psychopharmacological Agents That May Be Useful in the Treatment of Canine Behavioral Diagnoses—cont'd

Psychopharmacological Agent	Dosage Information
Fluoxetine (capsules: 10, 20 mg; solution: 5 mg/mL)*	0.5-1 mg/kg PO q12-24h × 6-8 wk to start
Flurazepam (capsules: 15, 30 mg)	0.1-0.5 mg/kg PO q12-24h as appetite stimulant
Fluvoxamine (tablets: 25, 50, 100 mg)	1 mg/kg PO q12-24h × 6-8 wk to start
Gabapentin (capsules: 100, 300, 400 mg; tablets: 600, 800 mg; solution: 250 mg/5 mL)	2-5 mg/kg PO q12h at the lower end of recommendations; 10-20 mg/kg PO q8-12h at the higher end of recommendations (there are usually so few side effects—serious or minor—that starting at the higher end of the dosage range is fine; capsule size may affect decisions
Hydrocodone (tablets: 5 mg; solution: 1 mg/mL)	0.25 mg/kg PO q8-12h
Hydroxyzine (tablets: 10, 25, 50 mg; capsules: 25, 50 mg)	0.5-2.2 mg/kg PO q8-12h
Imipramine (tablets: 10, 25, 50 mg; capsules: 75, 100, 125, 150 mg)	2.2-4.4 mg/kg PO q12-24h; 1-2 or 2-4 mg/kg PO q12-24h (start low)
Lithium (tablets/extended release: 450 mg; capsules: 150, 300, 600 mg)	6-12 mg/kg PO q12h
Lorazepam (tablets: 0.5, 1.0, 2.0 mg; intravenous or intranasal solutions: 2 or 4 mg/mL)	0.02-0.1 mg/kg PO q8-12h
Memantine (tablets: 5, 10 mg; solution: 2 mg/mL)	0.3-0.5 mg/kg PO q12h to start; up to 1.0 mg/kg
Methylphenidate (tablets: 5, 10, 20 mg; extended release: 20 mg)	≥5 mg/**dog** for a small dog PO q12h; 20-40 mg/**dog** for a large dog PO q12h
Naloxone (injectable: 0.02, 0.4, 1 mg/mL)	11-22 µg/kg SC, IM, IV
Naltrexone (tablets: 50 mg)	2.2 mg/kg PO q12-24h
Nicergoline (tablets: 5, 10, 30 mg)*	0.25-0.5 mg/kg PO q24h
Nortriptyline (capsules: 10, 25, 50, 75 mg; solution 10 mg/5 mL)	1-2 mg/kg PO q12h
Oxazepam (tablets: 15 mg; capsules: 10, 15, 30 mg)	0.2-1.0 mg/kg PO q12-24h
Paroxetine (tablets: 10, 20, 30, 40 mg; suspension: 10 mg/5 mL)	0.5-1 mg/kg PO q24h × 6-8 wk to start
Pentazocine (injectable: 30 mg/mL) + naloxone (0.02, 0.4, 1 mg/mL)	50 mg pentazocine + 0.5 mg naloxone/**dog** PO q12h
Phenylpropanolamine (tablets: 50 mg)*	1.0-2.0 mg/kg PO q8h; up to 4.0 mg/kg PO 12h
Pindolol (tablets: 5, 10 mg)	0.125-0.25 mg/kg PO q12h (2.5-5 mg/medium-large **dog**) PO q12-24h to start
Propranolol (tablets: 10, 20, 40, 60, 80, 90 mg; capsules/extended release: 60, 80, 120, 160 mg)	0.2-1.0 mg/kg PO q8h; ≥5 mg/**dog** PO q8h for small dogs; 10-20 mg/**dog** PO q8h for large dogs; can give up to 3 mg/kg if give q12h
Propentofylline (tablets: 50, 100 mg)	3 mg/kg PO q8h; 2.5-5 mg/kg PO q12h
Protriptyline (tablets: 5, 10 mg)	0.2-0.5 mg/kg (5-10 mg/**dog**) PO q12-24h (narcolepsy)
Selegiline (Anipryl; Selgian) (tablets: 5, 10, 15, 30 mg; capsules: 5 mg)*	0.5-1.0 mg/kg PO q24h × 6-8 wk to start; some dogs may take up to 2 mg/kg PO q24h
Sertraline (tablets: 25, 50, 100 mg)	1.0 mg/kg PO q24h to start; can increase to 2+ mg/kg PO q24h if monitoring for serotonin-based side effects is excellent and ongoing
Trazodone (tablets: 50, 100 mg)	1.7-9.5 mg/kg PO q8-24h; start with 2-3 mg/kg PO q24h and increase if needed and effective
Triazolam (tablets: 0.125, 0.5 mg)	0.01-0.1 mg/kg PO as needed; as high as 0.125-1.0 mg/kg PO q12h

BZD, Benzodiazepine; IM, intramuscularly; IV, intravenously; PO, orally (per os); SC, subcutaneously.
*Veterinary label for some canine and feline conditions; label depends on country and species. Please note the range of the dosages listed for TCA, SSRIs, et cetera may be lower than commonly cited. Above these dosages, serotonin augmenting medications may cause increased arousal and agitation, usually associated with increased heart rate (which clients can monitor). Should these signs be seen with increasing dose, it is wise to decrease the dose to the level where the arousal does not do not occur, and if additional treatment effects are needed, consider possible polypharmacy.

Log for medication

Patient's name:

Date medication was provided or refilled	Name of medication	Dose	Amount provided	Number of refills	Weight of pet	Comments/notes about beneficial effects/undesirable or side effects with date
EXAMPLE: 1 July 2014	fluoxetine	1 20-mg cap every 24h	30 caps	3	48 pounds/21 kg	21 July 2014 HR=76 (was 70) bpm, eating well, seems to not react to as many triggers, sleeps more deeply

Fig. 10-6 Sample log to monitor behavioral medications taken by a specific patient (a client version of this is included with the client handout, "Protocol for Using Behavioral Medication Successfully").

Integration of all of these treatment modalities into modern veterinary medicine is a truly "holistic" approach that will benefit the veterinarian as much as it benefits patients and clients.

The answers to the questions that clients often ask, which were noted earlier in this chapter at the beginning of the medication section, are provided in Table 10-17 and in the client handout, "Protocol for Using Behavioral Medication Successfully." Medication dosages are listed in Table 10-18 for cats and Table 10-19 for dogs. A client log for monitoring medication use is shown in Figure 10-6. A client version of this log is included with the "Protocol for Using Behavioral Medication Successfully."

Supplemental Materials

References

[A].

Adamec RE. Behavioral and epileptic determinants of predatory behavior in the cat. Can J Neurol Sci 1975a;2:457-466.

Adamec RE. The neural basis of prolonged suppression of predatory attack. I. Naturally occurring physiological differences in the limbic systems of killer and non-killer cats. Aggr Behav 1975b;1:315-330.

Adamec RE. Hypothalamic and extrahypothalamic substrates of predatory attack: suppression and the influence of hunger. Brain Res 1976a;106:57-69.

Adamec RE. The interaction of hunger and preying in the domestic cat (Felis catus): an adaptive hierarchy? Behav Biol 1976b;18(2): 263-272.

Adamec RE. Does kindling model anything clinically relevant? Biol Psychiatry 1990a;27:249-279.

Adamec RE. Role of the amygdala and medial hypothalamus in spontaneous feline aggression and defense. Aggr Behav 1990b;16: 207-222.

Adamec RE, Stark-Adamec C, Livingston KE. The development of predatory aggression and defense in the domestic cat (Felis catus): III. Effects on development of hunger between 180 and 365 days of age. Behav Neural Biol 1980a;30:435-447.

Adamec RE, Stark-Adamec C, Livingston KE. The development of predatory aggression and defense in the domestic cat (Felis catus). II. The development of aggression and defense in the first 164 days of life. Behav Neural Biol 1980b;30:410-434.

Adamec RE, Stark-Adamec C, Livingston KE. The development of predatory aggression and defense in the domestic cat (Felis catus). I. Effects of early experience on adult patterns of aggression and defense. Behav Neural Biol 1980c;30:389-409.

Adamec RE, Stark-Adamec C, Livingston KE. The expression of an early developmentally emergent defensive bias in the adult domestic cat (Felis catus) in non-predatory situations. Appl Anim Ethol 1983;10:89-108.

Adler L, Adler H. Ontogeny of observational learning in the dog (Canis familiaris'). Devel Psychobiol 1977;10: 267-272.

Agrawal HC, Fox MW, Himwich WA. Neurochemical and behavioral effects of isolation-rearing in the dog. Life Sciences 1967;6: 71-78.

Amat J, Aleksejev RM, Paul E, Watkins LR, Maier SF. Behavioral control over shock blocks behavioral and neurochemical effects of later social defeat. Neuroscience 2010;165:1031-1038.

Amat M, Manteca X, Mariotti VM, Ruiz JL, Fatjó J. Aggressive behavior in the English cocker spaniel. J Vet Behav: Clin Appl Res 2009;4:111-117.

Anand BK, Brobeck JR. Hypothalamic control of food intake in rats and cats. Yale J Biol Med 1951; 24:123-140.

Anderson RS. Obesity in the dog and cat. In: The Veterinary Annual 11, Eds. Grunsell CSG, Hill FWG. John Wright & Sons, Bristol, 1973:182-186.

Anseeuw E, et al. for the NAVC PGI Behavioral Medicine Course. Handling cats humanely in the veterinary hospital. J Vet Behav: Clin Appl Res 2006;1:84-88.

Appleby D. Socialization and habituation. In: The Behaviour of Dogs and Cats, Ed. Fisher J. Stanley, Paul and Company, Ltd., Random House, London:24-40, 1993.

Appleby MC. The probability of linearity in hierarchies. Anim Behav 1983;31:600-608.

Apps PJ. Home ranges of feral cats on Dassen Island. J Mammol 1986;67:199-200.

Araujo JA, De Rivera C, Either JL, Lansberg GM, Denenberg S, Arnold S, Milgram NW. Anxitane® tablets reduce fear of human being in a laboratory model of anxiety-related behavior. J Vet Behav: Clin App Res 2010:5:268-275.

Araujo JA, Landsberg GM, Milgram NW, Miolo A. Improvement of short-term memory performance in aged beagles by a nutraceutical supplement containing phosphatidylserine, Ginko biloba, vitamin E, and pyroxidine. Can Vet J 2008;49:379-385.

Archer J. The behavioural biology of aggression. Cambridge University Press, New York, 1988.

Arhant C, Bubna-Littitz H, Bartels A, Futschik A, Troxler J. Behaviour of smaller and larger dogs: effects of training methods, inconsistency of owner behaviour and level of engagement in activities with the dog. Appl Anim Behav Sci 2010;123, 131–142.

Arnold LE, Kirilcuk V, Corson SA, Corson EO. Levoamphetamine and dextroamphetamine: differential effect on aggression in hyperkinesis in children and dogs. Am J Psychiatry 1973;130: 165-170.

Asa CS, Mech LD, Seal US, Plotka ED. The influence of social and endocrine factors on urine-marking by captive wolves. Horm Behav 1990;24:497-509.

Aust U, Range F, Steurer M, Huber L. Inferential reasoning by exclusion in pigeons, dogs, and humans. Anim Cogn 2008;11:587-597.

[B].

Bacon WD. Aversive conditioning in neonatal kittens. J Compar Physiol Psychol 1973;83:306-313.

Bacon WD, Stanley W. Effects of deprivation levels in puppies on performance maintained by a passive person reinforcer. J Compar Physiol Psychol 1963;56:783-785.

Bacon WD, Stanley W. Avoidance learning in neonatal dogs. J Compar Physiol Psychol 1970;71:448-452.

Baerends A, Stewart CN, Warren JM. Pattern of social interaction in cats (Felis domesticus). Behaviour 1957;11:56-66.

Baerends-van Roon JM, Baerends G. The Morphogenesis of the Behavior of the Domestic Cat: With a Special Emphasis on the Development of Prey-Catching. North Holland Press, Amsterdam, 1979.

Bagshaw CS, Ralston SL, Fisher H. Behavioral and physiological effect of orally administered tryptophan on horses subjected to acute isolation stress. Appl Anim Behav Sci 1994;40:1–12.

Bamberger M, Houpt KA. Signalment factors, comorbidity, and trends in behavior diagnosis in dogs: 1,644 cases (1991-2001). J Am Vet Med Assoc 2006;229:1591-1601.

Barratt ED. The use of anticonvulsants in aggression and violence. Psychopharmacol Bull 1993;29:75-81.

Barrett P, Bateson P. The development of play in cats. Behaviour 1978;66:106-120.

Barrette C. The "inheritance of dominance," or an aptitude to dominate. Anim Behav 1993;46:591-591.

Bateson P. The development of play in cats. Appl Anim Ethol 1978;4:290.

Bateson P, Mendel M, Feaver J. Play in the domestic cat is enhanced by the rationing of the mother during lactation. Anim Behav 1990;40:514-525.

Bateson P, Turner DC. Questions about cats. In: The Domestic Cat:The Biology of Its Behaviour. Eds. Turner DC, Bateson P. Cambridge University Press, Cambridge, 1988:193-201.

Bateson P, Young M. Separation from the mother and the development of play in cats. Anim Behav 1981;29:173-180.

Bateson P. How do sensitive periods arise and what are they for? Anim Behav 1979;27:470-486.

Battaglia C. Periods of early development and the effects of stimulation and social experiences in the canine. J Vet Behav: Clin Appl Res 2009;4:203-210.

Bauer EB, Smuts BB. Cooperation and competition during dyadic play in domestic dogs. Canis familiaris. Anim. Behav. 2007;73:489–499.

Baumgartner A, Pinna G, Hiedra L, Gaio U, Hessenius C, Campos-Barros A, Eravci M, Prengel H, Thoma R, Meinhold H. Effects of lithium and carbamazepine on thyroid hormone metabolism in rat brain. Neuropsychopharm 1997;16:25-41.

Beach FA, Gilmore RW. Responses of male dogs to urine from females in heat. J Mammol 30:391-392, 1949.

Bear MF, Connors BW, Pradiso MA. Neuroscience: Exploring the Brain, 2nd edition, Lippincott Williams and Wilkins, Baltimore, 2001:269.

Beata C, Beaumont-Graff E, Coll V, Cordel J, Marion M, Massal N, Marlois N, Tauzin J. Effect of alpha-casozepine (Zylkene) on anxiety in cats. J Vet Behav: Clin Appl Res 2007b:2:40-46.

Beata C, Beaumont-Graff E, Diaz C, Marion M, Massal M, Marlois N, Muller G, Lefranc C. Effects of alpha-casozepine (Zylkene) versus selegiline hydrochloride (Selgian, Anipryl) on anxiety disorders in dogs. J Vet Behav: Clin Appl Res 2007a;2:175-183.

Beato M, Chávez S, Truss M. Transcriptional regulation by steroid hormones. Steroids 1996;61:240-251.

Beaver BV. Feline Behavior: A Guide for Veterinarians. WB Saunders, Philadelphia, 1980, 1992.

Beaver BV. Problems and values associated with dominance. Vet Med Sm Anim Clin 1981:76:1129-1131.

Beaver BV. Hormone therapy for animals with behavioral problems. Vet Med Sm Anim Clin 1982;77:337-338.

Beaver BV. Canine aggression. Appl Anim Behav Sci 1993;37:81–82.

Beaver BV, Terry ML, LaSagna CL. Effectiveness of products in eliminating cat urine odors from carpet. J Am Vet Med Assoc 1989;194:1589-1591.

Beck AM. The Ecology of Stray Dogs: a Study of Free-Ranging Urban Animals. York Press, Baltimore, MD, 1973.

Beck AT. Cognitive Therapy and the Emotional Disorders. International Universities Press, Madison, CT, 1975.

Becker RF, King JE, Markee JE. Studies on olfactory discrimination in dogs: II. Discriminatory behavior in a free environment. J Comp Physiol Psychol 1962:55;773–780.

Beerda B, Schilder MBH, van Hooff JARAM, de Vries HW. Manifestations of chronic and acute stress in dogs. Appl Anim Behav Sci 1997;52:307–319.

Beerda B, Schilder MHB, Van Hooff JARAM, de Vries HW, Mol J. 1998. Behavioural, saliva cortisol and heart rate responses to different types of stimuli in dogs. Appl Anim Behav Sci 1998;58:365–381.

Beerda B, Schilder MHB, Van Hooff J, de Vries HW, Mol J. 2000. Behavioural and hormonal indicators of enduring environmental stress in dogs. J. Appl. Anim.Welf. Sci. 2000;9:49–62.

Bekoff M. The development of social interaction, play, and metacommunication in mammals: an ethological perspective. Q Rev Biol 1972;47:412-434.

Bekoff M. Social play in coyotes, wolves and dogs. J Biosci 1974;24:225–230.

Bekoff M. Social communication in canids: evidence for the evolution of a stereotyped mammalian display. Science 1977;197:1097-1099.

Bekoff M. Ground scratching by male domestic dogs: a composite signal. J Mammol 1979a;60:847-848.

Bekoff M. Scent-marking by free-ranging domestic dogs: olfactory and visual components. Biol Behav 1979b;4:123-139.

Belkin M, Yinon U, Rose L, Reisert I. Effect of visual environment on refractive error of cats. Doc Ophthalmol 1977;42:433-437.

Bell C, Abrams J, Nutt D. Tryptophan depletion and its implications for psychiatry. Br J Psychiatry 2011;178:399-405.

Benbernou N, Tacher S, Robin S, Rakotomanga M, Senger F, Galibert F. Functional analysis of a subset of canine olfactory receptor genes. J Hered 2007;98:500-505.

Bernstein P, Strack M. Home ranges, favored spots, time-sharing patterns and tail usage by fourteen cats in the home. ABCN 1993;10(3):1-3.

Bernstein PL, Strack M. A game of cat and house: spatial patterns and behavior of 14 domestic cats (Felis catus) in the home. Anthrozoös 1996;9(1):25-39.

Bernston GG, Beattie MS, Walker JM. Effects of nicotinic and muscarine compounds on biting attacks in cats. Pharmacol Biochem Behav 1976b;5:235-239.

Bernston GG, Hughes HC, Beattie MS. A comparison of hypothalamically induced biting attack with natural predatory behavior in the cat. J Compar Physiol Psychol 1976a;90:167-178.

Bernston GG, Leibowitz SF. Biting attack in cats: evidence for central muscarinic medication. Brain Res 1973;52:366-370.

Bernston GG, Micco DJ. Organization of brainstem behavioral systems. Brain Res Bull 1976;1:471-483.

Bernstein IS. Dominance: the baby and the bathwater. Behav Brain Sci 1981;4:419-457.

Berry SJ, Ewing LL, Coffey DS, Strandberg JD. Effect of age, castration, and testosterone replacement on the development and restoration of canine benign prostatic hyperplasia. The Prostate 1986;9:295-302.

Biben M. Predation and predatory play behavior of domestic cats. Anim Behav 1979;27:81-94.

Bielsky IF, Young LJ. Oxytocin, vasopressin, and social recognition in mammals. Peptides 2004; 25:1565-1574.

Bienvenido M-N, Belmaker M, Bar-Yosef O. The large carnivores from 'Ubeidiya (early Pleistocene, Israel): biocronological and biogeographical implications. J Human Evol 2009;56:514-524.

Bisaz R, Sandi C. The role of NCAM in auditory fear conditioning and its modulation by stress: a focus on the amygdala. Genes Brains Behav 2010; 9:353-364.

Blackwell EJ, Twells C, Seawright A, Casey R.A.. The relationship between training methods and the occurrence of behavior problems, as reported by owners, in a population of domestic dogs. J Vet Behav: Clin Appl Res 2008;3:207-217.

Bolhuis JJ, Fitzgerald RE, Dijk DJ, Koolhaas JM. The corticomedial amygdale and learning in an agonistic istuation in the rat. Phys Behav 1984;32:575-579.

Borchelt PL. Aggressive behavior of dogs kept as companion animals: classification and influence of sex, reproductive status and breed. Appl Anim Ethol 1983;10:45–61.

Borchelt PL. Development of behaviour in the dog during maturity. In: Nutrition and Behavior of Dogs and Cats, Ed. Anderson RS. Pergamon Press, New York,1984:189-197.

Born J, Lange T, Kern W, McGregor GP, Bickel U, Fehm HL. Sniffing neuropeptides: A transnasal approach to the human brain. Nat Neurosci 2002;5:514 –516.

Bosch G, Beerda B, Beynen AC, van der Borg J, van der Poel FB, Hendriks WH. Dietary tryptophan supplementation in privately owned mildly anxious dogs. Appl Anim Behav Sci 2009;121:197–205.

Bosch G, Beerda B, Hendriks WH, van der Poel AFB, Verstegen MWA. Impact of nutrition on canine behaviour: current status and possible mechanisms. Nutr Res Rev 2007;20:180-194.

Boyd R, Silk JB. A method for assessing cardinal dominance ranks. Anim Behav 1983;31:45-58.

Boyko AR, Boyko RH, Boyko CM, Parker HG, Castelhano M, Corey L, Degendardt JD, Auton A, Hedimbi M, Kityou R, Ostrander EA, Schoenebeck J, Todhunter RJ, Jones P, Bustamante CD. Complex population structure in African village dogs and its implication for inferring dog domestication history. Proc Natl Acad Sci USA 2009;106:13903–13908.

Bradshaw J, Cameron-Beaumont C. The signaling repertoire of the domestic cat and its undomesticated relatives. In: The Domestic Cat: The Biology of Its Behaviour, 2nd Edition. Eds. Turner DC, Bateson P. Cambridge University Press, Cambridge, UK, 2000:67-94.

Bradshaw JWS. The Behaviour of the Domestic Cat. CAB International, Wallingford, England, 1992.

Bradshaw JWS, Brown SL. Behavioral adaptations of dogs to domestication. In: Pets, Benefits and Practice, Ed. Berger IH. British Veterinary Association Publications, London UK, 1990:18-24.

Bradshaw JWS, Natynczuk S, Macdonald DW. Potential for applications of anal sac volatiles in domestic dogs. In: Chemical Signals in Vertebrates, Eds. Macdonald DW, Natynczuk SE. Oxford University Press, Oxford, UK, 1990: 640-644.

Bradshaw JWS, Nott HMR. Social and communication behavior of companion dogs. In: The Domestic Dog: The Biology of Its Behavior, Ed. Serpell JA. Cambridge University Press, Cambridge, UK, 1992: 115-130.

Brammeier S et al. for the NAVC PGI Advanced Behavior Course. Good trainers: how to identify one and why this is important to your practice of veterinary medicine. J Vet Behav: Clin Appl Res 2006;1:47-52.

Branchey L, Branchey M, Shaw S & Lieber CS. Depression, suicide, and aggression in alcoholics and their relationship to plasma amino acids. Psychiatry Res 1984;12:219–226.

Breitschwerdt EB. Feline bartonellosis and cat scratch disease. Vet Immun Immunopath 2008;123:167-171.

Broadhurst CL, Cunnane SC, Crawford M. Rift Valley lake fish and shellfish provided brain-specific nutrition for early Homo. Br J Nutr 1998;79:3-21.

Brodey RS, Goldschmidt MA, Rozel JR. Canine mammary gland neoplasm. J Am Anim Hosp Assoc 1983;19:61-90.

Brown AM, Ransom BR. Astrocyte glycogen and brain energy metabolism. Glia 2007;55:1263-1271.

Brown KA, Buchwald JS, Johnson JR, Mikolich DJ. Vocalization in the cat and kitten. Devel Psychobiol 1978;11:559-570.

Brown TM, Skop BP, Mareth TR. Pathophysiology and management of the serotonin syndrome. Annals Pharmcother 1996;30:527–33.

Brunner HG, Nelen M, Breakefield XO, Ropers HH, van Oost BA. Abnormal behavior associated with a point mutation in the structural gene for monoamine oxidase A. Science 1993;262:578-580.

Bryan JN, Keeler MR, Henry CJ, Bryan ME, Hahn AW and Caldwell CW. A population study of neutering status as a risk factor for canine prostate cancer. The Prostate 2007;67:1174-1181.

Buck L, Axel R. A novel multigene family may encode odorant receptors: a molecular basis for odor recognition. Cell 2004;65:175–187.

Buck LB. The molecular architecture of odor and pheromone sensing in mammals. Cell 2000;100:611—618.

Buck LB. Olfactory receptors and odor coding in mammals. Nutr Rev 2004;62s3:S184-188.

Burgess PR, Perl ER. Cutaneous mechanoreceptors and noci-ceptors. In: Handbook of Sensory Physiology. Vol. II: Somatosensory Systems, Ed. Iggo A. Springer-Verlag, New York, NY, 1973: 29-78.

Burt WH. Territoriality and home range concepts as applied to mammals. J Mammol 1943;24:346-352.

Bush WW, Barr CS, Stecker MM, Overall KL, Bernier NM, Darrin EW, Morrison AR. Diagnosis of rapid eye movement sleep disorder with electroencephalography and treatment with tricyclic antidepressants in a dog. J Am Anim Hosp Assoc 2004;40:495-500.

[C].

Cadieu E, Neff NW, Quignon P, Walsh K, Chase K, Parker HG, VonHoldt BM, Rhue A, Boyko A, Byers A, Wong A, Mosher DS, Elkahloun AG, Spady TC, André C, Lark KG, Cargill M, Bustamante CD, Wayne RK, Ostrander EA. Coat Variation in the Domestic Dog Is Governed by Variants in Three Genes. Science 2009;326:150-153.

Cafazzo S, Natoli E. The social function of tail up in the domestic cat (Felis silvestris catus). Behav Proc 2009;80:60-66.

Cairns RB, Hood KE, Midlam J. On fighting in mice: is there a sensitive period for isolation effects? Anim Behav 1985;33:166-180.

Çakiroglu D. Meral Y, Sancak AA, Cifti G. Relationship between the serum concentrations of serotonin and lipids and aggression in dogs. Vet Rec 2007;161:59–61.

Cambridge AJ, Tobias KM, Newberry RC, Sarkar DK. Subjective and objective measurements of postoperative pain in cats. J Am Vet Med Assoc 2000;217:685-690.

Camps T, Amat M, Mariotti VM, Le Brech S, Manteca X. Pain-related aggression in dogs: 12 clinical cases. J Vet Behav: Clin Appl Res 2012;7:99-102.

Cannas S, Frank D, Minero M, Godbout M, Palestrini C. Puppy behavior when left home alone: changes during the first few months after adoption. J Vet Behav: Clin Appl Res 2010;5:94-100.

Carlsson ML. On the role of cortical glutamate in obsessivecompulsive disorder and attention-deficit hyperactivity disorder, two phenomenologically antithetical conditions. Acta Psychiatr Scand 2000;102:401–413

Carlstead K, Brown JL, Monfort SL, Killens R, Wildt DE. Urinary monitoring of adrenal responses to psychological stressors in domestic and nondomestic felids. Zoo Biol 1992;11:165-176.

Carlstead K, Brown JL, Strawn W. Behavioral and physiological correlates of stress in laboratory cats. Appl Anim Behav Sci 1993;38:143-158.

Caro TM. Relations between kitten behavior and adult predation. ZeitTierpsychol 1979;51:158-168.

Caro TM. The effects of experience on the predatory patterns of cats. Behav Neural Biol 1980a;29:1-28.

Caro TM. Effects of the mother, object play, and adult experience on predation in cats. Behav Neural Biol 1980b;29:29-51.

Caro TM. Predatory behavior and social play in kittens. Behaviour 1981a;76:1-24.

Caro TM. Sex differences in the termination of social play in cats. Anim Behav 1981b;29:271-279.

Caro TM. Predatory behavior in domestic cat mothers. Behaviour 1980c;74:128-148.

Carola V, Gross C. BDNF moderates early environmental risk factors for anxiety in mouse. Genes Brains Behav 2010;9:379-389.

Carter AP, Chen C, Schwartz PM, Segal RA. Brain-derived neurotrophic factor modulates cerebellar plasticity and synaptic ultrastructure. J Neurosci 2002;22:1316-1327.

Carter GC, Scott-Moncrieff JC, Luescher AU, Moore G. Serum total thyroxine and thyroid stimulating hormone concentrations in dogs with behavior problems. J Vet Behav: Clin Appl Res 2009;4: 230–236.

Cases O, Seif I, Grimsby J, Gaspar P, Chen K, Pournin S, Müller U, Aguet M, Babinet C, Shih J, de Maeyer E. Aggressive behavior and altered amounts of brain serotonin and norepinephrine in mice lacking MAOA. Science 1005;268:1763-1766.

Casey BJ, Castellanos FX, Giedd JN, Marsh WL, Hamburger SD, Schubert AB, Vauss YC, Vaituzis AC, Dickstein DP, Sarfatti SE, Rapoport JL: Implication of right frontostriatal circuitry in response inhibition and attention-deficit/hyperactivity disorder. J Am Acad Child Adolesc Psychiatry 1997; 36:374–383.

Castonguay TW. Dietary dilution and intake in the cat. Physiol Behav 1981;27:547-549.

Castroviejo-Fisher S, Skoglund P, Valadex R, Vilà C, Leonard J. Vanishing native American dog lineages. BMC Evol Biol 2011;11:73. doi:10.1186/1471-2148-11-73.

Center SA, Elston TH, Rowland PH, Rosen DK, Reitz BL, Rodan I, House J, Bank S, Lynch LR, Dring LA, Levy JK. Fulminant hepatic association associated with oral administration of diazepam in 11 cats. J Am Vet Med Assoc 1996;209:68-625.

Chamberlain B, Ervin FR, Pihl RO, Young SN. The effect of raising or lowering tryptophan levels on aggression in vervet monkeys. Pharmacol Biochem Behav 1987;28:503–510.

Chamberlain SR, Blackwell AD, Fineberg NA, Robbins TW, Sahakian BJ. The neuropsychology of obsessive compulsive disorder: the importance of failures in cognitive and behavioural inhibition as candidate endophenotypic markers. Neurosci Biobehav Rev 2005;29:399–419.

Chapman BL, Voith VL. Behavioral problems in old dogs: 26 cases (1984-1987). J Am Vet Med Assoc 1990;196:944-946.

Chesler P. Maternal influence in learning by observation in kittens. Science 1969;166:901-902.

Christie L-A, Opii WO, Head E, Araujo JA, De Rivera C, Milgram NW, Cotman CW. Effects of acetyl-L-carnitine and lipoic acid supplementation on cognition in aged beagles. J Vet Behav: Clin Appl Res 2010;5:160.

Ciribassi J, Luescher A, Pasloske KS, Robertson-Plouch C, Zimmerman A, Kaloostian-Whittymore L. Comparative bioavailability of fluoxetine after transdermal and oral administration to healthy cats. Am J Vet Res 2003;64:994–998.

Clancy EA, Moore AS, Bertone ER. Evaluation of cat and owner characteristics and their relationships to outdoor access of owned cats. J Am Vet Med Assoc 2003;222:1541-1545.

Clark GI, Boyer WN. The effects of dog obedience training and behavioral counselling upon the human-canine relationship. Appl Anim Behav Sci 1993;37:147-159.

Clough G. Environmental effects on animals used in biomedical research. Biol Rev 1982;57:487-523.

Cloutier S, Newberry RC, Cambridge AJ, Tobias KM. Behavioural signs of postoperative pain in cats following onychectomy or tenectomy surgery. Appl Anim Behav Sci 2005;92:325-335.

Cohen JA, Fox MW. Vocalizations in wild canids and possible effects of vocalization. Behav Proc 1976;1:77-92.

Colgan P. Animal Motivation, Chapman and Hall, London. 1989.

Collard RR. Fear of strangers and play behavior in kittens with varied social experience. Child Develop 1967;38:877-891.

Collier S. Breed specific legislation and the pit bull terrier: Are the laws justified? J Vet Behav: Clin Appl Res 2006;1:17–22.

Collins S. Tail Talk: Understanding the Secret Language of Dogs. Chronicle Books, San Francisco, CA, 2007.

Compaan JC, van Wattum G, de Ruiter AJH, van Oortmerssen GA, Koolhaas JM, Bohus B. Genetic differences in female house mice in aggressive response to sex steroid hormone treatment. Physiol Behav 1993;54:899-902.

Conway CM, Christiansen MH. Sequential learning in non-human primates. Trends Cog Sci 2001;12:539-546.

Cooley DM, Beranek BC, Schlittler DL, Glickman NW, Glickman LT, Waters DJ. Endogenous gonadal hormone exposure and bone sarcoma risk. Cancer Epidemiol Biomarkers Prev 2002; 1434-1440.

Cooper-Kazaz R, Apter JT, Cohen R, Karagichev L, Muhammed-Moussa S, Grupper D, Drori T, Newman ME, Sackelm HA, Glaser B, Lerer B. Combined treatment with sertraline and liothyronine in major depression. Arch Gen Psychiatry 2007;64:679–688.

Corbett LK. Feeding ecology and social organization of wild cats (Felis silvestris) and domestic cats (Felis catus) in Scotland. PhD Thesis, University of Aberdeen, Scotland,1979. Cited in: The Domestic Cat: The Biology of its Behaviour, Eds. Turner DC, Bateson P. Cambridge University Press, Cambridge, 1988: 25.

Cornelissen JMR, Hopster H. Dog bites in The Netherlands: a study of victims, injuries, circumstances and aggressors to support evaluation of breed specific legislation. Vet J 2010;186:292-298.

Corson SA, Corson EO. Constitutional differences in physiological adaptation to stress and distress. In: Psychopathology of Human Adaptation, Ed. Serban G. Plenum Press, New York, 1976:77-94.

Corson SA, Corson EO, Decker RE, Ginsburg BE, Trattner A, Connor RL, Lucas LA, Panksepp J, Scott JP. Interaction of genetics and separation in canine hyperkinesis and in a differential response to amphetamines. Pav J Biol Sci 1980;15:5-11.

Corson SA, Corson EO, Kirilcuk V. Tranquilizing effects of D-amphetamine on hyperkinetic untrainable dogs. Fed Proc 1971;30:206.

Cotman CW, Berchtold NC, Christie L-A. Exercise builds brain health: key roles of growth factor cascades and inflammation. Trends Neurosci 2007;30:464-472.

Cotman CW, Head E, Muggenburg BA, Zicker S, Milgram NW. 2002. Brain aging in the canine: a diet enriched in antioxidants reduces cognitive dysfunction. Neurobiol Aging 23:809-818.

Cottam N, Dodman NH. Comparison of the effectiveness of a purported anti-static cape (the Storm Defender®) vs. a placebo cape in the treatment of canine thunderstorm phobia as assessed by owners' reports. Appl Anim Behav Sci 2009;119:78-84.

Coyle JT, Puttfarcken P. Oxidative stress, glutamate, and neurodegenerative disorders. Science 1993;262:689-695.

Cracknell NR, Mills DS. A double-blind placebo-controlled study into the efficacy of a homeopathic remedy for fear of firework noises in the dog (Canis familiaris). Vet J 2008;177:80–88.

Cracknell NR, Mills DS. An evaluation of owner expectation on apparent treatment effect in a blinded comparison of 2 homeopathic remedies for firework noise sensitivity in dogs. J Vet Bheav: Clin Appl Res 2011;6:21-30.

Cramer PE, Cirrito JR, Wesson DW, Lee CYD, Karlo JC, Zinn AE, Casali BT, Restivo JL, Goebel WD, James MJ, Brunden KR, Wilson DA, Landreth GE. ApoE-directed therapeutics rapidly clear β-amyloid and reverse deficits in AD mouse models. Science 2012;335:1503-1506.

Crowell-Davis SL, Seibert LM, Sung W, Parthasarathy V, Curtis TM. Use of clomipramine, alprazolam, and behavior modification for treatment of storm phobia in dogs. J Am Vet Med Assoc 2003; 222:744–748.

Cummings BJ, Satou T, Head E, Milgram NW, Cole GM, Savage MJ, Podlisny MB, Selkoe DH, Siman R, Greenberg BD, Cotman CW. Diffuse plaques contain C-terminal Aβ$_{42}$ and not Aβ$_{40}$: Evidence from cats and dogs. Neurobiol Aging 1996;17:653-659.

Cupp CJ, Jean-Philippe C, Kerr WW, Patil AR, Perez-Camargo G. Effect of nutritional interventions on longevity of senior cats. Int J Appl Res Vet Med 2006;4:34-50.

Curtis TC. Human-directed aggression in the cat. Vet Clin NA: Sm Anim Pract 2008;38:1131-1143.

Curtis TM, Knowles RJ, Crowell-Davis SL. Influence of familiarity and relatedness on proximity and allogrooming in domestic cats (Felis catus). Am J Vet Res 2003;64:1151-1154.

[D].

Dards JL. The behaviour of dockyard cats: interactions of adult males. Appl Anim Ethol 1983;10:133-153.

Davidson MG, Baty KT. Anaphylaxis associated with intravenous sodium fluorescein administration in a cat. Prog Vet Comp Ophthalmol 1991;1:127–128.

Davis M. Neurobiology of fear responses: the role of the amygdala. J Neuropsychiatry Clin 1997;9:382-402.

Davis M. Are different parts of the extended amygdala involved in fear and anxiety? Biol Psychiatry 1998;44:1239-1247.

Davis RG. Olfactory psychophysical parameters in man, rat, dog, and pigeon. J Comp Physiol Psychol 1973;85:221-232.

Deag JM, Manning A, Lawrence CE. Factors influencing the mother-kitten relationship. In: The Domestic Cat: The Biology of Its Behavior, Eds. Turner DC, Bateson P. Cambridge University Press, Cambridge, UK: 23-39, 1988.

De Bellis MD, Keshavan MS. Sex differences in brain maturation in maltreatment-related pediatric posttraumatic stress. Neurosci Biobehav Rev 2003;27:103-117.

De Bellis MD, Keshavan MS, Beers SR, Hall J, Fustaci K, Masalehdan A, Noll J, Boring AM. Sex differences in brain maturation during childhood and adolescence. Cerebral Cortex 2001;11:552-557.

de Boer JN. The age of olfactory cues functioning in chemocommunication among male domestic cats. Behav Proc 1977;2:209-225.

De Keuster T, Lamoureux J, Kahn A. Epidemiology of dog bites: a Belgian experience of canine behaviour and public health concerns. Vet J 2006;172, 482–487.

De Keuster T, Moons C, De Cock I. Dog bite prevention – how a Blue Dog can help. Eur J Comp Anim Pract 2005:15:137–139.

de Meester R, De Bacquer D, Vermeire S, Peremans K, Coopman F, Planta D, Audenaert K. A preliminary study on the use of the socially acceptable behavior test as a test for shyness/confidence in the temperament of dogs. J Vet Behav: Clin Appl Res 2008;3: 161-170.

de Meester RH, Pluijmakers J, Vermeire S, Laevens H. The use of the socially acceptable behavior test in the study of temperament of dogs. J. Vet. Behav.: Clin. App.l Res. 2011;6:211-224.

DeNapoli JS, Dodman NH, Shuster L, Rand WM, Gross KL. Effect of dietary protein content and tryptophan supplementation on dominance aggression, territorial aggression, and hyperactivity in dogs. J Am Vet Med Assoc 2000;217:504-508.

Denenberg S, Landsberg GM. Effects of dog-appeasing pheromones on anxiety and fear in puppies during training and on long-term socialization. J Am Vet Med Assoc 2008;233:1874–1882.

Dennis JC, Allgier JG, Desouza LS, Eward WC, Morrison EE. Immunohistochemistry of the canine vomeronasal organ. J Anat 2003; 202:515-524.

De Porter TL, Landsberg GM, Araujo JA, Eithier JL, Bledso DL. Haromonease Chewable Tablets reduces noise-induced fear and anxiety in a laboratory canine thunderstorm situation: a blinded and placebo controlled study. J Vet Behav: Clin Appl Res 2012;7: 225-232.

De Quervain DJF, Aerni A, Schelling G, Roozendaal B. Glucocorticoids and the regulation of memory in health and disease. Front Neuroendocrinol 2009;30:358-370.

Derr M. How the Dog Became the Dog. The Overlook Press, NY, 2012.

Dewey CW. A Practical Guide to Canine and Feline Neurology. Google Books, www.books.google.com, 2008.

Dienel GA, Cruz NF. Astrocyte activation in working brain: energy supplied by minor substrates. Neurochem Intl 2006;48: 586-595.

Diskin SJ, Hou C, Glessner JT, Attiyeh EF, Laudenslager M, Bosse K, Cole K, Mossé YP, Wood A, Lynch JE, Pecor K, Diamond M, Winter C, Wang K, Kim C, Geiger EA, McGrady PW, Blakemore AIF, London WB, Shaikh TH, Bradfield J, Grant FA, Li H, Devoto M, Rappaport ER, Hakonarson H, Maris MM. Copy number variation at 1q21.1 associated with neuroblastoma. Nature 2009;459:987-991.

Dodds WJ. How to test, interpret thyroid function. Veterinary Practice News April 2011: 52.

Dodman NH, Aronson L, Cottam N, Dodds JW. The effect of thyroid replacement in dogs with suboptimal thyroid function on owner-directed aggression: A randomized, double-blind, placebo-controlled clinical trial. J Vet Behav: Clin Appl Res 2013;8: http://dx.doi.org/10.1016/j.jveb.2012.12.059.

Dodman NH, Karlsson EK, Moon-Fanelli A, Galdzicka M, Perloski M, Shustr L., Lindblad-Toh K, Ginns EI. A canine chromosome 7 locus confers compulsive disorder susceptibility. Molec Psychiatry 2010;15:8-10.

Dodman NH, Knowles KE, Shuster L., Moon-Fanelli AA, Tidwell AS, Keen CL. Behavioral changes associated with suspected complex partial seizures in bull terriers. J Am Vet Med Assoc 1996;208: 688-691.

Dodman NH, Reisner IR, Shuster L, Rand WM, Luescher UA, Robinson I, Houpt KA. Effect of dietary protein content on behavior in dogs. J AmVet Med Assoc 1996;208:376-379.

Dodman NH, Shuster L, Court MH. Use of a narcotic antagonist in the treatment of a stereotypic behavior pattern (crib-biting) in the horse. Am J Vet Res 1987;48:311-319.

Dodman NH, Shuster L, Court MH, White SD. Behavioral effects of narcotic antagonists. J Assoc Vet Anesthetists 1988a;15:56-64.

Dodman NH, Shuster L, Court MH. Use of a narcotic antagonist (nalmefene) to suppress self-mutilative behavior in a stallion. JAVMA 1988b;192:1585-1586.

Döring D, Roscher A, Scheipl F, Kuchenhoff H, Erhard MH. Fear-related behavior of dogs in veterinary practice. Vet J 2009; 182:38-43.

Dorries KM, Adkins-Regan E, Halpern BP. Sensitivity and behavioral responses to the pheromone androstenone are not mediated by the vomeronasal organ in domestic pigs. Brain Behav Evol 1997;49:53–62.

Doty RL, Dunbar I. Attraction of beagles to conspecific urine, vaginal, and anal sac secretion odors. Physiol Behav 1974;12:825-833.

Driscoll CA, Clutton-Brock J, Kitchener AC, O'Brien SJ. The taming of the cat. Sci Am 2009;June:68-75.

Drobatz KJ, Smith G. Evaluation of risk factors for bite bounds inflicted on caregivers by dogs and cats in a veterinary teaching hospital. J Am Vet Med Assoc 2003;223:312-316.

Drobbie AK. Patient monitoring equipment: problems of interference and electrical safety. Proc Roy Soc Med 197;66:39-40.

Duffy DL, Hsu Y, Serpell JA. Breed differences in canine aggression. Appl Anim Behav Sci 2008;114, 441-460.

Dulac C. Sensory coding of pheromone signals in mammals. Curr Opionion Neurobiol 2000;10:511-518.

Dulac C, Axel R. A novel family of genes encoding putative pheromone receptors in mammals. Cell 1995;83:195-206.

Duman R. Role of neurotrophic factors in the etiology and treatment of mood disorders. Neuromolecular Med 2004; 5:11–25.

Duman RS. Novel therapeutic approaches beyond the serotonin receptor. Biol Psychiatry 1998;44:324-335.

Duman RS, Heininger GR, Nestler EJ. A molecular and cellular theory of depression. Arch Gen Psychiatry 1997;54:597-606.

Duman RS, Monteggia LM. 2006. A neurotrophic model for stress-related mood disorders. Biol. Psychiatry 2006;59, 1116–1127.

Dumas C. Object permanence in cats (Felis catus): an ecological approach to the study of invisible displacements. J Comp Psych 1992;106:404-410.

Dunbar I. Olfactory preferences in dogs: the response of male and female beagles to conspecific odors. Behav Biol 1977;20:471-481.

Dunbar I. Olfactory preferences in dogs: the response of male and female beagles to conspecific urine. Biol Behaviour, 1978;3: 273-286.

Dunbar I, Buehler M. A masking effect of urine from male dogs. Appl Anim Ethology 1980;6:297-301.

Dunbar I, Carmichael M. The response of male dogs to urine from other males. Behav Neural Biol 1981;31: 465-470.

Dunn AJ. Changes in plasma and brain tryptophan and brain serotonin and 5-hydroxyindoleacetic acid after footshock stress. Life Sci 1988;42:1847–1853.

Dysart LMA, Coe JB, Adam CL. Analysis of solicitation of client concerns in companion animal practice. J Am Vet Med Assoc 2011;238:1609-1615.

[E].

Ebert D, Haller RD, Walton ME. Energy contribution of octanoate to intact rat brain metabolism measured by 13C nuclear magnetic resonance spectroscopy. J Neurosci 2003;23:5928-5935.

Egenvall A, Bonnett BN, Öhagen P, Olson P, Hedhammar Å, von Euler H. Incidence and survival after mammary tumors in a poplation of over 80,000 insured female dogs in Sweden from 1995 to 2002. Prev Vet Med 2005;69:109-127.

Egenvall A, Hagman R, Bonnett BN, Hedhammar Å, Olson P, Lagerstedt A-S. Breed risk of pyometra in insured dogs in Sweden. J Vet Intern Med 2001;15:530-538.

Ehrlich I, Humeau Y, Grenier F, Ciocchi S, Herry C, Luthi A. Amygdala inhibitory circuits and the control of fear memory. Neuron 2009;62:757–771.

Eichelmann B. Neurochemical studies of aggression in animals. Psychopharmacol Bull 1977a;13:17-19.

Eichelmann B. Catecholamines and aggressive behavior. In: Neuroregulators and Psychiatric Disorders, Ed. Usdin E. Oxford University Press, New York, NY, 1977b: 146-150.

Eigenmann JE, Eigenmann RY. Influence of medroxyprogesterone acetate (Provera) on plasma growth hormone levels and on carbohydrate metabolism, part I. Acta Endocrinol (Copenh) 98:599-602, 1981a.

Eigenmann JE, Eigenmann RY. Influence of medroxyprogesterone acetate (Provera) on plasma growth hormone levels and on carbohydrate metabolism, part II. Acta Endocrinol (Copenh) 98:602-608, 1981b.

Elliot O, Scott JP. The development of emotional distress reactions to separation in puppies. J Genetic Psychol 1961;99:3-22.

Ewer RF. Further observations on suckling behaviour in kittens, together with some general considerations of the interrelations of innate and acquired responses. Behaviour 1961;18:247-260.

Ewer RF. The Carnivores. Ithaca, New York. Cornell University Press, 1973.

[F].

Fagen R. Animal Play Behaviour. Oxford University Press, Oxford, UK, 1981.

Fahey GC, Barry KA, Swanson KS. Age-related changes in nutrient utilization by companion animals. Ann Rev Nutr 2008;28: 425-445.

Fahnestock M, Marchese M, Head E, Pop V, Milgram NW, Cotmann CW. BDNF increases with behavioural enrichment and an antioxidant diet in the aged dog. Neurobiol Aging 2012;33:546-554.

Falk SA, Woods NF. Hospital noise – levels and potential health hazards. NEJM 1973;289: 774-781.

Faragó T, Pongrácz P, Range F, Virányi Z, Miklósi Á. 'The bone is mine': affective and referential aspects of dog growls. Animal Behav 2010;79: 917-925.

Farhoody P, Zink MC. Bheavioral and physical effects of spaying and neutering domestic dogs (Canis familiaris). Unpublished summary of a Masters thesis, Hunter College, New York, NY, 2010.

Fatjó J, Amat M, Mariotti VM, Ruiz de la Torre JL. Analysis of 1040 cases of canine aggression in a referral practice in Spain. Journal of Veterinary Behavior 2007; 2:158-165.

Fatjó J, Stub C, Manteca X. Four cases of aggression and hypothyroidism in dogs. Vet Rec 2002;151:547–548.

Fay RR. Hearing in Vertebrates: A Psychophysics Data Book, Hill-Fay Associates, Winnetka, IL, 1988.

Feaver J, Mendl M, Bateson P. A method for rating the individual distinctiveness of domestic cats. Anim Behav 1986;34:1016-1025.

Feddersen-Petersen D. Some interactive aspects between dogs and their owners: are there reciprocal influences between both inter- and intraspecific communication. Appl Anim Behav Sci 1994;40:78.

Feldman HN. Maternal care and differences in the use of nests in the domestic cat. Anim Behav 1993;45:13-23, 1993.

Feldman HN. Methods of scent marking in the domestic cat. Can J Zool 1994;72:1093-1099.

Felthous AR, Kellert SR. Childhood cruelty to animals and later aggression against people: a review. Am J Psychol 1987;144: 710–717.

Ferdowsian HR, Durham DL, Johnson CM, Brüne M, Kimwlel C, Kranendonk G, Otali E, Akugizibwe T, Mulcahy JB, Ajarova L. Signs of generalized anxiety and compulsive disorders in chimpanzees. J Vet Behav: Clin Appl Res 2012;7:353–361.

Ferris CF, Delville Y. Vasopressin and serotonin interactions in the control of agonistic behavior. Psychoneuroendocrinol 1994;19: 593-601.

Ferris CF, Delville Y, Miller MA, Dorsa DM, De Vries GJ. Distribution of small vasopressinergic neurons in golden hamsters. J Comp Neurol 1995;360:589-598.

Ferris CF, Potegal M. Vasopressin receptor blockade in the anterior hypothalamus suppresses aggression in hamsters. Physiol Behav 1988;44:235-239.

Finco DR, Adams DD, Crowell WA, Stattelman AJ, Brown SA, Barsanti JA. Food and water intake and urine composition in cats: influence of continuous versus periodic feeding. Am J Vet Res 1986;47:1638-1642.

Firth AM, Haldane SL. Development of a scale to evaluate postoperative pain in dogs. J Am Vet Med Assoc 1999;214:651–659.

Flannigan G, Dodman NH. Risk factors and behaviors associated with separation anxiety in dogs. J Am Vet Med Assoc 2001;219: 460-466.

Fonberg E. Various relationships between predatory dominance and aggressive behavior in pairs of cats. Aggressive Behav 1985;11: 103-114.

Fonnum F. Glutamate: a neurotransmitter in mammalian brain. J Neurochem 1984;42:1-11.

Foster JA, Morrison M, Dean SJ, Hill M, Frenk H. Naloxone suppresses food/water consumption in the deprived cat. Pharmacol Biochem Behav 1981;14:419-421.

Fox MW. Behavioral effects of rearing dogs with cat during the critical period of socialization. Behav 1969;35:273-280.

Fox MW. Integrative Development of Brain and Behavior in the Dog. University of Chicago Press, Chicago, IL, 1971.

Fox MW. The behaviour of cats. In: The Behaviour of Domestic Animals, 3rd edition, Ed, Hafez ESE. Williams & Wilkins, Baltimore, MD, 1975: 410-436.

Fox MW, Bekoff M. The behaviour of dogs. In: The Behaviour of Domestic Animals, 3rd edition, Ed. Hafez ESE. Williams & Wilkins, Baltimore, MD, 1975: 370-409.

Fraile IG, McEwen BS, Pfaff DW. Comparative effects of progesterone and alphaxalone on aggressive, reproductive and locomotor behaviors. Pharm Biochem Behav 1988;30:729-735.

Frank D, Beauchamp G, Palestrini C. Systematic review of the use of pheromones for treatment of undesirable behavior in cats and dogs. J Am Vet Med Assoc 2010;236: 1308-1316.

Frank D, Minero M, Cannas S, Palestrini C. Puppy behavior when left home alone: a pilot study. Appl Anim.Behav Sci 2007;104: 61–70.

Frazer-Sisson DE, Rice DA, Peters G. How cats purr. J Zool 1991; 223:67-78.

Freedman DG, King JA, Elliot O. Critical periods in the social development of dogs. Science 1961;133: 1016-1017.

Fuller JL. Experiential deprivation and later behavior. Science 1967;158:1645-1652.

[G].

Gadow KD, Nolan EE, Sverd J, Sprafkin J, Paolicelli L. Methyl-phenidate in aggressive-hyperactive boys: I. Effects on peer aggression in public school settings. J Am Acad Child Adolesc Psych 1990;29:710-718.

Galac S, Knol BW. Fear-motivated aggression in dogs: patient characteristics, diagnosis and therapy. Anim Welf 1997;6:9-15.

Gallo PV, Werboff J, Knox K. Protein restriction during gestation and lactation: development of attachment behavior in cats. Behav Neural Biol 1980;29:216-223.

Gallo PV, Werboff J, Knox K. Development of home orientation in offspring of protein-restricted cats. Develop Psychobiol 1984;17: 437-449.

Galton F. The first steps towards the domestication of animals. Trans Ethnolog Soc London 1865;3:122-138 (cited in Clutton-Brock J. A Natural History of Domesticated Mammals, Cambridge University Press/BMNH, UK, 1987.)

Gamble MR. Sound and its effects on laboratory animals. Biol. Rev. 1982;57:395-421.

Gartlan JS. Structure and function in primate society. Folia Primatologica 1968;8:89-120.

Gazit I, Terkel J. Domination of olfaction over vision in explosives detection by dogs. Appl Anim Behav Sci 2003a;82:65-73.

Gazit I, Terkel J. Explosives detection by sniffer dogs following strenuous physical activity. Appl Anim Behav Sci 2003b; 81:149-161.

Germonpré MM, Lázničková-Galetová M, Sablin M. Paleolithic dog skulls at the Gravettian Předmostí site, the Czech Republic. J Arch Sci 2012;39:84-202.

Germonpré M, Sablin MV, Stevens RE, Hedges REM, Hofreiter M, Stiller M, Després VR. 2009. Fossil dogs and wolves from Palaeolithic sites in Belgium, the Ukraine and Russia: osteometry, ancient DNA and stable isotopes. Journal of Archaeological Science 2009;36:473–490.

Ghaffari MS, Khorami N, Marjani M, Aldavood J. Penile self-mutilstion as an unusual sign of a separation-related problem in a cross-breed dog. JSAP 2007;48:651-653.

Giger U, Jezyk PF. Diagnosis of inherited diseases in small animals. In: Current Veterinary Therapy. XI. Small Animal Practice, Eds. Kirk RW, Bongura JS. WB Saunders, Philadelphia, PA, 1992:18-22.

Gillman PK. A review of serotonin toxicity data: Implications for the mechanisms of antidepressant drug action. Biol Psychiat 2006;59: 1046-1051.

Gillman PK. Triptans, serotonin agonists, and serotonin syndrome (serotonin toxicity): a review. Headache 2010;50:264-272.

Gilor S, Gilor C. Common laboratory artifacts caused by inappropriate sample collection and transport: how to get the most out of a sample. TCAM: Clin Path Hematology 2011;26(2):109-118.

Giorgi M, Del Carlo S, Saccomanni G, Łebkowska-Wieruszewska B, Kowalski CJ. Pharmacokinetic and urine profile of tramadol and its major metabolites following oral administration of immediate release capsules administration in dogs. Vet Res Comm 2009b;33: 875-885.

Giorgi M, Saccomanni G, Łebkowska-Wieruszewska B, Kowalski C. Pharmacokinetic evaluation of tramadol and its major metabolites after single oral sustained tablet administration in the dog: a pilot study. Vet J 2009b;180:253-255.

Glessner JT, Wang K, Cai G, Korvatska O, Kim CE, Wood S, Zhang H, Estes A, Brune CW, Bradfield JP, Imielinski M, Frackelton EC, Reichert J, Crawford EL, Munson J, Sleiman PMA, Chiavacci R, Annaiah K, Thomas K, Hou C, Glaberson W, Flory J, Otieno F, Garris M, Soorya L, Klei L, Piven J, Meyer KJ, Anagnostou E, Sakurai T, Game RM, Rudd DS, Zurawiecki D, McDougle CJ, Davis LK, Miller K, Posey DJ, Michaels S, Kolevzon A, Silverman JM, Bernier R, Levy SE, Schultz RT, Dawson G, Owley T, McMahon WM, Wassink TH, Sweeney JA, Nurnberger JI, Coon H, Sutcliffe JS, Minshew NJ, Grant SFA, Bucan M, Cook EH, Buxbaum JD, Devlin B, Schellenberg GD, Hakonarson H. Autism genome-wide copy number variation reveals ubiquitin and neuronal genes. Nature 2009;459:569–573.

Gobbi M, Mennini T. Release studies with rat brain cortical synaptosomes indivate that tramadol is a 5-hydroxytraptamine uptake blocker and not a 5-hyrdroxytraptamine releaser. Eur J Pharmacol 1999;370:23-26.

Godbout M, Frank D. Persistence of puppy behaviors and signs of anxiety during adulthood. J Vet Behav Clin Appl Res 2011;6:92.

Godbout M, Palestrini C, Beauchamp G, Frank D. Puppy behavior at the veterinary clinic: a pilot study. J Vet Behav: Clin Appl Res 2007;2:126-135.

Goericke-Pesch S, Georgiev P, Antonov A, Albouy M, Wehrend A. Clinical efficacy of a GnRH-agonist implant containing 4.7 mg deslorelin, Suprelorin®, regarding suppression of reproductive function in tomcats. Theriogenology 2011;75:803-810.

Gogolla N, Caroni P, Lüthi A, Herry C. Perineuronal nets protect fear memories from erasure. Science 325:1258-1261, 2009.

Goodwin D, Bradshaw JWS, Wickens SM. Paedomorphosis affects agonistic visual signals of domestic dogs. Anim Behav 1997;53:297-304.

Gordon F, Jukes MGM. Dual organization of the exteroceptive components of the cat's gracile nucleus. J Physiol 1964;139:385-399.

Gosling LM. A reassessment of the function of scent marking in territories. Ethology 1982;60:89-118.

Gould E, Tanapat P. Stress and hippocampal neurogenesis. Biol Psychiatry 1999;46:1471-1479.

Grandin T, Deesing MJ, Struthers JJ, Swinker AM. Cattle with hair whorl patterns above the eyes are more behaviorally agitated during restraint. Appl Anim Behav Sci 1995;46:117-123.

Graves TK. When normal is abnormal: Keys to laboratory diagnosis of hidden endocrine disease. TCAM: Clinical Pathology and Hematology 2011;26(2):45-51.

Gray M, Granka JM, Bustamante, CD, Sutter NB, Boyko AR, Zhu L, Ostrander EA, Wayne RK. Linkage disequilibrium and demographic history of wild and domestic canids. Genetics 2009;181: 1493-1505.

Green HL, Rafterty EB, Gregory IC. Ventricular fibrillation threshold of healthy dogs to 50Hz current in relation to earth leakage currents of electromedical equipment. Biomed Eng 1972;7:408-141.

Green MK, Rani CSS, Josh IA, Soto-Piña AE, Martinez PA, Frazer A, Strong R, Morilak DA. Prenatal stress induces long term stress vulnerability, compromising stress response systems in the brain and impairing extinction of conditioned fear after adult stress. Neuroscience 2011;192:438-451.

Green S, Marler P. The analysis of animal communication. In: Handbook of Behavioral Neurobiology 3, Social Behavior and Communication, Eds. Marler P, Vandenbergh JG. Plenum Press, New York, NY, 1979:73-158.

Greenblatt DJ, Shader RI, Abernethy DR. Drug-therapy: current status of benzodiazepines. NEJM 1983;309:344–358.

Greenblatt DJ, Shader RI, Divoll M, Harmatz JS. Benzodiazepines: a summary of pharmacokinetic properties. Br J Pharm 1981;11 (Suppl):11S–16S.

Griffith CA, Steigerwald ES, Buffington T. Effects of synthetic facial pheromone on behavior of cats. JAVMA 2000;217:1154-1156.

Grigg EK, Pick L, Nibblett B. Litter box preference in domestic cats: covered versus uncovered. J Fel Med Surg 2013; DOI: 10.1117/1098612X12465606.

Grimmett A, Sillence MN. Calmatives for the excitable horse: a review of L-tryptophan. Vet J 2005;170:24-32.

Grint NJ, Alderson B, Dugdale AHA. A comparison of acepromazine-buprenorphine and medetomidine-buprenorphine for preanesthetic medication of dogs. J Am Vet Med Assoc 2010;237: 131-1437.

Grohmann K, Dickomeit MJ, Schmidt MJ, Kramer M. Severe brain damage after punitive training technique with a choke chain collar in a German shepherd dog. J Vet Behav: Clin Appl Res 2013;8: http://dx.doi.org/10.1016/j.jveb.2013.01.002.

Gruen ME, Sherman BL. Use of trazodone as an adjunctive agent in the treatment of canine anxiety disorders: 56 cases (1995-1997). J Am Vet Med Assoc 2008;233:1902-1907.

Gunn-Moore DA, Cameron ME. A pilot study using synthetic feline facial pheromone for the management of feline idiopathic cystitis. J Feline Med Surg 2004;6:133–138.

Gunn-Moore DA, McVee J, Bradshaw JM, Pearson GR, Head E, Gunn-Moore FJ. Ageing changes in cat brains demonstrated by beta-amyloid and AT8-immunoreactive phosphorylated tau deposits. J Feline Med Surg 2006 8:234-242.

Gunn-Moore D, Moffat K, Christie L-A, Head E. Cognitive dysfunction and the neurobiology of ageing in cats. JSAP 2007;48: 546-553.

Gunter R. The absolute threshold for vision in the cat. J Physiol 1951;114:8-15.

Gurski JL. Interaction of separation discomfort with contact comfort and discomfort in the dog. Dev Psychobiol 1980;13:463-467.

Guyot GW, Cross HA, Bennett TL: Early social isolation in the domestic cat: responses during mechanical toy testing. Appl Anim Ethol 1983;10:109-116.

[H].

Hailman JP. Optical Signals: Animal Communication and Light. Indiana University Press, Bloomington, IN,1977.

Hajszan T, Dow A, Warner-Schmidt JL, Szigeti-Buck K, Sallam NL, Parducz A, Leranth C, Duman RS. Remodeling of hippocampal spine synapses in the rat learned helplessness model of depression. Biol. Psychiatry 2009;65:392-400.

Hallgren A. Mother and pups. ABCN 1990;(3)1-2.

Hallgren A. Spinal anomalies in dogs. ABCN 1992;9(3):3-4.

Hamner CE, Jennings LL, Sojka NJ. Cat (Felis catus L.) spermatozoa requires capacitation. J Repro Fert 1970;23:477-480.

Hansen BD. Assessment of pain in dogs: veterinary clinical studies. ILAR J 2003;44:197-205.

Hansen BD, Hardie EM, Carroll GS. Physiological measurements after ovariohysterectomy in dogs: What's normal? Appl Anim Behav Sci 1997;51:101-109.

Hardie EM, Hansen BD, Carroll GS. Behavior after ovariohysterectomy in the dog: What's normal? Appl Anim Behav Sci 1997;51:111-128.

Hare B, Brown M, Williamson C, Tomasello M. The domestication of social cognition in dogs. Science 2002;298:1634-1636.

Hare B, Call J, Tomasello M. Communication of food location between human and dog (Canis familiaris). Evol Commun 1998;2:137-159.

Hare B, Tomasello M. Domestic dogs (Canis familiaris) use human and conspecific social cures to locate hidden food. J Comp Psychol 1999;113:173-177.

Harrington FH, Mech LD. An analysis of howling response parameters useful for wolf packs censusing. J Wildlife Manag 1982;46: 686-693.

Harris VS, Sachs BD. Copulatory behavior in male rats following amygdaloid lesions. Brain Res 1975;86:514-518.

Harrison J, Buchwald J. Aging changes in the cat P300 mimic the human. Electroencephalography Clin Neurophys 1985;62: 227-234.

Hart BL. Behavioral effects of long-acting progestins. Feline Practice 1974a;4:8-11.

Hart BL. Gonadal androgen and sociosexual behavior of male mammals: a comparative analysis (review). Psychol Bull 1974b;81 (7):383-400.

Hart BL. Problems with objectionable sociosexual behavior of dogs and cats: therapeutic use of castration and progestins. Comp Contin Edu Pract Vet 1979c;1:461-465.

Hart BL. Physiology of sexual function. Vet Clin North Am: Sm Anim Pract 1974d;4:557-571.

Hart BL. Feline Behavior. A Practitioner Monograph. Veterinary Practice Publishing, Santa Barbara, Calif, 1980.

Hart BL. Olfactory tractotomy for control of objectionable urine spraying and urine marking in cats. J Am Vet Med Assoc 1981;179:231-234.

Hart BL, Barrett RE. Effects of castration on fighting, roaming and urine spraying in adult male cats. J Am Vet Med Assoc 1973;163:290-292.

Hart BL, Cliff KD, Tynes VV, Bergman L. 2005. Control of urine marking by use of long-term treatment with fluoxetine or clomipramine in cats. J Am Vet Med Assoc 2005;226:378-382.

Hart BL, Leedy M. Identification of source of urine stains in multi-cat households. J Am Vet Med Assoc 1982;180:77-78.

Hart BL, Leedy MG. Female sexual response in male cats facilitated by olfactory bulbectomy and medial preoptic anterior hypothalamic lesion. Behav Neurosci 1983;97:608-614.

Hart BL, Leedy MG. Analysis of the catnip reaction: mediation by olfactory system, not vomeronasal organ. Behav Neurol Biol 1985;44:38-46.

Hart BL, Voith VL. Changes in urine spraying, feeding and sleep behavior of cats following medial preoptic-anterior hypothalamic lesions. Brain Res 1978;145:406-409.

Haskins R. A causal analysis of kitten vocalization: an observational and experimental study. Anim Behav 1979;27:726-736.

Hatch RC. Effect on drugs on catnip-induced (Nepeta cataria) pleasure behavior in cats. Am J Vet Res 1972;33:143-155.

Hauser MD, Newport EL, Aslin, RN. Segmentation of the speech stream in a non-human primate: statistical learning in cotton-top tamarins. Cognition 2001;78, B53-B64.

Head E, Moffat K, Das P, Sarsoza F, Poon WW, Landsberg G, Cotman CW, Murphy MP. β-amyloid deposition and tau phosphorylation in clinically characterized aged cats. Neurobiol Aging 2005;26:749-763.

Head E, Nukala VM, Fenoglio KA, Muggenburg BA, Cotman CW, Sullivan PG. Effects of age, dietary, and behavioral enrichment on brain mitochondria in a canine model of human aging. Exp Neurol 2009;220:171-176.

Head E, Pop V, Vasilevko V, Hill MA, Saing T, Sarsoza F, Nistor M, Christie LA, Milton S, Glabe C, Barrett E, Cribbs D. A two-year study with fibrillar β-Amyloid (Aβ) immunization in aged canines: effects on cognitive function and brain Aβ. J Neurosci 2008;28:3555-3566.

Heath SE, Barabas S, Craze PC. Nutritional supplementation in cases of cognitive dysfunction—A clinical trial. Appl Anim Behav Sci 2007;105:284-296.

Hegerl U, Bottlender R, Gallinat J, Kuss H J, Ackenheil M, Moller HJ. The serotonin syndrome scale: first results on validity. Eur Arch Psychiatry Clin Neurosci 1998;248: 96–103.

Hellyer P, Rodan I, Brunt J, Downing R, Hagedorn JE, Robertson SA. AAHA/AAFP pain management guidelines for dogs and cats. J Am Anim Hosp Assoc 2007;43:235-248.

Hellyer PW, Uhrig SR, Robinson NG. Canine Acute Pain Scale and Feline Acute Pain Scale. Colorado State University Veterinary Medical Center, Fort Collins, CO, 2006: www.cvmbs.colostate.edu/ivapm/professionals/members/drug_protocols/painscale-caninenobandagesPAH.pdf.

Hemmer H. Gestation period and postnatal development in felids. Carnivore 1979;2:90-100.

Henessy MB, Williams MT, Miller DD, Douglas CW, Voith VL. 1998. Influence of male and female petters on plasma cortisol and behaviour: can human interaction reduce the stress of dogs in a public animal shelter? Appl Anim Behav Sci 1998;61:63–77.

Herman LM, Richards DG, Wolz JP. Comprehension of sentences by bottlenosed dolphins. Cognition 1984;16:129–219.

Herman BH, Hammock MK, Egan K, Arthur-Smith A, Chatoor I, Werner A: Role for opioid peptide in self-injurious behavior dissociation from autonomic nervous system function. Dev Pharmacol Ther 1989;12:81-89.

Hernander L. Factors influencing dogs' stress level in the waiting room at a veterinary clinic. SLU Student report 190, 2008; 29 pp; ISSN 1652-280X.

Herron ME, Lord LK. Use of and satisfaction of pet owners with a clinical behavior service in a companion animal specialty referral practice. J Am Vet Med Assoc 2012;241:1463-1466.

Herron ME, Shofer FS, Reisner IR. Survey of the use and outcome of confrontational and non-confrontational training methods in client-owned dogs showing undesired behaviors. Appl Anim Behav Sci 2009;117;47-54.

Hewson CJ, Conlon PD, Luescher UA, Ball RO. The pharmacokinetics of clomipramine and desmethylclomipramine in dogs: parameter estimates following a single oral dose and 28 consecutive daily oral doses of clomipramine. J Vet Pharm Ther 1998;21: 214–222.

Hiby EF, Rooney NJ, Bradshaw JWS. Dogtraining methods: their use, effectiveness and interaction with behaviour and welfare. Anim Welf 2004;13:63–69.

Hinde RA. The biological significance of territories in birds. The Ibis 1956;98:340-369.

Hinde RA. The nature of aggression. New Society 1967;9:302-304.

Hinde RA. Animal Behaviour. 2nd Edition. McGraw-Hill, New York, NY, 1970.

Hirai T, Kojima S, Shimada A, Umermura T, Sakai M, Itakurat C. Age-related changes in the olfactory system of dogs. Neuropath Appl Neurobiol 1996;22:531-539.

Hirsch B, Dubose C, Jacobs HL. Dietary control of food intake in cats. Physiol Behav 1978;20:287-295.

Hofmeister EH, Chandler MJ, Read MR. Effects of acepromazine, hydromorphone, or an acepromazine-hydromorphone combination of the degree of sedation in clinically normal dogs. J Am Vet Med Assoc 2010;237:1155-1159.

Holland CT. Successful long term treatment of a dog with psychomotor seizures using carbamazepine. Austral Vet J 1988;65:389-392.

Holton L, Reid J, Scott EM, Pawson P, Nolan A. Development of a behaviour-based scale to measure acute pain in dogs. Vet Rec 2001;148:525-531.

Holton LL, Scott EM, Nolan AM, Reid J, Welsh E. Relationship between physiological factors and clinical pain in dogs scored using a numerical rating scale. J Small Anim Pract 1998a;39:469-474.

Holton LL, Scott EM, Nolan AM, Reid J, Welsh E, Flaherty D. Comparison of three methods used for assessment of pain in dogs. J Am Vet Med Assoc 1998b;212:61-66.

Holy TE. Wake up and smell the conspecific! Trends Neurosci 2003;26:463-465.

Hopkins SG, Schubert TA, Hart BL. Castration of adult male dogs: effects on roaming, aggression, urine spraying, and mounting. JAVMA 1976;168:1108-1110.

Hotez PJ, Wilkins PP. Toxocariasis: America's most common neglected infection of poverty and a helminthiasis of global importance? Neglect Trop Dis 2009;3(3):1–4.

Houpt KA. Ingestive behavior problems of dogs and cats. Vet Clin North Am: Sm Anim Pract 1982;12(4):683-692.

Houpt KA. Domestic Animal Behavior for Veterinarians and Animal Scientists, 2nd edition. Iowa State University Press, Ames, Iowa, 1991.

Howe LM, Slater MR, Boothe HW, Hobson HP, Holcom JL, Spann AC. Long-term outcome of gonadectomy performed at an early age or traditional age in dogs. J Am Vet Med Assoc 2001;218:217–221.

Howell S.R., Hicks DR, Scatina JA, Sisenwine SF. Pharmacokinetics of venlafaxine and O-desmethylvenlafaxine in laboratory animals. Xenobiotica 1994;24:315-327.

Hsu Y, Serpell JA. Development and validation of a questionnaire for measuring behavior and temperament traits in pet dogs. J Am Vet Med Assoc 2003;223, 1293-1300.

Hughes D, Moreau RE, Overall KL, Van Winkle TJ. Acute hepatic necrosis and liver failure associated with benzodiazepine therapy in six cats: 1986-1995. J Vet Emerg Crit Care 1996;6:13-20.

Hurni H, Rossbach W. The laboratory cat. In: The UFAW Handbook on the Care and Management of Laboratory Animals, 6th Edition, Ed. Poole TB. Longman Scientific and Technical: Harlow, 1987: 476-492.

Hydbring-Sandberg E, von Walter LW, Höglund K, Svartberg K, Swenson L, Forkman B. Physiological reactions to fear provocation in dogs. J Endocrinol 2004;180:439-448.

[I].

Iggo A. Cutaneous receptors with a high sensitivity to mechanical displacement. In: Touch, Heat, and Pain, Eds. de Reuck AVS, Knight J. CIBA Foundation, London, UK, 1966: 237-256.

Immelmann K, Beer C. A Dictionary of Ethology. Harvard University Press, Cambridge, MA, 1989.

Issel-Tarver L, Rine J. Organization and expression of canine olfactory receptor genes. PNAS 1996; 93:10897–10902.

Izawa M, Doi T, Ono Y. Grouping patterns of feral cats (Felis catus) living on a small island in Japan. Japan J Ecol 1982;32:373-382.

[J].

Jackson LA, Perkins BA, Wenger JD. Cat-scratch disease in the United States. Am J Public Health 1993;83:1707-1711.

Jacobsen KL, DePeters EJ, Rogers QR, Taylor SJ. Influences of stage of lactation, teat position and sequential milk sampling on the composition of domestic cat milk (*Felis catus*). J Anim Physiol a Anim Nutri 2004;88:46-58.

Jagoe A, Serpell J. Owner characteristics and interactions and the prevalence of canine behavior problems. Appl Anim Behav Sci 1996;47:31-42.

James W. Dominant and submissive behavior in puppies as indicated by food intake. J Genetic Psychol 1949;75:33-43.

Janczak AM, Pedersen LJ, Rydhmer L, Bakken M. Relation between early fear- and anxiety-related behaviour and maternal ability in sows. Appl. Anim. Behav. Sci. 2003;82:121–135.

Janczak AM, Bakken M, Braastad BO. A cautionery note regarding the use of nutritional L-tryptophan to alter aversion-related behavior in mice. Appl Anim Behav Sci 2001;72:365-373.

Jankowski AJ, Brown DC, Duval J, Gregor TP, Strine LE, Ksiazek LM, Ott AH. Comparison of effects of elective tenectomy or onychectomy in cats. J Am Vet Med Assoc. 1998;213:370-373.

Jensen RA, Davis JL, Shnerson A. Early experience facilitates the development of temperature regulation in the cat. Devel Psychobiol 1980;13:1-16.

John E, Chesler T, Barrett F, Victor I. Observational learning in cats. Science 1968;159:1489-1491.

Johnson WE, Eizirik E, Pecon-Slattery J, Murphy WJ, Antunes A. The late Miocene radiation of modern felidae: a genetic assessment. Science 2006;311:73-77.

Johnston SD, Root Kustritz MV, Olson PNS. Canine and Feline Theriogenology. Philadelphia: WB Saunders, 2001:80-87.

Jonas JM, Hearron AE Jr. Alprazolam and suicidal ideation: a meta-analysis of controlled trials in the treatment of depression. J Clin Psychopharmacol 1996;16:208-211.

Jones E, Coman BJ. Ecology of the feral cat (*Felis catus L.*) in South-Eastern Australia. III. Home ranges and population ecology in semi-arid North West Victoria. Austral Wildlife Res 1982: 409-420.

Juarbe-Diaz SV, Houpt KA. Comparison of two antibarking collars for treatment of nuisance barking. JAAHA 1996;32:231-235.

Junaidi A, Williamson PE, Cummins JM, Martin GB, Blackberry MA, Trigg TE. Use of a new drug delivery formulation of the gonadotropin-releasing hormone analogue Deslorelin for revisable long term contraception in dogs. Repro Fert Devel 2003;13:317-322.

Jurek J, McCauley L. Physical rehabilitation and senior pets. Clinician's Brief 2011;9.

[K].

Kalman DS, Feldman S, Feldman R, Schwartz HI, Krieger DR, Garrison R. Effect of a proprietary *Magnolia* and *Phellodendron* extract on stress levels in healthy women: a pilot, double-blind, placebo-controlled clinical trial. Nutr J 2008;7:11 doi:10.1186/1475-2891-7-11.

Kalmus H. The discrimination by the nose of the dog of the individual human odours and in particular the odours of twins. Brit J Anim Behav 1955;3:25-31.

Kaminski J, Call J, Fischer J. Word learning in a domestic dog: evidence for "fast mapping". Science 2004;304:1682-1683.

Kanarek RB. Availability and caloric density of the diet as determinants of meal pattern in cats. Physiol Behav 1975;15:611-618.

Kantelip JP, Duchene-Marullaz P, Delaigue-Farbry R, Eschalier A. Comparison of the effects of propranolol, pindolol, oxprenolol and acebutolol on atrioventircular conduction in unanesthetized dogs. Br. J Clin Pharmacol 1982;13(Suppl 2):159S-166S.

Karsh EB. Factors influencing the socialization of cats to people. In: The Pet Connection: Its Influence on our Health and Quality of Life, Eds. Anderson RK, Hart BL, Hart LA. University of Minnesota Press, Minneapolis, MN, 1984: 207-215.

Karsh EB. The effects of early handling on the development of social bonds between cats and people. In: New Perspectives on our Lives with Companion Animals, Eds. Katcher AH, Beck AM. University of Pennsylvania Press, Philadelphia, PA, 1983a: 22-28.

Karsh EB. The effects of early and late handling on the attachment of cats to people. In: The Pet Connection, Conference Proceedings, Eds. Anderson RK, Hart BL, Hart L. Globe Press, St. Paul, MN, 1983b.

Karsh EB, Turner DC. The human-cat relationship. In The Domestic Cat: the Biology of its Behaviour. Edited by Turner DC, Bateson P, Cambridge University Press, Cambridge, UK;1988:159-178.

Kato M, Miyajo K, Ohtani N, Ohta M. Effects of prescription diet on dealing with stressful situations and performance of anxiety-related behaviors in privately owned anxious dogs. J Vet Behav: Clin Appl. Res 2012;7:21-26.

Katz RJ, Thomas E. Effects of para-chlorophenylalanine upon brain stimulated affective attack in the cat. Pharmacol Biochem Behav 1976;5:391-394.

Kaufmann JH. Social relations of adult males in a free-ranging band of rhesus monkeys. In: Social Communication Among Primates, Ed. Altman SA. University of Chicago Press, Chicago, IL, 1967: 73-78.

Kemper DL, Schiefele P, Clark JG. Canine brainstem auditory evoked responses are not clinically impacted by head size or breed. Physiol Behav 2013;110-111:190-197.

Kemppainen RJ, Birchfield JR. Measurement of total thyroxine concentration in serum from dogs and cats by use of various methods. Am J Vet Res 2006;67:259-265.

Kendall K, Ley J. Cat ownership in Australia: barriers to ownership and behavior. J Vet Behav: Clin Appl Res. 2006;1:5-16.

Kerby G, Macdonald DW. Cat society and the consequences of colony size. In: The Domestic Cat: the Biology of its Behavior, Ed Turner DC, Bateson PPG. Cambridge University Press, Cambridge. 1988:67-81.

Kessler M R, Turner DC. Stress and adaptation of cats (*Felis silvestris catus*) housed singly in pairs and in groups in boarding catteries. Anim Welf 1997;6:243-254.

Kiley-Worthington M. The tail movements of ungulates, canids and felids with particular reference to their causation and function as displays. Behaviour 1976;1-2:69-114.

Kiley-Worthington M. Animal language? Vocal communication of some ungulates, canids and felids. Acta Zoologica Fennica 1984;171:83–88.

Kim HH, Yeon SC, Houpt KA, Lee HC, Chang HH, Lee, HJ. Effects of ovariohysterectomy on reactivity in German Shepherd dogs. Vet J 2006;172:154–159.

Kim JJ, Diamond DM. The stressed hippocampus, synaptic plasticity and lost memories. Nat. Rev. Neurosci. 2002;3:453–462.

Kimura K, Ozeki M, Juneja LR, Ohira H. L-theanine reduces psychological and physiological stress responses. Bio. Psychol. 2007;74: 39-45.

King J, Simpson B, Overall KL, Applby D, Pageat P, Ross C, Chaurand JP, Heath S, Beata C, Weiss AB, Muller G, Paris T, Bataille BG, Parker J, Petit S, Wren J. Treatment of separation anxiety in dogs with clomipramine. Results from a prospective, randomized, double-blinded, placebo-controlled clinical trial. J Appl Anim Behav Sci 2000a;67:255-275.

King JE, Becker RF, Markel JE. Studies on olfactory discrimination in dogs. III. Ability to detect human odour trace. Anim Behav 1964;12:311-315.

King JN, Maurer MP, Altman B, Strehlau G. Pharmacokinetics of clomipramine in dogs following single-dose and repeated-dose oral administration. Am J Vet Res 2000b;61:80–5.

King JN, Overall KL, Appleby D, Simpson BS, Beata C, Chaurand CJP, Heath SE, Ross C, Weiss AB, Muller G, Bataille BG, Paris T, Pageat P, Brovedani F, Garden C, Petit S. Results of a follow-up investigation to a clinical trial testing the efficacy of clomipramine in the treatment of separation anxiety in dogs. Appl Anim Behav Sci 2004b; 89:233-242.

King JN, Steffan J, Heath SE, Simpson BS, Crowell-Davis SL, Harrington LN, Weiss A-B, Seewalkd W. Determination of the dosage of clomipramine for the treatment of urine spraying in cats. J Am Vet Med Assoc 2004a;225:881–887.

King T, Hemsworth PH, Coleman GJ. 2003. Fear of novel and startling stimuli in domestic dogs. Appl. Anim. Behav.Sci. 2003;82: 45–64.

Kirsch P, Esslinger C, Chen Q, Mier D, Lis S, Siddhanti S, Gruppe H, Mattay VS, Gallhofer B, Meyer-Lindenberg A. Oxytocin modulates neural circuitry for social cognition and fear in humans. J Neurosci 2005;25:11489-11493.

Kleiman D. Scent marking in the canidae. Symp Zool Soc Lond 1966;18:167-177.

Kling A, Orbach J, Schwartz NB, Towne JC. Injury to the limbic system and associated structures in cats. Arch Gen Psychiatry 1960;3:391-420.

Knol BW, Egberink-Alink ST. Androgens, progestagens and agonistic behavior: A review. Vet Q 1989a;11:94-101.

Knol W, Egberink-Alink ST. Treatment of problem behaviour in dogs and cats by castration and progestagen administration: A review. Vet Q 1989b;11:102-107.

Knowles RJ, Curtis TM, Crowell-Davis Sl. Correlation of dominance as determined by agonistic interactions with feeding order in cats. Am J Vet Res 2004;65:1548-1556.

Kobelt AJ, Hemsworth PH, Barnett JL, Coleman GJ, Butler KL. The behavior of Labrador retrievers in suburban backyards: the relationship between the backyard environment and dog behavior. Appl Anim Behav Sci 2007;106:70-84.

Koenig R. Modeling the nonthyroidal illness syndrome. Curr Opin Endocrinol Diabetes Obes 2008;15:466-469.

Kogan LR, Schoenfeld-Tacher R., Simon AR. Behavioral Effects of Auditory Stimulation on Kenneled Dogs. J Vet Behav: Clin Appl Res 2012;7:268-275.

Kolb B, Nonneman AJ. The development of social responsiveness in kittens. Anim Behav 1975;23:368-374.

Komtebedde J, Hauptman J. Bilateral ischiocavernosus myectomy for chronic urine spraying in castrated male cats. Vet Surg 1990;19:293-296.

Kongara K, Chambers P, Johnson CB. Glomerular filtration rate after tramadol, parecoxib and pindolol following anesthesia and analgesia in comparison with morphine in dogs. Vet Anaesth Analgesia 2009;36:86-94.

Konrad KW, Bagshaw M. Effects of novel stimuli on cats reared in a restricted environment. J Compar Physiol Psychol 1970;70:157-164.

Koopmans SJ, Ruis M, Dekker R, van Diepen H, Korte M and Mroz Z. Surplus dietary tryptophan reduces plasma cortisol and noradrenaline concentrations and enhances recovery after social stress in pigs. Physiol Behav 2005;85, 469-478.

Kostarczyk E, Fonberg E. Heart rate mechanisms in instrumental conditioning reinforced by petting in dogs. Physiol. Behav. 1982; 28:27-30.

Kovach JK, Kling A. Mechanisms of neonate sucking behaviour in the kitten. Anim Behav 1967;15:91-101.

Krettek JE, Price JL. A description of the amygdaloid complex in the rat and cat with observations on intra-amygdaloid axonal connections. J Comp Neurol 1978;178:255-279.

Krishnan V, Nestler EJ. The molecular neurobiology of depression. Nature 2008;455:894-902.

Kronen PW, Ludders JW, Hollis NE, Moon PF, Gleed RD, Koski S. A synthetic fraction of feline facial pheromones calms but does not reduce struggling in cats before venous catheterization. Vet Anaesth Analg 2006;33:258-265.

Kuczenski R, Segal DS, Cho AK, Melega W. Hippocampus norepinephrine, caudate dopamine and serotonin, and behavioral responses to the stereoisomers of amphetamine and methamphetamine. J Neurosci 1995;15:1308-1317.

KuKanich B, Papich MG. Pharmacokinetics of tramadol and the metabolite O-desmethyltramadol in dogs. J Vet Pharmacolo Ther 2004;27:239-246.

KuKanich B, Papich MG. Pharmacokinetics and antinociceptive effects of oral tramadol hydrochloride administration in Greyhounds. Am J Vet Res 2011;72:256-162.

Kuo ZY. The genesis of the cat's response to the rat. J Comparative Psychol 1930;11:1-35.

Kuo ZY. Studies on the basic factors in animal fighting: VII. Inter-species co-existence in mammals. J Genetic Psychol 1960;97:211-225.

Kuribara H, Stavinoha WB, Maruyama Y. Behavioural pharmacological characteristics of honokiol, an anxiolytic agent present in extracts of Magnolia bark, evaluated by an elevated plus-maze test in mice. J Pharm Pharmacol. 1998;50:819-826.

Kuribara H, Stavinoha WB, Maruyama Y. Honokiol, a putative anxiolytic agent extracted from magnolia bark, has no diazepam-like side-effects in mice. J Pharm Pharmacol 1999;51:97-103.

Kuwabara N, Seki K, Aoki K. Circadian, sleep, and brain temperature rhythms in cats under sustained daily light-dark cycles and constant darkness. Physiol Behavior 1986;38:283-289.

[L].

Labuschagne I, Phan KL, Wood A, Angstadt M, Chua P, Heinrichs M, Stout JC, Nathan PJ. Oxytocin attenuates amygdale reactivity to fear in generalized social anxiety disorder. Neuropsychopharm 2010;35:2403-2413.

Lagerström MC, Rogoz K, Abrahamsen B, Persson E, Reinius B, Nordenankar K, Ölund C, Smith C, Mendez JA, Chen Z, Wood JN, Wallén-Mackenzie A, and Kullander K. VGLUT2-Dependent Sensory Neurons in the TRPV1 Population Regulate Pain and Itch. Neuron 2010;68:529–542.

Lainesse C, Frank D, Beaudry F, Doucet M. Effects of physiological covariables on pharmacokinetic parameters of clomipramine in a large population of cats after a single oral administration. J Vet Pharmacol Therap 2007a;30:116-126.

Lainesse C, Frank D, Beaudry F, Doucet. Comparative oxidative metabolic profiles of clomipramine in cats, rats and dogs: preliminary results from an *in vitro* study. J Vet Pharmacol Therap 2007b;30:387-393.

Lainesse C, Frank D, Meucci V, Intorre L, Soldani G, DOucet M. Pharmacokinetics of clomipramine and desmethylclomipramine after single-dose intravenous and oral administration in cats. J Vet Pharmacol Therap 2006;29:271-278.

Lakhan SE, Vieira KF. Nutritional therapies for mental disorders. Nutr J 2008;7:2. doi: 10.1186/1475-2891-7-2.

Lana SE, Rutteman GR, Winthrow SJ. Tumors of the mammary gland. In: Withrow and MacEwen;s Small Animal Clinical Oncology. 4th edition, Eds. Wonthrow SJ, Vail DM. Elsevier, St. Louis, MO, 2007:619-636.

Landau HG. On dominance relations and the structure of animal societies: I. Effects of inherent characteristics. Bull Math Biophys 1951;13:1-19.

Landsberg GM, Melese P, Sherman BL, Neilson JC, Zimmerman A, Clarke TP. Effectiveness of fluoxetine chewable tablets in the treatment of canine separation anxiety. J Vet Behav: Clin Appl Res 2008;3:12-19.

Landsberg GM, Wilson AL. Effects of clomipramine on cats presented for urine marking. J Amer Anim Hosp Assoc 2005;41: 3-11.

Lane R, Baldwin D. Selective serotonin reuptake inhibitor-induced serotonin syndrome: review. J Clin Psychopharm 1997;17:208-221.

Lanfumey L, Mongeau R, Cohen-Salmon C, Hamon M. Corticosteroid-serotonin interactions in the neurobiological mechanisms of stress-related disorders. Neurosci Biobehav Rev 2008;32:1174-1184.

Lange-Asschenfeldt C, Weigmann H, Hiemke C, Mann K. Serotonin syndrome as a result of fluoxetine in a patient with tramadol abuse: plasma level-correlated symptomology. J Clin Psychopharm 2002;22:440-441.

Lasley SM, Thurmond JB. Interaction of dietary tryptophan and social isolation on territorial aggression, motor activity, and neurochemistry in mice. Psychopharmacology 1985;87:313–321.

Lauder, JM, Liu J, Devaud L, Morrow AL. GABA as a trophic factor for developing monamine neurons. Persp Devel Neurobiol 1998;5:247–259.

Leathwood PD. Tryptophan availability and serotonin synthesis. Proc Nutr Soc 1987;46:143–156.

Leaver SDA, Reimchen TE. Behavioural responses of Canis familiaris to different tail lengths of a remotely-controlled life-size dog replica. Behaviour 2008;145:377-390.

LeDoux JE. Emotion circuits in the brain. Annu Rev Neurosci 2000;23:155–184.

LeDoux JE, Cicchetti P, Xagoraris A, Romanski LM. The lateral amygdaloid nucleus: sensory interface of the amygdala in fear conditioning. J Neurosci 1990;10:1062-1069.

Lee HY, Shepley M, Huang C-S. Evaluation of off-leash dog parks in Texas and Florida: a study of use patterns, user satisfaction and perception. Landscape Urban Planning 2009;92:314-324.

Lefebvre D, Diederich C, Delcourt M, Giffroy JM. The quality of the relation between handler and military dogs influences efficiency and welfare of dogs. Appl Anim Behav Sci 2007;104:49-60.

Lehman MN, Winans SS. Vomeronasal and olfactory pathways to the amygdale controlling male hamster sexual behavior: autoradiographic and behavioral analyses. Brain Res 1982;240:27-41.

Lekcharoensuk C, Osborne CA, Lulich JP. Epidemiologic study of risk factors for lower urinary tract diseases in cats. J Am Vet Med Assoc 2001;218:1429-1435.

Lenroot RK, Gogtay N, Greenstein DK, Wells EM, Wallace GL, Clasen LS, Blumenthal JD, Lerch J, Zijdenbox AP, Evans AC, Thompson PM, Giedd JN. Sexual dimorphism of brain developmental trajectories during childhood and adolescence. NeuroImage 2007;36:1065–1073.

Leonard JA, Wayne RK, Wheeler J, Valadez R, Guillen S, Vilà C. Ancient DNA evidence for old world origin of new world dogs. Science 2002;298:1613–1616.

Lesch KP, Mössner R. Genetically driven variation in serotonin uptake: is there a link to affective spectrum, neurodevelopmental, and neurodegenerative disorders? Biol Psychiatry 1998;44:179–192.

Levine MS, Lloyd RL, Fisher RS, Hull CD, Buchwalkd NA. Sensory motor and cognitive alterations in aged cats. Neurobiol Aging 1987;8:253-263.

Lewis MJ, Williams DC, Vite CH. Evaluation of the electroencephalogram in young cats. Am J Vet Res 2011;72:391-197.

Leyhausen P. The communal organization of solitary mammals. Symposium of the Zoological Society of London 1965;14:249-263.

Leyhausen P: Cat Behavior: the Predatory and Social Behavior of Domestic and Wild Cats. Garland STPM Press, New York, NY, 1979.

Liberg O. Spacing patterns in a population of rural free-roaming domestic cats. Oikos 1980;35:336-349.

Liberg O. Courtship behaviour and sexual selection in the domestic cat. Appl Anim Ethol 1983;10:117-132.

Liberg O, Sandell M: Spacial organisation and reproductive tactics in the domestic cat and other felids. In: The Domestic Cat: The Biology of Its Behavior, Eds. Turner DC, Bateson P. Cambridge University Press, Cambridge, UK, 1988: 83-98.

Liberg O, Sandell M, Pontier D, Natoli E. Density, spatial organization and reproductive tactics in the domestic cat and other felids. The Domestic Cat: the Biology of its Behaviour. 2nd Edition. Edited by Turner DC, Bateson P, Cambridge University Press, Cambridge, UK, 2000:119-148.

Liman ER. Sex and the single neuron: pheromones excite. Trends Neurosci 2001;24:2-3.

Lin DY, Zhang SZ, Block E, et al. Encoding social signals in the mouse main olfactory bulb. Nature 2005;434:470–477.

Lindblad-Toh K, Wade CM, Mikkelsen TS, Karlsson EK, Jaffe DB, Kamal M, Clamp M, Chang JL, Kulbokas EJ, Zody MC, Mauceli E, Xie X, Breen M, Wayne RK, Ostrander EA, Ponting CP, Galibert F, Smith DR, deJong PJ, Kirkness E, Alvarez P, Biagi T, BrockmanW, Butler J, Chin CW, Cook A, Cuff J, Daly MJ, DeCaprio D, Gnerre S, Grabherr M, Kellis M, Kleber M, Bardeleben C, Goodstadt L, Heger A, Hitte C, Kim L, Koepfli KP, Parker HG, Pollinger JP, Searle SMJ, Sutter NB, Thomas R, Webber C, Lander ES. Genome sequence, comparative analysis and haplotype structure of the domestic dog. Nature 2005;438:803-819.

Linnoila MI, Virkkunen M. Aggression, suicidality, and serotonin. J Clin Psychiat 1992;53(10, Suppl.):46-51.

Lipman AG. Analgesic drugs for neuropathic and sympathetically maintained pain. Clin Geriatr Med 1996;12:501-15.

Lippi G, Massimo F, Montagnana M, Salvagno GL, Poli G, Guidi GC. Quality and reliability of routine coagulation testing: can we trust that sample? Blood Coag Fibrinolysis 2006;17;513-519.

Lippi G, Salvagno GL, Brocco G, Guidi GC. Preanalytical variability in laboratory testing: influence of the blood drawing technique. Clin Chem Lab Med 2005;43:319-325.

Lisberg AE, Snowdon CT. The effects of sex, gonadectomy and status on investigation patterns of unfamiliar conspecific urine in domestic dogs, Canis familiaris. Anim Behav 2009;77:1147-1154.

Lisberg AE, Snowdon C. Effects of sex, social status and gonadectomy on countermarking by domestic dogs, Canis familiaris. Anim Behav 2011;81:757-764.

Lockwood R, Rindy K. Are "Pit Bulls" different? An analysis of the Pit Bull Terrier controversy. Anthrozoös 1987;1:2–8.

Lore R, Eisenberg F. Avoidance reactions of domestic dogs to unfamiliar male and female humans in a kennel setting. Appl Anim Behav Sci 1986;15:261-266.

Lossius MI, Taubøll E, Mowinckel P, Gjerstad L. Reversible effects of antiepileptic drug on thyroid hormones in men and women with epilepsy: a prospective randomized double-blind withdrawal study. Epilepsy Behav 2009;16:64-68.

Love M, Overall KL. Dogs and children: how anticipating relationships can help avoid disasters. J Am Vet Med Assoc 2001;219:446-453.

Lowe SE, Bradshaw JWS. Ontogeny of individuality in the domestic cat in the hoe environment. Anim Behav 2001;61:231-237.

Lu J, Sherman D, Devor M, Saper CB. A putative flip–flop switch for control of REM sleep. Nature 2006;441:589-594. doi:10.1038/nature04767.

Lubin FD, Roth TL, Sweatt JD. Epigenetic regulation of dbnf gene transcription and consolidation of fear memory. J Neurosci 2008;28:10576-10586.

Lucki I, Ashutosh D, Mayorga AJ. Sensitivity to the effects of pharmacologically selective antidepressants in different strains of mice. Psychopharmacology 2001;155:315–322.

Luescher AU, Reisner IR. Canine aggression towards familiar people: a new look at an old problem. Vet Clin NA: Sm Anim Pract 2008;38:1107-1130.

Luiten PGM, Koolhaas JM, de Boer S, Koopmans SJ. The cortical-medial amygdala in the central nervous system organization of agonistic behavior. Brain Res 1985;332:283-297.

Luo M, Fee MS, Katz LC. et al. Encoding pheromonal signals in the accessory olfactory bulb of behaving mice. Science 2003;299:1196–1201.

[M].

Macdonald DW, Apps PJ. The social behavior of a group of semi-dependent farm cats, Felis catus: a progress report. Carnivore Gen Newsletter 1978;3:256-268.

Macdonald DW, Apps PJ, Carr GM, Kerby G. Social dynamics, nursing coalitions, and infanticide among farm cats, Felis catus. Adv Ethol (Suppl Ethology) 1987;28:1-64.

MacDonald K, MacDonald TM. The peptide that binds: a systematic review of oxytocin and its proscial effects in humans. Harv Rev Psychiatry 2010;18:1-21.

MacDonald ML, Rogers QR, Morris JG. Nutrition of the domestic cat, a mammalian carnivore. Ann Rev Nutr 1984;4:52l-562.

MacDonald ML, Rogers QR, Morris JG. Aversion of the cat to dietary medium-chain triglycerides and caprylic acid. Physiol Behav 1985;35:371-375.

Maeda H. Effects of septal lesions on electrically elicited hypothalamic rage in cats. Physiol Behav 1978;21:339-343.

Maes M, Lin AH, Bonaccorso S, Goosens F, Van Gastel A, Pioli R, Delmeire L, Scharpé S, 1999. Higher serum prolyl endopeptidase activity in patients with post-traumatic stress disorder. J Affect Disorders 1999;53:27–34.

Maggi RG, Mozayeni R, Pultorak EL, Hegarty BC, Bradley JM, Correa M, Breitschwerdt EB. Bartonella spp. Bacteremia and rheumatic symptoms in patients from Lyme-disease endemic region. Emerging. Infect. Dis. 2012;18:783-791.

Magistretti PJ. Role of glutamate in neuron-glia metabolic coupling. Am J Clin Nutr 2009;90(suppl);875S-890S.

Mahmood I, Green MD, Fisher JE. Selection of the first-time dose in humans: comparison of different approaches based on interspecies scaling of clearance. J Clin Pharmacol 2003;43:692-697.

Maksymowicz K, Marycz K, Czogała J, Jurek T. Refutation of the stereotype of a "killer dog" in light of the behavioral interpretation of human corpses biting by domestic dogs. J Vet Behav Clin Appl Res 2011;6:50-56.

Mandrioli R, Mercolini L, Raggi MA. Benzodiazepine metabolism: an analytical perspective. Curr Drug Metab 2008;9:827-844.

Marder AR. Psychotropic drugs and behavior therapy. Vet Clin North Am: Sm Anim Pract 1991;21:329-342.

Mariti C, Gazzano A, Moore, JL, Baragli P, Chelli L, Sighieri C. Perception of dogs' stress by their owners. J Vet Behav: Clin Appl Res 2012;7:213-219.

Mariti C, Ricci E, Carlone B, Moore JL, Sighieri C, Gazzano A. Dog attachment to man: a comparison between pet and working dogs. J Vet Behav: Clin Appl Res 2013;doi:10.1016/j.jveb.2012.05.00.

Markl H. Manipulation, modulation, information, cognition: some of the riddles of communication. In: Experimental Behavioral Ecology and Sociobiology, Eds. Hölldobler B, Lindaur M. Sinauer, Sunderlin, MA, 1985:163-194.

Maros K, Dóka A, Miklósi Á. Behavioural correlation of heart rate changes in family dogs. Appl Anim Behav Sci 2008;109:329–341.

Marshall-Pescini S, Valsecchi P. Petak I, Previde EP. Does training make you smarter? The effects of training on dogs' performance (Canis familiaris) in a problem solving task. Behav Process.2008;78:449–454.

Marston LC, Bennett PC, Coleman GJ. What happens to shelter dogs? An analysis of data for one year from three Australian shelters. J Appl Anim Welf Sci 2004;7:27–47.

Marston LC, Bennett PC, Coleman GJ. What happens to shelter dogs? Part 2. Comparing three Melbourne welfare shelters for non-human animals. J Appl Anim Welf Sci 2005;8:25-45.

Martin F, Taunton A. Perceived importance and integration of the human-animal bond in private veterinary practice. J AmerVet Med Assoc 2006;228:522-527.

Martin KM. 2010. Effect of clomipramine on the electrocardiogram and serum thyroid concentrations of healthy cats. J Vet Behav: Clin Appl Res 2010;5:123-129.

Martin P. The 4 whys and wherefores of play in cats: a review of functional, evolutionary, developmental, and causal issues. In: Play in Animals and Humans, Ed. Smith PK. Basil Blackwell, Oxford, UK, 1984:71-94.

Martin P, Bateson P. The ontogeny of locomotor play behaviour in the domestic cat. Anim Behav 1985;33:502-510.

Martin P, Bateson P. Behavioral development in the cat. In: The Domestic Cat: The Biology of its Behaviour, Eds. Turner DC, Bateson P. Cambridge University Press, Cambridge, UK, 1988:9-22.

Martin WR, Eades CG, Thompson WO, Thompson JA, Flanary HG. Morphine physical dependence in the dog. J Pharmacol Exp Ther 1974;189:759-771.

Masek P, Heisenberg M. Distinct memories of odor intensity and quality in Drosophila. PNAS 2008;105:15985-15990.

Masserman JH, Siever DW. Dominance, neurosis, and aggression: an experimental study. Psychosomatic Med 1944;6:7-16.

McCobb EC, Patronek GJ, Marder A, Dinnage JD, Stone MS. Assessment of stress levels among cats in four animal shelters. J Am Vet Med Assoc 2005; 226:548-555.

McConnell J, Kirby R, Rudloff E. A retrospective study on the use of acepromazine maleate in dogs with seizures. J Vet Emerg Crit Care 2007;17:262–7.

McConnell PB. Acoustic structure and receiver response in domestic dogs, Canis familiaris. Anim Behav 1990;39:897-904.

McConnell PB, Baylis JR. Interspecific communication in cooperative herding: Acoustic and visual signals from human shepherds and herding dogs. Zeit Tierpsychol 1985;67:302-328.

McCune S. Temperament and welfare of caged cats. Doctoral Dissertation, University of Cambridge, Cambridge, UK, 1992.

McCune S. The impact of paternity and early socialization on the development of cat's behaviour to people and novel objects. Appl Anim Behav Sci 1995;45:109-124.

McCune S, Stevenson J, Fretwell L., Thompson A, Mills DS. Ageing does not significantly affect performance in a spatial learning task in the domestic cat (Felis silvestris catus). Appl. Anim. Behav. Sci. 2008;112:345-356.

McDevitt L. Control Unleashed: Creating a Focused and Confident Dog. Clean Run Press Productions/CRP, 2007.

McEwen BS, Magarinos AM. Stress and hippocampal plasticity: implications for the pathophysiology of affective disorders. Hum Psychopharmacol 2001;16, S7–S19.

McGowan PO, Sasakil A, D'Alessio AC, Dymov S, Labonte B, Szyf M, Turecki G, Meaney MJ. Epigenetic regulation of the glucocorticoid receptor in human brain associates with childhood abuse. Nature Neurosci 2009;12:342-348.

McGreevy P, Grassi TD, Harm AM. A strong correlation exists between the distribution of retinal ganglion cells and nose length in the dog. Brain Behav Evol. 2004;63:13-22.

McGregor IS, Haargreaes GA, Apfelbach R, Hunt GE. Neural correlates of cat odor-induced anxiety in rats: region-specific effects of the benzodiazepine midazolam. J Neurosci 2004;24:4134–4144.

McKinley PE. Cluster analysis of the domestic cat's vocal repertoire. Unpublished doctoral dissertation. University of Maryland, College Park. 1982.

Mehlman PT, Higley JD, Faucher I, Lilly AA, Taub DM, Vickers J, Suomi SJ, Linnoila M. Low CSF 5-HIAA concentrations and severe aggression and impaired impulse control in nonhuman primates. Am J Psychiatry 1994;151:1485-1491.

Meier GW. Infantile handling and development in Siamese kittens. J Compar Physiol Psychol 1961;54:284-286.

Meier GW, Stuart JL. Effects of handling on the physical and behavioral development of Siamese kittens. Psychol Rep 1959;5:497-501.

Meier M, Turner DC. Reactions of home cats during encounters with a strange person: evidence for two personality types. J Delta Soc 1985;2:45-53.

Meints K, De Keuster T. Brief report: don't kiss a sleeping dog: the first assessment of the 'The Blue Dog' bite prevention program. Journal Pediatric Psychology 2009;34:1084–1090.

Mellen JD. The effects of hand-raising on sexual behavior of captive small felids using domestic cats as a model. In: AAZPA Annual Conference Proceedings. American Association of Zoological Parks and Aquariums. Wheeling, WV. 1988:253-259.

Melzack R. The role of early experience in emotional arousal. Ann NY Acad Sci 1968;159:720-730.

Melzack R, Scott TH. The effects of early experience on the response to pain. J Comp Physiol Pyschol 1957;50:155-161.

Melzer S, Michael M, Caputi A, Eliava M, Fuchs EC, Whittington MA, Monyer H. Long-range-projecting GABAergic neurons modulate inhibition in hippocampus and entorhinal cortex. Science 2012;335:15506.

Mendl M. The effects of litter-size variation on the development of play behaviour in the domestic cat: litters of one and two. Anim Behav 1988;36:20-34.

Mendl M. Performing under pressure: stress and cognitive function. Appl Anim Behav Sci 1999;65:221–244.

Meneses A. 5-HT system and cognition. Neurosci Biobehav Rev 1999;23:1111-1125.

Mertens P. Canine Aggression. In: BSAVA Manual of Canine and Feline Behavioral Medicine, Eds. Horwitz D, Mills, D, Heath S. BSAVA, Gloucester, UK, 2002:195-215.

Mertl-Millhollen A, Goodmann P, Klinghammer E. Wolf scent marking with raised-leg urination. Zoo Biology 1986;5:7-20.

Miklósi Á, Polgardi R, Topál J, Csányi V. Intentional behaviour in dog-human communication: an experimental analysis of "showing" behaviour in the dog. Anim Cog 2000;3:159-166.

Miklósi Á, Topál J, Csányi V. Comparative social cognition: what can dogs teach us? Anim Behav 2004; 67: 995–1004.

Milgram NW, Head E, Muggenburg B, Holowachuk D, Murphey H, Estrad J, Ikeda-Douglas C, Zicker SC, Cotman CW. Landmark discrimination learning in the dog: effects of age, an antioxidant fortified food, and cognitive strategy. Neurosci Biobehav Rev 2002;679-695.

Milgram NW, Head E, Zicker SC, Ikeda-Douglas CJ, Murphey H, Muggenburg B, Siwak C, Tapp D, Cotman CW. Learning ability in aged beagle dogs is preserved by behavioral enrichment and dietary fortification: a two-year longitudinal study. Neurobiol Aging 2005;26:77-90.

Milgram NW, Head E, Zicker SC, Ikeda-Douglas C, Murphey H, Muggenberg BA, Siwak CT, Tapp PD, Lowry SR, Cotman CW. Long-term treatment with antioxidants and a program of behavioral enrichment reduces age-dependent impairment in discrimination and reversal learning in beagle dogs. Exper Gerontol 2004;39:753-765.

Milgram NW, Ivy GO, Head E, Murphy MP, Wu PH, Ruehl WW, Yu PH, Durden DA, Davis BA, Paterson IA, Boulton AA. The effect of L-deprenyl on behavior, cognitive function, and biogenic amines in the dog [review]. Neurochem Res 1993;18: 211-1219.

Miller DD, Staats SR, Partlo C, Rada K. Factors associated with the decision to surrender a pet to an animal shelter. J Am Vet Med Assoc 1996;209:738-742.

Miller PE, Murphy CH. Vision in dogs. J Am Vet Med Assoc 1995; 207:1623-1634.

Mills DS, Ramos D, Gandia Estellés M, Hargrave C. A triple blind placebo-controlled investigation into the assessment of the effect of dog appeasing pheromone (DAP) on anxiety related behavior of problem dogs in the veterinary clinic. Appl Anim Behav Sci 2006;98:114–126.

Minckley BB. A study of noise and its relationship to patient disdcomfort in the recovery room. Nurs Res 1968;17:247-250.

Mitsui S, Yamamoto M, Nagasawa M, Mogi K, Kikusui T, Ohtani N, Ohta M. Urinary oxytocin as a noninvasive biomarker of positive emotion in dogs. Horm Behav 2011;60:239-243.

Moe L. Population-based incidence of mammary tumors in some dog breeds. J Reprod Fertil Suppl 2001;57:439-443.

Moelk M. Vocalizing in the house cat: a phoenetic and functional study. Am J Psychol 1944;57:184-205.

Moelk M. The development of friendly approach behavior in the cat: a study of kitten-mother relations and the cognitive development of the kitten from birth to eight weeks. In: Advances in the Study of Behavior 10th, Ed. Rosenblatt J. Academic Press, NY, 1979:164-224.

Moffat KS, Landsberg GM, Beaudet R. Effectiveness and comparison of citronella and scantly spray bark collars for the control of barking in a veterinary hospital setting. J Am Anim Hosp Assoc 2003;39:343-348.

Molnár C, Kaplan F, Roy P, Pachet F, Pongrácz P, Dóka A, Miklósi Á. Classification of dog barks: a machine learning approach. Anim Cogn 2008;11:389–400.

Molnár C, Pongrácz P, Dóka A, Miklósi Á. Can humans discriminate between dogs on the base of the acoustic parameters of barks? Behav. Process 2006;73:76–83.

Molnár C, Pongrácz P, Faragó T, Dóka A, Miklósi Á. Dogs discriminate between barks: the effect of context and identity of the caller. Behav Proc 2009;82:198–201.

Mongillo P, Adamelli S, Bernardini M, Fraccaroli E, Marinelli L. Successful treatment for abnormal feeding behavior in a cat. J Vet Behav: Clin Appl Res 2012;7:390-393.

Moon-Fanelli AA, Dodman NH. Description and development of compulsive tail chasing in terriers and response to clomipramine treatment. J Am Vet Med Assoc 1998;212:1252-1257.

Moon-Fanelli AA, Dodman NH, Cottam N. Blanket and flank sucking in Doberman pinschers. J Am Vet Med Assoc 2007;231:907-912.

Morey DF. The early evolution of the domestic dog. Am Sci 1994:82;336–347.

Mos J, Olivier B. Quantitative and comparative analyses of proaggressive actions of benzodiazepines in maternal aggression of rats. Psychopharmacol 1989;97:152-153.

Mos J, Olivier B, van Oorschot R. Behavioural and neuropharmacological aspects of maternal aggression in rodents. Aggress Behav 1990;16:145-163.

Moulton DG, Ashton EH, Eayers JT. Studies in olfactory acuity. 4. Relative detectability of n-aliphatic acids by the dog. Anim Behav 1960;8:117-128.

Moyer KE. Kinds of aggression and their physiological basis. Communications Behav Biol 2(A):65-87, 1968.

Mugford RA. External influences on the feeding of carnivores. In: The Chemical Senses and Nutrition, Eds. Kare MR, Maller O. Academic Press, New York, NY, 1977:25-50.

Mula M. Anti-convulsants-antidepressants pharmacokinetic drug interactions: The role of the CYP450 system in psychopharmacology. Curr Drug Metab 2008;9:730-737.

Murphree OD, Dykman RA, Peters JE. Genetically determined abnormal behavior in dogs: results of behavioral tests. Conditional Reflex 1967;1:199-205.

Murphree OD, Peters JE, Dykman RA. Behavioral comparisons of nervous, sable, and cross-bred pointers at ages 2, 3, 6, 9, and 12 months. Conditional Reflex 1969:4:20-23.

Murphy MD, Larson J, Tyler A, Kvam V, Frank K, Eia C, Bickett-Weddle D, Flaming K, Baldwin CJ, Petersen CA. Assessment of owner willingness to treat or manage diseases of dogs and cats as a guide to shelter animal adoptability. J Am Vet Med Assoc 2013;242:46-53.

Murrell JC, Hellebrekers LJ. Medetomidine and dexmedetomidine: a review of cardiovascular effects and antinociceptive properties in the dog. Vet Anaesth Analgesia 2005;32:117-127.

[N].

Natoli E. Behavioral responses of urban feral cats to different types of urine marks. Behaviour 1985;94:234-243.

Natoli E, Baggio A, Pontier D. Male and female agonistic and affiliative relationships in a social group of farm cats (Felis catus L.). Behav Proc 2001;53:1370143.

Natoli E, de Vito E. The mating system of feral cats living in a group. In: The Domestic Cat: The Biology of Its Behaviour, Eds. Turner DC, Bateson P. Cambridge University Press, Cambridge, UK, 1988: 99-108.

Natoli E, de Vito E. Agonistic behaviour, dominance rank, and copulatory success at a large, multi-male feral cat, Felis catus L, colony in central Rome. Anim Behav 1991;42:227-241.

Natynczuk S, Bradshaw JW, Macdonald DW. Chemical constituents of the anal sacs of domestic dogs. Biochem System Ecol 1989;17:83-87.

Neff WD, Diamond IP. The neural basis of auditory discrimination. In: Biological and Biochemical Basis of Behavior, Eds. Harlow HF, Woolsey CN. University of Wisconsin Press, Madison, WI, 1958: 101-126.

Neilson JC. Feline house soiling: Elimination and marking behaviors. Vet Clin NA: Sm AnimPract 2003;33:287-301.

Neilson JC, Hart BL, Cliff KD, Ruehl WW. Prevalence of behavioral changes associated with age-related cognitive impairment in dogs. J Am Vet Med Assoc 2001;218:1787-1791.

Neitz J, Geist T, Jacobs GH. Color vision in the dog. Vis Neurosci 1989;3:119–125.

Netto WJ, van der Borg JA, Slegers JF. The establishment of dominance relationships in a dog pack and its relevance for the man-dog relationship. Tijdschr Diergeneeskd 1992;117 Suppl 1:51S-52S.

Nicastro N. Perceptual and acoustic evidence for species-level differences in meow vocalizations by domestic cats (Felis catus) and African wild cats (Felis silvestris lybica). J Comp Psychol 2004;118:287-296.

Nicastro N, Owren MJ. Classification of domestic cat (Felis catus) vocalizations by naive and experienced human listeners. J Comp Psychol 2003;117:44–52. doi:10.1037/0735-7036.117.1.44.

Nippak PMD, Mendelson J, Muggenburg B, Milgram NW. Enhanced spatial ability in aged dogs following dietary and behavioural enrichment. Learn Mem 2007;87:610-623.

Norris AM, Laing EJ, Valli VEO, Withrow SJ, Macy DW, Ogilvie GK, Tomlinson J, McCaw D, Pidgeon G, Jacobs RM. Canine bladder and urethral tumors: a retrospective of 115 cases (1980-1985). J Vet Int Med 1992;6:145-153.

Notari L, Mills DS. Possible behavioural effects of exogenous corticosteroids on dog behaviour: a preliminary investigation. J Vet Behav: Clin Appl Res 2011;6:321-327.

Nutter FN, Levine JF, Stoskopf MK. Reproductive capacity of free-roaming domestic cats and kitten survival rate. J Am Vet Med Assoc 2004;225:1399-1402.

[O].

O'Farrell V, Peachey E. Behavioural effects of ovariohysterectomy on bitches. Journal of Small Animal Practice 1990;31, 595–598.

Ogata N, Dodman NH. The use of clonidine in the treatment of fear-based behavior problems in dogs: an open trial. J Vet Behav: Clin Appl Res 2010;6:130-137.

Ogata N, Hashizuma C, Momozawa Y, Masuda K, Kikusui T, Takeuchi Y, Mori Y. Polymorphisms in the canine glutamate transporter-1 gene: identification and variation among five dog breeds. J Vet Med Sci 2006;68:157-159.

Ogle CW, Lockett MF. The urinary changes induced in rats by high pitched sounds (2 kcyc/sec). J Endocrinol 1968;42:253-260.

Ohl F, Arndt SS, van der Staay J. Pathological anxiety in animals. Vet J 2008;175:18-26.

Olender T. The olfactory receptor universe—from whole genome analysis to structure and evolution. Genet Mol Res 2004;3: 545-553.

Olney JW. Neurotoxicity of NMDA receptor antagonists: An overview. Psychopharm Bull 1994;30:533-540.

Opii W, Joshi G, Head E, Milgram NW, Muggenburg BA, Klein JB, Piece WM, Cotman CW, Butterfield DA. Proteomic identification of brain proteins in the canine model of human aging following a long-term treatment with antioxidants and a program of behavioral enrichment: relevance to Alzheimer's disease. Neurobiol Aging 2008;29:51-70.

Orihel JS, Fraser D. A note on the effectiveness of behavioural rehabilitation for reducing inter-dog aggression in shelter dogs. Appl Anim Behav Sci 2008;112:400-405.

Orotolani A. Spots, stripes, tail tips and dark eyes: predicting the function of carnivore colour patterns using the comparative method. Biol J Linn Soc 1999;67:433-476.

Osella MC, Re G, Badino P, Bergamasco L, Miolo A. Phosphatidylserine (PS) as a potential nutraceutical for canine brain aging: A review. J Vet Behav: Clin Appl Res 2008;3:41-51.

Overly B, Shofer FS, Goldschmidt MH, Shere D, Sorenmo KU. Association between ovariohysterectomyand feline mammary carcinoma. J Vet Intl Med 2005;19:560-563.

Overall KL. Animal behavior case of the month. Use of fluoxetine (Prozac) to treat complicated interdog aggression. J Am Vet Med Assoc 1995a;206:629-632.

Overall KL. Animal behavior case of the month. Intrasexual interdog aggression in two pugs. J Am Vet Med Assoc 1995b;207:305-307.

Overall KL. Sex and aggression. Canine Practice. 1995c;20(3):16-18.

Overall KL. Clinical Behavioral Medicine for Small Animals. Mosby, St. Louis, 1997.

Overall KL. Animal Behavior Case of the Month: Treatment of a complicated case of separation anxiety. J Am Vet Med Assoc 1998;212:1702-1704.

Overall KL. Dogs as "natural" models of human psychiatric disorders: assessing validity and understanding mechanism. Prog Neuropsychopharmacol Biol Psychiatry 2000;24:727-276.

Overall KL Pharmacological treatment in behavioral medicine: the importance of neurochemistry, molecular biology, and mechanistic hypotheses. Vet J 2001;162:9-23.

Overall KL. Veterinary behavioural medicine: a roadmap for the 21st century. The Veterinary Journal 2005a;169:130-143.

Overall KL. Mental Illness in Animals. In Well-being in Animals. Edited by McMillan F, ISU Press, Ames, IA, 2005b:127-143.

Overall KL. Veterinary behavioural medicine: a roadmap for the 21st century. The Veterinary Journal 2005;169:130-143.

Overall KL. Guest Editorial: Working bitches and the neutering myth: Sticking to the science. The Veterinary Journal 2007;173:9-11.

Overall KL. That dog is smarter than you know: advances in understanding canine learning, memory, and cognition. TCAM 2011;26:1-9.

Overall KL, Arnold SA: Olfactory neuron biopsies in dogs: a feasibility pilot study. Appl Anim Behav Sci 2007;105:351-357.

Overall KL, Burghardt WF. 2006. Discussion round table: terminology think tank. J Vet Behav: Clin Appl Res 2006;1:29-32.

Overall KL, Dunham AE. Clinical features and outcome in dogs and cats with obsessive-compulsive disorder: 126 cases (1989-2000). J Am Vet Med Assoc 2002;221:1445-1452.

Overall KL, Dunham AE. Personal View: Homeopathy and the curse of the scientific method. The Veterinary Journal 2009;180:141-148.

Overall KL, Dunham AE, Frank D: Frequency of nonspecific clinical signs in dogs with separation anxiety, storm/thunderstorm phobia, and noise phobia, alone or in combination. J Am Vet Med Assoc 2001;219:467-473.

Overall KL, Dunham AE, Frank D, Seksel K, Ash-Mahoney C. Dominance aggression: are females still younger? Proceedings American Veterinary Society of Animal Behavior (AVSAB) meeting, New Orleans, LA, July 1999.

Overall KL, Love M. Dog bites to humans: demography, epidemiology, and risk. J Am Vet Med Assoc 2001;218:1-12.

Ovodov ND, Crockford SJ, Kuzmin YV, Higham TFG, Hodgins GWL, van der Plicht. A 33,000-Year-Old Incipient Dog from the Altai Mountains of Siberia: Evidence of the Earliest Domestication Disrupted by the Last Glacial Maximum. PLoS ONE 2011;6(7): e22821. doi:10.1371/journal.pone.0022821

[P].

Paape SR, Shille VM, Seto H, Stabenfeldt GH. Luteal activity in the pseudopregnant cat. Biol Reprod 1975;13:470-474.

Packer C, Gilbert DA, Pusey AE, O'Brien SJ. A molecular genetic analysis of kinship and cooperation in african lions. Nature 1991;351:562-565, 1991.

Packwood J, Gordon B. Stereopsis in normal domestic cat, Siamese cat and cat raised with alternating monocular occlusion. J Neurophysiol 1975;38:1485-1499.

Pal SK. Play behaviour during early ontogeny in free-ranging dogs (Canis familiaris). Appl Anim Behav Sci 2010;126:140-153.

Palestrini C, Minero M, Cannas S, Berteselli G, Scaglia E, Barbieri S, Cavallone E, Puricelli M, Servida F, Dall'Ara P. Efficacy of a diet containing caseinate hydrolysate on signs of stress in dogs. J Vet Behav: Clin Appl Res 2010;5:309-317.

Palestrini C, Minero M, Cannas S, Rossi E, Frank D. Video analysis of dogs with separation-related behaviors. Appl Anim Behav Sci 2010;124:61-67.

Palestrini C, Previde EP, Spiezio C, Verga M. Heart rate and behavioural responses of dogs in the Ainsworth's strange situation: a pilot study. Appl. Anim. Behav. Sci. 2005;94:75–88.

Panaman R. Behavior and ecology of free-ranging female farm cats (Felis catus L.) Zeit Tierpsycol 1981;56:59-73.

Pang J-F, Kluetsch C, Zou X-J, Zhang A, Luo L-Y, Angleby H, Ardalan A, Ekström C, Sköllermo A, Lundeberg J, Matsumura S, Leitner T, Zhang Y-P, Savolainen P. mtDNA data indicate a single origin for dogs south of Yangtze River, less than 16,300 years ago, from numerous wolves. Molec Biol Evol 2009;26:2849-2864.

Panksepp J. Commentary on the possible role of oxytocin in autism. J Autism Dev Disord 1993;23:567–569.

Papich MG. Drug compounding for veterinary patients. AAPS J 2005;7:E281-287.

Parker HG, Kim LV, Sutter NB, Carlson S, Lorentzen TD, Malek TB, Johnson GS, DeFrance HB, Ostrander EA, Kruglyak L. Genetic structure of the purebred domestic dog. Science 2004;304:1160-1164.

Parthasarathy V, Crowell-Davis, SL. Relationship between attachment to owners and separation anxiety in pet dogs (Canis lupis familiaris). J Vet Behav: Clin App Res 2006;1:109-120.

Passanisi WC, Macdonald DW. Group discrimination on the basis of urine in a farm cat colony. In: Chemical Signals in Vertebrates, Vol 5, Eds. Macdonald DW, Muller-Schwarze D, Natynczuk SE. Oxford University Press, Oxford, UK, 1990:336-345.

Patel KN, Dong X. An Itch To Be Scratched. Neuron 2010;68: 334-339.

Patronek GJ, Glickman LT, Beck AM, McCabe GP, Ecker C. Risk factors for relinquishment of cats to an animal shelter. J Am Vet Med Assoc 1996;209:582-588.

Patronek GJ, Slavinski SA. Animal bites. J Am Vet Med Assoc 2009;234:336-345.

Pauli AM, Bentley E, Diehl KA, Miller PE. Effects of the application of neck pressure by a collar or harness on intraocular pressure in dogs. J Am Anim Hosp Assoc 2006;42:207-211.

Pavlov IP. Conditioned Reflexes. An Investigation of the Physiological Activity of the Cerebral Cortex. Oxford University Press, London, UK, 1927.

Pawlowski AA, Scott JP. Hereditary differences in the development of dominance in litters of puppies. J Compar Physiol Psychol 1956;49:353-358.

Pellis SM, O'Brien DP, Pellis VC, Teitelbaum P. Escalation of feline predation along a gradient from avoidance through "play" to killing. Behav Neurosci 1988;102:760-777.

Pellerin L, Bouzier-sore, A-K, Aubert A, Serres S, Merle M, Costalat R, Magistretti PJ. Activity-dependent regulation of energy metabolism of astrocytes: an update. Glia 2007;55:1251-1262.

Peremans K, Audenaert K, Coopman F, Blanckaert P, Jacobs F, Otte A, Verschooten F, Bree H, Heeringen K, Mertens J. Estimates of regional cerebral blood flow and 5-HT2A receptor density in impulsive, aggressive dogs with 99mTc-ECD and 123I-5-I-R91150. Eur J Nuc Med Mol Imaging 2003;30:1538-1546.

Peremans K, Audenaert K, Hoybergs Y, Otte A, Goethals I, Gielen I, Blankaert P, Vervaet M, van Heerigen C, Dierckx R. The effect of citalopram hydrobrombide on 5-HT2A receptors in the impulsive-aggressive dog, as measures with ^{123}I-5-I-R91150 SPECT. Eur J Nucl Med Mol Imaging 2005;32:708-716.

Peters A, Schweiger U, Pellerin L, Hubold C, Oltmanns KM., Conrad M, Schultes B., Born J, Fehm, HL. The selfish brain: competing for energy resources. Neurosci Biobehav Rev 2004;28:143–180.

Peters RP, Mech LD. Scent-marking in wolves. Am Sci 1975; 63:628-637.

Peterson ME. The effects of megestrol acetate on glucose tolerance in growth hormone secretion in the cat. Res Vet Sci 1987;42: 354-357.

Peterson ME, Gamble DA. Effects of non-thyroidal illness on serum thyroxine concentrations in cats: 494 cases. J Am Vet Med Assoc 1988;197:1203-1208.

Peterson ME, Melián C, Nichols R. Meaurement of serum total thyroxine, triiodothyronine, free thyroxine, and thyrotropin concentrations for diagnosis of hypothyroidism in dogs. J Am Vet Med Assoc 1997;211:1396-1402.

Peterson ME, Melián C, Nichols R. Measurement of serum concentrations of free thyroxine, total thyroxine, and total triiodothyronine in cats with hyperthyroidism and cats with nonthyroidal disease. J Am Vet Med Assoc 2001;218:529-536.

Petkov CI, Taglialatela JP. Primate neuroscience and ethology — an enduring union? Curr Biol 2010;20: R501-R503.

Pettijohn T, Wong T, Elert P, Scott JP. Alleviation of separation distress in three breeds of young dogs. Devel Psychobiol 1977;10: 373-381.

Phan KL, Fitzgerald DA, Nathan PJ, Tancer ME. Association between amygdale hyperactivity to harce faces and severity of social anxiety in generalized social phobia. Biol Psychiatry 2006;59:424-429.

Pickar D, Vartanian F, Bunney WE, Maier HP, Gastpar MT, Prakash R, Lideman R, Belyaev BS, Tsutsulkovskaja MVA, Jungkunz G, Nedopil N, Verhoeven W, van Praag H. Short-term naloxone administration in schizophrenic and manic patients. A World Health Organization Collaborative Study. Arch Gen Psychiatry 1982;39:313-319.

Pierantoni L, Albertini M, Pirrone F. Prevalence of owner-reported behaviours in dogs separated from the litter at two different ages. Vet Rec 2011;169;468 doi: 10.1136/vr.d4967.

Pilley JW, Reid AK. Border collie comprehends object names as verbal referents. Behav Proc 2011;86:184-195.

Pitman DL, Ottenweller JE, Natelson BH. Plasma corticosterone levels during repeated presentation of two intensities of restraint stress: Chronic stress and habituation. Physiol Behav 1988;43: 47-55.

Pizzorusso T. Erasing fear memories. Science 2009;325:1214-1215.

Platt SR, Randell SC, Scott KC, Chrisman CL, Hill RC, Gronwall RR. Comparison of plasma benzodiazepine concentrations following intranasal and intravenous administration of diazepam to dogs. Am J Vet Res 2000;61:651-654.

Plutchik R. Individual and breed differences in approach and withdrawal in dogs. Behaviour 1971;40:302-311.

Podberscek AL, Blackshaw JK. Dog attacks on children: report from two major city hospitals. Austral Vet J 1991a;68:248-249.

Podberscek AL, Blackshaw JK, Beattie AW. The behavior of laboratory colony cats and their reactions to a familiar and unfamiliar person. Appl Anim Behav Sci 1991b;31:119-130.

Podberscek AL, Serpell JA. Environmental influences on the expression of aggressive behavior in English cocker spaniels. Appl Anim Behav Sci 1997;52:215-227.

Pollard JS, Baldock MD, Lewis RFV. Learning rates and use of visual information in five animal species. Austral J Psychol 1971;23:29-34.

Polsky R. Can aggression in dogs be elicited through the use of electronic pet containment systems? J Appl Anim Wel Sci 2000;3:345-358.

Pongrácz P, Miklósi Á, Kubinyi E, Curobi K, Topál J, Csányi V. Social learning in dogs: the effect of a human demonstrator on the performance of dogs in a detour task. Anim Behav 2001;62:1109-1117.

Pongrácz P, Miklósi Á, Kubinyi E, Topál J, Csányi V. Interaction between individual experience and social learning in dogs. Anim Behav 2003;63:595-603.

Pongrácz P, Molnár C, Miklósi Á. Acoustic parameters of dog barks carry emotional information for humans. Appl Anim Behav Sci 2006;100:228-240.

Pongrácz P, Molnár C, Miklósi Á, Csányi V. Human listeners are able to classify dog barks recorded in different situations. J. Comp. Psychol. 2005;119:136–144.

Pop V, Head E, Hill M-A, Gillen D, Berchtold NC, Muggenburg BA, Milgram NW, Murphy MP, Cotman CW. Synergistic effects of long-term antioxidant diet and behavioral enrichment on β-amyloid load and non-amyloidogenic processing in aged canines. J Neurosci 2010;30:9831-9839.

Porter RJ, Gallagher P, Watson S, Young AH. Corticosteroid-serotonin interactions in depression: a review of the human evidence. Psychopharmacology (Berl) 2004;173:1– 17.

Premack D. Toward empirical behavior laws. I. positive reinforcement. Psychol Rev 1959;66:219–233.

Prymack C, McKee LJ, Goldschmidt MH, Glickman LT. Epidemiological, clinical, pathologic and prognostic characteristics of splenic hemangiosarcoma and splenic hematoma in dogs: 217 cases (1985). J Am Vet Med Assoc 1988;193:706-712.

Pryor PA, Hart BL, Bain MJ, Cliff KD. Causes of urine marking in cats and effects of environmental management on frequency of marking. J Am Vet Med Assoc 2001;219:1709-1713.

Pryor PA, Hart BL, Cliff KD, Bain MJ. Effects of a selective serotonin reuptake inhibitor on urine spraying behavior in cats. J Am Vet Med Assoc 2001;219:1557-1561.

Pypendop BH, Ilkiw JE. Pharmacokinetics of tramadol, and its metabolite O-desmethyl-tramadol in cats. J Vet Pharmacol Ther 2008;31:52-59.

[Q].

Quaranta A, Siniscalchi M, Vallortigara G. Asymmetric tail-wagging responses by dogs to different emotive stimuli. Curr Biol 2007;17:R199-201.

Quignon P, Giraud M, Rimbault M, Lavidne P, Tacher S, Morin E, Retout E, Valin AS, Lindblad-Toh K, Nicolas J, Galibert F. The dog and rat olfactory receptor repertoires. Genome Biol 2005;6:R83, (doi:10.1186/gb-2005-6-10-r83).

Quignon P, Kirkness E, Cadieu E, Touleimat N, Guyon R, Renier C, Hitte C, André C, Fraser C, Galibert F. Comparison of the canine and human olfactory receptor gene repertoires. Genome Biol 2003;4:R80 (http://genomebiology.com/2003/4/12/R80).

[R].

Radinsky L. Evolution of the felid brain. Brain Behav Evol 1975;11:214-254.

Radosta LA, Shofer FS, Reisner IR. Comparison of thyroid analytes in dogs aggressive to familiar people and in non-aggressive dogs. Vet J 2012;192:472-475.

Radtke KM, Ruf M, Gunter HM, Dohrmann K, Schauer M, Meyer A, Elbert T. Transgenerational impact of intimate partner violence on methylation in the promoter of the glucocorticoid receptor. Transl Psychiatry 2011;1:e21 doi:10.1038/tp.2011.21.

Raichle ME, Minton MA. Brain work and brain imaging. Ann Rev-Neurosci 2006;29:449-476.

Raihani G, González D, Arteaga L, Hudson R. Olfactory guidance of nipple attachment and suckling in kittens of the domestic cat: inborn and learned responses. Devl Psychobiol 2009;51: 662-671.

Ralls K. Mammalian scent marking. Science 1971;171:443-449.

Randall W, Lasko V. Body weight and food intake rhythms and their relationships to the behavior of cats with brainstem lesions. Psychosomatic Sci 1968;11:33-34.

Randall W, Swenson RW, Parsons V, Elbin J, Trulson M: The influence of seasonal changes in light on hormones in normal cats and in cats with lesions of the superior colliculi and pretectum. J Interdisciplin Cycle Res 1975;6:253-266.

Rang HP, Dale MM, Ritter JM, Flowere RJ, Henderson G. Rang and Dale's Pharmacology, 7th Edition. Elsevier, St. Louis, MO, 2012.

Range F, Horn L, Virany Z, Huber L. The absence of reward induces inequity aversion in dogs. PNAS 2009;106:340–345.

Range F, Leitner K, Virany Z. The influence of the relationship and motivation on inequity aversion in dogs. Soc Just Res 2012; 25:170-194.

Rauschecker J, Marler P, Eds. Imprinting and Cortical Plasticity. John Wiley & Sons, New York, NY, 1987.

Re S, Zanoletti M, Emanuele E. Aggressive dogs are characterized by low omega-3 polyunsaturated fatty acid status. Vet Res Comm 2008;32:225-230.

Re S, Zanoletti M, Emanuele E. Association of inflammatory markers elevation with aggressive behavior in dogs. J Ethology 2009;27: 31-33.

Rees P. The ecological distribution of feral cats and the effects of neutering a hospital colony. In: The Ecology and Control of Feral Cats. Ed. Universities Federation for Animal Welfare. UFAW. Potters Bar, England.1981:12-22.

Reger MA, Henderson ST, Hale C, Cholerton B, Baker LD, Watson GS, Hyde K, Chapman D, Craft S. Effects of (β-hydroxybutyrate on cognition in memory-impaired adults. Neurobiol Aging 2004;25:311-314.

Regnery R, Martin M, Olson J. Naturally occurring ''Rochalimaea henselae'' infection in domestic cat. Lancet 1992;340:557–558.

Reich MR, Ohad, DB, Overall KL, Dunham AE. Electrocardiographic assessment of antianxiety medication in dogs and correlation with drug serum concentration. J Am Vet Med Assoc 2000; 216:1571–1575.

Reichler IM, Hubler M, Jöchle W, Trigg TE, Piché CA, Arnold S. The effect of GnRH analogs on urinary incontinence after ablation of the ovaries in dogs. Theriogenology 2003;60:1207-1216.

Reid J, Scott M, Nolan A. Development of a short form of the Glasgow Composite Measure Pain Scale (CMPS) as a measure of acute pain in the dog. Vet Anaesth Analgesia 2005;32:7.

Reiger I. Scent rubbing in carnivores. Carnivore 1979;2:17–25.

Reis DJ. Brain monamines in aggression and sleep. Clin Neurosurg 1971;18:471-502.

Reis DJ. The chemical coding of aggression in the brain. Advances Behav Biol 1974;10:125-150.

Reisner IR, Erb HN, Houpt KA. Risk factors for behavior related euthanasia among dominant-aggressive dogs: 110 cases (1989-1992). J Am Vet Med Assoc 1994;205:855-863.

Reisner IR, Hollis NE, Erb EN, Quimby FW. Friendliness to humans and defensive aggression in cats: the influence of handling and paternity. Physiol Behav 1994;55:1119-1124.

Reisner IR, Mann JJ, Stanley M, Huang YY, Houpt KA. Comparison of cerebrospinal fluid monoamine metabolite levels in dominant-aggressive and non-aggressive dogs. Brain Res 1996;714:57–64.

Rème CA, Kern DV, Hofmans J, Halsberghe C, Mombiela DV. Effect of S-adenosylmethionine tablets on the reduction of age-related mental decline in dogs: a dounle-blinded, placebo-controlled trial. Vet Ther 2008;9:69-82.

Remmers JE, Gautier H. Neural and mechanical mechanisms of feline purring. Respir Physiol 1972;16:351-361.

Rescorla RA, Wagner AR. A theory of Pavlovian conditioning: Variations in the effectiveness of reinforcement and nonreinforcement, Classical Conditioning II, Edited by Black AH, ProkasyWF, Appleton-Century-Crofts, New York, NY,1972.

Reynolds JN, Maitra R. Propofol and flurazepam act synergistically to potentiate GABA$_A$ receptor activation in human recombinant receptors. Eur J Pharmacol 1996;314:151-156.

Richards JE. Respiratory sinus arrhythmia predicts heart rate and visual responses during visual attention in 14–20 week old infants. Psychophysiology 1985;l22:101–108.

Riss J, Cloyd J, Gates J, Collins S. Benzodiazepines in epilepsy: pharmacology and pharmacokinetics. Acta Neurol Scand 2008;118:69-86.

Riva J, Marelli SP, Redaelli V, Bondiolotti GP, Sforzini E, Santoro MM, Carenzi C, Verga M, Luzi F. The effects of drug detection training on behavioral reactivity and blood neurotransmitter levels in drug detection dogs: a premilinary study. J Vet Behav: Clin Appl Res 2012;7:11-20.

Riva J, Marelli SP, Redaelli V, Sforzini E, Luzi F, Bondiolotti GP, Di Mari E, Verga M. Effect of training on behavioral reactivity and neurotransmitter levels in drug detection dogs. J Vet Behav: Clin Appl Res 2010;5:38-39.

Roberts T, McGreevy P, Valenzuela M. Human induced rotation and reorganization of the brain of domestic dogs. PLoS ONE 2010;5(7):e11946. doi:10.1371/journal.pone.0011946.

Robin S, Tacher S, Rimbault M, Vaysse A, Dréano S, André C, Hitte C, Galibert F. Genetic diversity of canine olfactory receptors. BMC Genomics 2009;10:21 doi:10.1186/1471-2164-10-21.

Robinson I. Behavioural development of the cat. In: The Waltham Book of Dog and Cat Behaviour, Ed. Thorne C. Pergamon Press, Oxford. 1992:53-64.

Robinson SR. Ontogeny of the area centralis in the cat. J Comp Neurol 1987;255:50–67.

Rodan I, Sundahl E, Carney H, Gagnon A-C, Heath S, Landsberg G, Seksel K, Yin S. AAFP and ISFM feline-friendly handling guidelines. JFMS 2011;13:364-375.

Romand R, Ehret G. Development of sound production in normal, isolated, and deafened kittens during the first postnatal months. Dev Psychobiol 1984;17:629–649.

Romans CW, Conzemius MG, Horstman CL, Gordon WJ, Evans RB. Use of pressure platform gait analysis in cats with and without bilateral onychectomy. Am J Vet Res 2004; 65: 1276-1278.

Romatowski J. Jugular veinipuncture for blood sample collection in cats. J Am Vet Med Assoc 2012,240;806-807.

Rooney NJ, Bradshaw JWS. An experimental study of the effects of play upon the dog–human relationship. Appl Anim Behav Sci 2002;75:161–176.

Rooney NJ, Bradshaw JWS. The effects of play upon dominance and attachment dimensions of the dog–owner relationship. J Appl AnimWelf Sci 2003;6:67–94.

Rooney NJ, Bradshaw JWS. Breed and sex differences in the behavioural attributes of specialist search dog—a questionnaire survey of trainers and handlers. Appl Anim Behav Sci 2004;86;123–135.

Rooney NJ, Bradshaw JWS, Robinson IH. Do dogs respond to play signals given by humans? Anim. Behav 2001;61:715-722.

Rooney NJ, Cowan S. Training methods and owner-dog interactions: links with dog behaviour and learning ability. Appl Anim Behav Sci 2011;132:169-177.

Rooney NJ, Gaines SA, Bradshaw JWS. Behavioural and glucocorticoid responses of dogs (Canis familiaris) to kennelling: investigating mitigation of stress by prior habituation. Physiol Behav 2007;92:847–854.

Rooney N, Gaines S, Hiby E. A practitioner's guide to working dog welfare. J Vet Behav: Clin Appl Res 2009;4:127-134.

Roozendaal B, Hahn EL, Nathan SV, de Quervain DJF, McGaugh JL. Glucocorticoid effects on memory retrieval require concurrent noradrenergic activity in the hippocampus and basolateral amygdala. J. Neurosci 2004;24:8161-8169.

Roozendaal B, Okuda S, Van der Zee EA, McGaugh JL. Glucocorticoid enhancement of memory requires arousal-induced noradrenergic activation in the baso lateral amygdala PNAS 2006;103: 6741-6746.

Rosado B, Garcia-Belenguer S, Leon M, Chacon G, Villegas A, Palacio J. Blood concentrations of serotonin, cortisol and debydroepiandrosterone in aggressive dogs. Appl Anim Behav Sci 2010;123:124-130.

Rosado B, Garcia-Belenguer S, Palacio J, Chacon G, Villegas A, Alcalde AI. Serotonin transporter activity in platelets and canine aggression. Vet J 2010;186:104-105.

Rosecrans JA, Watzman N, Buckley JP. The production of hypertension in male albino rats subjected to experimental stress. Biochem Pharmacol 1966;15:1707-1718.

Roselli CE, Resko JA. Testosterone regulates aromatase activity in discrete brain areas of male rhesus macaques. Biol Reproduction 1989;40:929-934.

Rosenbaum JF, Fava M, Hoog, Ascroft RC, Krebs WB. Selective serotonin reuptake discontinuation syndrome: a randomized clinical trial. Biol Psychiatry 1998:44:77-87.

Rosenblatt JS. Stages in the early behavioural development of altricial young of non-primate animals. In: Growing Points in Ethology, Eds. Hinde RA, Bateson PPG. New York: Cambridge University Press, 1976:345-383.

Rosenblatt JS, Turkewitz G, Schneirla TC. Early socialization in the domestic cat as based on feeding and other relationships between female and young. In Determinants of Infant Behavior, Ed. Foss BM. London: Methuen & Co., Ltd. 1961:51-74.

Rosenblatt JS, Turkewitz G, Schneirla TC. Development of suckling and related behavior in neonate kittens, In: Roots of Behavior, Ed. Bliss EL. Hoeber, New York, NY. 1962:198-210.

Roshier AL, McBride EA. Veterinarians' perception of behaviour support in small animal practice. Vet REC 2012a, doi: 10.1136/vr.101124.

Roshier AL, McBride EA. Canine behaviour problems: dicussions between veterinarians and dog owners during annual booster consultations. Vet REC 2012b, doi: 10.1136/vr.101125.

Rothschild AJ. Disinhibition, amnestic reactions, and other adverse reactions secondary to triazolam: a review of the literature. J Clin Psychiatry 1992;53(suppl):69-79.

Rothschild AJ, Shindul-Rothschild JA, Viguera A, Murray, Brewster S. Comparison of the frequency of behavioral disinhibition on alprazolam, clonazepam, or no benzodiazepine in hospitalized psyschiatric patients. J Clin Psychopharmacol 2000;20:7-11.

Roudebush, P, Zicker SC, Cotman CW, Milgram NW, Muggenburg BA, Head E. Nutritional management of brain aging in dogs. J Am Vet Med Assoc 2005;227:722-728.

Rowell TE. A quantitative comparison of the behaviour of a wild and a caged baboon group. Anim Behav 1967;5:499-509.

Rowell TE. The Social Behavior of Monkeys. Penguin, Harmondsworth, 1972.

Rowell TE. The concept of social dominance. Behav Biol 1974;11:131-154.

Ru G, Terracini B, Glickman LT. Host-related risk factors for canine osteosarcoma. Vet J 1998; 156:31–39.

[S].

Sacks JL, Sattin RW, Bonzo SE. Dog bite-related fatalities from 1979 through 1988. JAMA 1989;262:1489–1492.

Sadzuka Y, Sugiyama T, Suzuki T, Sonobe T. Enhancement of the activity of doxorubicin by inhibition of glutamate transporter. Toxicol. Lett. 2001;123:159–167.

Saetre P, Lindberg J, Leonard JA, Ilsson K, Pettersson U, Ellegran H, Bergström TF, Vilà C, Jazin E. From wild wolf to domestic dog: gene expression changes in the brain. Mol Brain Res 2004;126:198-206.

Salazar I, Sánchez-Quinteiro P. A detailed morphological study of the vomeronasal organ and the accessory olfactory bulb of cats. Microsc Res Tech. 2011;74:1109-20. doi: 10.1002/jemt.21002.

Sales G, Hubrecht R, Peyvandi A, Milligan S, Shield B. Noise in dog kennelling: Is barking a welfare problem for dogs? Appl Anim Behav Sci 1997;52:321-329.

Salman MD, Hutchison J, Ruch-Gallie R, Kogan L, New JC, Kass PH, Scarlett JM. Behavioral reasons for relinquishment of dogs and cats to 12 shelters. J Appl Anim Welf Sci 2000;3:93-106.

Salman MD, New J, Scarlett JM, Kass PH, Ruch-Gallie R, Hetts S. Human and animal factors related to relinquishment of dogs and cats in 12 selected animal shelters in the United States. J. Appl Anim Welf Sci 1998;1:207-226.

Salmeri KR, Bloomberg MS, Scruggs SL, Shille V. Gonadectomy in immature dogs: Effects on skeletal, physical, and behavioral development. J Am Vet Med Assoc 1991;198:1193-1203.

Salter M, Pogson CI. The role of tryptophan 2,3-dioxygenase in the hormonal control of tryptophan metabolism in isolated rat liver cells. Effects of glucocorticoids and experimental diabetes. Biochem J 1985;229:499–504.

Sam M, Vora S, Malinc B, Ma W, Novotny MV, Buck LB. Odorants may arouse instinctive behaviours. Nature 2001;412:142. doi:10.1038/35084137.

Sanguinetti-Morelli D, Angelakis E, Richet H, Davoust B, Rolain JM, Raoult D. Seasonality of cat-scratch disease, France, 1999–2009. Emerg Infect Dis 2011;17:705–707.

Sano T, Nishimura R, Mochizuki M, Sasaki N. Effects of midazolam-butorphanol, acepromazine-butorphanol and medetomidine on an induction dose of propofol and their compatibility in dogs. J Vet Med Sci 2003;65:1141-3.

Santarelli L, Saxe M, Gross C, Surget A, Battaglia F, Dulawa S, Weisstaub N, Lee J, Duman R, Arancio O, Belzung C, Hen R. Requirement of hippocampal neurogenesis for the behavioral effects of antidepressants. Science 2003;301:805-809.

Sapolsky RM. Depression, antidepressants, and the shrinking hippocampus. PNAS 2011;98:12320–12322.

Sarter M, Markowitsch HJ. Involvement of the amygdala in learning and memory: A critical review, with emphasis on anatomical relations. Behav Neurosci 1985;99:342-380.

Sartor LL, Trepanier LA, Kroll MM, Rodan I, Challoner L. Efficacy and safety of transdermal methimazole in the treatment of cats with hyperthyroidism. J Vet Intern Med 2004;18:651-655.

Savaskan E, Ehrhardt R, Schulz A, Walter M, Schächinger H. Post-learning intranasaloxytocin modulates human memory for facial identity. Psychoneuroendocrin 2008;33:368-374.

Savolainen P, ZhangYP, Luo J, Lundeberg J, Leitner T. Genetic evidence for an East Asian origin of domestic dogs. Science 2002;298:1610-1613.

Sawyer LS, Moon-Fanelli AA, Dodman NH. Psychogenic alopecia in cats: 11 cases (1993-1996). J Am Vet Med Assoc 1999;214L7174.

Scahill L, Chappell PB, Kim YS, Schultz RT, Katsovich L, Shepherd E, Arnsten AFT, Cohen DJ, Leckman JF. A placebo-controlled study of guanfacine in the treatment of children with tic disorders and attention deficit hyperactivity disorder. Am J Psych 2001;158:1067-1074.

Scarlett JM, Salman MD, New J, Kass PH. Reasons for relinquishment of companion animals in U.S. animal shelters: selected health and personal issues. J Appl Anim Welf Sci 1999;2:41-57.

Schafe GE, Nader K, Blair HT, LeDoux JE. Memory consolidation of Pavlovian fear conditioning: a cellular and molecular perspective. Trends Neurosci 2001;24:540-546.

Schalke E, Stichnoth J, Ott S, Jones-Baade R. Clinical signs caused by the use of electric training collars on dogs in everyday life situations. Appl Anim Behav Sci 2007;105:369-380.

Schatzberg AM, Nemeroff CB. The American Psychiatric Publishing Textbook of Psychopharmacology, 3rd Edition, Washington, DC, 2004.

Scheifele P, Martin D, Clark JG, Kemper D, Wells J. Effect of kennel noise on hearing in dogs. Am J Vet Res 2012;73:482-489.

Schemera B, Blumsack JT, Cellino AF, Quiller TD, Hess BA, Rynders PE. Evaluation of otoacoustic emissions in clinically normal alert puppies. Am J Vet Res 2011;72:295-301.

Schenkel LR. Submission: its features and function in the wolf and dog. Amer Zool 1967;7:319-329.

Schilder MB, van der Borg JA. Training dogs with help of the shock collar: short and long term behavioural effects. Appl Anim Behav Sci 2004;85:319-334.

Schilder MGH, Netto WJ. On punishment and aggression. ABCN 1991;8(3):2-3.

Schipper LL, Vinke CM, Schilder MBH, Spruijt BM. The effect of feeding enrichment toys on the behaviour of kennelled dogs (Canis familiaris). Appl Anim Behav Sci 2008;114:182-195.

Schmidt HD, Duman RS. The role of neurotrophic factors in adult hipoocampal neurogenesis, antidepressant treatments and animal models of depressive-like behavior. Behav Pharmacol 2007;18:391-418.

Schmidt HD, Duman RS. Peripheral BDNF produces antidepressant-like effects in cellular and behavioral models. Neuropsychopharmacology 2010;35: 2378-2391.

Schmidt PM, Chakraborty PK, Wildt DE. Ovarian activity, circulating hormones and sexual behavior in the cat. II. Relationships during pregnancy, parturition, lactation, and the postpartum estrus. Biol Reprod 1983;28:657-671.

Schneider BM, Dodman NH, Maranada L. Use of meantime in treatment of canine compulsive disorders. J Vet Behav: Clin Appl Res 2009;4:118-126.

Schneider R, Dorn CR, Taylor DO. Fctors influencing canine mammary cancer development and postsurgical survial. J Natl Cancer Inst 1969;43:1249-1261.

Schneirla TC, Rosenblatt JS, Tobach E. Maternal behavior in the cat. In: Maternal Behavior in Mammals, Ed. Rheingold HR. New York: John Wiley. 1963:122-168.

Schoon A, Groth Berntsen T. Evaluating the effect of early neurological stimulation on the development and training of mine detection dogs. J Vet Behav: Clin Appl Res 2011;6:150-157.

Schwartz MA, Koechlin BA, Postma E, Palmer S, Krol G. Metabolism of diazepam in rat, dog, and man. J Pharm Exper Ther 1965; 149:423–35.

Schwartz S. Separation anxiety syndrome in cats: 136 cases (1991-2000). J Am Vet Med Assoc 2002;220:1028-1033.

Scorza FA, Cavalheiro EA, Arida RM, Terra VC, Scorza CA, Riberio MO, Cysneiros RM. Positive impact of omega-3 fatty acid supplementation in a dog with drug-resistant epilepsy: A case study. Epilepsy Behav 2009;15:527-528.

Scott JP. The process of primary socialization in canine and human infants. Monograph Soc Res Child Devel 1963;28:1-47.

Scott JP, Fuller JL. Genetics and the Social Behavior of the Dog. University of Chicago Press, Chicago, 1965.

Sechzer JA, Brown JL. Color discrimination in the cat. Science 1964;144:427-429.

Segall S. Opium addiction in the dog. J Am Vet Med Assoc 196;144:603-604.

Segurson SA, Serpell JA, Hart BL. Evaluation of a behavioral assessment questionnaire for use in the characterization of behavioral problems of dogs relinquished to animal shelters. J Amer Vet Med Assoc 2005;227:1755–1761.

Seitz PFD. Infantile experience and adult behaviour in animal subjects: age of separation from mother and adult behavior in the cat. Psychosom Med 1959;21:353-378.

Seksel K. Training Your Cat, Hyland House, Australia, 2001.

Seksel K, Lindemann MJ. Use of clomipramine in the treatment of anxiety-related and obsessive-compulsive disorders in cats. Aust Vet J 1998;76:317-321.

Seksel K, Lindemann MJ. Use of clomipramine in treatment of obsessive-compulsive disorder, separation anxiety and noise phobia in dogs: a preliminary, clinical study. Aust Vet J 2001;79:252-256.

Seligman ME. Phobias and preparedness. Behav Ther 1971;2:307–320.

Selye H. The concept of stress as it appears in 1952. Brux Med 1952;32:2383-2392.

Sentürk S, Yalçin E. Hypocholesterolaemia in dogs with dominance aggression. J Vet Med Series A. Physiol Path ClinMed 2003;50:339–342.

Serpell JA, Hsu Y. Development and validation of a novel method for evaluating behavior and temperament in guide dogs. Appl Anim Behav Sci 2001;72:347-364.

Shaikh MB, Dalsass M, Siegal A. Opioidergic mechanisms mediating aggressive behavior in the cat. Aggr Behav 1990;16:191-206.

Shepherd K. The Canine Commandments. Broadcast Books, Bristol, UK, 2007.

Shell LG. Feline hyperethesia syndrome. Feline Pract 1994;22:10.

Sherman BL, Gruen ME, Meeker RB, Milgram B, DiRivera C, Thomson A, Clary G, Hudson L. The use of a T-maze to measure cognitive-motor function in cats (Felis catus). J Vet Behav: Clin Appl Res 2013;8:32-39.

Sherman CK, Reisner IR, Taliaferro LA, Houpt KA. Characteristics, treatment, and outcome of 99 cases of aggression between dogs. Appl Anim Behav Sci 1996;47:91–108.

Shoblock JR, Sullivan EB, Maisonneuve IM, Glick SD. Neurochemical and behavioral differences between d-methamphetamine and d-amphetamine in rats. Psychopharmacology 2003;165:359-369.

Shore ER. Returning a recently adopted companion animal: adopters' reasons for and reactions to the failed adoption experience. J Appl Anim Welf Sci 2005;8:187-198.

Shore ER, Girrens K. Characteristics of animals entering an animal control or humane society shelter in a midwestern city. J Appl Anim Welfare Sci 2001;4:105-116.

Shore ER, Peterse CL, Douglas DK. Moving as a reason for pet relinquishment: a closer look. J Appl Anim Welf Sci 2003;6:39-52.

Shuler CM, DeBess EE, Lapidus JA, Hedberg K. Canine and human factors related to dog bite injuries. J Amer Vet Med Assoc 2008;232:542–546.

Shyan MR, Fortune KA, King C. Bark parks—a study on interdog aggression in a limited-control environment. JAAWS 2003;6:25-32.

Siegel A, Pott CB. Neural substrate of aggression and flight in the cat. Prog Neurobiol 1988;31:261–283.

Siegel A, Shaikh JB. The neural bases of aggression and rage in the cat. Aggr Violent Behav 1997;2:241–271.

Sih A, Bell A, Johnson JC. Behavioral syndromes: an ecological and evolutionary overview. Trends Ecol Evol 2004;19:372–378.

Simko J, Horacek J. Carbamazepine and risk of hypothyroidism: a prospective study. Acta Neurologica 2007;116:317-321.

Simpson BS, Papich MG. Pharmacologic management in veterinary behavioral medicine. Vet Clin North Am: Small Anim Pract 2003;33:365-404.

Simpson BS, Landsberg GM, Reisner IR, Ciribassi IR, Horwitz D, Houpt KA, Kroll TL, Luescher A, Moffat KS, Douglass G, Robertson-Plouch C, Veenhuizen MF, Zimmerman A, Clark TP. Effects of Reconcile (fluoxetine) chewable tablets plus behaviour management for canine separation anxiety. Vet Therapeutics 2007;8:18-31.

Simonson M. Effects of maternal malnourishment, development, and behavior in successive generations in the rat and cat. In: Malnutrition, Environment, and Behavior, Ed. Levisky DA. Cornell University Press: Ithaca, NY. 1979:133-148.

Singh L, Lewis AS, Field MJ, Hughes J, Woodruff GN. Evidence for involvement of the brain cholecystokinin B receptor in anxiety. PNAS USA 1991;88:1130-1133.

Siwak CT, Tapp PD, Head E, Zicker SC, Murphey HL, Muggenburg BA, Ikeda-Douglas CJ, Cotman CW, Milgram NW. Chronic antioxidant and mitochondrial cofactor administration improves discrimination learning in aged but not young beagles. Prog Neuro-Psychopharm Biol Psych 2005;29: 461-469.

Siwak-Tapp CT, Head E, Muggenburg BA, Milfram NW, Cotman CW. Region specific neuron loss in the aged canine hippocampus is reduced by enrichment. Neurobiol Aging 2008;29:39-50.

Slabbert JM, Rasa OAE. Observational learning of an acquired maternal behavior pattern by working dog pups: an alternative training method? Appl Anim Behav Sci 1997;53:309-316.

Slabbert JM, Rasa OA. The effect of early separation from the mother on pups in bonding to humans and pup health. J S Afr Vet Assoc 1993;64:4-8.

Slotnick B, Restrepo D, Schellinck H, Archbold G, Price S and Lin W. Accessory olfactory bulb function is modulated by input from the main olfactory epithelium. Eur J Neurosci 2010;31:1108–1116.

Smirnova T, Laroche S, Errington ML, Hicks AA, Bliss TVP, Mallet J. Transsynaptic expression of a presynaptic glutamate receptor during hippocampal long-term potentiation. Science 1993b;262: 433-436.

Smirnova T, Stinnakre J, Mallet J. Characterization of a presynaptic glutamate receptor. Science 1993a;262:430-433.

Smith BA, Jansen GR. Brain development in the feline. Nutr Rep Int 1977a;16:487-495.

Smith BA, Jansen GR. Maternal undernutrition in the feline: brain composition of offspring. Nutr Rep Int 1977b;16:497-512.

Smith BA, Jansen GR Maternal undernutrition in the feline: behavioral sequelae. Nutr Rep Int 1977c;16:513-526.

Smith DW, Gong BT. Scalp-hair patterning: Its origin and significance relative to early brain and upper facial development. Teratology 1974;9:17-34.

Smith KS, Berridge KC, Aldridge JW. Disentangling pleasure from incentive salience and learning signals in brain reward circuitry. PNAS 2011;108:E255-E264. Doi: 10.1073/pnas.1101920108.

Smith WJ. Message, meaning and context in ethology. Am Nat 1965;99:405-509.

Smith WJ. The Behaviour of communicating. An Ethological Approach. Harvard University Press, Cambridge, MA, 1997.

Soderstrom H, Blennow K, Manhem A, Forsman A. CSF studies in violent offenders. I. 5-HIAA as a negative and HVA as a positive predictor of psychopathy. J Neural Trans 2001;108:869–878.

Sohn RS, Ferrendelli JA. Anticonvulsant drug mechanisms. Phenytoin, phenobarbital, and ethosuximide and calcium flux in isolated presynaptic endings. Arch Neurol 1976;33:626-629.

Song Z, Wixted JT, Hoplins RO, Squires L. Impaired capacity for familiarity after hippocampal damage. PNAS 2011;108: 9655-9660.

Sorenmo KU, GoldschmidtM, Shofer F, Goldkamp C, Ferracone J. Immunohistochemical characterization of canine prostatic carcinoma and correlation with castration status and castration time. Vet Comp Oncol 2003;1:48–56.

Sorenmo KU, Shofer FS, Goldschmidt MH. Effect of spaying and timing of spaying on survival of dogs with mammary carcinoma. J Vet Intern Med 2000;14:266-270.

Sowell ER, Thompson PM, Holmes CJ, Jernigan TL, Toga AW. *In vivo* evidence for post-adolescent brain maturation in frontal and striatal regions. Nature Neurosci 1999;2:859–861. doi: 10.1038/13154.

Spain CV, Scarlett JM, Houpt KA. Long-term risks and benefits of early-age gonadectomy in dogs. JAVMA 2004;224:380-387.

Spencer L. Behavioral services in a practice lead to quality relationships. J Am Vet Med Assoc 1993;203:940-941.

Spinka M, Newberry RC, Bekoff M. Mammalian play: training for the unexpected. QuartRev Biol 2001;76:141e.

Sprague RH, Anisko JJ. Elimination patterns in the laboratory beagle. Behaviour 1973;47:257-267.

Steigerwald ES, Martin S, Philip M, Podell M. Effects of feline immunodeficiency virus on cognition and behavioral function in cats. J Acquired Immune Def Syn Human Retrovir 1999;20:411-419.

Steiss JE, Schaffer C, Ahmad HA, Voith VL. Evaluation of plasma cortisol levels and behaviour in dogs wearing bark control collars. Appl Anim Behav Sci 2007;106:96-106.

Sternbach H. The serotonin syndrome. Am J Psychiatry 1991;148:705-713.

Steur ER. Chemical and surgical castration of male dogs: behavioral effects. Doctoral Thesis University of Utrecht, Utrecht, Holland, 2011.

Stogdale L, Delack JB. Feline purring. Comp Cont Educ Pract Vet 1985;7:551-553.

Stowers L, Marton TF. What is a pheromone? Mammalian pheromones reconsidered. Neuron 2005;46:699–702.

Studinski CM, L-A Christis, Araujo JA, Burnham WM, Head, Cotman CW, Milgram NW. Visuospatial function in the beagle dog: An early marker of cognitive decline in a model of human aging and dementia. Neurobiol Learn Mem 2006;86:197-204.

Studzinski CM, MacKay WA, Beckett TL, Henderson ST, Murphy MP, Sullivan PG, Burnham WM. Induction of ketosis may improve mitochondrial function and decrease steady-state amyloid-β precursor protein (APP) levels in the aged dog. Brain Res 2008;1226:209-217.

Sung W, Crowell-Davis SL. Elimination behaviour patterns of domestic cats (*Felis catus*) with and without elimination behaviour problems. Am J Vet Res 2006;67:1500-1504.

Sutter NB, Eberle MA, Parker HG, Pullar BJ, Kirkness EF, Kruglyak L, Ostrander E. Extensive and breed-specific linkage disequilibrium in *Canis familiaris*. Genome Res 2004;14:2388-2396.

Sutter NB, Ostrander EA. Dog star rising: the canine genetic system. Nature Reviews Genetics 2004;5:900-910.

Suzuki S, Yamatoya H, Sakai M, Kataoka A, Furushiro M, Kudo S. Oral administration of soybean lecithin transphosphatidylate phosphatidylserine improves memory impairment in aged rats. J. Nutr 2001;131:2951–2956.

Svartberg K., Tapper I., Temrin H., Radesäter T., Thorman S.. Consistency of personality traits in dogs. Anim Behav 2005;69:283-291.

Svenningsson P, Chergui K, Rachleff I, Flajolet M, Zhang X, El Yacoubi M, Vaugeois J-M, Nomikos GG, Greengard P. Alterations in 5-HT1B receptor function by p11 in depression-like states. Science 2006; 311:77-80.

Swanson KS, Vester BM, Apanavicius CJ, Kirby NA, Schook LB. Implications of age and diet on canine cerebral cortex transcription. Neurobiol Aging 2009;30:1314-1326.

Syme GJ. Competitive orders as measures of social dominance. Anim Behav 1974;22:931–940.

Szetei V, Miklósi Á, Topál J, Csányi V. When dogs seem to lose their nose: an investigation on the use of visual and olfactory cues in communicative context between dog and owner. Appl Anim Behav Sci 2003;83:141-153.

[T].

Tacher S, Quignon P, Rimbault M, Dreano S, Andre C, Galibert F. Olfactory receptor sequence polymorphism within and between breeds of dogs. J Hered 2005;96:812–816.

Taglialatela JP, Russell JL, Schaeffer JA, and Hopkins WD. Communicative signaling activates 'Broca's' homolog in chimpanzees. Curr Biol 2008;18:343-348.

Taha AY, Henderson ST, Burnham WM. Dietary enrichment with medium chain triglycerides (AC-1203) elevates polyunsaturated fatty acids in the parietal cortex of aged dogs: implications for treating age-related cognitive decline. Neurochem Res 2009; 34: 1619-1625.

Taheri S, Zeitzer JM, Mignot E. The role of hypocretins (orexins) in sleep regulation and narcolepsy. Ann Rev Neurosci 2002;25: 283-313.

Takeuchi Y, Ogata N, Houpt KA, Scarlett JM. Difference in background and outcome of three behavior problems of dogs. Appl Anim Behav Sci 2001;70:297–308.

Takeuchi Y, Uetsuka K, Murayama M, Kikuta F, Takashima A, Doi K, Nakayama H. Complementary distributions of amyloid-β and neprilysin in the brains of dogs and cats. Vet Pathol 2008; 45:455-466.

Tami G, Gallagher A. Description of the behaviour of domestic dog (*Canis familiaris*) by experienced and inexperienced people. Appl Anim Behav Sci 2009;120:159-169.

Tan PL, Counsilman JJ. The Influence of weaning on prey-catching behaviour in kittens. Zeit Tierpsycol 1985;70:148–164.

Taubøll E, Gjerstad L. Comparison of 5 alpha-pregnan-3 alpha-ol-20-one and phenobarbital on cortical synaptic activation and inhibition studied in vitro. Epilepsia 1993;34:228-35.

Taylor AM, Reby D, McComb K. Human listeners attend to size information in domestic dog growls. J Acoustical Soc Amer 2008;123:2903–2910.

Taylor AM, Reby D, McComb K. Context-related variation in the vocal growling behaviour of the domestic dog (*Canis familiaris*). Ethology 2009;115: 905–915.

Taylor AM, Reby D, McComb K. Size communication in domestic dog, Canis familiaris, growls. Anim Behav 2010;79:205-210.

Tenter AM, Heckeroth AR, Weiss LM. Toxoplasma gondii: from animals to humans. Int J Parasitol 2000;30:1217-1258.

Teske E, Naan EC, van Dijk EM, Van Garderen E, Schalken JA. Canine prostate carcinoma: epidemiological evidence of an increased risk in castrated dogs. Mol Cell Endocrinol 2002;197:251-255.

Thesen A, Steen JB, Døving KB. Behaviour of dogs during olfactory tracking. J Exp Biol 1993;180:247–251.

Thompson WR, Heron W. The effects of restricting early experience on the problem-solving capacity of dogs. Can J Psychol 1954;8:17-31.

Thorne CJ. Feeding behavior in the cat – recent advances. J Sm Anim Pract 1982;23:555-562.

Thornton WE. Tricyclic antidepressant and cardiovascular drug interactions. Am Fam Physician 1979;20(1):97-9.

Tobias KM, Marioni-Henry K, Wagner R. A retrospective study on the use of acepromazine maleate in dogs with seizures. J Am Anim Hosp Assoc 2006;42:283-289.

Tod E, Brander D, Waran N. Efficacy of dog appeasing pheromone in reducing stress and fear related behaviour in shelter dogs. Appl Anim Behav Sci 2005;93:295–308.

Tompkins DC, Steigbigel RT. *Rochalimaea's* role in cat scratch disease and bacillary angiomatosis. Ann Intern Med 1993;118:388-390.

Toner BS, Miller DI. Olfactory discrimination of individual human odors using experienced tracking police and work dogs. Anim Behav Consult Newsletter 1993;10(4):2-4.

Topál J, Miklósi Á, Csányi V. Dog-human relationship affects problem solving behavior in dogs. Anthrozoös 1997;10:214-224.

Topál J, Miklósi Á, Csányi V, Dóka A. Attachment behavior in dogs (*Canis familiaris*): a new application of Ainsworth's (1969) strange situation test. J Comp Psychol 1998;112:219–229.

Torda A. Toxoplasmosis. Are cats really the source? Aust Fam Physician 2001;30:743-747.

Tóth L, Gácsi M, Topál J, Miklósi A. Playing styles and possible causative factors in dogs' behavior when playing with humans. Appl Anim Behav Sci 2008;114:473-484.

Truss M, Beato M. Steroid hormone receptors: interaction with deoxy-ribonucleic acid and transcription factors. Endocr Rev 1993;14:459-479.

Trut LN. Experimental studies of eary canine domestication. In: The Genetics of the Dog, Ed. Ruvinsky A, Sampson J. CABI Publishing, UK, 2001: 15-41.

Tucker AO, Tucker SS. Catnip and the catnip response. Econ Bot 1988;42:214–231.

Tulving E. Episodic memory: from mind to brain. Annu Rev Psychol 2002;53:1–25.

Turner DC. Cat behaviour and the human–cat relationship. Animal Famil 1988;3:16–21.

Turner DC. The ethology of the human-cat relationship. Swiss Arch Vet Med 1991;133:63-70.

Turner DC, Feaver J, Mendl M, Bateson P. Variations in domestic cat behavior toward humans: a paternal effect. Anim Behav 1986;34:1980-19822.

Turner DC, Meister O. 1988, Hunting behavior of the domestic cat. In: The Domestic Cat: The Biology of Its Behavior, Ed. Turner DC, Bateson P. Cambridge University Press, Cambridge. 1988:111-121.

Turner DC, Mertens C. Home range size, overlap and exploitation in domestic farm cats. Behaviour 1986;99: 22-45.

Turner EH, Loftis JM, Blackwell AD. Serotonin a la carte: supplementation with the serotonin precursor 5-hydroxytryptophan. Pharmacol Ther 2006;109:325–38.

[U].

Uchida Y, Moon-Fanelli AA, dodman NH, Clegg MS, Keen CL. Serum concerntrations of zinc and copper in bull terriers with lethal acrodermatitis and tail-chasing behavior. Am J Vet Res 1997;58:808-810.

[V].

Väisänen MA-M, Valros AE, Hakaoja E, Raekallio MR, Vainio OM. Pre-operative stress in dogs – a preliminary investigation of behavior and heart rate variability in healthy hospitalized dogs. Vet Anaesth Analgesia 2005;32:158-167.

Våge J, Fatjó J, Menna N, Amat M, Nydal RG, Lingaas F. Behavioral characteristics of English Cocker Spaniels with owner-defined aggressive behavior. JVet Behav: Clin Appl Res 2008;3:248-254.

Våge J, Wade C, Biagi T, Fatjó J, Amat M, Lindblad-Toh K, Lingaas F. Association of dopamine- and serotonin-related genes with canine aggression. Genes Brain Behavior 2010;9:372-378.

van den Berg SM, Heuven HCM, van den Berg L, Duffy DL, Serpell JA. Evaluation of the C-BARQ as a measure of stranger-directed aggression in three common dog breeds. Appl Anim Behav Sci 2010;124:136–141.

van der Borg JAM, Beerda B, Ooms M, Silveira de Souza A, van Hagen M, Kemp B. Evaluation of behavior testing for human directed aggression in dogs. Appl Anim Behav Sci 2010;128:78-90.

van Hall G, Stromstad M, Rasmussen P, Jans O, Zaar M, Gam C, Quistorff B, Secher NH, Nielsen HB. Blood lactate is an important energy source for the brain. J Cerebral Blood Flow Metab 2009;29:112-1129.

Vandenbergh JG. The effects of gonadal hormones on the aggressive behaviour of adult golden hamsters (Mesocricetus auratus). Anim Behav 1971;19:589-594.

Verberne G, de Boer J. Chemocommunication among domestic cats, mediated by the olfactory and vomeronasal senses. I. Chemocommunication. Z Tierpsychol 1976;42:86-109.

Vermeire S, Audenaert K, Dobbeleir A, De Meester R, Vandermeulen E, Waelbers T, Peremans K. Regional cerebral blood flow changes in dogs with anxiety disorders measured with SPECT. Brain Imaging Behav 2009;3:342-349.

Vermeire S, Audenaert K, Dobbeleir A, Vandermeulen E, Waelbers T, Peremans K. A Cavalier King Charles dog with shadow chasing: Clinical recovery and normalization of the dopamine transporter binding after clomipramine treatment. J Vet Behav: Clin Appl Res 2010;5:345-349.

Vilà C, Maldonàdo JE, Wayne RK. Phylogenetic relationships, evolution, and genetic diversity of the domestic dogs. J Hered 1999;90:71–77.

Vilà C, Savolainen P, Maldonado JE, Amorim IR, Rice JE, Honeycutt RL, Crandall KA, Lundeberg J, Wayne RK. Multiple and ancient origins of the domestic dog. Science 1997;76:1687–1689.

Villablanca JR, Olmstead CE. Neurological development of kittens. Dev Psychobiol 1979;12:101-127.

Vochteloo JD, Koolhaas JM. Medial amygdala lesions in male rats reduce aggressive behavior: interference with experience. Physiol Behav 1987; 41: 99-102.

Voith VL, Borchelt PL. Diagnosis and treatment of dominance aggression in dogs. Vet Clin North Am Small Anim Pract 1982;12:655-663.

Voith VL, Wright JC, Danneman PJ. Is there a relationship between canine behavior problems and spoiling activity, anthropomorphism, and obedience training? Appl Anim Behav Sci 1992;34:263-272.

Volpe JJ. The Neurology of the Newborn. Saunders/Elsevier, St. Louis, 2008:97-98.

VonHoldt BM, Pollinger JP, Lohmueller KE, Han E, Parker HG, Quignon P, Degenhardt JD, Boyko AR, Earl DA, Auton A, Reynolds A, Bryc K, Brisbin A, Knowles JC, Mosher DS, Spady TC, Elkahloun A, Geffen E, Pilot M, Jedrzejewski W, Greco C, Randi E, Bannasch D, Wilton A, Shearman J, Musiani M, Cargill M, Jones PG, Qian Z, Huang W, Ding ZL, Zhang YP, Bustamante CD, Ostrander EA, Novembre J, Wayne RK. Genome-wide SNP and haplotype analyses reveal a rich history underlying dog domestication. Nature 2010;464:898-902.

[W].

Waagepetersen HS, Sonnewald U, Schousboe A. The GABA paradox: multiple roles as metabolite, neurotransmitter, and neurodifferentiative agents. J Neurochem 1999;73:1335–1342.

Wada N, Hori H, Tokuriki M. Electromyographic and kinematic studies of tail movement in dogs during treadmill locomotion. J. Morphol. 2003;217:105-113.

Walker DB, Walker JC, Cavnar PJ, Taylor JL, Pickel DH, Hall SB, Suarez, J.C.. Natualistic quantification of canine olfactory sensitivity. Appl. Anim. Behav. Sci. 2006;97:241-254.

Waller GR. Metabolism of plant terpenoids. Prog Chem Fats Other Lipids 1969;10:153-238.

Walther FR. Artiodactyla. In: How Animals Communicate, Ed. Sebeok TA. Indiana University Press, Bloomington, IN, 1977:655-714.

Wang K, Zhang H, Ma D, Bucan M, Glessner JT, Abrahams BS, Salyakina D, Imielinso M, Bradfield JP, Sleiman PMA, Kim CE, Hou C, Frackelton E, Chiavacci R, Takahashi N, Sakurai T, Rappaport E, Lajonchere CM, Munson J, Estes A, Kirvatska O, Piven J, Sonnenblick LI, Alvarez Retuerto AI, Herman EI, Dong H, Sweeney JA, Brune CW, Cantor RM, Bernier R, Gilbert JR, Cuccaro ML, McMahon WM, Miller J, State MW, Wassink TH, Coon H, Levy SE, Schultz RT, Nurnberger JI, Haines JL, Sutcliffe JS, Cook EH, Minshe NJ, Buxbaum JD, Dawson G, Grant SFA, Geschwind DH, Pericak-Vance MA, Schellengery GD, Hakonarson H. Common genetic variants on 5p14.1 associate with autism spectrum disorders. Nature 2009;459:528-533.

Ware WA, Hopper DL. Cardiac tumors in dogs: 1982-1995. J Vet Intl Med 1999;13:95-103.

Warner MH, Beckett GJ. Mechanisms behind the non-thyroidal illness syndrome: an update. J Endocrinol 2010;205:1-13.

Warner-Schmidt JL, Vanover KE, Chen EY, Marshal JJ, Greengard P. Antidepressant effects of selective serotonin reuptake inhibitors (SSRIs) are attenuated by antiinflammatory drugs in mice and humans. PNAS 2011;108:9262-9267.

Warren JM, Levy SJ. Fearfulness in female and male cats. Anim Learn Behav 1979;7:521-524.

Weaver ICG, Diorio J, Sickl JR, Szyf M, Meaney MJ. Early environmental regulation of hippocampal glucocorticoid receptor gene expression: characterization of intracellular mediators and potential genomic target sites. Annals NY Acad Sci 2004;1024:182-212.

Wedekind KJ, Zicker S, Lowry S, Paetau-Robinson I. 2002. Antioxidant status of adult beagles is affected by dietary antioxidant intake. J Nutr 2002;132:1658S-60S.

Wedge MK. The truth behind tramdol and antidepressants: An interaction of concern? CJP/RPC 2009;142:71-74.

Wedl M, Bauer B, Gracey D, Grabmayer C, Spielauer E, Day J, Kotrschal K. Factors influencing the temporal patterns of dyadic behaviours and interactions between domestic cats and their owners. Behav Proc 2011;86:58-67.

Wells DL. A review of environmental enrichment for kennelled dogs, Canis familiaris. Appl Anim Beh Sci 2004;85:307-317.

Wells DL. The effect of videotapes of animals on cardiovascular responses to stress. Stress Health 2005;21:209-213.

Wells DL, Graham L, Hepper PG. The influence of auditory stimulation on the behaviour of dogs housed in a rescue shelter. Anim Welf 2002;11:385-393.

Wells DL, Hepper PG. Male and female dogs respond differently to men and women. Appl Anim BehavSci 1999;61:341-349.

Welt T, Englemann M, Renner U, Erhardt A, Müller MN, Landgraf R, Holsboer F, Keck ME. Temazepam triggers the telease of vasopressin into the rat hypothalamic paraventricular nucleus: novel Insight into benzodiazepine action on hypothalamic–pituitary–adrenocortical system activity during stress. Neuropsychopharmacology 2006; 31:2573–2579.

Wemmer C, Scow K. Communication in the Felidae with emphasis on scent marking and contact patterns. In: How Animals Communicate, Ed. Sebeok TA. Indiana Univ. Press, Bloomington. 1977;749-766.

Wenzel BM. Tactile stimulation as reinforcement for cats and its relations to early feeding experiences. Psychol Rep 1959;5:297-300.

West M. Social play in the domestic cat. Amer Zool 1974;14:427-436.

West MJ. Play in domestic kittens. In: The Analysis of Social Interactions, Ed. Cairns, RB. Lawrence Erlbaum: Hillsidem New Jersey. 1979:179-193.

Westropp JL, Kass PH, Buffington CAT. Evaluation of the effects of stress in cats with idiopathic cystitis. Am J Vet Res 2006;67:731-736.

Wilson M, Warren JM, Abbott L. Infantile stimulation, activity, and learning by cats. Child Devel 1965;36:843-853.

Winslow CN. Observations of dominance-subordination in cats. J Genet Psychol 1938;52:425-428.

Winslow CN. Social behavior of cats. II. Competitive, aggressive and food-sharing behavior when both competitiors have access to the goal. J Comp Psychol 1944;37:315-326.

Wismer TA. Antidpressant drug overdoses in dogs. Vet Med 2000;95:520-525.

Wittenberg GM, Tsien JZ. An emerging molecular and cellular framework for memory processing by the hippocampus. Trends Neurosci 2002;25:501-505.

Wolf M, van Doorn SG, Leimar O, Weissing FJ. Life-history trade-offs favour the evolution of animal personalities. Nature 2007;447:581–584.

Wolfle TL. Understanding the role of stress in animal welfare: Practical Considerations. In: The Biology of Animal Stress – The Principles and Implications for Animal Welfare, Eds. Moberg GP, Mech JA. CABI Publishing, Wallingford, UK, 2000:355-368.

Wolpe J. The Practice of Behavior Therapy. Pergamon Press, Oxford, UK, 1969.

Wolski TR. Social behavior of the cat. Vet Clin North Am: Small Anim Pract 1982;12:693-706.

Wright JC, Amoss RT. Prevalence of house soiling and aggression in kittens during the first year after adoption from a humane society. J Am Vet Med Assoc 2004;224:1790–1795.

Wrubel KM, Moon-Fanelli A, Maranda LS, Dodman NH. Interdog household aggression: 38 cases (2006-2007). J Am Vet Med Assoc 2011;238:731–740.

Wyrwicka W. Imitation of mother's inappropriate food preference in weanling kittens. Pavlov J Biol Sci 1978;13:55-72.

[Y].

Yamane A. Male reproductive tactics and reproductive success of the group living cat (*Felis catus*). Behav Proc 1998;43:239-249.

Yau JLW, Noble J, Hibbert C, Rowe WB, Meaney MJ, Morris RGM, Seckl JR. Chronic treatment with the antidepressant amitriptyline prevents impairments in water maze learning in aging rats. J Neurosci 2002;22:1436-1442.

Yehuda R, Boisoneau D, Mson JW, Giller EL. Relationship between lymphocyute glucocorticoid receptor number and urinary-free cortisol excretion in mood, anxiety, and psychotic disorder. Biol. Psychiatry 1993;34:18-25.

Yehuda R, LeDoux J. Response variation following trauma: a translational neuroscience approach to understanding PTSD. Neuron 2007;56:19-32.

Yeon SC, Kim YK, Park SH, Lee SS, Lee SY, Suh EH, Houpt KA, Chang HH, Lee HC, Yang BG, Lee HJ. Differences between vocalization evoked by social stimuli in feral cats and house cats. Behav Proc 2011;87:183-9. doi: 10.1016/j.beproc.2011.03.003.

Yerkes RM, Dodson JD. The relation of strength of stimulus to rapidity of habit-formation. J Comp Neuro Psychol 1908;18:459–482. http://psychclassics.yorku.ca/Yerkes/Law/.

Yin S. A new perspective on barking in dogs (*Canis familiaris*). J Comp Psychol 2002;116:189-193.

Yin S. Low Stress Handling, Restraint and Behavior Modification of Dogs & Cats. Cattledog Publishing, Davis, CA, 2009.

Yin S, McCowan B. Barking in domestic dogs: context specificity and individual identification. Anim. Behav. 2004;68:343-355.

Yokota S, Ishikura Y, Ono H. Cardiovascular effects of paroxetine, a newly developed antidepressant, in anesthetized dogs in comparison with those of imipramine, amitriptyline and clomipramine. Jap J Pharm 1987:45:335–42.

Young MS. The evolution of domestic pets and companion animals. Vet Clin North Am: Sm Anim Pract 1985;15:297-309.

Young MS. Aggressive behavior. In: Clinical Signs and Diagnosis in Small Animal Practice, Ed. Ford RB. Churchill Livingstone, New York. 1988:135-150.

Yuan C, Mehendale S, Xiao Y, Aung HH, Xie J-T, Ang-Lee MK. The gamma-aminobutyric acidergic effects of valerian and valerenic acid on rat brainstem neuronal activity. Anesth Analg 2004;98:353–358.

Yudofsky SC, Silver JM, Jackson W, Endicott J, Williams D. The Overt Aggression Scale for the objective rating of verbal and physical aggression. Am J Psychiatry 1986;143:35-39.

Yudofsky SC, Silver JM, Schneider SE. Pharmacologic treatment of aggression. Psychiatric Annals 1987;17:397-407.

[Z].

Zajeka J, Fawcett J, Amsterdam J, Quitkin F, Reimherr F, Rosenbaum J, Michelson D, Beasley C. Safety of abrupt discontinuation of fluoxetine:a randomized, placebo-controlled study. J Clin Psychiatry 1998;18:193-197.

Zangwill KM, Hamilton DH, Perkins BA, Regnery RL, Plikaytis BD, Hadler JL, Cartter ML, Wenger JD. Cat scratch disease in Connecticut: Epidemiology, risk factors, and evaluation of a new diagnostic test. N Engl J Med 1993;329:8-13.

Zhang C, Hua T, Zhu Z, Luo X. Age-related changes in structures in cerebellar cortex of cat. J Biosciences 2006;31:55-60.

Zhang H-H, Sampogna S, Morales FR, Chase MH. Age-related changes in hypocretin (orexin) immunoreactivity in the ct brainstem. Brain Res 2002;l930:206-211.

Zulch HE, Mills DS, Lambert R, Kirberger RM. The use of tramadol in a Labrador retriever presenting with self-mutilation of the tail. J Vet Behav: Clin Appl Res 2012;7:252-258.

How to Use These Handouts and Protocols

It is impossible for the author of a textbook to know what is known by anyone who reads the text. Because of this, all the questionnaires and client handouts provided are extremely detailed.

Permission to Evaluate and Treat

Veterinarians frequently ask about consent forms for treatment. Because of the nature of behavioral cases, consent should be sought for permission to *evaluate and treat*. During the behavioral exam, some treatments may be discussed or implemented and behavioral techniques that can change the behavior of the dog or cat may be employed to learn if the dog or cat can do them, or if they affect the dog's or cat's behavior. A consent form that covers all of this and explains something about the appointment can prevent misunderstandings and help to create and manage reasonable expectations.

Questionnaires

There are two types of questionnaires: the "short" survey questionnaire for regular and universal use, and the long basic history questionnaire.

"Short" Survey Questionnaire

The "short" survey questionnaire is intended to be used at each visit so that you can learn if any of the common behaviors that signal the onset of true behavioral problems have appeared between visits. By using these forms at each visit, veterinarians will be able to ask the same questions in the same way to ensure some consistency in patterns of responses, and the information gained will allow veterinarians and their staffs to intervene early and in an organized and cogent manner in addressing potential or real behavioral concerns.

Behavioral issues in some guise are still responsible for the death, abandonment, or relinquishment of more pets than is any other class of problems. Behavioral problems are most easily prevented or treated early in their development.

The routine use of these short questionnaires creates the first step for organizing your practice as a "behavior-centered practice" that places the welfare and needs of the pets for whom you care as your primary concern.

As you learn more about behavior and the types of responses to the short form that characterize your patient population and demographic, you may be able to shorten the form. Some veterinarians with a lot of behavior training have four questions that they ask all clients, and a shorter form may work for you. Please remember that you have a staff and associates who may vary greatly in their knowledge of veterinary behavior and behavioral medicine. The short form of the questionnaire ensures that everyone has the same high level of baseline information available to inform their decisions and treatment advice. Patient populations differ and by adapting an extant questionnaire you can maintain thoroughness and quality.

Basic History Questionnaire

The long basic history questionnaire is for use in understanding true behavioral complaints and problems. After reviewing the short survey questionnaire, you may decide that the clients would benefit from a behavioral consultation. The clients would then complete this basic history questionnaire.

Depending on your routine intake forms, you may be able to delete some of the information about the clients. As you become more practiced in assessing problematic behaviors, you may decide to shorten these forms.

These forms have the advantage of being informed by decades of clinical experience by multiple specialists. Virtually all specialists use some version of an exhaustive history form, in part, because they need *a valid and legal record of the behavior consultation*. If you start to use these questionnaires for truly distressed clients and/or patients, you will see that they make clear patterns that are helpful to you for both diagnosis and treatment, and that may provide insight into etiology and sensitive issues that may require redress.

Because these long questionnaires require specific answers *not* influenced by personal opinion, you will also be able to use them to evaluate progress in treatment, and some of the potential causes of that. *Do not neglect the opportunity to explore open-ended answers or elaborations to whichever questions are relevant.* Not only is much of the useful information needed to successfully implement treatment in these discussions, but these discussions solidify good client relationships. The people who successfully help their pet through behavioral problems will seek care for complex medical problems as the pet ages. *Time spent on behavior and behavioral history taking is a superb investment.*

Client Handouts

For every condition and most situations discussed in this text there is an accompanying client handout. The pronouns used for dogs in these handouts are "he" or "she," not "it," and one randomly selected sex is used throughout the handout because "he and/or she" is cumbersome. Dogs and cats are living beings, so the interrogative pronoun "who" is used.

These handouts are organized into the following groups:
- Foundation protocols for use in *cats and dogs*
- Discharge instructions *specifically for dogs*
- Second tier of behavior modification protocols for *cats and dogs*
- Protocols for understanding and treating specific conditions in *cats*
- Protocols for understanding and treating specific conditions in *dogs*
- Protocols for treating specific conditions that affect *both dogs and cats*
- Protocols for using medication for *both dogs and cats*
- Protocols for understanding miscellaneous behaviors in *dogs and cats*
- Protocols for preventing problems for *dogs*
- Protocols for preventing problems for *cats*
- Protocols for preventing problems for *both dogs and cats*
- Resources

Within each group, each client handout is geared toward helping the client understand the specific behavioral concern while providing information about the strategies that can be used to improve the pet's behavior or redress the concerns/problems. For each topic, the handout explains what the condition is and how it usually develops, and makes an attempt to convey the distressed dog's or cat's perspective so that the clients can have a compassionate response to treatment and management.

These handouts are intended to give veterinarians and other professionals the dialog and words that they may not otherwise have to communicate about behavioral pathology and its redress. Veterinary training does not teach us to communicate with our patients or our clients. These handouts provide a patient and client tested, practical framework for discussions and explanations that can lead to successful and humane outcomes.

- Some of these handouts explain normal dog and cat behavior because clients often do not know what normal is (e.g., the **Protocol for Basic Manners Training and House Training for New Dogs and Puppies**).
- Some of these handouts contain specific and detailed behavior modification protocols that require the clients to behave in certain ways in order to teach their dogs and cats different behaviors (e.g., the **Protocol for Deference**; the **Protocol for Generalized Discharge Instructions for Dogs with Behavioral Concerns**; the **Protocol for Handling "Special-Needs Pets" During Holidays and Other Special Occasions**).

Regardless of the type of client handout, all of these handouts are written in plain English with *the client* as the intended audience. The content of these handouts *mirrors the information* in the text provided for veterinarians. Each of these handouts is referenced in the text with respect to specific conditions/problems/concerns, and cluster of handouts may be noted to be useful for intervention in specific problems.

Because no author can know how much either the veterinarian or client knows—or how well they communicate what they know with each other—these handouts err on the side of caution and assume that no one knows anything. *These handouts can be used as roadmaps for the veterinary staff to find the language and thought process to successfully communicate with their clients about behavioral concerns.* This is essential because most veterinary schools still offer no formal training programs in veterinary behavioral medicine and our patients suffer for that decision.

You can use most of these handouts to prevent and treat behavioral problems. You will want to give some of these handouts from the prevention and resource categories to anyone with a new dog/puppy or cat/kitten (e.g., the **Protocol for Teaching Cats and Dogs to "Sit," "Stay," and "Come"**; the **Protocol for the Introduction of a New Pet to Other Household Pets; Resources for Information, Tools, Books, Products and Other Help**).

Some of these handouts will allow your staff to successfully demonstrate the use of tools that will help most dogs (e.g., the **Protocol for Choosing Collars, Head Collars, Harnesses, and Leads**). Some of these handouts will benefit any client at certain life stages (e.g., the **Protocol for Introducing a New Baby and a Pet; the Protocol for Teaching Kids—and Adults—to Play with Dogs and Cats**).

All of these handouts are intended to keep dogs and cats healthy and happy and alive, so that they can become long-term patients in your practice. Providing humane, scientifically based care for pets with behavioral problems can make you wealthy and wise and help to keep you and your staff engaged. Happier, better behaved patients lower everyone's stress level. Appropriate use of these handouts will help.

How to Use the Handouts

You have three choices for how to use these handouts:

1. Hand them to clients and suggest that they read them.
2. Review key points with your clients and highlight areas on which you particularly wish them to concentrate.
3. Have someone on your staff—and it could be you—go over the handouts in detail to ensure that the clients understand them and have no questions. This also provides the opportunity to customize some of the recommendations for that particular patient and to provide some demonstrations.

However you choose to use them, these handouts give you the opportunity to have a real, ongoing, and beneficial dialog with your clients about the dogs and cats they love.

For the three foundation protocols (the **Protocol for Deference;** the **Protocol for Teaching Your Dog to Take a Deep Breath and Use Other Biofeedback Methods as Part of Relaxation;** the **Protocol for Relaxation: Behavior Modification Tier 1**), there is an accompanying video, *Humane Behavioral Care for Dogs: Problem Prevention and Treatment,* that explains and demonstrates the techniques and principles addressed in the handouts. Your clients would benefit from having their own copy of this video. This video may also help to explain the protocols to your staff and to any training professionals with whom you collaborate to help solve your clients' toughest problems.

Used appropriately, these handouts and the video will focus all of us and our best efforts on meeting the most common unmet need experienced by our patients: humane behavioral care and intervention. When we put the behavioral welfare needs of our patients first, all of us will have more fun.

Carpe diem!

LISTING OF CLIENT HANDOUTS AND QUESTIONNAIRES FOUND IN TEXT AND ON THE ACCOMPANYING WEBSITE

Questionnaires

- Permission to Evaluate and Treat
- Short Survey Questionnaire to Be Used at All Visits to Monitor Behavioral Changes in Cats
- Short Survey Questionnaire to Be Used at All Visits to Monitor Behavioral Changes in Dogs
- Basic History Questionnaire—Cats
- Basic History Questionnaire—Dogs

Client Handouts

Foundation protocols for use in *cats and dogs*

- Protocol for Deference
- Protocol for Teaching Your Dog to Take a Deep Breath and Use Other Biofeedback Methods as Part of Relaxation
- Protocol for Relaxation: Behavior Modification Tier 1

Discharge instructions *specifically for dogs*

- Protocol for Generalized Discharge Instructions for Dogs with Behavioral Concerns
- Protocol for Handling and Surviving Aggressive Events

Second tier of behavior modification protocols for *cats and dogs*

- Tier 2: Protocol for Teaching Your Dog to Uncouple Cues About Your Departures from the Departure
- Tier 2: Protocol for Desensitizing and Counter-Conditioning a Dog or Cat from Approaches from Unfamiliar Animals, Including Humans
- Tier 2: Protocol for Desensitization and Counter-Conditioning Using Gradual Departures
- Tier 2: Protocol for Desensitization and Counter-Conditioning to Noises and Activities That Occur by the Door
- Tier 2: Protocol for Desensitizing and Counter-Conditioning Dogs to Relinquish Objects
- Tier 2: Protocol for Desensitizing Dogs Affected with Impulse Control Aggression

Protocols for understanding and treating specific conditions in *cats*

- Protocol for Understanding and Treating Cats with Elimination Disorders and Elimination Behaviors That Concern Clients
- Protocol for Understanding and Treating Play Aggression in Cats
- Protocol for Understanding and Treating Feline Aggressions with an Emphasis on Intercat Aggression
- Protocol for Understanding, Managing and Treating Impulse Control/Status-Related Aggression in Cats

Protocols for understanding and treating specific conditions in *dogs*

- Protocol for Understanding and Treating Canine Panic Disorder
- Protocol for Understanding and Treating Dogs with Noise and Storm Phobias
- Protocol for Understanding and Treating Generalized Anxiety Disorder
- Protocol for Understanding, Managing, and Treating Dogs with Impulse Control Aggression
- Protocol for Understanding and Treating Dogs with Fear/Fearful Aggression

- Protocol for Understanding and Managing Dogs with Aggression Involving Food, Rawhide, Biscuits, and Bones
- Protocol for Understanding and Treating Dogs with Interdog Aggression
- Protocol for Understanding and Treating Dogs with Protective and/or Territorial Aggression
- Protocol for Understanding and Treating Dogs with Separation Anxiety

Protocols for treating specific conditions that affect *both dogs and cats*

- Protocol for Understanding and Treating Redirected Aggression in Cats and Dogs
- Protocol for Understanding and Treating Obsessive-Compulsive Disorder
- Protocol for Understanding and Helping Geriatric Animals
- Protocol for Preventing and Treating Attention-Seeking Behavior
- Protocol for Treating Fearful Behavior in Cats and Dogs

Protocols for using medication for *both dogs and cats*

- Protocol for Using Behavioral Medication Successfully
- Generalized Guidelines for Using Alprazolam for Noise and Storm Phobias, Panic, and Severe Distress
- Informed Consent Statements for the Most Commonly Used Medications

Protocols for understanding miscellaneous behaviors in *dogs and cats*:

- Protocol for Understanding and Managing Odd, Curious, and Annoying Canine Behaviors

- Protocol for Understanding Odd, Curious, and Annoying Feline Behaviors

Protocols for preventing problems for *dogs*

- Protocol for Choosing Collars, Head Collars, Harnesses, and Leads
- Protocol for Handling "Special-Needs Pets" During Holidays and Other Special Occasions
- Protocol for Basic Manners Training and Housetraining for New Dogs and Puppies
- Protocol for Assessing Pain and Stress in Dogs

Protocol for preventing problems for *cats*

- Protocol for Assessing Pain and Stress in Cats

Protocols for preventing problems for *both dogs and cats*

- Protocol for Introducing a New Baby and a Pet
- Protocol for the Introduction of a New Pet to Other Household Pets
- Protocol for Teaching Cats and Dogs to "Sit," "Stay," and "Come"
- Protocol for Teaching Kids—and Adults—to Play with Dogs and Cats
- Protocol for Choosing Toys for Your Pet
- Protocol for Activities for Clients to Practice with Puppies and Kittens

Resources

- Resources for Information, Tools, Books, Products, and Other Help

PERMISSION TO EVALUATE AND TREAT

Permission to evaluate and treat cats and dogs for behavioral complaints, concerns, problems and pathologies

A history form (provided) will need to be completed before we can evaluate your cat/dog. The information you provide on this form and during the appointment is considered confidential. Please keep a copy of the history form for your own records.

If you have had any behavioral evaluations or physical/laboratory exams done elsewhere it would be helpful if we had a copy before your appointment.

You may also be asked to provide a video and/or photos of your dog or cat. We request these because it is the best way to see the behaviors that concern you within the context of everyday life. The video should:
- Show the behavior(s) about which you are concerned, excepting any injurious behavior
- Give a brief tour of the dog's or cat's environment (house/apartment and yard)
- Show any other relevant facets of the patient's life (e.g., where your dog or cat sleeps, sits, eats, drinks, walks, plays, interaction with other animals, et cetera)

If aggression with injury is one of the complaints, ***please do not provide a video of the cat or dog biting someone, and do not put the cat or dog in a situation where any aggression may be provoked.*** If aggression is a concern, other behaviors will be indicative of it.

Videos and/or photos may also be taken during the appointment. Any videos/photos used to evaluate the patient become part of the record and may be used anonymously in all modes of teaching (including teaching staff or other clients) and/or research.

The appointment will start with your dog on a lead and/or your cat on a lead and harness or in a carrier. Further management of all interactions with humans and/or other animals is at the discretion of the clinician. This policy helps to keep everyone as safe as possible and distress the patient as little as possible.

Behavior appointments can be lengthy and the amount of time we schedule for the initial appointment and the plan for the appointment(s) will be explained when you schedule the appointment. By completing these forms and signing below, you give permission for us to evaluate, assess, formulate a treatment plan, and treat your cat or dog. You will receive a written copy of the discharge instructions and treatment plan, and we encourage you to comply with our recommendations and to ask questions at any time.

The evaluation, assessment, and treatment plan do not represent a guarantee of successful treatment. Few behavioral problems are truly cured, and responsible management is a factor for every patient.

If your dog or cat is aggressive, you should know the following:
- Any animal who is aggressive for any reason can do serious damage and harm.
- Special precautions must be taken to ensure that everyone is safe. These precautions may include some form of confinement (e.g., gates, crates) or the use of leads, harnesses, head collars, and/or muzzles.
- Proof of current rabies vaccination, where required by law, should accompany your completed history forms.
- Seeking treatment for a behavioral problem and/or treating a behavioral problem is not a substitute for adherence to local laws.
- Owning a cat and/or dog carries with it responsibilities, including responsibility/potential liability for any damage the dog and/or cat does to people or property. This responsibility is not changed/transferred by seeking behavioral help.
- Problems involving pathological behaviors, including aggression, are never cured but they can be well treated and managed, to the point where the dog or cat lives a happy, safe life. Failure to manage and treat these problems may lead to euthanasia. Even as a last resort, the death of a pet is an outcome that everyone would seek to avoid, if at all possible. *The point of this appointment is to provide humane care that allows your dog or cat to live a long and happy life.*

If you have any questions about this form or this history form, please ask. Clear communication helps produce the best outcomes.

Name of person responsible for the cat and/or dog: _____

Signature: _____

Date: _____

SHORT SURVEY QUESTIONNAIRES TO BE USED AT ALL VISITS TO MONITOR BEHAVIORAL CHANGES IN CATS

This short survey questionnaire can be used at **any and all visits** to check if the clients have any questions or complaints about their cat.

You have to remember that the clients might not even know that they have questions or complaints because they do not know what "normal" is. Also, if anything, myths about breeds, behavior, nature, and nurture are far more insidious in the client community than in the veterinary community. These questionnaires, when used at each visit, together with the other more detailed and specific tools provided, will tell you if further information is necessary and hint at some of the underlying factors contributing to the problems.

Clients may be uncomfortable with a behavior, but not know how to ask if it is abnormal. These questionnaires will give clients the vocabulary and opportunity to discuss their pet's behaviors with their veterinarian in an efficient, consistent, and meaningful way.

If you know nothing about veterinary behavioral medicine, these short questionnaires will walk you through most of what you will need to ask. If you are experienced in asking about behavioral issues, you can shorten these questionnaires considerably. The complete and detailed version is attached here because authors have no way of knowing what readers know.

Survey questionnaire about general cat behaviors—to be used at all visits:

1. Client(s):	2a. Today's date: ____ /____/____ 2b. Cat's date of birth: ____ /____/____ ☐ Estimated ☐ Known
3. Patient's name:	4a. Breed: 4b. Weight: _____ lb/_____ kg 4c. Sex: ☐ M ☐ MC ☐ F ☐ FS 4d. If your cat is castrated or spayed [neutered], at what age was this done? _____ weeks/months (circle)
5a. Age in weeks at which your cat was adopted? 5b. How many owners has your cat had? 5c. How long have you had this cat?	a. _____ weeks/months (circle) b. ☐ 0 ☐ 1 ☐ 2 ☐ 3 ☐ 4 ☐ 5+ ☐ Unknown c. _____ months

6a. Is your cat (please circle):
    a. Indoor, only
    b. Outdoor, only
    c. Indoor/outdoor
	6b. How many litterboxes does your cat have:
	☐ 0 ☐ 1 ☐ 2 ☐ 3 ☐ 4 ☐ 5+
	6c. What types of litter do you use?
	
	6d. How often do you change the litterbox completely?
	_____ times weekly/monthly (circle)
	6e. How often do you scoop the box?
	_____ times daily/weekly (circle)

7a. Does your cat leave urine or feces outside the litterbox?	☐ Yes ☐ No ☐ Don't know If you answered yes, a. Urine—Where specifically? b. Feces—Where specifically? c. Both—Where specifically?
7b. Does your cat "spray"?	☐ Yes ☐ No ☐ Don't know If you answered yes, where specifically?
8. Do you have any concerns, complaints, or problems with urination in the house now?	☐ Yes ☐ No If you answered yes, (a) Where is the cat urinating that you find undesirable (list all areas)? (b) How many times per week is the cat urinating in places you find undesirable? (c) At what time of day is the urination occurring? (d) Is the pattern different on days when you are home and days you are not home? (e) Are you at work during the hours when the cat urinates? (f) How many times per day does your cat usually urinate when he or she is not urinating in places you find undesirable?
9. Do you have any concerns, complaints, or problems with defecation in the house now?	☐ Yes ☐ No If you answered yes, (a) Where is the cat defecating that you find undesirable (list all areas)? (b) How many times per week is the cat defecating in places you find undesirable? (c) At what time of day is the defecation occurring?

	(d) Is the pattern different on days when you are home and days you are not home? (e) Are you at work during the hours when the cat defecates? (f) How many times per day does your cat usually defecate when he or she is not defecating in places you find undesirable?
10. Does your cat destroy any objects or anything else by chewing, sucking, or eliminating on them (e.g., furniture, rugs, clothes, et cetera) now?	☐ Yes ☐ No If you answered yes, what objects specifically does the cat destroy? Please list all of them and note which are destroyed when you are home or not home—please note if they destroy at both times—tick both columns:

Object	When home	When gone
	☐	☐
	☐	☐
	☐	☐
	☐	☐

11. Does your cat mouth, bite, suck, or nip anything or anyone?	a. ☐ Yes ☐ No If you answered yes, to whom is this behavior directed? b. Is this a problem for you? ☐ Yes ☐ No
12. Does your cat exhibit any vocalization about which you are concerned?	☐ Yes ☐ No If you answered yes, what is/are the vocalization(s) and when do they occur:

Vocalization	Situation in which it occurs
a. Yowling	
b. Growling	
c. Meowing	
d. Hissing	

13. Does your cat show any signs of hissing, growling, or biting?	☐ Yes ☐ No If you answered yes, what does the cat do and when does he or she do it?

Sign	Situation in which it occurs
a. Hissing	
b. Growling	
c. Biting	

14. Have you ever been concerned that your cat is "aggressive" *to people*?	☐ Yes ☐ No If you answered yes, why?
15. Have you ever been concerned that your cat is "aggressive" *to cats*?	☐ Yes ☐ No If you answered yes, why?
16. Have you ever been concerned that your cat is "aggressive" *to animals other than cats*?	☐ Yes ☐ No If you answered yes, why?
Does your cat hunt or prey on other animals?	☐ Yes ☐ No If you answered yes, which animals and where?

17. Has your cat ever bitten or clawed anyone, regardless of the circumstances?	☐ Yes ☐ No If yes, what happened?
18. Has your cat had any changes in sleep habits?	☐ Yes ☐ No If you answered yes, what are these changes?
19. Has your cat had any changes in eating habits?	☐ Yes ☐ No If you answered yes, what changes have occurred?
20. Has your cat had any changes in locomotor behaviors or the ability to get around or jump on the bed, et cetera?	☐ Yes ☐ No If you answered yes, what changes have occurred?
21. Has anyone ever told you that they were afraid of your cat?	☐ Yes ☐ No If you answered yes, what did they say?
22. Has anyone every told you that your cat was ill-mannered?	☐ Yes ☐ No If you answered yes, why—what did the cat do that made them say this?
23. Do you have any concerns about your cat's grooming behaviors?	☐ Yes ☐ No If you answered yes, a. Little to no grooming b. Sucking c. Chewing d. Licking e. Self-mutilation/sores f. Barbering/trimming g. Plucking out clumps of hair
24. Is the cat exhibiting any behaviors about which you are concerned, worried, or would like more information?	☐ Yes ☐ No If you answered yes, please list these behaviors below:

SHORT SURVEY QUESTIONNAIRES TO BE USED AT ALL VISITS TO MONITOR BEHAVIORAL CHANGES IN DOGS

This short survey questionnaire can be used at **any and all visits** to check if the clients have any questions or complaints about their dog.

You have to remember that the clients might not even know that they have questions or complaints because they do not know what "normal" is. Also, if anything, myths about breeds, behavior, nature, and nurture are far more insidious in the client community than in the veterinary community. These questionnaires, when used at each visit, together with the other more detailed and specific tools provided, will tell you if further information is necessary and hint at some of the underlying factors contributing to the problems.

Clients may be uncomfortable with a behavior, but not know how to ask if it is abnormal. These questionnaires will give clients the vocabulary and opportunity to discuss their pet's behaviors with their veterinarian in an efficient, consistent, and meaningful way.

If you know nothing about veterinary behavioral medicine, these short questionnaires will walk you through most of what you will need to ask. If you are experienced in asking about behavioral issues, you can shorten these questionnaires considerably. The complete and detailed version is attached here because authors have no way of knowing what readers know.

Survey questionnaire about general dog behaviors—to be used at all visits:

1. Client(s):	2. Date:
3. Patient:	4a. Breed: _____ 4b. Weight: _____ lb/_____ kg 4c. Sex: ☐ M ☐ MC ☐ F ☐ FS 4d: If your dog is castrated or spayed [neutered] at what age was this done? _____ weeks/months (circle)
5. Age in weeks at which your dog was definitively house-trained (e.g., no accidents in the house). If you adopted your dog as an adult and the dog was house-trained, just put in the adoption age.	_____ weeks ☐ My dog is not really house-trained

6. Does your dog "mark" with urine or feces?	☐ Yes ☐ No
	☐ I don't know
	☐ Not sure—I don't know what marking is
	If you answered yes,
	    a. Urine—where specifically?
	    b. Feces—where specifically?
	    c. Both—where specifically?

7. Do you have any concerns, complaints, or problems with urination in the house now?	☐ Yes ☐ No

8a. Do you have any concerns, complaints, or problems with defecation in the house now?	☐ Yes ☐ No
	If you answered yes,
	    (a) Where is the dog defecating that you find undesirable (list all areas)?
	
	    (b) How many times per week is the dog defecating in places you find undesirable?
	
	    (c) At what time of day is the defecation occurring?
	
	    (d) Is the pattern different on days when you are home and days you are not home?
	
	    (e) Are you at work during the hours when the dog defecates?
	
	    (f) How many times per day does your dog usually defecate when he or she is not defecating in places you find undesirable?

8b. Does your dog experience periodic bouts of diarrhea?	☐ Yes ☐ No
9. Did your dog destroy any objects that were not toys while teething?	☐ Yes ☐ No ☐ Unknown If you answered yes, what objects specifically did the dog destroy?
10. Does your dog destroy any objects or anything else (doors, windows, et cetera) *now*?	☐ Yes ☐ No If you answered yes, what objects specifically does the dog destroy? Please list all of them and note which are destroyed when you are home or not home—please note if they destroy at both times—tick both columns:

Object	When home	When gone
	☐	☐
	☐	☐
	☐	☐

11. Does your dog mouth anything or anyone?	☐ Yes ☐ No If you answered yes, what or whom does the dog mouth? Is this a problem for you? ☐ Yes ☐ No
12. Does your dog exhibit any vocalization about which you are concerned?	☐ Yes ☐ No If you answered yes, what is/are the vocalization(s) and when do they occur?

Vocalization	Situation in which it occurs
a. Barking	
b. Growling	
c. Howling	
d. Whining	

13. Does your dog show any signs of growling, barking, snarling, or biting?	☐ Yes ☐ No If you answered yes, what is/are the sign(s) and when do they occur?

Sign	Situation in which it occurs
a. Barking	
b. Growling	
c. Snarling	
d. Biting	

14. Have you ever been concerned that your dog is "aggressive" *to people*?	☐ Yes ☐ No If you answered yes, why?
15. Have you ever been concerned that your dog is "aggressive" *to dogs*?	☐ Yes ☐ No If you answered yes, why?
16. Have you ever been concerned that your dog is "aggressive" *to animals other than dogs*?	☐ Yes ☐ No If you answered yes, why?
17. Has your dog ever bitten anyone, regardless of the circumstances?	☐ Yes ☐ No If you answered yes, what happened?
18. Has your dog had any changes in sleep habits?	☐ Yes ☐ No If you answered yes, what are these specifically?
19. Has your dog had any changes in eating habits?	☐ Yes ☐ No If you answered yes, what are these specifically?
20. Has your dog had any changes in locomotor behaviors or its ability to get around or jump on the bed, et cetera?	☐ Yes ☐ No If you answered yes, what are these specifically?
21. Has anyone ever told you that they were afraid of your dog?	☐ Yes ☐ No If you answered yes, what did they say?
22. Has anyone every told you that your dog was ill-mannered?	☐ Yes ☐ No If you answered yes, why—what did the dog do that made them say this?
23. Is the dog exhibiting any behaviors about which you are concerned, worried, or would like more information?	☐ Yes ☐ No If you answered yes, please list these behaviors below:

Basic history questionnaire—Cats

The questionnaire that follows focuses on all aspects of your cat's behavior and health issues that could contribute to any behavioral concerns. To interpret this information in the most detailed possible light, it would be helpful for you to list your cat's weight and your cat's body condition score. If you do not know your cat's body condition score, please go to the websites listed to see the scoring systems routinely used.

Cat's weight: _____ kg or _____ lb

Body condition score/BCS: _____

www.pet-slimmers.com/shapecat.htm
www.purina.com/cat/weight-control/bodycondition.aspx

Please complete the pages below as accurately as possible.

1. Client(s):	2a. Today's date: ___ / ___ / ___ 2b. Cat's date of birth: ___ / ___ / ___ ☐ Estimated ☐ Known
3. Patient's name:	4a. Breed: 4b. Weight: _____ lb/ _____ kg 4c. Sex: ☐ M ☐ MC ☐ F ☐ FS 4d: If your cat is castrated or spayed [neutered] at what age was this done? _____ weeks / months (circle)

5a. Age in weeks at which your cat was adopted?
 5b. How many owners has your cat had?
 5c. How long have you had this cat?
 5d. Where did you get this cat?
	a. _____ weeks/months (circle)
	 b. 0 1 2 3 4 5+ unknown
	 c. _____ months
	 d. 1. Serious show breeder
	   2. Breeder who doesn't show
	   3. Found
	   4. SPCA/Humane Society
	   5. Found (or cat found you)
	   6. Friend
	   7. Bred from one of your cats
	   8. Other—please specify:

6a. Is your cat (please circle):
   a. Indoor, only
   b. Outdoor, only
   c. Indoor/outdoor
	6b. How many litterboxes does your cat have:
	   ☐ 0 ☐ 1 ☐ 2 ☐ 3 ☐ 4 ☐ 5+
	 6c. What types of litter do you use? _____
	 _____
	 6d. How often do you change the litterbox completely?
	   _____ times weekly/monthly (circle)
	 6e. How often do you scoop the box?
	   _____ times daily/weekly (circle)

7a. Does your cat leave urine or feces outside the litterbox?
 	
 7b. Does your cat spray?
	☐ Yes ☐ No ☐ Don't know
	 If you answered yes,
	   a. Urine—where specifically?
	   b. Feces—where specifically?
	   c. Both—where specifically?
	 ☐ Yes ☐ No ☐ Don't know
	 If you answered yes, where specifically?

8. Do you have any concerns, complaints, or problems with urination in the house now?	☐ Yes ☐ No If you answered yes, (a) Where is the cat urinating that you find undesirable (list all areas)? _____ _____ _____ (b) How many times per week is the cat urinating in places you find undesirable?

	(c) At what time of day is the urination occurring?
	(d) Is the pattern different on days when you are home and days you are not home?
	(e) Are you at work during the hours when the cat urinates?
	(f) How many times per day does your cat usually urinate when he or she is not urinating in places you find undesirable?
9. Do you have any concerns, complaints, or problems with defecation in the house now?	☐ Yes ☐ No If you answered yes, (a) Where is the cat defecating that you find undesirable (list all areas)? _____ _____ _____ (b) How many times per week is the cat defecating in places you find undesirable? (c) At what time of day is the defecation occurring? (d) Is the pattern different on days when you are home and days you are not home? (e) Are you at work during the hours when the cat defecates? (f) How many times per day does your cat usually urinate when he or she is not urinating in places you find undesirable?
10. Did your cat destroy any objects while teething?	☐ Yes ☐ No ☐ Unknown If you answered yes, what objects specifically did the cat destroy? Please list all of them and note which, if any, you had given the cat as toys or to play with by putting a * next to them.
11. Does your cat destroy any objects or anything else by chewing, sucking, or eliminating on them (e.g., furniture, rugs, clothes, et cetera) now?	☐ Yes ☐ No If you answered yes, what objects specifically does the cat destroy? Please list all of them and note which are destroyed when you are home or not home—please note if they destroy at both times—tick both columns:

Object	When home	When gone
	☐	☐
	☐	☐
	☐	☐
	☐	☐

12. Does your cat mouth, bite, suck, or nip anything or anyone?	☐ Yes ☐ No a. If you answered yes, what or whom does the cat mouth? b. If you answered yes, does the cat: bite, suck, mouth, nip, lick, or chew? (Please circle) c. Is this a problem for you? ☐ Yes ☐ No
13. Does your cat exhibit any vocalization about which you are concerned?	☐ Yes ☐ No If you answered yes, what is/are the vocalization(s) and when do they occur?

Vocalization	Situation in which it occurs
a. Yowling/'barking'	
b. Growling	
c. Howling	
d. Hissing	
e. Other—please specify:	

14. Does your cat show any signs of growling, yowling, hissing, or biting?	☐ Yes ☐ No If you answered yes, what is/are the sign(s) and when do they occur? <table><tr><td>**Sign**</td><td>**Situation in which it occurs**</td></tr><tr><td>a. Yowling</td><td></td></tr><tr><td>b. Growling</td><td></td></tr><tr><td>c. Hissing</td><td></td></tr><tr><td>d. Biting</td><td></td></tr></table>
15. Have you ever been concerned that your cat is "aggressive" to people?	☐ Yes ☐ No If you answered yes, why?
16. Have you ever been concerned that your cat is "aggressive" to cats?	☐ Yes ☐ No If you answered yes, why?
17. Have you ever been concerned that your cat is "aggressive" to animals other than cats?	☐ Yes ☐ No If you answered yes, why?
18. Does your cat hunt or prey on other animals?	☐ Yes ☐ No If you answered yes, which animals and where?
19. Has your cat ever bitten or clawed anyone, regardless of the circumstances?	☐ Yes ☐ No If you answered yes, what happened?
20. Has your cat had any changes in sleep habits?	☐ Yes ☐ No If you answered yes, what are these, specifically?
21. Has your cat had any changes in eating habits?	☐ Yes ☐ No If you answered yes, what are these, specifically?
22. Has your cat had any changes in locomotory behaviors or ability to get around or jump on the bed, et cetera?	☐ Yes ☐ No If you answered yes, what are these, specifically?
23. Has anyone ever told you that they were afraid of your cat?	☐ Yes ☐ No If you answered yes, what did they say?
24. Has anyone ever told you that your cat was ill-mannered?	☐ Yes ☐ No If you answered yes, why? What did the cat do that made them say this?
25. Do you have any concerns about your cat's grooming behaviors?	☐ Yes ☐ No If you answered yes, a. Little to no grooming b. Sucking c. Chewing d. Licking e. Self-mutilation/sores f. Barbering/trimming g. Plucking out clumps of hair
26. Is the cat exhibiting any behaviors about which you are concerned, worried, or would like more information?	☐ Yes ☐ No If you answered yes, please list these behaviors below:

27. Please list the people, including yourself, currently living in the household now.

	NAME	SEX	AGE	RELATIONSHIP (Self, husband, wife, mother-in-law, etc.)	OCCUPATION
1.				SELF *	
2.					
3.					
4.					
5.					
6.					
7.					

* Self means the person completing questionnaire.

28. Please list all the animals (include all pets, even non-cats) in the household.

Name	Order obtained	Type/Breed	Sex: M MC F FS	Age obtained in months	Age now in months	Any medical illness?	Any behavioral illness?
						☐ Yes ☐ No	☐ Yes ☐ No
						☐ Yes ☐ No	☐ Yes ☐ No
						☐ Yes ☐ No	☐ Yes ☐ No
						☐ Yes ☐ No	☐ Yes ☐ No
						☐ Yes ☐ No	☐ Yes ☐ No
						☐ Yes ☐ No	☐ Yes ☐ No

29. If any of these pets have been identified as having a medical problem, please specify what the problem is: _____

30. If any of these pets have been identified as having a behavioral problem, please specify what the problem is: _____

31. Please describe, in detail, how you prepare to leave the house when the cat will be left alone. Do you ignore the cat, do you seek him or her out and say goodbye, do you make a fuss, et cetera?_____

_____

_____

32. What does your cat do as you prepare to leave? _____

_____

33. Please list your cat's behavioral concerns and let us know how much of a problem you consider the behavior.

Complaint #	Specific complaint/problem	Very serious?	Serious?	Not serious?
1				
2				
3				
4				
5				

For the complaints numbered above, please estimate the frequency of occurrence of the undesirable behavior:

Complaint 1: ☐ Daily ☐ Weekly ☐ Monthly	Percent of time that animal is in situation and during which undesirable behavior occurs: ☐ Less than 25% ☐ 25%-50% ☐ 51%-75% ☐ 76%-100%	Complaint 2: ☐ Daily ☐ Weekly ☐ Monthly	Percent of time that animal is in situation and during which undesirable behavior occurs: ☐ Less than 25% ☐ 25%-50% ☐ 51%-75% ☐ 76%-100%
Complaint 3: ☐ Daily ☐ Weekly ☐ Monthly	Percent of time that animal is in situation and during which undesirable behavior occurs: ☐ Less than 25% ☐ 25%-50% ☐ 51%-75% ☐ 76%-100%	Complaint 4: ☐ Daily ☐ Weekly ☐ Monthly	Percent of time that animal is in situation and during which undesirable behavior occurs: ☐ Less than 25% ☐ 25%-50% ☐ 51%-75% ☐ 76%-100%

Complaint 5:	Percent of time that animal is in situation and
☐ Daily	during which undesirable behavior occurs:
☐ Weekly	☐ Less than 25%
☐ Monthly	☐ 25%-50%
	☐ 51%-75%
	☐ 76%-100%

Please describe the last three or four events in which you felt that your pet's behavior was problematic. Please include the relevant circumstances and what your response was. You can append additional sheets, if you wish.

34. If your pet has what you perceive to be a problem, why have you kept the pet despite this problem?

35. Are you concerned that you may have caused the problem?   ☐ Yes   ☐ No
36. Do you feel guilty about this problem?   ☐ Yes   ☐ No
37. Have you considered finding another home for this pet?   ☐ Yes   ☐ No
38. Have you considered euthanasia (putting your cat 'down'/to 'sleep')?   ☐ Yes   ☐ No

On the issue of biting:

39. How many total bites has your cat inflicted **on any human**?   0   1   2   3   4   5   >5
40. How many **bites to humans** broke the skin?   0   1   2   3   4   5   >5
41. How many **bites to humans** were reported, and to whom?
    (i.e., local authorities, hospital, Humane Society, et cetera.) Number reported: 0   1   2   3   4   5   >5
    Reported to:

42. Was there legal action taken as a result of any **bite to humans**?   ☐ Yes   ☐ No
43. How many total bites has your cat inflicted on any **cat/dog/other animal**?   0   1   2   3   4   5   >5
44. How many bites to **cats/dogs/other animals** broke the skin?   0   1   2   3   4   5   >5
45. How many **bites to cats/dogs/other animals** were reported, and to whom?
    (i.e., local authorities, hospital, Humane Society, et cetera.) Number reported: 0   1   2   3   4   5   >5
    Reported to:

46. Was there legal action taken as a result of any bite to **cats/dogs/other animals**?   ☐ Yes   ☐ No
47. Has the frequency or the intensity of the occurrence of the behavior changed
    since the problem started?   ☐ Yes   ☐ No
    If so, how and when?

48. Please provide a brief outline of the chronological development of the problem, including any significant incidents that you think we should know.

49. Duration of problem: _____ days _____ months _____ years
50. Age of the cat when he or she first began showing signs of the problem:
51. Do you know if the parents engage in similar behaviors as presented animal?
    ☐ Yes, they did   ☐ No, they didn't   ☐ Don't know
    If so, what behaviors were exhibited by whom?

52. Do you know if any littermates are engaging in same behaviors?
    ☐ Don't know   ☐ No, they aren't   ☐ Yes, they are
    If so, what behaviors were exhibited by whom?

53. What are you feeding your cat and when are you feeding him/her? Please be specific. If you meal-feed, please let us know the brand names and times. If you leave out food free choice, please give us the brand name. If you give treats, what kind and when? As we learn more about potential effects of diet on behavior this information is important.

Elimination history: We know that you have already answered some questions about your cat's elimination behaviors. Here, we ask specific information that may be relevant to better understanding your cat.

	Box 1	Box 2	Box 3	Box 4
1. How many litterboxes are available for the cat(s)? _____				
2. Is the box covered?				
3. What are the sizes of the boxes?				
4. Where are the boxes?				
5. How deep is the litter in each of the boxes?				
6. Are liners ever used?				
7. If liners are used, are they scented?				
8. List all the types of litter used for each box (names/brands, please).				
9. Are any of the litters used scented?				
10. Does the cat respond differently to any of the above styles of boxes or litters, or sizes of box and depths of litters?				
11. How frequently is the litter changed?				
12. How frequently is the litter scooped?				
13. How frequently is the litterbox washed and replaced?				
14. Are deodorants used in the cleaning process?				
15. How many cats actually share a litterbox?				

16. What does the cat do in the litterbox?: does he get in, does he stand outside, does he dig in or out, et cetera?

17. Is the cat ever allowed outside?
   a. Free access—cat door
   b. Indoor only or primarily
   c. Outdoor only or primarily
   d. Outdoor on lead, supervised, enclosed area, et cetera

18. Does the cat eliminate in the presence of other animals or people, or is the elimination behavior secret?

  a. eliminates where no one can see   b. eliminates in the presence of humans or other animals

19. Will the cat immediately use a freshly cleaned litterbox?

  a. always   b. sometimes   c. never

20. Has the cat ever had any variation in whether or not it covers its feces or urine, and is any of that variation associated with the presence or absence of any other situation or cat?

21. Does the cat ever vocalize while he or she eliminates?

  a. always   b. sometimes   c. never

22. Will the cat spray against the back of a covered litterbox?

  a. always   b. sometimes   c. never

23. Does your cat ever use a shower, bath tub, or tile floor for elimination?

  a. always   b. sometimes   c. never

24. What other areas are ever used for elimination? Please provide a complete list with locations, substrate (e.g., wood floor, chair, rug, et cetera) and frequency of use.

Aggression screen for cats:
KEY: NR = No reaction; S = Stare; B = Bite; H = Hiss, howl, growl, vocalize (not purr); SW = Swat/scratch; P = Piloerect/arch/puff up; TS = Switch or twitch tail; WD = Withdraw; NA = Not applicable.

This screen can be used in three ways: (1) to note the presence or absence, at any time, of any of the behaviors; (2) to keep as a log about the baseline behavior, noting how many times the behavior occurs, given the number of times it is attempted, per unit time (i.e., per week); and (3) to keep a log about frequencies of the occurrence behaviors, given the number of times the circumstance has been encountered, during treatment so that these numbers can be compared with (2). Please note if the reaction is consistent in style, or only directed toward one person, or only present in one restricted circumstance. If using this screen only for the first use, note if the cat has been worsening in intensity or frequency in any category.

Please note: we want to know what your cat does when you routinely interact with her—if you don't know how your cat would react in the following circumstances, please do not try to find out because you may provoke the cat.

	NR	S	B	H	SW	P	TS	WD	NA
1. Take cat's food dish with food									
2. Take cat's empty food dish									
3. Take cat's water dish									
4. Take food (human) that falls on floor									
5. Take real bone									
6. Take food treat									
7. Take toy									
8. Human approaches cat while eating									
9. Another cat approaches cat while eating									
10. Human approaches cat while playing with toys									
11. Another cat approaches cat while playing with toys									
12. Dog approaches cat while eating									
13. Dog approaches cat while playing with toys									
14. Human walks past cat in doorways									
15. Human approaches/disturbs cat while sleeping									
16. Cat approaches/disturbs cat while sleeping									
17. Step over cat									
18. Push cat off bed/couch									
19. Reach toward cat									
20. Reach over head									
21. Put on harness or collar									
22. Push on shoulders or rump									
23. Pet cat when in lap									
24. Pet cat when not in lap									
25. Towel when wet									
26. Bathe cat									

	NR	S	B	H	SW	P	TS	WD	NA
27. Groom cat's head									
28. Groom cat's body									
29. Trim cat's nails									
30. Put on nail caps									
31. Stare at									
32. Stranger enters room									
33. Cat in yard—person passes									
34. Cat in yard—dog passes									
35. Dog enters room where cat is									
36. Human physically carries cat									
37. Cat in vet's office									
38. Cat in boarding kennel									
39. Cat in groomers									
40. Cat yelled at									
41. Cat physically punished—hit									
42. Squirrels, cats, small animals approach									
43. Cat sees another cat through window									
44. Cat sees squirrels, birds, dogs through window									
45. Human approaches cat who is at top of stairs									
46. Cat removed from hiding place									
47. Human body parts move under covers on bed									
48. Crying infant									
49. Playing with 2-year-old children									
50. Playing with 5- to 7-year-old children									
51. Playing with 8- to 11-year-old children									
52. Playing with 12- to 16-year-old children									

Stereotypic and ritualistic behavior sheets

Please complete this form **only** if the cat is showing any repetitive, ritualistic behaviors **that you find troublesome or about which you are concerned.**

1. Which of the following categories below fits your cat's behavior?

Check as many categories that apply to the cat's behavior. Then check the best description that relates to the selected behavior.

a. ☐ Grooming	☐ Chewing self ☐ Biting self ☐ Licking self ☐ Plucking hair from self ☐ Barbering/trimming hair on self ☐ Sucking self ☐ Continuously doing any of these behaviors *to another individual*. Please explain:
b. ☐ Hallucinatory	☐ Staring and attending to things that are not there ☐ Tracking things that are not there ☐ Pouncing on or attacking things that are not there
c. ☐ Consumptive	☐ Consuming rocks ☐ Consuming dirt or soil ☐ Consuming other objects ☐ Eating, licking, sucking or chewing wool or fabric, rugs, furniture, et cetera ☐ Licking or gulping air
d. ☐ Locomotory	☐ Circling/spinning ☐ Tail-chasing ☐ Freezing
e. ☐ Vocalization	☐ Rhythmic vocalization ☐ Howling ☐ Growling

Please indicate the appropriate answer (Yes/No/Uncertain) for each of the following questions. Please feel free to add any information that you think might be helpful. If you choose *yes*, please describe in detail what is ongoing and, if relevant, who or what might be involved. If no one is home often enough to know or the cat cannot be reliably observed, please choose *uncertain*.

	Yes	No	Uncertain
2. Was there a change in the household or an event associated with the development of the behavior?			
3. Is there any time of day when the behavior seems more or less intense?			
4. Is there a person or another pet in the presence of whom the behavior seems more intense?			
5. Does the cat respond to its name or seem aware of its surroundings while in the midst of the behavior?			
6. Is the cat aware that you are calling him/her? If yes, how can you tell?			
7. Can you convince the cat to stop the behavior by a. Calling him or her			
b. Using physical restraint			
8. List the kinds of things (i.e., noises, treats, toys), if any, that will interrupt the behavior once it has started.			
9. Is there a location in which the cat prefers to perform the behavior? If so, where?			
10. For ingestion, list what types of objects are consumed. Be as specific as possible—what type of rug or sweater fabric (e.g., cotton only, merino wool only, all natural fabrics, et cetera)?			
11. Does any event or behavior routinely occur immediately before the behavior begins? If you answer yes, what occurs?			
12. Does any event or behavior routinely occur immediately after the behavior ceases? If you answer yes, what occurs?			
13. Has the cat's general behavior changed in any way since the onset of the atypical behavior (i.e., the cat is more or less aloof, aggressive, withdrawn, playful, et cetera)? If you answer yes, please let us know what the change is.			
14. Has the cat's diet recently been changed? If yes, what is the change?			
15. How old do you think your pet was when its ritualistic behavior began?	Age in months _____		
16. Did anyone else in the cat's family exhibit these or similar behaviors?			
17. Is there a pattern to the behavior? What are the duration, frequency, characteristics of the events themselves?	Duration: ☐ days. ☐ weeks. ☐ months Pattern: After meals, in AM, et cetera (please specify)		

Questionnaire to evaluate behaviors of old cats. Please complete this section *ONLY* if your pet is elderly or if your complaints have to do with possible age-related changes

Behavior screen for age associated changes:

1. Locomotory/ambulatory assessment (tick **only one**)
   - ☐ a. No alterations or debilities noted
   - ☐ b. Modest slowness associated with change from youth to adult
   - ☐ c. Moderate slowness associated with geriatric aging
   - ☐ d. Moderate slowness associated with geriatric aging plus alteration or debility in gait
   - ☐ e. Moderate slowness associated with geriatric aging plus some loss of function (e.g., cannot climb stairs)
   - ☐ f. Severe slowness associated with extreme loss of function, particularly on slick surfaces (may need to be carried)
   - ☐ g. Severe slowness, extreme loss of function, and decreased willingness or interest in locomoting (spends most of time in bed)
   - ☐ h. Paralyzed or refuses to move

2. Appetite assessment (may tick **more** than **one**)
   - ☐ a. No alterations in appetite
   - ☐ b. Change in ability to physically handle food
   - ☐ c. Change in ability to retain food (vomits or regurgitates)
   - ☐ d. Change in ability to find food
   - ☐ e. Change in interest in food (may be olfactory, having to do with the ability to smell)
   - ☐ f. Change in rate of eating
   - ☐ g. Change in completion of eating
   - ☐ h. Change in timing of eating
   - ☐ i. Change in preferred textures

3. Assessment of elimination function (tick **only one** in **each** category)
   - a. Changes in frequencies and "accidents"
     - ☐ 1. No change in frequency and no "accidents"
     - ☐ 2. Increased frequency, no "accidents"
     - ☐ 3. Decreased frequency, no "accidents"
     - ☐ 4. Increased frequency with "accidents"
     - ☐ 5. Decreased frequency with "accidents"
     - ☐ 6. No change in frequency, but "accidents"

   - b. Bladder control
     - ☐ 1. Leaks urine when asleep, only
     - ☐ 2. Leaks urine when awake, only
     - ☐ 3. Leaks urine when awake or asleep
     - ☐ 4. Full-stream, uncontrolled urination when asleep, only
     - ☐ 5. Full-stream, uncontrolled urination when awake, only
     - ☐ 6. Full-stream, uncontrolled urination when awake or asleep
     - ☐ 7. No leakage or uncontrolled urination, all urination controlled, but in inappropriate or undesirable location
     - ☐ 8. No change in urination control or behavior

   - c. Bowel control
     - ☐ 1. Defecates when asleep
       - Formed stool   Diarrhea   Mixed (Circle appropriate answer, if this occurs, please)
     - ☐ 2. Defecates without apparent awareness
       - Formed stool   Diarrhea   Mixed (Circle appropriate answer, if this occurs, please)
     - ☐ 3. Defecates when awake and aware of action, but in inappropriate or undesirable locations
       - Formed stool   Diarrhea   Mixed   (Circle appropriate answer, if this occurs, please)
     - ☐ 4. No changes in bowel control

4. Visual acuity—how well do you think the cat sees? (tick **only one**)
   - ☐ a. No change in visual acuity detected by behavior—appears to see as well as ever
   - ☐ b. Some change in acuity **not** dependent on ambient light conditions
   - ☐ c. Some change in acuity dependent on ambient light conditions
   - ☐ d. Extreme change in acuity **not** dependent on ambient light conditions
   - ☐ e. Extreme change in acuity dependent on ambient light conditions
   - ☐ f. Blind

5. Auditory acuity—how well do you think the cat hears? (tick **only one**)
   - ☐ a. No apparent change in auditory acuity
   - ☐ b. Some decrement in hearing—not responding to sounds to which the cat used to respond
   - ☐ c. Extreme decrement in hearing—have to make sure the cat is paying attention or repeat signals or go get the cat when called
   - ☐ d. Deaf—no response to sounds of any kind

6. Play interactions—if the cat plays with **toys** (other pets are addressed later), which situation best describes that play? (tick **only one**)
   - ☐ a. No change in play with toys
   - ☐ b. Slightly decreased interest in toys, only
   - ☐ c. Slightly decreased ability to play with toys, only
   - ☐ d. Slightly decreased interest and ability to play with toys
   - ☐ e. Extreme decreased interest in toys, only
   - ☐ f. Extreme decreased ability to play with toys, only
   - ☐ g. Extreme decreased interest and ability to play with toys

7. Interactions with humans—which situation best describes that interaction? (tick **only one**)
   - ☐ a. No change in interaction with people
   - ☐ b. Recognizes people but slightly decreased frequency of interaction
   - ☐ c. Recognizes people but greatly decreased frequency of interaction
   - ☐ d. Withdrawal but recognizes people
   - ☐ e. Does not recognize people

8. Interactions with other pets—which situation best describes that interaction? (tick **only one**)
   - ☐ a. No change in interaction with other pets
   - ☐ b. Recognizes other pets but slightly decreased frequency of interaction
   - ☐ c. Recognizes other pets but greatly decreased frequency of interaction
   - ☐ d. Withdrawal but recognizes other pets
   - ☐ e. Does not recognize other pets
   - ☐ f. No other pets or animal companions in house or social environment

9. Changes in sleep/wake cycle (tick **only one**)
   - ☐ a. No changes in sleep patterns
   - ☐ b. Sleeps more in day, only
   - ☐ c. Some change—awakens at night and sleeps more in day
   - ☐ d. Much change—profoundly erratic nocturnal pattern and irregular daytime pattern
   - ☐ e. Sleeps virtually all day, awake occasionally at night
   - ☐ f. Sleeps almost around the clock

10. Is there anything else you think that we should know?

Basic history questionnaire—Dogs

The questionnaire that follows focuses on all aspects of your dog's behavior and health issues that could contribute to any behavioral concerns. To interpret this information in the most detailed possible light it would be helpful for you to list your dog's weight and your dog's body condition score. If you do not know your dog's body condition score, please go to the websites listed to see the scoring systems routinely used.

Dog's weight: _____ kg or _____ lb

Body condition score/BCS: _____

www.pet-slimmers.com/shapedog.htm
www.purina.com/dog/weight-and-exercise/bodycondition.aspx

Please complete the pages below as accurately as possible.

1. Pet's name	
2. Owner/client's name	
3. Kennel name (if applicable)	
4. Owner's address	
5. Owner's home phone number	
6. Owner's office phone number	
7. Owner's fax number	
8. Owner's e-mail address	
9. Breed of dog	
10. Sex of dog	
11. Has this dog been neutered?	☐ Yes ☐ No
12. How old, in months, was the dog when neutered?	_____ months
13. What was the reason for neutering?	
14. Any behavioral changes after neutering?	☐ Yes ☐ No If yes, what?
15. Has this dog been bred?	☐ Yes ☐ No
16. If you have not yet bred this dog, do you plan on breeding him or her?	☐ Yes ☐ No
17. Any behavioral changes after breeding?	☐ Yes ☐ No If yes, what?
18. Describe your dog's coat color	
19. Dog's date of birth	Day: _____ Month: _____ Year: _____
20. Dog's age at completion of this questionnaire, in months	_____ months
21. How old was your pet when you first acquired him or her, in months?	_____ months
22. Has this pet had other owners?	☐ Yes ☐ No If so, how many? ☐ 0 ☐ 1 ☐ 2 ☐ 3 ☐ 4 ☐ 5+ ☐ Unknown Why was pet given up?
23. How long have you had this dog, in months?	_____ months

24. Where did you get this pet?	a. Stray/found b. Breeder—serious show/performance breeder c. Breeder—backyard breeder d. SPCA/Humane shelter e. Breed rescue service f. Newspaper adoption ad (not breeder) g. Pet store h. Friend i. Other (Please explain)
25. Why did you get this dog?	
26. When was your dog last vaccinated?	
27. When was your last complete veterinary check up?	
28. Does this dog have any physical problems that your veterinarian has noted?	☐ Yes ☐ No If so, what specifically?
29. Is your dog taking any medication for any of the medical problems discussed above?	☐ Yes ☐ No If so, what specifically?
30. Is your dog taking heartworm preventative?	☐ Yes ☐ No If so, brand:
31. Is your dog taking flea or tick preventative?	☐ Yes ☐ No If so, brand:
32. What food (brand names, amounts, and schedules) is your dog fed?	
33. What treats does your dog get (brand names, amounts, and schedules)	
34. Does your dog get anything else to eat?	☐ Yes ☐ No If so, what specifically?
35. How is your dog exercised/maintained?	This dog is (please check all that apply): ☐ a. Allowed to run free, unsupervised ☐ b. Fenced/kenneled/run ☐ c. Leash walked ☐ d. Outside, unleashed but supervised ☐ e. Indoors only ☐ f. Outdoors only
36. How many walks does your dog get daily, and how long are these walks?	# walks _____ Average length in minutes_____
37. How many play sessions does your dog get daily?	
38. How many training sessions does your dog get daily?	
39. How often is your dog groomed?	
40. How is your dog kept when you leave him or her alone?	☐ a. free in house ☐ b. free outdoors ☐ c. indoor kennel/run ☐ d. outdoor kennel/run ☐ e. crate indoors ☐ f. crate outdoors or garage ☐ g. behind a gate or door in house ☐ h. other (please specify)

41. What percentage of the 24 h day does your pet spend inside?	_____ % inside
42. What percentage of the day does your pet spend outside?	_____ % outside
43. What kind of a living situation do you have?	☐ a. Apartment ☐ b. Townhouse/condominium ☐ c. House with small yard ☐ d. House with large yard ☐ e. Farm
44. Has your household changed since acquiring this pet?	☐ Yes ☐ No If so, how? ☐ a. Death of human in family ☐ b. Death of pet in family ☐ c. Divorce ☐ d. Marriage ☐ e. Baby born ☐ f. Child moved ☐ g. Pet added ☐ h. Family moved ☐ i. Family schedule changed (lost or gained jobs) ☐ j. Other
45. Do you know how many animals were in this pet's litter?	☐ Yes ☐ No # _____ females # _____ males
46. Are any litter mates affected with any **medical** problems?	☐ Yes ☐ No
47. Are any litter mates affected with any **behavioral** problems?	☐ Yes ☐ No ☐ Don't know If yes, what specifically?
48. Why did you choose **this specific animal** from the litter?	
49. Why did you choose **this specific breed**?	
50. Have you owned this particular breed before?	☐ Yes ☐ No
51. Have you owned pets before?	☐ Yes ☐ No
52. Have you owned dogs before?	☐ Yes ☐ No
53. Have you owned cats before?	☐ Yes ☐ No
54. Have you owned birds before?	☐ Yes ☐ No
55. Where does your pet sleep? (Please check all that apply; we know pets move at night.)	☐ a. In or on your bed ☐ b. On his/her own bed in your bedroom ☐ c. In a crate in your bedroom ☐ d. On a bed in another room ☐ e. In a crate in another room ☐ f. On the floor next to your bed ☐ g. In another room, voluntarily, anywhere he or she wants ☐ h. In another room, because he/she is locked from your bedroom ☐ i. Anywhere he/she wants
56. What is your dog's obedience school/training history?:	☐ a. No school—trained yourself ☐ b. Puppy kindergarden ☐ c. Group lessons—basic ☐ d. Group lessons—advanced ☐ e. Private trainer at house ☐ f. Private trainer—sent to trainer ☐ g. Agility ☐ h. Flyball ☐ i. Specialty training (hunting, herding, et cetera); please specify

57. Age when dog started lessons/training in months:	_____ months
58. How did the dog do in obedience school/training?	
59. Who took the dog to training?	
60. Does the dog have any obedience titles?	☐ Yes ☐ No

61. How well does this dog do with the following cues/ "commands"/requests?

	Perfect	OK, needs work	Badly
a. Sit			
b. Stay			
c. Down/lie down			
d. Wait			
e. Heel			
f. Fetch			
g. Leave it/drop it			
h. Take it			
i. Other (please specify)			

62. Please list the people, including yourself, currently living in the household now.

NAME	SEX	AGE	RELATIONSHIP (Self, husband, wife, mother-in-law, etc.)	OCCUPATION
1.			SELF *	
2.				
3.				
4.				
5.				
6.				
7.				

* Self means the person completing questionnaire.

63. Please list all the animals (include all pets, even non-dogs) in the household.

Name	Order obtained	Breed	Sex: M MC F FS	Age obtained in months	Age now in months	Any medical illness?	Any behavioral illness?
						☐ Yes ☐ No	☐ Yes ☐ No
						☐ Yes ☐ No	☐ Yes ☐ No
						☐ Yes ☐ No	☐ Yes ☐ No
						☐ Yes ☐ No	☐ Yes ☐ No
						☐ Yes ☐ No	☐ Yes ☐ No
						☐ Yes ☐ No	☐ Yes ☐ No
						☐ Yes ☐ No	☐ Yes ☐ No
						☐ Yes ☐ No	☐ Yes ☐ No
						☐ Yes ☐ No	☐ Yes ☐ No

64. If any of these pets have been identified as having a medical problem, please specify what the problem is:
_____

65. If any of these pets have been identified as having a behavioral problem, please specify what the problem is:
_____

66. Please describe, in detail, how you prepare to leave the house when the dog will be left alone. Do you ignore the dog, do you seek him or her to say goodbye, do you make a fuss, et cetera? _____
_____
_____

67. What does your dog do as you prepare to leave? _____
_____

68. If your dog has a behavior problem(s), please list them and let us know how much of a problem do you consider the behavior. Please tick relevant degree of concern.

Complaint #	Specific complaint/problem	Very Serious?	Serious?	Not serious?
1				
2				
3				
4				
5				

For the complaints numbered above, please estimate the frequency of occurrence of the undesirable behavior:

Complaint 1: Percent of time that animal is in situation and during which undesirable behavior occurs:
☐ Daily
☐ Weekly
☐ Monthly
☐ Less than 25%
☐ 25%-50%
☐ 51%-75%
☐ 76%-100%

Complaint 2: Percent of time that animal is in situation and during which undesirable behavior occurs:
☐ Daily
☐ Weekly
☐ Monthly
☐ Less than 25%
☐ 25%-50%
☐ 51%-75%
☐ 76%-100%

Complaint 3: Percent of time that animal is in situation and during which undesirable behavior occurs:
☐ Daily
☐ Weekly
☐ Monthly
☐ Less than 25%
☐ 25%-50%
☐ 51%-75%
☐ 76%-100%

Complaint 4: Percent of time that animal is in situation and during which undesirable behavior occurs:
☐ Daily
☐ Weekly
☐ Monthly
☐ Less than 25%
☐ 25%-50%
☐ 51%-75%
☐ 76%-100%

Complaint 5: Percent of time that animal is in situation and during which undesirable behavior occurs:
☐ Daily
☐ Weekly
☐ Monthly
☐ Less than 25%
☐ 25%-50%
☐ 51%-75%
☐ 76%-100%

69. If your dog has what you perceive to be a problem, why have you kept the dog despite this problem?

70. Are you concerned that you may have caused the problem? ☐ Yes   ☐ No

71. Do you feel guilty about this problem? ☐ Yes   ☐ No

72. Have you considered finding another home for this pet? ☐ Yes   ☐ No

73. Have you considered euthanasia (putting your pet to sleep)? ☐ Yes   ☐ No

On the issue of biting:

74. How many total bites has your dog inflicted on any **human**? 0 1 2 3 4 5 >5

75. How many bites to **humans** broke the skin? 0 1 2 3 4 5 >5

76. How many bites to **humans** were reported, and to whom? (i.e., local authorities, hospital, humane society, etc.) Number reported: 0 1 2 3 4 5 >5
Reported to:

77. Was there legal action taken as a result of any bite to **humans**? ☐ Yes   ☐ No

78. How many total bites has your dog inflicted on any **dog**? 0 1 2 3 4 5 >5

79. How many bites to **dogs** broke the skin? 0 1 2 3 4 5 >5

80. How many bites to **dogs** were reported, and to whom? (i.e., local authorities, hospital, Humane Society, et cetera.) Number reported: 0 1 2 3 4 5 >5
Reported to:

81. Was there legal action taken as a result of any bite to **dogs**? ☐ Yes   ☐ No

82. Has the frequency or the intensity of the occurrence of the behavior changed since the problem started? ☐ Yes   ☐ No
If so, how and when?

83. Please provide a brief outline of the chronological development of the problem, including any significant incidents that you think we should know.

84. Duration of problem: _____ days _____ months _____ years

85. Age of animal when first began showing signs of the problem: _____

86. Do you know if the **parents** engage in **similar behaviors** as presented animal?

☐ Yes, they did   ☐ No, they didn't   ☐ Don't know

If so, what behaviors were exhibited by whom?

87. Does the client know if any **littermates** are engaging in same behaviors?

☐ Don't know   ☐ No, they aren't   ☐ Yes, they are

If so, what behaviors were exhibited by whom?

88. Does your dog exhibit **periodic diarrhea or gastrointestinal distress**?

☐ Yes   ☐ No   ☐ I don't know

Separation anxiety and noise phobia/reactivity screen

The first set of these questions deals with an "actual absence"—the client actually leaves the house and the dog is either alone or totally without the client. The second set deals with "virtual absence"—the client is home, but not accessible because the door is closed or the dog is barricaded in another room. The questions are the same for each, but please answer both.

Check **NO** if the dog does not react in the listed circumstance.

Check **UNKNOWN** if you don't know.

Check **YES** if the dog reacts. Please evaluate the extent of the reaction from the list below.

IF **YES**:
- 100% of the time = always
- <100% of the time, but > 60% = more often than not
- 40%-60% of the time = about equally
- 0% of the time but < 40% = less often than not

Behaviors during an **ACTUAL** absence

BEHAVIOR	YES	DON'T KNOW	NO
1. Destructive behavior when separated from client.	☐ 100% of the time ☐ <100% but > 60% ☐ 40%-60% of the time ☐ > 0% but < 40%		
2. Urination when separated from client.	☐ 100% of the time ☐ <100% but > 60% ☐ 40%-60% of the time ☐ > 0% but < 40%		
3. Defecation when separated from client.	☐ 100% of the time ☐ <100% but > 60% ☐ 40%-60% of the time ☐ > 0% but < 40%		
4. Vocalization when separated from client.	☐ 100% of the time ☐ <100% but > 60% ☐ 40%-60% of the time ☐ > 0% but < 40%		
5. Salivation when separated from client.	☐ 100% of the time ☐ <100% but > 60% ☐ 40%-60% of the time ☐ > 0% but < 40%		
6. Panting when separated from client.	☐ 100% of the time ☐ <100% but > 60% ☐ 40%-60% of the time ☐ > 0% but < 40%		
7. If the answer is YES for any of the above responses, what is the timing of the onset of behaviors (if known)? a. ☐ Within 5 minutes b. ☐ More than 5 minutes, but less than 30 minutes c. ☐ More than 30 minutes, but less than 1 hour d. ☐ More than 1 hour, but less than 3 hours e. ☐ Only after several hours			

Behaviors during a **VIRTUAL absence**

BEHAVIOR	YES	DON'T KNOW	NO
8. Destructive behavior when separated from client	☐ 100% of the time ☐ <100% but > 60% ☐ 40%-60% of the time ☐ > 0% but < 40%		
9. Urination when separated from client	☐ 100% of the time ☐ <100% but > 60% ☐ 40%-60% of the time ☐ > 0% but < 40%		
10. Defecation when separated from client	☐ 100% of the time ☐ <100% but > 60% ☐ 40%-60% of the time ☐ > 0% but < 40%		
11. Vocalization when separated from client	☐ 100% of the time ☐ <100% but > 60% ☐ 40%-60% of the time ☐ > 0% but < 40%		
12. Salivation when separated from client	☐ 100% of the time ☐ <100% but > 60% ☐ 40%-60% of the time ☐ > 0% but < 40%		
13. Panting when separated from client	☐ 100% of the time ☐ <100% but > 60% ☐ 40%-60% of the time ☐ > 0% but < 40%		

14. If the answer is YES for any of the above responses, what is the timing of the onset of behaviors (if known)?
   a. ☐ Within 5 minutes
   b. ☐ More than 5 minutes, but less than 30 minutes
   c. ☐ More than 30 minutes, but less than 1 hour
   d. ☐ More than 1 hour, but less than 3 hours
   e. ☐ Only after several hours

Reactions to noise

BEHAVIOR	YES	DON'T KNOW	NO
1. Reaction during thunderstorms. Type of response—please check all that apply: ☐ Salivate ☐ Hide ☐ Defecate ☐ Tremble ☐ Urinate ☐ Destroy ☐ Escape ☐ Freeze ☐ Pant ☐ Will not eat food/treats ☐ Pace ☐ Pupil dilation ☐ Vocalize (bark, whine, growl, howl)	☐ 100% of the time ☐ <100% but > 60% ☐ 40%-60% of the time ☐ > 0% but < 40%		
2. Reaction to fireworks. Type of response—please check all that apply: ☐ Salivate ☐ Hide ☐ Defecate ☐ Tremble ☐ Urinate ☐ Destroy ☐ Escape ☐ Freeze ☐ Pant ☐ Will not eat food/treats ☐ Pace ☐ Pupil dilation ☐ Vocalize (bark, whine, growl, howl)	☐ 100% of the time ☐ <100% but > 60% ☐ 40%-60% of the time ☐ > 0% but < 40%		
3. Reaction to gunshots. Type of response—please check all that apply: ☐ Salivate ☐ Hide ☐ Defecate ☐ Tremble ☐ Urinate ☐ Destroy ☐ Escape ☐ Freeze ☐ Pant ☐ Will not eat food/treats ☐ Pace ☐ Pupil dilation ☐ Vocalize (bark, whine, growl, howl)	☐ 100% of the time ☐ <100% but > 60% ☐ 40%-60% of the time ☐ > 0% but < 40%		

BEHAVIOR	YES	DON'T KNOW	NO
4. Reaction to **other noises.** Type(s) of noise(s) (vacuum cleaners, leaf blowers, weed whackers, dump trucks, sirens, alarm systems, etc.): Type of response—please check all that apply: ☐ Salivate ☐ Hide ☐ Defecate ☐ Tremble ☐ Urinate ☐ Destroy ☐ Escape ☐ Freeze ☐ Pant ☐ Will not eat food/treats ☐ Pace ☐ Pupil dilation ☐ Vocalize (bark, whine, growl, howl)	☐ 100% of the time ☐ <100% but > 60% ☐ 40%-60% of the time ☐ > 0% but < 40%		

5. How frequently in terms of *weeks* do noise events such as thunder, fireworks, or gunshots occur in the dog's environment?

a. Never 0%	b. Occasionally > 0% but < 50% Once a week or so	c. Regularly 50% but < 100% A few times a week	d. Frequently 100% At least multiple times a week

6. Has this dog ever been treated for noise sensitivities or phobias? If so, with what, please?

7. Does your dog react to other aspects of storms?			
a. Wind	☐ Yes	☐ No	☐ Uncertain
b. Darkness	☐ Yes	☐ No	☐ Uncertain
c. Ozone	☐ Yes	☐ No	☐ Uncertain
d. Barometric pressure	☐ Yes	☐ No	☐ Uncertain
e. Rain	☐ Yes	☐ No	☐ Uncertain

Aggression screen

KEY: NR=No reaction; S=Snarl (noise); L=Lift lip (can see corner teeth); B=Bark (aggressive, **not** an alerting bark); G=Growl (**not** a play growl); SP=Snap (no connection with skin); BT=Bite (connects with skin, regardless of damage); WD=Withdraw or avoid; NA=Not applicable (animal has never been in that situation)

This screen can be used in three ways:
(1) To note the presence or absence, at any time, of any of the behaviors
(2) By the clients to keep as a log about the baseline behavior, noting how many times the behavior occurs, given the number of times it is attempted, per unit time (i.e., per week)
(3) To keep a log about frequencies of the occurrence behaviors, given the number of times the circumstance has been encountered, at different intervals during treatment so that these numbers can be compared with those in (2)

Please note if the reaction is consistent in style, or only directed toward one person, or only present in one restricted circumstance. If using this screen only for the first use, note if the dog has been worsening in intensity or frequency in any category.

	NR	S	L	B	G	SP	BT	WD	NA
1. Take dog's food dish with food									
2. Take dog's empty food dish									
3. Take dog's water dish									
4. Take food (human) that falls on floor									
5. Take rawhide									
6. Take real bone									
7. Take biscuit									
8. Take toy									
9. Human approaches dog while eating									
10. Dog approaches dog while eating									
11. Human approaches dog while playing with toys									
12. Dog approaches dog while playing with toys									
13. Human approaches/disturbs dog while sleeping									
14. Dog approaches/disturbs dog while sleeping									
15. Step over dog									
16. Push dog off bed/couch									
17. Reach toward dog									

	NR	S	L	B	G	SP	BT	WD	NA
18. Reach over head									
19. Put on leash									
20. Push on shoulders									
21. Push on rump									
22. Towel feet when wet									
23. Bathe dog									
24. Groom dog's head									
25. Groom dog's body									
26. Stare at									
27. Take muzzle in hands and shake									
28. Push dog over onto back									
29. Stranger knocks on door									
30. Stranger enters room									
31. Dog in car at toll booth									
32. Dog in car at gas station									
33. Dog on leash approached by dog on street									
34. Dog on leash approached by person on street									
35. Dog in yard—person passes									
36. Dog in yard—dog passes									
37. Dog in vet's office									
38. Dog in boarding kennel									
39. Dog in groomers									
40. Dog yelled at									
41. Dog corrected with leash									
42. Dog physically punished—hit									
43. Someone raises voice to owner in presence of dog									
44. Someone hugs or touches owner in presence of dog									
45. Squirrels, cats, small animals approach									
46. Bicycles, skateboards									
47. Crying infant									
48. Playing with 2-year-old children									
49. Playing with 5- to 7-year-old children									
50. Playing with 8- to 11-year-old children									
51. Playing with 12- to 16-year-old children									

Previous Treatment Questionnaire

This questionnaire is designed to help us evaluate any role previous treatment may play in either your dog's problems or in their resolution. We would like you to answer two types of questions. The first set focuses on general, global approaches recommended. The second set, which is a fairly lengthy tick list, focuses on specific actions recommended. Please complete these tables to the best of your ability, and if our lists are not complete, or you feel that an explanation is warranted, please complete the "comment" section at the bottom. Even if you think that your dog is problem-free it would be extraordinarily helpful if you also completed this questionnaire so that we can compare dogs with problems to dogs without problems. Thanks!

Table 1: Global, general approaches recommended

	Suggested ° = Yes	By whom	Attempted ° = Yes	Outcome
1. Obedience class				
2. Private trainer				
3. Send to a shelter				
4. Place in another home				
5. Kill or euthanize				

	Suggested ° = Yes	By whom	Attempted ° = Yes	Outcome
6. Take to board certified behaviorist (ACVB)				
7. Agility trainer				
8. Consult your vet				
10. Consult a non-veterinary behavior consultant				
11. Make into working dog (e.g., guard, herding, hunting, etc.)				

Table 2: It's helpful if we know what treatments, tricks, or strategies clients have tried or have had recommended to them to alter their dogs' behaviors or to help shape better behaviors. Please tick the items below if they were suggested and or attempted. Please let us know who suggested that you try the activity noted, and the outcome if you attempted it. Please remember that you may have chosen not to try something that was suggested. Alternatively, you may have tried something that was not suggested, so please let us know what this was and the outcome at the bottom of the form.

	Suggested ° = Yes	By whom	Attempted ° = Yes	Outcome
1. Stare at or "stare down"				
2. Grab by jowls and shake				
3. Get an additional dog as a companion for this one				
4. Step on leash or choke collar and force down				
5. Blow in nose or face				
6. Buy different types of dog toys (e.g., Kongs, etc.)				
7. Metal choke collar				
8. Prong collar				
9. Halti, head collar, or Gentle Leader				
10. Harness				
11. No pull or Sporn harness				
12. Martingale collar				
13. Scruffy Guider				
14. Fabric choke collar				
15. Electronic or shock collar controlled by owner				
16. Electronic or shock collar controlled by trainer				
17. Electronic or shock collar– remote control or bark activated				

	Suggested ° = Yes	By whom	Attempted ° = Yes	Outcome
18. Citronella collar				
19. Citronella spray				
20. Throw a tin or can of pennies				
21. Water pistol				
22. Whistle				
23. Foghorn				
24. Hit dog with hand				
25. Use a blow torch				
26. Hit dog with empty plastic soda bottle				
27. Hit dog with whiffle ball bat				
28. Hit dog with leash				
29. Hit dog with chain				
30. Hit dog with board, plank, or baseball bat				
31. Hit dog under chin				
32. Step on dog's toes				
33. Knee dog in chest / belly				
34. Kick dog				
35. Bite dog				
36. "Alpha roll" [hold spread eagle on back]				
37. "Dominance down" [hold down on side, legs extended, head flat]				
38. Growl at dog				
39. Yell or scream at dog				
40. Long down				
41. Sit and wait				
42. "Time out" [if you do this let us know where and how, and for how long]				

	Suggested ° = Yes	By whom	Attempted ° = Yes	Outcome
43. Praise for good behavior				
44. Crate				
45. Kennel outdoors				
46. Fenced yard				
47. Invisible fence				
48. Isolate somewhere in house [if you do this, please let us know where and for how long]				
49. Board at vet's or kennel (which, please)				
50. Use whip on dog				
51. Chain				
52. Cattle prod				
53. "String up" or hang by leash and collar—all 4 feet off ground				
54. "String up" or hang by leash and collar—only front feet off ground				
55. Pop and jerk leash				
56. Yank or pull on leash				
57. Tie up physically				
58. Tie out or stake on very short lead hooked to wall or floor				
59. Muzzle				
60. Increase exercise				
61. Increase play				
62. Give treats for good behavior				
63. Deprive of food				
64. Throw against wall				
65. Beat with your fists				
66. Shove dog's nose/face into urine, feces, or destruction				
67. Use scat mats or other electronic avoidance systems				
68. Calming cap				
69. Thundershirt or Anxiety Wrap				
70. Doggles or eyeshades				

	Suggested ° = Yes	By whom	Attempted ° = Yes	Outcome
71. Anything else that was recommended or tried?				

Comments?

Stereotypic and ritualistic behavior history

This section of the history form is to be completed *only* if your dog is showing any repetitive, ritualistic behaviors **that you find troublesome or about which you are concerned.** If your dog is not doing this, you do not have to complete this form.

This first section focuses on a description and categorization of your dog's behavior(s).

---

1. Which of the following categories below fits your dog's behavior?

Tick as many categories that apply to the dog's behavior. Then tick the best description that relates to the selected behavior. If needed, please provide an explanation.

a. ☐ Grooming	☐ Chewing self ☐ Biting self ☐ Licking self ☐ Plucking hair from self ☐ Barbering/trimming hair on self ☐ Sucking self ☐ Continuously doing any of these behaviors to *another individual*. Please elaborate: ☐ Other, please explain:
b. ☐ Hallucinatory	☐ Staring and attending to things that are not there ☐ Tracking things that are not there ☐ Pouncing on or attacking things that are not there ☐ Other, please explain:
c. ☐ Consumptive	☐ Consuming rocks ☐ Consuming dirt or soil ☐ Consuming other objects ☐ Eating, licking, sucking, or chewing wool or fabric, rugs, furniture, et cetera ☐ Licking or gulping air ☐ Other, please explain:
d. ☐ Locomotory	☐ Circling/spinning ☐ Tail-chasing ☐ Freezing ☐ Other, please explain:
e. ☐ Vocalization	☐ Rhythmic barking ☐ Howling ☐ Growling ☐ Other, please explain:

This next section focuses on *patterns* of behaviors. Please indicate the appropriate answer (YES/NO/UNCERTAIN) for each of the following questions. Please feel free to add any information that you think might be helpful. You can add additional pages if needed.

	YES	NO	UNCERTAIN
2. Was there a change in the household or an event associated with the development of the behavior?	*If yes, please describe in detail.*		
3. Is there any time of day when the behavior seems more or less intense?	*If so, please describe in detail what is usually going on at that time of day.*		No one is home often enough to know.
4. Is there a person or another pet in the presence of whom the behavior seems more intense?	*If yes, who is this and what is their association to the pet?*		

	YES	NO	UNCERTAIN
5. Does the dog respond to its name or seem aware of its surroundings while in the midst of the behavior?			
6. Is the dog aware that you are calling him/her?	*If yes, how can you tell?*		
7. Can you convince the dog to stop the behavior by:			
a. Calling him or her			
b. Using physical restraint			
8. List the kinds of things (i.e., noises, treats, toys), if any, that will interrupt the behavior once it has started.			
9. Is there a location in which the dog prefers to perform the behavior?	*If yes, where?*		
10. For ingestion, list what types of objects are consumed. Be as specific as possible—what type of rug or sweater fabric?			
11. Does any event or behavior routinely occur immediately before the behavior begins?	*If so, what?*		
12. Does any event or behavior routinely occur immediately after the behavior ceases?	*If so, what?*		
13. Has the dog's general behavior changed in any way since the onset of the atypical behavior (i.e., the dog is more or less aloof, aggressive, withdrawn, playful, et cetera)?	*If so, please specify?*		
14. Has the dog's diet recently been changed?	If so, what specifically was the change?		
15. How old do you think your pet was when its ritualistic behavior began?	Age in months _____		
16. Did anyone else in the dog's family exhibit these or similar behaviors?			
17. Is there a pattern to the behavior? What are the duration, frequency, characteristics of the events themselves?	Duration: Days Weeks Months Pattern: After meals, in AM, et cetera (please specify)		

Finally, familial patterns of this condition have been documented so if you can provide a pedigree for this dog, it would be extremely helpful and informative. If you are able to provide a pedigree please label the dogs in it with the following code:

KA – Known affected
KU – Known unaffected
TA – Tentatively or possibly affected
TU – Tentatively or possibly unaffected
AO – Affected with another behavioral problem

Any blank dogs will be assumed to have no known behavioral information.

For this condition, affected relatives do not have to have the same form of the condition to be considered affected. In other words, some dogs may suck themselves whereas others follow fences or chase their tails. If you know what any other affected dogs do, please let us know.

☐ I am attaching a pedigree for this dog.
☐ There is a pedigree available for this dog but it is not attached.
☐ No pedigree is available for this dog.

Thank you for your help in providing as much information as possible.

Questionnaire to evaluate behaviors of old dogs

This section of the history form is to be completed *only* if your dog is older (> 7 years for larger dogs and > 10 years for smaller ones) so that we can assess changes associated with aging. If your dog is not elderly or you have no complaints that could be associated with age, you do not have to complete this form. If you are uncertain, please complete the form.

Behavior screen for age associated changes:

1. Locomotory/ambulatory assessment (tick **only one**)
   - ☐ a. No alterations or debilities noted
   - ☐ b. Modest slowness associated with change from youth to adult
   - ☐ c. Moderate slowness associated with geriatric aging
   - ☐ d. Moderate slowness associated with geriatric aging plus alteration or debility in gait
   - ☐ e. Moderate slowness associated with geriatric aging plus some loss of function (e.g., cannot climb stairs)
   - ☐ f. Severe slowness associated with extreme loss of function, particularly on slick surfaces (may need to be carried)
   - ☐ g. Severe slowness, extreme loss of function, and decreased willingness or interest in locomoting (spends most of time in bed)
   - ☐ h. Paralysed or refuses to move

2. Appetite assessment (may tick **more** than **one**)
   - ☐ a. No alterations in appetite
   - ☐ b. Change in ability to physically handle food
   - ☐ c. Change in ability to retain food (vomits or regurgitates)
   - ☐ d. Change in ability to find food
   - ☐ e. Change in interest in food (may be olfactory, having to do with the ability to smell)
   - ☐ f. Change in rate of eating
   - ☐ g. Change in completion of eating
   - ☐ h. Change in timing of eating
   - ☐ i. Change in preferred textures

3. Assessment of elimination function (tick **only one** in **each** category)
   a. Changes in frequencies and "accidents"
      - ☐ 1. No change in frequency and no "accidents"
      - ☐ 2. Increased frequency, no "accidents"
      - ☐ 3. Decreased frequency, no "accidents"
      - ☐ 4. Increased frequency with "accidents"
      - ☐ 5. Decreased frequency with "accidents"
      - ☐ 6. No change in frequency, but "accidents"

   b. Bladder control
      - ☐ 1. Leaks urine when asleep, only
      - ☐ 2. Leaks urine when awake, only
      - ☐ 3. Leaks urine when awake or asleep
      - ☐ 4. Full-stream, uncontrolled urination when asleep, only
      - ☐ 5. Full-stream, uncontrolled urination when awake, only
      - ☐ 6. Full-stream, uncontrolled urination when awake or asleep
      - ☐ 7. No leakage or uncontrolled urination, all urination controlled, but in inappropriate or undesirable location
      - ☐ 8. No change in urination control or behavior

   c. Bowel control (Circle appropriate answer, if this occurs, please)
      1. Defecates when asleep

         Formed stool   Diarrhea   Mixed

      2. Defecates without apparent awareness

         Formed stool   Diarrhea   Mixed

      3. Defecates when awake and aware of action, but in inappropriate or undesirable locations

         Formed stool   Diarrhea   Mixed

      4. No changes in bowel control

4. Visual acuity—how well do you think the dog sees? (tick **only one**)
   - ☐ a. No change in visual acuity detected by behavior—appears to see as well as ever
   - ☐ b. Some change in acuity **not** dependent on ambient light conditions
   - ☐ c. Some change in acuity dependent on ambient light conditions
   - ☐ d. Extreme change in acuity **not** dependent on ambient light conditions
   - ☐ e. Extreme change in acuity dependent on ambient light conditions
   - ☐ f. Blind

5. Auditory acuity—how well do you think the dog hears? (tick **only one**)
   - ☐ a. No apparent change in auditory acuity
   - ☐ b. Some decrement in hearing—not responding to sounds to which the dog used to respond
   - ☐ c. Extreme decrement in hearing—have to make sure the dog is paying attention or repeat signals or go get the dog when called
   - ☐ d. Deaf—no response to sounds of any kind

Questionnaire to evaluate behaviors of old dogs

6. Play interactions—if the dog plays with **toys** (other pets are addressed later), which situation best describes that play? (tick **only one**)
   - ☐ a. No change in play with toys
   - ☐ b. Slightly decreased interest in toys, only
   - ☐ c. Slightly decreased ability to play with toys, only
   - ☐ d. Slightly decreased interest and ability to play with toys
   - ☐ e. Extreme decreased interest in toys, only
   - ☐ f. Extreme decreased ability to play with toys, only
   - ☐ g. Extreme decreased interest and ability to play with toys

7. Interactions with humans—which situation best describes that interaction? (tick **only one**)
   - ☐ a. No change in interaction with people
   - ☐ b. Recognizes people but slightly decreased frequency of interaction
   - ☐ c. Recognizes people but greatly decreased frequency of interaction
   - ☐ d. Withdrawal but recognizes people
   - ☐ e. Does not recognize people

8. Interactions with other pets—which situation best describes that interaction? (tick **only one**)
   - ☐ a. No change in interaction with other pets
   - ☐ b. Recognizes other pets but slightly decreased frequency of interaction
   - ☐ c. Recognizes other pets but greatly decreased frequency of interaction
   - ☐ d. Withdrawal but recognizes other pets
   - ☐ e. Does not recognize other pets
   - ☐ f. No other pets or animal companions in house or social environment

9. Changes in sleep/wake cycle (tick **only one**)
   - ☐ a. No changes in sleep patterns
   - ☐ b. Sleeps more in day, only
   - ☐ c. Some change—awakens at night and sleeps more in day
   - ☐ d. Much change—profoundly erratic nocturnal pattern and irregular daytime pattern
   - ☐ e. Sleeps virtually all day, awake occasionally at night
   - ☐ f. Sleeps almost around the clock

10. Is there anything else you think we should know?

PROTOCOL FOR DEFERENCE

Overview

This protocol is one of three foundation protocols that will help ensure that **any** dog—even one *without* behavioral concerns—has a better, less confusing, and less anxious relationship with people. This protocol will also help cats, even though they should not be viewed as small, fuzzy dogs, as discussed below.

This protocol is a set of instructions that allows dogs to:
- Begin to learn to be calm
- Learn that they can ask questions of people
- Learn that they can get guidance about what is expected or whether they need worry if they just sit calmly

Together, these three points teach the dog that they learn better, feel safer and have more control in creating favorable interaction if they are calm.

These three points make this program completely different from "leadership," "earn to learn," "nothing in life is free," and other similar programs. Unlike these other programs, the **Protocol for Deference** is based on understanding and using innate dog social and cognition systems, and it uses the dog's ability to ask questions.

All dogs should be raised with this protocol beginning in early puppyhood. Using this protocol as part of the dog's daily life from early puppyhood will prepare the dog's brain to learn, and to learn in a manner that will minimize behavioral problems.

The Very Short Version of This Program

This basic program asks dogs to do one thing: sit calmly and look at the human whenever anything is desired or needed. That's it! Sitting is a deferential behavior for dogs, and if the dog is quiet, calm, relaxed, and looking at the human, the dog is receptive to any information that the human can share with the dog. That's it.

To learn why being receptive to information is important and why it works so well, read further. If you are content to just know that sitting calmly for all interactions will help your dog, you can stop reading here!

Longer Version of the Program

Canine Social Systems

Dogs have social systems that are very similar to those of humans:
- Dogs live in extended family groups.
- Dogs have extensive and extended parental care.
- Dogs will work as a group or a family to help care for the offspring and nurse their young prior to feeding them semi-solid, then solid, food.
- Dogs use play as one form of developing social skills where they learn to make mistakes successfully.
- Dogs communicate extensively vocally and non-vocally.
- Most importantly, dogs have a social system that is based on deference to others and that governs different roles in different contexts.

This understanding of normal dog behavior is at odds with the myths about dog behavior, many of which focus on dogs "struggling" for "dominance." Please ignore those myths. They are not only proving to be wrong whenever data have been collected, but they often result in unkind behavior toward dogs and render situations dangerous for humans.

Fights for status or control are notoriously **rare** among wild canids, including wolves. The same is true for humans. Unless the situation involves abnormal or severely stressed social conditions (e.g., famine, war, too many individuals and too few resources, mental health crises, et cetera), most human social relations are structured by negotiation and deference to others, rather than by violence. The same pattern holds for dogs. In fact, in both dog and human interactions, violence is often regarded as a symptom that something has gone wrong.

What do we mean by "deference"? Deference occurs when social individuals assess an ongoing situation and wait calmly to get input from another member of the group before pursuing another set of behaviors or social interactions.

Deference-based systems mean that:
- "Hierarchies," or the repeatable pattern of relationships each individual has with others are fluid and flexible depending on context;
- The individual to whom others defer may differ depending on the social circumstances; and
- Status and circumstances are not absolute.

For example, a human child may defer to his parents' requests, but then be the individual on the playground to whom other children defer. Dogs are similar: a dog may always adhere to instructions given by one spouse but not the other. This is because the dog has different relationships with each spouse.

Much has been written about dogs viewing their human families as their packs. It's important to remember that "pack" is just a word to describe a social grouping of canines, like "pod" describes a group of whales, and "gaggle" describes a group of geese.

True canine "packs" are composed of animals born into the social group, making them more closely related to each other than they are to most animals in another pack. This **does not** describe the situation in anyone's household because no human gave birth to their dog. Furthermore, most multi-dog households are made up of unrelated dogs, many of whom come into the household as young adults, or adults, not newborn puppies. Quite simply, pet households do not meet the definition for a "pack." The way most dogs live in human households is almost the "anti-pack": relationships are imposed upon resident dogs every time a new animal is added. If we understand this difference, deferential relationships will help us understand how relationships between dogs in households can change with time.

The problem for our dogs with our careless usage is that there is a value judgment within the word "pack." Humans have misused the concept in two ways:
1. by saying that they and their dogs are part of the same social group or "pack" when, actually, dogs have different relationships with dogs than they do with humans and
2. by assuming that—because they and their dogs are a "pack"—the humans must be the "leaders of the pack" and that they must show behaviors that are meant to maintain the social rank of everyone in the household.

Both of these assumptions are wrong, and they have caused us to behave badly toward animals who share their lives with us. Instead, it is important to know that while we care for dogs, they know that we are not dogs, and their relationships with dogs and humans will differ. We can better understand the complex interdependent relationship between dogs and humans by letting go of the "pack" concept.

Dogs are social and, like other social species, will communicate when they are uncertain or needy to other members of their group. This means that they are well adapted to look to their people for guidance. Dogs often become problems for their people when they cease to look to people for guidance, or if they never do this, or if they cannot do this.

To successfully understand and use this protocol you must understand that, although they do not have verbal speech, *dogs ask questions.* Sometimes they do this by offering a series of behaviors and wait for the change in human response, sometimes they do this by vocalization, sometimes they do this by pestering us by pawing, and sometimes they sit quietly and look at us. This protocol capitalizes on the last behavior because it is the one that gives us the time and space to exchange information with our dogs.

What's the Protocol for Deference?

The **Protocol for Deference** is the first step in both **preventing** problems associated with a lack of guidance and in **treating** all forms of behavioral problems. The keys to this program are simple:

- The dog must attend to the humans by quietly looking at or monitoring them for signals about which behaviors are accepted.
- The dog must relax when he does this.
- The humans must be clear in their signals.
- The humans must be reliable, reasonable, and humane.

All social animals create some form of rule structure for social interaction. Although cats have very different social systems than do dogs and people, the rule structure used to get information about varying situations from others is the same: Simply, you have to have the mental ability to pay attention and to send and receive information. This means that cats will also benefit from this program, although it is primarily written for dogs.

Clear communication is essential in social animals because it avoids an inefficient and potentially dangerous use of time (e.g., fighting). Every time there is uncertainty in a situation there is the potential for anxiety. Every time there is the potential for anxiety there is the chance to make a mistake in a behavioral response and to learn to reinforce that mistake. We want to avoid such uncertainty because by doing so we will minimize behavioral problems and maximize joyous, fun and loving relationships with our dogs.

Because dogs are so similar to us in so many ways, and so frequently look like they are hanging on our every word, we assume that they are complying with **our** rule structure and all its nuances. We need to understand that, while the ability to seek information from others is shared by all social species, we must learn how to do this with each new set of individuals. By using the tendency to defer—to seek information from others—we can ensure that we teach our dogs and cats how to exchange information with us in a nonviolent manner.

How Important Are Rule Structures?

All young animals need to learn the rule structures of their group, and they often do so by trial and error. Puppies need guidance in how to best communicate with humans to ensure their needs are met. Problem dogs need to have a consistent, benign, kind rule structure explicitly spelled out for them. If the dog knows a consistent rule or behavior that will get the attention of their people, they will then be receptive to guidance. Please note that "consistent" does not mean "rigid" or "unforgiving."

This pattern is a form of "discipline." People often confuse discipline, verbal or physical punishment, and violence or abuse. *The Protocol for Deference and all other behavioral protocols MUST be executed without violence or physical abuse,* or you will earn your pet's distrust. For most dogs, withdrawal of attention is a far more profound correction than is a physical "correction" or abuse. Abused dogs and those consistently mismanaged with physical punishment will either learn to override the punishment, or learn to seek it because punishment may be the only human contact they get.

What About Punishment?

Physical punishment can include some commonly recommended approaches to changing canine behavior:

- leash or collar "corrections" using a "choke" collar or a prong collar or any other tight, confining device,
- hitting the dog,
- walking the dog into a pole or tree to make him pay attention, and
- tying the dog so that he cannot move.

If these punishment techniques sound abusive, it's because most often they are.

The true definition of punishment doesn't require pain; it requires a stimulus sufficiently powerful that the undesirable behavior is abandoned by the dog **with the subsequent result** that the probability of the dog exhibiting the behavior **in the future** is lowered. The emphasized parts of the previous sentence are important because unless these conditions are met, the dog is not being "punished"—he is being injured mentally and, perhaps, physically.

Using Deferential Behaviors to Prevent Problems

The best way to handle undesirable behaviors is to prevent them. If we cannot prevent problematic behaviors we should just ignore the behaviors. By doing so we do not accidentally reward the dog with any of our behaviors associated with our reaction to the problem.

For example, if we forgot to take the puppy out after he ate, and he urinated on the carpet, it's too late to "correct," "punish," or interrupt him. He is done urinating and emptying the bladder is a self-rewarding behavior. Instead, just clean up and pay better attention to the dog's needs the next time. Think about this carefully. If you reach for the dog, show him the urine and yell at him, he will learn that you become erratic and scary when you show him his urine. He will **not** learn **not** to urinate on the rug.

Finally, we should be clear to the dog and tell the dog what behaviors **will** get the dog attention. It's utterly unfair to the dog to have him try to "guess" what it is that will get you to stop yelling at him and start loving him, yet these are the circumstances to which many dogs are reduced. We could tell someone a million times what *not* to do, but unless we tell them what we *want* them to do, they will still make mistakes. No one learns without knowing what is specifically expected as part of the successful task. So every time you use the word "no" you must try to couple it to offering the dog a replacement behavior. If the dog chews on the chair, you can say "no" only if you offer an alternative choice—a chew bone or the chance to come sit in front of you, look at you, and have a belly rub.

Core Steps for Deference

The three steps of (1) clear communication, (2) no punishment, and (3) ignoring undesirable behaviors are at the core of practicing deference.

How to Use This Protocol

The intent of this program is to:
- set a baseline of good behavioral interaction between the human and the dog and
- teach the dog that if he consistently is calm, quiet, attentive, and defers to his people, instruction, attention, and rewards will follow. In turn, the people learn to have realistic expectations for their pet and to signal clearly, calmly, and kindly to their pet.

This protocol also gives you permission to **not** be angry at your dog—instead, you can walk away. To have a great relationship with your pet you do **not** have to control his every move. The best dog–human relationships are the ones where clear signaling is involved—and good play almost guarantees this—and ones where both the dog's and human's needs are respected and met.

These goals must be accomplished in a safe, kind, passive manner, which is harder than most people realize.

If you are talking, reading, or watching TV and your dog comes to you and rubs, paws, or leans against you, you likely usually passively reach out and touch or pet the dog without asking the dog to sit and look at you first. The dog "controlled" the situation and got a response that rewarded him for pesky behaviors. The human was not aware of the association the dog made.

People have traditionally viewed such interactions as "contests": "dog, 1; human, 0." This is an adversarial translation of what really happened and it hides all the important information we need to have. Simply, if the dog is uncertain, anxious, concerned, or worried about the rules of the interaction, getting attention from people in a context of concern and anxiety makes that anxiety worse because it is passively reinforced (See Box 1 for a listing of behaviors that are associated with anxiety in dogs). By attending to the dog and asking him to defer to you by sitting when he requests attention, you have avoided accidentally rewarding problematic behaviors and ensured that you reward calm ones.

BOX 1

Nonspecific Signs of Anxiety

- Urination
- Defecation
- Anal sac expression
- Panting*
- Increased respiration and heart rates
- Trembling/shaking*
- Muscle rigidity (usually with tremors)
- Lip licking
- Nose licking
- Grimace (retraction of lips)
- Head shaking
- Smacking or popping lips/jaws together
- Salivation/hypersalivation
- Vocalization (excessive and/or out of context)
  - Frequently repetitive sounds, including high pitched whines,* like those associated with isolation
- Yawning
- Immobility/freezing or profoundly decreased activity*
- Pacing and profoundly increased activity*
- Hiding or hiding attempts
- Escaping or escape attempts
- Body language of social disengagement (turning head or body away from signaler)
- Lowering of head and neck
- Inability to meet a direct gaze

- Staring at some middle distance
- Body posture lower (in fear, the body is extremely lowered and tail tucked)
- Ears lowered and possibly droopy because of changes in facial muscle tone
- Mydriasis
- Scanning
- Hyper-vigilance/hyper-alertness (may only be noticed when touching or interrupting a dog or cat; they may hyper-react to stimuli that otherwise would not elicit this reaction)
- Shifting legs
- Lifting paw in an intention movement
- Increased closeness to preferred associates
- Decreased closeness to preferred associates
- Profound alterations in eating and drinking (acute stress is usually associated with decreases in appetite and thirst, chronic stress is often associated with increases)
- Increased grooming, possibly with self-mutilation
- Decreased grooming
- Possible appearance of ritualized or repetitive activities
- Changes in other behaviors including increased reactivity and increased aggressiveness (may be non-specific)*

The most commonly recognized signs of anxiety identified via questionnaire by clients.

This exercise is simple but the mindfulness involved is not.

Humans need to understand that they are **always** signaling to the dog whether they intend to or not and that dogs read nonverbal signaling better than people do. Given this, you must assess if your response is rewarding the particular behavior that you think it is. Here's a hint: if the dog is getting peskier or more worried, you are not reading the signaling situation correctly. You can re-set the social situation and ensure that you are correctly understanding it and providing helpful information, if you ask the dog to sit for just a second and look at you. The dog will understand that you are clarifying the signals for him. In fact, dogs do this, themselves, when among other dogs.

In this program, under no circumstance can you touch, love, or otherwise interact with your dog unless your dog is attending to you, sits, and deferentially awaits attention. *This is not about "control," "leadership," or "mastery" of the dog—it's about increasing the chance that you can signal clearly to the dog, that you have the dog's undivided attention while signaling, and that you are actually rewarding the behaviors that you desire.* Because dogs naturally defer to other dogs by sitting or lying down and looking at them, we can have them defer to us and be ready to take their cues from our signals by having the dog sit. Both dogs and humans may need to learn how to do all of this. Once everyone knows the rules, dogs will come to a human, sit quietly and receive love or instructions and all of this will take place within seconds. Dogs and humans who comply with this protocol generally interact more, have more fun and have a better relationship than those who do not use the protocol. In fact, you will find that your dog initiates more interactions and seeks to interact with you in more contexts.

Some simple guidance:

- The *sit* does not have to be and should not be prolonged. It can be as short as seconds as long as the dog's bottom is on the ground and the dog is looking quietly at the person. Even a wiggling 5-week-old puppy can sit—butt flush to the ground for a few seconds—and look at you. Puppies can even learn to sit and attend to you (look at you for cues, make eye contact, look happy and attentive while being quiet) in exchange for a food treat. As soon as the puppy sits, say "Good girl (boy)!" and give a tiny treat of something special.
- "Special" means that the treat is not something they get every day. "Treat-only" dog biscuits, tiny pieces of cheese, dried chicken, a tiny dab of cream cheese, et cetera will interest most dogs and signal that something special and good is coming up. The currency for dogs is access to you and your love. Treats can be a physical manifestation of love. As soon as the puppy's bottom is on the ground, praise and pet the pup, tell him he is brilliant, and give the treat.

For a dog who already knows how to sit the only problem is going to be reinforcing sitting while being calm for **everything** that the dog wants.

The Rule

The dog must sit and be quiet and—this is the essential part—look to you and attend to you for cues about whether her behavior is appropriate, in order to have access to **anything** and **everything** she wants for the rest of her life! This includes sitting for:

- food and feeding,
- treats,
- love,
- grooming,
- being able to go out—and come in,
- having the leash, halter, or harness put on,
- having her feet toweled,
- being **invited** onto the bed or sofa (if desired),
- playing games,
- playing with toys,
- having a tick removed,
- having a wound checked,
- being petted or loved,
- attention, and
- anything!

Remember, the dog must sit long enough to obtain the information she needs or to accomplish the task. Sitting by the door may be short; sitting to remove a tick will be longer.

If the dog is older or arthritic, she might be more comfortable lying down. The point is to cease being in motion and to calmly attend to the human for information.

Remember that you minimize the chance of miscommunication if each side is attending to the other. Sitting calmly allows the dog to do this.

The **Protocol for Deference** provides dogs with a rule that allows them to seek, and then take, guidance and help. *All dogs should learn this and *no* dog is too old to learn this.*

Using the **Protocol for Deference** *will not* take away a dog's spunk, fire, or individuality. It *will* allow you to have a far better relationship with the dog and to modulate any behaviors you view as problematic, while protecting the dog. This good relationship is critical if the dog is about to put himself in a potentially injurious position, like jumping out of the car in a parking lot. Also, people notice that when they don't have to struggle with the dog to get into or out of the house, when they don't get mauled while feeding the dog, and when they can regain their space on the sofa or bed just by asking the dog to come to them and sit, life with dogs is pleasurable, instead of a struggle.

What do deferential behaviors and the **Protocol for Deference** do to treat or prevent problem behaviors?

- Sitting and deferring for everything the dog wants, forever, reinforces the innate social structure of the dog and teaches him to look to his people for cues about the appropriateness of his or her behavior. You must respond by giving the dog your quiet, undivided attention and providing the information he needs or requests.
- Deferential behaviors can act as a form of mini "time out": they give the dog respite from a situation so that it does not have to get worse. The dog can learn that if he responds to a person's request to sit, that the person will help him or her decide what the next best behavior is. This is a great relief to dogs that are anxious about appropriate responses (i.e., many dogs with behavioral problems).
- Deferential behaviors allow the dog to calm down. A sitting dog is less reactive than one that is tearing around, so these behaviors allow the dog to couple a verbal cue, a behavior, and the physiological response to that behavior. All of this will have a calming effect.
- Deferential behaviors minimize the chance that any individual in the interaction is misunderstanding it, and allow the interaction to move forward in a clear and kind way.
- Deferential behaviors, when consistently reinforced, will allow the dog to anticipate what is expected. This is a very humane rule structure.

Points to Remember

- Starting immediately, the dog must ask for everything that he wants for the rest of his life, if you do not automatically anticipate the dog's wishes and needs. The dog does this by quietly sitting and staying for a few moments while looking to you for information (deferring to you). The important part here is the quiet, receptive attention to you. Sitting is helpful because it acts as a "stop" signal.
- The dog is requested to sit by using his name and then saying "Sit." The dog's name and a request to sit can be repeated every 3 to 5 seconds as needed. This is not an obedience class exercise—by using the dog's name and repeating your request if the dog is paying attention to you, you will reassure and refocus an anxious dog. Please do not think that if the dog does not comply with your every wish instantaneously that he is being "defiant"—*your relationship with your pet does not have to and shouldn't be an adversarial one*—the dog may just need time to become calm enough to sit, or the dog may be confused about what you really want because of past interactions. Some dogs are so shocked that they can actually be praised for just sitting and being calm that the idea takes a little getting used to. *Give the dog the mental space he needs to attend to and respond to you.*
- If the dog resists or refuses to comply or acts confused or anxious—*walk away from the dog.* The dog will eventually follow you. When the dog appears or demands attention, ask him to sit as prescribed above. If the dog resists—*walk away from the dog.* Sooner or later this dog will try sitting—a natural canine information-gathering behavior—as a way to learn if this is what you want. You just have to outlast the dog. Do not use the dog's lack of compliance as an excuse to get angry: the dog's intent is not to make you angry—the dog may not be able to perform the request yet because of anxiety or fear. If you persist in calm, clear instructions the dog's behavior will change. Talk to concerned dogs in a calm tone that lets them know that they can sit for attention at any time.
- As soon as the dog sits, reward him with praise. A food reward will hasten the process for a dog that doesn't know how to sit. The next step is to teach the dog "stay" (see **Protocol for Teaching "Sit," "Stay," and "Come"**). Please remember that the dog must stay until released. Because the point of this protocol is to enforce deference in a way that will allow the dog to generalize being calm now to being calm in other situations, quick releases are desired. Later, if you wish, you can practice long stays and downs as part of an overall relaxation and behavior modification program (see **Protocol for Relaxation: Behavior Modification Tier 1**). The **Protocol for Relaxation** is a necessary part of the treatment program for dogs with true behavior problems.
- Watch for subtle, pushy, defiant, anxious, distressed, uncertain behaviors that the dog may exhibit. Expect that you and the dog will occasionally make mistakes—don't fight with the rest of the family about it. This will not help the dog. Remember that dogs read body language far better than you do and they are watching you all the time. They could be watching for an opportunity to escape or for a signal from you that tells them if they have to worry. Use that watchful behavior, and shape it into using more deferential behaviors. As soon as your dog can sit and look at you, you will want to add the second of the three foundation programs: **Protocol for Teaching Your Dog to Take a Deep Breath and Use Other Biofeedback Methods as Part of Relaxation.**
- Please remember that everyone in the household must be consistent and work with the dog. Children need to be monitored to ensure their safety and to help them to avoid teaching the dog the wrong behavior. Children must understand the difference between a food salary and a bribe, and **must be taught not to tease the dog.** Dangling food out in front of a dog at a distance is an invitation to get up and lunge, and very young children may not realize that they are doing this. Open, flat hands are the best way to offer food to dogs.
- Reward the dog. This should be fun for everyone.

Note the Following

- You can and should use the dog's name—this will get her to attend to you. You can use the name frequently, unlike in obedience, *as long as she is paying attention to you.* In fact, her name should be her cue to orient toward you. If she doesn't look at you immediately, put the treat near your eye. You need her to focus. If you have unintentionally taught the dog to ignore her name, you will have to start with a new verbal cue and couple it with putting the treat to your eye to get the dog to look at you for the verbal cue.
- Repeat your request after a few seconds if the dog is not paying attention to you. Again, this is not obedience—the dog needs your reassurance and may need help focusing on you. If you have taught the dog to ignore her name, the new verbal cue you have chosen may take a few repetitions for the dog to learn. As the dog improves or learns more, you will repeat their request signals less frequently and at greater intervals. This is what those who study learning call a "shaping behavior": We can learn something by gradually approximating it and being rewarded for progressively closer approximations.
- Reward the dog appropriately. Eventually, the food treats will appear less predictably. At the outset the dog needs everything you can do to help her.
- Remember to use one or two words consistently as a releaser ("All done!," "That's it!," "Bellissimo!," et cetera). Then remember that if you use those words while talking to the dog, the dog will get up, so choose words the dog is not going to hear all the time. If the dog gets up before release, ask the dog to stay and stay again, and wait 3 to 5 seconds before release. This will prevent Jack-in-the-box behavior.
- Don't expect even the best-behaved dog to be able to pay attention to you, be calm, and respond to your request if pandemonium surrounds the dog. You cannot expect dogs to be fully responsive in stressful, noisy, confusing environments unless they are specifically taught to do so, as are service dogs.

As the dog becomes more experienced and masters staying at a short distance, *gradually* increase the distance between you and the dog. ***Do not*** go from getting the dog to stay within 1 meter of you to walking across the room. The temptation for the dog to get up and follow you will be great and all you have done is to provoke conflict and anxiety in the dog. This will defeat your goal. A more detailed approach that reinforces stay is found in the **Protocol for Relaxation: Behavior Modification Tier 1**.

If you would like, you can do this on a lead, using a head collar, which may help some dogs to sit. See the handout on head collars (**Protocol for Choosing Collars, Head Collars, and Harnesses**) before deciding to do this.

A Cautionary Word on Food Treats

Remember, the treats are to be used as a salary or reward—*not as a bribe.* If you bribe a dog or cat you are sunk before you start. *Bribes* come *before* the dog executes the desired behavior to lure him away from an undesirable behavior; *rewards* come *in exchange* for a desirable behavior. It is often difficult to work with a problem dog that had learned to manipulate bribes, but there are creative ways around this, often involving head collars.

First, find a food that the dog likes, and that he does not usually experience. Suggestions include boiled, slivered chicken or tiny pieces of cheese. Boiled, shredded chicken can be frozen in small portions and defrosted as needed. Individually wrapped slices of cheese can be divided into tiny pieces (0.5 × 0.5 cm) suitable for behavior modification through the plastic, minimizing waste and mess. Whatever you choose, the following are guidelines:

- Foods that are high in protein *may* help induce changes in brain chemistry that help the dog to relax, so choose a protein treat over a carbohydrate one.
- Dogs should not have chocolate because it can be toxic to dogs.
- Some dogs do not do well with treats that contain artificial colors or preservatives.
- Dogs with food allergies or those taking medications that are monoamine oxidase inhibitors may have food restrictions (some cheeses, for dogs taking MAOIs = Anipryl, PrevenTics collars).
- Dog biscuits and kibble generally are not sufficiently interesting for learning new behaviors but some foods are so desirable that the dog is too stimulated by them to relax—you want something in between these two extremes.
- Treats should be tiny (less than half of a thumbnail) so that the dog or cat does not get full, fat, or bored with them.
- If the dog or cat stops responding for one kind of treat, try another.
- Do not let treats make up the bulk of the dog's diet—they need their normal, well-balanced ration.

The Reward Process

There is an art to rewarding dogs and cats with food treats. Learning to do so correctly will help the dog or cat to focus on the exercises and will keep everyone safe. If you keep prepared treats in a cup or bag behind your back, or in a treat bag at your waist, you always have easily available treats. By keeping only one or a few treats in your hand at a time you will be able to prevent dogs and cats from lunging for treats. The hand that you will use to reward your pet can then be kept behind your back so that the dog or cat doesn't stare at the food, or you can move your hand to your eye so that you can teach your pet to look at you. The food treat must be small—the focus of the pet's attention must be you, not the food. Bring your hand, with lightly closed fingers, to the dog, just under his mouth, and open your hand flat. You want to move quickly enough to ensure that your pet gets the reward a second or two after successfully completing the task, but not so fast or forcefully that you scare or threaten your pet.

Animals who have been hit or beaten may need to have the food treats gently dropped in front of them at first. Otherwise, they may shy from the hand with the treat.

When first starting the **Protocol for Deference** let the cat or dog smell and taste the reward so that he knows what the currency is. If your cat or dog is too terrified to approach, you can place a small amount of the treat on the floor.

If the dog or cat is too fearful or too aggressive to look at you for any extended period of time without fleeing or lunging, you can still ask him to "look," but you have to modify how this is done. In such cases, ask them to very briefly look at you and then reward them low and off to the side so that they are not confronted by directly facing you. There are a lot of myths about whether you should look at dogs. Ultimately, you need to be able to look at your dog or cat directly—it's how all mammals best gauge trust—but "looking" is not the same as "staring." Most of us would perceive a stare as a threat.

Quick Dos and Don'ts

- **Don't** "stare down" dogs. Normal dogs will look away, anyway, if you look scary enough, troubled dogs will think you are a threat—because you are—and their anxiety or aggression will worsen.
- **Do** look at the dog or cat. Looking someone directly in the eye is the best way to ensure that you are communicating well. Looking at a dog is different than staring. When you stare you don't move your eyes, you stiffen the muscles in your face, and your pupils likely dilate. This is a threat. Looking is much more relaxed and is important for clear communication in all mammals with decent eyesight.
- If the dog or cat begins to be aggressive when you casually look at him—**do** divert or move your gaze so that you can keep him in view with your peripheral vision, while not making direct eye contact. This will often lessen any aggression. It is *always* a bad idea to try to "out stare" or "stare down" any aggressive animal.
- If you have an animal who is too worried or aggressive to look at you, raise your hand, with the treat concealed, to your forehead while saying "look" then quickly, but fluidly so that you don't startle or threaten the animal, move your hand down and to the side so that the animal has to turn their head to have the now-exposed treat.
- If the dog is really a concern or if you don't feel comfortable, after they look at you, drop the treat to their side but in front of their face so that they can still sit and see you while being rewarded. This trick requires that you have good aim. In any case, as you are rewarding the dog or cat say, "good sit" so that the praise and treat are coupled. This way the praise will later act on its own to reinforce the behavior.
- **Do not** hold treats in fingertips: this is an invitation for an accidental bite. Please don't make your dog or cat responsible for that.

All of these steps are shown on the video **Humane Behavioral Care for Dogs: Problem Prevention and Treatment**. Please watch this video.

If kittens and puppies are raised with this program most will be delights. For those who will still have problems, the problems will be readily identifiable early on, and recognized because of the change in the pet's otherwise impeccable behavior. Good luck, and enjoy your charmingly behaved companion!

PROTOCOL FOR TEACHING YOUR DOG TO TAKE A DEEP BREATH AND USE OTHER BIOFEEDBACK METHODS AS PART OF RELAXATION

Dogs, like humans, cannot learn new behaviors if they are distressed. In fact, we all best produce the needed brain chemicals to make lasting memory if we are attentive enough to watch carefully but not so attentive that we are overly concerned. Most dogs about whom clients are concerned and/or who have truly pathological behavior are not calm enough to learn and use new information, especially if part of that information is learning to be calm.

The purpose of this short handout is to teach you how to teach your dog to take a deep breath and how to use other biofeedback tools to prepare your dog to relax so that the dog can learn how to change his behavior in a way that makes everyone happier.

The three important signaling tools used here that involve biofeedback are:
- "look,"
- "breathe," and
- petting a dog in a manner that avoids unhelpful arousal and encourages useful focus.

These three signaling tools are demonstrated in the video, *Humane Behavioral Care for Dogs: Problem Prevention and Treatment.*

Look

You will make the most progress with your dog if you work with this protocol together with the other two foundation behavior modification programs, the **Protocol for Relaxation: Behavior Modification Tier 1** and the **Protocol for Deference.** Both of these protocols require that your dog "look"— meaning look at and, preferably, make eye contact with you—and work best if your dog can hold his breath for a second or two.

The nine steps for teaching "look" are as follows:
1. First, you want to couple your dog's attention to the word when giving the dog a food reward. Start by holding the treat in your hand with fingers closed, palm up, and then opening the hand to deliver the treat. The open hand prevents shying in some fiercely treated dogs and also promotes treat delivery that is gentle for the human. Your first step in teaching deep breathing may be to teach the dog to take a treat calmly. Feel free to get professional help with teaching this. You will need to ensure that you are not triggering any signs of anxiety, as this will not help the dog to be calm (see Box 1).

BOX 1

Non-specific Signs of Anxiety

- Urination
- Defecation
- Anal sac expression
- Panting*
- Increased respiratory and heart rates
- Trembling/shaking*
- Muscle rigidity (usually with tremors)
- Lip licking
- Nose licking
- Grimace (retraction of lips)
- Head shaking
- Smacking or popping lips/jaws together
- Salivation/hypersalivation
- Vocalization (excessive and/or out of context)
  - Frequently repetitive sounds, including high pitched whines,* like those associated with isolation
- Yawning
- Immobility/freezing or profoundly decreased activity*
- Pacing and profoundly increased activity*
- Hiding or hiding attempts
- Escaping or escape attempts
- Body language of social disengagement (turning head or body away from signaler)
- Lowering of head and neck
- Inability to meet a direct gaze

- Staring at some middle distance
- Body posture lower (in fear, the body is extremely lowered and tail tucked)
- Ears lowered and possibly droopy because of changes in facial muscle tone
- Mydriasis
- Scanning
- Hyper-vigilance/hyper-alertness (may only be noticed when touched or interrupted; dog or cat may hyper-react to stimuli that otherwise would not elicit this reaction)
- Shifting legs
- Lifting paw in an intention movement
- Increased closeness to preferred associates
- Decreased closeness to preferred associates
- Profound alterations in eating and drinking (acute stress is usually associated with decreases in appetite and thirst, chronic stress is often associated with increases)
- Increased grooming, possibly with self-mutilation
- Decreased grooming
- Possible appearance of ritualized or repetitive activities
- Changes in other behaviors including increased reactivity and increased aggressiveness (may be non-specific)*

The most commonly recognized signs of anxiety identified via questionnaire by clients.

2. Start by giving the dog a treat so that he knows what the reward is and so that you can be sure the dog loves the treat. Remember that dogs work best for information about expectations. A really good treat tells them that their work with you will be appropriately rewarded.

3. Once you are sure that your dog likes the treat, take the treat in your hand, close your fingers over the treat so that only your fingers—not the treat—show and move it to your eye. See Photos 1 and 2.

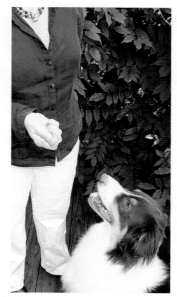

Photo 1 Fingers closed over treat in hand.

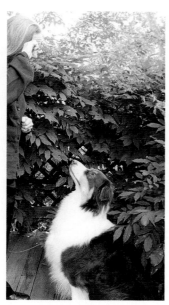

Photo 2 Distance to stand from the dog (Picasso) with the dog looking at a closed hand that is held near your eye.

4. When you get the treat to your eye, say "look."

5. As soon as the dog looks at your eyes, however briefly, tell him he is great and quickly move your hand with the treat down and open it flat under his chin so that he can have the treat.

6. Then, continue to practice the sequence above where you reward eye contact with the treat to further promote the coupling of the word "look" to actually looking up to your eye.

7. Next, reward better eye contact with a signal that draws the dog's attention to your eye (e.g., moving a finger to the eye while saying "look"). You can do this by hiding the food behind your curled index finger and thumb so that your dog is watching your finger and not the food. This action helps dogs to follow a target—your finger—not a lure—the treat. See Photo 3.

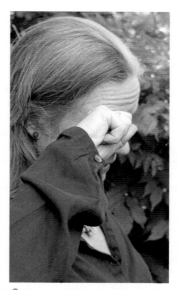

Photo 3 Fingers hiding treat brought to eye.

8. Ideally and ultimately, your dog should be able to respond to the nonverbal signal *and* to sit and relax when he sees your finger go to your eye. It takes practice to get this amount of progress but it's achievable within a few practice sessions. See Photo 4.

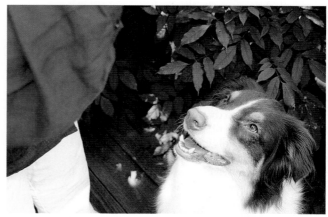

Photo 4 Picasso sitting and looking with relaxed face

9. Finally, as soon as you say the dog's name and begin to move your finger to your eye, your dog should sit and look at you.

A really smart dog figures out that we are working with deferential behaviors, and every time you say his name he will look at you and if you are close to him, he will sit. This is a desirable outcome because it means you are meeting his needs for information and you are communicating well.

Please note: If you are using these instructions for teaching "look" and "breathe" so that you can begin the **Protocol for Relaxation: Behavior Modification Tier 1,** please *go slowly* until you are sure that the dog responds as described above. *It is very easy to teach dogs to be obedient but more anxious if you rush any of these programs.*

The single biggest mistake that clients make in working with true behavior modification is that they move through the process too rapidly without paying attention to the dog's signals about whether he is calm, scared, or simply overwhelmed. It's best to pretend that all dogs have special needs and go slowly—there is no cost to going slowly enough so that the dog is always rewarded for clearly showing you he is calm and attentive.

On the other hand, *there is a huge cost in confusion and anxiety on the dog's part*—and frustration on the human's part—when the human goes too fast for that dog's particular comfort level. Frequent, short sessions are preferable to long, drawn-out sessions for both the client and dog. Working for a few minutes 4 to 5 times a day actually may help the dog to learn and use the behaviors better than would 1 to 2 long sessions. This work schedule also allows everyone to incorporate the behavior mod into everyday life.

Breathe

Heart rate, attentiveness, and respiratory rate are all linked. If we can teach humans or dogs to take slower, deeper breaths, they relax, their heart rate decreases, and they can be more attentive to focusing on the task at hand. These responses are all coupled to changes in hormonal and other chemical signals that shift the brain's and body's reactivity from a system ready to act on a threat to one ready to focus on learning, not reacting.

The first step for dogs is to teach them to hold their breath as a way to learn deep breathing and focus.

The trick to getting this to work is to teach the dog to breathe deeply and to incorporate this breathing into all encouraged deferential behaviors. Understanding how dogs breathe will help in understanding how we can teach them to hold their breath.

Dogs cannot simultaneously pant and smell or breathe through their nose, and they have alar folds/flaps on the sides of their nose that move up and out when they take a deep breath. This means that you can use the movement of these folds—the dilation of the nostrils—to indicate and confirm when the dog is holding her breath. With small or thin and short-coated dogs, you can also watch the ribcage to see if the rate at which it moves slows. The steps are as follows.

1. You can start to teach the dog to take a deep breath by asking the dog to sit and "look" at you for a food treat, as explained above. See Photo 5.
2. Next, as you quickly move the treat from your eye region (where it is hidden in your curled finger) and while the dog makes eye contact with you, stop moving your finger a few centimeters in front of the dog's nose without giving the treat. Say the word "breathe." See Photo 6. *If your dog is reactive or aggressive when food is available, you will want to watch carefully here to ensure that the dog remains*

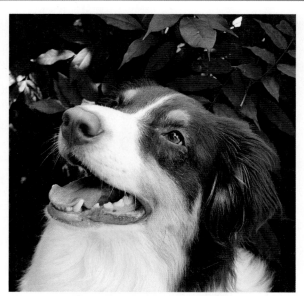

Photo 5 Picasso sitting and looking as he is beginning to relax and take a deep breath

calm. If the dog becomes more agitated, you will benefit from working with a professional (a trained, certified dog trainer or trained veterinary professional who uses only *force-free techniques; see the Pet Professional Guild website [www.pet professionalguild.com] for information) who can help you to desensitize the dog to food moving toward his nose.* If your dog doesn't know how to take food without grabbing it and is overly enthusiastic, but not aggressive, then don't give the dog the treat until he stops grabbing for it; the dog will learn not to grab.

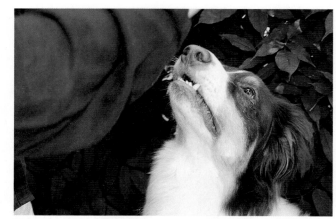

Photo 6 Changes in Picasso's mouth and nose as the treat is lowered to his face and he inhales.

3. The dog's nostrils will usually flare as he smells the treat, and because he cannot sniff something and pant at the same time, the dog will hold his or her breath. See Photo 7.
4. As soon as you see that the dog has held his breath and/or flared his nostrils, immediately deliver the treat with the phrase "good breathe, Picasso.[1]" See Photos 8 and 9. If your dog does not flare his nostrils, you will have to shape

---

[1]Picasso is the name of the dog in the photos; you should use your dog's name.

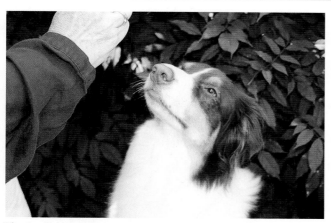

Photo 7 Nostrils begin to flare as Picasso closes his mouth and inhales in response to the request "breathe."

the flare. Simply reward any movement of the nostrils at first. Then reward the dog only when the nostrils are larger. Then, move toward only rewarding larger, flared nostrils once they are held still, round, and open. Most dogs can figure this out in a few minutes, but the changes can be hard to see. By only using positive rewards in this activity, mistakes are recoverable and it's okay that both the human and the dog are learning.

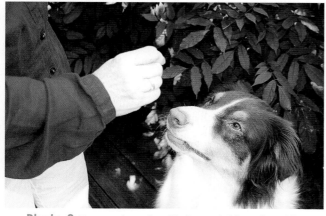

Photo 8 Deeper breath with flare of sides of nostrils.

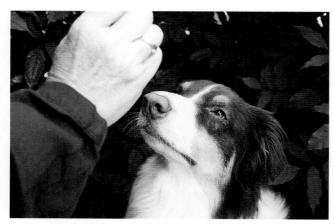

Photo 9 Deep breath and fully flared nostrils.

5. Practice this for a few minutes until you are certain that you know what you are looking for and that your dog is giving it to you. It can be difficult to see nostril flares in dark-faced dogs, but once you learn what a nostril flare looks like on your dog, you will know it.

6. As your dog gets better at responding to the "breathe" request, start to delay the provisioning of the treat a few seconds at a time.

7. Within a short while you will have a dog who holds his breath and slows his heart and respiratory rate, and so becomes more focused and relaxed. If you only reward the most focused and relaxed states, your dog will come along quite nicely.

It does not usually take more than 5 minutes to teach a dog to hold her breath, even if the dog is very hairy, making the nose tough to see (Photo 10, *A*) or the nose is dark (Photo 10, *B*), but it may take longer for you to recognize and encourage the behavior. You will need to be observant and quick, and not linger with presenting the food as an olfactory stimulus.

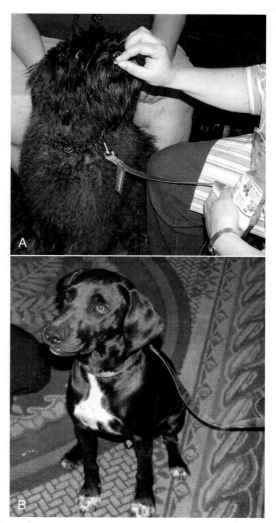

Photo 10 Naïve dogs being taught to "breathe" and flare their nostrils. Very hairy faces (**A**) and dark noses (**B**) often make it a bit harder for people to see the nostrils move, but veterinarians in this laboratory class had no difficulty.

If you videotape yourself, you will learn to teach the dog to take a deep breath upon request because you will see when the dog takes a breath and learn to look for the associated behaviors in your dog.

Here is a Youtube link that will help you to see how breathing and relaxation can help: www.youtube.com/watch?v=DIxELL4FkWI. This video was made by a client who taught the technique to her dog, and here the dog is using it to calm himself when she is not available to give him cues.

How to Pet a Thoughtful Dog

Finally, people pet their dogs, but few calm them by petting them. In fact, people usually arouse their dogs when petting them by petting in quick, short strokes all over the dog's head, face, and shoulders.

Instead, if we want a thoughtful, calm dog who looks to us for information that is helpful to him, we need to replace conventional petting with long, slow strokes, deep muscle pressure, and massage.

"Smart pet" instructions:

1. To start, the next time you touch your dog, don't move your hand. Instead, touch him and press firmly but gently. Most dogs will move into your hand.
2. Then, gradually, using constant, gentle pressure, move your hand from his head, down his neck, and slowly down his spine. If you move too quickly to be able to identify and count the vertebrae (back bones), you are going too fast (or the dog is too plump).
3. Then press and massage the front of your dog's chest in a circular motion. Concentrate on the area just above where the front legs attach. Use one hand at first until you get used to slow, firm pressure. Slowly extend your circular massage movements to the dog's shoulders and neck and work your way back down the dog.
4. The dog will relax if he is not worried about you (see Photo 11), there have been no traumatic handling experiences, and the dog has no painful conditions.

These "smart pet" instructions are demonstrated in the video, *Humane Behavioral Care for Dogs: Problem Prevention and Treatment.* For most dogs this type of petting really helps them to focus when needed because they learn what it is like to be calm and to be able to take in information when

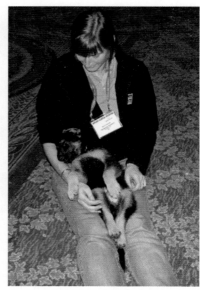

Photo 11 Puppy after being petted and massaged slowly.

calm. This type of handling and physical interaction also changes the dog–human relationship. The dogs get to have some seriously enjoyable downtime with their people and then seem more attentive to them in other circumstances.

What's After "Look," "Breathe," and "Pet"?

Enjoy the calm and use it to help promote the dog's ability to learn the other two parts of the foundation behavior modification protocols: the **Protocol for Relaxation: Behavior Modification Tier 1,** and the **Protocol for Deference.** These act as foundations for kind and humane rules by which you can guide your dog through more appropriate and desired behavioral responses.

If your dog has no behavior problems, these exercises will minimize the chance that any problems will develop.

But most importantly, these exercises will ensure that you and your dog understand each other's signals and needs. That's priceless!

PROTOCOL FOR RELAXATION: BEHAVIOR MODIFICATION TIER 1

This protocol contains the essential, basic behavior modification program on which all more complex programs using desensitization (DS) and counter-conditioning (CC) will be built. This protocol can be used for both cats and dogs. The protocol has the following sections:

1. Introduction
2. Starting Out: Roles for Spontaneous Reward and Using the "Shaping" Technique
3. Description of the Protocol for Relaxation: Tier 1
4. A Note About Food Treats
5. Understanding the Reward Process
6. Getting the Dog's or Cat's Attention
7. Avoiding Problems
8. The Format for the Protocol
9. The Protocol Task Sheets and Tips for Implementing These
10. Suggestions for Future Repetitions

There are 15 task sheets, enough to allow you to work steadily for *at least 2 weeks at the fastest recommended pace*. The speed with which you complete this behavior modification program with your pet depends entirely on your pet's response, as explained below. *There is no reward for speedy completion; however, the reward for successful completion is a happy, calm, less reactive and more interactive pet.*

1. Introduction

This program is the foundation program for all other behavior modification programs. You can see how this program should be done and learn about some pitfalls in the video, *Humane Behavioral Care for Dogs: Problem Prevention and Treatment.*

First, some advice: Please do not be afraid of the term "behavior modification." When most people hear this term they think of some complex set of exercises that will take hours a day. **Not so.** Behavior modification is nothing more than a set of exercises that lead to changes in behavior. You can practice these for 2 minutes 10 times a day, 5 minutes a day, 30 minutes a day, or 20 minutes twice a day—whatever works best for you and your pet.

A cautionary note is warranted: Please do not feel that you *should* do this. If you feel that this program is a troublesome imposition and a burden, you will not be able to use it as a tool that empowers you and makes your relationship with your pet better. *Please do not set a schedule you cannot keep, or one that makes you feel rushed or burdened.* Will your pet improve more slowly if you work less often and for shorter periods of time with the program? Yes. But if you resent working with your pet, feel that you should do so, and cram a long exercise into an already overburdened schedule, you will resent the program and your pet, and you will not do it correctly. Instead, work with a realistic schedule for you and work at your pet's pace. You will both be happier, and as your pet improves, you will be more willing to work with her.

Accordingly, you should realize that this **Protocol** can also be used as a *preventative* program for puppies and kittens. In fact, if everyone used the **Protocol for Deference,** the **Protocol for Teaching Your Dog to Take a Deep Breath (and Use Other Biofeedback Methods as Part of Relaxation),** and this **Protocol** as the rule structure for teaching puppies and kittens

or newly adopted cats and dogs appropriate behaviors, we would likely prevent most behavioral complaints, or recognize and treat concerns earlier. *The single biggest mistake that veterinarians and trainers make is to forget about the preventative use of these types of programs.*

Before your read further *please note* that this is **not** your typical "behavior mod" program. This program differs from most other behavior programs in that the behavior you are rewarding is subtle, and the better you get at rewarding the subtleties, the faster your dog or cat will improve.

The purpose of this **Protocol** is to teach the dog or cat to sit and stay *while relaxing* in a variety of circumstances. It's important that you understand that there is nothing magical about just sitting. Sitting is helpful because a sit acts as a "stop" signal understood by us, dogs, and cats, and it helps focus your pet on the task and on your signals. In dogs, sitting is a deferential behavior, and it's the rare dog who will not sit and then look to another individual for instructions or information about what is to come next. *However*—and this is a **huge** *however*—dogs can sit and look at you **and still be terrified or concerned.** If you reward the dog or cat when he is exhibiting any behavior other than a relaxed, calm pose, you have just inadvertently also rewarded anxiety, fear, and distress. This is *not* what you want to do. Because of this, your pet should be able to comply with the **Protocol for Deference** and the **Protocol for Teaching Your Dog to Take a Deep Breath (and Use Other Biofeedback Methods as Part of Relaxation)** before starting this protocol. If your dog or cat cannot sit and stay, see the **Protocol for Teaching Cats and Dogs to "Sit," "Stay," and "Come."**

2. Starting Out: Roles for Spontaneous Reward and Using the "Shaping" Technique

Before you start this program, learn what a relaxed facial and body expression in your pet looks like. Practice rewarding this expression. See the **Protocol for Teaching Your Dog to Take a Deep Breath (and Use Other Biofeedback Methods as Part of Relaxation)** for one approach. If you can only get the animal to look calm and relaxed for a few seconds at first, that's fine; you can gradually expand the time they stay relaxed by rewarding the behavior every time it occurs and while it is continuing to occur.

If you cannot get the "relaxed look" at all, go for one that is less distressed and then use a technique called "shaping." When you use shaping you continually reward behaviors that are better approximations of the behavior you want. When your pet backslides—and she will—please do not shriek at her. Instead, just ignore the anxious behaviors that are not going in the direction that you want (e.g., more relaxed). For example, if no matter what you do the dog's eyes are popping out of his head and he's panting, just walk away and quit. This is not an endurance test. Then, when the dog spontaneously exhibits calm behaviors, maybe even before he goes to sleep, reward *those* calm behaviors. Softly telling your pets that they are wonderful when they are already asleep is the least-used trick to improve their behavior, but it works! Don't startle them, don't pet them, just quietly commend them.

For very, very anxious dogs, before you can even start this program, you will have to spend a lot of time spontaneously rewarding the dog when he exhibits the relaxed behavior just in the context of everyday life. Only then will that dog be able to move on to having his behavior shaped in response to a request. Dogs should not be starting this **Protocol** until they can be and have been rewarded for a sufficient number of calm, spontaneous behaviors that they have learned are valued by you. Working consistently with the **Protocol for Deference,** especially when coupled with tangible rewards like food treats, will help speed this initial process.

3. Description of the Protocol for Relaxation: Tier 1:

The circumstances under which you will work with your pet in this **Protocol** change from very reassuring ones where you are present, to potentially more stressful ones where you are absent and acting pretty strangely. You may wish to tailor the program to your specific needs and lifestyle. Please remember that the point of the program is not to teach the dog or cat to sit; *sitting (or lying down, if the dog or cat is more comfortable) is only a tool.* The five main points of the program are to teach the dog or cat to:
1. relax,
2. attend to you for cues about the appropriateness of her current behavior **and** information about what is to come next,
3. defer to you,
4. enjoy earning a salary for an appropriate, desirable behavior, and
5. develop, as a foundation, a pattern of calm, relaxed behaviors that will then let her cooperate with future behavior modification (generally desensitization and counterconditioning).

This **Protocol** will act as a foundation for teaching the dog or cat context-specific appropriate behavior. The focus is to teach the dog or cat to rely on you for all the cues as to the appropriateness of his behavior so that he can learn not to react inappropriately.

4. A Note About Food Treats

This program utilizes food treats. Please read about the logic of using food treats in the **Protocol for Deference.** Remember, the treats are to be used as a salary or reward, not as a bribe. If you bribe a problem dog, you are sunk before you start. It is often difficult to work with a problem dog who has learned to manipulate bribes, but there are creative ways around this, some of which may involve head collars. Head collars are humane ways to prevent biting, to help the dog to focus on you, and to stop dogs from bolting away or jumping up. For more information about these, please see **Protocol for Choosing Collars, Head Collars, Harnesses, and Leads.**

First, find a food that your pet likes, but doesn't get all the time. Suggestions include boiled, slivered chicken, freeze-dried liver, and tiny pieces of cheese. Boiled, shredded chicken can be frozen in small portions and defrosted as needed. Individually wrapped slices of cheese can be divided into tiny pieces suitable for behavior modification through the plastic, minimizing waste and mess. Tinned shrimp can be drained and frozen individually in a plastic container, and then you can take out and defrost only what you need. Very young kittens and puppies will like salty, yeasty dabs (e.g., Vegemite, Marmite) that can be placed on their nose or lips. Whatever you choose, the following eight guidelines apply:
1. Foods that are high in protein may help induce changes in brain chemistry that help the dog to relax.
2. Dogs and cats should not have chocolate because it can be toxic to them.
3. Some dogs and cats do not do well with treats that contain artificial colors or preservatives, so you may wish to avoid semi-moist treats.
4. Dogs and cats with food allergies or those taking drugs that are monoamine oxidase inhibitors (MAOIs) may have food restrictions (e.g., some cheeses for dogs taking or using MAOIs such as Preventics Collars and Anipryl).
5. Dog biscuits generally are not sufficiently interesting for some of the work needed here, but some foods are so desirable that the dog is too stimulated by them to relax; you want something between these two extremes.
6. Treats should be tiny (less than one-half of a thumbnail) so that the dog or cat does not get full, fat, or "bored" with them.
7. If the dog or cat stops responding for one kind of treat, try another.
8. Do not let treats make up the bulk of the dog's or cat's diet; they need their normal, well-balanced ration.

That said, people have been reduced to tears because they have felt they cannot use treats to reward a dog or cat who is fat, and their veterinarian has warned them about the dangers of obesity. Obesity is not good, but by working with a veterinary nutritionist, a program that factors in food treats and minimizes weight gain can easily be created. For most pets, if they gain a little bit of weight, it's not tragic, they can lose it when they are better. Remember that behavioral problems will kill pets faster than will obesity. Sometimes in life we have to make some tradeoffs.

5. Understanding the Reward Process

There is an art to rewarding dogs and cats with food treats. Learning to do so correctly will help the dog or cat to focus on the instructions and will keep everyone safe. To prevent the dog from lunging for the food, keep the already prepared treats in a little cup or baggie behind your back, and keep one treat in the hand that you'll use to reward the dog. That hand can then either be kept behind your back so that the dog or cat doesn't stare at the food, or can be moved to your eye so that you can teach the dog to look happy and make eye contact with you. The food treat must be small so that the focus of the dog's or cat's attention is not a slab of food, but rather your cues. A treat that is the correct size can be closed in the palm of your hand just by folding it, and will not be apparent when held between the thumb and forefingers. When presenting the dog or cat with the treat, bring the hand, with a lightly closed fist, up quickly to the dog (*do not* startle the dog or cat), and turn your wrist to open your hand, as you say "Good boy!"

When first starting the program, let the dog or cat smell and taste the reward so that he knows what the reward for the work will be. If your pet is too terrified to approach, you can place a small amount of the treat on the floor. Then ask the dog to "sit"; if the dog or cat sits instantly, say "Good boy!" and instantly open your hand to give the treat while saying "stay." Two tips: (a) *whisper*—most troubled pets have experienced enough screaming to last a lifetime, and (b) use an "upbeat" voice with a lilt at the end—pets respond to tone and you will need to watch yours.

6. Getting the Dog's or Cat's Attention

If the dog or cat does not sit instantly, call his name again, and as soon as your pet looks at or attends to you, say "sit." If you cannot get your dog or cat to look at you and pay attention, don't keep saying "sit." If you continue to give a request that you cannot reinforce, all you will do is teach the recipient to ignore that your request. This isn't what you want.

If necessary, use a whistle or make an unusual sound with your lips to get your pet's attention. As soon as the dog or cat looks at you, say "sit." Use a cheerful voice. Some people find that they have to soften or lower their voice almost to a whisper to get the dog to pay attention to them. This is usually because, in the past, the dog or cat has had all "commands" delivered in a forceful voice, and that tone is now ignored.

If the dog or cat is looking at you but not sitting, approach and lessen the distance between the two of you, raise the treat gently to your eyes, and request "sit." Often just moving toward a dog helps that dog to sit. Not only have you decreased the distance between you, but now to look at your eyes the dog must raise his head, a behavior often accompanied by sitting. You can use these innate dog behaviors as long as you are careful. This means:

- Never force a growling dog to back up.
- Never corner a fearful dog or cat.
- Never continue to approach a dog or cat who is getting more aggressive the closer you come to her.

Remember that the point of this **Protocol** is to teach the dog or cat to relax and look to you for the cues about the appropriateness of his behavior. The dog or cat can't do this if she is upset.

If the dog still will not sit for your request, consider using a head collar (see **Protocol for Choosing Collars, Head Collars, Harnesses, and Leads**). **If your dog or cat is wearing a head collar or harness** you may be able to use a long-distance lead to help you request that the dog or cat "sit," by gently getting her attention. You must be able to reward your pet with a treat as soon as sitting occurs.

Cautionary Note

If your dog is aggressive, or if you are afraid to approach him, do not do any of these exercises off-lead until the dog is **perfect** on-lead. Please consider working with a good, modern, educated and certified dog trainer or veterinary professional to help you fit the dog with a head collar and work with the dog only on a lead. A head collar allows you to close the dog's mouth if the dog begins to be aggressive. This is an ideal "correction" because you have interrupted the dog's inappropriate behavior within the first few seconds of the onset of the behavior so that the dog can learn from the experience, if they are not made fearful.

Be gentle, but be consistent. Taking your anger or fear out on the dog will only make him worse. As soon as the dog responds to the halter and calmly sits, reward the dog, and

continue. Never reward a dog who is growling, lunging, barking, shaking, or urinating. These are all signs that the dog sees the situation as threatening and to continue may put his welfare at risk.

After the dog or cat sits for the first time, you are ready to begin the program. Remember the following four guidelines:

1. Use the dog's or cat's name to help her orient toward you and to pay attention. If this doesn't work, use a whistle or a sound to which your pet is not accustomed.
2. Once the dog or cat is attending to you (paying attention) say "sit" and give her 3 to 5 seconds to respond. If the dog or cat *does* sit, reward her instantly; if not, repeat the request to "sit" in the same calm, cheerful voice. You may want to experiment with voices to see the tonal qualities to which your pet best responds.
3. Do not worry about using the dog's name frequently or about repeating the commands if the dog responds. This is not obedience class; but if you later wish to take the dog to obedience, the dog will do well if she did well on these programs. Making the adjustment will not be a problem. In fact, your dog will likely be a star of the class!
4. Do not chase the dog or cat all over the room to try to get her to comply with your command. If necessary, choose a small room with minimal distractions, and use a leash with a head collar or harness. Please use leads, head collars, and harnesses kindly.

A sample behavior mod sequence might look like this:

"Bonnie—sit—(3-second pause)—sit—(3-second pause)— Bonnie, sit, look—(move closer to dog and move treat to your eye to encourage her to track the treat to your eye and "look")—sit— good girl! (treat)—stay—good girl—stay (take a step backward while saying "stay"—then stop)—stay Bonnie—good girl—stay (return while saying "stay"—then stop)—stay Bonnie—good girl (treat)—okay (the releaser and she can get up)!"

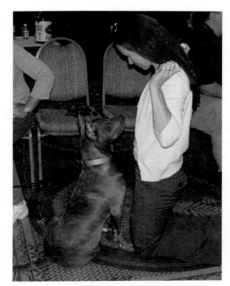

Teaching "sit" and "look" to a dog in laboratory class. Notice that the human moved closer and lower (by kneeling) to this dog to keep the dog focused on her. The dog is about to be given a treat which is enclosed in the human's left hand (a clicker is in the right hand).

Note that you talk non-stop to the dog or cat at the beginning of these programs. This type of talking is not allowed in obedience classes, but is desperately needed with inexperienced puppies and kittens and problem dogs and cats. These dogs and cats need all the cues that they can get. They need the constant guidance and reassurance of hearing your voice with clear instructions. These instructions and reassurances should occur in the context of shaping or gradually guiding their behavior towards more appropriate behaviors. You will have to learn to read subtle cues that your dog or cat is giving and using these to your advantage. You will find this easier to do than you believe. The one thing that you *absolutely cannot do* is to talk a continuous stream to the dog or cat *without receiving the context-appropriate responses* to your requests. If you just rush through everything you will only stress the dog or cat and teach him to ignore everything you say. This is not good. A corollary of this admonition is that it is necessary to use consistent terminology of brief phrases and to do so in an environment when no one else is carrying on long, loud, distracting conversations.

7. Avoiding Problems

Please do not push or pull on your dog or cat or tug on his collar to get him to sit. These types of behaviors can be viewed as scary or as threats by some dogs, especially, and may make them potentially dangerous. Use the methods discussed above. If you really feel that the dog will need some physical help in sitting, please use a head collar (and have someone who works with these dogs for a living present to help you).

Please do not wave your hands or the treat around in front of the dog or cat. This will just act as a distraction and confuse your pet. Part of the point of this program is to make your pet *calmer and less confused.* Excitable behavior on your part or unclear signals can make your dog or cat more anxious. This will not help. If you wish to add hand signal or clicker training to the skills your pet is now developing, please do so only after your pet has flawlessly mastered the program. Otherwise, you have just provided another level of complexity. It is unlikely that either you or your pet can handle all of those levels simultaneously if the reason that you are doing this is to treat a behavioral problem.

Please be calm. Your dog or cat will make mistakes. This doesn't have to reflect on you. Problem dogs and cats and new kittens and puppies require a lot of patience. The people who have had the most success with these animals using these protocols have been the people who work the hardest and the most consistently. Finally, it is difficult, but please leave your anger behind.

Please do not let your dog or cat become a jack-in-the-box. You must control the situation so that you can give appropriate direction, and you must do so by convincing the dog or cat to defer to you. If your pet gets up to get the treat every time it is offered, you have not made the rule structure clear. *We forget that so many of the behaviors that animals offer to us and other animals are offered as a way of getting information: they watch the response and learn from that. Your pets are always asking questions, and their answers are taken from your behaviors.* If you reward both sitting and popup behavior, you have just taught your pet that both sitting and reactive behaviors are your desired response. This is not what you want.

If the dog or cat pops up as you approach with the treat, ask yourself if you were too far away from the dog or cat when you offered the treat. If so, move closer to your pet. Ideally, your pet should be able to get the treat just by stretching out his neck. He should not have to get up. If you have a little dog or a kitten, this may mean that you have to squat down. Be careful if the dog or cat is aggressive as your face is now close to your pet.

If you are close enough for your pet to do the exercise properly and your pet still gets up, close your hand over the treat, and *softly and calmly* say "No." One advantage of holding the treat in the manner recommended above is that you can safely deny a dog or cat the treat at the last second if the dog acts inappropriately. Here, a soft and gentle "no" is a verbal marker for an incorrect response with notification that it will result in a lack of reward. Then gently ask your dog or cat to "sit" again. After your pet sits, say "stay," wait 3 to 5 seconds, say "stay" again, and THEN immediately give the treat. The two "stays" with the time period between them will serve to reinforce the concept that getting up is not part of the pattern of behavior that is rewarded. By twice asking your dog or cat to stay you are telling him that whenever he makes a mistake he has to do two things to recover from it. A sample sequence might look like this:

> "Susie—sit—(3- to 5-second pause)—sit—good girl!—stay—(start to give treat and dog gets up)—no (whispered)—(close hand over treat)—sit—stay—(3- to 5-second pause)—s-t-a-y (long, low sound; no shouting)—good girl!—s-t-a-y (long, low sound; no shouting)—(and give treat)—okay!" (dog is now allowed to get up).

Please do not tell the dog or cat that she is good if she is not. *Do not* reward shaking, growling, whining, or any other behavior that may be a component of the behavior on which you are trying to work. If you reward these behaviors you are only rewarding the underlying anxiety and sabotaging your own program. In fact, if you see these behaviors, your dog or cat is not ready for what you wish to teach. These are signs of stress and distress, and you need to go back to any calm interaction that can be rewarded without these signs appearing.

If the dog becomes impatient and barks at you for attention say "Ah, softly! (again, whisper) Quiet! (soft whisper, no anger)—stay—good girl—stay—good girl—(treat)—stay...." If a vocal signal is not sufficient to quiet the dog, please remember that a head collar can be pulled forward to close the mouth and abort the bark before it starts, so that your correction is appropriately timed. This technique may allow you to reward the dog for closing her mouth and for being quiet, but *you have to be gentle and ensure that she is not barking because she is distressed.*

Finally, if you accidentally drop a food treat and the dog or cat gets up to get it, don't correct the dog or cat. She didn't make a mistake. Any food that hits the ground is hers. Don't lunge and try to retrieve the treat, especially if your pet really cares about and protects food, as you will be bitten and/or scratched. Just consider the dropped treat a free one, and then restart the **Protocol** at the place where you dropped the treat.

The use of behavior modification as discussed here is fully covered and demonstrated in the videotape, *Humane Behavioral Care for Dogs: Problem Prevention and Treatment.*

8. The Format for the Protocol

This program was designed so that your dog or cat could learn from it without becoming stressed or distressed, and without learning to ignore the tasks because they were too predictable. The **Protocol** intersperses long activities with short ones. You may have to adjust some of these to your particular needs.

It is preferable to reward the dog or cat *only* for performing each task perfectly, but if this is not possible for your dog, you can use a "shaping" procedure. When shaping a behavior you first reward the dog for any behavior that approaches that indicated in the task. The *next* time you do the task the behavior should be closer to that which you desire in order to be rewarded. Steps to improvement can be quite small. *Don't rush a worried pet*—you will just make him worse. Done correctly, you will get your dog or cat to perform the task perfectly within a short time.

The **Protocol** is a foundation for later behavior modification protocols and techniques, including those involved in desensitizing and counter-conditioning your dog or cat to situations in which he reacts inappropriately, such as meeting another dog, greeting a child, entering a veterinary clinic, and getting into a car.

The numbered tasks can be used as one day's tasks, one week's tasks, or you can go at the dog's speed (which may be faster or slower). Some of the exercises are weird (asking you to run in circles or talk to people who don't exist), but can be very helpful in getting dogs to learn to relax in a variety of circumstances.

Before you can start the actual exercises you must practice with the dog or cat so that she can sit perfectly for 15 seconds without moving. Do this with food treats as described above. Once your pet can sit this way and look happy and as if they worshiped the ground you walk on, you are ready for the more challenging stuff!

Theoretically, the tasks are grouped in 15- to 20-minute units. As stated, your dog or cat may have to go more slowly, or may be able to go more quickly. *Please do not treat this*

Protocol as a competitive race. People who push their pets too quickly create additional anxiety problems for their pets. Watch your pet's cues. If your dog or cat really cannot perform an exercise or task, go back to one that he knows flawlessly, reward his excellent performance of that task, and stop. It's best if every member of the family works daily with the dog or cat, but it may be less anxiety provoking and more stimulating for the dog if this is done in three or four 5-minute segments, than in one long segment. Study the graphs below.

In Figure 1, you have a static model of normal vs. various versions of reactive dogs. When working with the **Protocol for Relaxation** you always want to keep your dog or cat below the level at which he or she starts to react. In Figure 2, the more real-world, continuous type of reaction is represented. It is clear why it is so hard to keep worried dogs and cats below the level at which they change from watchful and worrying to becoming truly reactive: They have a very narrow window of time over which they become distressed quickly. One of the goals of the **Protocol for Relaxation** is to stretch this window of time so that there is more time to intervene and less time spent reacting and on the way to reacting.

If everyone in the family cannot or will not work with the dog or cat, *the people who are not participating must not sabotage the program.* They *minimally* must comply with the **Protocol for Deference.** If family members cannot or will not do this, they should not be interacting with the dog or cat. If there is non-cooperation in the household, the dog or cat will not get as well as he can get. If that non-cooperation is deliberate, please consider family counseling. Often, pets are either responding to or further victimized by extant inter-personal problems in the household.

Please remember that the keys to success are consistency and appropriate rewards. This means that, although it may be more helpful to work 15 to 20 minutes 1 to 2 times per day, you should work for only as long as both you and the dog are enjoying and benefiting from the program. If this means that you use six 5-minute intervals to get through three or

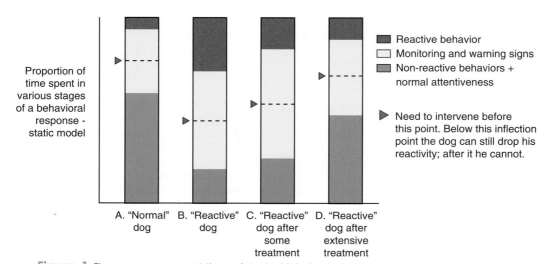

Figure 1 The *arrows* represent the point at which the behavior changes from being more watchful to being more reactive. If you want the dog or cat to become less reactive *(green areas)* you cannot reward any behaviors above this point, and should avoid anything that triggers such behaviors because fear and reactivity, like calm, are reinforced with practice.

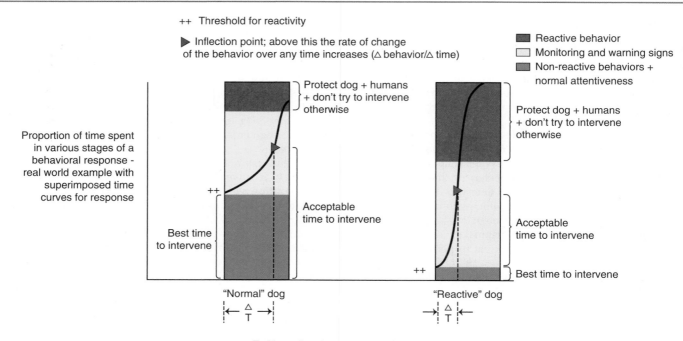

++ Threshold for reactivity

▶ Inflection point; above this the rate of change of the behavior over any time increases (△ behavior/△ time)

■ Reactive behavior
□ Monitoring and warning signs
■ Non-reactive behaviors + normal attentiveness

Proportion of time spent in various stages of a behavioral response - real world example with superimposed time curves for response

Protect dog + humans + don't try to intervene otherwise

Acceptable time to intervene

Best time to intervene

++

"Normal" dog
← △ →
    T

Protect dog + humans + don't try to intervene otherwise

Acceptable time to intervene

Best time to intervene

++

"Reactive" dog
→ △ ←
   T

△ T Time client has to convince dog not to react

Figure 2 In a continuous model of reactivity it is clear why you wish to keep the dog or cat below the threshold for reactivity, if possible, and why this is so difficult with a reactive dog or cat. It also should be clear why it is essential to keep the dog or cat below the level—the inflection point—at which the behavior changes from watchful to reactive.

four of the tasks, this is fine. Please do not end on a bad note. If the dog's behavior is deteriorating or his attention is dissipating, go back to one final, fun, easy exercise and *stop*. By pushing the dog or cat past his limits you will induce anxiety and your pet will backslide.

Once your pet is able to perform all of the tasks and exercises both on- and off-lead in one location (the living room), *repeat them all in other rooms and circumstances (the backyard or the park—use a lead here)*.

Please *make a list of all the things to which your pet reacts that distress you* and that you and your vet think are problematic. Then, incorporate these into your own, customized behavior mod program.

When the dog or cat is just terrific for all the tasks listed in all places with all household members, add your specific concerns using the slow and broken-down approach recommended in this program. Then, when your pet has succeeded in these situations, you are ready for **Tier 2** of the protocols, which focuses on your dog's or cat's specific problems.

If at any point you cannot get past one task, try breaking that task into two or three component parts. If this still doesn't help, call the veterinarian who recommended the program and who is working with the dog's behavior problems. The veterinarian will be able to help you discover where the problem lies. You can also video your work session with your pet. Chances are that you'll see exactly what the problem is and how to fix it. Please do not just continue, accepting suboptimal responses. The goal is to get your dog or cat better.

If you are not sure that your dog is improving, *measure the outcomes*. There are numerous ways to do this and they are not equally easy for all people.

- Video yourself and others working with the dog every day. Compare the same exercise each day, noting all of the postures that worry you and all of the postures that you think are good. Bring the video and your impressions to your vet.
- You can video the dog performing the behavior modification program once a week and compare specific behaviors by the week. Measures taken from the video may include the number of times the dog scanned the room, the number of times the dog licked his lips, the dog's respiratory rate, and the number of repeats of an exercise before the dog was calm and perfect for it. There are many, many things that you can measure, and if you are uncertain, ask your vet for guidance. Obviously, the best behaviors to monitor are those that indicate that your dog is distressed. If the behavior mod is successful, these should decrease with time.
- Count and record the seconds until the dog complies in a happy way. As the dog improves, these intervals should be shorter, but you need to ensure that the dog is happy.
- Have the dog repeat the exercise and have some criteria for how often the dog must be "perfect" in her position and calm before you can move on. In these types of measures, common assessments might include:
  - the dog succeeding 3 of 4 times during 4 repeats of the exercises over 2 days,
  - the dog succeeding 9 of 10 times during 1 or 2 repeats of the exercises on 1 day, and
  - the dog succeeding 8 of 10 times during 1 or 2 repeats of the exercises over 2 days.

Note the pattern here: In these types of measures you need a better success rate to advance over a short period of time than you do if you are going to advance more slowly over a period of days. These types of measures are common validity tools, and are most useful when the dog is learning something that has a clear end point.

Regardless of how you decide to measure your and your dog's progress, you should advance to the next steps only when there is true progress and when your dog has learned something helpful. If you are having trouble, get help from your vet and people who do this for a living.

Finally, please remember that your dog or cat will give you lots of cues about how they are feeling. This program differs from other behavior modification programs because of the emphasis on these signals. We are rewarding the physical changes associated with relaxation and happiness and so will also reward the underlying physiological states associated with this (parasympathetic part of the autonomic nervous system). This means that if the dog is relaxed—his body is not stiff; his jaws hang relaxed and are not tense; his ears are alert or cocked, but not rigid; his head is held gently at an angle; and his eyes are calm and adoring—you will be rewarding the nervous system responses that help your dog to learn. If you mistakenly reward fear, tension, aggression, or avoidance, you will not make as much progress. If it is easier for you and the dog or cat to be relaxed if the dog or cat is lying down, do that.

Good luck, and don't get discouraged. Many pets go through a period of a few days to a few weeks where they get worse before they get better. This is because they have a new rule structure to follow and they are trying to learn all the rules, while at the same time clinging to the rule structure that has worked for them in the past. As they discover they are rewarded for being relaxed and happy, their behavior will improve. These programs are harder on the people, in many ways, than they are on the dogs or cats. Stick with it!

9. The Protocol Task Sheets

These task sheets are meant to give you guidance, only. They are designed to take the approach of very, very, very gradual changes. Such tiny steps allow you to reward aspects of the behaviors that are good, without accidentally rewarding behaviors that are not so good. Built into these programs are the concepts of desensitization, where you stimulate the animal to a response but at a level below which they become distressed, and counter-conditioning, where you reward behaviors that are in direct opposition or contrast to those that are undesirable. If you open any applied text or article on learning, you will see similar programs. There is nothing magic or novel or original here. These tasks are those that are common to most dog and cat training and behavior modification programs, and you will see similar task sheets in a variety of training books. Please remember that what *is* different *here* is that you are rewarding the physical signals that underlie your pet's behavioral state. You are rewarding *only* relaxed, compliant behaviors. The tasks, themselves, involve only common situations in which pets may respond inappropriately or undesirably. Some of these situations may not be relevant to you, and others that are relevant may be missing. Please feel free to customize or alter this program, but do so using the pattern of approach used here (e.g., gradually work up to the task, frequent returns to something easier, always ending on a good note, et cetera).

The task is listed on the left. To the right is a space for you to make comments about how easy or hard the task was for the dog, how many times it had to be repeated, or other questionable behaviors that appeared during the task. You should discuss these with your veterinarian at your re-exam appointment.

Remember, after each task you are to verbally praise the dog or cat and reward him with a treat for perfect performance prior to going on to the next task. Each set of exercises is designed for a day or a block of time, and have warm-up and cool-down periods just like physical exercises.

At the first signs of any anxiety (e.g., lips retracted, pupils dilated, head lowered, ears pulled down and back, trembling, scanning, lip licking, avoidance of eye contact, hissing, growling, et cetera), move back to an exercise with which the dog or cat is more comfortable, or break down the exercise that produced these behaviors into smaller steps.

Antianxiety medications may help some dogs who otherwise are not able to succeed in this program. Please remember that if it's decided that medication could benefit your dog, you need to use it *in addition* to the behavior modification, not instead of it.

Task Sheets

Tips
1. Reward your pet after each successfully completed task.
2. Stop when either one of you is tired or concerned.
3. Pay attention to the parenthetical notes that suggest potentially worrisome tasks.

Task Set 1

Sit for 2 seconds
Sit for 5 seconds
Sit for 10 seconds
Sit while you take 1 step back and then return
Sit while you take 2 steps back and then return
→ **(Note: You may have problems here. If so, please make the steps smaller. At first, you may only be able to move 1 to 2 cm at a time.)**
Sit for 5 seconds
Sit for 10 seconds
Sit while you take 1 step to the right and then return
Sit while you take 1 step to the left and then return
→ **(Note: You may have problems here. If so, please make the steps smaller. At first, you may only be able to move 1 to 2 cm at a time.)**
Sit for 5 seconds
Sit for 10 seconds
Sit while you take 2 steps back and return
Sit while you take 2 steps to the right and return
→ **(Note: You may have problems here. If so, please make the steps smaller. At first, you may only be able to move 1 to 2 cm at a time.)**
Sit for 5 seconds
Sit for 10 seconds
Sit for 15 seconds
Sit while you take 2 steps to the left and return
→ **(Note: You may have problems here. If so, please make the steps smaller. You may have to find some intermediate distance between 1 and 2 steps.)**
Sit for 5 seconds
Sit for 10 seconds

Sit for ___ seconds
Sit wh___ you clap your hands softly once
Sit f___ seconds
Sit ___ 10 seconds
Sit ___ r 15 seconds
Sit while you take 3 steps back and return
→ (Note: You may have problems here. If so, please make the steps smaller. You may have to find some intermediate distance between 2 and 3 steps.)
Sit while you count out loud to 3
Sit while you count out loud to 5
Sit while you count out loud to 10
→ (Note: You may have problems here with all of the above. If so, whisper. Find a voice or sound to which your pet does not react. If you cannot do this now, come back to it later.)
Sit while you clap your hands softly once
Sit while you count out loud to 5
Sit while you count out loud to 10
→ (Note: You may have problems here with all of the above. If so, whisper. Find a voice or sound to which your pet does not react. If you cannot do this now, come back to it later.)
Sit while you count out loud to 5
Sit while you count out loud to 10
Sit while you count out loud to 20
→ (Note: You may have problems here. This is a big jump and voice modulation will be key.)
Sit while you take 3 steps to the right and return
→ (Note: If you had a problem with the counting your pet may be upset and you will have a problem with taking 3 steps. If so, try again with smaller, fewer steps and work your way up.)
Sit while you clap your hands softly twice
Sit for 3 seconds
Sit for 5 seconds
Sit while you take 1 step back and return
Sit for 3 seconds
Sit for 10 seconds
Sit for 5 seconds
Sit for 3 seconds

Task Set 2

Sit for 5 seconds
Sit for 10 seconds
Sit while you take 1 step back and return
Sit while you take 3 steps back and return
→ (Note: You may have problems here. If so, please make the steps smaller. You may have to find some intermediate distance between 1 and 3 steps.)
Sit for 10 seconds
Sit while you take 3 steps to the right and return
Sit while you take 3 steps to the left and return
→ (Note: You may have problems here. If so, please make the steps smaller or take fewer steps, then work up to 3 steps.)
Sit for 10 seconds
Sit while you take 3 steps to the right and clap your hands
→ (Note: You may have problems here. This is the first time you have combined 2 stimuli. If you have problems, break this step down into fewer steps and less sound and then gradually work your way up to this task.)
Sit while you take 3 steps to the left and clap your hands
Sit for 5 seconds

Sit for 10 seconds
Sit while you walk one-quarter of the way around the dog to the right
→ (Note: You may have problems here. If so, please make the distance smaller and work your way up g-r-a-d-u-a-l-l-y.)
Sit while you take 4 steps back
→ (Note: You may have problems here. If so, please make the steps smaller or fewer, then combine # of steps and distance.)
Sit while you walk one-quarter the way around the dog to the left
Sit for 10 seconds
Sit while you take 5 steps back from the dog, clapping your hands, and return
→ (Note: You may have problems here. If so, please make the steps smaller and fewer and then work your way back up to more and bigger steps.)
Sit while you walk halfway around the dog to the right and return
Sit while you walk halfway around the dog to the left and return
→ (Note: You may have problems here. If so, please make the distance smaller and work your way up g-r-a-d-u-a-l-l-y.)
Sit for 5 seconds
Sit for 10 seconds
Sit while you jog quietly in place for 3 seconds
Sit while you jog quietly in place for 5 seconds
Sit while you jog quietly in place for 10 seconds
Sit for 10 seconds
Sit while you jog one-quarter of the way around dog to right and return
Sit while you jog one-quarter of the way around dog to left and return
Sit for 5 seconds
Sit for 10 seconds

Task Set 3

Sit for 10 seconds
Sit for 15 seconds
Sit while you take 2 steps backwards and return
Sit while you jog 5 steps backwards from dog and return
→ (Note: This is a big increase for some dogs. You may have to take fewer or smaller steps.)
Sit while you walk halfway around the dog to the right and return
→ (Note: You may have problems here. If so, please make the distance smaller and work your way up g-r-a-d-u-a-l-l-y.)
Sit while you walk halfway around the dog to the left and return
Sit while you take 10 steps backwards and return
Sit for 5 seconds
Sit for 10 seconds
Sit for 15 seconds
Sit while you take 10 steps to the left and return
→ (Note: This is a huge increase in the # of steps. Feel free to work up to this and use smaller steps if you think your pet might be becoming more reactive.)
Sit while you take 10 steps to the right and return
→ (Note: This is a huge increase in the # of steps. Feel free to work up to this and use smaller steps if you think your pet might be becoming more reactive. Please also remember that if your pet reacted to the previous exercise, they

may react more for this one. Feel free to tailor the # of steps to your pet's abilities.)

Sit for 5 seconds

Sit for 10 seconds

Sit for 15 seconds

Sit for 20 seconds

Sit while you walk halfway around the dog to the right, clap your hands, and return

→ (Note: You are now adding distance and noise, following some tasks that may have caused your pet to be more reactive. If your pet is uncertain, please scale back distance, activities, and volume.)

Sit for 20 seconds

Sit while you walk halfway around the dog to the left, clap your hands, and return

Sit for 10 seconds

Sit while you jog 10 steps to the right and return

→ (Note: You are now adding distance, following some tasks that may have caused your pet to be more reactive. If your pet is uncertain, please scale back distance.)

Sit while you jog 10 steps to the left and return

Sit while you jog in place for 10 seconds

→ (Note: This is a new activity and may startle some pets. Feel free to use fewer steps and less exaggerated activity before working up to this.)

Sit for 5 second

Sit for 10 seconds

Sit for 15 seconds

Sit while you jog in place for 20 seconds

Sit for 10 seconds

Sit while you jog backwards 5 steps and return

→ (Note: This is a change in behavior. If your pet is reactive, please use fewer steps and behavior that is more familiar.)

Sit while you jog to the right 5 steps and return

Sit while you jog to the left 5 steps and return

Sit for 5 seconds while you clap your hands

Sit for 10 seconds while you clap your hands

Sit for 10 seconds

Sit for 5 seconds

Task Set 4

Sit for 5 seconds

Sit for 10 seconds

Sit while you jog backwards 5 steps and return

→ (Note: This is a relatively new activity and may startle some pets. Feel free to use fewer steps and less exaggerated activity before working up to this.)

Sit for 5 seconds

Sit for 10 seconds

Sit for 20 seconds

Sit while you jog halfway around the dog to the right and return

→ (Note: Feel free to make the distance smaller if your pet is reactive.)

Sit while you jog halfway around the dog to left and return

Sit while you move three-quarters of the way around the dog to the right and return

→ (Note: Feel free to make the distance smaller if your pet is reactive.)

Sit while you move three-quarters of the way around the dog to the left and return

Sit while you jog backwards 5 steps, clapping your hands and return

→ (Note: This is a new set of combinations and some pets will react. If so, scale back the # of steps and volume, or separate activities and do slowly and separately first before putting them together.)

Sit for 10 seconds

Sit for 15 seconds

Sit while you clap your hands for 20 seconds

→ (Note: This is a huge change. You may need to work up to clapping for this amount of time.)

Sit while you quickly move backwards 10 steps and return

→ (Note: This is a large # of steps. You may have to work up to them.)

Sit while you quickly move 15 steps backwards and return

→ (Note: This is a large # of steps. You may have to work up to them.)

Sit for 20 seconds

→ (Note: If your pet was previously reactive, you may need to work up to this amount of time again.)

Sit while you jog halfway around the dog to the right and return

Sit while you jog halfway around the dog to the left and return

Sit while you quickly walk 15 steps to the left and return

Sit while you quickly walk 15 steps to the right and return

→ (Note: Again, you may have to work up to the distance for the preceding exercises depending on the reactivity level of your pet. More reactive pets will require work with smaller increments.)

Sit for 20 seconds

Sit while you move three-quarters of the way around the dog to the right and return

Sit while you move three-quarters of the way around the dog to the left and return

→ (Note: Again, this is a change. Alter your behavior, if needed, depending on your pet's reactivity.)

Sit while you walk all the way around the dog

Sit while you walk approximately 20 steps to an entrance and return

Sit while you walk approximately 20 steps to an entrance, clapping your hands, and return

→ (Note: Again, this is a huge change. Alter your behavior, if needed, depending on your pet's reactivity.)

Sit while you walk around the dog, quietly clapping your hands and then return

Sit for 20 seconds

Sit while you quickly jog around the dog

→ (Note: Again, this is a change. Alter your behavior, if needed, depending on your pet's reactivity.)

Sit for 20 seconds

Sit for 10 seconds while you clap your hands

Task Set 5

Sit for 5 seconds

Sit for 15 seconds

Sit while you walk quickly 15 steps to the right and return

→ (Note: Again, this is a huge change in # and tempo. Alter your behavior, if needed, depending on your pet's reactivity.)

Sit while you walk quickly 15 steps to the left and return

Sit while you walk approximately 20 steps to an entrance and return

Sit while you walk approximately 20 steps to an entrance, clapping your hands, and return

Sit for 20 seconds

Sit while you walk around the dog, clapping your hands

Sit for 20 seconds

Sit for 10 seconds

Sit while you walk quickly backwards, clapping your hands, and return

→ **(Note: Again, this is a change. Alter your behavior, if needed, depending on your pet's reactivity.)**

Sit while you walk approximately 20 steps to an entrance and return

Sit while you walk approximately 20 steps to an entrance, clapping your hands, and return

Sit while you go to an entrance and just touch the doorknob or wall and return

Sit for 10 seconds

Sit while you walk quickly backwards, clapping your hands, and return

Sit while you walk approximately 20 steps to an entrance and return

Sit while you walk approximately 20 steps to an entrance, clapping your hands, and return

→ **(Note: Again, this is a change. Alter your behavior, if needed, depending on your pet's reactivity.)**

Sit while you go to an entrance and just touch the doorknob or wall and return

Sit for 20 seconds

Sit while you walk approximately 20 steps to an entrance, clapping your hands, and return

Sit while you go to an entrance and just touch the doorknob or wall and return

Sit for 10 seconds

Sit while the doorknob is touched or you move into entryway an return

→ **Note: Again, this is a change. Alter your behavior, if needed, depending on your pet's reactivity. Pets who worry about being left may stall here and you may have to work up to this. If your pet does stall, she may continue to be reactive for the next tasks, which should then be scaled back.)**

Sit for 10 seconds

Sit for 15 seconds while you clap your hands

Sit for 10 seconds while you jog in place

Sit for 5 seconds

Task Set 6

Sit for 10 seconds

Sit for 20 seconds while you jog back and forth in front of the dog

Sit for 15 seconds

Sit while you walk approximately 20 steps to an entrance and return

→ **(Note: Again, this is a change. Alter your behavior, if needed, depending on your pet's reactivity. Pets with problems surrounding departures may react more at entrances. Behave as recommended above, please.)**

Sit while you walk quickly backwards, clapping your hands, and return

Sit while you go to an entrance and just touch the doorknob or wall and return

Sit for 20 seconds while jogging

Sit while you walk around the dog

Sit while you walk around the dog clapping your hands

Sit for 15 seconds

Sit for 20 seconds

Sit for 30 seconds

Sit while you walk quickly backwards, clapping your hands, and return

Sit while you go to an entrance and just touch the doorknob or wall and return

→ **(Note: Again, this is a change. Alter your behavior, if needed, depending on your pet's reactivity. Pets with problems surrounding departures may react more at entrances. Behave as recommended above, please.)**

Sit while you open the door or go into the entrance for 5 seconds and then return

Sit while you open the door or go into the entrance for 10 seconds and then return

Sit for 30 seconds

Sit while you walk quickly backwards, clapping your hands, and return

Sit while you go to an entrance and just touch the doorknob or wall and return

Sit for 10 seconds

Sit while you go through the door or the entranceway and then return

Sit while you go through the door or the entranceway, clapping your hands and then return

Sit while you open the door or go into the entrance for 10 seconds and then return

Sit for 30 seconds

Sit while you disappear from view for 5 seconds and then return

→ **(Note: Again, this is a change. Alter your behavior, if needed, depending on your pet's reactivity. Pets with problems surrounding departures may react more here. Behave as recommended above, please.)**

Sit for 20 seconds

Sit for 10 seconds while you clap your hands

Sit for 5 seconds

Task Set 7

Sit for 10 seconds

Sit for 20 seconds while you clap your hands

Sit while you take 10 steps backwards and return

Sit while you walk around the dog

Sit while you go through the door or the entranceway and then return

→ **Note: Again, this is a change. Alter your behavior, if needed, depending on your pet's reactivity. Pets with problems surrounding departures may react more at entrances. Behave as recommended above, please.)**

Sit while you go through the door or the entranceway, clapping your hands and then return

Sit while you open the door or go into the entrance for 10 seconds and then return

Sit for 30 seconds

Sit while you disappear from view for 5 seconds and then return

Sit while you go through the door or the entranceway and then return

Sit while you go through the door or the entranceway, clapping your hands and then return

Sit while you open the door or go into the entrance for 10 seconds and then return

→ (Note: Again, these are changes and the preceding exercises all build on each other and become more provocative for some pets. Alter your behavior, if needed, depending on your pet's reactivity. Pets with problems surrounding departures may react more at entrances. Behave as recommended above, please.)

Sit for 10 seconds

Sit for 20 seconds

Sit for 30 seconds

→ (Note: Remember that if your pet is reactive, returning to even smaller time intervals is reassuring.)

Sit while you disappear from view for 10 seconds and then return

Sit while you disappear from view for 15 seconds and then return

Sit for 10 seconds

Sit for 15 seconds

Sit for 5 seconds while you clap your hands

Sit while you jog in place for 10 seconds

Sit while you jog three-quarters of the way to the right and return

Sit while you jog three-quarters of the way to the left and return

Sit while you go through the door or the entranceway, clapping your hands and then return

→ (Note: Again, this is a change. Alter your behavior, if needed, depending on your pet's reactivity. Pets with problems surrounding departures may react more at entrances. Behave as recommended above, please.)

Sit while you open the door or go into the entrance for 10 seconds and then return

Sit for 30 seconds

Sit while you disappear from view for 15 seconds and then return

Sit for 10 seconds

Sit for 5 seconds

Task Set 8

Sit for 10 seconds

Sit for 15 seconds while you jog and clap your hands

Sit while you back up 15 steps and return

Sit while you circle the dog and return

Sit while you disappear from view for 20 seconds and return

→ (Note: Again, this is a change. Alter your behavior, if needed, depending on your pet's reactivity. Pets with problems surrounding departures may react more at entrances. Behave as recommended above, please.)

Sit while you disappear from view for 25 seconds and return

Sit for 5 seconds

Sit for 5 seconds while you sit in a chair (placed 5 feet from the dog)

Sit for 5 seconds

Sit for 15 seconds while you jog and clap your hands

Sit while you back up 15 steps and return

Sit while you circle the dog and return

Sit while you disappear from view for 20 seconds and return

Sit while you disappear from view for 30 seconds and return

→ (Note: Again, this is a change. Alter your behavior, if needed, depending on your pet's reactivity. Pets with

problems surrounding departures may react more at entrances. Behave as recommended above, please.)

Sit for 5 seconds

Sit while you circle the dog and return

Sit while you disappear from view for 20 seconds and return

Sit while you disappear from view for 25 seconds and return

→ (Note: Again, this is a change. Alter your behavior, if needed, depending on your pet's reactivity. Pets with problems surrounding departures may react more at entrances. Behave as recommended above, please.)

Sit for 5 seconds while you sit in a chair near the dog

→ (Note: This is a new task and may provoke some pets. Work up to it as needed.)

Sit while you disappear from view for 10 seconds, sit in the chair for 5 seconds, and return

Sit for 10 seconds

Sit for 20 seconds while you jog and clap

Sit for 15 seconds while you run around

Sit for 10 seconds

Sit for 5 seconds while you turn around

Sit for 5 seconds while you sit in a chair near the dog

Sit while you disappear from view for 10 seconds, sit in the chair for 5 seconds, and return

Sit for 10 seconds

Task Set 9

Sit for 5 seconds

Sit for 10 seconds while you turn around

Sit for 5 seconds while you jog

Sit while you walk around the dog

Sit while you jog around the dog

Sit while you jog around the dog, clapping your hands

→ (Note: Again, this is a change. Alter your behavior, if needed, depending on your pet's reactivity.)

Sit while you jog twice around the dog

Sit for 10 seconds

Sit for 15 seconds while you clap your hands

Sit for 20 seconds

Sit while you move three-quarters of the way around the dog to the right and return

Sit while you move three-quarters of the way around the dog to the left and return

Sit while you disappear from view for 10 seconds and then return

Sit while you circle the dog and return

Sit while you disappear from view for 20 seconds and return

→ (Note: Again, this is a change. Alter your behavior, if needed, depending on your pet's reactivity. Pets with problems surrounding departures may react more at entrances. Behave as recommended above, please.)

Sit while you disappear from view for 25 seconds and return

Sit for 5 seconds while you sit in a chair near the dog

Sit while you disappear from view for 10 seconds, sit in the chair for 5 seconds, and return

Sit for 10 seconds

Sit while you bend down and touch your toes

Sit while you stretch your arms

Sit while you stretch your arms and jump once

Sit while you touch your toes 5 times

Sit while you stretch your arms and jump 3 times

Sit for 15 seconds

Sit for 10 seconds
Sit for 5 seconds

Task Set 10

Sit for 5 seconds and clap
Sit for 10 seconds while you touch your toes
Sit for 15 seconds while you sit in a chair
Sit while you walk quickly 15 steps to the right and return
→ **(Note: Pace changes may cause some pets to be more reactive. Alter your behavior as needed.)**
Sit while you walk quickly 15 steps to the left and return
Sit while you walk approximately 20 steps to an entrance and return
Sit while you leave the dog's view for 5 seconds and return
Sit while you leave the dog's view for 10 seconds and return
Sit while you leave the dog's view for 15 seconds and return
→ **(Note: Again, this is a change. Alter your behavior, if needed, depending on your pet's reactivity. Pets with problems surrounding departures may react more at entrances. Behave as recommended above, please.)**
Sit for 10 seconds
Sit for 5 seconds
Sit while you walk quickly 15 steps to the right and return
Sit while you walk quickly 15 steps to the left and return
Sit while you walk approximately 20 steps to an entrance and return
Sit while you leave the dog's view for 5 seconds and return
Sit while you leave the dog's view for 10 seconds and return
Sit while you leave the dog's view for 15 seconds and return
Sit while you leave the dog's view for 5 seconds, knock softly on the wall and return
→ **(Note: A new behavior may be provocative for some dogs.)**
Sit for 5 seconds
Sit while you leave the dog's view for 5 seconds and return
Sit while you leave the dog's view for 10 seconds and return
Sit while you leave the dog's view for 15 seconds and return
Sit while you leave the dog's view for 5 seconds, knock softly on the wall and return
Sit while you leave the dog's view, quickly knock softly on the wall and return
Sit for 5 seconds
Sit while you leave the dog's view for 10 seconds, knock softly on the wall and return
Sit for 10 seconds
Sit for 5 seconds

Task Set 11

Sit for 5 seconds
Sit for 10 seconds
Sit while you leave the dog's view, quickly knock softly on the wall and return
Sit for 5 seconds
Sit while you leave the dog's view for 10 seconds, knock softly on the wall and return
Sit for 30 seconds
→ **(Note: Again, this is a change. Alter your behavior, if needed, depending on your pet's reactivity. Pets with problems surrounding departures may react more at entrances. You have now combined leaving with other, provocative activities. Please alter your behavior as needed.)**
Sit while you leave the dog's view, ring the doorbell, and immediately return

Sit while you leave the dog's view, ring the doorbell, wait 2 seconds, and return
Sit for 30 seconds
→ **(Note: Again, this is a change. Alter your behavior, if needed, depending on your pet's reactivity. Pets with problems surrounding departures may react more at entrances. Behave as recommended above, please.)**
Sit while you leave the dog's view, ring the doorbell, and immediately return
Sit while you leave the dog's view, ring the doorbell, wait 5 seconds, and return
Sit for 30 seconds
→ **(Note: Again, this is a change. Alter your behavior, if needed, depending on your pet's reactivity. Pets with problems surrounding departures may react more at entrances. Behave as recommended above, please.)**
Sit while you leave the dog's view, ring the doorbell, and immediately return
Sit while you leave the dog's view, ring the doorbell, wait 10 seconds, and return
Sit for 5 seconds while you jog
Sit while you walk around the dog
Sit while you jog around the dog
Sit while you jog around the dog, clapping your hands
Sit while you jog twice around the dog
Sit for 10 seconds
Sit for 15 seconds while you clap your hands
Sit for 20 seconds
Sit while you move three-quarters of the way around the dog to the right and return
Sit while you move three-quarters of the way around the dog to the left and return
Sit while you disappear from view for 10 seconds and then return
Sit while you circle the dog and return
Sit for 10 seconds
Sit for 5 seconds

Task Set 12

Sit for 10 seconds
Sit for 5 seconds while you clap your hands
Sit for 15 seconds
Sit for 20 seconds while you hum
→ **(Note: This is a new behavior that some pets may find provocative.)**
Sit while you disappear from view for 20 seconds and return
Sit while you disappear from view for 25 seconds and return
Sit for 5 seconds while you sit in a chair near the dog
Sit while you disappear from view for 10 seconds, sit in the chair for 5 seconds, and return
Sit for 15 seconds
Sit for 20 seconds while you hum
Sit while you disappear from view for 20 seconds and return
Sit while you disappear from view for 25 seconds and return
Sit while you move three-quarters of the way around the dog to the right and return
Sit while you move three-quarters of the way around the dog to the left and return
Sit while you disappear from view for 10 seconds and then return
Sit while you circle the dog and return
Sit for 10 seconds

Sit while you leave the dog's view, quickly knock softly on the wall and return

Sit for 5 seconds

Sit while you leave the dog's view for 10 seconds, knock softly on the wall and return

Sit for 30 seconds

Sit while you leave the dog's view, ring the doorbell, and immediately return

→ **(Note: Again, this is a change. Alter your behavior, if needed, depending on your pet's reactivity. Pets with problems surrounding departures may react more at entrances. Behave as recommended above, please.)**

Sit while you leave the dog's view, ring the doorbell, wait 2 seconds, and return

Sit for 30 seconds

Sit while you leave the dog's view, say "hello," and return

→ **(Note: Again, this is a change. Alter your behavior, if needed, depending on your pet's reactivity. Pets with problems surrounding departures may react more at entrances. Behave as recommended above, please.)**

Sit while you leave the dog's view, say "hello," wait 3 seconds, and return

Sit for 10 seconds

Sit for 5 seconds

Task Set 13

Sit for 5 seconds

Sit for 15 seconds while you hum

Sit for 15 seconds while you hum and clap

Sit while you disappear from view for 20 seconds and return

Sit while you disappear from view for 25 seconds and return

Sit for 5 seconds while you sit in a chair near the dog

Sit while you disappear from view for 10 seconds, sit in the chair for 5 seconds, and return

Sit for 5 seconds

Sit for 10 seconds

Sit while you leave the dog's view, quickly knock softly on the wall and return

Sit for 5 seconds

Sit while you leave the dog's view for 10 seconds, knock softly on the wall and return

Sit for 30 seconds

Sit while you leave the dog's view, ring the doorbell, and immediately return

Sit while you leave the dog's view, ring the doorbell, wait 2 seconds, and return

Sit for 30 seconds

Sit while you leave the dog's view, say "hello," wait 5 seconds, and return

Sit while you leave the dog's view, knock or ring the bell, "hello," wait 5 seconds, and return

Sit for 30 seconds

→ **(Note: Again, this is a change. Alter your behavior, if needed, depending on your pet's reactivity. Pets with problems surrounding departures may react more at entrances. Behave as recommended above, please.)**

Sit while you leave the dog's view, say "hello," wait 5 seconds, and return

Sit while you leave the dog's view, knock or ring the bell, "hello," wait 5 seconds, and return

Sit for 20 seconds while you hum

Sit for 15 seconds while you clap

Sit for 5 seconds

Sit while you jog around the dog

Sit for 10 seconds while you clap and hum

Sit for 5 seconds while you jog in place

Sit while you jog around dog, humming

Task Set 14

Sit for 10 seconds

Sit for 10 seconds

Sit for 5 seconds while you hum and clap

Sit while you run around dog

Sit while you walk back and forth to door

Sit while you leave room and quickly knock or ring bell and return

Sit for 5 seconds

Sit for 10 seconds

Sit for 10 seconds

Sit for 5 seconds while you hum and clap

Sit while you run around dog

Sit while you walk back and forth to door

Sit while you leave room and quickly knock or ring bell and return

Sit for 5 seconds

Sit for 10 seconds

Sit while you leave the dog's view for 10 seconds, knock softly on the wall and return

Sit for 30 seconds

Sit while you leave the dog's view, ring the doorbell, and immediately return

Sit while you leave the dog's view, ring the doorbell, wait 2 seconds, and return

Sit for 30 seconds

Sit while you leave the dog's view, say "hello," wait 5 seconds, and return

Sit while you leave the dog's view, knock or ring the bell, say "hello," wait 10 seconds, and return

Sit for 30 seconds

Sit while you leave the dog's view, say "hello," wait 10 seconds, and return

Sit while you leave the dog's view, knock or ring the bell, say "hello," wait 10 seconds, and return

Sit for 20 seconds while you hum

Sit for 20 seconds

Sit for 5 seconds

Task Set 15

Sit for 10 seconds

Sit for 5 seconds

Sit for 15 seconds while you clap and hum

Sit while you leave the dog's view, knock or ring the bell, say "hello," talk for 10 seconds, and return

Sit for 20 seconds while you hum

Sit while you leave the dog's view, say "hello," invite the invisible person in, wait 5 seconds, and return

→ **(Note: Again, this is a change. Alter your behavior, if needed, depending on your pet's reactivity. Pets with problems surrounding departures may react more at entrances. Behave as recommended above, please.)**

Sit for 10 seconds

Sit for 5 seconds

Sit while you leave the dog's view, say "hello," invite the invisible person in, wait 10 seconds, and return

Sit while you leave the dog's view, say "hello," talk as if to someone for 5 seconds, and return

Sit for 5 seconds while you hum and clap

Sit while you run around dog

Sit while you walk back and forth to door

Sit while you leave room and quickly knock or ring bell and return

Sit for 5 seconds

Sit while you leave the room and knock or ring the bell for 3 seconds and return

Sit while you leave the room and knock or ring the bell for 5 seconds

Sit while you leave the room and talk to people who aren't there for 3 seconds

Sit while you leave the room and talk to people who aren't there for 5 seconds

Sit while you leave the room and talk to people who aren't there for 10 seconds

Sit while you run around the dog

Sit for 10 seconds while you sit in a chair

Sit for 30 seconds while you sit in a chair

Sit for 15 seconds while you jog and clap

Sit for 5 seconds

10. Suggestions for Future Repetitions

- Repeat all tasks in different locations.
- Repeat all tasks with all family members.
- Repeat all tasks with only every second or third being rewarded with a treat. (Remember praise!)
- Repeat with only intermittent treat reinforcement. (Remember praise!)
  Congratulations: You and your pet are now ready for Tier 2!

PROTOCOL FOR GENERALIZED DISCHARGE INSTRUCTIONS FOR DOGS WITH BEHAVIORAL CONCERNS

The following instructions/suggestions will help any dogs with a behavioral concern, regardless of a diagnosis.

Foundation for Understanding Behavioral Concerns

The vast majority of canine behavioral problems either include normal behaviors that humans don't like or 'don't understand, or anxiety-related concerns that comprise true behavioral diagnoses. The foundation for treating any canine behavioral concern relies on:

- understanding "normal,"
- identifying risk,
- communicating well with your dog,
- reading your dog's signals well, and
- meeting your dog's needs.

This handout will likely be accompanied by more specific instructions that will explain and make suggestions for how to best intervene for your dog's particular diagnosis. That said, all dogs—even lovely but bratty puppies—can benefit from some set of *baseline instructions* like those provided here.

What Behavior Modification Is and Is Not

Throughout these instructions we are going to use the phrase "behavior modification" (a.k.a. behavior mod) a lot. It's important that you understand what is meant by this term as used here.

Behavior mod is *not*:

- a learn-to-earn program,
- a nothing-in-life-is-free (NILIF) program,
- a sit-stay program,
- training,
- training by compulsion,
- abuse,
- discipline,
- a leadership program,
- a reconditioning program,
- doggie boot camp, or
- punishment (please do not even think of trying this).

True behavior modification is *a humane rule structure* that allows dogs to replace one set of rules that encourages reaction, with another set that allows the animal to relax and to take his cues from the contextual environment. True behavior modification involves clear signaling and learned trust from both participants, and reliability from humans.

Behavior modification is nothing more than the process of altering an animal's behavior. The classic response to having "behavior mod" recommended as part of a treatment plan is to say *"I don't have time for that."*

What is not generally understood is that *we engage in behavior modification either actively or passively every hour of the day and in everything we do.* The basic tenets of behavior modification treatment are not complex, and are put into action whether or not we consciously acknowledge or recognize that this is so. You are often unconsciously and accidentally employing principles associated with learning and behavior mod, and may be inadvertently doing an excellent job of reinforcing exactly the behaviors about which you are most distressed! This is especially easy for those of us who are very busy.

Learning occurs all the time, and we can shape the direction, rate and complexity of the learning process with conscious effort. This does **not** mean that you "must" engage in complex active behavior mod. It **does** mean that you can use small, relatively passive techniques to effect huge changes.

What Scares Us

People are also afraid of the terms used in behavior mod: desensitization (DS), counter-conditioning (CC), conditioned stimulus, et cetera. For those who do not use these terms daily they are jargon, but we can change our pets' behaviors without using these labels while still making use of the important concepts. The key to clear communication is to lose the jargon and concentrate on content.

Potential Problems for Changing Behavior

The problem with changing any behavior is threefold:

1. Inertia is a powerful force.
2. It can be difficult to break behaviors down into elements that require change.
3. Understanding how to change basic components can be difficult.

The difficulty lies in understanding exactly what is called for in the behavior modification technique of choice and in the timing of your response to the dog's behavior and communicatory gestures.

Before you can change your pet's behavior—or your own, with respect to your pet—you will need to recognize:

1. what normal signaling is,
2. what signals are associated with the behaviors you wish to change, and
3. what signals precede point 2.

In any situation there are three environments available for intervention that have the potential to be modified:

- The physical environment
- The behavioral environment
- The pharmacological environment

These environments are not independent. The key to understanding how dogs learn is to appreciate the complexity of interaction between these environments, and the importance of factors affecting temporal and intensity changes and interactions within these environments. If you wish to learn more about the pharmacological environment, please see the **Protocol for Using Behavioral Medication Successfully.**

Keys to Success

Keys to successful implementation of behavior modification include the following:

1. You are able to stop using any behaviors or behavioral sequences that promote, trigger, cause, encourage, or

correlate with any of the behaviors in the dog or cat that you wish to change.

2. You commit to clear signaling and a humane and possible set of rules by which you can interact with the cat or dog.

3. The signals in (2) have a canine or feline equivalent so that the dog or cat can understand and have the mental space to understand what you want.
   - For example, "sitting" in dogs and cats is a "stop" behavior. For dogs this is a deferential behavior that passes the job of giving the next signal back to the individual who encouraged the "sit." If you ask your dog to "sit," when he does so, he is now giving you the responsibility to provide him with the next useful piece of information.

4. The behavior mod—which is a true rule structure—should signal to the dog or cat what she can expect to happen next or it should teach her that she can look to you for all cues about the appropriateness of her behavior whenever she is concerned.

5. The reward structure—which is another rule structure—should be clearly defined and appropriately reinforced at all times. You will need to understand at the gut level that we teach best by rewarding every instance of appropriate behavior and that we retain what we have learned best by rewarding intermittently. You also need to understand that intermittent is **not** synonymous with "seldom."

6. Unless you wish to teach the dog or cat to fear you or that you are not trustworthy, **you MUST stop all punishment, shrieking, yelling, throwing things, et cetera, no matter how good it sometimes feels (for and to you—the dog and cat have a different opinion).**

Important Points About Behavior Mod That Should Go Without Saying, But Don't

The following important points regarding behavior modification exercises are those which are most frequently misunderstood by clients and vets, alike.

1. Behavior modification exercises are **not,** repeat **not,** obedience exercises.
   First, although sitting is part of obedience training, the goal of these programs is not just to have your dog sit, but to **relax** and be receptive to changing his behavior while doing so. It is critical that you understand and appreciate this difference. Dogs who are stressed or anxious cannot successfully learn a more appropriate behavior and they certainly cannot associate that behavior with having fun or with good things happening.
   Second, behavior modification is about changing the way the dog thinks about interactions by rewarding the physical cues associated with the underlying physiological state. Obedience training, while sharing many similarities with behavior modification, differs in the premise, interactive reward structure, goal, and outcome. Most of the dogs that undergo behavior modification have been through some form of training and most know how to sit. For a dog to do this successfully in a class (or even a show) situation, the dog does not have to be relaxed. For behavior mod to work as well as it can the dog *must* be relaxed.

2. **Relaxation is key here**—the sitting and staying is merely a facilitator for the relaxation response. There is no sense to having your dog sit and stay if he is panting, salivating,

his pupils are dilated, his ears are back, and he is clearly distressed. What on earth is your dog learning? It's simple: Your dog is learning to be more distressed—while sitting—and also teaching himself to become refractory to complex learning because of arousal of the hypothalamic-pituitary-adrenal axis. This is why old-fashioned, outmoded, and simplistic "sit-stay" programs so often fail: the dog sits, but is still distressed. *Good news: now that you understand this you can prevent such distress!*

3. You may have trouble with appropriate timing of rewards and "corrections." "Corrections" should be restricted to walking away from the dog or a quick, soft vocal signal that tells the dog he is behaving undesirably. The point of the "correction" is to interrupt the dog—not to "get even." Anyone who wants to "get even" may be at risk for potentially—albeit accidentally—exhibiting abusive behaviors that will make any dog worse.
   Dogs read nonvocal or body language far better than do most humans. It is easy for them to "subvert" the exercise and "shape" your behavior. Problem dogs have been doing this already, and such behaviors are **not** malicious. They **are,** however, behaviors that logically are exhibited by a confused, uncertain animal in an attempt to gain information about what can be expected—and what their response should be—within that context. Because we often attribute uncharitable "motivations" to our pets, someone from outside of the relationship needs to be able to comment on timing problems and to help us with our posture, tone, or quickness of praise or reward. Most of us are quite good at learning to do this, but may need help. Ask your veterinarian for help if you are unsure you are doing this correctly. There are trained and certified dog trainers and veterinary professionals who can help you and will only use humane and positive methods to do so.

4. What happens if behavior mod doesn't seem to be helping?
   If you are not seeing an improvement, or are having an actual problem, one or more of the following is true:
   - You are pushing the dog too hard, too fast (very common in today's hi-tech, faster-is-better world).
   - You are giving confusing signals.
   - Your timing is wrong.
   This is hard work—it is not magic. Make a video of you working with your dog and see if you can spot the problem. More often than not you will see something that you could improve. Seek help along the way. Certified Professional Dog Trainers (CPDT; www.ccpdt.org) often have a good demonstration dog and may be uniquely equipped to teach the practical implementation of behavior modification (contact the Association of Pet Dog Trainers [APDT]; www.apdt.com). One new organization, the Pet Professional Guild (www.petprofessionalguild.com), is devoted to completely force-free training.

A Few Words About Rewards

Most commonly used behavior modification programs employ praise and food treats or other rewards. The higher the quality of the treat—from the dog's viewpoint—the better will be the dog's response. A dog who might work for American cheese while on the property, might need dried liver when out in traffic. **No one goes to hell for using food treats,** but to hear people's reactions, you'd be certain this was the case.

The approach to behavior modification discussed here does **not** use hand signals **or** clickers. Clickers are unforgiving with respect to timing, and to ask you to read a problem pet's signals, monitor them constantly, teach them to sit and relax, **and** incorporate the clicker system into behavior mod, are not kind to you, and can further confuse the dog. If you are already masterful in the use of clicker training, you *can, but do not have to, use them* in these programs.

Hand signals are commonly used in obedience and can be useful for dogs and for us, but behavioral patients need every bit of help that they can get. Once the dogs master the programs, they will have no problems coupling the learned vocal cues to visual ones. Until then, these dogs should work in calm, quiet circumstances, without distraction, for vocal cues, and a consistent reward structure. Dogs can learn all the words for the "commands," signals, or requests that they will need for these programs.

Most importantly, hand signals at this stage will only ask the dog to distract their attention from the behavior modification process, and, for very aggressive dogs, such signals will put the person using them at risk. **Without exception, dangling body parts in front of an aggressive dog is not recommended, and will make the animal more anxious.** In a worst-case scenario, hand signals can be seen by the dog as threats.

Basic Instructions

1. Have all dogs in the household—regardless of whether they have problems—practice the passive behavior modification program, **Protocol for Deference.** Ask all dogs to sit for everything so that they are calm, focused on you, and so that you can reward this excellent, calm behavior.

   Try to reward your dog when he has his ears up, is looking at you, and is not panting. This is the first step in teaching a dog to calm and take a deep breath.

2. Teach your dog to breathe deeply as part of becoming calmer (see the **Protocol for Teaching Your Dog to Take a Deep Breath and Use Other Biofeedback Methods as Part of Relaxation**).

3. Your dog will learn everything faster if the same set of rules is applied to *all dogs in the household* and if he can model many of his behaviors on a dog who is not anxious or problematic. Recent research shows that dogs are very good at observational learning.

   Any program that can help treat a behavioral problem, can be used to prevent behavior problems. The earlier all dogs are taught rule structures that allow them to have their needs met in a humane partnership, the better.

4. Remember that developmental stages and social maturity matter. Dogs are physically immature until they are about 6 to 9 months of age and socially, "emotionally," and "intellectually" immature until approximately 12 to 18 months of age when social maturity *begins*. Changes in brain neurochemistry are associated with such changes in other species and these changes are likely in dogs. Additionally, changes in social interactions, signals, relationships, and ways of thinking accompany this change. Households are affected by the changes that go with social maturity. This may mean that more than one dog is undergoing social maturation at the same time in the household and that other canine, feline, and human relationships may not be unaffected. If household dogs learn to be calm together by using this program it will bode well for them as the youngsters pass through social maturity.

5. You will make the most progress if you work with the first part of the active behavior modification program: **Protocol for Relaxation: Behavior Modification Protocol Tier 1.** Before you can do this successfully you will need to ensure you and your dog can accomplish the **Protocol for Teaching Your Dog to Take a Deep Breath and Use Other Biofeedback Methods as Part of Relaxation.** The video *Humane Behavioral Care for Dogs: Problem Prevention and Treatment* shows you how to use these protocols.

6. Please note: The early parts of the behavior modification protocols are very easy to mess up. *GO SLOWLY.* The single biggest mistake that humans make in working with true behavior modification in dogs is that they move through the process too rapidly without paying attention to the dog's signals about whether he is calm or scared. Pretend that all dogs have special needs and go slowly; there is no cost to this, but a huge cost in confusion and anxiety on the dog's part and frustration on the human's part to going too fast.

7. Increase your dog's aerobic exercise. Tired dogs are happy dogs and they have ecstatic people! Think of the needs of your dog in terms of breed, age, and individual "temperament" or "personality." Young border collies from working lines are not good candidates for couch potato status. Meet the needs you identify in your dog. Suggestions for increasing your dog's exercise include leash walks, running with your dog, and playing with toys indoors and out. See the **Protocol for Choosing Toys for Your Pet** for some ideas.

8. Intellectual stimulation, clear and kind rules, and opportunities for dogs to know that they can succeed and will be rewarded for succeeding are important. As dogs begin to improve, become more attentive, and are calmer, clicker training for tricks or sports like agility can be terrific. Again, this is a place where humans tend to push their dogs too fast, too soon, so please be careful. And if you decide to engage in these activities, please ensure that you have discussed the dog's problems and needs with the organizer or instructor. Your dog may not be suitable for the class you had in mind, and it may not be suitable for him. Many dog clubs run smaller or quieter classes for needier dogs. Please be realistic; to not be realistic may be injurious to your dog, and your dog's well-being has to be your first concern.

9. You can also exercise your dog's brain whenever he is left alone, or when you cannot otherwise pay active attention to him (e.g., you are having a dinner party). Food puzzles like Roll-a-Treat Balls, Kongs, and Planet toys are just some of the growing number of food toys that will let the dog exercise his or her dexterity and cognitive skills and be rewarded immediately. Please remember, such toys are not substitutes for true behavioral treatment, and they will not fix dogs who are distressed when left alone. Distressed dogs cannot eat, but as they improve, if the treat is good enough they will begin to go after it.

These types of toys can also be used outside of the house to keep the dogs focused on you and to reward them for not worrying. Think of a toy that the dog really loves as a "security blanket," which, if carried on walks, not only shifts his focus but tells him that the world is a safer place.

Float toys in kiddie pools so that dogs can keep cool and play at the same time.

10. Please remember that most canine behavioral concerns are routed in anxiety. The key to fixing this is to anticipate where the dog may be uncertain and give her instructions that preempt her uncertainty. That's what behavior mod does for dogs—when done well it provides them with a humane set of rules with reasonable expectations. By using food treats, we also make use of the biofeedback aspect. The following patterns may help you to understand your dog.

   - Many dogs need to control their world as a way of addressing the uncertainty and anxiety in their world. When they cannot get instructions from context they may use "challenges" to provoke the environment and decide whether the person is a risk. If you can begin to think about when the dog will not have a choice, you'll be able to avoid any problems.

   - Some dogs can only function when the rules are clear; their world is all black and white. Our job is to teach them that shades of gray are okay.

   - Remember that frank aggression with many dogs is a last resort, but "last resort" is defined **by the dog's definition of last resort.** You may think the dog responded too quickly and so be tempted to use punishment. Please think carefully about this. *Punishment will only make the dog worse because the dog is already anxious, which is why she responded so quickly.* If the dog is now scared or hurt, she will make the association with her already worried mindset and become worse.

   - Please remember that the dogs are taking their cues from you. Think of it this way: If every event for them is about a set of rules that determine whether they react and you are anxious, your signal indicates that you are concerned. Does your signal that you are worried help to make them more anxious or less anxious? More anxious.

   - Please also remember that every time a dog with concerns acts inappropriately, the dog gets worse, and that worsening leaves the dog more uncertain.

11. Please remember that although the breed shapes the behavior—both appropriate and not—no dog is "aggressive" or "reactive" because he is a certain breed. Even when behavioral diagnoses and pathology run in family lines, not all members of the breed are affected by the pathology, so it would be wrong and inappropriate to label the problem a result of the breed, or a breed-associated trait. That said, when dogs with anxiety disorders show their anxiety, the anxiety tends to take the form of the behaviors for which they were selected. For example, you may see some of the classic herding and nipping behaviors in some herding dogs when they have some problem aggressions.

12. Anxiety disorders are about apprehension of future events or reactions and the behaviors we see are vigilance and scanning, increased or decreased locomotor activity (e.g., pacing), and autonomic hyper-reactivity (e.g., panting, salivating, increased heart rate, et cetera). Watch for behaviors like yawning, licking, scratching, increased vigilance and scanning, increased attentiveness and following, salivation, et cetera. These behaviors tell you that the dog is uncertain. Learn to read dog signaling. For example, dogs who snort will invariably do what you want them to do although they really don't want to do it. Please note that uncertainty and anxiety have nothing to do with love or needing love, or the behaviors that you may see as loving. Once these types of dogs improve, you will truly see how relaxed they can be when loving you—they will be less needy. Please do not interpret this as less loving. It's not. It's a healthier form of loving.

13. All dogs with behavioral concerns should be removed from provocative situations. Anticipating such situations is good, avoiding them is better. Remember that if you have videotaped and watched your dog and provided an accurate history, you will be able to identify all the circumstances in which he will react.

   The key to working with these situations is to always make sure that the dog is focused on you and calm before you ask the dog to do something. You should be giving your dog verbal signals that he can be calm and look to you, but remember that dogs need space to listen to you. A frantic dog cannot pay attention.

   In the beginning, when it is unlikely your verbal cues will get the dog to attend to you, don't talk to your dog if he is not stopped. Sitting is a stop signal in dogs, and unless your dog has the mental space to listen, he can only fail.

   If the dog cannot attend to you, don't scream, shout, throw things, or whack the dog—just walk away. This technique works because it gives the dog a choice—he can offer another behavior that you may prefer. If you struggle with a dog, that dog only has one choice and that's to react. By leaving, you allow the dog to come to you to ask for information. This is why it is so important to work with your dogs in controlled, non-provocative circumstances first. Dogs need to learn that they can seek information from humans when they are uncertain. We focus a lot on giving information to the dogs. We need to step back and also allow them to request information, if we are going to meet their needs.

14. Once your dog is working well with you in comfortable, non-provocative circumstances, you can start to walk and work with the dog in more provocative ones. The dog should always be on a lead and a harness or head collar, if possible, whenever you even have a hint that the dog could worry.

   When you anticipate that the dog might react, ask her to "look" and chat her up. Dogs take their cues from your tone of voice and the words with which they have learned to make associations. For anxious dogs you should be supplying almost continuous commentary so that they can learn that you will give them cues that tell them when they should worry and that this is almost never. Furthermore, by talking to your dog, you can frequently and instantly reward good behavior.

Use your dog's name—her name may be the first cue that allows her to sift through the noise of the crowd and focus on you. When people tell you that they have been told in obedience training that they shouldn't use the dog's name, gently explain to them that sporting contests are very different than building a helpful relationship. And if no one plays the national anthem when you walk your dog, you are not at a sporting event and you can use your dog's name—preferably, early and often—if your dog has not learned to tune it out. Don't worry that others on the street will think you are crazy for talking nonstop to your dog; it's not their well-being that's the issue.

15. Any time you are not going to be able to keep a direct eye on a dog that has behavioral concerns and there is **any** change to his rule structure, you must protect the dog by not allowing him to be part of the interaction. Dogs can be very comfortable in crates, behind locked doors, out of the way of traffic, et cetera. If you are having unpredictable guests—and the more worried you are about your dog, the more unpredictable your guests will seem—lock the dog **in** a room. Affix a latch at the very top of the door so that someone cannot accidentally open the door, and so that they have to think about what they are doing. Also, put a sign on the door that reminds people not to disturb the dog. This sounds like overkill, but it's not.

16. Many people carry on about how important it is to not allow your dog to be pushy (or "dominant"). This is another entrenched myth having to do with unclear terms and murkier understanding. Please remember that it is okay for a dog to be a pushy and assertive dog if he is also well mannered.

    This isn't about having "dominion" over the dog. It's about signaling clearly to the dog and being reliable so that they learn to take their clues about the appropriateness of their behaviors from you. Changing your pet's behavior is not about getting more control or dominion over them; it is about making them want to elicit certain behaviors from you. This requires that you be calm and clear in your signals.

    Problem pets have special needs, and although they can be difficult to manage, the vast majority of such pets improve. You can only address their individual needs if you let go of the useless and dangerous concepts of "dominance," "submission," "pack," and "alpha." Canine behaviors, like ours, are context dependent. This means that what works in some situations for some individuals won't be an option for others. Forcing the behaviors into unrealistic categories will get in the way of seeing the behaviors as they truly are and improving them. For more information on these issues, please see the American Veterinary Society of Animal Behavior (AVSAB) Dominance Position Statement (www.avsabonline.org/avsabonline/images/stories/Position_Statements/dominance%20statement.pdf) and the Dog Welfare Campaign position statement (www.dogwelfarecampaign.org/why-not-dominance.php).

    Please try to avoid all circumstances known to be provocative to your pet. This may mean a change in your lifestyle, but meanwhile you are not inadvertently

reinforcing an inappropriate behavior that your pet is exhibiting.

17. Get and use a head collar or a no-pull harness for all walks and all interactions with humans and dogs at gatherings or in any situation where people may try to get close to the dog. If you are uncertain how to use these, ask your veterinarian for help. Training videos are also available or you can call the manufacturer for help.
    - The use of a head collar makes a real difference in how these anxious dogs behave and in how concerned you are because head collars allow you to turn the dog's head away from another dog or a human, and close the jaws, if needed.
    - Proper use of head collars may prevent bites and will insure that any reactive dogs can be separated safely, should they get into a fight, and that worried dogs don't inadvertently provoke anything such as other humans or dogs.
    - Head collars can also be an enormous help during visits to the veterinarian: When used correctly you will need almost no restraint, and you will never need a muzzle. The less restraint, force, and concern that we can employ in veterinary practice, the better.

    No-pull harnesses cannot close a dog's mouth but can allow you to turn a dog away from a worrying situation and have some leverage that helps, rather than hurts, them.

18. The single most unexploited technique for good behavior is also among the most simple: **reward your dog for any spontaneously excellent behavior—like sleeping.** Any time your dog plops his butt down tell him he's wonderful. The flip side of this is that you cannot touch, talk, or interact with the dog until his butt is on the ground and he is attending to you. Remember that sitting acts as a "stop" signal in dogs, and you don't want to inadvertently reward bratty behaviors because the dog is otherwise engaged. This isn't about discipline; it's about ensuring that you are not accidentally rewarding anxious behaviors.

    Sometimes attention-seeking behaviors occur because the dog just wants attention, but when we are working with problem dogs, most of these behaviors are about neediness (see **Protocol for Attention-Seeking Behavior**). When understood in this way, guiding the dog into calmer, less reactive postures before petting makes complete sense. Then, if your dog is calm and you wish to do so, you can invite him into your lap, onto the sofa, et cetera, providing that you can also invite him to get off and he can easily and happily comply.

19. Most people don't think much about how to pet a dog. But we must remember that dogs are very tactile animals and unlike animals with speech (us) they communicate a lot by touching. Not all touching is the same. Please remember that when you pet or touch your dog, long, slow strokes are better than short rapid ones. You want everything in the dog's life to be about being calm. See the **Protocol for Teaching Your Dog to Take a Deep Breath and Use Other Biofeedback Methods as Part of Relaxation** for instructions.

20. When you decide to practice the active behavior mod (**Protocol for Relaxation: Behavior Modification Tier 1**), remember to start in a physical place where your dog will not consider the environment to be provocative. If your

dog is exhibiting any of the signs of anxiety before you start (vigilance and scanning, increased heart or respiratory rate, increased or decreased locomotor activity, puffing out or licking his lips, et cetera) you will only teach her to be more reactive—not less. Subtlety is important here.

21. Please remember that **anxious behaviors are associated with uncertainty.** Dogs are uncertain about what the rules are when they do not have enough consistent guidance. Most normal dogs learn not to worry either by watching humans or other dogs and by getting their information from the context. **By definition, dogs with behavioral concerns have an impaired ability to obtain information from the pattern of context, because to do so they would have to be able to inhibit their ability to react.** By asking your dog to look to you for all of his cues, or to touch your hand as a targeting exercise, you can prevent the development of worse anxiety-related pathology. Fear and anxiety are not exactly the same things, but they are related both behaviorally and neurochemically. The main difference between these two problems is that fearful dogs withdraw and signal their willingness to withdraw, whereas anxious dogs often provoke the situation to get information. Neither of them can easily get information from context, but the purely fearful dog finds it acceptable to not have the information and assume the worst; the anxious dog provokes or pushes to get information, which is now viewed through their troubled lens. Anxiety disorders factor into the rule structure: these dogs react and provoke instead of sitting back and getting their information from context. This also explains why any compulsion-based techniques are doomed to fail. Dogs with anxiety disorders provoke the environment—not because they are nasty, but because they have only one rule structure and that rule requires that they are ever-vigilant. Their default assumption is that everything is potentially a threat and they react by learning whether it is.

22. There is a lot of debate about the effects of (a) protein levels and behaviors, (b) dietary composition and behaviors, and (c) dietary additives, preservatives, et cetera and behavior. Unfortunately, there are few data. Some dogs clearly have problems with certain foods or additives. Anything that makes you feel ill makes you more reactive, and so dogs with behavioral concerns may be witchier when they feel less than topnotch. For dogs who are not heavily exercised or worked, the composition or quality of the protein may be more important than the amount, and decreasing protein may contribute to making the dog less reactive. Fortunately, there are enough commercially prepared diets that you can do your own experiments and see if different diets have any effect on any of the above for your dog.

23. We cannot always be perfect so we need to anticipate what we can do if the dog reacts.
    - The first most important task we need to accomplish is to avoid situations where our dogs react. If we fail, we cannot react roughly to our dog's problematic behaviors.
    - The second most important thing is to interrupt these behaviors—without rewarding them—as early in the inappropriate sequence as possible.
    - The third most important thing we can do is to look for a way to reward our dog quickly for a wholly appropriate and freely offered behavior. This pattern allows learning and recovery to occur and for our dogs to improve.

PROTOCOL FOR HANDLING AND SURVIVING AGGRESSIVE EVENTS

No one wishes to be victimized by an aggressive cat or dog, but bites are so common that more than 50% of all children 11 years of age and younger have been bitten by a cat or dog. Tables 1 and 2 contain information on developmental stages for dogs and children that can factor into bites, and warning signs in dogs that may indicate that they have concerns about children's behaviors. Table 3 is an injury scale that is an adaptation of those commonly seen in the literature.

Understanding which specific canine and feline behaviors indicate a potentially aggressive response and knowing how not to worsen an already bad situation can help people to avoid attacks by animals. If the person behaves appropriately, even if they are not able to avoid the attack, they can minimize the damage they experience during the attack. Because most serious bites to people that occur in the United States and Europe involve dogs, this handout focuses primarily on avoiding dog bites, but the information in it can be adapted to avoiding being injured by cats, too.

Everyone should know that fatal dog bites are rare, despite the amount of media attention they receive when they occur.

Regardless, for those who experience bites, injuries can be both physical and psychological, and may have long-term consequences.

- From the veterinary perspective, the most serious of these long-term consequences may involve attitudes that adversely affect people's willingness to get and care for pets.
- From the legal perspective, fear of dog bites and the accompanying public outcry has engendered a series of legislative initiatives that have nothing to do with the real risk that anyone will be bitten.

Accordingly, anything we can do to decrease the number of dog bites and to understand those that occur will help us to be better guardians of dogs, safer when we interact with dogs, and more humane in our overall approach to interactions between ourselves and dogs.

What Is Aggression?

Before we consider specific circumstances involving aggression, we should define it.

Aggression is best described as an appropriate or inappropriate, inter- or intraspecific, threat, challenge, or contest that ultimately results in either deference or combat, and in resolution.

The next few paragraphs explain each of the three parts of this definition in a way that will allow most people to evaluate whether the dog poses a risk.

1. *Aggression can be appropriate.*
   - If you are attacked, you would likely want your dog to growl and protect you.
   - If the dog is being tortured or injured, fighting back can be an appropriate response.

These are key considerations when dog bites are litigated and when decisions about a dog's behaviors are made. Every law regulating dogs has a provision for *biting as an appropriate behavior.* Yet people often do not consider that they are living with a carnivore who has an identical social system to theirs, but who uses her mouth in many cases where humans would use their hands. For example, the Labrador retriever who brings you the morning paper does not carry it in one paw and hop home three-legged—the dog carries the paper in his mouth.

If people are unwilling to realize that dog bites can be both appropriate and accidental, they likely have insufficient education or understanding to humanely raise and care for a dog.

Inappropriate aggression occurs when either the context is wrong or the degree of force is excessive. For example, most dogs shouldn't and don't savagely attack people when they are surprised or startled. If a dog did so—in the absence of any history of abuse—the behavior would be inappropriate because it's out of context and because the force used would be excessive. If a dog is startled, the person startling the dog might be gently grabbed because the dog is uncertain or afraid: In this case, a gentle grab would not be inappropriate in terms of force.

Whether this behavior is inappropriate in terms of context depends very much on the previous experience of the dog. If the dog is teased frequently, his response may be perfectly contextually appropriate. If the dog is deaf, he might startle quite easily, so using his mouth to gently stop someone and get more information would be wholly appropriate.

2. *"Interspecific" means between species, and "intraspecific" means within species.*

Interactions with those of the same species (dog–dog) may have different rules than those between species (dog–human, dog–cat), so it is important to evaluate the behavior within the context of those specific rules.

For example, dogs play very roughly with their mouths and paws when playing with other dogs. They also have fur and thick skin. Such behaviors—translated to humans in an unedited form—could be injurious to humans. Dogs usually play more gently with humans than they do with other dogs unless humans have been very foolish and have encouraged rough play. Often this happens because the human thinks the rough play was cute in the 10-pound puppy. Later, although the human actively taught the dog to play roughly, he finds the same behavior problematic in the 100-pound adult dog. Unfortunately, it is usually the dog, not the human, who pays for this error in judgment.

3. *Aggression can result in threats or in a contest and either can be paths to some form of resolution.*

Finally, in any altercation, someone ultimately defers and the tone is set for some kind of negotiated truce (e.g., a rule structure by which each side knows what to expect), or there is a battle to death. Because most of our signaling as social species is about learning what the rules are and then checking to make sure this is so, behavior modification should act as a rule structure that specifies context-dependent outcomes. This is exactly what the **Protocol for Deference** and the **Protocol for Relaxation** do: They specify rules by which everyone in the interaction can become more clear and reliable. These rules both treat aggression and help to prevent it.

The Unknown or Unfamiliar Dog

When one considers the potential to be bitten, dogs who are unknown to individuals pose a different set of problems than do those who are familiar to the victim. Most dogs who bite people in public places or in their communities are **not** true strays—they are owned by someone and may be a good pet

TABLE 1

Developmental Stages for Children and Their Effects on Dogs

Age of Child	Developmental Milestone(s)	Typical Child Behaviors Affecting Dogs	Typical "Normal" Dog Behavior	Diagnoses in Abnormal Dogs That Could Put Children at Risk
0-6 months	Reflexive behaviors Sitting up/creeping	New noises: crying, screaming, babbling New smells Grabbing fur, body parts of dogs	Sniffing Licking Avoidance, at first	Predatory aggression Fear aggression
6-24 months	Fine-motor skills improve Crawling/cruising Walking/running Curiosity-exploration	Increased noise/chaos Exploration of dog's body with hands, mouth, teeth	Freezing or avoidance Waiting for food	Fear Fear aggression Pain aggression Food-related aggression Possessive aggression
2-5 years	Autonomy-tantrums Gross/fine motor coordination improves Egocentricity Magical thinking/fantasizing Animism/anthropomorphism New friends enter household	Interactions with dog: • interrupt sleep/rest • fondling • chasing games • removal of toy/food • sharing human/dog food	More distant withdrawal Avoidance Offering of toy Soliciting food	Fear aggression Pain aggression Food-related aggression Possessive aggression Protective/territorial aggression Impulse-control aggression Fear Inappropriate herding behavior
5-9 years	Intense curiosity Experimentation Independence—decreased adult supervision Poor deductive/generalizing powers Desire for control	Interactions with dog: • Teasing • Reprimanding/punishing • Bossing • Roughhousing/tug of war	Curiosity Following Playing with toys Playing roughly Sleeping in specific child's room	Inappropriate play Fear aggression Pain aggression Possessive aggression Territorial/protective aggression Play aggression Impulse-control aggression Fear Inappropriate herding behavior Inappropriate play Play aggression
9-12 years	Increased peer influence Increased sense of responsibility Concrete operations Problem-solving Increased deductive/generalizing powers	Interactions with dog: • may take responsibility for feeding, grooming, exercising • increased teasing/rough play • abusive interaction may begin	Accompanying specific child Aerobic play Sleeping in specific child's room	Impulse-control aggression Fear aggression Play aggression Protective/territorial aggression

From Love M, Overall KL: Dogs and children: how anticipating relationships can help avoid disasters, J Am Vet Med Assoc 219:446–453, 2001.

TABLE 2

Warning Signs in Dogs That Can Indicate Distress Associated with Children

- Acute change in a dog's normal behavior (e.g., withdrawal or increased circling and patrol behavior; changes in amount or character of vocalization).
- Change in appetite, particularly if dog will only eat in the absence of the child, or if the dog suddenly shows food-guarding.
- Increased reactivity of pet (e.g., barking, growling, patrolling, lunging in new or lesser circumstances).
- Changes in sleeping/resting activity and locations.
- Changes in behaviors associated with behavioral diagnosis and increase in or appearance of gastrointestinal signs (vomiting, regurgitation, diarrhea) associated with stress.
- Signs of separation anxiety only when left with children (e.g., vocalization, destruction, elimination, salivation, increase or decrease in motor activity).
- Frank aggression—even without a specific diagnosis—in the presence of children.

From Love M, Overall KL: Dogs and children: how anticipating relationships can help avoid disasters, J Am Vet Med Assoc 219:446–453, 2001.

TABLE 3

Assessing Damage Done During Aggressive Events

The following scale is an adaptation of one widely used to assess damage caused by dogs during an aggressive event.

Severity Level	Threat or Bite Characteristics
1	Posturing, growling, lunging, or snarling behavior occurred without teeth touching skin (i.e., mostly mild agonistic, intimidation behavior). *Note: These behaviors may be completely normal.*
2	Teeth touched skin, but no puncture wounds greater than $\frac{1}{10}$ of an inch were inflicted. Marks or minor scratches from paws and nails (minor surface abrasions) may have been incurred. Abrasions more likely to be horizontal than vertical. *Note: These may be normal behaviors and no-to-minor injury may be normal. The extent of injury is often associated with the amount of movement of the individuals involved and their relative masses.*
3	Punctures were half the length of a canine tooth and resulted in 1 to 4 holes from a single bite. No tears or slashes were incurred, and the recipient was not shaken side to side. Lacerations are in a single direction. *Note: Movement and mass matter here because force = mass × acceleration. This consideration should factor into all interactions with dogs, including those involving play (dog–dog and human–dog).*
4	One to 4 holes from a single bite, with 1 or more holes deeper than half the length of a canine tooth. Deep bruising from prolonged pressure and contact results. Contact and punctures were incurred from more than the canine teeth. Tears, slash wounds, or both resulted, and shaking—as evidenced by lacerations in multiple directions—was involved. *Note: The extent of damage done in this circumstance may be affected by mass and movement, but also by dog morphology. Jaw size and mass and distribution of jaw muscles matter, and should be a consideration when evaluating to what extent any inhibition could have been involved.*
5	Multiple bites at severity level 4 or greater incurred in a concerted, repeated attack. *Note: The context in which this type of bite can occur matters, and dogs who are defending people have been known to exhibit these behaviors. In the absence of any justified context, these dogs are extremely dangerous.*
6	Any bite that resulted in death of any individual (dog, human, cat, et cetera). *Note: It is important to realize that dogs will hunt if hungry, and that accidental bites can have fatal consequences. This is the best justification for evaluating the appropriateness of the behavior given the context in which it occurs.*

Adapted from the Association of Professional Dog Trainers website (www.apdt.com): Dr. Ian Dunbar's dog bite scale. An assessment of the severity of biting problems based on an objective evaluation of wound pathology. www. apdt.com/veterinary/assets/pdf/ Ian Dunbar Dog Bite Scale.pdf. Accessed August 3, 2011; and Wrubel KM, Moon-Fanelli A, Maranda LS, Dodman NH: Interdog household aggression: 38 cases (2006-2007), J Am Vet Med Assoc 238:731–740, 2011.

for their people, but they are now acting as loose and free-ranging pets.

Some general information about the behavior of free-ranging dogs can help people to avoid bites.

- Dogs in groups may be more confident and more reactive than are single dogs.
- Single dogs may be more wary, but may still bite if cornered.
- Dogs become bolder and more confident if close to their home turf. Unfortunately, if the dog is unknown to the person, knowing where their home turf is can be difficult.
- Dogs can view stares as threats. No one should ever stare at an unfamiliar dog. Oblique, downward gazes allow humans to monitor the dog's behavior while not appearing as a threat.
- Dogs will chase individuals running away from them in one of two ways: as they would chase an intruder or as they would chase prey. In both cases, four-footed animals with large shearing teeth—your basic dog—has all the advantages. Please note that breed may affect how the dog chases: herding breeds may treat running humans as they would animals they are trying to round up and grab them in the same way. Accordingly, *people should not run in the presence of dogs they do not know.* In a situation involving an unfamiliar dog, dogs will almost always pursue someone who runs either away or toward them. If people cease to act like fleeing animals, active pursuit often stops. You have a much better chance of remaining uninjured if you slowly back away from unknown dogs, talk softly, and keep the dogs only in your peripheral vision.
- Children who shriek are far more liable to elicit active pursuit and biting than those who are quiet.
- Throwing stones, sticks, or anything else, or aggressively waving your arms at a dog that is pursuing you is far more likely to intensify the dog's aggression than it is to mollify the dog.
- Young children and older people are more at risk for serious injury than are adults. Individuals in both of these age groups are less likely to be able to successfully retreat from and fend off an attack because they may not be able to move in a coordinated manner, or because they cannot anticipate the event. In fact, the mortality rate for humans in these groups is much higher than for older children and adults who are not elderly and/or debilitated.
- Although it is inappropriate and incorrect to say that certain breeds are more aggressive than others, more damage does occur when larger breeds attack. The greater the size–person mismatch, the more damage that will be done. If the person attacked is a child, the chance of serious, and often fatal, injury increases.

Concerns for Children and Dogs

Children should be encouraged to *not* play with unfamiliar dogs. *Under no circumstance should children play with dogs that are not theirs unless they are supervised by a responsible adult.* This advice is as much for the *dog's protection* as it is for the child's.

Both children and dogs can be unpredictable and the interaction can occasionally be toxic. Many dogs only respond aggressively to a child after an extended period of rough

handling or frank abuse, but the dog will never get the benefit of the doubt.

Children may also not understand that the manner in which they are interacting with the dog is unacceptable and unkind for the dog. An adult needs to teach children appropriate behavior when handling pets. All adults should have a vested interest in protecting their dogs and their children.

Some children understand that what they are doing is provocative, and continue to do so *exactly* for this reason. In such cases, those involved should evaluate the child's behaviors in other circumstances. Animal/dog abuse and child abuse are tightly linked. Children who are exposed to abusers can learn to hone their abuse skills on their pets. Those in law enforcement know that the hallmark of many criminals is early animal abuse and torture. Early recognition and redress by veterinarians, trainers, teachers, those who have dogs, public health personnel, and social service personnel is an essential part of breaking the cycle of abuse. Local humane organizations can provide guidance should one have a question about the suitability of a child–dog interaction. Should the local humane organization be unable to provide such information, the Humane Society of the United States, in Washington, DC, sponsors a program called **First Strike,** which provides guidance in such situations (www.humanesociety.org/assets/pdfs/abuse/first_strike.pdf; www.animalsheltering.org/programs_and_services/first_strike).

If an unfamiliar or at-large dog approaches a child in a public place, the child should tell an adult immediately, and the adult should tell someone responsible for the maintenance of the open space. If the dog is clearly friendly and solicitous, the adult may make the decision to take the dog home, but any dog that is exhibiting any wariness or threat should be avoided if a child is present.

Threat postures in dogs include wide-legged stances with lowered heads, growling and baring of teeth, pupil dilation and staring, and piloerection. *Dogs who wag their tails are only indicating their willingness to interact: they are not communicating that they are friendly.* People should remember that interactions can be good or bad.

How to React If You Think That the Dog Might Be Aggressive

If one is approached by a worrisome dog, one should:

- Not stare at the dog; instead, look at them obliquely out of the corner of your eye.
- Back up SLOWLY, insuring that you do not trip over anything.
- Keep arms and legs to the side—do not flail arms or make sudden bolting movements.
- Talk calmly and soothingly to the dog in a low voice *if* this seems to calm the dog; if the dog intensifies its growl, clearly this was not a good idea.
- Hold oneself as tall as possible.
- Move as directly as possible to a safe area—inside a building or car, behind a truck, et cetera.
- If the human is holding anything, the object should be moved to the front of her body—if she can do so slowly—so that the object can be used as a shield for protection, should the animal lunge. Allowing the animal to take the

object, rather than a body part, can be a survival strategy.

It is no accident that this same advice is given in wilderness situations for handling the approach of wild carnivores, including mountain lions, bears, and wolves. It is good advice and will help here.

Do not assume that because the dog stands still that you can start to run. You can only run if you can get inside a building in 1 to 2 steps—dogs are that fast. Running will trigger a chase response in a dog, and to run you must turn your back on the dog. *Don't do it.* Dogs have 4 feet on the ground and no matter the size of the dog, she can almost always outrun a human. Dogs almost always can overpower or incapacitate a human if they launch an attack.

Following Up

If you successfully avoid an aggressive dog, you cannot just go on with your life. Once you are away from the dog, call for help and wait until it comes. The dog should be evaluated. It may just be someone's scared pet, but everyone in a community will benefit from the evaluation. If the dog is a lost, scared animal, the owners will need to be educated about the risks to stray dogs and how to more humanely maintain their pet.

Practice the above strategies with children. Please remember that children can understand this intellectually far more easily than they can actually put it into action. *For children to have an appropriate "gut" response, they will either have to be older (>12 years) or have practiced the strategies a lot.* Also teach children that if the dog is jumping for them, they should fall directly and silently to the ground, curl up in a ball, and cover their head with their hands and arms. Kids should be taught to look like armadillos when threatened by advancing dogs. This is also good advice for anyone who accidentally trips during the process of getting away from the dog.

Finally, if the dog makes contact with you, stay calm, stay silent, and *do not get into a tug of war over any of your body parts.* This last piece of advice is difficult to enact, but it is important. In situations involving actual bites from dogs, the majority of the damage is done when a person tries to pull their arm or other body part from the dog's mouth. The dog's innate response is to tighten their hold with their jaws and to shake the victim. These last two behaviors are the prime culprits in profound attacks that result in debility and death. Be calm; once the dog releases her grip, follow the above instructions and try to get away.

If children are grabbed by a dog, *do not* struggle with the dog for the child as the child will be further injured. Instead, look for something to throw over (a blanket) or at (a bucket of water) the dog to get the dog to stop the behavior. Be calm and quiet. Try to distract the dog. If you are successful with this advice the outcome may still be awful, but it will always be a lot worse if you get into a physical contest with the dog.

Known Dogs

Known dogs, in this context, are defined as dogs who are known to have an aggression problem and who may pose a risk to the people who live with them. For information on teaching children appropriate behavior when interacting with dogs who have no behavioral problems, please consider using the Blue Dog interactive DVD and booklet (www.thebluedog.org).

The first step in the treatment of any canine or feline aggression is to avoid *any* circumstances that are known to be associated with aggression. This means that you are responsible for protecting children and unsuspecting friends from your dog.

- If safety requires that the dog be banished when people come to visit, banish the dog. You will feel worse if your dog mauls a child than you will if the dog spends the day in the bedroom.
- If the visiting children are going to run free, the bedroom in which the dog is placed must be locked. The best lock is one that children cannot reach and that acts as a physical reminder to humanely protect the dog behind a locked door. This can be as simple as a hook-and-eye latch or a slip bolt placed at the very top of a door.
- Remember that kids, too, can be unpredictable. You should assume that if your dog has an aggression problem, you cannot take a chance with that aggression and with people whom the dog does not know. Dogs become more reactive when people are excited, and problem dogs, in particular, become more reactive in unfamiliar, noisy circumstances. Who cares if you never find out if the dog would have been good with the children? Minimize the cost of error and blunt your curiosity. A little common sense and a sane, disciplined approach can save a lot of heartbreak. Have an unyielding rule structure for managing and protecting your problem dog. For example, your rule might be, "When there is a child in my house the dog is always behind a locked door, the child is told not to approach the door and is monitored so that they do not do so."

You must protect yourself from your pet's aggressions by learning to give the pet cues that will encourage appropriate behavior. This means that you have to change your behavior in order to change the pet's behavior. Although it is true that you did not cause the pet's problem, you are responsible for managing it, and you are an essential part of fixing it. This means that if you know that your dog is more aggressive when he is allowed to sleep on your bed, the dog is no longer allowed to sleep on the bed unless you can ask the dog to get off the bed and lie down, **and** the dog complies willingly without complaint or threats. If you cannot ask the dog to get off the bed without being threatened, the dog cannot be in the bedroom because he will always be at risk.

If you know that the dog growls every time you groom or pet the dog, you must avoid grooming or petting until the dog can lie down and relax for this. Use of a head collar can hasten this response and render the dog safe. *Under no circumstances must you ever believe that in order to make progress in changing your pet's behavior do you have to put yourself at risk.* This is absolutely wrong.

Please remember that dogs read body language much better than we do and will pick up on any uncertainty. Whether they can smell "fear" is beside the point—aggressive dogs will exhibit aggression in the face of any uncertainty because it is scary for them. Here, it is important to really understand that almost all aggression in dogs and cats is based in underlying anxiety or uncertainty. This is not about winning or losing—it's about understanding the situation and doing as little harm as possible. So many canine aggressive behaviors are about obtaining information from the human about whether the human is a threat. If you hesitate, the dog can view this behavior as one signaling uncertainty or a potential threat and may provoke the situation further either to get additional information or to control you so that you cannot hurt the dog. If this sounds like some kind of strange, reverse logic, that's because it is: *by definition, dogs with aggressive and anxiety disorders are not normal. Expecting them to act as they are will only cause trouble.*

If you cannot be calm, confident, and patient when working with the dog, you will have a low probability of changing the dog's behavior. Each and every time that a dog or cat with a problem behavior exhibits the inappropriate or aggressive behavior, these behaviors are reinforced and become better "learned." Whether the behavior is normal or abnormal, desirable or undesirable, the pet learns how to do the behavior better with exposure, experience, and repetition. There is now excellent molecular evidence to support this pattern, and the fact that by doing so, the basic neurochemistry surrounding the response is also altered. Hence, avoidance is key.

If you do everything right and the dog still threatens you, back off just as is described above for unknown dogs. People who have dogs with *known aggression* problems have an advantage over the situation above, though: You can keep devices like blankets, water pistols, air horns, spray canisters, full seltzer bottles, et cetera near you or in the room where you interact with the dog so you can distract the dog or protect yourself. If you ask the dog to sit, whether part of a behavior modification program or not, and the dog begins to growl or otherwise become aggressive, you should gently try to get the dog to relax using verbal request. If this does not work, release the dog without a reward and slowly back away. It is far better to ignore the dog than to struggle to "win" or "dominate" the dog. You will succeed at doing neither.

If you are consistent, the dog will ultimately approach and be willing to exhibit deferential behaviors in exchange for a request. In extreme cases, this can take days. The dog has to learn that (a) no harm will come to him—that you are not a threat, (b) that you are consistent in providing information that you are nonthreatening when threatened, and (c) that if the dog exhibits appropriate and deferential behavior, such behaviors will be rewarded.

If the dog continues to threaten you and avoidance does not elicit deference, leave the dog alone in an enclosed area. Sometimes just letting the dog into the backyard can interrupt the aggression. It's perfectly acceptable to keep the dog behind a barrier for as long as is necessary for the dog to calm. This time may also help you to acknowledge and set aside feelings of hurt, fear, mistrust, and anger. Your dog has a problem and cannot be held to some of these standards.

If you are determined that the dog will get as well as he can, understanding that you might never have a "normal" dog, the dog will improve. This isn't magic: People who understand how abnormal and distressed the dog is have unconsciously vowed to protect themselves from the dog and the dog from popular opinion, and have made the decision to find a rule structure that will help the dog improve to the extent possible.

If your dog bites you, **freeze** and do not struggle with the dog—you will lose. Go limp, look away, become small and quiet, and slowly retreat at the first opportunity. Most severe damage is done as humans try to pull away from dogs that are biting. Most dogs do not repeatedly bite.

Remember that the term "bite" is usually poorly to un-defined. Dogs do not have hands and opposable thumbs. They cannot hold you to stop you with anything other than their teeth. Humans should not be complicit in making any injury worse than it needs to be.

It is normal to feel anger and a sense of disappointment and betrayal, but dogs with aggression problems cannot respond rationally to those feelings. Leave the dog alone to be quiet. Do not punish the dog physically no matter how angry or hurt you are—this will only make things worse. Get any required medical care, and then calmly approach the dog again using the deference and relaxation measures that the dog has been taught.

If you are either too fearful or hurt to do this, or you no longer want to work with the dog after such an event, the prognosis is poor. The vast majority of dogs can improve but there are not as many "special needs" homes as there are "special needs dogs." Please do not make any decision to relinquish the dog just after there has been a bite. Instead, if you are uncertain as to whether you can keep the dog, board the dog for a few days to see what it is like to be without the dog. Quarantine for bites—even for rabies vaccinated dogs—is 10 days. This is adequate time to observe the dog's behaviors and your feelings and capabilities, and to decide if the dog can humanely improve in your home. Interestingly, most dogs can improve, and the amount of improvement that they can experience is limited only by our understanding, ability to protect them, and investment of time and effort.

Poor prognosticators, however, include the following:
- people who want to blame the dog,
- people who have an idealized version of the dog and expect that the dog "should" behave in a specific manner,
- people who cannot or will not take the precautions recommended above or who cannot or will not learn to read the dog's signals,
- people with lots of other stressors in their life—these dogs can be, but don't have to be strains on marriages and family relationships,
- people who are caught in a cycle of anger and fighting within the family that always seems to revolve around the dog and the dog's behavior,
- people who have ill-behaved or unsupervised or unsupervisable young children,
- people who have a family member who wants the dog dead or out of the house,
- people who live in very reactive, unpredictable households and environments, and
- people who have seriously considered putting down the dog and entertain this thought in most or all discussions involving the dog.

Notice that all of these factors involve the people. One of the remarkable findings of an analysis of more than a decade of cases involving canine aggression is that no matter how awful the dog was, if the people were committed to helping the dog become less distressed, the dog improved. Furthermore, the single best indicator that the dog would be put down was that the people had seriously considered it. Dogs don't get a vote here, and these findings should give pause to everyone concerned about the well-being of dogs and the safety of their humans.

Finally, anyone who has dogs in the United States should keep a copy of their rabies certificate in a safe place. If your dog bites someone, the tag on his collar is not sufficient legal proof of definitive vaccination. That tag is important, and your dog should wear one, but it only indicates the year in which the vaccine was given. This year is imprinted on the tag, and the tags are encoded by color and shape for year, should the engraving become illegible. Different states/jurisdictions have different rules for age at first vaccination and frequency of vaccination. Additionally, there are annual and triennial vaccines. The reason the tag is not sufficient, should there be a problem, is that no one can tell if the dog had a 1- or a 3-year vaccine, and when in the calendar year that vaccine was given. This is why the certificate, which is dated and specifies the type of vaccine, is so important. The veterinarian who vaccinated your pet will almost always keep a copy of the certificate, but yours should be kept someplace safe, where you can find it if you need it. Some of the newer electronic tags will allow you to include this information, but it may still have to be verified by your vet. If you have a dog who is aggressive for any reason—even if she exhibits aggressive behavior only when protecting your house and you think this is normal and acceptable—you may wish to make a copy of the certificate and keep it at your office, while leaving the original at home.

In addition to the problem surrounding proof of rabies, anyone with a problematic pet (and actually anyone with a dog) needs to review her insurance coverage at least annually. Umbrella or catastrophic policies can be added to most home owners' or other coverage plans at a very low price if nothing disastrous has happened. If something disastrous should happen (e.g., your dog bites and injures someone, whether the bite was appropriate or not), these plans can preserve your financial security, and can act as a buffer so that your home owners' insurance is not canceled.

Liability and legal issues are awkward to consider, but important. Treatment is not a guarantee that a dog will not bite, but what is learned by both parties in the course of treatment can humanely minimize risk for everyone.

TIER 2: PROTOCOL FOR TEACHING YOUR DOG TO UNCOUPLE CUES ABOUT YOUR DEPARTURES FROM THE DEPARTURE

Why You Should *Not* Use This Protocol

This protocol should not be attempted unless you are extremely able to read your dog's signals and can ensure that you are only rewarding relaxed behaviors. If this is not the case, the risk with this protocol is that you will make your dog much, much worse, and sensitize her to all behaviors that are associated with leaving her alone.

How to Use This Protocol If You Think It Will Help

There are two components to *beginning* to teach dogs not to react anxiously when you leave them.

1. The first component involves resisting the normal tendency to reassure an unhappy dog, and instead, asking her to sit and to be calm (see the **Protocol for Deference** and the **Protocol for Relaxation: Tier 1**).
2. The second component involves teaching the dog to relax upon request **(Protocol for Teaching Your Dog to Take a Deep Breath and Use Other Biofeedback Methods as Part of Relaxation)** so that you can reward her for being calm while she gradually learns to be left alone (see the **Protocol for Separation Anxiety** and **Tier 2: Protocol for Desensitization and Counter-Conditioning Using Gradual Departures**).

Dogs who become distressed after you have left probably become distressed before you leave. You need to be alert for the behavioral cues that distress is occurring—panting, pacing, whining, digging, trembling, not eating, et cetera—and ensure that you do not inadvertently reward such cues by telling your dog that she is "okay," when she is clearly distressed. She knows she is not okay. In truth, you are only rewarding and reinforcing your dog for being anxious.

Using Triggers for Anxious Behaviors

If you wish to reverse this trend, you *may* be able to focus on triggers for your dog's anxious behaviors.

- Before your dog becomes distressed, make sure you reward her calm behaviors. Talk happily to her; massage her; if offered, rub her belly and chest very slowly. If you cannot do this without your dog panting or moving around, she was already distressed when you started. You cannot desensitize dogs to triggers or cues of their distress if you do not know what those triggers or cues are. *If your dog is already upset when you awaken, desensitizing her to "departure cues" may actually sensitize her to cues that signal your departure is approaching.*
- If you can interact in a truly calm way with your dog on a day when you know you will later leave, you may be able to teach her that she can divorce the cues or signals you give when you are about to leave from her anxiety at your departure.
- Make a list of all of the things that you do differently on days when you leave compared with days when you stay home. If setting the alarm is something that you only do on days that you leave, this may be the most important clue to the dog. This is a problem. Although you can

desensitize your dog to an alarm, the process will be complicated because the dog has an ongoing and prolonged state of arousal. Your best chance at intervening in this type of arousal is with medication.

- If you notice that your dog reacts *only* to other very timely signals—briefcases, keys, gym bags, certain items of clothing—start to go through the same routine that you use when leaving, but then sit down and watch television, read a book, or throw a toy for your dog. If you always go to the health club with a gym bag, pick up your gym bag and go make dinner. If you only wear high heels and makeup when you go to work, wear them, instead, on a Sunday, and spend the day by the fire reading the newspaper. You get the idea.
- All dogs are different. Some dogs only react when the keys are picked up, others only when the car is started, some because of the hour at which their people awake when going to work, and still others because of the presence of absence of a meal or a type of food. These are typical examples; your dog may respond to something different.
- Whatever specific event triggers anxiety in your dog needs to be uncoupled from your actual departure. If your dog becomes more relaxed when you practice uncoupling a cue, *reward her with praise and treats.* This is exactly what you want. However, if you do not think the dog is relaxing, or if you think that her anxiety is increasing, *please stop trying to desensitize her to departure cues.* You will be able to tell if you are making your dog worse or better by videotaping yourself working with your dog and watching her responses.
- The more lead time between the dog's first arousal cue and your departure, the more difficult teaching your dog to uncouple cues will be.
- You may also wish to use this program in reverse: uncouple the cues that you are staying home from staying home. For example, if you only eat breakfast on weekends when you stay home, start eating breakfast on weekdays. If you only wear jogging clothes on weekends, wear them to work and change there. Again, caution is urged. If your dog now starts to react to your jogging clothes or preparation of breakfast no matter what the day is, *please stop trying to desensitize her with departure cues.* You are making her more anxious.

Roles for Safety Cues

You may be able to condition your dog to relax when a safety signal is present. This tells the dog that something may happen, but because she recognizes the cue, she can and will be able to relax as practiced. Safety cues will likely help only mildly affected dogs, but they are worth practicing. As an example, you play a specific, easily recognizable piece of music, while practicing relaxation and breathing with your dog. Your dog learns that the music signals that she can now display the relaxed feeling taught by the relaxation and breathing exercises. You can then use this piece of music to help to teach the dog to relax when you are leaving (or, by remote control, when you are not there).

The anxiety induced by the specific event that your dog associates with your departure is often a self-fulfilling prophecy. If the dog can be taught not to become anxious in the first place, whether through use of medication or a safety cue, she can learn not to be anxious when you are gone. Please remember that what we know about anxiety indicates that it is a cascade phenomenon: Once you get upset, it is easier to become more upset, more quickly.

What Other Choices Do You Have?

If your dog worsens when you scramble cues and routines, please stop doing so. Talk to your veterinarian and consider doggie daycare, at home care, taking the pet with you to work when possible, et cetera. Meanwhile, continue to work with the active behavior modification protocols while your dog is taking medication. If your dog needs this protocol, you can return to it later, when she is better able to learn from it. With long-term medication and other work, you may learn that your dog figures out for herself that she doesn't have to worry about cues associated with leaving because she now can think more rationally about everything. If so, this is terrific!

Anti-anxiety medications may be essential for some dogs affected by separation anxiety, but please remember that medication is to be used **in addition** to the behavior modification, not instead of it.

TIER 2: PROTOCOL FOR DESENSITIZING AND COUNTER-CONDITIONING A DOG OR CAT FROM APPROACHES FROM UNFAMILIAR ANIMALS, INCLUDING HUMANS

This protocol is written primarily for dogs, but clever clients can adapt it for cats. It is intended to be started *after* the **Protocol for Deference,** the **Protocol for Teaching Your Dog to Take a Deep Breath and Use Other Biofeedback Methods as Part of Relaxation,** and the **Protocol for Relaxation: Behavior Modification Tier 1** have been successfully completed.

This protocol is intended to help animals who respond inappropriately (with uncertainty, fearfully, aggressively, or fearfully aggressively) to strange animals, primarily dogs, or people. The successful and useful execution of this protocol requires the cooperation of several people and, sometimes, another dog or cat. If your dog's problem involves other dogs, a second dog will be required. If your dog is very aggressive toward or fearful of other dogs, the first dog who works with your dog should be one to whom your dog is accustomed, and with whom he is comfortable or, at least, to whom he does not respond or react. Later, another dog, generally one not a member of the household and who will likely provoke the response we are seeking to treat, will be required.

It is best to set practice of these tasks in a T-shaped hallway. If you do not have a T-shaped hallway, your dog can be placed in a room off a hall, a few meters away from the door or entryway. The point of this physical restriction is to allow the dog, by using his peripheral vision, to see a stranger (the "approacher") for only a brief moment, at first. A momentary glimpse will generally not provoke the dog and so will lessen the dog's anxiety, allowing the desensitization techniques emphasized in **Tier 1** to be used.

Starting This Protocol

Ask the dog to sit and stay, or to lie down and stay, if this is more relaxing for the dog. Reward the dog for sitting or lying down, being calm and attending to you. Position the dog either in another room or in the stem of the T-shaped hallway. The dog should face the hallway where the person or dog will approach. The greater the distance between the dog and the door, the less the dog will be able to see of the approaching stranger, and the more "momentary" will be any glimpse of this person or dog. *See the accompanying illustration for an example of how to position everyone involved.*

Remember that with desensitization techniques we wish to teach dogs that they will be rewarded if they do not react to the person or animal approaching them. If we start at a level below that at which they will react, we can gradually work up to more challenging interactions.

If your dog is extremely anxious, move him away from the door/hallway and the person or dog acting as the "approacher." In this way, the "approacher" is within your dog's visual field for only a second or two, allowing you to reward him for not reacting. When you are sure that your dog can repeatedly look to you as the "approacher" passes, and truly relax (see the **Protocol for Teaching Your Dog to Take a Deep Breath and Use Other Biofeedback Methods as Part of Relaxation**), knowing that the "approacher" has passed, you can gradually move your dog closer to the door or hall. By moving your dog closer you expand his field of vision and allow him to have a longer period of exposure to the person or animal to whom he reacts.

Make sure that what you are rewarding is the dog remaining relaxed and being attentive to you. This is very different from just rewarding sitting.

As the "approacher" passes, your dog is permitted to quickly glance at him ("Look at that (LAT)" or some variant), but should not react inappropriately or anxiously by putting his hair up, whining, growling, barking, trembling, salivating, or looking distressed. **At all times the dog should look calm and relaxed.**

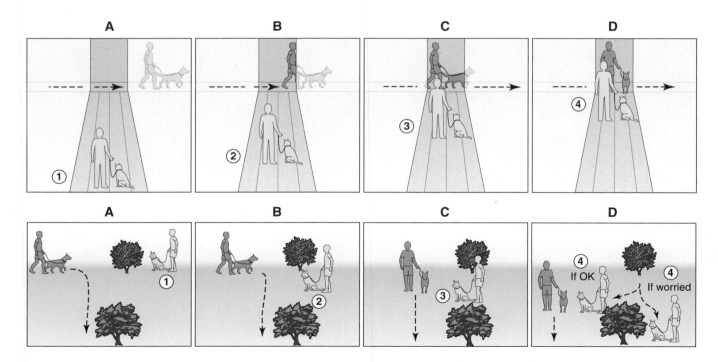

By asking your dog to take a deep breath and relax you will be able to monitor whether the "approacher" was too stimulating and provocative for the dog.

If your dog looks at the "approacher" for more than a moment, as soon as you say your dog's name (in a happy, upbeat voice), he should be able to look at you and relax. If he stares at the "approacher"—whether or not the "approacher" is visible—your dog may be concerned.

Things to Remember

Remember that a tone of voice that conveys that you are worried for the dog or angry that he is not instantaneously responding will increase the dog's anxiety. If you use these exercises in the gradual manner intended, your dog will eventually respond instantaneously to your request and look at you first to learn if the "approacher" is a threat. No distressed dog can do all of this at once in the beginning.

Remember that your dog must look at your face and eyes, not at the food rewards. Once your dog doesn't react at all you can make the rewards intermittent, but at the outset you will need to reward him every time he looks at you, and then periodically for not reacting.

Practice your timing so that you can deliver the rewards quickly. Ensure that you use your voice to praise him for good behavior as soon as you know that he may have reason to react but did not do so. To do this you will need to anticipate when the "approacher" will cross your dog's visual field, so communication with the people helping you is important.

Be very quick with the food rewards: As soon as the dog responds to your vocal request, reward him. *The potentially anxiety-provoking event—the movement of the "approacher"—should be timed to coincide with and take place during the reward phase of the exercise if you hope to benefit from the counter-conditioning aspects of this program.* Counter-conditioning programs require rewards for a behavior incompatible with that previously exhibited.

Varying the Tasks

If your dog continues to not react as exposure increases, vary the tasks by having the "approacher" come toward your dog from the side, and then, finally, from the back. Approaches from the back will cause more dogs to react than approaches from the front, so they are best left until your dog is really good at these exercises.

If cooperative strangers are not available, or if you want more practice, these exercises can be performed in shopping centers, parks, or other busy places using fortuitous strangers. Please remember to behave responsibly. You can only take advantage of these fortuitous, natural-setting situations if, **and only if, you have good control over your dog's head and he does not pose a risk to any dog or human.**

For dogs who need more help, a head collar can help you to remind your dog to look at you. Additionally, head collars and no-pull harnesses will prevent the dog from bolting if he becomes scared.

Special Hints for Dogs Who React to Other Dogs

This protocol and these exercises can be used for dogs who have problems with humans or with dogs. If you are using these exercises to help your dog learn not to react to dogs, you can make some changes that will help your dog.

- The person handling the "approacher dog" may or may not be known to your dog. If your dog worries a lot, using a known person may help.
- The "approacher dog" will always be accompanied by a human. If you start these exercises with the "approacher dog" on the far side of the human partnered with him, your dog will see that there is a human buffer between him and the "approacher dog." This may help calm him.
- After you and your dog have completed all the tasks with the "approacher dog" on the far side of your dog, repeat all of them with the dog on the near side to your dog.

If an unfamiliar dog is unavailable, you can first use another dog of your own, or use dogs who are behind fences or in the park, leashed. Please remember that other unknown dogs may have problems, too, and you need to not only protect other dogs from your dog, but you want to protect your dog from them. This is often not easy to do if any of the other dogs run free. Use sound judgment and err on the side of caution.

If your dog has problems only with a particular dog, or a particular class of dogs, start with a dog or class of dogs with which there is no problem and then, gradually, begin to use the problem dog. You may need to do so intermittently at first.

Final Considerations for Success

You will need the cooperation of lots of other people and dogs to be able to succeed in this protocol. You can get this cooperation by being cautious and ensuring that your dog can injure no one. Head halters can speed the rate at which the dogs can learn these exercises because they help to turn the dog's head before he becomes fully engaged in the upsetting behavior. This early interruption can prevent a cascade phenomenon of inappropriate behavior that can be hurtful to your dog's learning process. Head collars also provide an extra degree of protection for the "approacher dog," too, and should be used for both dogs in all circumstances where the problems exist between the dogs.

If you cannot find appropriate strangers (dogs or people) with which to practice the approaches, see if your veterinarian can arrange staged approaches at her practice, or if a trainer in your area is certified and trained to use these protocols. Trainers often have access to large spaces where staged encounters can occur. If you start to use these exercises under extremely controlled circumstances (e.g., your vet's office), you will eventually need to practice under less-controlled circumstances.

Every time you add a layer of complexity, please remember that at each step you are rewarding your dog for relaxing and being happy and confident while he does not react. You must ensure you do not reward a reactive dog who is sitting still.

If you have difficulty with any of the following tasks, break them down into simpler, smaller, more manageable tasks. Your dog's behavior will tell you what he can manage. *Do not make your dog more fearful. It is better to work for three 5-minute periods that your dog enjoys than for one 15-minute period where your dog becomes distressed.*

What We Hope to Accomplish

The intent of this program is to teach the dog that someone can walk quickly up to him, touch him while making noise, and keep going, without causing your dog distress.

If the problem is with another dog, the intent is to teach your dog that another dog can pause in front of him, sniff, and then pass without ensuing problems.

Will Medication Be Helpful?

Antianxiety medications may help some dogs who otherwise are not able to succeed in this program. Please remember that if it's decided that medication could benefit your dog, you need to use it **in addition** to the behavior modification, not instead of it.

Task Sheet Instructions

These tasks are meant to give you guidance only. They are designed to use very, very, very gradual changes. Such tiny steps allow you to reward aspects of the behaviors that are good, without accidentally rewarding aspects of behavior that are not so good.

Built into these programs are the concepts of desensitization (DS), where you teach the dog not to react to some situation by exposing him to the situation at a level below that needed to have him react and become distressed, and counterconditioning (CC), where you reward behaviors that are in direct opposition or contrast to those that are undesirable.

If you open any applied psychology text or article on learning, you will see similar programs. There is nothing magic or novel or original here; these tasks are those that are common to most dog and cat training and behavior modification programs, and you will see similar task sheets in a number of books, articles, and online sources.

Pease remember that what *is different here* is that you are rewarding the physical signs that the dog is less distressed or worried. You are rewarding *only* relaxed behaviors (review the **Protocol for Teaching Your Dog to Take a Deep Breath and Use Other Biofeedback Methods as Part of Relaxation**).

The tasks involve only common situations in which your dog may respond inappropriately or undesirably. Some of these situations may not be relevant to you, and others that are relevant may be missing. Please feel free to customize or alter this program, but please do so using the pattern of approach used here (i.e., gradually work up to the task, frequent returns to something easier, always ending on a good note, et cetera).

The task is listed on the left. There is space for you to make comments about how easy or hard the task was for the dog, how many times it had to be repeated, or other questionable behaviors that appeared during the task. You should discuss these with your veterinarian at your re-exam appointment.

Try grouping these tasks into segments that you work through in *no more than 15 minutes*. Shorter, calmer sessions will help the dog to better consolidate memory and learning.

If your dog is learning to approach another animal, they need not sniff or touch, but your dog should be able to stand there for 15-30 seconds and remain calm. This exercise has a real-life application since such scenarios are common when dogs receive veterinary care.

Dog's Task
The dog sits, stays, and relaxes when:
- An "approacher" passes quietly and quickly past the door or hall opening through which the dog can see

- An "approacher" passes quietly and at a moderate pace past the door or hall opening
- An "approacher" passes at a low pace past the door or hall opening and makes a slight noise (i.e., scuffing of feet)
- An "approacher" passes at a slow pace past the door or hall opening, making slightly more noise (i.e., the jangling of keys)
- An "approacher" passes the door or hall opening quickly and quietly
- An "approacher" passes the door or hall opening moderately quickly and quietly
- An "approacher" passes the door or hall opening slowly and making a slight noise
- An "approacher" passes the door or hall opening slowly and making more noise
- An "approacher" passes the door or hall opening quickly and quietly, veering toward the dog at the opening
- An "approacher" passes the door or hall opening moderately quickly and quietly, veering toward the dog at the opening
- An "approacher" passes the door or hall opening slowly and quietly, veering toward the dog at the opening
- An "approacher" passes the door or hall opening slowly, making a slight noise, veering toward the dog at the opening
- An "approacher" passes the door or hall opening quietly, veering toward the dog at the opening and pausing momentarily in the doorway
- An "approacher" passes the door or hall opening quietly, taking one very tiny step into the doorway and momentarily pausing
- An "approacher" passes the door or hall opening quietly, taking one brief step into the doorway, and pauses briefly, glancing at the dog
- An "approacher" takes 2 steps into the doorway or opening
- An "approacher" takes 2 steps into the doorway or opening and pauses briefly
- An "approacher" takes 2 steps into the doorway or opening, pauses briefly, and glances at the dog
- An "approacher" takes 3 steps into the doorway or opening
- An "approacher" takes 3 steps into the doorway or opening and pauses briefly
- An "approacher" takes 3 steps into the doorway or opening, pauses briefly, and glances at the dog
- An "approacher" walks quickly and quietly through the doorway and passes the dog
- An "approacher" walks quickly and quietly past the dog, and reaches slightly toward the dog
- An "approacher" walks quickly and quietly past the dog, and briefly reaches slightly closer to the dog
- An "approacher" walks quickly and quietly past the dog, briefly reaching slightly toward the dog
- An "approacher" walks moderately quickly past the dog, briefly reaching slightly more toward the dog
- An "approacher" walks slowly past the dog
- An "approacher" walks slowly, briefly reaching toward the dog
- An "approacher" walks slowly, briefly reaching slightly closer to the dog
- An "approacher" walks slowly, pausing briefly next to the dog
- An "approacher" walks slowly, pausing briefly next to the dog and glancing at him

- An "approacher" briefly pauses next to the dog, glances at him, and reaches slightly toward the dog
- An "approacher" briefly pauses, glances, and reaches slightly more toward the dog
- An "approacher" pauses and looks at the dog (DO NOT STARE) for 5 seconds
- An "approacher" pauses and looks at the dog (DO NOT STARE) for 10 seconds
- An "approacher" pauses and looks at the dog (DO NOT STARE) for 20 seconds
- An "approacher" pauses and looks at the dog (DO NOT STARE) for 30 seconds
- An "approacher" pauses and looks at the dog (DO NOT STARE) for 45 seconds
- An "approacher" pauses and looks at the dog (DO NOT STARE) for 1 minute
- An "approacher" pauses next to the dog for 1 minute, then reaches slightly toward the dog

- An "approacher" pauses for 1 minute, reaches closer to the dog, and almost touches the dog
- An "approacher" pauses for 1 minute, reaches closer to the dog, and touches the dog
- An "approacher" pauses for 1 minute, reaches down, and pets the dog

For Future Repetitions

- Repeat all tasks in different locations.
- Repeat all tasks with all family members.
- Repeat all tasks with only every second or third being rewarded with a treat. (Remember praise!)
- Repeat with only intermittent treat reinforcement. (Remember praise!)

TIER 2: PROTOCOL FOR DESENSITIZATION AND COUNTER-CONDITIONING USING GRADUAL DEPARTURES

Dogs with separation anxiety often begin to experience distress at the first indication that you will be leaving the dog's sight. The first set of protocols concentrated on reinforcing general relaxation and responsiveness to your vocal cues (see **Protocol for Deference, Protocol for Relaxation: Behavior Modification Tier 1** and **Protocol for Teaching Your Dog to Take a Deep Breath and Use Other Biofeedback Methods as Part of Relaxation**). For some dogs who are overly concerned about departure patterns, you may have practiced uncoupling cues for departure from the actual event. Remember that done too quickly or inappropriately, the latter may make dogs more anxious. This Tier 2 program concentrates on desensitizing and counter-conditioning the dog to actually being left alone for gradually longer periods, by teaching the dog that he can be calmer and will feel better when he does not become distressed. Ultimately, we want your dog to learn that he has some control over how he feels, and that distress need not be the only choice.

It is not sufficient that your dog does not bark or destroy something when left alone. The goal of this program is to reinforce relaxation and behaviors associated with actually feeling calm when left alone (i.e., happy looks, lowered heart rates, and slowed respiration). Once again, go slowly. It is particularly important that dogs with separation anxiety do not become stressed or made more anxious during this protocol. Speed is not a measure of success—behavior is. Remember to shape the dog's behavior by rewarding even the smallest, incremental hint that the dog is more relaxed than previously.

If at any time you notice outward physical and physiological signs that your dog is becoming anxious while working—panting, pacing, salivating, licking of the lips, scanning the environment, an unwillingness to sit still—break the suite of tasks on which you were working into smaller components. And give the dog a break from working. Research now shows that dogs consolidate and use more of what they have learned if they have some time off. So if you are having trouble working well with your dog one day, consider it a holiday and start again the following day. If, however, you continue to have difficulty, consider returning to your vet or veterinary behaviorist for additional help and suggestions.

Remember that outward physical and physiological signs of stress or anxiety are very variable and can also include an increased heart rate, lowered head with ears retracted, lips pulled back horizontally, dilated pupils, "redder" eyes with or without movement, shaking or shivering, whimpering or whining, and blowing in and out of "cheeks." If you see any of these signs, your dog is too distressed to effectively learn to change its behavior. Backtrack and return to a level at which your dog does not react inappropriately and can respond happily. Break the tasks with which he had difficulty into smaller components. All of the following tasks can be broken into smaller components. If you have trouble getting the dog through even smaller task lists, make sure you are continuing to reinforce the deep breathing. If doing this still does not help, you may be trying to move through all of this too quickly and might benefit from additional help from your vet, trainer, or veterinary behaviorist.

Everyone in the family who is involved with your dog must be able to successfully complete the program, so that the dog does learn to worry only about one person's absences, and so he can learn to generalize a relaxed response to being left.

When the program is completed in one physical location where your dog was able to remain, you are ready to start working with the dog in other locations: other rooms, indoors or outside, inside or outside a fence, et cetera.

Remember to use your dog's behavior to help you decide how to adapt the protocol for your dog's specific needs. If your dog is perfectly calm when left in a car but is distressed when someone leaves, start by practicing the tasks in the car. If the dog is calm when all but one person leaves the house but panics when that person leaves, start by practicing with departures involving people for whom your dog does not panic, working up to the person about whom the dog most worries. If your dog appears to keep a good calendar and does not become distressed when people leave on weekends, start by practicing the tasks in the protocol repeatedly on weekends.

Remember to shape your dog's behavior by rewarding even the smallest signal that it is more relaxed with each succeeding task. Be patient. Do not become angry. Do not punish the dog. Stop and return later if you are feeling stressed.

Note: As usual, for the following tasks always remember to physically return to the dog and stand in front of him so that you can give the reward after completing the task without accidentally encouraging the dog to get up and possibly become reactive.

Day 1: Dog's Task

- Sit quietly and calmly for 5 seconds
- Sit quietly and calmly for 10 seconds
- Sit quietly and calmly for 20 seconds
- Sit quietly and calmly while you take one step back
- Sit quietly and calmly while you take two steps back
- Sit quietly and calmly while you take one step to the side
- Sit quietly and calmly while you take two steps to the side
- Sit quietly and calmly while you take three steps back
- Sit quietly and calmly while you take three steps to the side
- Sit quietly and calmly while you walk around the dog
- Sit quietly and calmly while you take 10 steps backward and return
- Sit quietly and calmly while you go through the door or the entranceway and return
- Sit quietly and calmly while you open the door or go into the entrance for 10 seconds and return
- Sit quietly and calmly while you take one step to the side
- Sit quietly and calmly while you take two steps to the side
- Sit quietly and calmly while you take three steps back
- Sit quietly and calmly while you take three steps to the side
- Sit quietly and calmly while you walk around the dog

Day 2: Dog's Task

- Sit quietly and calmly for 20 seconds
- Sit quietly and calmly while you take 10 steps backward and return

- Sit quietly and calmly while you go through the door or the entranceway and return
- Sit quietly and calmly while you open the door or go into the entrance for 10 seconds and return
- Sit quietly and calmly for 30 seconds
- Sit quietly and calmly while you disappear from view for 5 seconds and return
- Sit quietly and calmly while you go through the door or the entranceway and return
- Sit quietly and calmly while you touch a doorknob
- Sit quietly and calmly while you rattle a doorknob
- Sit quietly and calmly while you turn the doorknob, but do not open the door
- Sit quietly and calmly while you touch a doorknob
- Sit quietly and calmly while you rattle a doorknob
- Sit quietly and calmly while you turn the doorknob, but do not open the door
- Sit quietly and calmly while you open the door a few centimeters and quickly close it
- Sit quietly and calmly while you open the door 0.25 meters (10 inches) and then close it
- Sit quietly and calmly while you open the door 0.5 meters (20 inches) and then close it
- Sit quietly and calmly while you walk back 10 steps
- Sit quietly and calmly while you rattle the doorknob
- Sit quietly and calmly while you open the door 0.5 meter (20 inches) and then close it
- Sit quietly and calmly while you open the door 1 meter (3.3 feet) and then close it
- Sit quietly and calmly while you step into the door but remain in view

Day 3: Dog's Task

- Sit quietly and calmly while you turn the doorknob, but do not open the door
- Sit quietly and calmly while you open the door a few centimeters and quickly close it
- Sit quietly and calmly while you open the door 0.5 meter (20 inches) and then close it
- Sit quietly and calmly while you open the door 1 meter (3.3 feet) and then close it
- Sit quietly and calmly while you step into the door but remain in view
- Sit quietly and calmly while you step into the doorway
- Sit quietly and calmly while you step through the doorway
- Sit quietly and calmly while you step through the doorway, close the door just slightly, and immediately return
- Sit quietly and calmly while you step through the doorway, close the door, wait 5 seconds, and return
- Sit quietly and calmly while you disappear from view for 10 seconds and return
- Sit quietly and calmly while you disappear from view for 15 seconds and return
- Sit quietly and calmly for 10 seconds
- Sit quietly and calmly for 15 seconds
- Sit quietly and calmly while you disappear from view for 15 seconds and return

- Sit quietly and calmly while you step through the doorway, close the door, wait 10 seconds, and return
- Sit quietly and calmly while you step through the doorway, close the door, wait 20 seconds, and return
- Sit quietly and calmly while you go out of the door and firmly close it
- Sit quietly and calmly for 20 seconds
- Sit quietly and calmly for 10 seconds
- Sit for 5 seconds

Day 4: Dog's Task

- Sit quietly and calmly for 10 seconds
- Sit quietly and calmly while you go out of the door and close it:
  - And wait 5 seconds
  - And wait 30 seconds
  - And wait 45 seconds
  - And wait 90 seconds
  - And wait 2 minutes
- Sit quietly and calmly while you go out of the door and close it:
  - And wait 3 minutes
  - And wait 4 minutes
  - And wait 5 minutes
  - And wait 7 minutes
  - And wait 10 minutes

Continue as above until your dog can sit quietly and relaxed while left alone for 30 minutes. If you video your dog when you are gone, you will have an objective assessment of whether the dog is improving. You can also monitor your dog from work using a webcam. All of these tools will make you more effective at helping your dog.

Generally, if a dog can be relaxed while left alone for 30 minutes, he will be able to relax when left alone for normal durations, prohibiting any startling or disastrous consequences. "Startling or disastrous consequences" can include storms for some dogs. *If your dog is afraid of storms and one occurs while your dog is left alone, relapse is possible.* Treat *all* of your dog's problems. Remember that anxious dogs have co-morbid conditions, meaning that, unless your dog's condition was diagnosed early in its development, he may have multiple conditions and all of them need to be treated.

If you let your dog's behavior be your guide, you will seldom go wrong!

For Future Repetitions

- Repeat all tasks in different locations.
- Repeat all tasks with all family members.
- Repeat all tasks with only every second or third task being rewarded with a treat. (Remember praise!)
- Repeat with only intermittent treat reinforcement. (Remember praise!)

Anti-anxiety medications may help some dogs who are otherwise unable to succeed in this program. Remember, if it is decided that medication could benefit your dog, you need to use *it in addition to the behavior modification, not instead of it.*

TIER 2: PROTOCOL FOR DESENSITIZATION AND COUNTER-CONDITIONING TO NOISES AND ACTIVITIES THAT OCCUR BY THE DOOR

Some dogs who cannot be left alone become anxious whenever any activity occurs by doors. Some dogs who are fearfully aggressive, or who are protectively or territorially aggressive, react whenever anyone comes to a door and rings the bell or knocks.

Because the reaction level at the door is a key component for the dog's increasing anxieties, you may need to work separately on desensitizing and counter-conditioning the dogs to noises and activities around the door. This protocol is designed to help you teach your dog to not react and, instead, to relax and be calm in such circumstances. As with the other protocols, it is expected that you have completed **Protocol for Deference** and **Protocol for Relaxation: Behavior Modification Tier 1.** You may benefit from using this protocol to help with the last part of **Tier 1.**

When working with this protocol you can place your dog in the middle of the room with his side facing the door. This will allow him to use peripheral vision, but will not direct him to focus all of his attention on the door. It is best to have two people to practice this protocol: one person acts as the "rewarder," and one acts as the "stranger." At the first pass, it is best if the stranger is a person with whom the dog is comfortable.

Remember that the point of this protocol is to teach the dog to relax, when given a cue to do so, despite someone being at the door. Some people prefer that the dog be permitted to give one or two barks as a warning before they are quiet. This may be possible, but it will depend on the dog. For some dogs, barking even twice can send them into a cascade of behavior that is undesirable and inappropriate.

Please remember, as with the Tier 1 behavior modification program, *it is not sufficient that your dog is sitting or lying quietly—he must not be showing any of the physical signs of underlying physiological stress (shaking, trembling, panting, salivating, increased heart rate, averted gaze and frequent eye movements, et cetera).* Relaxed animals can learn more easily and animals who enjoy the tasks learn faster. Experiencing true distress-reinforced fearful and associated reactive behaviors actively blocks the learning of the new behaviors you wish your dog to substitute for these.

When your dog is sitting or lying down and relaxed, give instructions to the stranger to begin to knock softly and briefly (see Task List below). You will want to review the plan with the stranger *before* you practice with the dog, so that you and the stranger can communicate without confusion. This will help prevent anxiety in your dog. You may find that the use of cell phones with ear pieces can help, but you will have to resist the tendency to talk more than minimally, because this will distract the dog, and your stranger will also have to keep talk to a minimum so that she is not a distraction for you.

As soon as you hear or anticipate that you will hear the knock, ask your dog to look at you. As soon as he looks at you, say "Good boy!" and reward him with a treat. If your dog glances quickly at the door, but otherwise does not appear to be upset, and either spontaneously returns his gaze to you, or responds immediately to a soft reminder signal from you (clicking your tongue, clearing your throat, softly saying your dog's name), reward your dog immediately.

If, instead, your dog reacts or stares at the door, call him to you, and move further away from the door so that he is not so close to the sound of the knocking. Then repeat the exercise by having the stranger knock more softly. If these changes do not help and your dog continues to react, remove him from the room, practice some tasks from **Tier 1** when the dog is calm enough to successfully do so, and start over at a softer level of knock, with even more distance between the dog and the door.

A head collar or no-pull harness may help if your dog is quickly reactive. If you can use a head collar you can hold the lead taut but not tight and as soon as your dog begins to bark, you can gently guide his head away from the door. This action may interrupt his behavioral sequence sufficiently for him to not experience the full arousal cascade. Dogs who cannot wear head collars can be turned by and get a tactile signal from a well-fitted harness. If you have worked to teach your dog that his response to the shift in the harness should be to look at you, a harness can work as well as a head collar. By gently turning your dog's head toward you and then immediately rewarding the dog for looking at you, you encourage your dog to look to you for cues about the expected behavior while also encouraging him to ignore the door.

Finally, if you have to remove your dog from the room, it's best if you can do so using a verbal request. Grabbing and dragging the dog from the door will teach the dog to avoid you. If your dog will not respond to a verbal request to come once he is upset, you will need a head collar to kindly and gently lead the dog toward a more appropriate behavior. If he is still upset and pulls on the head collar, you are not ready for this tier of the behavior modification. Go back and work on Tier 1 or break the earliest steps of this protocol that he could do into smaller segments.

It is best to work with a stranger who is not afraid of your dog. If you think that your dog's reaction will scare someone, or if your dog reacts particularly fiercely to certain people, please consider using a head collar when working with these exercises. In a worst-case scenario, a head collar will keep everyone safe. If your stranger is calm and not worried, your dog will be less aroused. If you are not worried, your dog will be less aroused.

For very reactive dogs, you may have to gradually work toward having the dog not react at the door while off-lead and without a head collar or harness. If this never happens, it is not a disaster. As long as you are with your dog you can use a head collar and a long distance lead to help your dog be less reactive at the door. Please do not leave a lead or head collar on a dog if you are not supervising the dog. He could injure himself or become entrapped and die.

If you do not have someone to help you practice the tasks, you can **still** participate in this behavior modification protocol. Make a tape recording of the tasks as listed, with appropriate pauses between each task, and start with the volume very low. As your dog improves, increase the volume. This strategy also works well for dogs who react more to the people on the other side of the door than they do to the sounds.

The following tasks will help you to teach your dog to react more appropriately when at the door. Please also remember that you can use a baby gate to keep the dog in a room away from the door so that you do not get into a contest of wills at an entryway. If your dog is less distressed under gated circumstances, you will be able to progress more quickly with the program, as the dog will not continue to learn from and reinforce his inappropriate behavior.

Finally, anti-anxiety medications may help some dogs who otherwise are not able to succeed in this program. Please remember that if it's decided that medication could benefit your dog, you need to use it **in addition** to the behavior modification, not instead of it.

Task Sheet Instructions

These tasks are meant to give you guidance, only. They are designed to use very, very, very gradual changes. Such tiny steps allow you to reward aspects of the behaviors that are good, without accidentally rewarding aspects of behavior that are not so good.

Built into these programs are the concepts of desensitization (DS), where you teach the dog not to react to some situation by exposing him to the situation at a level below that needed to have him react and become distressed, and counter-conditioning (CC), where you reward behaviors that are in direct opposition or contrast to those that are undesirable.

If you open any applied psychology text or article on learning, you will see similar programs. There is nothing magic or novel or original here; these tasks are those that are common to most dog and cat training and behavior modification programs, and you will see similar task sheets in a number of books, articles, and online sources.

Pease remember that what *is different here* is that you are rewarding the physical signs that the dog is less distressed or worried. You are rewarding *only* relaxed behaviors (review the **Protocol for Teaching Your Dog to Take a Deep Breath and Use Other Biofeedback Methods as Part of Relaxation**).

The tasks involve only common situations in which your dog may respond inappropriately or undesirably. Some of these situations may not be relevant to you, and others that are relevant may be missing. Please feel free to customize or alter this program, but please do so using the pattern of approach used here (e.g., gradually work up to the task, frequent returns to something easier, always ending on a good note, et cetera).

The task is listed on the left. There is space for you to make comments about how easy or hard the task was for the dog, how many times it had to be repeated, or other questionable behaviors that appeared during the task. You should discuss these with your veterinarian at your re-exam appointment.

Try grouping these tasks in groups that you work through in segments that last no more than 15 minutes.

Dog's Task

The dog sits, stays, and relaxes when:
- Stranger knocks briefly and softly
- Stranger knocks softly for 5 seconds
- Stranger knocks softly for 10 seconds
- Stranger knocks moderately and briefly
- Stranger knocks moderately for 5 seconds
- Stranger knocks moderately for 10 seconds
- Stranger knocks normally, briefly
- Stranger knocks normally for 5 seconds
- Stranger knocks normally for 10 seconds
- Stranger knocks loudly for 5 seconds
- Stranger knocks loudly for 10 seconds
- Stranger bangs on door briefly
- Stranger bangs on door for 5 seconds
- Stranger bangs on door for 10 seconds
- Stranger rings bell briefly
- Stranger rings bell for a normal length of time
- Stranger rings bell for 5 seconds
- Stranger knocks on door normally and turns knob
- Stranger opens door 2 cm
- Stranger opens door 5 cm
- Stranger opens door 10 cm
- Stranger opens door, steps into doorway, and then closes door (does not enter)
- Stranger opens door, steps through doorway into room, then exits
- Stranger opens door, enters room, closes door behind him

Once your dog can sit and stay while a family member or someone known to them can come to and through the door, repeat the task list with someone who is less familiar to the dog.

For Future Repetitions

- Repeat all tasks in different locations.
- Repeat all tasks with all family members.
- Repeat all tasks with only every second or third being rewarded with a treat. (Remember praise!)
- Repeat with only intermittent treat reinforcement. (Remember praise!)

TIER 2: PROTOCOL FOR DESENSITIZING AND COUNTER-CONDITIONING DOGS TO RELINQUISH OBJECTS

Some dogs have difficulty relinquishing objects about which they care. These objects can range from bones, whose value people can generally appreciate, to seemingly illogical objects like seeds harvested outside that the dog brings into the house. All dogs should be able to relinquish their possessions to their people upon request. This is a sign that the dog is willing to take information from his people, and it is a behavior that could save the dog's life someday if the object that he is fiercely protecting can hurt him. People should also be reasonable in their requests. This means that if we offer our dogs a giant knuckle bone, we shouldn't take it just because we can. And, if the dog is really aroused, no matter what he has, if it is not going to kill him now, we may want to just let him have it rather than contribute to worsening his aggression or getting anyone injured. Of course, this behavior mod protocol was designed with exactly the latter dog in mind.

Choose Your Coping Strategy

There are three strategies for dealing with a dog who exhibits possessive aggression and guards objects:

- Teach the dog that he does not have to worry about the object and can relinquish it freely **upon request.** This is the focus of this protocol.
- Omit the object(s) that trigger the possessive aggression from the dog's repertoire. If you choose to do this, and this is a perfectly rational choice, you have to ensure that you are consistent. This means that the object that the dog guards is truly and forever out of his repertoire. For dogs who are aggressive if given a bone, a form of food-related aggression, reasonable management may mean that the dog never experiences a bone.
- If you do not wish to avoid objects that the dog guards, or to teach him not to do so, you can only be kept safe by ignoring the dog when these objects are present. *This is a perfectly acceptable strategy if you can really do it, but most dogs are too worried about their objects to make this strategy practical.*

Remember that the goals of this program are twofold:

- You want to decrease your dog's anxiety if he is inappropriately protecting an object; by doing this we hope that your dog will learn that he does not have to guard the object.
- You want to minimize any danger to any person who may come in contact with your dog when he has an object he might protect. When dogs learn to behave appropriately, they become safer.

What Do You Need to Begin?

Prior to starting this tier of the behavior modification programs, all dogs should have successfully completed the **Protocol for Deference,** the **Protocol for Teaching Your Dog to Take a Deep Breath and Use Other Biofeedback Methods as Part of Relaxation,** and the **Protocol for Relaxation: Behavior Modification Tier 1.** Unless your dog has been able to calmly and happily complete these programs, she will be unable to complete this one.

To begin the tasks in this protocol, select an object in which the dog has no interest, such as a paperweight or a rock from outdoors. The object should have no value to your dog and should not frighten her.

Working Through This Protocol

Ask your dog to sit and stay, or to lie down and stay, and relax, and then place the object about 2 to 3 meters (6.5 to 10 feet) from her so that she can see it. Reward the dog for relaxing.

Instruct your dog to "stay" ("Stay, be a good girl, stay, good girl.") and then pick up and quickly return the object.

Return to your dog and reward her if she relaxed and didn't move.

Continue to pick up and replace the object, moving it progressively closer to your dog in a very gradual manner. Each time you pick up and replace the object remember to return to your dog and reward her if she is calm and relaxed (see the Task Sheets below).

What If the Dog Grabs the Object?

If at any point your dog picks up the object, ask her to "drop it." This is a request that all puppies should learn, and you can use this protocol to teach it to puppies. If your dog drops the object, tell her that she is good. Ask her to wait 5 to 10 seconds, and then reward her with a food treat when she is looking at you. This pattern will encourage her to look to you for instructions about how she should handle the object while not encouraging her to steal objects to get attention.

If your dog is unable or unwilling to drop the object after a second request, ignore her and walk away from her and the object. She will seek you out. When she does so, ask her to sit, and practice some of the exercises from the **Protocol for Relaxation: Behavior Modification Tier 1** without using any objects. This will remind her that your relationship is not adversarial and that behavior modification can be fun. Then start with the tasks in this protocol, again.

You may feel safer if you use a head collar to work with your dog. If your dog is wearing a head collar and she tries to grab you or the object, you can safely and kindly interrupt her, while continuing to reward her, when appropriate, for relaxing while sitting or lying down. If you are at all concerned about your ability to take an object directly from your dog, you should use a head collar for the first round of these exercises.

After your dog is able to sit quietly and relax even if the object is picked up from directly in front of her, select a different item with which to work. This next object should be one about which the dog cares slightly more than she did the first object. Repeat the entire protocol as listed in the task pages using this new object.

Then continue to repeat all of the tasks, sequentially selecting an item that is progressively more interesting to your dog until you get to the objects that you know have triggered a protective response in the past.

Finally, if your dog is able to go through the entire protocol and appear relaxed and happy when you pick up even the most valued of her items, you may wish to start to teach her "take it–drop it." This is another exercise that all puppies should learn. Again, start with objects in which your dog has a mild interest (e.g., a "broken" squeak toy that has no squeak) and proceed to objects in which your dog has a keen interest (e.g., a rope toy).

Consider using rawhides or real bones if, and only if, your dog is not aggressive around food. Teaching dogs who are aggressive to food to relinquish it is hard and may be risky. Think seriously about whether this is your bet choice. Consult the **Protocol for Understanding and Managing Dogs with Aggression Involving and Food, Rawhide, Biscuits, and Bones** to help you make your choice.

It is ideal to start puppies out by teaching them to relinquish rawhides, but if you begin to have problems with aggression, please talk to your veterinarian. It is always safer to deny dogs rawhides and real bones. Your dog will not be deprived if you do so.

Finally, remember that this protocol is an extension of the **Protocol for Relaxation: Behavior Modification Tier 1.** Everything that you learned about body language and non-verbal cues applies here, also. Remember that distressed dogs cannot learn or focus and may shake, tremble, whine, salivate, move their eyes from side to side, et cetera. For these protocols to work best, it is not sufficient that your dog just sits and stays. She must be relaxed while doing so. Dogs who learn to enjoy the exercises will progress at the fastest rate. If at any point your dog continues to have difficulty with the tasks, divide them into smaller units and continue. If your dog works best for three 5-minute periods, instead of one 15-minute period, use the shorter periods.

Anti-anxiety medications may help some dogs who otherwise are not able to succeed in this program. Please remember that if it's decided that medication could benefit your dog, you need to use it **in addition** to the behavior modification, not instead of it.

Task Sheet Instructions

These tasks are meant to give you guidance, only. They are designed to use very, very, very gradual changes. Such tiny steps allow you to reward aspects of the behaviors that are good, without accidentally rewarding aspects of behaviors that are not so good.

Built into these programs are the concepts of desensitization (DS), where you teach the dog not to react to some situation by exposing him to the situation at a level below that needed to have him react and become distressed, and counterconditioning (CC), where you reward behaviors that are in direct opposition or contrast to those that are undesirable.

If you open any applied psychology text or article on learning, you will see similar programs. There is nothing magic or novel or original here; these tasks are those that are common to most dog and cat training and behavior modification programs, and you will see similar task sheets in a number of books, articles, and online sources.

Please remember that what *is different here* is that you are rewarding the physical signs that the dog is less distressed or worried. You are rewarding *only* relaxed behaviors (review the **Protocol for Teaching Your Dog to Take a Deep Breath and Use Other Biofeedback Methods as Part of Relaxation**).

The tasks involve only common situations in which your dog may respond inappropriately or undesirably. Some of these situations may not be relevant to you, and others that are relevant may be missing. Please feel free to customize or alter this program, but please do so using the pattern of approach used here (i.e., gradually work up to the task, frequent returns to something easier, always ending on a good note, et cetera).

The task is listed on the left. There is space for you to make comments about how easy or hard the task was for the dog, how many times it had to be repeated, or other questionable behaviors that appeared during the task. You should discuss these with your veterinarian at your re-exam appointment.

Dog's Task

The dog sits, stays, and relaxes when:

- The object is placed on the floor 3 meters (10 feet) away from the dog; briefly retrieve and replace the object.
- The object is placed on the floor 2.5 meters (8 feet) away from the dog; briefly retrieve and replace the object.
- The object is placed on the floor 2 meters (6.5 feet) away from the dog; briefly retrieve and replace the object.
- The object is placed on the floor 1.5 meters (5 feet) away from the dog; briefly retrieve and replace the object.
- The object is placed on the floor 1 meter (3 feet) away from the dog; briefly retrieve and replace the object.
- The object is placed on the floor 0.5 meter (20 inches) away from the dog; briefly retrieve and replace the object.
- The object is placed on the floor 0.25 meter (10 inches) away from the dog; briefly retrieve and replace the object.
- The object is placed on the floor 10 centimeters (4 inches) away from the dog; briefly retrieve and replace the object.
- The object is placed on the floor 5 centimeters (2 inches) away from the dog; briefly retrieve and replace the object.
- The object is placed on the floor 2 centimeters away from the dog; briefly retrieve and replace the object.
- The object is placed on the floor, touching the dog's feet; briefly retrieve and replace the object.

For Future Repetitions

- Repeat all tasks in different locations.
- Repeat all tasks with all family members.
- Repeat all tasks with only every second or third being rewarded with a treat. (Remember praise!)
- Repeat with only intermittent treat reinforcement. (Remember praise!)

See the "Advanced section" that follows.

Advanced Section—and for All Puppies!

Have your dog sit and relax while you hold out a toy in which your dog is interested.

Put the toy directly under your dog's nose or gently in his mouth and say "Take it." Before the object can be fully grasped and the dog leaves, say "Good boy!" and then say "Drop it." Hold out a tiny treat as a reward. As soon as the dog drops the toy, reward him for giving it up, even if he never really grabbed it completely. Letting a toy go is easier for puppies if they have not fully grabbed it and started to shake it. Otherwise, the movement and "playback" character of the toy is so rewarding that they will not initially want to give it up.

Dog's Task

- For the first pass of this program use a toy that is not a favorite for your dog.
- For very reactive dogs you can start with a toy that the dog actually does not like, because if he doesn't "take it" you can still reward him for "drop it" as you move the toy away.
- Put the toy into your dog's mouth or, if he will take the toy, offer it with the request to "Take it" and let the dog hold it 1 second; then repeat the request to "Drop it," as above.
- Put the toy into your dog's mouth or, if he will take the toy, offer it with the request to "Take it" and let the dog hold it 2 seconds; then repeat the request to "Drop it," as above.
- Put the toy into your dog's mouth or, if he will take the toy, offer it with the request to "Take it" and let the dog hold it 3 seconds; then repeat the request to "Drop it," as above.
- Put the toy into your dog's mouth or, if he will take the toy, offer it with the request to "Take it" and let the dog hold it 4 seconds; then repeat the request to "Drop it," as above.
- Put the toy into your dog's mouth or, if he will take the toy, offer it with the request to "Take it" and let the dog hold it 5 seconds; then repeat the request to "Drop it," as above.

Repeat the exercise above with toys that the dog finds progressively more fascinating.

Final Words

Our goal is to ensure that when you request that your dog take an object, he does so and drops it upon request. If you are working with a puppy with no behavioral problems, this goal may be accomplished. However, if you are working with a troubled dog who cares about objects, this protocol may help you to define your dog's limitations. Some dogs may learn to give up everything except one toy. The advantage of learning about such limits is that you can protect your dog from situations that he cannot manage. Not all of us are capable of behaving in a way others consider perfect all of the time. If you learn of a limitation for your dog, it may be kindest to respect it.

TIER 2: PROTOCOL FOR DESENSITIZING DOGS AFFECTED WITH IMPULSE CONTROL AGGRESSION

Prior to desensitizing your dog to gestures or actions that may accidentally encourage him to exhibit aggression, you should have been working with the **Protocol for Deference,** the **Protocol for Teaching Your Dog to Take a Deep Breath and Use Other Biofeedback Methods as Part of Relaxation,** and the **Protocol for Relaxation: Behavior Modification Tier 1.** In addition, you should have been complying with the **Protocol for Impulse Control Aggression.** The purpose of this program is to begin to shape your dog's undesirable and reactive behaviors into behaviors that are less reactive, less risky, and more desirable.

At the outset of these tasks one person should be able to successfully request that your dog sit and stay, both on- and off-lead, in the same format as recommended in **Tier 1.** The dog should be calm and relaxed. If you cannot accomplish these two behaviors on- and off-lead with a calm dog, you are not yet ready for **Tier 2.**

The person giving the dog his cues/signals (the handler) will be the one responsible for rewarding appropriate behaviors with treats. Because your dog has already been through **Tier 1** of the program with this person, the dog should not view this situation as confrontational—the dog should be fully relaxed and happy to work with the programs. This is important because—please remember—these dogs can be dangerous. You cannot have anyone struggle for control with a dog who has an anxiety disorder because you will make your dog worse, not better. *Please go back and practice Tier 1 until you are sure that your dog is happily able to engage in the tasks involved.*

This protocol will help you to desensitize and counter-condition your dog to gestures that he may consider to be threats or challenges associated with control. For you to work successfully with this program, you have to accept that your dog's reactions, while odd, are not normal and are a function of his impairment/pathology. You cannot focus on the idea that this "should not be happening." It *is* happening and for this program to be successful you need to be able to recognize what will trigger an aggressive or concerned response by your dog. You will either avoid or desensitize your dog to these gestures or to their component parts.

This protocol requires the cooperation of a second person, the helper. It is *best* if your dog *does not react to* your first helper. It's *ideal* if your dog *likes* your first helper. We can add progressively more reactive helpers later.

The helper is to stand, or sit if the dog is less reactive when the helper sits, approximately 3 meters (10 feet) away from your dog, off to the dog's side. This means that your dog knows that the person is there and can see the person using peripheral vision, but that he can still attend to and focus directly on you or anyone else giving the cues. This distance was chosen because dogs who have successfully completed Tier 1 should be able to see the helpers from this distance, but not react to them. Being able to see the helper without reacting is the key in choosing distances at which you should work.

With one arm held at waist height, bent at the elbow, and with the palm of that hand facing the floor, the helper should start to make small circles in the air. As the dog learns to ignore this activity and relax while receiving treats as a reward for the relaxation, the helper will gradually make larger circles, move the circles from waist to shoulder height, approach the dog, make the gestures quicker, form the movements closer to the dog, and, eventually, reach down, press on the dog, and possibly very gently massage the dog, stretched out onto his side *with* (and only with) his cooperation. Some dogs will never allow you to manipulate their bodies, but may be able to offer all postures you would manipulate, if asked. That's absolutely fine. The entire point is to teach the dog that these pretty normal human behaviors are not threats.

Under no circumstance should anyone think that they have to force any dog onto his back. Forcing a dog onto his back is an unambiguous threat, and it is a foolish, dangerous exercise that can be damaging to most dogs. If you are never able to move your dog onto his side or back but he is no longer anxious and aggressive, do not be concerned—this is a success. You have to realize that dogs are in a vulnerable and invasive position when they are on their backs.

Please remember that punishment, restraint, and physical corrections all make these dogs worse because you have removed any uncertainty regarding their anxiety: If you exhibit force or punishment, you have proved to the dog that you are a threat!

This **Tier 2** program starts with the helper forming small circles close to his own body. While the dog sits quietly and attentively, and looks as happy as possible **(remember that unhappy or anxious dogs do not learn well and cannot change their behavior),** the size of the circles can be increased. If the dog remains relaxed, the helper can step closer to the dog, again decreasing the circle size. After the dog relaxes, the circle size is increased. Remember that larger gestures, closer to, or over the dog are potentially big threats to these dogs. By repeating the pattern of small circles—relaxation—larger circles—relaxation—approach—small circles—relaxation—larger circles—relaxation, the helper should be able to continue to approach the dog with the dog remaining calm.

You should all work to the point where your dog is able to sit quietly and remain attentive to the handler, while large circles are made over his head. Gradually, the helper will approach the dog and attempt to touch him and then push on him.

The program will talk you through all the necessary steps. Remember that the following six rules apply for this tier of the protocols, as for the others:

1. You are only to reward your dog when he reacts appropriately. Never bribe the dog. Reward the smallest indication of relaxation.
2. If your dog becomes distressed or anxious and cannot successfully complete some part of the program, back up and slowly work on the exercises with which the dog has problems. If your dog just cannot get past one suite of tasks, contact the veterinarian with whom you are working and ask for advice. A certified dog trainer who knows how to use these programs may also be helpful. Regardless, make sure that your dog ends on a positive note for each session.
3. Keep sessions short—a *maximum* of 15 to 20 minutes once or twice a day. If either you or you dog have trouble with

that time block, use shorter, but more frequent, sessions (5-minute sessions 6 to 8 times per day; 3-minute sessions 5 to 10 times a day; or as often as you can manage without feeling pressured). Shorter sessions may work better for some dogs.

4. If at any time you feel that your dog is becoming aggressive or you or your helper feel threatened, stop. Walk the dog around, reward small positive behaviors. Resume when everyone is calm. If your dog cannot regain his calm, that session is over.

5. If your dog appears to lose interest after a few days, make sure that you are rewarding him at the appropriate times in the response sequence. You may also need to change rewards at some point and use the natural tendency to be more interested in novel items. Video yourself to check on your timing and your dog's response to treats.

6. If you or your helper would feel safer or more comfortable with your dog on-lead, practice with him on-lead. It may be best to work with a head collar or no-pull harness because these tools allow you to gently redirect the dog. Well-fitted head collars can also help you to kindly close some dogs' mouths. If you use a halter or harness, hold the leash in one hand and reward with the other. If you choose to just use a leash attached to a collar, put it under your foot with a small amount of slack. This leaves both your hands free, but requires that you can quickly slip your other foot gently across the leash so that the dog's head is held away from you. **DO NOT slam the dog's head to the floor.** *If you have to slip your foot across the lead more than once, you are not ready for this Tier 2 program.* If you feel that you need this type of extreme control over the dog at all times, you are not ready for this Tier 2 program, and you should be using a head collar for all work with your dog.

During these tasks your dog should remain attentive to the handler, whether or not this is you, as the helper performs the potentially distracting activities. A brief glance at the helper is acceptable **if, and only if,** your dog is immediately responsive to a quick request to look back at the handler, **or** your dog, on his own, spontaneously returns his attention to the handler. Use his name as you see him turn toward the helper: "Sparky, look!" If you know that he will look at the helper at a certain point in the sequence, give him permission to do so: "Sparky, look at that! Good boy." Then immediately ask him to look back to you, and praise and reward. This sequence just taught the dog that he can take in information from the helper without worry and then can be rewarded for refocusing his attention. These are important and fairly advanced skills.

The helper is to form small circles close to his body. When the dog sits quietly and attentively, the circles are to be increased in size and speed. If the dog remains relaxed, the helper can step toward the dog, again returning to the smaller circle size that is less threatening. As your dog relaxes, the circle size should again be increased. It is sometimes helpful if the handler anticipates the next phase of the helper's actions and gets the dog's attention before he has time to become concerned. For example, as the helper steps forward, the handler could say "Sparky!" (use an upbeat tone) and reward the dog (if he behaves appropriately) **as** the helper makes her move. Go slowly. Large or quick gestures can be threats to these dogs. By going slowly, the helper will be able to

continue to approach the dog with progressively more complicated desensitization gestures.

Clients are often frustrated by this s-l-o-w approach. Don't be. Just remember that wherever you are in this tier of the program, there are tasks that came earlier that you would not have been able to execute without your commitment to desensitization and counter-conditioning. These desensitization programs are hard work for everyone. These programs will help your dog to get as well as he can get. They offer you an alternative to forever banishing the dog and protecting him from people, gestures, and environments that he finds provocative. Please remember that your job is to keep the dog as safe and happy as possible.

The helper will eventually be standing next to the dog. The circling hand should gradually be lowered until it just touches your dog's fur. If your dog permits this, the helper can gradually begin to apply more pressure to the dog with each pass of his hand. *Watch your dog carefully as the touching begins.* Many of these dogs who cope with their anxiety by controlling the behavior of others will tolerate gestures that do not involve physical contact, but will become aggressive at the least intimate contact. The handler is responsible for monitoring your dog's facial and eye gestures for any sign of concern. If anyone is concerned for any reason, back off. It is far wiser to not take any chances. You can always return to working at a less reactive level and gradually build to a more intimate level. *Remember to do no harm.*

The objective of this program is to gradually work up to the point where the helper can greet, pass, bump, and pet the dog without problems. Once this is possible, the entire program should be repeated in different rooms, indoors and out, and from different positions relative to the dog (behind the dog and, the more threatening position, in front of the dog). Everyone in the household should practice by acting as both the helper and the handler.

The ultimate hope is that people will be able to rush up and hug the dog. *Not all dogs will attain this level of behavioral change.* Caution is urged and some dogs may never be able to be hugged and surrounded by strangers. That's okay. Remember, your main obligation is to the dog's welfare, not to whatever others may think that they "should" be able to do to your dog. **One of the benefits of these programs is that you will become aware of gestures that signal the dog's limits and can decide whether you wish to attempt to modify these, or whether the dog will be happier with some protected limitations.**

Protocol Task Sheets

These tasks are meant to give you guidance only. They are designed to use very, very, very gradual changes. Such tiny steps allow you to reward aspects of the behaviors that are good, without accidentally rewarding aspects of behavior that are not so good.

Built into these programs are the concepts of desensitization (DS), where you teach the dog not to react to some situation by exposing him to the situation at a level below that needed to have him react and become distressed, and counter-conditioning (CC), where you reward behaviors that are in direct opposition or contrast to those that are undesirable.

If you open any applied psychology text or article on learning, you will see similar programs. There is nothing magic or novel or original here; these tasks are those that are common to most dog and cat training and behavior modification programs, and you will see similar task sheets in a number of books, articles, and online sources.

Please remember that what *is different here* is that you are rewarding the physical signs that the dog is less distressed or worried. You are rewarding *only* relaxed behaviors (review the **Protocol for Teaching Your Dog to Take a Deep Breath and Use Other Biofeedback Methods as Part of Relaxation**).

The tasks involve only common situations in which your dog may respond inappropriately or undesirably. Some of these situations may not be relevant to you, and others that are relevant may be missing. Please feel free to customize or alter this program, but please do so using the pattern of approach used here (i.e., gradually work up to the task, frequent returns to something easier, always ending on a good note, et cetera).

The task is listed on the left. There is space for you to make comments about how easy or hard the task was for the dog, how many times it had to be repeated, or other questionable behaviors that appeared during the task. You should discuss these with your veterinarian at your re-exam appointment.

Try grouping these tasks into segments that you work through in *no more* than 15 minutes.

Tasks

The dog sits, stays, and relaxes. The helper should:
- Make small circles at 3 meters (10 feet)
- Make large circles at 3 meters (10 feet)
- Make small circles at 2.5 meters (8 feet)
- Make large circles at 2.5 meters (8 feet)
- Make small circles at 2 meters (6.5 feet)
- Make large circles at 2 meters (6.5 feet)
- Make small circles at 1.5 meters (5 feet)
- Make large circles at 1.5 meters (5 feet)
- Make small circles at 1 meter (3 feet)
- Make large circles at 1 meter (3 feet)
- Make small circles at 0.5 meter (1.5 feet)
- Make large circles at 0.5 meter (1.5 feet)
- Make small circles at 0.25 meter (1 foot)
- Make large circles at 0.25 meter (1 foot)
- Bend at waist at 0.25 meter (1 foot) and make small circles above dog's head
- Bend at waist at 0.25 meter (1 foot) and make large circles above dog's head
- Make small circles immediately above dog's head
- Make large circles immediately above dog's head*
- Quickly and lightly brush dog's fur while circling above dog's back*
- Repeat the above and brush for a slightly longer time*
- Repeat, increasing pressure slightly*
- Repeat, with petting pressure*
- Press gently on the dog's shoulders*
- Press moderately on the dog's shoulders*
- Press firmly on the dog's shoulders*
- Press firmly on the dog's back*
- Keep increasing pressure on the dog until the dog is pushed to the ground*
- Massage neck, shoulders, and hips*
- Roll on to back so that belly is exposed*
- Massage belly, groin, and chest gently*

For Future Repetitions

- Repeat all tasks in different locations.
- Repeat all tasks with all family members.
- Repeat all tasks with only every second or third being rewarded with a treat. (Remember praise!)
- Repeat with only intermittent treat reinforcement. (Remember praise!)

---

*__Caution:__ These gestures can be viewed as threats by your dog. Observe the dog's signals carefully. Do not take risks. Not all dogs will succeed at the most advanced levels. This is fine. Frequent repetitions will often allow dogs to continue to improve.

PROTOCOL FOR UNDERSTANDING AND TREATING CATS WITH ELIMINATION DISORDERS AND ELIMINATION BEHAVIORS THAT CONCERN CLIENTS

The most common behavioral concerns reported by clients about their cats involve litterbox use. Complaints about litterbox use can often be prevented and usually be successfully treated if the client becomes good at observing their cat's behavior. The key to resolving **all** elimination concerns is to recognize and be able to identify the pattern in the choices the cat makes about elimination. If clients can do this, the problem will resolve. Otherwise, you need to know that *the single biggest reason why cats are relinquished or euthanized involves elimination behaviors that the client views as problematic*, whether or not these are true behavioral problem for the cat.

Concerns about litterbox use generally involve one or more of the following complaints:

- The cat doesn't use the box at all.
- The cat uses the box for either urine or feces, but not both.
- The cat eliminates right next to or on the box, but not in it.
- The cat uses the box, but doesn't cover urine or feces.

There is one final elimination concern that actually does not involve the issue of litterboxes: spraying. **Spraying** is the term for the set of behaviors where cats deposit urine against a vertical surface like a wall, the back of a couch, a closet door, et cetera. The behaviors involved in spraying include:

- backing up against or within a few centimeters of the vertical surface,
- arching the back slightly when moving toward the vertical surface,
- raising the tail so that it is almost straight up and can be seen from a distance, like a flag,
- treading or kneading with the feet, usually the front feet,
- waving or wiggling the tail, particularly the tip, and
- partly closing the eyes while moving the ears back.

Spraying of urine usually, but not always, follows these behaviors.

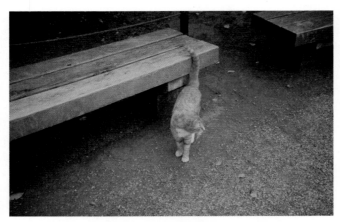

An intact male cat exhibiting all of the behaviors, as listed, that are involved in spraying. In addition, he is rubbing his tail base against the cedar bench. This cat did not spray.

Spraying can be a normal behavior. You may not want to hear this, but it's true. Both male and female cats can and will spray, as will neutered/desexed cats. Neutering can decrease or stop spraying if it has been occurring for only a short while or it is related solely to estrus cycles or responses to them,

and neutered cats spray less than do cats who have their ovaries and testicles. In part, these findings about neutering and spraying are likely associated with the unique feline mating system:

- Male cats advertise for females, and females would live within family groups of related females, given the choice.
- Males may mate with more than one female in the group and try to prevent, with varying success, other males from having access to "their" females.
- Because female cats are induced ovulators, meaning that they need to be hormonally stimulated to be able to become pregnant, the scent of male urine is particularly important in this context.

If you watch your cat it will be clear how important the sense of smell is to cats. Urine can be a currency of scent to cats and they use it to signal to each other. Because of this signaling, whenever spraying is involved it is absolutely critical that you work closely with your veterinarian to understand all the social relationships in the household, and in the vicinity of the houses where the cat lives. Chances are, spraying is a nonspecific sign of social disruption or distress and spraying will not resolve unless the social concerns are addressed. See the **Protocol for Understanding and Treating Feline Aggressions with an Emphasis on Intercat Aggression** for situations where addressing litterbox hygiene does not help.

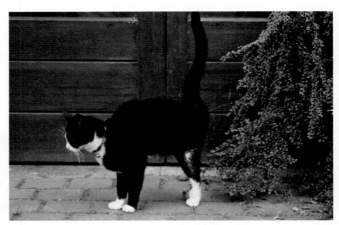

Cat spraying vegetation. (Photo courtesy of Anne Marie Dossche.)

Cats who do not use the box at all can be characterized or grouped by patterns of their elimination behaviors:

- The cat picks one class of objects on which to eliminate (e.g., blankets, bedding, bathmats, laundry, **or** in the shower, in the bathtub, on tile floors, in sinks, on linoleum, on wood). Note that here the types of surfaces—or substrates—on which cats eliminate are linked by texture. In the case of blankets, et cetera, the substrates chosen are all soft, and in the case of sinks, et cetera, all of the substrates chosen are smooth and cool to the touch. This problem is usually termed **"a substrate preference for elimination."**
- The cat picks one type of location in which to eliminate (e.g., under the dining room table, next to the box, on the

bathroom floor, by the window near your side of the bed, et cetera). This problem is generally termed **"a location preference for elimination."**

- The cat eliminates in a pattern that does not seem to be associated with how something feels, or where it is. When this happens it is extremely important that you consider two other possibilities:
  - that a medical problem is involved and
  - that the pattern of elimination is conveying information about concerns the cat has about the social environment.

In all of the above situations the cat could exhibit the problem for either urine or feces, or for both.

Finally, preferences can develop either innately, because the cat truly prefers some substrate other than the litter in the box, or they can develop after they learn to hate their litter or box. Cats who hate their litter, box, or something about the litter and box (e.g., **a substrate or location aversion**) will, by necessity, choose something else. Often these cats go through a period of sampling other locations or substrates, which may look like the cat is behaving in a random manner. This type of behavior is common early on in the development of the problem, but if the problem persists, the cats will ultimately choose a preferred substrate or location. **This is one reason why it is so important that you talk to your veterinarian—early and often—about your cat's behaviors.**

The steps below are designed to help resolve substrate and location **preferences** and substrate and location **aversions.** These steps are intended to help reinforce what litterbox use that most people consider appropriate, while also meeting the cat's social and personal hygiene needs. Please remember that the feline social system may also be having an effect on the behavior of a cat who is not using his litterbox—social interactions might be compounding the problem. You should watch for changes in relationships among the cats in your household, and also realize that changes in the canine and human relationships, schedules, and composition are all destabilizing influences on cats who like some degree of predictability. Accordingly, alterations of some social situations may be necessary to fully resolve an elimination problem.

Steps for Redressing Elimination Concerns:

1. Identify the problem. Approaches for handling a location versus substrate preference differ. Follow the cat around and see what the cat chooses in terms of area and substance on which to eliminate. If this doesn't work, videotape the cat while she is at the litterbox. If the videocamera is on a tripod, most cats will ignore it and you will be able to see what behaviors the cat uses when she explores the litterbox. You can then view this video with your veterinarian and identify normal and promising behaviors, and ones that indicate a problem. Also, please consider videotaping normal daily activities of your cat and her interactions with anyone else—feline or not—in the household. If you do this, you will see your cat through new eyes, and with the help of your veterinarian, will learn about the problem and what you can do to fix it.

2. Because cats are so good at smelling and identifying odor, the step you immediately need to take is to clean, clean, and then clean again. First cleanings should involve soaking the area with plain water (club soda or seltzer can also be used and may help urine that is deep into carpets to bubble to the surface). After soaking, blot the area. Repeat this until you can no longer detect even a trace of the scent of urine or feces on the towels that are used to blot the wet area. You will go through a lot of towels so consider using rags, disposable sponges, or paper towels. Remember, this is the baseline cleaning; repeat it more often if you can, because although you cannot smell the urine or feces, the cat will be able to do so. Once you think you are done, use a small blacklight (they are inexpensive) to go over all relevant areas: urine fluoresces. Continue to clean until you cannot detect it.

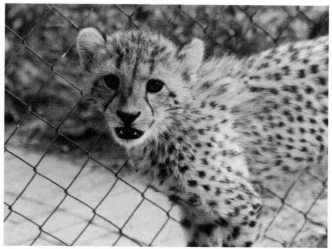

Cats are very good at detecting odor, and you may see your cat exhibiting this open-mouthed behavior when she sniffs around. This is a "Flehmen response." This behavior helps the cat to aerosolize and understand chemical composition of odors.

3. All affected areas must be cleaned with a good odor eliminator. The best odor eliminators have both enzymatic capabilities to break down or degrade the substances in the urine, while making it harder for the scents to aerosolize when the cat sniffs the area. These include Nature's Miracle (available at pet supply stores), FON (available at pet supply stores), PON (available at pet supply stores), Urine-Off (available online and off in numerous places), Get Serious! (www.getseriousproducts.com), Elimin-Odor (available from veterinarians), The Equalizer (available from veterinary supply companies), Anti-Icky Poo/AIP (www.antiickypoo.com), and KOE/AOE (broadly commercially available). The last four have a reputation for being particularly effective. Febreeze has also been noted to have good odor-elimination properties (e.g., if an odor eliminator is good the cat pays less attention than he otherwise would to the soiled area).

4. After cleaning, cover affected areas with heavy gauge plastic to both alter the tactile sensation for the cat and to prevent further penetration in the event of elimination.

5. Make the litterboxes appealing in a manner that meets the cat's needs.
   - Get multiple litterboxes, generally one more than there are cats. If you have more than five cats, this may

become problematic because large numbers of cats may render the olfactory stimulus too strong for many litterboxes to have more effect than would a half-dozen. Still, you should see how many boxes the cats willingly use and adjust your household to accommodate this number. Given the chance, the cats will tell you what they need.

- Place the litterboxes in a variety of locations. You should be guided in this by the choices your cat has already made. The places the cat chooses contain information about what the cat needs. Meet these needs. If the box is in a particularly awkward spot from your viewpoint, if the problem is a location preference, you will gradually be able to move the box (1 cm/day) once the cat has routinely used it for weeks. If you need to move the box for a party, both the cat and the box can be temporarily placed in a room in the house in which the cat is comfortable.
- Choose litterboxes of a style the cat likes. Humans often like covered and small litterboxes because they keep down dust and odor, but cats do not.
  - Cats actually prefer larger boxes; research shows that cats prefer a box that is 1.5 times the length of the cat.
  - Additionally, only very shy cats may prefer closed boxes; some cats don't like them because they enclose smells or make the cat feel trapped.
  - Consider the depth of the box. Cats that are small or arthritic need easy access, and large, shallow boxes may be the best overall choice here. Few, if any, commercial litterboxes meet these needs so consider using unlidded sweater boxes as litterboxes.
- Throw out the box and get a new one as soon as there are scratches in the bottom of the box. These scratches are hiding holes for odor. Cats have reputations for being fastidious. This means that they don't want to use a smelly litterbox any more than you would want to use a smelly toilet.
- Wash litterboxes at least weekly in very hot water. If you wish you can use a mild detergent if you rinse well. If you choose to use a disinfectant like bleach you must rinse, and rinse, and rinse. Strong, chemical smells are disliked by cats, and given their sense of smell, even a small odor will smell strong.
- Choose a litter that the cat likes. How do you know what the cat will like? Mimic the texture of the objects chosen.
  - If the cat is choosing soft fabrics use a litter that feels soft (e.g., potting soil; number 3 blasting sand; soft, clumpable litters; litters made from puffed up, recycled paper or wood; plant-based litters; et cetera). Some cats will use the now commercially available chucks, or soft paper fabric pads that are lined in plastic. These have the advantage over litters of not having any components that can adhere to a cat's fur. **This concern may be very important for long-haired cats.**
  - If the cat is choosing smooth, cool, well-drained substrates that reflect light, either put a small amount of litter in the box, use a cookie sheet or gardening tray as a box, or line the box with ceramic tiles and use no litter. If the cat restricts elimination to a shower or sink, you may just want to make the decision to clean these multiple times per day rather than have the cat sample and learn about areas that are not so easy to clean. In the wild, cats prefer open, well-drained, reflective surfaces, like clear sand, and they may not cover their urine or feces. **Not covering elimination products is often a normal behavior.** You should only be concerned if there has been a dramatic change.
- Remember that cats like soft, clean-smelling substances. This means that litter that holds on to odor will not be preferred by cats.
- Studies show that clumpable, recyclable litters may be terrific for humans but are not always so good for the cats. By reusing these litters we are actually stirring around and redistributing microscopic pieces of feces that come to coat the silicaceous grains. From the cat's perspective, these litter grains stink, even if there are clean grains interspersed among them.

6. **Litter should be scooped at least daily, and most litters should be dumped totally at least every-other-day.** The clumpable litters must also be scooped multiple times per day, but can be topped up and stirred. Still, given the findings about microscopic feces adhering to the grains, these litters should be dumped and replaced considerably more often than is discussed on their labels. Dump them every few days, and more often if more than one cat is using the box.

7. Not all cats prefer the same litter depth. Some cats like to dig in deeper areas but some don't like to bury their paws. Learn what your cat likes. One hint is that cats dig more in litters they like, whether or not they cover their urine and/or feces.

8. Mechanized litterboxes and other novel formats can and will be used by some cats, but the risk may be greater that the cat will not like these. These boxes are not for fearful cats or those who easily startle. Although they are most appealing because of ease of clean-up, we need to remember that the point of a litterbox is actually to meet the cat's needs.

9. Please remember that cats are not truly "trained" to litterboxes in the sense that we think of "housetraining" a dog. Seeking out a preferred substrate, digging, and covering urine or feces, if the cat chooses to do so, are behaviors that develop in kittens in the absence of human intervention. Accordingly, we cannot train cats with an elimination problem to use a litterbox; however, they can be encouraged to do so by taking the cat to the litterbox frequently, waiting with him, and praising him whenever he uses the box. Remember that elimination behaviors in ancestral cats may include urinating and defecating in different places, and seeking out reflective, open, well-drained substrates for elimination. Not all cats will cover their urine or feces and this can be **normal.**

10. If the cat is seen to squat outside the box, punishment or extreme startle will only make the cat more secretive about where or when she eliminates. If you use a gentle interruption and it occurs as the cat is beginning to eliminate (e.g., when she sniffs, circles, et cetera), such interruption may work to stop the cat from eliminating in the undesired spot. This will only work if you can then take

the cat to a preferred spot, have the cat use it, and praise the cat. Frankly, this sequence of behaviors is not highly likely. Given the amount of damage we can do by scaring a cat, we may wish to abandon this and related tactics. **Regardless, punishment after the fact is useless and physical punishment, including rubbing the cat's nose in the soiled area, should be avoided at all costs because it teaches the cats to avoid their people, and may also lead to physical or behavioral injury of the cat.**

11. Some cats may benefit from being confined to a restricted area at first. If you do this, make sure that the cat has the same choice of litters/boxes discussed above and that you pay **lots** of attention to the cat during its confinement. If this was a very social cat before confinement, confinement has to be arranged to meet the cat's social needs. If the behavior of the other cats in the household changes when one is isolated, this hints to a social problem that may need to be addressed as part of the therapy for the elimination disorder. Access to the rest of the house can be expanded once these cats are using litter appropriately in the confined area. It is important that the expanded access be closely supervised both because of the potential relapses and because of potential social problems that may not have been previously recognized. A bell attached to a break away collar can act as a reminder that supervision is necessary (Bear Bells, www.rei.com). Access should be gradually expanded; don't give the cat free access to the entire house all at once after 6 weeks of confinement. If the cat has truly learned and demonstrated a preference for a litter or box style, this will generalize to the rest of the house only if the reintroductions are gradual. Please remember that the number of boxes still has to be maintained at the increased number and all cleanliness rules still apply.

12. Take into account the way cats perceive scent and make this work for you.
    - Do not use plastic liners. Whether or not they are scented, they smell different to the cat. Cats also usually do not like the additional texture.
    - Do not use scented litters. Consider the cat's needs first. Scents that mask the scent of elimination products for you may be very upsetting to cats.
    - You can try placing a mint-scented bar of soap in an area the cat has soiled. Some cats will avoid it. Some won't, but you have done no harm.

13. Good hygiene for litterboxes can also contribute to good hygiene and healthcare for humans. Immunocompromised and other at-risk individuals need to take care in handling cat feces. See the following websites for more information: www.petsandparasites.org./cat-owners/; www.cdc.gov/parasites/toxoplasmosis/gen_info/pregnant.html.

14. Anti-anxiety medications may help some cats that are otherwise unable to succeed with this program. Please remember, if it is decided that your pet could benefit from anti-anxiety medication, you will need to use it in addition to the behavioral and environmental medication, above. All anti-anxiety medication should be used judiciously, and only after a thorough physical examination has been performed, and laboratory tests have determined that your cat is not unduly at risk from side effects of the drugs.

Tick List:

☐ I. General
- Scoop litterboxes daily.
- Dump litter at least every other day.
- Wash the litterbox in hot, ± mild soapy water once a week; use no ammonia products and make sure that the box is well rinsed and dried.
- Soak soiled areas with clear water and blot dry; repeat until NO scent is detectable to you, then repeat again.
- Clean soiled areas with an odor eliminator, repeat, and cover to prevent re-soiling.
- Take cat to the box often and praise for scratching and/or use.
- Provide one more box than the number of cats.
- Change litter types, depths, and box styles.
- Make sure that the box is at least 1.5 cat-lengths long.

☐ II. Location preferences
- Follow General instructions above.
- Place a scent deterrent in area (mint or deodorant scented soap).
- Place food and/or water dishes on the spot(s).
- Place a litterbox on the spot.

☐ III. Substrate preferences
- Follow General instructions above.
- Try different litters:
  - Types tried
    1. _____
    2. _____
    3. _____
    4. _____
- Try covered versus open boxes.
- Try different depths of litter.

☐ IV. Provide your veterinarian with routine information on your cat's behavior at every visit. This history tick list will help. Bring a completed copy to your veterinarian at each appointment.

The questionnaire below is a survey questionnaire that can be used at **any and all veterinary visits** to help you review subjects about which you might have questions. This questionnaire will also allow you to see if your pet's behaviors change over time. This questionnaire, when used at each visit, will tell you if further information is necessary and hint at some of the underlying factors contributing any problems that are identified. This questionnaire will also give you the vocabulary and opportunity to discuss your pet's behaviors with your veterinarian in an efficient, consistent, and meaningful way.

Survey questionnaire about general cat behaviors—to be used at all visits:

1. Client(s):	2a. Today's date: _____ /_____ /_____ 2b. Cat's date of birth: _____ /_____ /_____ ☐ Estimated ☐ Known
3. Patient's name:	4a. Breed: 4b. Weight: _____ lb/_____ kg 4c. Sex: ☐ M ☐ MC ☐ F ☐ FS 4d. If your cat is castrated or spayed [neutered], at what age was this done? _____ weeks/months (circle)
5a. Age in weeks at which your cat was adopted? 5b. How many owners has your cat had? 5c. How long have you had this cat?	a. _____ weeks/months (circle) b. ☐ 0 ☐ 1 ☐ 2 ☐ 3 ☐ 4 ☐ 5+ ☐ Unknown c. _____ months

6a. Is your cat (please circle):
   a. Indoor, only
   b. Outdoor, only
   c. Indoor/outdoor
	6b. How many litterboxes does your cat have:
	 ☐ 0 ☐ 1 ☐ 2 ☐ 3 ☐ 4 ☐ 5+
	 6c. What types of litter do you use?
	
	 6d. How often do you change the litterbox completely?
	 _____ times weekly/monthly (circle)
	 6e. How often do you scoop the box?
	 _____ times daily/weekly (circle)

7a. Does your cat leave urine or feces outside the litterbox? 7b. Does your cat "spray"?	☐ Yes ☐ No ☐ Don't know If you answered yes, a. Urine—Where specifically? b. Feces—Where specifically? c. Both—Where specifically? ☐ Yes ☐ No ☐ Don't know If you answered yes, where specifically?
8. Do you have any concerns, complaints, or problems with urination in the house now?	☐ Yes ☐ No If you answered yes, (a) Where is the cat urinating that you find undesirable (list all areas)? (b) How many times per week is the cat urinating in places you find undesirable? (c) At what time of day is the urination occurring? (d) Is the pattern different on days when you are home and days you are not home? (e) Are you at work during the hours when the cat urinates? (f) How many times per day does your cat usually urinate when he or she is not urinating in places you find undesirable?
9. Do you have any concerns, complaints, or problems with defecation in the house now?	☐ Yes ☐ No If you answered yes, (a) Where is the cat defecating that you find undesirable (list all areas)? (b) How many times per week is the cat defecating in places you find undesirable? (c) At what time of day is the defecation occurring?

	(d) Is the pattern different on days when you are home and days you are not home? (e) Are you at work during the hours when the cat defecates? (f) How many times per day does your cat usually defecate when he or she is not defecating in places you find undesirable?
10. Does your cat destroy any objects or anything else by chewing, sucking, or eliminating on them (e.g., furniture, rugs, clothes, et cetera) now?	☐ Yes ☐ No If you answered yes, what objects specifically does the cat destroy? Please list all of them and note which are destroyed when you are home or not home—please note if they destroy at both times—tick both columns:

Object	When home	When gone
	☐	☐
	☐	☐
	☐	☐
	☐	☐

11. Does your cat mouth, bite, suck, or nip anything or anyone?	a. ☐ Yes ☐ No If you answered yes, to whom is this behavior directed? b. Is this a problem for you? ☐ Yes ☐ No
12. Does your cat exhibit any vocalization about which you are concerned?	☐ Yes ☐ No If you answered yes, what is/are the vocalization(s) and when do they occur:

Vocalization	Situation in which it occurs
a. Yowling	
b. Growling	
c. Meowing	
d. Hissing	

13. Does your cat show any signs of hissing, growling, or biting?	☐ Yes ☐ No If you answered yes, what does the cat do and when does he or she do it?

Sign	Situation in which it occurs
a. Hissing	
b. Growling	
c. Biting	

14. Have you ever been concerned that your cat is "aggressive" *to people*?	☐ Yes ☐ No If you answered yes, why?
15. Have you ever been concerned that your cat is "aggressive" *to cats*?	☐ Yes ☐ No If you answered yes, why?
16. Have you ever been concerned that your cat is "aggressive" *to animals other than cats*? Does your cat hunt or prey on other animals?	☐ Yes ☐ No If you answered yes, why? ☐ Yes ☐ No If you answered yes, which animals and where?

17. Has your cat ever bitten or clawed anyone, regardless of the circumstances?	☐ Yes ☐ No If yes, what happened?
18. Has your cat had any changes in sleep habits?	☐ Yes ☐ No If you answered yes, what are these changes?
19. Has your cat had any changes in eating habits?	☐ Yes ☐ No If you answered yes, what changes have occurred?
20. Has your cat had any changes in locomotor behaviors or the ability to get around or jump on the bed, et cetera?	☐ Yes ☐ No If you answered yes, what changes have occurred?
21. Has anyone ever told you that they were afraid of your cat?	☐ Yes ☐ No If you answered yes, what did they say?
22. Has anyone every told you that your cat was ill-mannered?	☐ Yes ☐ No If you answered yes, why—what did the cat do that made them say this?
23. Do you have any concerns about your cat's grooming behaviors?	☐ Yes ☐ No If you answered yes, a. Little to no grooming b. Sucking c. Chewing d. Licking e. Self-mutilation/sores f. Barbering/trimming g. Plucking out clumps of hair
24. Is the cat exhibiting any behaviors about which you are concerned, worried, or would like more information?	☐ Yes ☐ No If you answered yes, please list these behaviors below:

PROTOCOL FOR UNDERSTANDING AND TREATING PLAY AGGRESSION IN CATS

Cats who are weaned early and then hand-raised by humans may never learn to temper their play responses. Social play in cats peaks early (2-9 weeks) and is replaced by weeks 10-12 with behaviors like pouncing that are involved in predatory behavior. Young cats engage in true social fighting by week 14.

Play aggression is usually associated with two risk factors:
- early weaning and an adaptive shift to more predatory behaviors and
- rough play with—and often initiated by—humans.

Kittens who are raised with their littermates and by their mother usually learn to modulate their play responses because other cats let them know what hurts. Kittens who are early-weaned/bottle-fed may not have had the experience of learning normal play behaviors from other cats. Kittens who never learned to sheathe their claws or inhibit biting in play may play too aggressively with people.

Because kittens are normally very playful and chase moving objects, people often play with them using their hands or feet. This is a mistake, especially if the kitten is early-weaned/bottle-fed and may already exhibit inappropriately aggressive play behaviors. While kittens may do little damage when they play aggressively, the same behaviors in an older and larger cat can do considerable damage. The best way to avoid learned play aggression is to encourage appropriate play with toys that ensure that even if the cat makes a mistake, she cannot injure you. See the **Protocol for Choosing Toys for Your Pet.**

Cat bites and scratches cause disease. They can be seriously dangerous to someone who is already ill, is immuno-compromised, or has poor circulation. You are not being mean by avoiding and redirecting your cat's play aggression. If anything, your relationship with your cat will improve.

Treatment Strategies:

Treatment of play aggression focuses on three major strategies:
1. avoiding the circumstances that encourage the cat to play in this manner,
2. being attentive to the behaviors that are associated with the play aggression and interrupting those, and
3. giving the cat a more appropriate outlet for her play and energy.

Tick List for Treating Play Aggression in Cats:

1. Never play roughly with your cat, and never use your hands or feet to play with your cat. These behaviors only teach your cat that you will play roughly, and she will respond with increasingly rough play. Do not:
   - play roughly with your hands,
   - wrestle with your cat,
   - grab her by her head and shake it,
   - move your hands back and forth so that your cat chases them, or
   - pull the cat's tail.
2. Do not physically punish or "correct" the cat by flicking her nose, pinching her neck, "scruffing" her, biting her, et

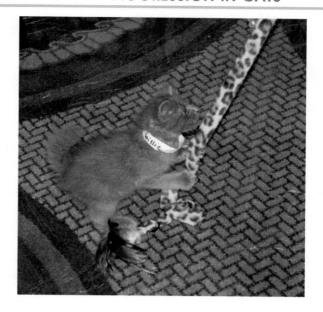

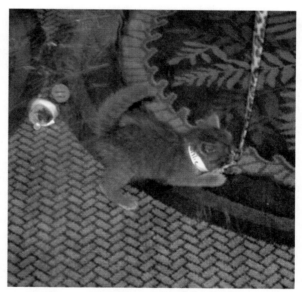

Notice that this rescue kitten has fiercely used his claws to "catch" the toy and then goes on to bite it. This is *exactly* why people should never play with kittens using their hands or other body parts. As early as possible, play should be directed to appropriate toys, like this one.

cetera. Your "corrections" will not be the same as those delivered by another cat, can severely injure your cat, and will teach your cat that you are truly a threat. Cats have extremely sensitive pressure receptors around their face and at the base of their teeth and can interact safely with kittens in ways humans cannot.

3. Learn to recognize the early signs of play aggression in your cat. Cats with play aggression hide behind doors or around banisters, crouching and waiting for any

movement. They will spring, using both teeth and claws, before quickly fleeing. Expect your cat to hide in these locations and beware. Redirect the cat to a more appropriate target by throwing a toy or a ball of crumpled paper, or with a feather toy. If you know that you cannot redirect your cat, carry a towel or light sheet or blanket that you can toss over her to safely maneuver her to an area where she cannot grab anyone.

4. Put a bell on a break-away collar (Bear Bells: www.rei.com). A bell is particularly helpful for cats who pounce on human body parts or clothing, and those who are adept at hiding and waiting for you to pass. Many of these cats hide under furniture and attack toes when you sit down and move your feet. The bell will let you know exactly where the cat is and will allow you to redirect the cat or protect yourself from her.

5. Whenever you play with your cat you must use a toy. If you do not use a toy, your cat will not learn to distinguish your body parts from items signaling play. If your cat misses the toy and grabs or scratches your hand or arm, stop the play. Walk away. If you wish to continue play, when your cat is calm, can sit and look at you (see the **Protocol for Deference** and the **Protocol for Teaching Cats and Dogs to "Sit," "Stay," and "Come"**).

6. Increase the amount of your cat's aerobic exercise. You can throw rolled-up tin foil or paper for her to bat around the room. You can rig a scratching post so that she gets a treat if she scratches energetically at the top of the post. If your cat likes catnip, you can use a toy system with catnip "mice" and springs that are attached to kitty condos. You can attach a toy to extendable, flexible, elastic roping that you tie to your waist so that wherever you walk, your cat can chase a moving toy.

7. If all else fails or if you are not averse to it and your cat is young or is a kitten, consider getting another cat. Another cat often provides the perfect foil for your cat's aggressive play, and may teach your cat to inhibit some of her more damaging behaviors. Try to select a cat who is outgoing. Adopting a mother and another kitten will give your cat a normal social group in which to mature (and you save the life of the mother). Do not choose a very young kitten who could be injured by your cat's rough play.

8. Make sure that you trim your cat's claws frequently. Your cat can trim her own claws if you cover a scratching post with sand paper and encourage her to use it. Logs, scratching posts, and tree branches can be good choices for cats to scratch. Reward and praise your cat whenever you see her scratching appropriate surfaces, especially ones that are not you.

9. If your cat persists in aggressive play, banish her to another room. When she is calm, let her out and redirect her play to toys. If she is again aggressive, repeat the

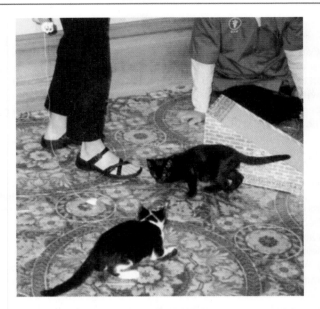

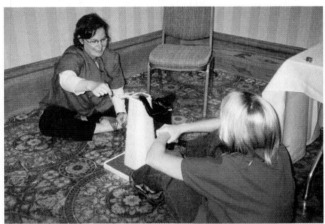

Two solutions for helping cats to keep their claws trimmed: the upper photo shows a commercially available version of an inclined plane covered in sandpaper; the bottom photo shows a scratching post covered with jute rope. Both of these can be incorporated into play with cats to encourage their use as "nail files."

banishment, release, and toy offer cycle. Most play is about attention so this strategy usually works.

10. If anyone is injured by your cat, seek immediate competent medical help. This is another reason to suggest that when adopting a kitten, clients should also take the mother, if possible. Otherwise, kittens should be brought into homes with other normal, healthy cats who can help them to modulate their feline responses, and teach them to play more gently.

PROTOCOL FOR UNDERSTANDING AND TREATING FELINE AGGRESSIONS WITH AN EMPHASIS ON INTERCAT AGGRESSION

Feline Aggression and Associations with Elimination Disorders

Feline social systems differ from those of dogs in many ways, and the history of cat and human associations is helpful in understanding these differences.

Cats were likely never truly "domesticated." Ancestral cats are not very different from modern cats in either size or habit. Cats have historically been found near and around human settlements, because where there are people there is stored food, and where there is stored food there are rodents. A mouse or a rat makes a single meal for the cat on the go. Accordingly, modern cats are solitary hunters who live in matrilineal (mother focused) social groups. Unlike the situation with dogs, we have not substantially altered anything about their social behavior until fairly recently. When we started to purpose-breed cats to develop cat breeds/breed fancy, we focused on changes in color, coat texture, coat length, tail or ear shape, et cetera, not on enhancing specific jobs that different breeds do, as was originally the case with dogs.

It is not surprising that the types of inappropriate aggression witnessed by clients differ from those seen in dogs and that they are understandable given the evolutionary context of feline social systems and the developmental context of sensitive periods.

Categorization of feline aggression is similar to that of canine aggression; differences in the manifestation of the aggressions may be attributable to differences in mating behaviors and differences in social relationships and "hierarchies." Feline aggression includes:

- aggression because of a lack of socialization,
- play aggression (also see the **Protocol for Understanding and Treating Play Aggression in Cats**),
- intercat aggression (main topic of this protocol),
- territorial aggression,
- fearful aggression (also see the **Protocol for Treating Fearful Behavior in Cats and Dogs**),
- maternal aggression,
- redirected aggression (also see the **Protocol for Understanding and Treating Redirected Aggression in Cats and Dogs**),
- predatory aggression, and
- impulse control (formerly "assertion or status-related") aggression (also see the **Protocol for Understanding, Managing, and Treating Impulse Control/Status-Related Aggression in Cats**).

Aggression Due to Lack of Socialization

Cats who have not had contact with humans prior to 3 months of age have missed sensitive periods important for the development of normal approach responses to people. Cats who are handled intensely and/or exposed to as many new things as possible between 2 and 7 weeks of age will have the best chance of dealing well with those stimuli. These patterns suggests that we did not domesticate cats. In dogs, where domestication is well established, the sensitive periods are long, flexible, and variable, a pattern thought to be a common sequela to domestication or a co-evolutionary process. Cats are more like captive wolves: If you don't handle them early, they do not develop easily into animals who enjoy handling.

Lack of early exposure to, and experience with, other cats may result in a lack of normal inquisitive and tolerant responses to other cats. Furthermore, total isolation from cats can have negative consequences for future interactions with humans. This constellation of deprivation scenarios may be contributory to many of the aggressions seen in urban, feral cats. These cats will never be normal, cuddly pets, although they may be fairly affectionate to one person or a small group of people who have worked with them over a period of time. If forced into a situation involving restraint, confinement, or intimate contact, these cats may become extremely aggressive.

Play Aggression

Cats who were weaned early and then hand-raised by humans may never have learned to temper their play responses. Social play in cats peaks early and is replaced by more predatory activities by weeks 10 to 12, and by social fighting by week 14. Cats who, as kittens, never learned to modulate their responses may play too aggressively with people. These cats may not have learned to sheathe their claws or inhibit their bite. This is another reason to suggest that when adopting a kitten, clients should also take the mother, if possible. Otherwise, kittens should be brought into homes with other normal, healthy cats who can help them to modulate their responses, and teach them to play more gently.

It is not clear if there is a component of learning about oral responses that is missing when cats are bottle-fed. Were the kitten to nurse too hard on the mother or hurt her in play, the mother would swiftly correct the kitten. We are unlikely to be able to issue corrections with good timing or with appropriate intensity. Concerns about injuring the kitten are not trivial.

The best ways to stop play aggression in cats include:
- Never play roughly with the cat.
- Never "correct" the cat using your hands or teeth. This "correction" will *not* be equivalent to what mom does.
- Redirect the cat's play to toys that are large enough that if the kitten makes a mistake, she bites or swats the toy and not your hand (see photos on the following page).

More detailed and specific advice can be found in the **Protocol for Understanding and Treating Play Aggression in Cats.**

Territorial Aggression

Territorial aggression can be exhibited toward other cats or people. Such cats may delineate their turf by patrol, chin rubbing, or spraying or non-spraying marking. *It should be noted that territorial concerns are attributed to feline aggressions far more often than is supported by the data.* Because of complex, transitive, feline social hierarchies, a cat who is aggressive to one housemate, may not be aggressive to another, and all of this occurs within the same "turf."

If the cat is defending and, or marking a turf, and the perceived offender crosses into it, threats and a fight may ensue. If part of the struggle involves social hierarchy, cats

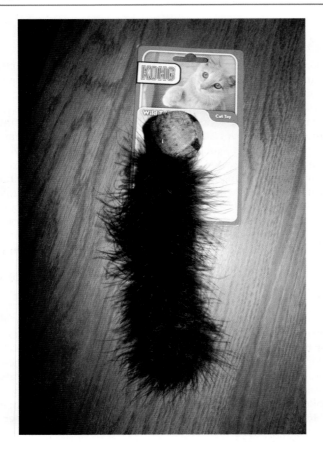

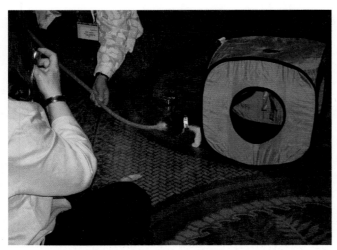

(Bottom) A toy that encourages aerobic play in a manner safe for humans and cats. *(Top)* An example of an appropriate toy for cats. This toy can be thrown so that the cat chased the "tail," not the human.

may lure or seek out their challengers and then attack after the "territory" has been "invaded." Because of the over-riding social component, territorial aggression can be difficult to treat without also treating the intercat aggression, which is usually the main problem, particularly if there is a marking

component. Any marking problem should act as a flag for a possible underlying aggressive situation. Environmental modification (including space sharing), behavioral modification (including setting non-overlapping times to share space), and pharmacological intervention are all treatment options; however, aggressions involving strong, underlying social strife are notoriously difficult to treat once pronounced. Ultimately, one cat may have to be placed in another home or be banished to another region of the property.

Fear/Fearful Aggression

There are "genetically friendly" cats and "genetically shy" cats. It is unclear the extent to which shy cats have the potential to become fearfully aggressive, but there are cats who, despite the best socialization possible, become aggressive whenever fearful. These cats also may become fearful without an apparent stimulus. Regardless, if threatened, any cat will defend himself. Depending on the type of treatment chosen, the cat can learn to become fearfully aggressive. Any intervention that makes a particular cat feel trapped will worsen fear aggression. This is why "flooding" is not recommended as a method to help fearful cats. "Flooding" is a technique that constrains two animals to be in each other's presence without the possibility of physical or behavioral escape. It will always make a very frightened cat worse, and any pathology worse.

If small children are involved, fear and fear aggression are serious conditions, because the children may not know how to appropriately respond to a cat who is crouching. Any animal who is cornered and cannot escape has the potential to attack. It is imperative that the cat not learn that his only recourse is aggression, as this could lead to the cat becoming aggressive in response to any approach. Behavior modification can be very effective early in the development of a fearful condition but you have to realize that it is developing.

Pharmacological intervention can be an especially useful addition to treating fearful and fearfully aggressive cats, because it may affect how reactive they become and how they learn.

Please be aware that it is not clear if any intervention can be successful if the condition is genetic. This does not mean you should not try to improve the quality of life for the fearful cat—you absolutely must do so—but intervention needs to focus more on management and avoidance than on changing the cat's global response to social interactions with humans. Please note, there is a full client handout to help with this serious problem: the **Protocol for Treating Fearful Behavior in Cats and Dogs.**

Maternal Aggression

Maternal aggression, as in dogs, may occur in the periparturient period, and may be normal behavior. Queens may protect nesting areas and kittens, and aggression in such situations may be appropriate. When aggression appropriate for protecting nest and kittens occurs, threats intended to thwart further approach are the rule. Attacks are rare. Such threats are usually directed toward unfamiliar individuals. When maternal aggression is a pathological problem, the aggression is directed toward known individuals who pose no threat. Avoidance is the strategy of choice, because a cornered queen can attack. As the kittens mature, the aggression—whether appropriate or not—usually resolves.

Redirected Aggression

Redirected aggression is seen in cats and dogs; however, it can be difficult to recognize in cats and may only be reported as incidental to another form of aggression. In redirected aggression, any interruption of an aggressive event between two parties by a third party results in redirection of the aggressive behavior to the third party or to another, uninvolved individual. It is important to realize that the interrupted aggressive event may only be a threat, so that the person (or animal) interrupting it may not realize what is occurring.

Cats appear to remain reactive for an extended period of time after being thwarted in an aggressive interaction, and if they continue to be reactive they can be quite hostile and potentially dangerous. Anyone who has a cat with redirected aggression needs to understand the potential risk and be aware of the subtle behaviors signaling the cat's increasing arousal and hostile intent. Because redirected aggression is often precipitated by another inappropriate behavior, it is essential to treat that behavior, as well. Treatment involves standard behavior modification techniques. If there is a socially mediated conflict within the household cats, some environmental modification may be necessary to decrease the extent to which the involved cats are capable of interacting. Clients should be encouraged to use inanimate objects (blankets, large pieces of cardboard, et cetera) to intervene between fighting animals. Use of objects minimizes danger to the clients and may have the benefit of aborting the behavior while teaching the cat that there are consistent, undesirable consequences to her inappropriate behavior. There is a separate, more detailed treatment handout on redirected aggression, **Protocol for Understanding and Treating Redirected Aggression in Dogs and Cats.**

Predatory Aggression

Predatory aggression in felines is similar to that in canines. Hallmarks of this aggression include stealth, silence, heightened attentiveness, body postures associated with hunting (slinking, head lowering, tail twitching, and pounce postures in cats), and lunging or springing at a "prey" item that exhibits sudden movement after a period of quiescence. Solitary predatory behavior is developed quite young in kittens (5 to 7 weeks of age), and cats can become proficient hunters by 14 weeks of age, especially if they are hungry.

Cats can exhibit appropriate, although sometimes undesirable, predatory behavior to small animals.

- Belling cats (Bear Bells: www.rei.com) can give some advance warning to small prey, but is not usually sufficient to avoid predation because of the element of stealth.
- Scat mats and indoor invisible fences are usually insufficient to deter a focused cat. No one should rely on such devices for protection of a victimized cat. *Aversive "treatments" like electronic mats can often make a reactive or aggressive cat more reactive or aggressive. There are also welfare and humane care issues involved in using these treatments and they are not recommended.*
- The best insurance for outdoor wildlife is to deny the cat access to them. In many parts of the world, this is becoming law as part of a strategy to protect endangered wildlife. Cat fences can fence either the cats or the wildlife in or out, giving both some ability to safely co-exist

(www.purrfectfence.com, www.catfencein.com, www.catterydesign.com).

Cats kept indoors live longer than outdoor cats and are healthier than are outdoor cats. Unfortunately, intellectual stimulation is often missing in the life of an indoor cat. This does not have to be the case and there are many clever ways to avoid having an under-stimulated, fat, unengaged cat. Food puzzles, active toys that respond when the cat moves them, and other animals are just a few suggestions. When taught to do so young, cats will happily walk on leashes and harnesses or be pushed in pet buggies. More information on this can be found in the **Protocol for Understanding and Managing Odd, Curious, and Annoying Feline Behaviors.**

It's important to distinguish *predatory aggression*, a diagnosis and abnormal manifestation of behavior, from *predatory behavior*, usually normal feline behavior, and contextually appropriate, if undesirable. There is a lot of variability in feline temperament regarding predatory inclinations. Some cats have no interest in hunting, whereas other cats make *inappropriate context distinctions about prey items.*

The latter situations become a concern if the prey item is the owner's foot or hand, or a young infant. Any cat who exhibits the pre-pounce behaviors described above in these contexts may be at risk for inappropriate predatory aggression. Cats have recurved teeth and claws so bites or scratches should always be taken seriously. If the injured human is very old, very young, ill, or immunocompromised, scratches and bites from cats must be viewed as serious risks for infection and be medically attended.

Concerns about true, predatory aggression (the pathological diagnosis) is another good reason to never leave young infants of any species alone when pets are present. The cat who regards an infant as a prey item usually ceases to do so once the infant has matured sufficiently to demonstrate normal postural responses (e.g., the puppy is independently and effectively mobile, the human infant sits up and looks like a human). Regardless, any kind of true feline predatory aggression is a potentially very dangerous situation and utmost caution is urged.

Impulse Control Aggression

Also called assertion or status aggression, impulse control aggression has been described as the "leave me alone bite" and most frequently occurs when the cat is being petted. The most similar situation in canines is also impulse control aggression (formerly "dominance" aggression); however, the divergent evolutionary history of canine and feline social systems argues that these are not homologous situations. These cats share with dogs with similar problems the need for control of the situation during a time of heightened reactivity. Given their different evolutionary histories, the mechanisms underlying the problem may be different for dogs and cats. Affected cats may be provoked by normal human behaviors. In other words, nothing you did provoked the cat intentionally; rather the cat becomes aroused when given attention and has a need to control when the attention starts and when it ceases. Some cats do this by biting and leaving, whereas the occasional cat will take your hand with its teeth, but not bite. Some biting can be severe.

Fortunately, you can learn to observe signs of impending aggression (staring, tail flicking, ears flat, pupils dilated, head hunched, claws possibly unsheathed, stillness or tenseness, low growl) and interrupt the behavior at the first sign of any of these by standing up and letting the cat fall from your lap. You can abandon the cat and refuse to interact until she is exhibiting an appropriate behavior.

Do not physically "correct" these cats, because the cat may view a physical correction as a threat, and it may further arouse and intensify her aggression. If your cat does not respond to passive control or to attempts to redirect her attention to a toy or other object, it is safer to protect yourself in a way that will stop the behavior (e.g., drop a blanket over the cat). This intervention should be the least aversive possible. Your goal is to interrupt your cat's behavior, not to teach her that you are a threat or someone to be feared.

If you can interrupt the behavior as it is starting, or, in a worst case scenario, within the first 30 to 60 seconds of the *onset* of the inappropriate behavior (which may be the pupil dilation and thoughts of stalking that the cat had when you sat on the sofa), you may encourage the cat to learn not to exhibit the behavior. However, if you scare the cat with your "interruption" you have done harm. Cats with this problematic aggression are never going to be hugely cuddly, although, if you can refrain from petting them, they may be willing to sit quietly on your lap for extended periods. Please note, there is a full protocol to help with this quite serious problem, **Protocol for Understanding and Treating Impulse Control Aggression in Cats.**

Intercat Aggression

"Normal," nonpathological aggression between cats is common only if the cats are toms. In most wild, feline social systems, few males mate with most of the females. The skewed sex ratio in the breeding population is induced and maintained by vigilance and aggression on the part of the males. There is an additional olfactory component of spraying and non-spraying marking that contributes to the aggression and relative "status." The aggression exhibited by males in these circumstances is classic and involves flattened ears, howling, hissing, piloerection, threats using eyes, teeth, and claws, and outright combat. Early neutering (prior to 12 months of age) decreases or prevents fighting by 90%. It is not clear if very early spaying and neutering programs would further reduce this, but given the hormonal facilitation of the aggression, one would hypothesize that this would be the case.

That said, **true intercat aggression, which is far more common and more likely than is territorial aggression, is pathological and is more commonly based on conflicts within social relationships/hierarchies than it is with sex.** Cats begin to become socially mature somewhere between 2 and 4 years of age. At this time, some cats may begin to challenge others. Problems arise when one cat will not accept lack of engagement by another cat. Responses include passive aggression (staring and posturing), active aggression (hissing, swatting, pouncing, biting), and marking. Cats who consider themselves as more equal are less likely to participate in overt and active aggression—expect covert and more passive aggression (Table 1 provides a sample format by which to understand the variants of this form of aggression). Intercat aggression is extremely complex, often subtle, and underappreciated.

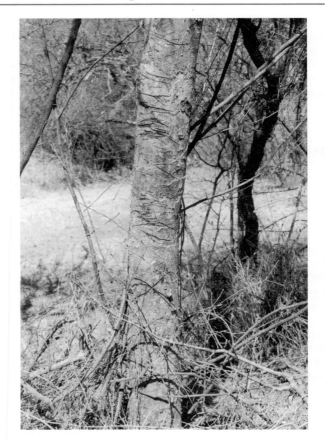

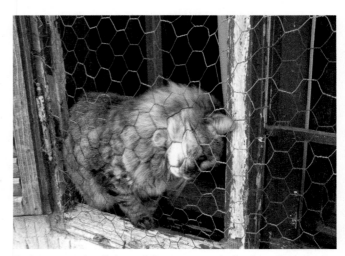

Cats can mark using scratches, as seen in the top photo, or by rubbing, as seen in the photo on the bottom. The tree at the top *(top photo)* sits between the area occupied by two groups of lions. Rubbing leaves an odor mark, and may leave an oily mark that is visible on a clean wall. Scratching leaves clear visual marks, in addition to the odor marks from foot glands.

Cats who are afraid of other cats can be afraid because they have been attacked, and may develop fearful behavior or fear aggression as sequelae. Fear can also develop without attack. Co-occurrence of diagnoses should alert clients and veterinarians to ask which came first.

Cats who react as if there is a challenge about social status when there is none are reacting inappropriately and out of

TABLE 1

Model for Thinking About Phenotypic Patterns of Feline Aggression

Potential Axes
- Overt vs. covert aggression
- Active vs. passive aggression
- Offensive vs. defensive aggression

Sample Scenarios
- Overt, passive, offensive aggression: confident cat staring when another enters room
- Overt, passive, defensive aggression: less-confident cat leaving room or backing up and withdrawing into smaller space, tail tucked, vocalizing
- Covert, passive, defensive aggression: vanquished or less-confident cat marking with mystacial glands in boundary areas or areas from which cat had been displaced
- Covert, active, offensive aggression: vanquished or less-confident cat marking with urine or feces in boundary areas or areas from which cat had been displaced
- Overt, active, offensive aggression: chase and attack using teeth and accompanied by vocalization by resident cat toward new cat in environment
- Overt, active, defensive aggression: attack or response using hitting and or swatting while leaning back or avoiding further pursuit
- Covert, active, defensive aggression: withdrawal and marking of restricted area by victim cat
- Covert, passive, offensive aggression: displacement or theft of "bully" or higher ranking cat's toys, bed, food, or hidden copulations (?), accompanied by non-elimination marking

context. If there is a challenge (staring, blocking, hackles up, hissing, swatting, growling, et cetera) of any kind, a reaction might be appropriate, but it is important to remember that as is true for people, many normal social behaviors in cats have rules. If one cat responds to another cat's stare or approach by leaving, it would then be an inappropriate social response for the staring cat to track down the cat who, appropriately, turned and left, and subject that cat to more aggression and more overt aggression. When this happens you know you have a problem. Most aggression in cats is far more subtle than it is in dogs, and because of this, may be more damaging to household situations.

Most intercat aggression occurs between housemates, and it may occur more commonly between different sex housemates, in contrast with dogs. Also, because feline systems are matrilineal, aggression may only become apparent after the loss of a "matriarch" or cat fulfilling this role. It is not unusual for cats to have lived in relative harmony together for 2 years before there are problems because the development of these problems reflects the intrinsic change that all social animals experience when they become socially mature.

Challenges can involve staring, vocalizing, or outright aggression. Cats can start with staring and escalate to overt aggression. Regardless, it is important to treat the problem as soon as it becomes apparent. The longer that the problem is allowed to persist, the worse the cats will get.

In profound cases of intercat aggression, the situation is not simple. This is especially true if multiple cats are in the household because cats form coalitions. This means that a cat who has been neutral to another specific cat may change her behavior depending on the addition or loss of new cats and the shifting of coalitions. Also, these relationships are not absolute. They change with age, health, and, most importantly, with context.

The behaviors associated with these relationships can be affected by the people who are present and by how those people interact with them. Some relationships apply only to feeding and sleeping orders. A cat who challenges one cat may not care about another cat in the household that, to all outward appearances, seems to act the same and be the same age and sex. Chances are they are not acting identically, and it is in the subtleties that the problems with the relationship occur.

Treatment of Intercat Aggression

Treatment of intercat aggression focuses on keeping everyone safe, and on setting and maintaining a new social arrangement where no one has to sustain constant threats. Generally, reinforcement (attention, play, treats, praise, et cetera) is given to the cat who is behaving most appropriately. You can most easily determine this by videotaping your cats and working with your veterinarian to understand what's going on between the cats. Identification of problem cats and those who are really normal is actually pretty easy if you can watch the cats in an unbiased manner. This is the advantage of videotape over real-time. The specifics of treatment follow.

- First, **never physically punish these cats.** All you will do is to raise their level of distress, and they might feel that they have to fight you off. Clients are often injured when disciplining or separating fighting animals. You could make a bad situation worse by further causing the involved cats to be reactive and to learn that you are a threat.
- Second, if at all possible, never reach between two fighting animals. Most people have good intentions and want to separate fighting animals to prevent injury to them, but if you place your body parts between the animals, you may be accidentally injured.
- If you know that you have a problem with your cats, watch them like a hawk any time they are together and keep cardboard, a broom, a bucket of water, a hose, a bottle of unopened club soda or seltzer, or a blanket handy. These are all "remote control" items that you can use to separate the cats safely. If no small children, high-strung humans, or nervous animals are in the house, a loud noise, like that generated by a foghorn, can also help to separate the animals *for whom nothing else works*, but this should be a last resort and is an indication that the cats' aggression is seriously out of control. **Screaming by humans, particularly young humans, will worsen the situation.**
- Generally, once the cats are apart, they start to calm down, and you can remove the aggressor. The aggressor should be locked in a neutral area with water, a litterbox, and, if they will eat, some food. You will have to plan ahead and be careful about how you will provision your cat, and ensure

that she is kept enclosed until she is truly calm. Please remember that **cats can stay reactive for 24 to 48 hours** and that you may have to banish them while still protecting yourself. By removing the victim, instead of the aggressor, you may enhance the "helplessness" of the victim in the eyes of the aggressor. You don't want to do this, if possible. Still, it is important to remember that any animal who is injured hurts and is frightened. Frightened animals can bite you without being malicious. Avoid potential bites by transporting cats to be separated using blankets and boxes.

Basic Treatment Tips and Tick List

1. First, keep all cats involved in the intercat aggression separated at all times when not supervised. If you are able to identify the aggressor, the aggressor cat should be confined to the less-desirable room (a spare bedroom, rather than your bedroom; a pen in the heated, well-lit basement, rather than the kitchen where the dogs are fed). All other cats should have free range. Again, watch for changes in coalitions that may not be in the direction that you find helpful!

2. Bell the cats with different sounding bells (Bear Bells: www.rei.com). Breakaway collars that will come apart if they snag on furniture or other objects are now widely available and are a safe option for attachment of bells in all environments. If the cats are loose, you must be willing to supervise them. The bell will tell you when the aggressor is approaching and when the problem animals are close together. The bell will also alert the victim cat that the aggressor is approaching. The cats can have a chance to approach each other **if and only if** you are confident that you can control them long-distance, and prevent any injury. Please remember that **injury can be physical or behavioral.** Of these, **the behavioral injury may be worse for many cats who learn to live in constant terror.** If you do not feel that you can control interactions, you must separate the cats in a manner that prevents fighting and covert threats such as stares or urine marks.

3. Choose an order in which to reinforce the cat based on identifying which cat is behaving the most appropriately. **Remember that reinforcement is not about rewarding the pushiest, most "dominant" cat;** it's about rewarding the cat who is most appropriate so that all the cats get the message that obnoxious behaviors are not rewarded, but calm, nonthreatening ones are.
   - Reinforcing the chosen cat has active and passive components. First, separate the cats as discussed above. Second, enforce the concept that the cat being threatened has the right to exist by feeding him first, letting him out before the others (if the cats go out), giving him a treat or toy first, playing with him first, grooming him first, et cetera.
   - **You are not imposing a "rank" order on these cats;** instead, you are encouraging the normal types of social deference that would be exhibited by cats under normal conditions. By reinforcing an appropriately behaved cat, you encourage the normal fluidity of the social system.
   - You can also more passively encourage the aggressor to understand that the victim has some status by allowing the victim to sleep in a crate in your room, on a bed there, or on your bed, while the other cat is banished to a room or crate outside your room. This has nothing to do with beds and "spoiling" and everything to do

with the fact that access to preferred spots or to attention is a currency.
   - Regardless of how you decide to work with the cats, each cat needs daily individual attention. The cat who is being reinforced should always get the attention first, in the presence of the other cat if this can be done quietly, and without threats or overt aggression. If necessary, restrain the inappropriate cat using a harness.
   - Treatment is about both understanding the neurochemical changes that occur with learning and repeated exposure, and about becoming humane. To do this, we must begin to see the world from the cat's point of view, which minimally requires that we let go of labels that may say more about us and our need than they do about the cat's behavior.s about rewarding the cat who is most appropriate so that all the cats get the message that obnoxious behaviors are not rewarded, but calm, nonthreatening ones are.

4. Use harnesses with cats, if they are going to be together. Harnesses give you a quick way to intervene if you need it, while gradually reintroducing the cats to each other when there is no attention being given. For example, watch TV while both cats sit quietly, secured at a distance where they can see each other, but not lunge, and connect.
   - If the cat who has been problematic stares at the cat you are trying to reinforce, gently turn his head away from the other cat and toward you so that he can take his cues from you.
   - If the cat who you are trying to reinforce stares at the other, ignore him if the other cat doesn't react.
   - If the other cat does react, interrupt the reaction by asking the staring cat to look at you. If this does not work, or if the aggression intensifies, remove the most aggressive cat and banish him.
   - If the cat who you are trying to reinforce stares at the other cat and the other cat looks away, reward them both with food treats—that is exactly the type of fluid and flexible behavioral relationship you are trying to reinforce.

5. Anti-anxiety medications may help or may be required for some cats who otherwise are not able to succeed in this program (Table 2). Please remember that if it's decided that medication could benefit your cat, you need to use it **in addition** to the behavior modification, not instead of it.
   - Benzodiazepines, although humanly abusable, can be excellent drugs for some cats who have combined elimination/aggression problems because of underlying nonspecific anxiety that results in a decrease in outgoing behavior in the affected cat. Clients should be advised to watch for any signs associated with liver disease, although these are extraordinarily rare. At low dosages, benzodiazepines act as mild calming agents, facilitating daytime activity by tempering excitement. At moderate dosages they act as anti-anxiety agents, facilitating social interaction in a more proactive manner. At high dosages they act as hypnotics, facilitating sleep. Ataxia and profound sedation usually only occur at dosages beyond those needed for anxiolytic effects. Note that the duration of action of the parent compound, diazepam, and its intermediate metabolite, nordiazepam (N-desmethyldiazepam) in cats is 5.5 hours and 21 hours, respectively. For this reason, it is

TABLE 2

Useful Medications (Brand Names Are Those in the United States)

- Alprazolam (Benzodiazepine; Xanax): for the victim, primarily, to make more outgoing and friendlier; for the aggressor if aggression is secondary to anxiety about interaction and increased friendliness will help
- Amitriptyline (TCA; Elavil): for the victim or aggressor with nonspecific anxiety
- Nortriptyline (TCA; Pamelor): for the victim or aggressor with nonspecific anxiety and sedation with amitriptyline
- Clomipramine (TCA; Clomicalm): for the victim or aggressor with more specific anxiety
- Buspirone (NSA; BuSpar): for the victim, only; may make more outgoing and situation resolves with some overt aggression
- Fluoxetine, paroxetine (SSRI; Prozac, Paxil): for more specific anxieties involving outburst (fluoxetine) and social (paroxetine) anxieties

best to choose benzodiazepines that do not use this intermediate metabolite (e.g., oxazepam, alprazolam).

- Tricyclic antidepressants (TCAs) act to inhibit serotonin and norepinephrine (NE) re-uptake, and can be useful for some cats that spray, some who are averse to or anxious about their litterbox, and cats who are experiencing anxiety about their social situation. Drugs of choice include amitriptyline and its active intermediate metabolite, nortriptyline, and clomipramine. Knowledge of intermediate metabolites can be important: Animals experiencing sedation or other side effects with the parent compound may do quite well when treated with the intermediate metabolite alone. For example, cats who become sedated or nauseous when treated with amitriptyline may respond well when treated with nortriptyline at the same dose as the former has twice the NE re-uptake effect of the latter.

- Partial 5-HT$_{1A/B}$ agonists (e.g., buspirone) have few side effects, do not negatively affect cognition, allow rehabilitation by influencing cognition, attention, arousal, and mood regulation, and may aid in treating aggression associated with impaired social interaction. Because buspirone may make cats more outgoing and assertive, you may have overt aggression where it previously did not occur, as part of the outcome of changing social interactions.

- The selective serotonin reuptake inhibitors (SSRIs) (fluoxetine, paroxetine, sertraline, and fluvoxamine) are derivatives of TCAs. These compounds have a long half-life, and after 2 to 3 weeks, plasma levels peak within 4 to 8 hours. Because these medications act to induce receptor conformation changes, an action that can take 3 to 5 weeks, treatment must continue for a minimum of 6 to 8 weeks before a determination about efficacy can be made. Most of the SSRI effects are a result of highly selective blockade of the reuptake of 5-HT$_{1A}$ into presynaptic neurons.

- Newer treatments involving synthetic pheromonal analogues (e.g., Feliway in spray or diffuser form) have not been subject to the type of rigorous, blinded scientific testing to demonstate an effect. Few good, scientific studies have been conducted, and the need for such studies is more critical in this situation than in those involving some oral medications because the mechanism of action of pheromonal analogues is often asserted, but remains little tested and unknown. In the few studies that provide reliable information, effects are minimal and may involve some lowering of overall reactivity.

PROTOCOL FOR UNDERSTANDING, MANAGING AND TREATING IMPULSE CONTROL/STATUS-RELATED AGGRESSION IN CATS

Overview of the Role for Social Systems in This Diagnosis

Cats do not have social systems that are identical to those of dogs or humans, but they still have a system where some individuals have relatively different status than others. Usually, any conflicts about controlling status occur only with other cats. Occasionally, some cats will exhibit behaviors usually seen only with cats in social contexts involving humans. This situation is similar, but likely not identical, to that seen in dogs diagnosed with impulse control aggression. This problem has been termed assertion or status-related aggression, but may be more appropriately termed feline impulse control aggression.

Patterns of Behavior Exhibited by the Cat

Some cats have been described as disliking attention or as rejecting petting ("the leave-me-alone bite"). The problem with this description is that, as is true for dogs with impulse control aggression, these cats often seek people out and monitor their behaviors. For affected cats, rejecting attention by biting is the most obvious sign of the pathology. If you watch these cats, you will usually note that the affected cat stares at you and that you often—consciously or not—avoid the cat's stare. Some of these cats constantly block access to furniture or to pathways, like doors and hallways, in a similar way that they would block access to another cat about whom they were concerned.

Some of these cats rub everywhere a particular person has been or rub (or even spray!) the people whom they monitor and attempt to control. Some cats never display any aggressive behaviors, but may exhibit the same marking behaviors in the context of including humans and cats in the same social group. Scent marking, alone, is not sufficient to make a diagnosis of impulse control aggression. Impulse control aggression is about control or access to control of the human by the cat, and scent marking may be only one aspect of this condition.

Cats with impulse control aggression actively solicit attention by jumping into someone's lap, and then biting if they are petted or shifted. Unlike the friendly, solicitous cat who is calm, relaxed, and attentive without being forceful when seeking attention from humans, cats with impulse control aggression are tense, forceful, vigilant, and watchful, and become more aroused and reactive as they seek and receive attention. Cats with exaggerated impulse control/status-related aggression may lie on their people, batting at them to make them settle in positions that the cat controls, and then biting the people if they do not do this, or if they move. These pathological cats are good at both passive and active control of human behavior.

This is a confusing diagnosis, especially in the developing stages, because sometimes these cats appear to enjoy petting until they reach a threshold where they become so reactive that they will savage the person attempting to cuddle them. As the condition progresses, the threshold for their reactivity lowers, and even short petting sessions may be provocative for them.

Any intense need to control others in any species is pathological.

When your cat initiates petting, she might tolerate touching if there is no manipulation like cuddling or moving. These human behaviors may be viewed by the cat as an attempt at control.

For some cats, any petting will be met with frank aggression, usually biting. Once the impulse control aggression is fully developed, these cats seldom swat with their claws first, a behavior that often accompanies most normal forms of feline antagonistic behavior. Instead, these cats become stiff, may twitch their tail, erect the hair down their back and tail, put their ears back, dilate their pupils, unsheathe and flex their claws, growl, and bite. All of these behaviors will occur in close proximity to each other, seemingly mirroring their enhanced neurochemical reactivity.

The Unique Case of the Cat's Brain and Reactivity

The pathological need to control occurs despite—not because of—the behaviors of the human, strongly suggesting that these cats cannot read, process, or act on information about whether there is a truly contextual threat to them in social situations involving humans. Like dogs, their response to this pathological anxiety is to control and preempt any responses that they find uncertain. The form that these impulsive responses take is a result of a peculiarity of the feline brain that allows cats to remain aroused for prolonged periods of time (24 to 48 hours) and to become extremely quickly aroused. Cats have been used as a model for seizure activity in humans because the cells in the *hypothalamus*, the region responsible for triggering an initial threat or stress response, are stimulated easily and they recruit other cells, quickly making these cats extremely reactive. The same underlying mechanism may result in impulse control aggression.

As is true for dogs, anxiety-related conditions in cats become fully developed at social maturity. Cat social systems are composed of extended family groups and matrilineal systems that may promote a slightly older age for social maturity (probably between 2 and 4 years). Clients are often unable to understand why the cat "changed." He "changed" because his brain chemistry changed as he moved through social maturity, a pattern seen in all social species studied.

Helping the Cat

The key to controlling impulse control aggression is the same for dogs and cats: You cannot allow the cat to have control, *and* you have to remove or address the need for pathological control. This is tougher than it sounds, because most of the cat's behaviors may have been so passive that you may not have recognized these behaviors as aggressive. The tick list below provides specific guidance about how to alter these behaviors. The key to treating these cats is to provide clear, reliable, humane rule structures that ensure that interactions with humans are predictable to the cat, and safe for the human.

These cats may never be cuddly (and you would be well advised to never expect them to be so), but they can learn to live harmoniously in the household, and will usually do well with a cat that *is* cuddly.

Finally, please remember that these cats are ***potentially very dangerous.*** Cats with profound impulse control/status-related aggression will become reactive when they are uncertain about social interactions where the human is not actually focusing on the cat (e.g., when the human is talking on the phone). Because affected cats become so uncertain and reactive at these times, they will bite humans without preamble, and then often run away. Affected cats behave in this way because it's the rule that they use to avoid their own anxiety and to control their own reactivity about uncertainty. If we create an alternative rule structure that specifies how and when cats will get attention in a humane way we can change their behaviors, keep ourselves safe, and create a safer and richer relationship with our cats.

Tick List for Avoiding and Treating Impulse Control Aggression in Cats

1. Avoid all situations in which you know that the cat might react inappropriately. Do not view this as "giving into the cat." View it as a necessary and humane step to keep the cat's brain chemistry as non-reactive as possible.

2. Be suspicious of these cats when they jump into your lap. Watch them carefully. At the first sign of any unsheathed claws, tensing of muscles, twitching of tail, movement of ears, or rippling of back, stand up and let the cat fall from your lap. Do not reach for, pick up, or push these cats from your lap. These actions by you will be treated as a confirmation by the cat that you are a threat and need to be controlled, so you will be bitten. This all happens within seconds. *If you do not think that you can monitor your cat if she jumps into your lap, do not allow her to jump into your lap.*

3. If your cat does not give a lot of warning of impending reactivity, keep with you at all times a blanket, a bottle of water, or something else that will interrupt his behavior. Whatever you choose to carry, please remember that:
   * You wish to protect yourself.
   * By interrupting your cat early in the process of becoming aggressive, he will not be able to "practice" and improve his aggressive behaviors.
   * You wish to keep the cat's reactivity at the lowest level possible so that the cat does not stay reactive for a long period of time; in this way he will not learn how to become more reactive.
   * You do not wish to scare or threaten the cat; this will just convince him that you are a threat and not to be trusted.

   Accordingly, you need to use the lowest level of "stimulus" that will stop the cat. You want him to refocus his attention and abandon the aggression. By covering your cat with a blanket, you may be able to safely put him in another, neutral room where he can calm. Only when he is calm—and this may take 24 to 48 hours—can you release your cat and calmly and patiently interact with him. Do not pet him. Talk softly to him and ensure that he is nonreactive before any of your interactions progress further. Use food and praise to reward calm cats who are lying or sitting down and not staring at you.

4. If your cat appears calm in your lap, you can give her one to two pets. You, not the cat, always have to terminate the attention and regulate the amount of attention as part of the new rule structure that will increase the predictability of your behavior and the outcome of the interaction for the cat. Do not get involved in a love-fest—you are putting yourself at risk. Cease petting your cat ***before*** she reacts.

5. *If you are too fearful of your cat to do the above, do not interact with her.* Do not feel guilty. Your cat will benefit from not having to interact in uncertain circumstances.

6. Use a breakaway collar and put a bell on it (Bear Bells: www.rei.com) so that you know where your cat is at all times. Monitor his movements. Do not let your cat surprise you by attacking you as you pass a doorway or come around a corner. Remember that under these conditions the cat has incomplete information and will be more reactive. If you know where the cat is you can invite him to come to you, to sit and be calm, and to accompany you calmly by using treats and praise (see the **Protocol for Deference**). If you cannot yet ask the cat to come calmly with you, carry your blanket at all times and use it to interrupt aggression and prevent injury.

7. Do not let your cat control your access to anything. Ask the cat to move from the location and come to you for a treat. If your cat will not work for treats—he may be too reactive for this—try throwing a toy that he will chase. If your cat will not move, either abandon the cat so that there is no longer any value to the cat in controlling your access to the area or, if you must have access, use a blanket, broom, cardboard box, et cetera, to gently move the cat. Do not use your hands or feet to move the cat; the cat will see these behaviors as a challenge (the broom may also be seen as a challenge) and the cat will become more reactive, not less reactive. When you consider how reactive your cat is in such situations, there may be very few circumstances where you feel you must have immediate access to the area the cat is controlling. This is a good decision because it minimizes risk to you and to the cat.

8. You can teach your cat to do tricks that require the cat to defer to you in exchange for small food rewards (tiny pieces of tinned shrimp or sardines, boiled chicken livers, shredded boiled chicken) (See the **Protocol for Deference** and the **Protocol for Relaxation: Behavior Modification Tier 1**). Decide what you want the cat to do (e.g., lie down, or reach up and touch your hand with his paw). *If you do not feel safe teaching these behavior modification protocols and offering treats, consider clicker training your cat and rewarding his appropriate behaviors by tossing him tiny treats. If your cat is a picky eater, keep him a little hungry by offering smaller meals so that you can practice the behavior modification exercises frequently.*

   If at any time your cat's pupils dilate, her ears go back, or she shows any of the other signs discussed above, cease interaction. Wait until your cat comes to you for attention before interacting again, and ask her to sit and calm for a treat. If she again becomes reactive, move away as discussed above.

9. If your cat rubs against you and marks you, remove yourself from the situation after one to two rubs. This way you have participated in the social interaction where chemical information is exchanged, but you have not allowed your cat to become so reactive that she must control you.

10. Remember that dogs and cats do not have identical social systems. Their behaviors can differ although they may exhibit similar signals. If you are more familiar with dogs than with cats, watch your cat's specific behaviors.

11. Most of these cats are so persistent and distressed that they would benefit from anti-anxiety medication. Because of the impulsive nature of this condition and the uniquely feline pattern of recruiting many neurons quickly in reactive responses, medication may be the most humane choice. All medication should be used in addition to, not instead of, behavioral and environmental modification.

12. If you do not wish to monitor the cat, isolate him when you cannot or will not be able to work with him. This can be as simple as closing a door. Ensure that the room where the cat is enclosed has water, a litterbox, and, depending on the length of time you expect the cat to be there, some food.

13. Please remember that some cats are more aroused when in the presence of some herbs (catnip, garden mints). If your cat becomes more aroused, you will want to avoid exposure to these herbs.

14. *Left untreated,* some of these cats can become too dangerous to keep in some households. If that is the case, very few of them can go to another, very special home. Please do not turn these cats loose on the streets.

15. *If anyone is scratched or bitten by your cat seek competent medical help immediately. Cats have curved teeth and claws. Cat bites and scratches become infected easily and can be dangerous.*

PROTOCOL FOR UNDERSTANDING AND TREATING CANINE PANIC DISORDER

Overview of Panic Disorder

Canine panic disorder (PD) is characterized by a profound reaction to specific external or internal stimuli, and to some memory of these stimuli and how they made the dog feel. The stimuli could be visual, could involve a sound, taste or smell/odor, or could involve a pattern of social behaviors or signals. In some cases the dog appears to react only to a memory or perception of how a certain circumstance made her feel in the past. We cannot know what dogs "perceive," but we do know that dogs have excellent memories and the same brain architecture and function as do humans, so when we see behaviors consistent with true panic, even if the stimuli are not present, we need to consider that the memory of these stimuli, or the memory of the sensation that the stimuli may have caused, could be what is distressing the dog. One of the most problematic and recognized triggers for PD in dogs is entrapment, or its perception.

What Are the Signs of Panic Disorder?

The classic signs of PD are an extreme version of the signs seen in true phobias, including noise and storm phobia. Signs shown by the dog include intense avoidance of or attempts to escape from the situation that is distressing them. Specific and commonly seen signs are all associated with arousal of the sympathetic ("fight or flight") branch system of the autonomic nervous system (ANS) and may include:

- urination,
- defecation,
- vocalization,
- salivation,
- trembling/shaking,
- increased and unfocused motor activity,
- decreased motor activity or freezing,
- random destruction, and
- escape behaviors.

How Is Panic Disorder Different from a Phobia?

A trigger or focus of most phobias can be identified. This may not be true for PD. PD is triggered internally, and even when a trigger is identified, the *panic appears to be associated with the memory or perception of how some event caused the dog to feel, and it may not matter if the trigger is present.* Because PD is associated with memory or perception, avoidance of and withdrawal by the dog from the stimulus/trigger, as we see in fear and phobias, is just not possible. Our memories follow us.

Dogs with PD may be incapable of accepting any external information that could keep them safe or calm. The hallmark of PD is that these dogs have decreased sensitivity to pain and social stimuli, and so can do themselves great harm. These dogs experience these profound, non-graded, extreme responses in a way that is—externally—out of context to the environment or stimulus that provoked them.

If your dog has experienced one panic event, her risk of future events increases. This pattern is probably a result of what happens in a profoundly reactive region of the brain called the *amygdala*, where adaptive fear memories are quickly

formed. When something goes wrong, the result is a dog with a *pathological response to the memory or perception of an experience* who panics under such circumstances.

What Else Should You Watch for?

PD is a classic example of a co-morbid condition. This means that it occurs with another anxiety-related condition. Only very rarely is a dog seen with PD and no other anxiety-related condition, but it can happen. PD is more commonly diagnosed in dogs who also suffer from fear, noise reactivity or phobia, separation anxiety, generalized anxiety disorder (GAD), and/or obsessive-compulsive disorder (OCD).

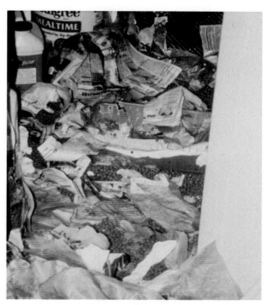

Random destruction in a pantry that occurred during a panicky event when a dog was left alone. None of the food was eaten; severely distressed individuals cannot eat.

PD may be the result of "entrapment" that is real or imagined. Dogs who are crated can panic because they cannot "escape."

- It is not surprising that a dog who may have been entrapped in a crate during a fire in the house could panic when crated. Everyone would consider that response to be normal.
- Most dogs who exhibit PD when crated, gated, kenneled, or otherwise enclosed, have *not* experienced anything external that is awful or threatening. For the vast majority of dogs who experience PD when confined, nothing happened to them in their crate, *except* that they could not leave.

These dogs cannot be confined because to do so would be to force them to experience PD. These dogs have been known to kill themselves in the process of trying to escape whatever confined them.

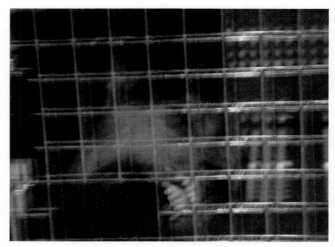

Dog panicking and biting at crate.

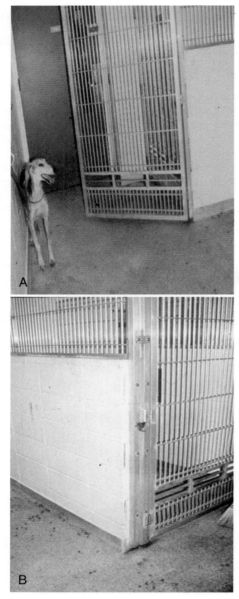

A dog who panicked when kenneled. She urinated, broke her claws (see blood on wall), and crashed into and spilled her food (B). Notice that she was still panting when the photo was taken (A).

Do Dogs Suffer from Posttraumatic Stress Disorder and Could Canine Posttraumatic Stress Disorder Be a Special Case of Panic Disorder?

The answer to this question is "maybe." Canine posttraumatic stress disorder (C-PTSD) is best described as a profound, nongraded, extreme response manifested as intense avoidance, escape, or anxiety, and associated with the sympathetic branch of the ANS in response to exposure to an identifiable, untenable (from the patient's perspective) stimulus or situation that the individual was unable to avoid or from which escape was impossible when these behavioral and physical signs were first felt. *Confirming behaviors can include mania or catatonia concomitant with decreased sensitivity/responsiveness to pain or social*

stimuli. Once the response is established, repeated exposure to any aspect of the original circumstance that triggered the original response, or that triggers a memory of the original response, results in an invariant pattern characteristic for that patient.

For a diagnosis of PTSD to be made, the response must be characteristic, the triggering event must be known and truly and profoundly traumatic or associated with some aspect of the trauma (and this could be an odor), and the response must only occur in a circumstance where some aspect of the triggering event is perceived by the dog.

In most pet dogs these criteria are difficult, but not impossible, to meet. A number of military dogs have met the criteria for this diagnosis, as have some pet dogs.

How Can We Treat Panic Disorder?

PD is a serious and debilitating behavioral condition that must be treated as soon as it is noticed. Anyone who uses a crate, gate, or kennel should inspect it daily for any signs that the dog may have tried to escape. If the dog was simply trying to leave, most of the damage may be concentrated around the locking mechanism. If the dog panicked, the damage is not so focused and rational.

If you are not sure whether your dog is panicking, videotape her when she is engaging in the behavior you think is a concern. Most modern video cameras are small and can easily record long videos in the event that you are not home when the dog may be panicking. If you show the video to your veterinarian, you will have provided extremely helpful information that will help with the design of a good treatment program.

If your dog panics when enclosed, treatment must involve finding a way to contain her safely without triggering the PD. For dogs who react to crates or runs, a larger crate or run will not suffice. Because so much of this condition is about how the dog "perceives" her world, you will get your best information about what distresses your dog by watching her. In some cases, day boarding or doggie daycare may be the best option.

Teaching the dog to begin to relax as soon as she feels the onset of a bout of panic is key to successful treatment. It is unlikely that you will be able to attain this goal without medication.

Depending on your dog's overall arousal level, how easily the PD is triggered, your ability to recognize and intervene before the trigger provokes the PD and whether other co-morbid conditions are involved, your dog will also need a daily medication, usually a selective serotonin reuptake inhibitor (SSRI) or a medication in a related class. For successful treatment to occur, we need to be able to:

- recognize and prevent the reaction to the trigger, even if it is internal,
- abort any panic attack that occurs, and
- raise the dog's threshold for reaction.

This three-part strategy generally requires the use of medication on both a daily and as-needed basis.

Medications that are most effective in breaking through and preventing the panicky events that characterize PD include:

- alprazolam, the panicolytic benzodiazepine (see the **Generalized Guidelines for Using Alprazolam for Noise and Storm Phobias, Panic, and Severe Distress**),
- other benzodiazepines, including clonazepam, for dogs who do not respond well to alprazolam,
- gabapentin, a compound that looks like the inhibitory transmitter, gamma-aminobutyric acid (GABA), but which is not active, and

- medications that affect central control of heart rate, like clonidine.

For more information on these and other medications please see the **Protocol for Using Behavioral Medication Successfully.**

Medication will allow you to help your dog attain a level of normalcy or calm that will permit her to learn to become more relaxed. This is the first step in learning to not react to her triggers, whether they are external or internal.

Your dog should start to work with the three foundation behavior modification protocols as soon as possible: the **Protocol for Deference,** the **Protocol for Teaching Your Dog to Take a Deep Breath and Use Other Biofeedback Methods as Part of Relaxation,** and the **Protocol for Relaxation: Behavior Modification Tier 1.** For some dogs, "as soon as possible" will be immediately, but for other dogs some response to medication will first be needed so that the dog is sufficiently calm to effectively learn new behaviors. One of the advantages of the newer behavioral medications is that *they actually speed the rate at which dogs acquire new behaviors through behavior modification.* Dogs affected with PD suffer so much that this is very good news.

PROTOCOL FOR UNDERSTANDING AND TREATING DOGS WITH NOISE AND STORM PHOBIAS

Overview of the Problem

Noise and storm/thunderstorm phobias are relatively common in dogs and may vary in commonness and intensity based on geographic location and frequency and severity of the noises. Not all reactions to storms are the same—some involve avoidance behaviors, some involve fear, and some involve outright panic. Not all noises are perceived to be the same to dogs. Some dogs can tolerate fireworks, but not storms or gunfire. Some dogs can tolerate gunfire, but not city noise, backfires of cars, or noises made by plastic bags or metal trash cans. Some noise-phobic dogs flee at the crackle of a fireplace or the alarm on a refrigerator or clothes dryer. It is extremely helpful to ensure that you know all the noises to which your dog reacts and that you share this list with your veterinarian.

If you are not sure what noises upset your dog, watch carefully. Videoing the dog in a number of environments and when you are not home will also help. Knowing whether dogs react to noise and to which noises they react is essential for the dog's well-being. Research shows that noise reactions often co-occur with other anxiety-related disorders that would otherwise not have been diagnosed. A tendency to react to noise may predispose dogs to other conditions. There is some evidence that the genes associated with noise reactivity in dogs appear to affect how dogs process information so early intervention is the humane solutions.

The key to treating these types of phobic reactions is to address them early in their ontogeny or development. **Left untreated, these types of problems—virtually without exception—become worse.** We now know that there are inherited forms of noise reactivity and phobias, and that herding dogs are often affected. If you know that at least one parent reacted to storms and, or other noises, expect the chances that the pup will react to be great, and look for early signs that may put the pup at risk. The same tools we use to treat noise reactivity and noise phobia can help prevent it from developing further if caught early in a dog with a known familial risk.

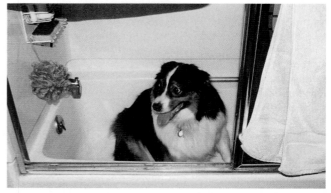

This Australian shepherd differs from the one below, who paces during storms. Instead, this dog freezes and tries to escape lightening.

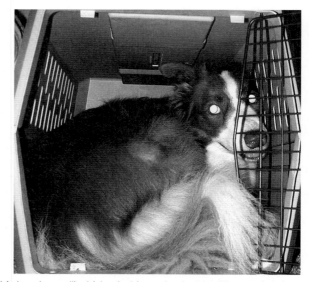

This border collie hides in his crate, but is still completely panicked. (Photo courtesy of Melanie Chang.)

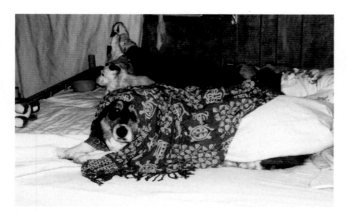

This Australian shepherd has been treated with a benzodiazepine, so she can hide and rest under a sheet rather than endlessly pace.

Noise Reactivity and Its Association with Other Anxiety-Related Conditions

Data indicate that if a dog has storm or noise phobia he may be more at risk for the development of separation anxiety, generalized anxiety disorder, panic disorder and, possibly, other anxiety-related conditions. The signs of noise phobia and separation anxiety can be the same: trembling, salivation, defecation, urination, destruction, escape, panting, vocalization, pupil dilation, cringing, et cetera. Not all dogs exhibit all signs, and not all dogs exhibit their signs with equal intensity. Some signs cluster together more frequently than others, although the neurochemical significance of this is currently unknown. We **do** know that the more signs the animal exhibits, and the longer the phobia has been ongoing, or the more profound the dog's reaction, the worse the case.

This handout discusses treatment for noise and storm phobias. Because of the commonness of these conditions, and the general lack of information available, this handout is more technical than most other handouts and contains information that clients can best use in consultation with their veterinarian.

Behavioral Approaches to Treatment

Treatment focuses on altering the dog's response to the stimuli by teaching the dog the competing behavior of relaxing. This part of the behavior modification requires that the dog is not inadvertently rewarded for his fearful or anxious response. For example, even if the dog is cringing under the bed and panting, *clients should not tell the dog that it is "okay," and they should not pet the dog.*

- First, it is not "okay," and the dog knows it. Most dogs associate the word "okay" with a behavior that is encouraged and rewarded. Telling them it is "okay" when it is not will confuse the dog and leave her without a clear road map of what is expected. As a result, the dog could become more anxious, although this is clearly an unintended consequence.
- Petting the dog can act in the same way as telling the dog that it is "okay." Petting is a reward; unfortunately, what is being rewarded is the anxious behavior. This is not what the client intends, but it can be what the dog learns. We also have to consider the possibility that for some dogs the petting is just one more stimulus that adds to an overly "noisy," stimulating, mental environment that will make the dog unhappier and worse.

So what can someone who wishes to help the dog do? *Watch the dog and learn what behaviors of yours, if any, calms the dog.*

- Try either leaving the dog alone in a space that is as calm and quiet as possible, if she is not at risk for injury, or just stay quietly by the dog. Quiet association can provide solace and security without accidentally rewarding the dog.
- And instead of petting the dog, just put *gentle continuous pressure,* either with an arm or the whole body, on the dog. This pressure works in most mammals to calm general arousal. If permitted by the dog, you can lean on or against the dog and you will likely feel the dog exhale and the muscles begin to relax. Obviously, if the dog becomes more frantic, you have learned that this is a dog who needs to be left alone or just subject to soft touching.
- Crates may help some animals who like their crate and who voluntarily go there as a place to relax. In this case, a blanket draped over a crate may help these dogs. Dogs who dislike being crated will learn to fear the crates if they are forced to be in one during a storm. They will feel trapped, and the entrapment factor will make their phobia and panic worse.
- Sometimes, darker rooms, closets, rooms without windows, spaces under desks are sought by dogs who are distressed. Provide these opportunities and see if the dog calms. If she is calmer, you have one tool for helping your dog through her distress.

- Dog runs—almost without exception—will make storm phobic dogs worse, because the dogs cannot escape, feel fully surrounded by the storm, and, if there is a roof, it is usually of a material that makes the sounds odder and louder. Clients who keep their dogs outdoors may not even know if their dog reacts to storms until the dog runs away, breaks through the run, or breaks her teeth and otherwise injures herself attempting escape. Simple containment is not a solution for this very debilitating diagnosis.
- There are anecdotal reports of successful use of "calming caps" and "anxiety wraps." "Calming caps" alter what the dog can see and apply some mild pressure to the head and face. They are not suitable for aggressive dogs who cannot be manipulated, for dogs who cannot stand having anything over their face, or for those who will panic if they cannot see something. The "anxiety wraps" (www.anxietywrap.com, www.thundershirt.com) are meant to function very much like putting gentle but constant physical pressure on a dog would. Neither of these tools can easily be put on a dog who is thrashing around. Whether these tools are helpful has not really been rigorously tested, but some clients may wish to try them and collect the data for their dog. Repeated use may be somewhat helpful for some dogs.
- One trendy addition to the list of tools available is the Storm Defender Cape (www.stormdefender.com). This wraparound, belted cape seeks to decrease the dog's exposure to static electricity that may be associated with some storms. The principle being used here is that of a Faraday cage, where a mesh grid, usually copper, blocks transmission of static electricity. All MRI units, for example, have Faraday cages built into their walls and doors. The cape does not cover the dog's head, legs, or tail, so coverage is incomplete. The extent to which the dog may benefit may depend on the trigger for the dog's reactivity, the dog's body size, and the type of storm. One study showed that a "placebo cape" was just as effective as the brand name cape, suggesting that paying attention to the dog's needs and/or allowing the dog to feel snug may help.

Using Behavior Modification Rationally

Most active behavior modification involves desensitization (DS; gradual exposure to the stimulus or sound at a level below which the patient reacts; the sound volume is slowly increased over days or weeks as the dog continues to not react) and counter-conditioning (CC; rewarding the dog for not reacting with a stimulus like a food treat that competitively interferes with the dog's ability to react), or some combination of the two. The **Protocol for Deference** and the **Protocol for Relaxation: Behavior Modification Tier 1** are really plans for how to conduct basic desensitization and counter-conditioning. You can use these basic behavior mod plans with a program that involves exposing dogs to noises to which they react. Few quantitative studies examining the effects of this form of behavior modification on noise phobias exist, but *the general impression is that these types of desensitization programs, by themselves, don't work well for dogs with fully established phobias.* If the reaction to the noise or storm has just started, exposure to these sounds using tapes, records, or CDs and an excellent stereo or quadraphonic sound system that can mimic some of the vibrational changes *might* work. Sources for these recordings change frequently, but CDs of natural events are available at some nature-themed stores or similar online sites, and there are many sources of a variety of noises from storms to explosions available online for those willing to search, and many of these have been produced with the intent of using them to desensitize dogs.

However, if the reaction to noise is severe, or has been ongoing a long time, exposure to recordings of noises and storms, alone, is unlikely to help and **may do further harm to the dog. Under no circumstance should anyone continue to expose a dog to these recordings if the dog remains at the same level of distress or becomes more distressed.** In some cases, as dogs begin to improve with drug treatment, exposure to sound recordings can be added and can help, but caution is urged regarding searches for quick fixes—there are none.

That said, devices that alter the dog's perception of the environment may help. Eye shades that permit either no light (useful for intense lightning storms and fireworks) or diffuse light can help some dogs to relax. If this is true, tinted Doggles or those with mesh may help (www.doggles.com) (see Figure A, below). Ear protection for dogs is also available in the form of Mutt Muffs® (www.muttmuffs.com) (see Figure B, below). Some dogs can gain relief from the use of any basic eye mask, like those used by humans on plane flights, that prevents them from seeing flashes of light. Because these fit loosely, most dogs do not resist them. Dogs should become used to these when not distressed (see Figures C and D, below). Any set of reactions that can be diminished will help the dog to improve, overall.

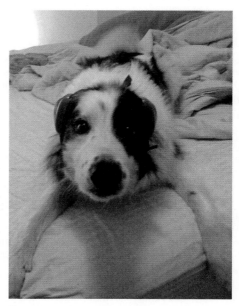

Figure B Muttmuffs. (Photo courtesy of Angelica Steinker.)

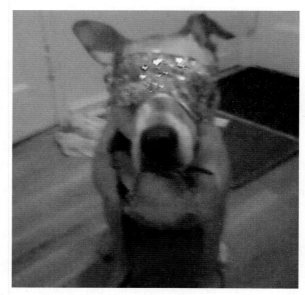

Figure C Human eye shades adapted for use on a dog. (Photo courtesy of Christina Shusterich.)

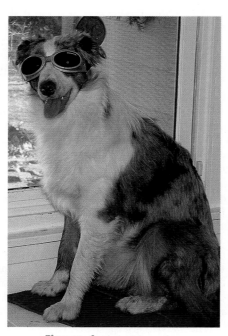

Figure A Tinted Doggles.

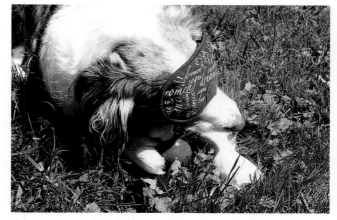

Figure D Accustoming dogs to human eye shades using an activity the dog enjoys.

Treatment Involving Medication

The most common, modern treatments for noise phobias involve drug treatment with medications designed to reduce or abort anxiety and panic. Most of the medications used are members of the class of drugs known as benzodiazepines, although alpha-agonists like clonidine and medications that affect serotonin like trazodone are being used more often. These drugs can have some drawbacks, including the potential induction of physiological dependence and the subsequent abuse that can follow. Dogs cannot open the bottles of medication by themselves so both abuse of and physiological dependence on benzodiazepines are avoidable, but there are some households that should not have benzodiazepines present. However, if used rationally for a dog who has had a complete physiological and laboratory evaluation that revealed no abnormalities, the benefits of this class of medication can be great and the risks few.

The list of medications commonly used to treat storm and noise phobias focuses primarily on benzodiazepines that can be given by mouth: diazepam, clorazepate, lorazepam, and alprazolam, with alprazolam being the drug of choice.

These medications are usually given "as needed," which is generally interpreted to be every 4 to 6 hours, the approximate half-life of many of the benzodiazepines. Instructions for how to use benzodiazepines, in general, and alprazolam, specifically are found in the handout, **Generalized Paradigm for Using Alprazolam for Noise and Storm Phobias, Panic, and Severe Distress.**

For dogs who react poorly to benzodiazepines, or who may not respond to them at all, some success has been reported for treatment of noise reactivity using clonidine, a medication that acts to block some of the cardiac reactivity that accompanies a panicky response.

The key to getting these medications to work is to get them into the dog **before** there are any behavioral, physical, or physiological signs of distress. For storm-related phobias, clients need to learn what the trigger for their dog is because it *may not* be the noise per se. Triggers can include flashes of light, noise, atmospheric pressure changes, ozone levels, et cetera. There are now a number of tools that can help clients monitor storms, including barometers, but the most useful might be Doppler radar. There are many weather programs that will download to laptops or handheld devices and can be set to alert you to certain atmospheric clues.

Regardless of the dog's cue, the client must get the drug into the dog **before** the dog begins to react to the stimulus. Accordingly, it may be good advice to recommend that the dog should be medicated if there is a 50% chance or greater of a storm and/or if the barometer is dropping.

The medications above are listed in order of duration from longer to shorter action of the parent compound. That said, no one wants a sedated or incoordinated dog and some of these medications (diazepam and clorazepate) are more likely to sedate dogs than are others (alprazolam). Alprazolam lacks an intermediate metabolite found in the other two medications that makes patients sleepy, so it is a better choice for most dogs. If people need very-long-acting benzodiazepines, medications like clonazepam, often used for some types of seizures and for sleep disorders, may be beneficial as it has a very long half-life (the amount of time it takes for one-half of the medication to leave your system).

Because so many of these medications produce another medication after passing through the liver, knowing the half-lives of both functional compounds and the individual dog's response to the medication may help you to know how frequently you need to provide medication for your dog. Benzodiazepines can be terrific medications, but they vary hugely in effect from one individual to the next. This lack of predictable effect is one reason why benzodiazepines are not used as often as they once were.

Clonidine, a centrally acting alpha$_{2A}$-adrenergic receptor agonist, is a hypotensive that lowers blood pressure by decreasing the amount of blood pumped and the tone or resistance of blood vessels. Clonidine is increasingly used in situations in which either the benzodiazepine and/or combinations of tricyclic anti-depressants/selective serotonin reuptake inhibitors have failed or are insufficient, and in dogs who are so hyperreactive that decreasing their sympathetic tone and arousal associated with noradrenaline/norepinephrine will help. Clonidine and other alpha-agonists show promise in treating dogs with profound noise phobia and panic disorders. Like benzodiazepine, it can be used as needed, and is generally given 30 to 90 minutes before the anticipated event. Unlike alprazolam, it does not lyse the panic and so cannot interrupt ongoing distress.

What About the Dogs Who Have Noise Phobia *and* Another Anxiety-Related Condition?

The goal of treatment of noise phobias and reactivity is not to sedate the dog; the goal is to stop the dog's distress while keeping the dog as normal as possible. These medications can be used on an "as-needed" basis in addition to the "maintenance medications," the tricyclic antidepressants (TCAs) and selective serotonin reuptake inhibitors (SSRIs). In fact, we now know that many dogs with separation anxiety also react to noises, and most animals that react to noises are at risk for developing some other anxiety. **If both of these or any other co-morbid conditions are not treated, the dog will not improve.**

For example, many dogs with separation anxiety will need a TCA or SSRI daily, and only need alprazolam if there is a storm, whereas others have a component of panic to their response to being left. In this case, the dog will also need alprazolam any time he is left, preferably **before** he begins to become distressed. This may mean that some dogs get some alprazolam every time the alarm goes off. If the medication and dosage are helping the dog, this is a good idea, but assessment is critical. For dogs who have other concomitant anxieties or anxiety-related problems or for those noise-phobic dogs who are profound, maintenance medication designed to lower the animal's overall reactivity and anxiety and to raise the threshold for a reaction involving panic is recommended. This means treating the dog on a daily basis with a TCA or SSRI.

Again, you must be able to assess the dog to see if the medication is making the dog worse (more incidents, greater intensity), better (fewer incidents, lesser intensity), or having no effect. By keeping daily logs and routinely videotaping the dog you will be able to note changes in many anxiety-related behaviors including destruction, elimination, self-mutilation, and barking. Panting and more subtle behaviors might require that you are present to observe them.

Regardless, pick some subset of the behaviors that the dog exhibits when distressed and monitor these for change. The information you gain will help you manage the dog's medication.

Finally, there is even some benefit to giving a benzodiazepine to the dog after they have already reacted. This won't abort the attack, but may shorten it and may also prevent the consolidation of some short-term memory about how terrible the experience was. Alprazolam is truly "panicolytic," in other words, something that cuts through panic and can and should be given during a storm or panic attack. It's important to remember that we all learn to panic or become anxious the more often it happens, so the humane thing to do is to use medication every time it's needed.

Clearance of these drugs is through liver (hepatic glucuronidation pathways) and kidney (renal) excretion, so knowing that the pathways are not impaired is important if we are to avoid side effects and minimize risk. We can learn about the animal's ability to metabolize the drugs by taking a blood sample and looking at serum kidney and liver enzymes. All TCAs affect the reuptake of both serotonin and norepinephrine, and the extent to which they do this for each catecholamine depends on the specific TCA. The effect that is desirable is the one associated with reuptake inhibition for serotonin; anxiety has been associated with low levels of serotonin. The SSRIs primarily affect serotonin, and most are relatively specific for one class of receptor thought to be involved in many anxiety-related conditions, the $5HT_{1A}$ subtype receptor.

As is true with humans, no one medication works for everyone and three or four medications or medication combinations may need to be tried before one that is successful is identified. Unfortunately, because of the amount of time needed to determine that a medication is not helpful to the dog, you may need 4 to 6 months to try different medications or medication combinations. By playing the odds of the patterns discussed above, we may find which medication may work more quickly. You should be engaged in behavior modification programs designed to teach the dog a more relaxed response while treating or trying to treat your dog with medication.

Lifelong maintenance medication may be necessary; some of these animals may have a true deficit of serotonin or an altered serotonin functioning in the same way diabetics can have a deficit of insulin. We generally ask clients to keep the dog on the drug for the amount of time it took to get the dog as perfect as possible, plus 30 days, and then wean the dog from the medication at the rate it took for the dog to improve. This translates to 4 to 6 months of treatment, minimally. If medication is long-term or lifelong, annual physical and laboratory evaluations are useful. There appear to be no side-effects of long-term treatment in healthy animals.

Remember that this entire discussion assumes that the client is also doing the relevant behavior modification. There are no quick fixes, and indiscriminate use of drugs leads to treatment failures.

More detailed information and advice on the use of these medications is found in the handout, **Protocol for Using Behavioral Medication Successfully.**

Summary

- Treatment of the noise/storm phobic dog with medication *before* the expected noise or storm, especially when combined with general behavior modification designed to teach the dog to relax while avoiding inadvertent reassurance of abnormal and undesirable behaviors, can be successful.
- As with most problems involving panic and anxiety, the earlier we can intervene, the greater the chance of success.
- Please remember that this is a condition that will require a degree of management, including anticipating when the dog is likely to be exposed to a scary noise (e.g., the use of online weather programs and Doppler radar), and protecting the dog while they continue to improve (e.g., using eye shades, head phones, rooms without windows where the dog feels secure, et cetera).
- For some dogs treatment is lifelong, and for some dogs it will be short-term.
- Phobias, once present, are extremely difficult to completely obliterate because the memory of a phobic response can trigger another panicky response.
- In reality, it doesn't matter if the dog always has the potential to react throughout his life, if we can ensure that we can alleviate the distress the dog feels whenever the noises that scare the dog occur. For the vast majority of dogs, we can now alleviate the fear and panic experienced during a noise phobic event, and that's a very good place to start.

PROTOCOL FOR UNDERSTANDING AND TREATING GENERALIZED ANXIETY DISORDER

Overview of Generalized Anxiety Disorder

Generalized anxiety disorder (GAD) is defined as consistent exhibition of increased autonomic hyperreactivity (increased heart rate, increased respiratory rate, changes in gastrointestinal activity, and dilated/enlarged pupils associated with distress), increased motor activity, and increased vigilance and scanning that interferes with a normal range of social interaction, *and* that occurs in the absolute absence of what would be considered a truly provocative stimulus. In other words, these dogs or cats are reactive before any noticeable stimulus or trigger sets them off, and they do not easily habituate to or learn to ignore anything that arouses them.

Situations in which dogs react when exposed to new social stimuli (dogs, cats, humans) may reflect an animal version of social anxiety. Caution is urged because closer inspection may indicate that the human or animal is just another unfamiliar stimulus, so that the criteria for GAD are met. This distinction is important because behavior modification will need to address all reactive situations.

The danger with this diagnosis is that it is very specific, but could easily and carelessly be made in the absence of critical thought or incomplete history. To some extent any dog or cat who reacts inappropriately in any circumstance could be said to be exhibiting generalized anxiety, but for the conditions of this diagnosis to be met, the focus of the stimulus must be general, not specific, and the behaviors aren't directed toward a discrete or limited set of conditions (e.g., other dogs, being left alone, et cetera). These animals may destroy during one of their bouts of extreme distress, but not during another, and there is no true pattern focusing on destruction itself. GAD should be a diagnosis of last resort, not first, and your dog's or cat's characteristically anxious signs should be present under conditions where any of these signs would have subsided in a "normal" or nonsymptomatic animal. This is one condition where a truly exhaustive history is needed.

GAD is a diagnosis that may also include general reactivity to unfamiliar individuals (animal or human). Whether this is the equivalent of human, social anxiety disorder, is difficult to know because of the dependent nature of dogs on people. Dogs who worry about social interactions also tend to react to new environments, physical, auditory, and olfactory stimuli, et cetera, and so meet the criteria for GAD. The distinction between GAD and what has been called "social anxiety disorder" may be less important in terms of treatment because the medications and behavior modification used to treat GAD will also help social anxieties. However, *understanding that reactive dogs can generalize their responses to a variety of situations, left untreated, is essential.* You will need to watch for changes in severity of response during treatment, and should watch to see if the number of categories in which your dog responds increases, decreases, or stays the same.

Finally, these cats and dogs appear to never truly relax, although they may be more relaxed and appear happy in totally predictable and protected physical and social environments. This pattern can make assigning the diagnosis of GAD difficult in some circumstances.

It's also important to ensure that your dog or cat is not suffering from any medical concern because the signs associated with GAD are truly nonspecific. In fact, an animal in pain can look exactly like an animal with GAD. You may note that your dog's or cat's wariness is way out of proportion to other pets' "startle" responses, that the patient is a light sleeper and awakes and startles easily, and that the intensity of the response is out of proportion to the stimulus.

Many dogs and cats with GAD also exhibit conditions for which their people may have already sought help, for example, frequent vomiting, frequent diarrhea, "itchiness" and scratching, rashes, et cetera. Many animals diagnosed with chronic or intermittent diarrhea associated with irritable bowel syndrome (IBS) may also have some anxiety-related condition. Unless the veterinarian is accustomed to looking for behavioral conditions, she may not think to ask about anxieties, and so will miss the flag that IBS provides for early diagnosis of anxiety. *You need to ensure that you know what normal is, and that you are persistent and forthright in reporting any and all behaviors that you find worrisome. Helping dogs and cats with behavioral problems requires a good dialog with your veterinarian and sometimes some gentle persistence from you if your veterinarian has had little or no training in behavioral medicine.*

Treatment of Generalized Anxiety Disorder

It's actually easier to use behavior modification if the focus to which the animal reacts is discrete (one or two things). The more circumstances in which an animal reacts, the more difficult and lengthy behavioral treatment will be. Because animals with GAD generalize their anxieties, they can also be encouraged, with time, work, and usually medication, to group sets of anxious situations together so that they improve by leaps rather than an infinite set of baby steps.

GAD is the one condition that absolutely requires that you be able to recognize progressively calmer behaviors, and the physical signs that correlate well with underlying physiological states indicating a calmer response. These signs of calm *must* be rewarded. It's sometimes hard to do this because if you are too excited, the cat or dog begins to worry again. Rewards here should be directed at encouraging continued calm. This means that grooming, if the animal likes it, massage, and slow petting with gentle pressure should be encouraged. The foundation behavior modification programs, the **Protocol for Deference**, the **Protocol for Teaching Your Dog to Take a Deep Breath and Use Other Biofeedback Methods as Part of Relaxation**, and the **Protocol for Relaxation: Behavior Modification Tier 1**, are essential for these pets. These programs likely will provide these pets with the only rule structure that they can understand—except the one that tells them to always worry. These behavior mod programs, if practiced correctly, will allow you to "break through" the anxiety and allow your pet to experience a different way of looking at the world. As your dog or cat improves, he will continually rely on what he learned in these programs so that he can react less.

Because good, aerobic exercise correlates with decreases in some forms of anxiety in humans, we have reason to believe that the same correlation may hold for cats and dogs. Dogs are easier to exercise than cats, but the trick with cats is to find the right stimulus. For many anxious cats, complex toys will be too noisy and unpredictable, but chasing a feather may be just right. Anything that can increase the aerobic component of your pet's activity without triggering anxiety should be included.

By definition, it's almost impossible to avoid all the triggers for GAD. If you can identify three or four of the most provocative stimuli for your pet (e.g., traffic, sudden movement, vacuum cleaners, et cetera) and avoid those while working with calming gestures and the behavior mod, your pet may begin to be able to ignore certain stimuli. Once there is at least one former trigger that your pet can ignore, it's possible to have hope that he will continue to improve. Again, improvement often comes in clusters, and you need to prepare for the "drought" when little improvement seems possible.

A lot has been written in the popular press about the roles for canine and feline "pheromones" for improving behavior. These compounds are not true pheromones. They are derived from natural waxy secretions that may contain compounds that stimulate animals to be more social. There are few controlled studies on these products, and no one knows how or if they function. It is possible that if they function they do so by encouraging a calming effect. If you are reasonable in your expectations and don't mind the expense, for some cases involving anxiety, these products may appear to be useful, but we know so little about how or if they work that their use is not truly based on evidence.

Once fully established, it's unlikely that any animal can recover from GAD without medication. In fact, it may be inhumane to ask them to try to do so because we humans have a pretty steep learning curve before we can work well with the behavior modification protocols. Medications of choice are usually the selective serotonin re-uptake inhibitors (SSRIs). The SSRIs most commonly and successfully used are paroxetine (Paxil) and sertraline (Zoloft). If true panic is involved, a "panicolytic" medication that stops the panic, like the benzodiazepine alprazolam (Xanax), may be needed. Panicolytic drugs should be used as needed to stop or prevent truly crippling events, in combination with daily use of an SSRI. Because SSRIs take a minimum of 3 to 5 weeks to cause changes in proteins made in brain cells, patience is truly a virtue during treatment. In this interval, you may find that they need to use benzodiazepines more often (4 to 6 times a day). That's fine as long your dog or cat is not simply being sedated.

The ideal treatment for long-term management of GAD involves daily sessions where relaxing is emphasized, regular practice of the behavior modification protocols, and appropriate use of medication. Medication is likely to be lifelong, although the dose may be decreased with time. Because GAD is one of the conditions that is often co-morbid (i.e., occurs) with other behavioral conditions, you may need to work especially hard to avoid and then desensitize your dog or cat to provocative stimuli. Any reduction in the signs of GAD is generally a signal that the other conditions can resolve and largely be controlled, also.

PROTOCOL FOR UNDERSTANDING, MANAGING, AND TREATING DOGS WITH IMPULSE CONTROL AGGRESSION

Anxiety and Aggression

The most common behavioral problems for dogs involve anxiety. Among the common anxiety disorders are those associated with aggression, including fear aggression, and the diagnosis discussed here, impulse control aggression. This condition was previously known as "dominance aggression," and the name of the diagnosis is still debated, although the condition and its recognition are not.

Dogs who are fearfully aggressive use distance-increasing strategies as their first choice to deal with humans and other animals whom they fear, and these dogs signal from long distances their fear through facial and body signals and vocalizations. Fearfully aggressive dogs continue to withdraw while threatening as long as is possible, and are only aggressive when they have no other choices, or when the opportunity to "chase" those they fear by nipping from behind.

Dogs with impulse control aggression do not withdraw from social situations involving humans, and instead seek them out and approach, *decreasing* the distance between themselves and the human focus of their concern. Dogs with impulse control aggression appear compelled to monitor such interactions. Paradoxically, rather than providing them with more information that could calm them, such interactions usually increase the anxiety of dogs with impulse control aggression. Impulse control aggression is best defined as abnormal, inappropriate, out-of-context aggression (threat, challenge, or attack) consistently exhibited by dogs toward people under any circumstance involving passive or active control of the dog's behavior or the dog's access to the behavior. Any intensification of any aggressive response from the dog upon any passive or active correction or interruption of the dog's behavior or the dog's access to the behavior confirms the diagnosis.

In summary, fearfully aggressive dogs back away from situations that those with impulse control aggression would approach. Fearfully aggressive dogs respond aggressively and out of context to behaviors initiated by those they fear, but dogs with impulse control aggression initiate the interactions, themselves, in situations where they may not have even been the focus of the human involved, and which are inappropriate given the human's behaviors.

The Diagnostic Label

"Impulse control aggression" has variously been called "dominance aggression," "impulsive aggression," and "conflict aggression." Here, we have chosen the label of "impulse control aggression" because it is the most informative. Some of the concerns about the other labels are that all aggressions can appear "impulsive," external "conflict" is at the heart of all aggressions, and internal "conflict" is rooted in anxiety and uncertainty, making these labels less clear and informative. There are at least two broad forms of this condition: a truly impulsive one, and one that can become seemingly impulsive when attempts by the dog to address his own anxiety by controlling people's actions fail.

The label of "dominance aggression" allowed relatively easy recognition of the set of dogs who shared this diagnosis, but the concept of "dominance" as applied to pet dogs is flawed and it has encouraged techniques that are dangerous to owners and dogs, alike, and unfair and often abusive to dogs. For more information on this issue see the **Protocol for Generalized Discharge Instructions for Dogs with Behavioral Concerns,** the American Veterinary Society of Animal Behavior's (AVSAB) Dominance Position Statement (www.avsabonline.org/avsabonline/images/stories/Position_Statements/dominance%20statement.pdf) and the Dog Welfare Campaign Position Statement (www.dogwelfarecampaign.org/why-not-dominance.php).

What This Condition Involves

In some areas of the world, the relative frequency of impulse control aggression has been greatly decreased because at least one form of it has a clearly heritable basis. Not breeding dogs in affected family lines has decreased the frequency of the condition for some families/breeds.

Any dog who is aggressive for any reason can be potentially dangerous to humans. Dogs with impulse control aggression can be particularly dangerous because their problem is rooted in a struggle with people over control of all aspects of the social environment. **This struggle is not because most of these dogs are mean and malicious.** Instead, they struggle and provoke people because this is the only way they can get information from and about the social environment and interactions. Dogs with any form of this diagnosis are unable to sit back and take the cues about the appropriateness of their behavior from the contextual environment. They also are unable to distance themselves from people about whom they are unreasonably concerned. Most of these dogs' people have not done anything malicious to them, are not deliberately provoking the dog, and are usually not even aware that their behaviors may be provocative to any dog. Some of the behaviors to which the dogs are most reactive are behaviors that are similar to those seen in rough play or social challenges with other dogs (e.g., reaching over the dog's neck or back, standing over the dog), but affected dogs are usually good with other dogs, and no correlation has been shown between this diagnosis and those pertaining to other animals.

Because the pattern of the dog's reactivity may depend on that dog's relationship with individual people *plus* his threshold for reactivity at that time, people may view these dogs as "unpredictable." Once people understand the pattern of the dog's behaviors, these dogs no longer seem "unpredictable."

By definition, impulse control aggression is a manifestation of *inappropriate, out-of-context responses to specific situations related to, or access to, control.* These dogs are very different from those who are pushy or assertive. Pushy and assertive dogs are usually confident and do a good job of reading contextual cues. Many people prefer pushy, assertive dogs because they work well in competitive obedience and trial situations, and because some people feel that these dogs are "personality plus." Being pushy or assertive does not mean that the dog has impulse control aggression.

Dogs with impulse control aggression have a focus on control that is *abnormal* and out of context. A normal and confident dog might stand in your way by the door because he wants attention or because he wants to go with you. If you do not give him attention or take him with you, he is disappointed but accepting. A dog with impulse control aggression stands in your way at the door because he is anxious and realizes that doors can signal changes in social contexts or interactions, and he must monitor all potential changes. When he is uncertain about whether the change will affect him, he provokes the situation—by stiffening and blocking you, by grabbing you—in an attempt to get information. Part of the pathology often involves a further misunderstanding of the response received.

Because dogs with impulse control aggression have problems with all forms of social control—even forms that their people do not intend, like reaching over them or petting them—it is imperative that you do the best job possible in recognizing and aborting even subtle behaviors associated with the dog's inappropriate responses, no matter how irrational these responses seem. These dogs cannot just sit back and get information from observing the patterns in the social context because they have a problem and are abnormal. These dogs function by provoking or deforming the social environment, getting information from the response to their behaviors, and moving forward event by event. Clients are often concerned that this makes no sense. If the dog's response made sense, given the context, the dog would be normal, and not have a behavioral problem. By definition, then, these dogs behave bizarrely under circumstances that would not provoke an ordinary, "normal" dog.

There are at least two broad forms of impulse control aggression: (a) a truly impulsive one, and (b) one that can become seemingly impulsive when attempts by the dog to address his own anxiety by controlling people's actions fails.

The Second Group of Impulsive Dogs

- Dogs in the second and more common group of dogs with impulse aggression use behavioral challenges to deform the social environment and get information about risk. Most dogs ask questions through observations and solicitous behaviors—these dogs are impaired in those abilities. Dogs with impulse control aggression can be particularly dangerous because their problem is rooted in a struggle with people over control of all aspects of the social environment. **This struggle is not because most of these dogs are mean and malicious.** Instead, they struggle and provoke people *because this is the only way they can get information from and about the social environment and interactions.*
  - Dogs with any form of this diagnosis are unable to sit back and take the cues about the appropriateness of their behavior from the contextual environment. Here, dogs use provocative behaviors to get information.
  - They also are unable to distance themselves from people about whom they are unreasonably concerned.
  - Most of these dogs' people have not done anything malicious to them, are not deliberately provoking the dogs, and are usually not even aware that their behaviors may be provocative to any dog.
  - Some of the behaviors to which the dogs are most reactive are behaviors that are similar to those seen in rough play or social challenges with other dogs (e.g., reaching over the dog's neck or back, standing over the dog), but

affected dogs are usually good with other dogs, and no correlation has been shown between this diagnosis and those pertaining to other animals.
- Because the pattern of the dog's reactivity may depend on that dog's relationship with individual people **plus** his threshold for reactivity at that time, people may view these dogs as "unpredictable." Once people understand the pattern of the dog's behaviors, these dogs no longer seem "unpredictable."
- These dogs are so uncertain of their relationships with humans that every time the human exhibits a behavior that *might* be construed to be a "challenge" or "threat," the dog pushes back to learn:
  - whether the human is a threat,
  - which human behaviors are offered in response to the dog's "threat," and
  - whether the human's response depends on context.
- Accordingly, dogs with this form of aggression may victimize only certain groups of people.
- Dogs with impulse control aggression have a focus on control that is *abnormal* and *out of context*. A normal and confident dog might stand in your way by the door because he wants attention or because he wants to go with you. If you do not give him attention or take him with you, he is disappointed but accepting. A dog with impulse control aggression stands in your way at the door because he is anxious and realizes that doors can signal changes in social contexts or interactions, and he must monitor all potential changes. When he is uncertain about whether the change will affect him, he provokes the situation—by stiffening and blocking you, by grabbing you—in an attempt to get information. Part of the pathology often involves a further misunderstanding of the response received.

The First Group of Impulsive Dogs— Truly Impulsive Dogs

- Truly impulsive dogs are always anxious and always uncertain. Depending on the other stimuli contributing to their arousal they may be more or less likely to react at different times.
- Dogs who are truly impulsive (the first group) may also use the rule structure above, but the extent to which they react may depend on their overall response to all stimuli at that time, rather than on a specific behavior that caused them to react. In other words, there is an internal aspect of heightened arousal and reactivity that may be independent of the social environment.
- The dogs in this group of truly impulsive dogs seem more unpredictable than the dogs in the second group (although the same stimuli provoke them) because at times they are better able to control their impulsivity.
- If clients pay attention to these dogs they realize that they are never fully relaxed and always anxious, even if they are attempting to seek interactions with humans which are usually viewed as calming (e.g., petting).
- These dogs act as if they are always trying to control their reactivity and to find some way to not react. When they are unable to do so we see the impulsive, aggressive explosions.

By definition, impulse control aggression is a manifestation of *inappropriate, out-of-context responses to specific situations related to, or access to, control.* These dogs are very different from those who are pushy or assertive. Pushy and assertive dogs are usually confident and do a good job of reading contextual cues. Many people prefer pushy, assertive dogs because they work well in competitive obedience and trial situations, and because some people feel that these dogs are "personality plus." Being pushy or assertive does not mean that the dog has impulse control aggression.

This is a very discrete definition of impulse control aggression and has the advantage of not coupling the challenge to food (food-related aggression), toys (possessive aggression), or space (territorial aggression). These aggressions can all be correlates of impulse control aggression and when associated with it, may be indicative of a more severe situation. The keys here are control and access. Most of the problems with diagnosing the condition arise from the human's misunderstanding of canine social systems, canine signaling, and canine anxieties associated with endogenous uncertainty about contextually appropriate responses.

This diagnosis cannot be made on the basis of a onetime event. The behavior, once it begins, will become more visible and consistent, but data on early signs, patterns of change with experience, and changes in intensity are lacking.

Some of these dogs, especially those in the second group, only victimize very forceful humans, because by "disciplining" the dog verbally or physically the human has convinced the dog that the human is a threat. In contrast, some of these dogs only victimize uncertain people or those who are less certain with or more worried about the dog. In this case, the dog continues to provoke these people because their uncertainty makes it hard for the dog to clearly understand the rules for the interaction, and they push further to get clearer information about how they are to interact with these people.

Patterns of Behavior for Dogs with Impulse Control Aggression

If we understand that abnormal aggression is an anxiety disorder, we can use the dog's patterns of aggressive responses to help us treat them. The patterns of problematic behaviors that these dogs use are actually a rule structure that the dog is using to deal with his world.

Normal dogs also use rule structures and we recognize these based on patterns of behavior (e.g., you pick up your car keys and the dog sits by the door; you get a food toy, the dog goes to his crate; you pick up a food dish, the dog sits and waits for it to be placed in front of him; you pick up the dog's leash and he barks and jumps around). *For dogs with behavioral diagnoses the rule structures, themselves, are pathological.* Because of this, the rule structure may be hurting the dog (e.g., he mutilates himself as part of his obsessive-compulsive disorder or when panicking and trying to escape from a storm). Pathological rule structures do not make the dog's world or his interactions in it any easier to negotiate.

The behaviors affected dogs use represent a rule structure that has basically gone wrong. The dog tries to use a set of rules for interaction, but these rules fail to help his anxiety or to make more sense of the situation. Most good and benign rules in normal situations make things clearer and help us all to be

less reactive, but in pathological situations, the "rules" make things less clear and cause the dog to be more reactive.

Because a need for control is such a clear rule, we can treat these dogs by substituting a more benign rule that removes the dog's need for control by providing him with information about what will happen next and what the expected response should be.

Specific Behaviors That May Cause an Aggressive Response

As part of the scenario involving control, dogs with impulse control aggression dislike any form of passive or active, or social or physical control: being pushed from a sofa or a bed, being stared at (and they may misinterpret benign eye contact as a stare; remember that these dogs are not normal, so they misinterpret otherwise "normal" signals), having their shoulders or back pushed on, reaching over their head (even if this is only to put on a leash), "corrected" verbally or with a leash, et cetera. *Virtually all dogs affected with impulse control aggression will intensify their aggression if physically punished.* This response makes sense: prior to the interaction the dog was not sure if the human was a threat; now, if the dog is physically punished or threatened, the dog is certain that the "threat" of the human is real, and intensified aggression can be his only response.

Many of these dogs are subtle and will cause you to redirect your activities: these dogs will lie in front of doors or furniture so that you avoid those areas. These dogs often lean against or put a paw on you at any opportunity, but you learn not to touch them, because if you do, they become aggressive.

Because these behaviors are also associated with attention-seeking behavior in normal dogs, clients often ask how they can be certain that their "normal" dog is not showing signs of becoming "problematic" by using these behaviors. The key distinction is that the pathological dog is always seeking information, whereas the pesky dog may just be seeking contact and comfort. You can learn to carefully test and evaluate whether the response is appropriate given the specific context. If the dog is leaning against you just to get attention, you should be able to physically move him without the dog becoming aggressive. This may be too risky a test for some dogs who are thought to be severely affected with impulse control aggression, so look for more subtle cues. Dogs who are leaning on you to be close or for attention do not stiffen, open their eyes, and then move so that they are again touching or pressing on you as most dogs with impulse control aggression will. Dogs who are seeking closeness will usually respond to verbal cues to get off or down, and then use solicitous behavior (turning their head on their side, rolling over, whining, wagging their tail, putting their ears loosely back, et cetera) to get you to attend to them. Dogs with impulse control aggression may "talk back," become stiffer, or become aggressive. Oddly, they seldom growl or vocalize as a precursor to lunging, but may do so as they grab someone. **Caution is urged.**

Victims of Impulse Control Aggression

Not all household members may be equally victimized by these aggressive dogs.
- Young children are often perceived as a threat by some of these dogs because they are at the same eye level as the dog and their "staring" is seen by the dog as a threat.

- The more compliant person in the household may be victimized more frequently than the person who is firm with the dog, because the dog is clear about the intent of the person who is clear about rules for social interactions. The dog needs to push to get the required information to make social decisions, and uncertain people—from the dog's perspective—make the dog's concern worse.
- Conversely, some of these dogs know that they can compliant people are never threats, and so do not challenge them. These dogs challenge the person who is more forceful because they worry that threats could be involved. Impulse control aggression is a highly variable condition.

Can Impulse Control Aggression Be Treated?

It's important to remember that any dog who is aggressive for any reason can be potentially dangerous. The first rule in treating aggressive dogs must be to take all precautions to keep people safe. *These same precautions will also keep the dog safe.* If the treatment employed for these dogs is humane and aimed at addressing their anxiety disorders, the vast majority of these dogs will improve to the extent that few people will even realize that the dog has a problem.

How Important Is Age and Developmental Stage with Impulse Control Aggression?

Impulse control aggression almost always develops at *social maturity (~18 to 24 months of age; range: 12 to 36 months)*. This is why your dog seemed perfectly normal as a puppy and then at about 2 years of age seemed to "suddenly" change. Although the majority of dogs who suffer from this form of pathological aggression are male, this condition is not controlled by hormones, although hormones may affect the form the aggression takes and the presence of testosterone may exacerbate the aggression. Testosterone can make a dog more reactive, but does not *per se* cause aggression of any kind. The fact that this aggressive condition occurs most often at social maturity is another hint that you did not "cause" the problem.

Females can also be affected by this condition and when they are affected they are often young (8 months of age or less), suggesting that the mechanism for the aggression may be related to *in utero* factors, rather than to the social maturity factors that affect most of the patients with this condition.

The key to treating all aggressive dogs, and especially dogs with impulse control aggression, is to avoid all the circumstances in which the dog might be "provoked" to react inappropriately. This means that you have to be a good observer of your dog so that you can avoid anything that the dog thinks is provocative, no matter how foolish this may seem.

For example, if your dog growls whenever you stare at him, do not stare. Think about using his troubled logic: If you stare at the dog you are asking the dog to respond to your challenge (the stare) with a challenge. He has no choice. Whereas if you walk away, you are telling him you are not a threat. You are not "giving in" to the dog; you are avoiding a confusion you know the dog will experience and you are keeping yourself and the dog safe.

As you progress through the behavior modification protocols discussed below you will gradually teach the dog that if he defers to you and looks to you for guidance, he will get attention and information that will help him replace his reactive rules with less-reactive rules. Later you will desensitize the dog to situations in which he responds inappropriately. You cannot do all of this at once. Please do not even try. **Remember that every time a dog has an *inappropriate response*, three things happen:**

1. The dog reinforces his aggressive response at the level of molecular learning.
2. You reinforce your associations with the experience of the inappropriate behavior simply because it continues to happen.
3. The dog backslides because he is upset by an aggressive event. Most dogs act as if they find the circumstance of their exhibition of aggression traumatic: they realize that something untoward happened, but cannot escape it. *Remember that these dogs are not "disobeying" you; they are behaving this way because they are abnormal and need help.*

The safest strategy in dealing with any aggressive dog, particularly those with this condition, is to **only** give the dog attention when he defers to you. See the **Protocol for Deference**. This is a simple rule that generalizes to every situation in which the dog can ever find himself. This rule will help to enforce the very types of behavior that not only help your dog, but that you desire. *By using this simple rule, the dog learns to look to you for the cues about the appropriateness of his behavior, learns that you are reliable and trustworthy, and learns that he can be less anxious in social systems when there are humane rules.* With time, then, these dogs can lead happy, safe, and humanely interactive lives. We also benefit by becoming more understanding and humane in our behavior toward all dogs.

Tick List of Actions to Take to Treat Impulse Control Aggression

1. Make a list of all of the situations in which your dog reacts. These are the situations you must avoid. The following are some common situations to avoid. You have watched your dog so you should be able to add other situations in which your dog reacts:
   - reaching for or pulling on the dog's collar,
   - pulling on the dog's legs,
   - pushing the dog down,
   - pushing the dog from the sofa or the bed,
   - yelling at the dog or pulling his legs,
   - disturbing the dog while he is sleeping or resting,
   - stepping over or on the dog,
   - pushing back if the dog paws at or jumps on you,
   - playing aggressively with the dog,
   - trying to take a toy from the dog's mouth,
   - allowing the dog on your lap where he can press on your head or shoulders, and
   - physically punishing the dog.
2. Now that you know all the situations in which the dog can react, you need a plan to deal with them. Consider these options:
   - Do not reach for or pull on the dog's collar; instead, ask the dog to come to you and sit, tell him he is good.
   - Do not pull on the dog's legs; instead, ask the dog to sit or lie down, and reward him when he does so.

- Do not push the dog down; instead, turn away and let the dog slide from you, then ask him to sit and tell him he is good.
- Do not push the dog from the sofa or the bed; instead, move away from the bed/sofa and ask the dog to come off the bed/sofa and out of the room, then close the door.
- Do not yell at the dog; instead, speak softly and calmly, or not at all. The dog will offer behaviors, reward the good ones.
- Do not disturb the dog while he is sleeping or resting; instead, talk to the dog to wake him up and when he is fully awake ask him to come to you and sit, and reward him.
- Do not step over or on the dog; instead, go around the dog or, if you cannot, ask him to get up and come to you, ask him to sit, and tell him he is good.
- Do not push back if the dog paws at or jumps on you; instead, fold your arms, ignore him, and walk away. If he follows you, ask him to sit, and reward him when he does so.
- Do not play aggressively with the dog; instead, play by throwing toys or balls and allowing the dog to retrieve them. Throw a new toy every time he brings back the old one.
- Do not try to take a toy from the dog's mouth; instead, ask the dog to drop the toy, reward him when he does, and offer him another toy so that you do not have to reach in front of him.
- Do not allow the dog on your lap where he can press on your head or shoulders; instead, ask him to get down. If he doesn't do this, stand up and slowly leave or have someone else call him, and do not let the situation occur in the future.
- Do not physically punish the dog. You may be angry, but anger will make him worse; walk away until you are both calm, then ask him to sit and reward him when he does.

3. If necessary, walk your dog only on a head collar. All head collars will allow you to control the direction of the dog's body and allow you to more safely control the dog. Depending on the shape of the dog and the type of head collar, some will allow you to close the dog's mouth. Warn your friends and neighbors that head collars are not muzzles. Explain that these will help keep your dog calmer and safer.

4. Play *only* with toys, not your hands. These dogs, by definition, have trouble with fine contextual distinctions. Help them. Make the difference between your hand and a potential threat and toy and assured play clear. See the **Protocol for Choosing Toys for Your Pet** for some guidance.

5. Do not let your dog sleep on your bed if you cannot ask him to get off and have him comply. Do not allow your dog to sleep in your bed if he becomes aggressive when you bump into him while you are asleep. For some dogs, this means that you may not even be able to let the dog sleep in the bedroom. This minimizes the potential for an inadvertent threat when you are sleepy and least able to anticipate problem behavior. Remember that your movements are less predictable to your dog when you are asleep, and all of our thresholds for reactivity are lessened

when we are asleep. Accordingly, if you startle your dog, the response may be explosive. Again, the key is to set your dog up to succeed, not to fail.

6. Feeding time may be a reactive situation. Many dogs with impulse control aggression may also have food-related aggression (most dogs with food-related aggression *do not* have impulse control aggression). If necessary, feed your dog in a separate room with the door closed in order to avoid any aggressive incidents. If you have small children, you should be able to lock the door. If you like to give your dog table scraps, all scraps should be placed in the dog's dish. Your dog is not allowed to beg at the table, and must sit and wait at all times before approaching his dish. If you cannot safely do these things, please put your dog behind a locked door or gate while you eat. Please do not feed your dog from the table if he does become aggressive around food, because this creates a potentially explosive and difficult to control situation. See the **Protocol for Understanding and Managing Dogs and Aggression Involving Food, Rawhide, Biscuits, and Bones** for more help.

7. ***Do not physically punish your dog!*** You will convince your dog that you are a threat and untrustworthy, and he will become more aggressive. If your dog stiffens, growls, or lunges, you may softly tell him "no" to interrupt the situation. If your dog has learned that the word "no" is a punisher with bad associations, please do not use it. You wish to interrupt the dog to lower his arousal, not punish him to raise his arousal. Any word or sound to which he calmly attends can be an interrupter. You can do this by asking your dog to come into another room and sit, or by leaving him. If your dog is wearing a head collar, gently pull the collar forward to close his mouth, softly say "no," then lead him from the inciting event quickly. If it is necessary to remove your dog from the room or from a situation, wait for the dog to become calm, then practice a few of the sitting and breathing exercises so that he realizes he must act appropriately to get "good" attention. See the **Protocol for Teaching Your Dog to Take a Deep Breath and Use Other Biofeedback Methods as Part of Relaxation** for more information. Remember that the preferred choice is to avoid any aggressive events. Most people find it easier to ignore the dog than to distract him, so this may be a safer and more effective tactic.

8. Please warn your friends and neighbors that any aggressive dog is potentially dangerous, and for this reason they must comply with your instructions to minimize danger to the dog and to themselves. This may mean that they are not to open the door to the room where you have placed your dog. This may mean that you will only bring your dog to the party on a head collar when everyone is calm and that no one can reach toward him. See the **Protocol for Handling "Special-Needs Pets" During Holidays and Other Special Occasions** for help.

9. If you are working with one of the behavior modification programs with your dog and he persists in challenging or ignoring you—stop. You both need a break. Either put your dog in another room and leave him alone, or leave the room he is in and leave him alone (and for this reason you may wish to work only in rooms that have doors or gates). By separating yourself from your dog you have removed his ability to control any part of the situation

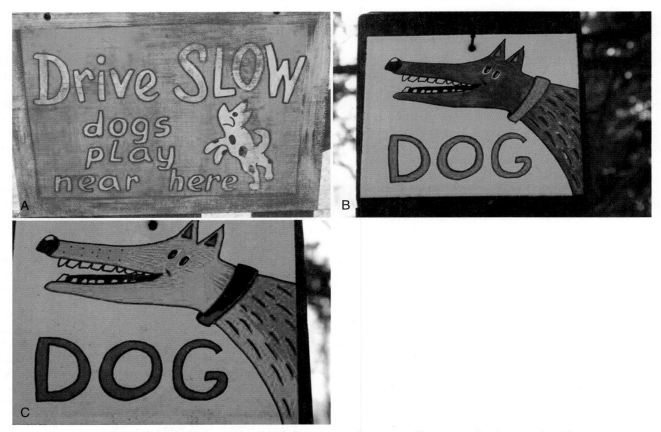

All three of these "Dog on Premises" signs are on the same driveway gate. Anyone should have the expectation that at least one dog lives on the property.

and provided him with the opportunity to become less reactive and anxious.

10. Get a "Dog on Premises" sign, or make a sign that announces that there is a dog living on the property. This is not an admission of a dangerous dog, but it is a civically responsible reminder that a dog is on the property. Anyone who has a dog should have such a sign.

11. Once your dog has successfully and happily completed the **Protocol for Deference, Protocol for Teaching Your Dog to Take a Deep Breath and Use Other Biofeedback Methods as Part of Relaxation,** and the **Protocol for Relaxation: Behavior Modification Tier 1,** you can move on to desensitizing him to gestures that may still startle him **(Tier 2: Protocol for Desensitizing Dogs Affected with Impulse Control Aggression).** You may need help with any or all parts of these programs. Talk to your vet to see if anyone in the practice is trained in behavioral modification techniques. If not, look for a good, kind and certified dog trainer who understands true behavior modification (in the United States, www.ccpdt.org and www.petprofessionalguild.com).

12. When your dog is as improved as everyone thinks is possible, please continue to reinforce appropriate behaviors for the rest of your dog's life. Lapses invariably result in regression. These dogs have anxiety disorders; they will always need good, clear information. We don't cure aggression, but we do a good job of controlling it. Dogs with impulse control aggression are not normal, but can learn to behave normally.

13. Anti-anxiety medications are likely a good idea for any dog with impulse control aggression and may help some dogs who otherwise are not able to succeed with the behavior modification programs. Please remember that medication is to be used *in addition* to the behavior modification, not instead of it. The biggest benefit of antianxiety medication for these dogs is that it enhances the rate at which new behaviors are able to be acquired.

Good luck! If you are calm, understand that your dog is abnormal, and work to humanely give the dog clear cues about expectations, your relationship will improve and the dog will surprise you with how well he can get.

PROTOCOL FOR UNDERSTANDING AND TREATING DOGS WITH FEAR/ FEARFUL AGGRESSION

Fear aggression is one of the most commonly diagnosed canine behavioral conditions. Dogs who are fearfully aggressive are often called "fear biters." Many fearfully aggressive dogs do not bite, but growl or bark aggressively in situations that upset them. Such situations can include approaches from other dogs, approaches from all people, approaches from children, approaches from people or dogs in specific places, interactions involving a certain kind of noise, et cetera.

In some cases, dogs become fearfully aggressive because they have been excessively punished or abused. Puppies who are physically punished for housetraining accidents can become fearfully aggressive.

Some dogs who are fearfully aggressive have not had any bad experiences—they are naturally anxious and fearful. These dogs are not normal, but can respond well to treatment.

Fearfully aggressive dogs generally react inappropriately when they feel intruded upon and worsen if they feel cornered. They do not actually have to **be** intruded upon or cornered to feel this way. When behavioral diagnoses are involved it is important that we understand the situation **from the dog's perspective.**

Merely approaching a dog that is fearfully aggressive can be sufficient to intensify his aggressive response. Many dogs continually threaten by barking, growling, or snarling, but do not bite. Such behaviors can be accompanied by postures that include slinking, lowering or tucking of the tail, ears pulled horizontally back, and piloerection (hair standing on end) over the regions of their neck and shoulders, hips, and tail. Some of these dogs will urinate or salivate while exhibiting aggressive behaviors.

If you are good at understanding canine behavior, you will understand that all of these behaviors signal that the dog does not wish to interact. These behaviors are all designed to remove the dog from an active social interaction. Please *do not view these behaviors as "submissive behaviors." These dogs are not "submitting" to you so that you can do whatever you want with them.* Instead, they are telling you that they are unable to interact calmly and that they feel threatened. This may not seem like a rational response to you, but it doesn't have to be rational. Such responses are an indicator that the dog needs help. The dog is giving you a lot of information and by understanding these signaling associations, outright aggression can often be avoided.

Patterns of Biting

Just because a dog has never bitten before does not mean that he will not do so. By definition, each dog who bites had to bite for a "first time." If you know that a dog has bitten, you actually have a lot of useful information. You know that the dog may feel sufficiently distressed to bite, and you know the circumstances in which this has happened. Hence, you can avoid bites.

Fearfully aggressive dogs often bite from behind, when the interaction is ending. These dogs will often grab someone when the person turns away from the dog. These dogs may not intend to bite: The grab may be intended to stop the human from changing behavior and doing something that the dog thinks is worrying. After these dogs have bitten, they often back up immediately. Remember that fearfully aggressive dogs try to avoid interactions, so in this context the backing up makes sense.

Please do not think that this pattern of behavior guarantees that fearfully aggressive dogs will *not* bite from the front: Biting from the front is their only recourse if they are cornered. Such dogs will *feel* cornered if they have no other means of escape. Situations that can make fearfully aggressive dogs feel cornered include when the dog is crated, when he is under a table, when he is in a corner, and when he is under a blanket.

Remember that aggressions are anxiety disorders and any time the dog has less control over his behavior or cannot monitor everyone else's behaviors, he will become more fearful and reactive.

The Role of Small Children

There is a special class of fearful aggression that can develop in households with small children. This type of fearful aggression is usually directed toward children who are 2 to 5 years of age. Because these children are very active, they may fall on the dog when playing and unintentionally hurt the dog. Older or ill dogs may be particularly at risk from young children because older dogs do not move quickly and may have physical ailments like arthritis or chronic/ periodic ear infections that are painful if someone grabs them or falls on them. If the dog begins to associate pain or discomfort with the presence of the child, and the child continues to pursue interaction with the dog, the dog may act aggressively out of fear of being hurt again. In the case of the dog with periodic ear infections, you may think that the dog has always acted appropriately in the past, and so may not understand why the dog "suddenly" snapped at the child until you realize that the dog's ears are, again, severely infected.

Children of all ages should be taught age-specific appropriate behaviors for interacting with pets. No child should be allowed to tug on any animal's ears or tails. Children should learn to play with all animals using toys—not their body parts. Children should learn to respect that pets are another species and that because of that they may not always understand that the child did not mean to hurt them. Children should learn to respect that animals have teeth and claws and can use those to defend themselves. Until the parent is positive that both the dog and the child are safe together they should not be left alone, unsupervised. **No exceptions.** For help with teaching your child safe, appropriate and fun ways to interact with dogs see *The Blue Dog.* The Blue Dog video is a product of the Blue Dog Trust (www.thebluedog.org). In the United States, it is available from the American Veterinary Medical Association (AVMA) for a nominal charge (www.avma.org/bluedog). The DVD is accompanied by an excellent booklet for caregivers and a website with supporting materials for parents, teachers, and other groups is being developed.

Treatment

The treatment of fear/fearful aggression involves treating both the fear and the aggression.

Because these dogs are already fearful, it is important that nothing in the course of treatment worsen this fear. These dogs **are not the same** as those that are just fearful without being aggressive. Dogs that are fearfully aggressive are potentially dangerous to the animals or people in whose presence they exhibit this response and must be treated with appropriate respect and caution.

The following tick list covers the steps necessary to help fearfully aggressive dogs learn to be both less fearful and less aggressive.

Tick List

1. Do not reach toward the dog, especially if the dog is cornered or if there is no way that she can escape from or avoid you (e.g., when she is under a table or in a crate). Instead, call the dog to you and ask her to sit and relax. When the dog relaxes, give her a treat. If you need help with teaching sitting or relaxing see the **Protocol for Deference** and the **Protocol for Teaching Your Dog to Take a Deep Breath and Use Other Biofeedback Methods as Part of Relaxation.**

2. Do not disturb the dog when she is resting. This could startle and frighten her. Instead, call the dog to you and ask her to sit and relax. When the dog relaxes, give her praise and a treat.

3. *Never* physically "correct" or punish the dog. Physical correction scares these dogs and will make them worse. Furthermore, punishment teaches them that their aggressive response is the correct one because it was met with aggression, and it teaches the dog that you are a threat. This is not what you want.

4. Consider using a snugly fitting head collar that will allow you to close the dog's mouth, if needed. Once the dog is fitted with this, the head collar can also be used indoors, when the dog is supervised. With a head collar you have the option of stopping any snapping or biting by closing the dog's mouth (rendering the dog safer) and then taking her safely from the room, away from the inciting event. Remember to reward your dog when she is calm. If your dog does not calm, ignore her.

5. Try to avoid any and all situations in which your dog may react aggressively.

6. Do not tell your dog it is "okay" when she becomes aggressive. It is *not* okay, either for you or her, and she knows it. You may be trying to reassure the dog, which is understandable, but you are only reinforcing the inappropriate behavior and, or confusing her by using a signal that is associated with feeling of calm or happiness that is impossible for the dog at this moment in time.

7. Please warn your friends and neighbors that any dog who is aggressive can be potentially dangerous. Please ask them to cooperate with you and avoid situations that may distress your dog. Emphasize to your friends and anyone who meets your dog that you need for them to listen to you *so that they can help the dog get better.* These requests may be as simple as not reaching toward the dog to pet her. When your friends come to visit, please consider placing your dog in another room, behind a locked door (see the **Protocol for Handling "Special-Needs Pets" During Holidays and Other Special Occasions**). Once everyone has settled down, your dog may be introduced to the people **if and only if:**
   - The dog has been quiet in the area in which she was placed.
   - The dog appears to have a happy interest in coming out of that area.
   - The dog can be introduced on a head collar.
   - The dog successfully sits and waits at your request (see **Protocol for Deference: Basic Program**).
   - Your friends agree to let your dog approach them and then to request that she sit and relax for a verbal request, and they agree that they will not reach for and startle the dog. You must have reliable, trustworthy friends who will listen to you for this plan to work.

   If the dog and the visitors can do all of these things, the visitors can reward the dog with small treats. This will also help your dog to learn not to react in such situations.

8. Minimize or avoid sudden movements or loud noises.

9. When your dog approaches any visitor—canine or human—she should be asked to sit, breathe, and relax. Humans should be requested not to stare at your dog, especially if they do so silently. Such stares can be interpreted as threats. It is okay to talk to your dog and look around the room or location normally, if the dog is calm. Take your cues from the dog.

10. If small children are involved, interaction with your dog should be allowed **only** when supervised. The dog should **always** be on a head collar and the children should practice asking your dog to sit before giving her attention. If the small children are visitors, your dog should be placed in another room behind a **locked door** (install a hook-and-eye at the very top where kids cannot reach) prior to the arrival of the small guests. This will:
    - protect the children,
    - save the dog from being placed in the situation of potentially making a mistake that could cost your dog her life, and
    - save the dog much anxiety.

    The dog should always have a "safe" room or area that is away from the situations (i.e., children) that are associated with her fearful aggression. This area should be comfortable and should **not** be used as punishment. Remember that the humane interests of the dog should always come first.

11. If the problem involves individuals in your home or situations that occur in the house, please put a bell around the dog's neck so that you know where she is (Bear Bells: www.rei.com). This will allow you to monitor the dog's movements and to either avoid or correct any inappropriate behaviors.

12. Get a "Dog on Premises" sign, or make a sign that announces that there is a dog living on the property. This is not an admission of a dangerous dog, but it is a civically responsible reminder that a dog is on the property. Anyone who has a dog should have such a sign.

13. After you have completed **Protocol for Deference: Basic Program** and **Protocol for Relaxation: Behavior**

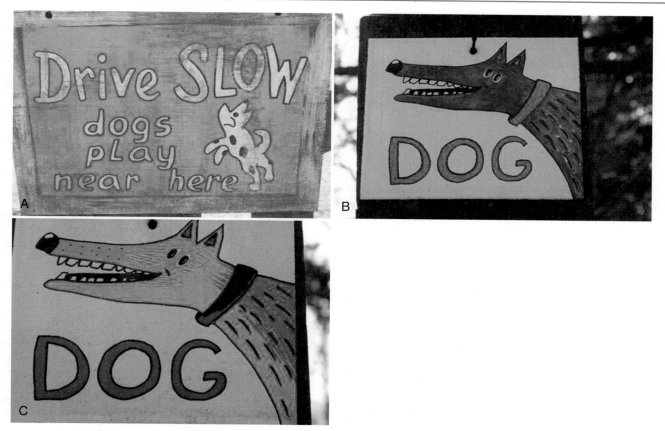

All three of these "Dog on Premises" signs are on the same driveway gate. Anyone should have the expectation that at least one dog lives on the property.

Modification Program Tier 1, you will begin **Tier 2,** which will focus on desensitizing the dog to the situations in which she reacts.

As with other conditions, many of the dogs with fear aggression can benefit from antianxiety medication. Antianxiety medication is not a substitute for the use of treatment with behavior modification, but medications augment such treatment and may speed the rate at which dogs learn new behaviors. For dogs who experience fear aggression in the absence of any abuse, medication may be an especially humane choice because the dog may never have been neurochemically normal.

PROTOCOL FOR UNDERSTANDING AND MANAGING DOGS WITH AGGRESSION INVOLVING FOOD, RAWHIDE, BISCUITS, AND BONES

This handout is designed to help you understand how problem behaviors involving food develop and how to avoid incidents of aggression. This handout discusses the two groups of dogs for whom behaviors around food are often misunderstood:

1. new puppies who are not yet exhibiting any problematic or worrisome behaviors around food and
2. older dogs who are exhibiting frank and troubling behaviors associated with food.

This handout also discusses the special case of puppy mill/farm dogs who never had enough food or the right nutrients, and the difference in handling aggression when given food toys versus meals.

What Dogs Eat

Myths about feeding dogs are almost as numerous as myths about dog behavior. Dogs are omnivorous, but with strong carnivore tendencies. This means that they may choose meat, but will also opportunistically supplement their diet with fruits, berries, and herbs. If given the chance, dogs will scavenge. Although scavenging is a public health problem in cities, it is interesting to note that scavenging garbage is one of the major ways wolves find food in some areas of Europe!

Because of the perception of dogs as obligate carnivores many people think that their dogs **must** have bones or rawhides, pigs' ears, pizzle sticks, cows' hooves, et cetera. It is **not** necessary for dogs to have any of these food treats for the dog to be well nourished; however, most dogs will value these treats. How much they value items like bones depends on many factors: their prior experience, their ease of access, how the dogs have historically been fed, social factors in the household, et cetera. These factors can contribute to these types of food items being valued and protected. When dogs protect food treats they can become aggressive. Food-related aggression may be restricted only to very special treats like these, may occur only occasionally or consistently, and may be directed towards humans or other animals.

"Resource Guarding" and the Special Case of Food

Food-related aggression is often lumped under the category of "resource guarding," but most dogs who react aggressively in the presence of some class of food do not inappropriately guard or protect other "resources" (toys, humans, beds, et cetera). In fact, the concern here is that "resource guarding" can commonly be viewed as a variant of normal behavior, or as a management-related problem that will respond to basic training. True food-related aggression is pathological and poses safety concerns for some households.

New Puppies Without Problematic Behaviors Involving Food

Feeding and Nourishing Pups When They Are Still with Mom

Puppies should learn early in life that they do not have to compete over food. This means that when the pups are first experiencing semisolid food (3 to 5 weeks of age) they should be fed from multiple dishes, or ones with central wells that help disperse the pups, ensuring that one pup does not control all the food.

- If one puppy is becoming a lot fatter than the other pups, or one puppy is a lot thinner than the others, breeders should be suspicious of behaviors at the food dish that may facilitate unequal feeding patterns.
- In extreme cases, plump, pushy puppies may need to be fed separately so that they do not learn to control access to food.
- Thin puppies may need more protection at feeding time or may simply need more food. Puppy metabolisms can vary and good breeders understand that they have to meet the individual puppy's needs.

Problems with Pet Store and Puppy Mill/Farm Puppies

Pet store and puppy mill/farm puppies (and virtually **all** dogs sold in pet stores in the United States **are puppy mill dogs**) are seldom fed in a manner that prohibits competition for food. Puppy mill/farm and pet store puppies are almost never assessed to see if their individual needs are met. As a result, puppy mill/farm and pet store puppies may be overrepresented in the population of young puppies and dogs who may have been food or nutrient deprived and who worry about having access to food.

Research shows that deprived puppies, like puppy mill/farm puppies, may have received inadequate nutrition *in utero* and in their first 2 months of life, resulting in impaired brain development and greater behavioral reactivity. If you know that you have adopted a puppy mill/farm or pet store puppy, please ensure that you feed them a high-quality puppy food that has been supplemented with docosahexanoic acid (DHA), the fatty acid that is most often lacking in their early diets and feeding strategies.

Please remember that these puppies usually are forced to compete for less-than-adequate levels of food. Once adopted, by feeding them often, even with small amounts of food, you can teach them that food will be available when they need it. For those young pups who hover over a food dish—empty or full—because they are so worried that they will miss their feeding opportunity, keeping a small amount of kibble available in a large number of locations may help them to learn that they do not have to worry that food will disappear. Obviously, if this strategy worsens the puppy's aggression or causes other pets in the house to eat too much, this intervention will not work for you. Instead, consider offering numerous, very tiny, protected meals throughout the day

How Often Do Puppies Need to Be Fed?

Frequent feedings are best because puppies will learn that when they are hungry there will be enough food. Puppies should be fed approximately 4 times a day from the time they start solid food through 5 to 6 weeks of age, then at least 3 times a day through 12 to 16 weeks of age, then at least twice a day through adulthood. Feeding an adult dog twice a day gives structure to the dog's day, allows the dog to eat on a schedule that approximates the family schedule, and allows the dog to be fed less food at once, which may improve the health of some dogs.

Additionally, some dogs who have relatively mild concerns about whether they will have enough food become more reactive when hungry. Feeding these dogs 2 or 3 times a day reduces their reactivity.

Recent research on canine brain development supports allowing the puppy to stay with the mother past the time when the mother is ready to wean the pup, which occurs somewhere in the 6- to 8-week range. Puppies continue to benefit from the nutrients provided by their mother's milk and by the social and learning environments she provides through at least 8.5 weeks of age.

Treats or Bones and Puppies

Once puppies are successfully eating solid food, they can have treats or, in some cases, bones. If puppies are given treats or bones, all puppies must be included. Puppies must be monitored and sometimes separated so that they do not fight. Treats/bones should never just be thrown into a group of puppies. No one puppy should be permitted to control access to all the treats or to all food, or to threaten littermates to get access to treats or food. If puppies are given fewer treats/bones than there are puppies, the pups will fight over the treat/bone. Research shows that if there are fewer bones than puppies, puppies structure a "hierarchy" by fighting over the bone. This is exactly what we do **not** want to encourage with our pets. *Puppies who do not have to fight for food, bones, or treats spend more time in play and social behaviors,* and do not learn to hone their fighting skills in the presence of food.

Teaching Puppies to Sit for Their Food and to Be Calm While Eating

No puppy who is old enough to be adopted is too young to learn to sit (See **Protocol for Deference**). The *earliest a puppy should be adopted into a new home is between 8 and 8.5 weeks* of age. Being allowed to live with their brothers, sisters, and mother through 8 weeks of age makes puppies more socially stable, makes them easier to house-train, improves their immunological health (they fight infections better), and allows them to respond to new environments with less stress and fear. Puppies as young as 4 to 5 weeks of age can learn to sit for a few seconds for a food treat, and excellent breeders take advantage of this. *Breeders should start to request that pups sit for treats and for feedings at this age.*

Having dogs sit for all food and treats will accomplish three things:

1. The dogs will start to learn to be calm before eating and when they want anything—the food dish is not going to come down until the individual dog is quiet.
2. The dogs will learn that physically contesting each other for food does not work, and, in fact, is associated with not getting the food.
3. Breeders can shift problematic coalitions either by preferentially feeding in a certain order, or feeding in a random and changing order. If there are no problem aggressions within the litter, feeding in a random and changing order is preferable because then the dogs will learn that humans are reliable and will feed them whether they are fed first or last.

Feeding the Puppy in His New Home

Once in his new home, the puppy should be taught to sit for all food treats (rewards for behavioral protocols, biscuits, and bones, et cetera). Puppies should learn to "wait" before the dish or treat is placed in front of them. Puppies have short attention spans and should not be asked to sit or wait long, and they should never be forced to sit. As they mature, they can be asked to wait for increasingly longer periods of time, but starting with 1 to a few seconds is reasonable. The easiest way to do this is as follows.

- You should ask the dog to sit.
- As you pick up the food, say "sit," and once the dog sits, say "wait." The pup only has to wait a second or two. If you do not know how to teach a dog or puppy to sit, please read the handout **Protocol for Teaching Cats and Dogs to "Sit," "Stay," and "Come."**
- As you put the dish/treat down say "okay," a signal that tells the dog it is okay to get up, and leave the dog to finish. If the dog gulps food, you may wish to hold the dish while the dog eats, frequently asking him to "sit" and "wait" while you add a bit more food so that you can help him to eat more slowly.
- If the puppy becomes excited every time the dish is slightly withdrawn, even if empty, only small amounts of food should be placed in the dish at any one time, and the dog should have to calm slightly before getting the food. Refilling the dish frequently but with tiny amounts will give you the opportunity to repeat the "sit, wait, okay" sequence frequently, and will help the puppy to reinforce his own appropriate behavior in response to these requests. Because the dog gets food when he complies with your requests, he will learn them quickly.

After the dog learns "wait" you can start teaching the dog to sit and to allow you to take the dish—whether or not the dog is done eating. This can be important because at some point you may need to get the dog's dish back while there is still food in it. The easiest way to do this is to hand-feed the dog the small amounts discussed above, and say "wait." If needed, you can *gently* restrain the dog by placing a hand softly on the chest. Move the dish away for a short while, get the dog to look quickly up at you ("Magda, look!"), and then **quickly** say "good girl" **and reward the dog with the food.**

What If the Puppy Worries When You Take the Food Dish?

If the dog has problems with waiting—and a problem is anything from wiggling and not looking at you to growling—teach the dog to sit and wait for an empty dish. Practice taking the dish and giving it back frequently at intervals that vary from a few to 30 seconds. Then, once the dog is perfect, start to add food to the dish. At first let the dog lick a small amount from your hand while your hand is in the dish, then add the food directly to the dish, always practicing "wait" and taking the food away, finally working up to the point where you can take the dish from the dog using the requests "sit" and "wait" when the dish contains food and is on the ground.

If the puppy still growls or becomes very worried about you taking the food or dish away, consider feeding the dog undisturbed, in a protected place. Puppies who become agitated when you have done nothing unkind to them may have had very awful early experiences, may have been undernourished *in utero,* may not have had the right kind of food early in life, or may be developing some problems. *By struggling with them, you will only make them worse.* By protecting them, you may gain their trust and help them to learn that they can rely on you.

Puppies and New Types of Food Items

Remember that new food items are naturally desirable, and a puppy who has been wonderful for presentation and removal of puppy chow might not be so wonderful for the presentation and removal of boiled chicken. Anticipate such problems and only offer tiny amounts of new food in the manner recommended above.

Older Dogs

Aggression When Food Is Present

Food-related aggression is a problem with some dogs. When a dog has food-related aggression, the dog guards their food, treats, rawhides, and/or real bones from other dogs or from people. Some dogs will guard and become aggressive when given any amount or any type of food, and others will become aggressive only when given something that they really value (e.g., a lamb shank). It is not unusual for dogs who are not aggressive when fed their routine meals to show aggression regarding special treats or foods and food toys.

Food-related aggression can be associated with other problem aggressions, but is a valid diagnostic category on its own.

If your dog is only aggressive around food, but does not challenge or become aggressive to you or someone else in other contexts, please do not assume that the dog's response to food is not problematic. Any inappropriate or undesirable canine aggression can cause a person to be maimed or killed. The presence of food is ubiquitous in our life and may be a particular problem for children who either carry food with them or who smell like food because they eat so frequently. Your choice is to either treat the food-related aggression or to manage it. Ignoring it is not a safe choice.

For many people, and especially for those with children in the house, deciding to manage rather than actively treat any food-related aggression can be a sane choice that will render your pet safe and loving.

Managing Food-Related Aggression

Food-related aggression can be quite variable.
- Some dogs will begin to growl softly as soon as they sense a human approaching and increase the intensity of their growl as people approach.
- Some dogs will growl while shaking and gulping their food.
- Some dogs will stare at anyone who is within their view while they are eating and snarl.

The safest resolution for all of these behaviors involves the same strategy: **if possible, feed the dog where he is undisturbed.**

Why Should We Suggest Leaving the Dog Undisturbed?

Food-related aggression may be tightly coupled to survival skills that have been honed over years of evolutionary time and treating it *safely* may be something that requires more effort than the average person is willing to expend.

Not treating the aggression IS NOT the same as ignoring it. A conscious, conscientious, and responsible decision to **not** treat food-related aggression means that:
- The people involved understand that the behavior is abnormal, undesirable, and dangerous.
- They do not wish to work with the dog to change the behavior.
- They will avoid eliciting the behavior at all costs so that they are safe and so that they do not help the dog to reinforce the undesirable response.

The decision to not treat food-related aggression, as described above, is an active, conscious choice. This is **not** the same as tolerating a dog who growls when he is fed. If you tolerate the growl, you are actually passively reinforcing or encouraging the inappropriate behavior. Dogs, like people, hone their skills every time they are allowed to exhibit a certain behavior, even if this behavior is inappropriate. If you do not wish to actively teach the dog a more suitable behavior than aggression in the presence of food, *or* if you cannot or are too afraid to work with the dog, you must ensure that you and the dog avoid all circumstances in which the dog will become aggressive.

How Can We Avoid Triggering Aggression Associated with Food?

Practicing avoidance of any situation that would trigger the food-related aggression includes the following steps:
1. The dog is fed at discrete times from a dish and is either kept sequestered until the dish is placed on the floor, at which point the dog is given access to the food **and** the humans leave, **or** the dog is asked to sit, stay, and wait until the dish is put down. The dog does not approach the dish until released ("Okay!") **and** the humans leave. Some dogs are fine when people are present, but react aggressively when other dogs or cats are present. They, too, must follow this first step.
2. The dog is **never** fed from the table or fed scraps when food is being prepared.
3. The dog is **always** behind a barrier (a locked gate, a locked door, or in a locked crate) when people are eating or preparing food. Yes, this **does** mean that the dog is banished from the family barbecues; however, this is safer than permitting the dog to be present.

   Please remember that the anxiety level of the people will decrease dramatically if they are not worried that the dog might bite. If people are stressed or distressed because they are concerned about the potential for a dangerous event to occur, they will have little patience for the dog and will be less understanding of the dog's special needs. Put the dog in another space and do not feel guilty.
4. Any treats (dog biscuits, table scraps) must be placed in the dog's bowl, in a room where the dog is undisturbed, and must be of a nature where the dog can finish them in one session. Being able to finish the treats or special food in one session is particularly important for dogs who guard food. If you know that your dog hoards and protects biscuits, even biscuits may be deleted from the dog's repertoire unless the dog can finish them within a few minutes of being given them. This is essential if the dog hides his biscuits in sofas, et cetera, because you will not know where the dog has stashed his treats and

will inadvertently be victimized by his hidden caches of food.

5. Some dogs respond aggressively **only** to **very**-high-quality treats such as bones, rawhides, pig ears, pizzle sticks, cow hooves, or chew sticks. If these **cannot** be finished in one setting (and most cannot), the simplest, easiest solution is to remove them from the dog's repertoire **forever**. This is not cruel, injurious, or deprivation for the dog—it is good common sense. Yes, the dog is forbidden to experience something that other dogs have and that he would find enjoyable; however, this cost is small when compared with the guilt you would feel if a child's skull were crushed because the child came between the dog and a bone. If dogs inappropriately protect food items, people must be responsible for insuring that they do not set the dog up to fail. This is a particular risk when small children are involved: even if the dog is behind a closed door with a rawhide, the child could open the door and pay profoundly for doing so.

Clearly, it is easy to avoid situations that provoke food-related aggression, and in most circumstances, this is a far preferable choice to treating the problem. *This aggression should only be treated if you can guarantee that you can always control the dog's access to food.* If you cannot do this (and *no household with children can do this*), you should not even entertain the notion of treating the aggression. Instead, it is preferable to believe that such aggression will occur when the opportunity is provided, and that it must and can be avoided.

If You Want to Treat the Food-Related Aggression and Can Do So Safely, What Do You Do?

Treatment of food-related aggression involves the same strategy outlined above for puppies (see *Feeding the Puppy in His New Home*): Gradually expose the dog to small amounts of food that is not terrifically valued, and follow this with increased amounts and quality of the food as the dog relaxes and does not respond. These are basic desensitization (DS) and counter-conditioning (CC) techniques with which a good, humane, trained/certified dog trainer can help.

You can start by hand feeding the dog small amounts of dog food. All food will come only from your hand and only when the dog is lying down, is quiet, and is calm. *If you are too fearful to do this, please do not even consider treating the aggression. Instead, please practice avoidance.* It's a better decision for you and for the dog, and the dog will trust you because of it.

If you wish to treat the dog, once the dog can accept all food from your hand without any aggression, fear, snatching or gulping, start to touch and then stroke the dog while feeding. Again, you must do this very, very gradually. With time, this should continue until you can massage the dog while providing food. The dog must be calm. Getting the dog to this stage could take months, and it may never occur in some dogs. *For these dogs, practicing avoidance is best.* If the dog trembles or gulps, avoiding and managing his food-related aggression may be kinder to him than treating it.

After the dog relaxes when touched and fed, you can introduce a dish as discussed above in the puppy section. At first a small amount of food should be offered. The dog should be taught "sit, wait, okay" and can only have the food when you say "okay." After the dog has finished the small amount of food, the dog should sit or lie down and wait while you reach for the dish, refill it, and replace it. *If the dog growls or lunges*

at any point in the sequence, you need to leave the dog alone and return to try again only when the dog is calm. If you do not wish to continue to try to teach the dog that you can take his food, please consider that a good decision. Manage and avoid his aggression.

If the dog gets up, you must move the food to where the dog cannot see it and repeat the sequence of "sit, stay, wait." You may have to do this many times before the dog responds appropriately, but that is far better than allowing the dog to become aggressive. If you do not feel you have the patience to pursue such a repetitious course, please do not treat the aggression. Instead, use avoidance to control the problem. This is a responsible, humane choice.

Finally, once you can fill, offer, reach for, get, and refill the food dish, you are ready to start practicing leaving the dog and returning while the dog is eating. At first you should only move a few centimeters from the dog and then return. The dog should never react aggressively or by shaking, whining, or cringing. If the dog shows any of these behaviors, you can try to repeat the movement more slowly until the dog is calm. Alternatively, you can just decide to protect the dog and manage his reactions.

The goal is to be able to put the dish down, leave the room, return, request that the dog sit (when the dish still has food), take the dish, and have the dog relax throughout. This can take months to accomplish and may never be wholly successful. If this plan is unsuccessful, you will at least have learned the dog's limits and you should be able to calmly accept that you have to control any potential danger (i.e., **avoid the situation**).

What About Special Food Items Like Rawhides and Real Bones?

You can repeat the above for any food-related substance to which the dog reacts: dog food, rawhides, real bones, or scraps. Please note: real bones and rawhides often elicit a much more exaggerated response than does any food in a dish. If you doubt your ability or desire to work successfully with the dog, just avoid the situation. Dogs do not require rawhides to be happy.

Anyone deciding to work with a dog with food-related aggression may feel more secure doing so if the dog is fitted with a head collar. These may help you to quickly, humanely, and safely close the dog's mouth, avoiding any untoward events. If you think that a head collar might help you, please see the **Protocol for Choosing Collars, Head Collars, Harnesses, and Leads.** If you feel you *need* a head collar, please think about whether avoiding the problem is a better choice.

Final Advice

It is perfectly all right, and quite sensible, for someone to decide that they do not wish to work with a dog who has food-related aggression, and, instead, choose avoidance. No one should feel guilty for this decision, and if the dog is worried about food, it is much kinder to feed him under conditions where he need not worry. Please remember that dealing with food-related aggression is not about "not letting the dog get away with it," "controlling the dog," or "dominating the dog." In fact, it's about protecting the dog and treating the dog humanely so that he can enjoy his food and his life with you and those you love.

PROTOCOL FOR UNDERSTANDING AND TREATING DOGS WITH INTERDOG AGGRESSION

Interdog aggression—the global term for truly problematic aggression between dogs—can be highly variable, but it generally appears at social maturity (approximately 18 to 24 months of age in dogs; range: ~12 to 36 months). Changes in social relationships *also* occur in dogs *who are not affected by problem aggressions,* and these changes occur during this same developmental time period. During the period of social maturity all social animals experience huge upheavals in neurochemistry, so it is not surprising that this is when we fully appreciate truly problematic social interactions.

Interdog aggression is more common between, but not restricted to, dogs of the same sex. Interdog aggression appears to be about social relationships between the dogs and how the affected or aggressor dog perceives relative social status or role, and his control over that status/role.

Interdog aggression can occur between dogs who are unknown to each other and/or between dogs who are known to each other. When threats or fighting are seen in dogs who are *unknown* to each other, it is important to rule out two reasons for the fighting other than interdog aggression:

1. normal behavior, which may involve some posturing, especially as dogs get to know each other, and
2. problematic behavior involving fear or fear aggression.

Neither of these is our concern in this protocol. For fearful dogs see the **Protocol for Understanding and Treating Dogs with Fear/Fearful Aggression.**

True Interdog Aggression

True interdog aggression usually involves household dogs who may have gotten along in the past without outright fighting, but who experience a profound change in their relationships as one or both of them moves through social maturity. The most commonly seen pattern may be the one where a young dog is becoming socially mature, and where the older dog is having difficulty with the accompanying behavioral changes and altered social behaviors shown by the younger dog.

Roles for Development

Very few dogs are aggressive to other dogs because they never learned how to interact with them when they were young, although this can happen. The vast majority of dogs affected by interdog aggression have had experience with other dogs that has been good and normal. Most dogs displaying interdog aggression have been part of the household since they were puppies and their behaviors are reported to have changed.

Dogs focus primarily on their parents and littermates until they are approximately 5 to 8 weeks of age, at which point they become very receptive to interaction with people. Puppies form loose social groupings that have relatively predictable interactions within the litter, and these social groups and interactions are maintained both by some agonistic or forceful behavior (posturing, vocalizing, and snapping) and by active and passive deference by the other pups (rolling on the back with or without urinating, or looking away).

The few studies that have been done on puppy social behavior indicate that these puppyhood social patterns appear to have no association with the relative interactions of the animals when they reach social maturity. Hence, these puppy patterns should not be associated with any later interdog aggression. It *is* conceivable (but probably rare) that some dogs who never see other dogs when they are puppies might have some problems relating to other dogs; however, these problems are often related to fear, not to the actual interaction with the other dogs. See the **Protocol for Understanding and Treating Dogs with Fear/Fearful Aggression** for information about these dogs.

The overwhelming majority of dogs who have problems with interdog aggression have a problem with changing social interactions and relationships, or in understanding these interactions, and have had no known untoward experiences as puppies. Most clients report that these dogs were "good" with the dogs with whom they are now fighting when younger, although we have very few detailed data about whether they were truly "good" or whether there were earlier problems that did not rise to the level of fighting. More detailed research will likely reveal some earlier problems with some aspect of signaling, communication or play ability that was misunderstood. The neurochemical shift that drives social maturity would make such problems worse.

The Complex Issue of Sex

Interdog aggression is *not* associated with sexual maturity (~6 to 9 months of age), although there is a role for testosterone in some forms of interdog aggression and in normal contests between intact dogs.

Testosterone can stimulate dogs to roam and mark with urine. These two behaviors take dogs into the path of other dogs, increasing the chances for potential conflict between two dogs who do not live in the same household. Testosterone may also facilitate fighting: intact (entire/non-castrated) dogs react quickly, react at a higher level overall, and take longer to calm down. These types of fights are not usually seriously injurious fights, and some sparring may be normal behavior for intact male dogs who are following estrus females. However, if an intact male dog is affected with true interdog aggression, the testosterone may facilitate the aggression. People with intact male dogs should know of these concerns.

Castration (removal of the testicles) may greatly decrease roaming, urine marking, and fighting between dogs, and has been reported to diminish all of these in approximately 60% of all dogs with such problems. *However, it is important to remember that all behaviors have learned components.*

- Just because a hormone may facilitate the development of one form of aggression does not mean that diminishing that hormone will simply fix the problem.
- If a dog has been exhibiting a series of behaviors for a long time (i.e., years) that dog has learned about the behavioral patterns and his response.
- Simply removing the hormones that help that response does not affect the learned component.
- Use of behavior modification will be needed to alter the learned component and we use behavior mod to change how dogs respond to other dogs.

The situation with intact (entire/non-spayed) females is not so simple, and few good data have been collected.

- Hormonal cycling does not appear to facilitate aggression between females in the same sense that testosterone facilitates aggression between normal or problematic males; however, clients often report that many intact bitches experience "mood" changes prior to and during estrus (heat).
- Many bitches also experience changes in appetite and activity levels during or preceding their heat cycles. If there were some mild status- or communication-related problems between the females in the household, they might be exaggerated at such times.
- If there is an intact male in the house, he might become highly interested in one of the females, and further disrupt the social rule structure that has allowed everyone to peacefully co-exist.
- Finally, some females become more social and solicitous when in heat.

There are few studies that have looked in-depth at any association between female hormones and aggression, but those that have done so indicate that female hormones *do not* seem to play a large role in interdog aggression.

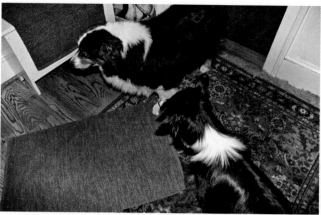

The dog at the lower right is meeting the dog at the top of the photo for the first time. Her automatic response to new dogs is to threaten them. In her case, she does this to find out whether they will pose a risk to her. The dog at the top knows this, and gives the correct response: he stops and averts his gaze.

Why Dogs React to Other Dogs

Dogs who react to *unknown dogs* generally do so for two reasons: they are either afraid of them or they act as if they perceive, with or without cause, that the other dog represents a social threat.

Dogs who are afraid of other dogs can be spontaneously afraid of them, or they can be afraid because they have been attacked, and may develop fearful behavior or fear aggression as sequelae. Co-morbidity of diagnoses should alert clients, veterinarians and handlers to ask which came first.

One function of any challenging or threatening behavior is to provoke a situation to learn if there is a risk to the individual displaying the behavior. *Dogs ask questions to gain information*, and one way they do so can involve a threat. Humans often misinterpret these aspects of canine signaling. We need to think about interpreting "dog behaviors" in terms of what they mean *for the dog*. A growl may be given to learn if the other dog will growl back or pick up a toy: the dog doing the growling clarifies the intent of the interaction by watching the response of the dog at whom he growled.

Dogs who react as if there is a challenge about social status or relationships when there is none are reacting inappropriately and out of context. If there is a challenge (staring, hackles up, paw on shoulders, growling, snarling, snapping) of any kind, a reaction might be appropriate, but it is important to remember that, as for people, *normal social behaviors* in dogs have rules. If the approaching dog just stares at your dog and your dog goes for his throat, refusing to let go even when the other dog is whimpering and has rolled over, the approaching dog is behaving appropriately—your dog is not.

We can understand and help these dogs if we pay attention to the *context* of the interaction.

The Common Versions of Interdog Aggression

Most reported interdog aggression occurs between housemates, and it occurs more commonly between same-sex housemates. Females are overrepresented in case studies of dogs with interdog aggression. It is not unusual for two dogs to have lived in relative harmony together for 2 years before there are problems. **These problems are not generally due to "inappropriate or incomplete early socialization" or to some abuse the dogs experienced.** The development of these problems reflects the intrinsic change that all social animals experience when they become socially mature.

One of the more common of the scenarios for interdog aggression within a household involves the younger dog, who was fine as a puppy, but now that he is becoming socially mature, new behaviors are tried out and what the older dog sees as "challenges" have become common. Normal dogs would not view such "challenges" as true threats and would negotiate the changes in the younger dog's behavior as he moves from puppy-like behaviors, through more assertive and sometimes uncertain behaviors, through calm and mature behaviors that will characterize the dog as an adult.

Dogs who are the aggressors in interdog aggression have difficulty with these transitions. We now believe that it may be likely that the aggressor was never truly completely "normal" as a pup, and that there is a definite role for worsening behavior associated with changes in brain neurochemistry as the dogs move through social maturity.

Challenges can include:
- blocking access to a bed or crate,
- lying on or in front of a couch or chair (blocking access),
- them on the other dog,
- stealing the other dog's biscuits, rawhides, or toys,
- blocking access to the other dog's food,
- shoving past the other dog to get out or in a door or car first,
- using halls, doorways, and steps as situations to control the other dog and his access to areas or escape from them,
- ritualized displays, including where the challenger approaches the other dog nose to shoulder,
- staring,
- vocalizing (aggressive barks, snarls, growls), and
- frank aggression.

These behaviors can all occur alone or in combination, and may be self-limiting or can escalate within a few minutes to outright aggression with grabbing and biting.

It is important to treat the problem as soon as it becomes apparent. The longer that the problem is allowed to persist, the worse the dogs will get.

Classic Presentations of Interdog Aggression

Some examples of classic presentations of interdog aggression will make clear the importance of four skillsets that normal dogs should possess: (a) reading signals correctly; (b) correctly processing/understanding the information in those signals; (c) make an appropriate plan based on the signals received, read, and processed; and (d) acting appropriately and signal an action or plan based on the original situation.

- One commonly seen version of interdog aggression involves a problematic younger dog who suddenly "challenges" the fairly normal dog in the contexts above. As a normal dog, the older dog does not wish to fight and tries to deescalate the situation by walking away from many of the situations. The younger dog continues to threaten the older dog, despite the fact that the older dog is always signaling that this is not necessary. Here we do not know if the younger dog can adequately read the social signals, or if he can understand and process the signals, or whether he can act appropriately on these signals.
- The older dog can be the aggressor and may be having difficulty with the behavioral changes associated with social maturity that the younger dog is exhibiting, despite any threats or challenges from the younger or new dog. Here the older dog read the signals correctly, but does not find the change of the pup into another adult acceptable.
- Sometimes the younger dog is just trying out some of the behaviors that develop with age (pushing on another dog), and may not be the least bit aggressive, but the older dog perceives the younger dog's behaviors as a serious problem and becomes aggressive. Here the older dog is reading the signals within the broad context inappropriately.

It is likely that the specific pathology differs in all three of the above situations. Regardless, by managing the environment, working with behavior modification and using medication as needed, we can improve the lives for both the humans and the dogs in most situations. To do this, we need to understand the patterns to the extent possible.

Generally, regardless of age, the dog that is challenged responds in one of four ways:

1. She unambiguously displays deferential behavior and shows the other dog that she is not interested in fighting; for example, the challenged dog rolls onto her back and may urinate, looks away, waits for the other dog to give the next set of social signals and instructions.
2. The challenged dog fights back, "wins" or "loses," and that outcome is accepted by both dogs.
3. Both dogs jockey for "status" and each is unwilling to concede status to the other. This means that fights continue to erupt and generally become more violent. Daily interactions may also contain more passive challenges.
4. One dog concedes to the other or pre-empts any aggressive behavior by offering deferential behaviors, but the other dog is still aggressive.

In situations 3 and 4, the aggression continues and may become prolonged, confusing, and dangerous.

The tricky situation is situation 4. Here, *the immediate aggression resolves, but the process of resolution is still dangerous because a pathological aggressor will ultimately not accept continued deferential behaviors from the other dog*—the aggressor wants the other out of the household.

Whether this is a response to an evolutionary pattern gone awry is unknown, but in free-ranging and wild dog groups, most males disperse at social maturity or help the related females in the group, and most females work closely socially with the females most related to them, often mothers, aunts, and cousins. Our living situation with our dogs does not consider this evolutionary pattern. Because our dogs do not grow up in their own extended family groups, the way we live with them may contribute to the pathology in susceptible dogs. Interdog aggression between dogs in the same household most often involves females, and this could be one reason why that is the case. That said, we have likely selected dogs over time to get along with others, and should recognize these problem behaviors, regardless of ultimate cause, as pathological.

Most people assume that when dogs fight they do so because one dog is pushy and just doesn't respect the dog who is the "top dog." *** Please do not assume that this is so; to do so is the single most common error made in managing fighting dogs.*** In fact, unless the aggression is transient and rare, this is likely *the exceptional situation*, and by thinking that dogs who fight are "normal," you are probably putting your dogs at risk for injury or death.

Identifying the Relative Aggressors and Victims

You can best learn whether your dogs fall into any of the scenarios, above, by following them around with a video camera and obtaining video on normal, daily interactions. In this way, patterns of association and space use will be clear. Videos allow you to share true behavioral data with your veterinarian, specialist and trainer so that you can get adequate help for your dogs. Once you understand which behaviors are normal and which are problematic you should be able to identify the relative victims (defensively aggressive dogs) and the relative aggressors (offensively aggressive dogs). Although most of the behavior modification could be helpful without correct identification of victims versus aggressors, you will be much more successful in preventing, anticipating and fixing problem interactions if you understand each dog's relative role.

If you have more than two dogs, you may have an advantage in learning about the relationships between your dogs. A third dog often acts as a "mediator" dog.

- If you have a mediator dog, he will be watchful of the interactions of the other dogs.
- The mediator dog often chooses to accompany one dog; this tends to be the victim dog (the one who may be exhibiting defensive aggression).
- The mediator dog often physically comes between the aggressor and the victim, turning the victim away from any active or passive threats from the aggressor.
- The mediator dog often blocks the view of or access to the victim dog.

Dogs read dog signaling better than humans do. If you have one of these helpful and "supranormal" dogs in your household as a mediator, you are fortunate. She will help you to identify relative victims and aggressors and will provide guidance about whether the changes you have made are helping. If you are not sure whether one of your dogs plays this role, review photos and video of your dogs; you will often be able to see the protective behaviors discussed above in action.

Some mediator dogs are so good at what they do that you may not appreciate how hard they were working until they can no longer protect the victim. Do not be surprised if these dogs try to pull the aggressor from the victim if there is a true fight.

Myths About Hierarchy, Dominance, and "Alpha"

Much has been written about ranking your dogs numerically, determining who is "alpha" and about "dominance." Most misunderstanding about canine signaling and social systems would vanish if we realized that the commonly used description of "dominance" is *not* synonymous with any aggression, including "dominance"/impulse control aggression and interdog aggression. "Dominance" may not even be synonymous with hierarchical standing.

"Dominance" has been defined in the original scientific literature as an individual's ability to maintain or regulate access to some resource. It is a description of the regularities of winning or losing contests over those resources, is not to be confused with status, and does not need to confer priority of access to resources. *Status, in contrast, is generally defined by the ease of frequency of engendering deferential behaviors from others.* It is important to keep labels separate from concepts. We often label dogs as "dominant" without giving any thought to the actual concept of dominance as it's defined. We would do better by deleting these "loaded" terms from our vocabulary and instead discuss what the dog is actually doing. If the dog is pushy, say so; if the dog is able to quell disputes among dogs and is automatically deferred to by other dogs, just say so.

Paradigms involving such hierarchical judgments usually fail because they encourage adversarial relationships, but they *especially* fail in profound cases of interdog aggression.

Interdog aggression is associated with relationships between dogs and their reactions—right or wrong—to threats and about the form of social interactions. These relationships between dogs are not absolute. They change with age, health, and, most importantly, context.

The manifestations of these relationships can be affected by the people who are present and by how those people interact with their dogs. Some relationships apply only to feeding and sleeping orders. Because dog social relationships and organization, like those of people, are not linear, the amount of aggression exhibited may depend on which dogs were where when. A dog who challenges one dog may not care about another dog in the household who, to all outward appearances, seems to act the same and be the same age and sex. Chances are they are not acting identically, and it is in the subtleties that the problems with the relationship occur.

Aggression as an Anxiety Disorder

Dogs who exhibit out-of-context or inappropriate responses to other dogs actually suffer from anxiety disorders: They cannot adequately assess the risk associated with the other dog and so provoke the situation in an attempt to get more information or to preempt any challenges.

Obviously, such out-of-context threats are not viewed favorably by most other dogs, who learn that the dog threatening or attacking them is unreliable. *With repeated exposure to aggressive interactions, both dogs in the interaction become more anxious and reactive and, often, more aggressive.*

A perfectly normal dog can become the aggressor if he perceives that the only way to not be hurt is to stop the other dog before the attack occurs. This is why it is so important to get as much information as possible about the way the dogs interacted over time.

Treating These Problematic Relationships

Treatment of interdog aggression focuses on setting and maintaining a new set of social relationships that will *relieve everyone's uncertainty and, most importantly, keep everyone safe.*

Generally, "reinforcement" is given to the dog who is best able to contribute to a stable social environment by behaving most appropriately, given the context. This may be the younger, the larger, the more physically fit, the more confident dog, but it certainly does not have to be this dog. If you have a "mediator dog," he will identify the dog behaving most appropriately for you: This is the dog the mediator dog is protecting and for whom he is running interference.

Some important cautions must be issued about working with these dogs:

- Never physically punish these dogs. All you will do is to raise their level of distress, and they might feel that they have to fight you off. Their reaction to punishment could be fear, pain, or redirected aggression. None of these are good choices, and you could make a bad situation worse.
- If at all possible, never reach between two fighting dogs. Most people have good intentions and want to separate fighting dogs to prevent injury to them. If you place your body parts between the dogs, the dogs might, accidentally, mistake you for the other dog and injure you. When this happens, the dogs usually withdraw, but the damage is already done. Instead, if you know that you have a problem with your dogs, watch them carefully any time they are together and keep cardboard, a broom, a bucket of water, a hose, a full, unopened bottle of seltzer or club soda, or a blanket handy. These are all "remote control" items that you can use to separate the dogs safely. If no small children, high-strung humans, or nervous animals are in the house, a loud noise, like that generated by a foghorn, may also help to separate the animals, but this will usually only work once. **Screaming by humans—particularly by young humans—will worsen the situation.**
- Generally, once the dogs are apart they start to calm down and you can remove the aggressor to a neutral spot behind a closed door. Removing the victim if the aggressor is unrestrained may enhance the helplessness of the victim in the eyes of the aggressor.
- Remember that any injured animal hurts and is frightened. These animals can bite you without being malicious. Avoid

this by transporting injured dogs using blankets and loose muzzles if they need veterinary care.

- Disregard all common myths about the "dominant" dog and "dominance," and, instead, watch the dogs to learn which dog is behaving most appropriately, given the context. Then, *reward the dog behaving most appropriately given the circumstances*, regardless of breed, sex, age, physical condition, or size. You may wish to read the following online position statements by members of groups devoted to humane behavioral care for pet dogs: www.avsabonline.org/avsabonline/images/stories/Position_Statements/dominance%20statement.pdf, www.dogwelfarecampaign.org (www.dogwelfarecampaign.org/why-not-dominance.php).

Basic Treatment Tick List

When Outdoors:

1. Only walk dogs together on leads who can get along. A lead automatically prohibits an anxious dog from leaving and victims of interdog aggression can be further victimized when they are constrained to stay close to the aggressor while on lead.
2. If you are walking the dogs as a group, make sure that if there is a dog that is "out in front" that dog is the one whose right to exist in an unmolested manner you are trying to reinforce. You do not want to be accidentally rewarding a walking order that the dogs understand to be associated with threats to one or more dogs.

    Under normal circumstances dogs should not need to care about who is in front of whom. If you are having these types of struggles on walks, your canine household has issues that need to be addressed. If you are unsuccessful in gently requesting that the pushier dog step back, consider some trial separations of the dogs to see if one dog blossoms when not harassed. If this happens, you need to work with the situation immediately.

    Remember that in anxiety-related conditions, like interdog aggression, many of the provocative behaviors are exhibited to gain information, and that part of the pathology may be that the dog is incapable of interpreting the response in all but the worse light for the victim. Also, abnormal dogs may misinterpret the behavior of a dog who pulls out in front of the others: to the normal dog, such behavior may just indicate that the dog is following a scent; to an abnormal dog the dog who pulled out in front may be seen as a deliberate threat.

    If you must walk dogs together and you have a "mediator dog," that dog should be between the victim and the aggressor.

3. If the dogs are traveling in the car, the aggressor must be gated in the far back of the car or crated in the back. The other dogs should be in seatbelts or crates in more forward regions of the car. You may need to cover the aggressor's crate or gate if he takes the opportunity of being close to them to stare at the other dogs.
4. If your dog only reacts to other dogs on the street, avoid the other dogs until you have completed **Protocol for Deference** and **Protocol for Relaxation: Behavior Modification Tier 1** and can begin **Tier 2: Protocol for Desensitizing and Counter-Conditioning a Dog (or Cat) from Approaches from Strangers.**

5. If possible, always walk your aggressor dog on a head collar, not a harness. At the first sign of any inappropriate behavior, ask the dog to sit and relax. Using the head collar, close the dog's mouth. If the dog still reacts, turn him around immediately, and ask him to sit and relax. If the dog still reacts, remove the dog from the situation as quickly as possible. Use the head collar to close the dog's mouth and lead him to a place where he can sit and relax. This will help whether your dog reacts to unfamiliar dogs on the street or the dogs with whom he is being walked. Please remember that dogs who only react to unfamiliar dogs can redirect their aggression to these dogs to others with whom they are walked. A head collar is the simplest all-around preventive solution. See the **Protocol for Choosing Collars, Head Collars, Harnesses, and Leads** for suggestions.
6. If your dog threatens or attacks dogs outside of the household on the street be aware that *this response may not be associated with interdog aggression—the response may be associated with fear.* Please discuss this possibility with your veterinarian. Automatically assuming that all dogs who show aggression to other dogs are either normal or nasty condemns dogs who are uncertain or fearful to a life of never getting the help they need.

When Indoors

1. Keep all dogs involved in the interdog aggression separated at all times when not supervised. Keeping unknown dogs on the street separate is easy. Keeping dogs separate within a household is difficult and requires thought, tangible plans, and possibly a written map or floor plan. If you able to identify the dog who is the aggressor, confine the aggressor to the less-desirable room (a spare bedroom; a pen in the heated, well-lit basement or garage). All other dogs should have free range. If more than one dog is actively problematic, all the problem dogs should be confined, and the non-problem dogs can be left loose. If everyone is a problem, they should all be kept in crates where they cannot see each other or threaten each other.
2. Bell the dogs with different sounding bells that you can distinguish (Bear Bells: www.rei.com). If you cannot distinguish the sounds, bell only the aggressor. The bell will tell you when the aggressor is approaching and when the problem dogs are close together. The dogs who have been victimized by the aggressor can also use the bell to monitor the aggressor's movements and avoid interaction. Dogs who are having problems with each other can have a chance to approach each other *if and only if* you are confident that you can control them long-distance, and prevent any injury. Please remember that injury can be physical or behavioral. Of these, the behavioral injury may be worse for many dogs who learn to live in constant terror. If you do not feel that you can adequately monitor the dogs when loose, or that you cannot read the dogs' signals well enough to relax, that's fine. You now have three choices:
   a. one or both dogs are crated,
   b. one dog is behind a baby gate, and
   c. the dogs are each on harnesses or head collars and restrained so that they cannot get to each other.
   Again, please remember that dogs who are separated but who are staring at each other are not "mentally" separated. The dog who is being threatened can be trapped

by crates, gates, and leads. Do not let this happen. These dogs can only be together under the conditions listed above if neither one of them visually or physically threatens the other. Also, if a dog is afraid of crates or cannot exhibit normal behaviors when in them, please do not crate that dog. Feeling entrapped makes such dogs more anxious and reactive and will worsen your situation.

3. Choose an order in which to reinforce the dogs based on identifying which dog is behaving the most appropriately. **Remember that reinforcement is not about rewarding the pushiest, most "dominant" dog.** It's about rewarding the dog who is most appropriate so that all the dogs get the message that obnoxious/abnormal behaviors are not rewarded, but calm, nonthreatening ones are. This type of reward-based reinforcement works because it mimics canine social systems and uses deferential behaviors to get attention and other "currencies." When reinforcing the most appropriate dog, feed that dog first, give her attention first, give her access to the yard first, et cetera. You can get hints about what will be most successful from the dogs' behaviors, as follows:

a. For example, you have two dogs and the younger one has begun to passively challenge the older, the older is snarling, and most of the time the younger backs off. The older one is larger and stronger than the younger, just as healthy, and not that different in age. Reinforce the older over the younger. The younger dog here is likely normal, but just too pushy, and can learn how to have a better relationship with his companion once the threats subside.

b. The older dog perceives a threat from the younger, but the younger isn't really doing anything active. The older is weaker than the younger, and although the younger is sweet, she is huge. Reinforce the younger dog and make sure that the older receives needed attention, including tasks he can still accomplish, so that the shift in relative social relationships is more fluid. The younger dog is actually behaving the most appropriately of the two dogs, and if you work with both dogs the older dog can learn that she is not a threat. You cannot reward the older dog because then you would be telling him that his out-of-context aggressions—and his perception that he must exhibit such aggressions— are acceptable when they are not. Please remember the role of exercise in reactivity: If the younger dog is not getting enough aerobic exercise she will be a brat, and pester the older dog. One solution here would be to find a play group of young, rambunctious dogs for the younger dog so that she is tired when she comes home to her older companion.

c. The younger dog is actively pushing around or challenging the older and is becoming very aggressive. The older is fighting back and the younger is meeting the challenge. The older is arthritic, and weaker, but the dogs are fairly evenly matched in size. It will break your heart, but reinforce the younger dog and see what happens. If the younger dog then recalibrates her response to the older dog, you'll be fine. If the younger dog is normal and just provoking the social system around her as part of the social learning that occurs as dogs (and humans) enter social maturity, the younger

dog will become less aggressive. *However, if the older dog does not respond to the aggression of the younger dog with another aggressive threat and the younger dog continues to threaten, you have a problem.* This behavior is abnormal and out-of-context, and the time to deal with it in the manner discussed in this handout for true aggression is *now*. Again, remember to meet the older dog's mental, physical, and behavioral needs, even if it means changes in your behavioral interactions.

d. One of the dogs—regardless of age—perceives a challenge and exhibits behaviors consistent with deferential or disengaged behaviors (e.g., turning the head or neck away, ceasing motion or other activity, turning the body away, displaying the ventral neck or the groin, tucking the tail, et cetera), but the aggressor/challenger doesn't seem to care. The last time the challenged dog rolled over on her back the other dog moved in for the "kill," and attacked the more passive dog's belly and neck. *CAUTION: This is the true problem scenario, and it is almost always misunderstood and mishandled!* Reinforce the challenged (deferential) dog. This may be very difficult to execute successfully, but if you are not able to give this dog some status (regardless of her age) so that the aggressive dog realizes that this dog has a right to exist, she will be a terrific victim. *Remember that it is abnormal to respond to a deferential behavior with a threat. By definition, aggression that occurs when the recipient is signaling that they are not a threat is inappropriate and out-of-context. DO NOT ASSUME THAT THE DOGS WILL NOT INJURE EACH OTHER.* These dogs can seriously disable or kill each other in such circumstances. If the dog that is deferring cannot hold the "status" in a way that encourages the aggressive dog to back down—and she may be doing everything right—you will either have to keep the dogs continuously separated or find one of the dogs another home. If you decide to place the challenger, that dog can only go to a home where he will be the single dog. You do not know if this dog will behave in the same manner to another dog in a new home, but in the interest of the welfare of all of the dogs you should assume that this could be the case and minimize the cost of error.

4. Reinforcing the chosen dog has active and passive components. First, separate them as discussed above. Second, enforce the concept that the dog being threatened has the right to exist by feeding him first, letting him out before the other dog(s), giving him a treat or toy first, walking first, playing with him first, grooming him first, et cetera. Make sure you understand what is really being said here— this is **not** about "dominance." It's actually about providing a clear set of rules that provide information about which dog should serve as the model for the other dogs' behaviors. Because misunderstandings are so injurious to dogs, a short discussion about what "status" means is warranted.

a. **You are not imposing a "rank" order on these dogs:** instead, you are encouraging the normal types of social deference that would be exhibited by dogs under normal conditions. Unfortunately, myths about dog–dog relations are so ingrained that we have come to believe that dogs seize control and force others to wait for them. Nothing could be more wrong. By reinforcing

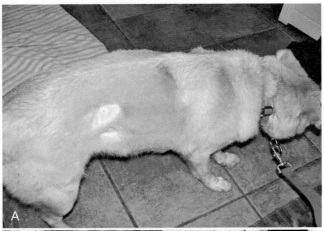

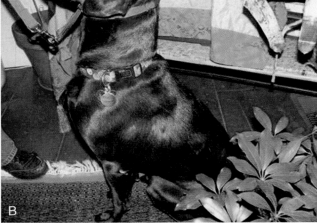

A common pattern of wounds resulting from interdog aggression involving another dog in the household.

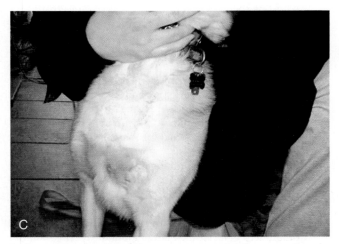

As the aggression intensifies, aggressors also focus on the victim's chest and neck.

an appropriately behaved dog you encourage the normal fluidity of the social system and can then reward the aggressive dog for not reacting.

b. You can also more passively encourage the aggressor to understand that the victim has some status by allowing the victim to sleep in a crate in your room, on a bed there, or on your bed (if you like this and the dog never growls at you while you are sleeping), while the other dog is banished to a room or crate outside your room. This has nothing to do with beds and "spoiling" and everything to do with the fact that access to preferred spots or to attention is a currency for dogs.

5. Regardless of how you decide to work with the dogs, each dog needs daily individual attention. The dog that is being reinforced should always get the attention first, in the presence of the other dog if this can be done quietly and without threats or overt aggression. If necessary, restrain the inappropriate dog using a harness.

6. Fit all dogs with a head collar, or a good no-pull harness, and gradually reintroduce them to each other when there is no attention being given. For example, watch TV while they both sit quietly, secured at a distance where they can see each other, but not lunge, and connect. If the dog that has been problematic stares at the dog you are trying to reinforce, gently turn his head away from the other dog and toward you so that he can take his cues from you. If the dog that you are trying to reinforce stares at the other, ignore her if the other dog doesn't growl. If the other dog does growl, interrupt the dogs by asking them to look at you. If this does not work, or if the aggression intensifies, remove the most aggressive dog and banish him. If the dog that you are trying to reinforce stares at the other dog and the other dog looks away, reward them both with food treats—that is exactly the type of fluid and flexible behavioral relationship you are trying to reinforce.

7. Make sure that you have followed **Protocol for Deference, the Protocol for Teaching Your Dog to Take a Deep Breath and Use Other Biofeedback Methods as Part of Relaxation,** and the **Protocol for Relaxation: Behavior Modification Tier 1.** The next phase will focus on desensitizing the dogs to each other. This will be true whether your dog reacts to dogs within the household or to strange dogs on the street (see **Tier 2: Protocol for Desensitizing and Counter-Conditioning a Dog or a Cat from Approaches from Strangers** and **Protocol for the Introduction of New Pets** [the principles are the same]).

In this world view, *treatment is about both understanding the neurochemical changes that occur with learning and repeated exposure, and about becoming more humane.* To do this, we must begin to see the world from the dog's point of view, which minimally requires that we let go of labels that may say more about us and our need, than they do about the behavior. The situation with interdog aggression demonstrates why we need to be more mindful of terminology, issues, and approaches that can inadvertently do more harm than good.

Antianxiety medications may help some dogs who otherwise are not able to succeed in this program, and are routinely required for serious aggression. Please remember that if it's decided that medication could benefit your dog, you need to use it **in addition** to the behavior modification, not instead of it.

PROTOCOL FOR UNDERSTANDING AND TREATING DOGS WITH PROTECTIVE AND/OR TERRITORIAL AGGRESSION

Dogs who have problems with protective or territorial aggression protect people or places regardless of whether there is actually a threat. Because there is no, true contextual threat, this aggression represents an inappropriate, out-of-context response, and one that is potentially dangerous to the person or other animal that the dog perceives is trespassing.

In contrast, a dog who behaves appropriately takes her cues as to the appropriateness of her behavior from her people or from the context. When a normal dog is unsure as to whether a threat exists, she may give a low-level threat (a bark or a growl). By behaving this way, dogs ask questions about whether they need to worry. A normal dog makes her decision about whether there is a threat based on the response to her provocative vocalization. In other words, dogs seek information and clarity about what's really going on. This is one reason why it is foolish to bark back at or growl at a barking or growling dog: the dog correctly perceives your response as an out-of-context, and perhaps threatening, answer and then the dog becomes more aggressive.

Roles for Appropriate Protective Behaviors

Clients often find protective and territorial behaviors desirable in their dogs, and want the dogs to protect them and their property. If there truly is a threat (an attack or a break-in), dogs treated for problem protective or territorial aggression will still react to repel the intruder. It is almost impossible to teach dogs to act in an *appropriately* protective manner unless they show signs of interest in doing so. Scaring or threatening normal dogs, or rewarding pathologically aggressive dogs, will **not** make them good protectors.

Once the dog appears to be willing to protect, those traits can be enhanced through training. The problem is that *appropriate* protection and *inappropriate* protective aggression are very different circumstances. Clients are often concerned that if they control their dog's inappropriate, out-of-context protective or territorial aggression that their dog will no longer protect them or their property if there is a threat. *This is not true,* and it is kinder and safer to everyone to take action to ensure that the dog learn not to react inappropriately.

Dogs can protect people or animals in their household from other people and/or other animals (protective aggression), or they can protect a space (crate, car, yard, room, house) from other animals and/or people (territorial aggression). The dog's behavior becomes problematic because **the dog responds as if there is a threat when none exists.** For example, when someone hugs you in the presence of your dog, and your dog threatens the person hugging you, this is an inappropriate and out-of-context aggression. Your dog is using the same behavior that he would use to repel an intruder, but there is no intruder.

Abuse Concerns

Some dogs react inappropriately even if no one touches their person. Sometimes dogs will start to growl if their person stops to talk to someone on the street. Clients often report that these dogs do not react if the client does not acknowledge the presence of the passerby, while other clients complain that if their dog even sees another person on the street they begin to react. Both behaviors are a part of a continuum of problematic behavior. In either case, the person that the dog threatens can be a total stranger (a delivery person) or someone known to the dog, but not well (the client's cousin). The reasons for such aggression may lie in the dog's past history, or the dog may be developing difficulty reading and understanding social cues.

In rare cases, the dog will inappropriately protect one household member from another. This situation sometimes arises when child or familial abuse is involved. Dogs who are not sure whether the threat is real may protect the child against being yelled at or hit by the parent. If no physical abuse of the pet or child is or has been involved, the response is undesirable, exaggerated, and inappropriate.

One of the requirements of treatment for the dog will be to find ways to correct the child that do not put the dog in the position of threatening the individual doing the correcting. On the other hand, if abuse has been involved, an aggressive response can be a learned survival tactic.

Roles for "Turf"

It is widely believed that dogs are "territorial" animals and that they will protect their turf (bed, crate, house, yard, et cetera). Animals will often protect such areas, but usually do so by marking and posturing, rather than by threats and violence. These situations are seldom truly about "turf." Such situations are usually about whether the behavior is appropriate or not.

- The dog who responds to another dog who walks past his unoccupied bed by growling, snarling, and lunging, without first posturing, staring, or waiting to see if the other dog takes the bed is acting out-of-context: he perceived a threat where there was none.
- The dog who guards the front of his crate from the children by pacing and scanning is acting inappropriately: there is no threat.
- The dog who is loose in the yard and snarls frantically at anyone who comes into the yard, has a problem, but how troubling it is will very much depend on her previous experience and the neighborhood circumstances. In some neighborhoods, this behavior will have been encouraged.
- The dog who will not let anyone enter the house, and who positions herself by the door so that she can lunge and snap at anyone who attempts to enter is not exhibiting appropriate behavior.
- Some dogs will be fine with strangers when off-lead, but will vigorously protect their people when on-lead.
- Some dogs are fine in the yard, but become extremely aggressive when they are put behind a fence. This makes sense; fences leave no doubt as to the extent of their property. If the dog is naturally protective, the fence provides a barrier to patrol. For appropriately behaved dogs, their behavior will be shaped by whether they know who is approaching the fence and how the approacher is behaving. For inappropriately behaved dogs, the fence signals that everyone is a threat.

Usually, dogs who exhibit protective or territorial *aggression*—in contrast to protective or territorial *behavior*, which may well be normal—are doing so because they are unsure whether there is a problem. This uncertainty causes them to be anxious in any a threat to space or individuals may exist. Protective and territorial aggression is a diagnosis of pathology, not a normal behavior.

General Patterns

Dogs with protective and territorial aggression can be perfectly appropriately behaved in other circumstances. If no one approaches these dogs on the street, these dogs can be terrific with the family. If no one enters the yard, or if the dog is in the house when someone enters the yard, they can be terrific. Some dogs who defend their yards or beds are perfectly fine and nonreactive to the same dogs or people when the dog is not in the yard. Protective and territorial aggression can have extremely variable patterns associated with them; however, both share in common the demonstration by the dog of the out-of-context, inappropriate, exaggerated, preemptive defense behaviors **in the absence of a true threat.**

The best improvement is seen for dogs whose people can identify discrete situations in which the dog will respond inappropriately.

The first step in the treatment process is to avoid situations which trigger the dog's reaction. For example, if the dog growls at anyone who approaches his crate, must he have a crate? Clear thinking will make management of this problem possible.

To change your dog's behavior, we will teach the dog that he does not have to be on guard all the time. To do this, we will use the **Protocol for Deference,** the **Protocol for Teaching Your Dog to Take a Deep Breath and Use Other Biofeedback Methods as Part of Relaxation,** and the **Protocol for Relaxation: Behavior Modification Tier 1.** Only after your dog has successfully completed these protocols will he be able to learn that he does not have to react in protective and territorial ways (**Tier 2: Protocol for Desensitizing and Counter-Conditioning a Dog or Cat from Approaches from Unfamiliar Animals, Including Humans**).

The tick list below is designed to help you to control or avoid basic and common situations in which most dogs with these problems will react.

Tick List of Tasks

1. Avoid any and all situations that may elicit the aggressive behavior. If you cannot instantly stop your dog from reacting aggressively by asking him to stop and come to you, he should not be in that situation. For example, if you cannot answer the door without having your dog bark and growl, and without having to cling to your dog's collar while he snarls and snaps, *your dog cannot go to the door with you.* Simply tell the person on the other side of the door to wait a minute and place the dog in another room behind a closed and locked door or in his crate until the person has left or is well settled into the house. If you know this pattern will regularly occur, consider posting a note near the door that explains that there may be a brief delay before you answer and open the door.

2. When enclosing dogs with territorial and protective aggression, you must use locks. Simply closing a door is not sufficient for a dog who is convinced that there is a threat to his people or property. The simplest locks are hooks-and-eyes that can be placed at the very top of every door, inside and out. Children cannot reach these and adults will or should think twice before opening them. If you know very persistent adults, please put a note on the door below the lock that tells them why you have chosen to protect your dog by locking him in the room.

3. Some people want to be able to take their dog to the door expressly for protection. As your dog improves, this will be a task that your dog will be expected to negotiate without inappropriate reaction. To expect him to do so at the outset of treatment is unrealistic. If you cannot instantly abort the aggressive behavior using a verbal request, consider a well-fitting head collar for all situations in which your dog might react. These may allow you to interrupt the dog as he begins to react inappropriately, close the dog's mouth humanely, rendering the dog safer, and can help you to remove the dog from the situation without an intensification of his aggression. All of these facets are critical for the dog's learning process. The head collar can be worn indoors so that dogs can be stopped at doors, or stopped as people within the household pass by. Do not leave head collars, or any other device on which any animal can become hung, on the dog when you are not directly supervising him. See the **Protocol for Choosing Collars, Head Collars, Harnesses, and Leads** for suggestions. If your dog cannot be fitted for a head collar a good, no-pull harness will give you leverage to help maneuver the dog more safely.

4. Please make sure that you warn your neighbors that a head collar is not a muzzle. This means that the dog can still bite if no tension is on the lead. Use of head collars still permits *appropriately* protective aggression. Do not make excuses for inappropriate aggression. For problem dogs, inappropriate aggression is far more common than appropriate aggression; do not rationalize a potentially dangerous situation.

5. If the dog growls or lunges, calmly say "no" or whatever word you wish to use to act as a flag that the response was inappropriate and the interaction is over, and disrupt the situation by leaving, and so removing you as an object of protection, or by bringing the dog into another room where he can be enclosed. For dogs who may also have impulse control aggression, which can co-occur with protective and territorial aggression, grabbing the dog when he reacts can put the client at risk. These dogs should be wearing head collars so that the risk can be minimized.

6. Dogs can be let out of a room in which they have been placed **only** under the following circumstances:
   a. the dog is quiet and calm and
   b. the dog, when released, willingly and perfectly performs a few exercises from the **Protocol for Relaxation: Behavior Modification Tier 1,** thus demonstrating his willingness to defer to you and to remain calm and attentive.
   If the visitor is still present, the dog can be introduced to them if:
   a. he is on a head collar,
   b. the visitor **does not** solicit the dog, instead letting the dog come to them, and

c. when the dog comes to the visitor, the visitor requests that the dog sit, the dog complies, and the visitor verbally praises the dog, but otherwise ignores him.

If these circumstances are not possible, the dog should stay securely protected behind a locked door.

7. Please warn your neighbors and friends that *any dog who is aggressive for whatever reason can be dangerous* and that it is important that they comply with your instructions to minimize danger to the dog and to themselves. *Please emphasize that such compliance will help the dog to improve.* This is also true for dogs who are protective or territorially aggressive with other dogs. In such circumstances, the other dog must also be able to respond appropriately.

8. Sudden arm gestures or motions, including shaking hands and reaching over fences, may be perceived as a threat to dogs with protective aggression. Caution people to avoid such gestures and be alert for potential problems so that you can avoid having the dog react.

9. If your dog continues to bark, growl, or to ignore you in any circumstance, **and** working through a series of behavior modification tasks that the dog knows well does **not** help him to relax, put him in another room. **Do not physically punish the dog.** Taking attention from these dogs is one of the most effective and safest "disciplinary" actions you can take. Dogs need space to think, and some time alone may be helpful. As soon as the dog is quiet or subdued he can be released, but you must ensure that he can sit and be calm when loose.

10. If your dog exhibits territorial aggression only when you are in the house, make sure that the dog is placed behind a secure door when any repair person comes. This should also hold true for a friend's visit if you cannot enforce the instructions above.

11. If your dog exhibits territorial aggression only when you are not present, **never** leave this dog in a situation where he can have or obtain access to delivery people, et cetera.

12. **No dog with territorial aggression should ever be left alone, loose outside.** Fences actually put these dogs more at risk and make them more aggressive because the dog has a clear and defendable boundary. *Invisible fences, which rely on electric shock, are the worst possible fence for these dogs.* Shocks will make these dogs more, not less wary. Because they are "invisible," humans do not know where the boundaries are and so may be very easily victimized by the dogs.

13. If your dog has territorial or protective aggression, and he is with you in a fenced yard, ensure no one can enter a gate without your permission.

14. If you decide to build a pen or run for your dog, make sure that it is not near any side walks, driveways, service areas (propane tanks), doorways, or any other areas to

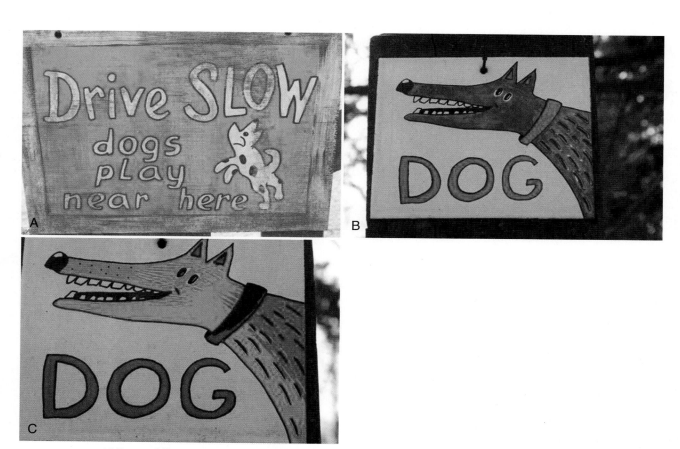

All three of these "Dog on Premises" signs are on the same driveway gate. Anyone should have the expectation that at least one dog lives on the property.

which strangers might need or have access. Remember that a run will become something to protect. Unless you can protect your dog from what he will consider intruders, a run will make him worse.

15. If your dog protects his crate, bed, or eating area, and you cannot guarantee that he will be left alone, exclude others from these areas with baby gates or doors. If your dog protects these spots from another pet in the house, do not leave them alone together, unsupervised. Always ensure that they are separated, behind secured doors, when not supervised, **and** place the dog that is being territorial in a place that is a less desirable area (e.g., a spare room, rather than your bedroom) that is not as defendable or worthy of defense. The pet who is behaving appropriately should always have free rein and be able to move, unimpeded, throughout the rest of the house. You may have to move the area in which you keep your dog frequently so that they do not begin to feel that it, too, is something to protect.

16. Get a "Dog on Premises" sign, or make a sign that announces that there is a dog living on the property. This is not an admission of a dangerous dog, but it is a civically responsible reminder that a dog is on the property. Anyone who has a dog should have such a sign.

17. If you have a dog that you know is protective and/or territorially aggressive and small children come to visit, lock the dog away from the child. Children can be unpredictable and may inadvertently provoke an aggressive dog. *Do not talk yourself into taking the chance.*

18. Please do not use any form of physical punishment. You'll make the dog worse and less predictable because you will appear unpredictable and a threat.

19. Please remember that by fixing your dog's problem aggressions we will not remove any appropriate protective behaviors.

20. Please consistently practice and enforce **Protocol for Deference** and **Protocol for Relaxation: Behavior Modification Program Tier 1.** When you and your dog have successfully completed **Tier 1,** you will be ready to move on to the relevant components of **Tier 2: Protocol for Desensitizing and Counter-Conditioning a Dog to Approaches from Strangers** and **Tier 2: Protocol for Desensitizing and Counter-Conditioning to Noises and Activities That Occur by the Door.**

Antianxiety medications may help some dogs that otherwise are not able to succeed in this program. Please remember that if it's decided that medication could benefit your dog, you need to use it **in addition** to the behavior modification, not instead of it.

PROTOCOL FOR UNDERSTANDING AND TREATING DOGS WITH SEPARATION ANXIETY

Dogs with separation anxiety traditionally exhibit a number of behaviors associated with distress when they are left alone (a "real" absence). The rarer dog exhibits these signs if she is denied access to you (a "virtual" absence). These clingy dogs very likely form a discrete subset of dogs affected with separation anxiety, and may have other problems that may not be relevant for many dogs with separation anxiety. The rarest subset of these dogs has been said to be "hyper-attached": affected dogs always are within touching distance of their human and will experience distress with increasing distance or if they cannot see or touch their humans, although they are not truly "separated."

Non-specific Signs of Separation Anxiety

Common signs of the distress experienced by dogs affected with any form of separation anxiety include:

- destruction of objects in the house,
- destruction of the house,
- vocalization (whining or ritualistic barking, howling, or yipping),
- urination,
- defecation,
- vomiting,
- salivation,
- continuous pacing, and
- complete inactivity/freezing behaviors (sometimes while staring at the door).

Patterns of Distress

For dogs who become distressed during "real" absences, the amount of time that they can be left alone without becoming distressed can be extremely variable. In profound cases of separation anxiety, dogs can be left alone for no more than minutes before they panic and exhibit these behaviors associated with anxiety. In such cases, it is important to realize that *panic is a co-varying or associated diagnosis* and that to successfully treat the dog with separation anxiety, you will have to also treat the panic. This is important because the medications that are used to treat panic are different from those used to treat anxiety-related conditions. If both panic and separation anxiety are issues, you will need to use both types of medication, in addition to expanded behavior modification, to treat both conditions.

In many cases of separation anxiety, the inappropriate behavior is only apparent after a schedule change. For instance, the dog may be fine until 5:30 or 6:00 at night when you are accustomed to coming home. If your schedule changes and now they are not home until 7:30, the dog may start to panic at 6:00 o'clock.

There are changes that appear spontaneously in some older dogs that may be associated with an old age onset version of separation anxiety. In this case, for no apparent reason, a dog who has been able to be left alone for all his life can no longer be left alone. When left, these dogs now appear confused and distressed, and may exhibit any of the behaviors listed above.

In some cases, the dog is only distressed if one particular person leaves, whereas in other cases the dog is fine as long as some human—any human, known or unknown—is in the house.

Oddly, studies show that the presence of cats or other dogs does not seem to have an effect on whether the dog is distressed or not.

In some cases, the fear of being left alone can be associated with horrific events. These events include being caught in a fire, or being in the house when a burglary was attempted, or being stuck in the house when an alarm system went off. Dogs, in these situations, may have a worse experience than dogs for whom separation anxiety develops more gradually, and may benefit at the outset from stronger medications.

Most separation anxiety in dogs appears to be "idiopathic," meaning that we don't understand what's causing it. It's likely that these dogs are truly abnormal in their reactivity at some neurochemical level.

Dogs who are at risk for separation anxiety include those rescued from humane shelters, those rescued from lab situations, those rescued from the street, and those who have spent extended periods of their life in kennels, or with one older, housebound person. That said, some dogs who have experienced stable upbringing may still develop separation anxiety as their brain chemistry changes during social maturation (approximately 1 to 2 years of age).

It's important to realize that dogs who have spent time in humane shelters—recycled pets—may have a higher incidence of separation anxiety than is found in the dog population as a whole, not because shelters induce such problems, but because dogs with behavior problems are at huge risk for being abandoned or dumped in a shelter. For these dogs, the uncertainty of their state is likely to worsen any anxiety, and dogs who have experienced rehoming multiple times may have had their uncertainty strongly reinforced.

As is true for most behavioral problems, we have no idea what the true incidence of separation anxiety is in the general population. It's likely that there are many dogs who are at risk, but show no signs of the condition because they are never left alone. In this case, our estimates of the numbers of dogs affected will be artificially low.

The steps below are designed to teach these dogs that they do not have to be anxious, scared, or fearful, and they do not have to have panic attacks when they are left alone. Please remember, separation anxiety can be extremely variable across dogs: many dogs may respond favorably if given a smaller space where they can feel secure, while others will panic if put in a crate. *If the dog panics when put in an enclosed space or in a crate, no matter how big or comfortable the space or crate is, or what room it is in, please do not force the dog to be crated or confined.* You will make the situation *worse.*

Some dogs can be left in a room and be comfortable, but will panic if truly "enclosed." Please observe and video your dog and ensure that the manner in which you contain her for safety isn't accidentally making the anxiety worse.

Step 1: Behavior Modification

The first step of this program that is designed to teach dogs to not be anxious when left alone involves teaching the dog to take all cues from you (**Protocol for Deference**). As your

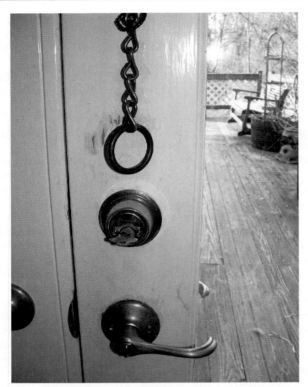

Some of the first signs of damage associated with separation anxiety may be seen on doors.

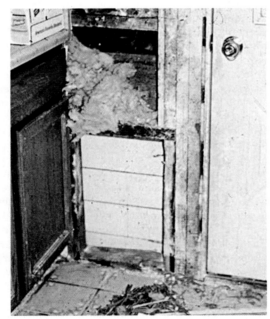

Serious destruction can be involved when a dog with separation anxiety panics.

dog learns the **Protocol for Deference,** he can learn to relax using the **Protocol for Teaching Your Dog to Take a Deep Breath and Use Other Biofeedback Methods as Part of Relaxation.** Your dog will need to be able to successfully learn from both of these protocols before he can start the first tier

of the active behavior modification program (**Protocol for Relaxation: Behavior Modification Tier 1**).

These programs are designed to teach the dog to look at you, to be calm, and then to "sit or lie down," "stay," and "relax" while you engage in a variety of behaviors, some of which may ultimately be upsetting to the dog, in a benign and protected circumstance. Once the dog can do all of these behaviors perfectly for every person in the household in each room in the house without reacting, and he can do the same behaviors outside and remain calm, your dog may be noticeably improved. Many dogs are so improved that their people are happy. Some dogs will benefit from additional tiers of active behavior modification.

Before focusing on the more complex behavior mod programs, please understand that the **Protocol for Deference** is designed to teach the dog that he has to "sit" (or lie down if this is physically more comfortable for the dog) and "stay" and look happy and relaxed. If the dog is truly relaxed, the dog is always praised or rewarded. This is harder than it sounds.

The difficult part of this program involves ensuring that you do not ***accidentally*** reward small, anxious behaviors. Please remember that dogs with separation anxiety are anxious. *These dogs are not just anxious in situations in which they are left alone, they are probably anxious in a variety of contexts, and it is important to be able to distinguish behaviors that signal anxiety from those that do not.* Once you can do this, you can reward the calm behaviors and ignore those that signal anxiety.

The single most important step in the treatment of any of these dogs is also the most commonly skipped step: *reward the dog whenever the dog is calm, even if this calmness is spontaneous and not requested by you.* The more relaxed behaviors you can encourage the dog to incorporate into daily life, the better off everyone will be. This means that you should even reward the dog when he is sleeping or napping as these are variants of calm behaviors.

You will make progress most quickly if everyone practices the behavior modification programs at least daily. If you can practice more often, the dog will improve more quickly. Most of us do not have 30 minutes at a time to practice, but we can engage in five or six 3- to 5-minute sessions of work with the dog daily. Working for at least a few minutes every day to help the dog relax is extremely important. Finally, if you are unable to get everyone in the household to work with the dog, you must ensure that no one is sabotaging your efforts. Not participating is different from active interference with helping the dog to learn to relax.

Your dog may benefit from the **Protocol for Gradual Departures: Behavior Modification Tier 2,** a second tier of behavior modification program for dogs with separation anxiety. This program involves teaching the dog that he can be left alone for gradually increasing increments of time without experiencing distress. Unfortunately, there are two problems with this approach that are usually not discussed.

- For many dogs who become panicky, leaving is not the problem. The problem is the panic and that may start as soon as their human signals in any way that they may leave the dog that day (e.g., a wakeup alarm goes off; most people only set alarms on days when they must leave). Teaching these dogs to relax as you go in and out of a door is not addressing their issue. If these dogs are already aroused when you try to teach them not to worry about people going through doors, you can actually make these dogs worse.

- Relaxation is essential if you wish the dog to improve. Most people focus on the dog's ability to sit and not destroy something or bark when teaching them gradual departures. Unfortunately, this means the dog is becoming sensitized to the departures but not able to show the behaviors associated with distress. In short, the dog becomes worse and suffers more.

If we know that the dog's distress is triggered by the departure, we can accurately monitor the dog's responses to this program, and if we can see a benefit, this tier of the behavior modification may be useful.

Step 2: Enclosing and Protecting the Dog When Left—Safety First

If possible—and only if the dog is happy enclosed—crate the dog or isolate her in a small room when you are not at home. This has less to do with making the dog feel "safe"—something often stated but never proved—than it does with minimizing damage and protecting the dog. Make sure that the crate and the room are puppy proof. There should be:

- no dangling cords,
- no exposed electric outlets, and
- no open areas of water, such as a toilet, in which a dog can drown.

Unless they destroy and ingest bedding, please make sure they have a blanket and/or bedding, water, toys, and a biscuit.

Should You Use a Crate?

Dogs who do not go willingly into their crates and seem happy to be there should not be contained in crates. What the human may perceive as secure, the dog could perceive as entrapment. If the dog's crate is left open when everyone is home and the dog chooses to spend time in it with the door open, chances are that the dog will be content when the door is closed. Regardless, all dogs left in crates should periodically be videoed. No dog who exhibits real or increasing signs of true distress should be forced to remain in a crate. Dogs have been known to break all of their teeth and nails in attempts to escape crates. Increasing the size of the crate or changing the style is generally not sufficient to render the dog content because the issue is that the dog feels entrapped and panics.

Never leave a collar, a head collar, a lead, or a harness on a dog while in a crate or run. Any dog can catch any collar on a crate and strangle to death. This tragic outcome may be more likely to occur with anxious dogs because they are often moving in unpredictable directions.

Anything that can be destroyed and ingested—or that you cannot bear to have destroyed—should be taken out of the room. If necessary, Plexiglas can be placed against and secured to the walls so that if the dog does become upset, no further damage is done. Please remember that once the dog starts to do damage, it is possible that the damaging behavior becomes self-perpetuating.

Never, *ever*, use the crate as punishment. Crates and safe rooms must be areas where the dog is content and feels secure.

Step 3: Providing Stimulation and Information for the Dog When Left

Make sure that the crate or safe room is in a brightly lit, temperature-controlled area. No dog is going to enjoy being thrown in a dank, dark garage just because that is the easiest place to clean up. Leave on a TV, CDs or a radio, and lights for the dog while you are gone.

Give the dog a fresh food toy when you leave (see the **Protocol for Choosing Toys for Your Pet**). Food toys will not "fix" a dog with separation anxiety, but they are good monitors of improvement in the dog's distress. Distressed dogs cannot eat. If the food toy is something that your dog would love were you present, you will be able to tell when the dog is beginning to improve because some of the food will be gone.

Make use of a signal that tells the dog when you are within 15 to 30 minutes of your arrival home (a light and a radio on a timer).

If the dog can learn to respond to this signal through short departures over the weekend, you can use it in the behavior modification program. You can try this by setting a light and timer on and coming into a room where the dog is sitting and relaxing for short periods. Every time you come in, the light should come in. Every time you leave, you reset it. If you can work with the dog to the point where you can leave the dog and have her remain calm for 15 to 30 minutes after the signal comes on, you may be able to use this as a signal throughout the day to cue the dog to relax. To implement this strategy of using the signal as a cue for relaxation correctly you will likely need help from a professional trainer (see www.petprofessionalguild.com or www.apdt.com for a list of Certified Professional Dog Trainers).

Step 4: Alternative Coping Strategies for Dogs Who Must Be Left

- Because some dogs only react inappropriately when one specific person leaves the house, consider whether it is possible to have that person take the dog to work. If the dog is otherwise well mannered and clean, this is becoming a more popular option.
- If it is not possible to take the dog with you, consider using a doggie daycare center, a pet sitter, or asking whether your veterinarian or kennel offers day boarding.
- If you only go out to shop, learn if your dog is distressed when left alone in the car. Many dogs who cannot be left alone in a house or apartment *can* be left alone in a car. The car seems to signal to them that the trips are short and you always return. There is also a lot of additional stimulation for them when in a car, and if they are not distressed they may benefit from it. Do not leave the dog alone in the car unless you are positive the dog will not destroy it. If you are going to use this coping strategy, please ensure that the dog travels safely in the car and is left safely in the car. No dog should be left in any situation where he can overheat or become excessively chilled. Please remember that when it is 80° F, the inside temperature in a car often reaches 140° F to 160° F. At such temperatures, dogs can die within 15 minutes.
- Many dog walkers are now offering multiple daily visits—with or without some behavior mod practice—as one of their services. This strategy works well for dogs who can go 3, but not 4, hours without attention.

Step 5: Bringing the Outside World and Its Information to the Dog Who Is Left Alone

Some dogs do best if they can observe the outside world.

- If your crate can be placed by French, sliding glass, or patio doors, the dog will do better than if he only has a wall to look at all day. If dogs can be calm enough to look at the outside world, having access to it will provide them with a needed and secure pattern and mental stimulation. Please ensure that as the sun moves the dog cannot overheat. Dogs who are crated cannot get up and move away if they are too warm.
- If you have an outdoor run that is sturdily enclosed (and has a roof) and is in a location where no one can steal or abuse the dog, some of these distressed dogs do much better if they are outside. This is certainly an option worth investigating. There are now numerous heated beds, dog houses or shelters, and water dishes that are commercially available that would allow people to comfortably have their dog remain in a run in colder climates. Putting a dog in an outside run should not be viewed as a "containment strategy." It is not. Instead, if the dog can be happier and calmer in the run *and does not feel entrapped* by this, an outdoor run can be one helpful aspect of a larger treatment program.

Step 6: Should You Try to Teach About "Departure Cues"?

If you can identify cues that tell your dog you are going to be leaving, you *may* be able to desensitize the dog to those cues. If you wish to try this you can read how to do so in the **Protocol for Teaching Your Dog to Uncouple Cues About Your Departure from the Departure.** Things that dogs use as cues often include putting on makeup, grabbing your briefcase, dressing in a suit, setting an alarm, getting up at 6 o'clock in the morning and putting on "real clothes" immediately, picking up your keys, et cetera. You can desensitize the dog to any or all of those cues.

- In other words, pick up your keys and don't go anywhere, put on makeup and high heels on the weekend, leave for your legal practice wearing a jogging suit, go out a different door than you usually do, change your pattern of things that you do prior to leaving.
- Start to water the plants before you leave instead of rushing out the door.

Anything you can do to decouple the cues the dog uses as a signal for your departure with the dog's actual initiation of anxiety-based behaviors (e.g., pacing, panting, whining, pupil dilation, movements of ears, frequent solicitation of attention, hiding, jumping up and down in solicitation of behavior) may help *if, by uncoupling these cues from your departure, the dog is calmer.*

If you work intently on these cues over a couple of weekends, you *may* totally uncouple them in a relatively short period of time. For dogs with fairly mild separation anxiety that is triggered only by the cue, this will help. For this to work you need to be able to note that a specific behavior is decreasing in form, in intensity or in frequency. If you cannot measure changes in the behavior or you do not see these changes going in the right direction, caution is urged in using this technique.

Please be aware that you can also sensitize dogs to these cues and teach them that now the cues are unreliable. Instead of helping your dog, your dog now begins to worry more and all the time and *you have made your dog worse.* Please monitor your dog's behaviors using a written log, a video, or both so that you can see whether what you are attempting is making the dog better or worse.

Also, please remember that in profound cases of separation anxiety, the cues may matter less than the actual absence. In this case, desensitizing the dog to cues associated with departure may not generalize to not being distressed when left. If you have to decide how to spend your time, spend it teaching the dog that being left is okay.

Step 7: When Medication Can Help

Finally, *the vast majority of these dogs will require some form of antianxiety medication to improve.* This is the humane choice. Most of the anti-anxiety medications have rather limited side effects, but tremendous benefits. If you are worried or dislike the idea of medication, you can certainly work with the dog using only behavior modification at first. This will actually give you a good baseline of the dog's behaviors against which you can compare later changes, with or without medication. But if the dog worsens at any point, or if his improvement stops, please consider adding medication to his treatment plan.

After you are through with the first tier of the behavior modification program, your dog may be placed on the second tier designed to get her to not react to gradual departures. At that point, we can always reassess the need for medication, but usually starting dogs out on anti-anxiety medication provides us with a real edge at any time. In all of the placebo-controlled double-blind studies, medication has been shown to speed the rate of recovery over that achieved with behavior modification alone, and dogs treated with medication have been shown to acquire the behavior mod more quickly.

Please remember that if your dog has any component of panic in their presentation of the signs of separation anxiety, you will need to give them an antipanic medication approximately 2 hours before you leave, as needed, in addition to their daily medication for anxiety. This sounds like a lot of medication, but because the classes of drugs (panic: benzodiazepines or centrally acting alpha-agonists; anxiety: tricyclic antidepressants [TCAs] or selective serotonin reuptake inhibitors [SSRIs]) act synergistically or together, you may need less of each medication, overall, to get a better effect.

In most, but not all cases, dogs can be weaned from the antipanic medication, even though they may stay on the anti-anxiety medication (see **Protocol for Using Behavioral Medication Successfully**).

Please note that many dogs with separation anxiety also have noise phobias and/or other anxiety-related conditions and unless **all** of these conditions are treated, none will improve to the extent possible. Noise and storm phobias may be types of panic conditions, and so will generally benefit from the same types of medication when given on an "as-needed" basis.

Outcomes

Dogs with separation anxiety can improve to the point where no one realizes that they have had a problem. Some of these dogs may always watch humans differently. Some of these dogs are more prone to other conditions like panic, generalized anxiety disorder (GAD), and noise/storm phobias. If any of these other conditions are also issues they must be treated.

Treatment may be lifelong, and if there are changes in the household—a human or dog dies, people move away—the dog may experience a relapse. As with all behavioral conditions, early intervention is really important. If the social or physical change in the household is a planned change (e.g., a

marriage), please talk to your veterinarian about anticipating this change and adjusting medication and behavioral care so that the dog moves through this period of transition as painlessly as possible.

The table below will help you to assess the extent to which your dog is affected and to monitor changes in behavior as improvement occurs. If you complete this table once or twice a week as soon as you note the problem, the effect of absences and of treatment will be apparent.

Daily/Weekly Schedule for Dogs with Separation Anxiety

Day/Date:

Absence #/Time Left	Maintenance Style	Amount of Time Left	Signs Noted
Absence 1 Time:	a. Left free b. Crated c. Confined in room d. Left outside—dog house or run e. Left outside—fenced f. Outside—free/unrestrained g. Other—please note:	a. Less than 5 minutes b. 5-10 minutes c. 10-20 minutes d. 20-30 minutes e. 30 minutes—1 hour f. 1-2 hours g. 2-4 hours h. 4-6 hours i. 6-8 hours j. More than 8 hours	a. None b. Urination c. Defecation d. Destruction e. Vocalization f. Salivation g. Other—please note:
Absence 2 Time:	a. Left free b. Crated c. Confined in room d. Left outside—dog house or run e. Left outside—fenced f. Outside—free/unrestrained g. Other—please note:	a. Less than 5 minutes b. 5-10 minutes c. 10-20 minutes d. 20-30 minutes e. 30 minutes—1 hour f. 1-2 hours g. 2-4 hours h. 4-6 hours i. 6-8 hours j. More than 8 hours	a. None b. Urination c. Defecation d. Destruction e. Vocalization f. Salivation g. Other—please note:
Absence 3 Time:	a. Left free b. Crated c. Confined in room d. Left outside—dog house or run e. Left outside—fenced f. Outside—free/unrestrained g. Other—please note:	a. Less than 5 minutes b. 5-10 minutes c. 10-20 minutes d. 20-30 minutes e. 30 minutes—1 hour f. 1-2 hours g. 2-4 hours h. 4-6 hours i. 6-8 hours j. More than 8 hours	a. None b. Urination c. Defecation d. Destruction e. Vocalization f. Salivation g. Other—please note:

PROTOCOL FOR UNDERSTANDING AND TREATING REDIRECTED AGGRESSION IN CATS AND DOGS

Redirected aggression is more common in cats than it is in dogs, and it is often intensely serious. Redirected aggression occurs when one individual is thwarted in her access to some behavior in which she is attempting to engage, and she then responds by becoming aggressive toward the individual who thwarted her. There is no evidence that one sex of dog or cat is affected more often than the other.

The individual responsible for preventing or interrupting access to the behavior may have done so deliberately, but with consequences that were not anticipated. One example of redirected aggression involves the dog who is chasing the cat. The client stops the dog from chasing the cat and the dog redirects the aggression to the client. In such cases, where there are no physical barriers that thwart the continuation of the aggression, it is very important to distinguish true redirected aggression from an accidental bite. An accidental bite is one that occurs to a person or animal simply because they found themself between fighting animals. In *accidental* bites, the biting cat or dog generally releases the person or other animals as soon as he realizes that he made a mistake. This is not true for redirected aggression, which may be quite fierce.

In situations where redirected aggression occurs, the individual responsible for preventing or interrupting access to the behavior may have done so inadvertently, and may not know of the interruption. For example, a playing dog could run through an interaction between two other dogs, disrupting it, and be grabbed by one of the dogs.

Redirected aggression can also occur when an inanimate object prevents access to the behavior in which the aggressor wishes to engage. The classic example of redirected aggression in cats involves two cats who are sitting in a window. Unknown to one of the cats, the other cat sees a third cat outside. Because the aroused cat cannot have access to the one that is outside and because this lack of access increases his agitation, he redirects his aggression to his housemate. *Redirected aggression involves both an aggressive response that is related to the social system AND—this is very important—the thwarted ability to resolve the "perceived" or actual social conflict.*

In redirected aggression, the animal acts as if "angry" at the individual who interrupted her behavior, and pursues this individual as the new victim of the aggression.

Because redirected aggression occurs relatively frequently in cats, this protocol is written primarily with cats in mind, but it can be easily adapted to dogs by applying the same principles and guidelines.

One of the key points of this protocol is to understand that the *victims* of redirected aggression can suffer a *profound decline in their quality of life*. This point is mentioned early because it is so important to understand that this is a complex condition and that everyone involved may require treatment.

Redirected aggression can be difficult to diagnose because the circumstances that precipitate it are not often witnessed. Accordingly, the people watching the redirected event, unless it is directed toward them, think that the primary problem is inter-animal (interdog or intercat) aggression.

Redirected aggression is potentially a *very* dangerous problem; the recipient of the aggression seldom anticipates it and is usually traumatized by the aggression because it appears so out of context to them. Please remember that the trigger for redirected aggression may not be obvious or visible to the ultimate target of the aggression, worsening the situation. Using the example above, if the cat who is attacked was asleep, he did not see the third cat pass the window, and so now the attack on him seems completely random. Unexplained, seemingly random adverse outcomes are associated with profound behavioral trauma and helplessness.

Unfortunately, redirected aggression can be so contextually inappropriate, so unexpected, and so traumatic that the recipient of the aggression becomes instantly and intensely fearful of the aggressor. This aggression can change the entire social relationship structure in the household and cause the victim to hide and become withdrawn. If the aggressor has had a problem with the victim in the past, this provides a good opportunity to further victimize that individual. If the victim is a cat, full-blown intercat aggression can then develop. If the recipient of the redirected aggression fights back, fighting back can either start or exaggerate an already existent cycle of intercat aggression.

It is not necessary that the aggressor *continue* to be aggressive in order for the victim to be fearful; the context is so sudden and inappropriate that a recipient can learn to be fearful based on *one* exposure.

Similarly, the aggressor may, with only one experience, learn to associate his inability to pursue an individual or circumstance in which he was initially thwarted with the presence of the housemate. In this case, every time the aggressor sees the housemate, regardless of whether, for example, the outdoor cat is present, he experiences the same full-blown set of behaviors as when the initial event occurred. No wonder the feline housemate now hides from the aggressor!

Treatment of redirected aggression is very difficult. In addition to the checklist, below, you will need to employ **all** of the relevant procedures found in **Protocol for Understanding and Treating Feline Aggressions with an Emphasis on Intercat Aggression** and **Protocol for Understanding and Treating Dogs with Interdog Aggression**. Caution is critically important here. These animals are not acting normally and can injure another individual.

Tick List:

☐ 1. Identify the primary source of the cat's or dog's initial upset.
- If your cats sit in the window, look outside for signs of an intruder cat (e.g., smells of urine, buried feces, paw prints, spraying against the window, nose prints on the glass, et cetera). Do anything you can to prevent the circumstances in which the initial aggression occurred from reoccurring (e.g., put a lace curtain in the window, ask your neighbors to keep their cat in).
- If you know that the aggression has happened when the dog is "corrected" for chasing the cat, separate them so that the chase cannot happen. Try to ensure that the precipitating stimulus is eliminated from the behavioral environment.

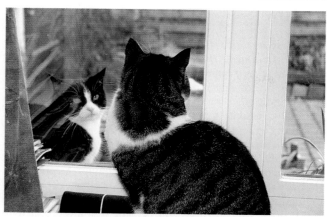

The ideal situation that could precipitate redirected aggression: the inside cat could not directly respond to a threat by the outside cat, and if another cat was sitting nearby indoors, that third cat could be victimized by redirected aggression. (Photo courtesy of *Anne Marie Dossche*.)

☐ 2. Using closed doors and/or crates/gates that prohibit one pet from seeing the other, separate the individuals involved in the redirected aggression **when not supervised.** Make sure that the victim or recipient of the aggression has the most freedom to roam or to select a preferred resting spot.

☐ 3. Reward the aggressor for ignoring the victim. Praise him and/or use food treats.

☐ 4. Make sure that the victim has attention first and that each cat or dog gets 5 to 10 minutes of individual, calming attention (grooming, massage) alone each day.

☐ 5. Adhere to instructions in the **Protocol for the Introduction of a New Pet to Other Household Pets.** Start as if these two have never known each other.

☐ 6. Bell the aggressor (Bear Bells: www.rei.com) and watch him like a hawk. Interrupt the aggressor at the first signs of any aggression, including staring. If just the aggressor's presence seems to frighten the victim or recipient of the aggression, banish the aggressor. Try to make sure that the recipient sees you do this.

☐ 7. *Redirected aggression is so horrific for most cats and some dogs that each of the animals involved requires anti-anxiety medication.* In the case of redirected aggression in cats, the medications chosen for each cat are usually different because the sought-after effects are different (rendering one cat less fearful while rendering the other less reactive and aggressive). Remember that these medications are adjuvants to, *not substitutions for,* behavioral and environmental modification.

☐ 8. If after months of effort and compliance nothing is helping, please consider placing one of the dogs or cats in another home. This is a horrible condition to treat, it may have a high relapse rate, and it may be safer to place one of the pets in another home. Because the problem is wrapped up in a specific complex circumstance, finding a new home is a good option, because it totally alters the circumstance. If this is truly not an option, and it is understandable that it may not be, you can have these pets live completely separately in the same house with some serious effort.

☐ 9. If the patient involved in the redirected aggression is a dog, please remember that canine redirected aggression can be associated with impulse and control aggression. Please ensure that this is not also a problem, and if it is, treat it (see **Protocol for Impulse and Control Aggression**).

PROTOCOL FOR UNDERSTANDING AND TREATING OBSESSIVE-COMPULSIVE DISORDER

Understanding Obsessive-Compulsive Disorder

Obsessive-compulsive disorder (OCD) (also sometimes called compulsive disorder [CD]) can afflict both cats and dogs, although the factors contributing to it appear to differ between species. OCD is defined as repetitive, stereotypic motor, loco-motory, grooming, ingestive, or hallucinogenic behaviors that occur out of context to their normal occurrence, or in a frequency or duration that is in excess of that required to accomplish the ostensible goal. We can be fairly certain that this diagnosis can be confidently made if these behaviors also occur in a manner that interferes with the animal's ability to otherwise normally function in his social environment.

One can debate whether animals can obsess because we cannot directly confirm that they do so. The way we learn if humans obsess, or whether there is a component of repetitive thoughts to their condition, is to ask them, an avenue of inquiry that is simply not available for dogs and cats. If we watch afflicted dogs and cats carefully, we can see in their own responses to these abnormal behaviors that they perceive and experience concern, so it's likely that they can and do obsess as part of this disorder. In fact, it may be the obsessional part of this condition that drives the compulsive or motor part. Any discussion of what dogs or cats can and cannot do needs to account for divergent evolutionary histories for animals that rely heavily on structured language and those that do not.

It's important that we acknowledge this **cognitive component** of the condition because unless we work to change it, we may be able to suppress the behaviors but not the animal's desire or need to do them. When this happens, the behaviors may be less annoying for the humans who have to live with the animals, but the cats and dogs still suffer. If we can extrapolate from what we believe about humans, this type of "mental" suffering may even be more debilitating than that associated with physical pain.

It's important that we distinguish nonspecific behaviors that may be quirky from the true diagnostic criteria required to make this diagnosis. The issue of intensity of action can help here: Whether a behavior is excessive or a manifestation of OCD may be a determination of degree. Careful description and recording of behaviors using tick lists, narrative descriptions of the behavior and its durations, and videos could provide data that would permit evaluation of the extent to which such behaviors may lie on a continuum.

As for any behavioral condition, it is *essential* that you keep notes on actual behaviors, on the intensity of the condition, and on duration of each bout (seconds, minutes, hours) so that you and your veterinarian can understand if the cat or dog is becoming better or worse with time and treatment. In fact, if you and your veterinarian are unsure of whether the behaviors truly meet the criteria for making a diagnosis of OCD, any uncertainty can usually be resolved by comparing changes over time. In this age of video equipment, you can supplement the descriptive logs and tick lists with videos taken in similar situations over time. This will allow everyone to see if the behaviors have changed in intensity, duration, or some basic qualitative feature (e.g., the dog is spinning in tighter circles with the tail more tightly wrapped).

Almost no fully developed cases of OCD will improve without treatment that includes medication, so accurate diagnosis is very important. The behavioral changes seen in OCD can be non-specific and may be shared by a number of other conditions. For example, some OCDs can resemble seizure-like activity that may be associated with epilepsy. By definition, epileptic or seizure-like activity is stereotypic, but it may not meet the criteria for OCD. This is why very explicit and specific diagnostic criteria that first rule out underlying medical conditions are needed for behavioral conditions. That said, there are huge areas of overlap between behavioral and neurological conditions that are currently poorly understood. What we call these will become less important than what drives them in the future as we understand more about the genetics and molecular biology of behavior.

Patterns of Behaviors

From studies of patients who meet the stated diagnostic criteria for OCD and who have been treated for the condition, we understand some basic patterns that will help you work with affected dogs and cats.

- Both dogs and cats appear to exhibit both *sporadic* and *heritable* forms of OCD. This means that some animals can develop OCD when no other family member has ever shown a hint of it (the sporadic form) and that some animals who develop OCD will come from families where multiple members are also affected.
- As is also true for humans, the form of the OCD differs between family members. This means that if one dog chases shadows, another may run fences, and if one cat licks her fur, another may suck on plastic.
- Finally, some breeds are over-represented among animals exhibiting OCD. The data on breeds are so incomplete that it would be really inappropriate for you to think that we fully understand the associations, but we know that Siamese cats, when they exhibit OCD, tend to chew on or suck fabrics (and it is likely that chewing and sucking differ at the neurochemical level), that when German shepherds develop OCD, they chase their tails and circle, and that rottweilers and dalmatians who are affected chase or run from things that are not there (hallucinations).

Because of the unfortunate tendency for people to assume that breeds in dogs mean that behavior is deterministic, it is critical that we recognize normal breed-associated behaviors and evaluate them carefully before assuming either that the behavior requires treatment or that it is normal and does not require treatment. For example, a border collie who comes from working lines and fetches balls all day long likely does not have OCD. The dog can be asked to stop and although she doesn't want to do so, she will. The less her needs are met, the more likely that the behaviors will strike people as extreme. However, you will be able to distinguish normal from abnormal: if play with the dog is intensified and she becomes less extreme, she does not have OCD.

Conversely, a border collie or sheltie who circles may suffer needlessly because people believe that "all shelties/border collies circle." *If the dog cannot be called out of the behavior, if it's out of context (most shelties and collies stop circling if they play with other dogs), or an increase in stimulation and exercise makes no difference, and the dog is distressed, regardless of breed biases, it's important to consider that the dog likely has OCD.*

As in most things, cats are different. For all dogs and cats with OCD, which is truly an anxiety disorder, household, environmental, and social stresses will all worsen their condition. If there are human divorces, marriages, moves, loss or gain of jobs, the addition of children or other pets, the loss of pets, et cetera, OCD that is well controlled may become dysregulated, and untreated OCD may worsen. For cats, however, regardless of whether the form is sporadic or heritable, social stress acts as a trigger. This is *not* the case for dogs, although any stressor will be a risk factor for making the condition worse in dogs.

- For dogs, OCD appears to correlate with the onset and period of social maturity that begins somewhere between 18 and 24 months of age. At this time neurochemistry begins to change, and it is likely those changes are encoded genetically. Something goes awry in what's translated and dogs begin to worsen. Left untreated the dogs continue to decline, although there are groups of dogs who worsen quickly and groups of dogs who worsen slowly.
- For cats, the onset of the condition also appears to coincide with social maturity (~2 to 4 years of age), but a social trigger is almost always involved. Frequently, this trigger is the addition of a new cat, or a change in the behavior of one of the resident cats as the patient reaches social maturity.

This means that if you know that your dogs or cats come from lines where OCD has been demonstrated or is suspected, and you add new cats to the household, you should be aware that your pets may be more at risk, and you can seek help as early in the development and expression of the condition as possible.

Treatment of Obsessive-Compulsive Disorder

Like all anxiety-related conditions, the earlier in the course of the condition that the patient is diagnosed and treated, the better. Even when behaviors are abnormal, practice allows the animal to improve how well they perform those behaviors. Accordingly, one step in the treatment of these problems is to interrupt the behavior and redirect the animal to a behavior that is (a) pleasurable and (b) directly contradictory to the OCD behavior in which they are engaged. This means that every time the cat starts to lick intensely, she is distracted with a fishing toy and play. Such behaviors are directly competitive with those exhibited in the OCD and are enjoyable to the cat.

If the OCD is fully developed by the time a diagnosis is made, even the first step of interrupting the behavior is likely to be impossible for you to successfully execute. The reason medication is so important in the treatment of this condition is that the medication allows external instruction to penetrate the fog of the obsessions. The medications that are most efficacious in this condition include the tricyclic antidepressant, clomipramine (Anafranil/Clomicalm) and the selective serotonin reuptake inhibitor, fluoxetine (Prozac/Reconcile).

Neither of these is licensed for use in cats or dogs for the treatment of OCD in the United States, but this is not the case in other countries. For more information on these medications, and medication in general see the **Protocol for Using Behavioral Medication Successfully.** Once the medication begins to allow the animal to be calmer and less anxious, which generally starts within a few weeks of treatment, interruption of the undesirable and damaging behaviors should be easier. Once you become accustomed to the joint task of gently and humanely interrupting the troublesome behavior and directing the pet to something that is competitive but fun, you will find this easier to do and the cat or dog will improve.

Once you are able to successfully interrupt the problem behaviors, you can start active behavior modification. Active behavior modification for OCD involves teaching the animal behaviors that actually encourage relaxation **and** that prohibit the animal from engaging in the OCD-related behavior. For some dogs who want to chase their tails, this may mean that they are encouraged to lie down completely flush with the ground with their head and neck stretched out. When the dog stretches out and takes a deep breath he gets a terrific food treat. If the cat has to lick, she can be encouraged instead to sit and rub into someone's hand. The intent of this type of active behavior mod is to help teach the animals that when they are rewarded for the physical signs that correlate with changes in underlying physiological state, they will feel not just the pleasure of the reward, but relief from the condition. This is a form of biofeedback for dogs and cats. If done correctly and consistently, the dogs and cats will learn that when they become distressed, they can alleviate that distress by exhibiting these competitive and relaxing behaviors. This is a lot of work, but if you can do it well, it will make a huge difference in the life of the dog or cat, and may allow you to decrease the amount of medication the pet requires. Clients can model the behavior mod they use here after that discussed in the **Protocol for Relaxation: Behavior Modification Tier 1** and **Protocol for Teaching Your Dog to Take a Deep Breath and Use Other Biofeedback Methods as Part of Relaxation.**

Long-term treatment is almost always the rule in OCD. This means that medication and behavior mod will be lifelong. Expect this. If the condition has been recognized very early it's possible that this will not be so, but realistic expectations are helpful for successful management of canine and feline OCD. As animals age, alterations, generally decreases in medication, may be possible or needed. If any of the stressors discussed occurs, more intensive behavior mod, changes in medication doses, or the addition of another anti-anxiety or anti-panic drug may be needed temporarily, but if ever there was a condition where you should be encouraged to "stay the course" with respect to treatment, this is it.

If you understand that you can manage OCD, you will become less distressed with the ups and downs of the condition and your pet will benefit. This is one condition where the humane aspects cannot be over-emphasized and where you benefit from understanding what it means to have a "special-needs" pet.

PROTOCOL FOR UNDERSTANDING AND HELPING GERIATRIC ANIMALS

Overview of What "Geriatric" Means

We all age, and some of us do it a lot better than others. The same is true for cats and dogs. Cats can be considered middle-aged starting somewhere between 8 and 9 years and entering old age and considered "geriatric" when they are 13 or so.

For dogs the issue is more complex because the larger the dog the shorter the life. This association has yet to be well explained, but there is some association between size and cell growth that may be important. If you have a toy breed, they may follow a cat-like pattern. If you have a medium-size breed (25 kg), the dog is middle-age somewhere by 7 to 8 years and becomes old by 10 to 11 years. Larger breeds are middle-age by 6 years and old by 8 or 9 years. Thinner dogs live longer than fatter ones and may age differently.

As is true for humans, aging for dogs and cats has never been a more palatable experience, but we need to understand the combined physical and behavioral needs of aging to insure the healthiest outcome. The following situations discuss changes that can be made to enhance the lives of aging dogs and cats.

Play and Exercise

People assume that their dogs and cats slow down and won't play as they age. This assumption is wrong, and will become self-fulfilling unless the clients change their own behaviors. The best way to prepare for a successful and healthy old age is to prepare for a successful and healthy adulthood.

Play with your dogs and cats throughout their life, and encourage them to play with other animals. Let the older animal set the pace for play and be mindful of things like arthritis that might make it harder for the dog to catch a ball or a cat to chase after a feather. Accommodate these needs by adjusting your play style. If you have pets who loved to run or swim as youngsters, but cannot because of arthritis, consider learning to use treadmills and therapeutic swimming pools or water treadmills as a form of play. These tools can be found in facilities that practice canine and feline rehabilitation.

Swimming is as good for dogs and cats as it is for people. Physical therapy for health and to address injury or aging is still not common for pets, but there are centers that offer canine or feline swimming. These facilities are ideal in that they have life vests, have created pools where animals will not panic and where they can feel their footing, et cetera. You can create the same types of environments at home with some effort.

If you have access to a pool that's deep enough for swimming you can "swim" with your older dog or cat.
- Fit a life jacket to the pet.
- Get in the pool.
- Have someone gently hand you the pet.
- Shepherd the dog or cat around the pool encouraging leg movement. Do not let your pet become tired or scared.
- Hand or gently haul the pet from the pool (some canine life jackets come with handles for this purpose), and towel dry.

If you start with short swims, the pet can and will work up to more aerobic and strengthening activities if they enjoy the water. If possible, do what hydrotherapy facilities do: heat the pool.

If you cannot do this, pets *can* go into hot tubs, *if and only if:*
- the temperature is moderate—you will not find it warm enough—and not at its maximum (remember that dogs and cats have hair that acts as insulation; we do not have that hair),
- the jets are off,
- no chlorine or other treatment product is involved,
- the pet is supervised (which means *you are in the tub with them*),
- the time spent in the tub is short,
- you do gently perform range-of-motion exercises with their limbs, and
- the pet cannot become chilled when taken from the tub.

Also, pet hair clogs filter systems. You'll need a plan to deal with this.

Please be aware that older dogs and cats who are blind, who suffer from severe arthritis, or who suffer from advancing dementia fall into and drown in pools every year. This can be prevented with adequate supervision and fences.

Leash Walking

All dogs and cats—yes, and cats—benefit from leash walking. Leash manners are best taught when the animals are babies. If cats become accustomed to harnesses and leashes when they are young they will be willing to exercise on a lead when they are older.

Mental stimulation is part of exercise. When your pets go for a leash walk they are not just exercising their legs—they also are exercising their nose, brain, and social skills. All of these need stimulation. New data on humans shows that exercise provides for muscle health, but also has far-reaching benefits on how well neurons in the brain function.

We need to remember that, no matter what their age, *animals left in a yard by themselves neither get the exercise they want and need, nor do they get the mental stimulation that is beneficial to them.* In fact, such animals may be lacking social contact. If you doubt that dogs left outside are not getting what they need or want, videotape your dog the next time he is alone in the yard. The dog is not as active as he would be, were you there. Studies show that more than 75% of dogs left in yards spend almost all of their time by the door.

Outdoor cats may get more exercise and stimulation than dogs, but fewer outdoor cats make it to old age than do indoor cats. The same is true for dogs who free-range. People who wish their cats to be able to go outside for social and olfactory stimulation may wish to install a cat fence or some other containment system to decrease the chance of injury or death (see www.catsondeck.com, http://habitathaven.com, http://catnet.stanford.edu, www.kittyfence.com, www.catfence.com, www.purrfectfence.com). Such systems allow cats and some dogs to explore and enjoy the outside world in a humane manner.

That said, all animals who can walk can benefit from some form of leash walking, and all animals should be comfortable on a lead.

Accommodating Old Age Changes with Leads and Harnesses

As dogs and cats age they may experience arthritic changes in their neck and spine. Accordingly, the lead and collar style you have used for the youngster may not be appropriate for an elderly animal. Regardless, the tools you choose should do no harm. This is the best argument for choosing head collars and harnesses as restraint and guidance devices throughout life. More information on these choices can be found in the handout, **Protocol for Choosing Collars, Head Collars, Harnesses, and Leads.**

Speed and Distance

As the dog or cat slows they will still enjoy slightly more sedate leash walks. It's the client's job to learn what the distance limit is and prepare for it, either by knowing when to turn around, or having a car or cart available to take the dog or cat home. Very elderly dogs and cats may miss exploring the olfactory and social environment. A well-padded cart, wagon, or wheel barrow can redress this concern if it is well oiled and maintained and gently pulled. Commercial strollers for cats and dogs are now available and can be terrific for providing stimulation. Strollers are particularly beneficial for older, arthritic dogs who live with young dogs because they allow everyone to go on the same walk. If you include the older dog in these outings, he will blossom and become more interactive in other situations.

For dogs who may no longer be walking on more abrasive surfaces like roads and walkways, you may wish to trim the hair on their feet and between their toes to prevent them from slipping on tile or wood flooring. If you use small, electric clippers, trimming hair is safe and easy. You may also wish to lightly trim hair around the vulva and anus so that it is easy for the older dog to stay clean. Never trim a dog to the skin, even if you are trimming them because they swim a lot. Dogs use hair to both keep warm and cool down, so shaving them bald is not a good idea.

Work for Dogs

If your pet is accustomed to doing a job for you on their walks (e.g., carrying the mail or a newspaper) ensure that they can still do this comfortably. This means ensuring that their teeth aren't hurting and their neck is not so arthritic that carrying the object causes pain. Dogs and cats will endure horrible pain to please, and we often do a less-than-adequate job of assessing pain. If your pet cannot carry their usual package, make a new package that the pet is able to carry. This could be a lighter paper, a toy, or some other object that is light and allows them to participate in your life.

Running with Other Dogs or Cats at Play Groups

If your dog or cat enjoyed running or playing with other animals as a youngster, they will not want to give this up in old age. Play with a member of your own species is also a terrific form of physical and mental stimulation where nonvocal signals conveying concern or level of ability/debility will be easily recognized. You will have to pick your play group or playmates.

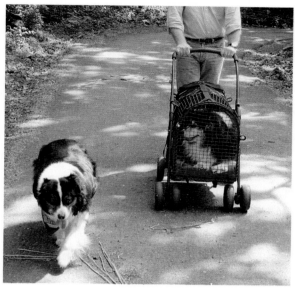

Tess, 14 years old and in buggy, was unable to go on the long walks the other dogs would take multiple times a week. Rather than leave her alone for hours at a time, the buggy allowed her to experience novel and complex stimuli, use different muscles, have the company of the other dogs (here accompanied by Flash) and smell the world as she passed through it.

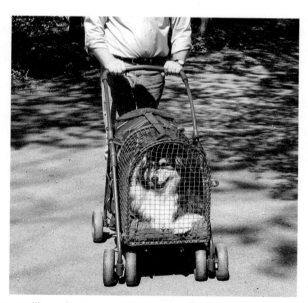

The positive effect on Tess of such stimulation is clear in her engaged and relaxed facial expression. Dogs of her age and debility are too often left alone where they resort to sleep, in the absence of cognitive stimulation.

Companions who are evenly matched by temperament, ability, and size are even more important the older the dog or cat gets. You do not want your older pet to be injured or frightened during play with other dogs and cats. Puppies can be a great boon to an older animal and can encourage them to play quite energetically. Please remember, though, that some puppies play too roughly or too long for the older pet. If you monitor the play and redirect the puppy to other play as the older pet tires, everyone will benefit.

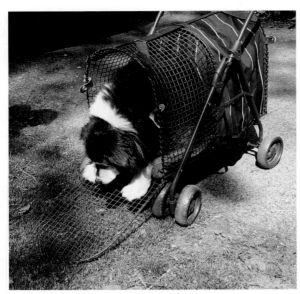

This buggy has a directional system where the dog enters from the back and leaves from the front. Notice that Tess is leaving onto soft, firm footing (the wheels of the buggy are locked).

Smaller groups or pairs of animals—always supervised—are ideal. Make sure that you always carry water and dishes, towels, and a few treats to reward good behavior. Watch to ensure that your pet is not becoming exhausted: stumbling, deep, erratic panting, and moving away from other animals are all signs of this.

If your pet is not ready to leave, but needs a rest, take the dog or cat away from the others, offer them water, wipe them down with a damp towel, if needed, and have them lie down on the towel, blanket or cooling bed that you have provided. Sometimes watching other dogs or cats play is enough.

If you fear that there is any risk of heat exhaustion, buy and carry with you one of the newer cooling vests, bandanas, or pads. These products contain a gel that acts as a surface coolant. Please remember that dogs and cats sweat only through their nose and paws and lose heat primarily by panting. Panting does not always meet the pet's needs, and this is especially true for very young or very old animals and for those who have a medical condition. *If your dog or cat becomes uncoordinated and does not seem to be able to pay attention to or recognize you at any time, take her to your veterinarian immediately. Heatstroke is an emergency. Place cool, wet cloths on their belly and head and travel quickly.*

Be prepared to carry or provide transport for elderly pets who are tired.

Car Trips

Trips in cars will always be enjoyable, if the dog or cat enjoyed car trips as a puppy or kitten. Even a dog or cat who is deaf, blind, and arthritic will enjoy a car ride if they did so earlier in life. The tactile sensation of motion and air, the olfactory stimulation and the pure comfort of being included in their people's daily lives do not diminish with age. In fact, the value of these outings may increase as the animal loses access to other activities they may have enjoyed.

Cats are relatively easily picked up and placed in the car on a bed or blanking with a seatbelt through the harness, or in an open crate. Dogs will need more help. There are now a number of commercially available ramps that help dogs enter and exit cars and boats. Very arthritic dogs will still need support getting out of the car: going down is harder than going up and gravity is going to help them fall if they are unsteady. A supporting hand or harness can make all the difference. Once in the car, padding (a bed or blanket) and a seat belt, crate, or barrier is essential. Older dogs and cats move less easily and can only slowly compensate sudden changes. They must be protected during these trips, in the event of sudden stops.

Be aware that older animals may be more sensitive to temperature extremes, so dogs and cats who always went with you in the late fall and early summer may not be able to do so at this stage of life without suffering—perhaps fatally—from cold or heat that you did not think was extreme.

Pain and Very Aerobic Activities

Many people whose dogs participate in higher levels of obedience, agility, Frisbee, flyball, et cetera worry about aging, pain, and performance capabilities. Your first concern must be the well-being of the dog.

Aging can be viewed by the dog as a release from punishment if he has been unfortunate enough to have lived with someone who demanded perfection in a competitive activity, and for whom nothing is good enough. One hopes that most people reading this handout will not fall into that category.

If the dog really enjoys the activity but is increasingly struggling with jumps, catches, et cetera, consider massage, hydrotherapy (usually swimming), supplementation with nutraceuticals or specially formulated food, and/or antiinflammatory agents. The number of antiinflammatories available for dogs and cats is growing. These agents can be used to relieve and prevent discomfort (as with humans they are best used *before* the pain is felt), but should never be used to push the dog to a level of *performance* that the *human* demands. Periodically step back and ask yourself what is in the dog's best interest.

All competitive activities can be modified for older dogs: jumps can be lowered; Frisbees can be thrown horizontally and a shorter distance, as can balls; courses can be shorter; et cetera. Even herding dogs can get help: I've seen farmers drive elderly collies to the sheep who need to be moved, have the dog do what's needed, and then pick the dog up and put him back in the truck or cart. This way everyone's needs are met. Remember that if your pet worked in any capacity, he still needs to feel useful. The extent to which he needs to work to feel useful will vary between animals and your job, as your pet's ultimate caretaker, is to learn what will humanely work for your dog.

Support for the Failing: Carts and Slings

Physical instability and pain is linked to anxiety. Many animals who could get more exercise are afraid to do so either because they hurt or they are concerned that they will not be able to recover. The time to begin to use carts, slings, or manual help is before it is needed. Perhaps the dog needs to be supported in a sling or with a hand under her rump only occasionally to go up the stairs. Knowing that there is help, if needed, will not only allow the dog to continue to use stairs, but will allow the animal to develop a signal system with her human indicating which days require help. This signaling can be as simple for the dog as standing at the bottom of the stairs and looking up.

Likewise, carts don't have to be an "end-of-mobility" decision. Instead, they can provide support and mobility at times when the animal is weaker, but still cognitively be able to learn to use such support creatively. Investigate these options, which are growing for dogs and cats, before you need them. If you don't like the idea of carts and slings, one option as you, the human, ages is to only obtain dogs that are of a size that you are sure you can always carry.

Diet, Treats, and Eating

As pets age they may become "finicky." Fussy behavior may be the result of mouth or tooth pain or some change in digestive function. Here's where you need to ensure that your older animal is healthy. You should have a physical exam with complete lab work at least once a year when the animal becomes middle aged. Do not wait until your pet is ill—a baseline lab evaluation will allow your veterinarian to recognize changes early and to learn how long laboratory values have been out of whack. This information is critical for determining the type and quality of care your pet will receive as he ages. As animals become older, it may be reasonable to have checkups every 6 months. Ask your veterinarian.

If your pet needs professional dental care, do it as soon as possible. Dogs and cats who cannot chew their food experience a loss of pleasure from one of the most pleasurable activities of their lives. They also have gastrointestinal upset because the food is not well processed before getting to their intestines. You should have been brushing your cat's or dog's teeth all their lives, but if you have not, it's not too late to start, and there are many products that can facilitate this.

Depending on how well your dog or cat processes her food, you may wish to change diets with age. If your pet has a favored biscuit, she can likely still have this, although for some animals on protein-restricted diets, the protein in the biscuit will have to be factored into their overall diet. Talk to your veterinarian. Also, even if your dogs or cats lose teeth, they can still enjoy biscuits and food toys if there is no pain in their mouth.

A sudden change in eating behavior in an older animal warrants a visit to the veterinarian. This is one reason why you should watch your pets eat so that you know what normal is for your companion.

Diets and Supplements for Your Pet's Brain

All clients should be aware of the incredible developments that have occurred in the pet food industry in terms of supplements and foods specially formulated with antioxidants, the "antiaging" compounds. In controlled studies, these foods and supplements have been shown to increase a pet's willingness to be active, to retain cognitive abilities, to interact well and with enjoyment with humans and other animals, to sleep well with fewer disturbances, and to retain housetraining. These studies have all shown that the antioxidants

help, as does exercise and mental stimulation, but the largest effects are for the combination of the antioxidants and mental and physical stimulation. This will work for your pets, it should work for you, and you should do it!

Elimination Behaviors

As dogs and cats age they can become arthritic and confused, just like us. Pain and joint immobility can be associated with an unwillingness to eliminate as the dog or cat had previously. In some cases, this leads to a cycle of constipation followed by diarrhea. Fecal material that is retained continues to lose water to the colon. The feces then become hard and are difficult to defecate. As the intestinal tract fills, the urgency associated with this imbalance then leads to defecation of hard feces followed by diarrhea. Whether it causes pain or not, at some point the dog or cat will need to eliminate. By addressing the pain and mobility issues, we can prevent this messy cycle that upsets pets and clients, alike.

Regular exercise promotes regular digestion. Anti-inflammatory pain killers will allow pets to maintain or increase exercise as discussed above.

If water and food dishes are at head height, cats and dogs who have arthritic necks will be able to eat and drink without pain and so will eat and drink more normally. Water or broth can be added to all foods to make them easier to chew and swallow and to provide more water for digestion. In this age of microwaves, all feline and canine meals can be warmed to make them easier to chew and to aromatize the volatile compounds in the foods. Stimulating the sense of smell often increases intake.

Agents that address constipation can be regularly added to the meals of older animals. Psyllium, the same bulk-forming agent used for humans, if added to meals with water will make the feces softer and easier to pass. This is really important for animals whose hips are less mobile and hurt. For pennies a day, cats can have ¼ to ½ teaspoon of psyllium mixed into food, and dogs can have ½ to 2 teaspoons, depending on size, type of food, and activity level of the dogs.

As hips fail and pain increases, dogs and cats may be less able to control their urination. It may be too painful to maintain a full bladder, or it may not be neurologically possible to do so. There are a couple of simple changes that can be implemented that will make the pet's and client's lives easier.

- Dogs can be taken out for leash walks earlier. Don't wait for the dog's bladder to be full; let the dog empty his bladder before it's full. This preventive action will insure that if there is a leak, the leak will be small, and also that the dog will get more exercise and more stimulation, which will help them remember to eliminate when given the opportunity.

- Dogs can also be taught to use a canine litterbox and a number of versions of these are now commercially available. You will need to retrain the dog to a new substrate, so the client who is considering this option needs to do it while the dog is still capable of learning new associations. For very little dogs, or for dogs who are at high risk for hip dysplasia and other mobility problems, clients may wish to dual train their dogs to eliminate in these boxes and outside as usual. This is also a good recommendation for people who intend to travel with their dogs and stay in hotels.

- Dogs can be diapered. Long-haired dogs should be trimmed. If diapering is the choice the clients **must** be prepared to change the diaper often, clean and dry the dog, and apply an unscented cornstarch powder and/or petroleum jelly to creases and folds. Urine scalding and bed sores are considered signs of neglect and, or abuse in dogs, and they need not ever occur.
- There are medications that will help older dogs who have decreased bladder muscle tone, regardless of cause. Most of these medications involve phenylpropanolamine (PPA) or a similar compound, and can be used safely in dogs if laboratory and physical exam is performed and the clients maintain a good dialog with their veterinarian.
- Steps are a problem. Clients can either carry dogs or, if the dog is big, build ramps or use carriers that help support the dog to allow them access to the outside. Dog doors must be "handicapped accessible." This may mean removing the bottom lip and make them flush with the floor.
- For cats, litterboxes may need to be made lower. Cookie sheets or shorter litterboxes with the side cut out can help.
- Cats should not have to go any further than they easily can to find a litterbox. This may mean that the clients need one litterbox per room. Although less than aesthetically pleasing, this is not a difficult situation to maintain and the boxes can be removed and the cat placed in a smaller, provisioned area if the client wishes to have a party or guests who won't understand.
- Cats develop arthritis and hip dysplasia, also. This means that stairs can be a problem. If the cat has problems, she cannot be expected to go up and down stairs to eliminate, regardless of how she behaved in the past. A litterbox must be available where the cat stays. If cats had been previously accustomed to jumping up to a litterbox, perhaps to keep the box away from dogs, a new plan will have to be devised. Clients can be creative when they have to be.
- Cats who use cat flaps may need to have a flap that moves more easily and one that requires less of a step. Cat/dog doors that are flush with the floor, without lips, prevent tripping.

Sleeping

Changes in sleep cycles are common with age. When cognition begins to fail, the alterations become tremendously abnormal: animals pace aimlessly at night and sleep deeply during the day, the pacing may end with the animal in corners or vocalizing with no object of the vocalization apparent to the client, et cetera.

Good exercise and diet, and comfortable sleeping areas, may help older animals sleep better and more regularly. The dog or cat who may never have had a bed needs and deserves one in old age. Dogs and cats who are painful for any reason need beds with orthopedic grade foam or memory foam. All bedding should be washable. This is not only for the sake of the pet; anything that makes the client's life easier will help with the maintenance of the animal.

If the sleep changes are truly extreme, it's time to talk with your veterinarian about medication. There are commercially available cognitive enhancing and/or antianxiety agents that work. This is a quality-of-life issue, and medication can provide that quality.

Interactions with Other Animals

The longer animals can maintain relationships with other animals, the better. Most animals are very good at reading nonvocal signals and if they know the elderly cat or dog, they will not insist on impossible or painful interactions. In fact, clients could learn from watching how other cats and dogs treat their elderly companion.

The introduction of a younger animal to an older pet can be both a godsend and a bane. Pain-wracked cats and dogs, deep in the stages of terminal old age, will not have the physical or mental plasticity to tolerate endless invitations to play. However, having a younger animal around the elderly one can stimulate the old cat or dog mentally and physically in a good way. If the client does not also have an adult animal or another youngster who can take the brunt of the play, they may wish to consider getting one. Otherwise, the clients will have to wear out the youngster and protect the elderly pet from unwanted attention while ensuring that they also have the company and stimulation.

The ideal time to get a younger pet is as the older animal is entering late middle age. The 8-year-old dog who you thought would never play again not only will play, but will look like a puppy. Additionally, by acting in the role of "foster parent" to the new baby in the house, all mental faculties are well exercised. Another pet can add years to the life of the older animal, and improve its quality in ways we likely do not fully understand.

Stimulating the Nose and the Mind

The nerves responsible for the ability to smell—olfactory neurons—are unique in the world of nerves because they are only one cell away from the outside world in the olfactory epithelium within the nose. These neurons are replaced throughout life. When humans begin to suffer losses in their ability to think, we also note that they have an impaired sense of smell. Whether by stimulating smell we can enhance cognition is unknown, but in animals for whom their most complete information comes from scent, we must assume that the maintenance of the olfactory system is not independent from that of the cognitive system.

Some of the best play activity for older dogs and cats may involve stimulating their noses! Let your dog or cat use her nose.

- Encourage your pets to use food puzzles to get some of their daily caloric needs. You can create food puzzles using upended flower pots, rocks, and hollowed bones all placed on trays with food in the hidey holes.
- Take them on walks where you have hidden treats.
- Learn to use a "scent trail" or adopt some of the training dogs undergo for tracking to stimulate your older cat or dog.
- Use food toys where the pet has to work to get special food (assuming that the physical state of the animal is coupled to the difficulty of the toy). Food toys are commercially available and there is one to meet every dog's or cat's needs.
- Let dogs and cats explore the scent world outside. Take them to new areas where they can sniff new scents. The data show that dogs and cats sniff more when they are in unfamiliar environments, or when they are on trails that other animals pass.

Olfactory memory is some of the first memory we gain and some of the last we lose, so any play that can involve the sense of smell will be play that benefits the dog or cat!

If you are worried that, in the process of getting cognitive stimulation your older pet could become confused or wander and become lost, consider investing in a device that lets you know when they are a certain distance from you. There are now a number of these commercially available. They are equally suited to baby and older humans, and older dogs.

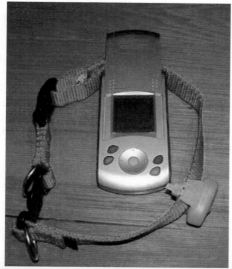

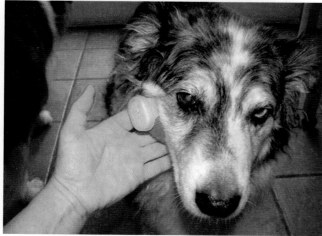

A commercially available locator system which uses a radio frequency tag that can be attached to a collar. The hand-held location (in silver, resting on the collar in the photo on the left) gives an auditory signal as the dog wanders from a pre-set distance and/or beeps as the device locates the dog.

Massage and Physical Manipulation

Dogs and cats can benefit from deep muscle massage and range-of-motion exercises, as do we as we age. Because canine and feline sizes and musculature vary considerably, talk to your veterinarian about the right kind of pressure to exert that does not cause pain or anxiety. Many massage therapists are now also willing to take canine patients or to teach clients

basic massage techniques. This has a dual benefit: Giving a massage can be almost as relaxing as getting one.

After injury, or as aging changes your dog's or cat's mobility, range-of-motion activities can help prevent or regain lost function. Limbs should be slowly but firmly moved through an entire cycle of movement. Before you can be successful at this you need to know how the limbs of dogs and cats naturally move. The time to best learn this is when your pet is young and more tolerant. Discuss with your veterinarian if this option can help your pet. If so, have your veterinarian demonstrate the range of motion and practice on a compliant animal first. Any animal who becomes fearful, resistant, or aggressive should be re-evaluated. Many cranky animals, in fact, become more docile because such activities decrease pain and stiffness. Remember to use anti-inflammatory medication if needed.

Manipulations: Ear, Teeth, Nails, and Coat Care

Any dog or cat who resented or fought maintenance care when young will tolerate it less when old. This is problematic because the older animal needs such care more than does a youngster.

- Overgrown nails will make it harder to walk on already painful joints.
- Untrimmed hair between the pads makes it easier to slip on smooth floors.
- Ear infections and waxy buildup will further compromise hearing.
- Bad, infected, and loose teeth will compromise nutrition.
- Mat of hair that hurt will make a dog or cat who is globally more painful overly reactive.

Old age is **not** the time to muscle an animal into some restraint posture and do everything, forcefully, at once. Actually, there probably never was a time when such force was a good idea, but it is a particularly bad idea for elderly animals. There are alternatives to restraint.

- Use a soft washcloth and delicious (canine or feline) toothpaste to work on one or two teeth a day. Give your dog or cat a couple of small treats while and after doing this.
- Trim one paw or a few nails on that paw at a time. Give your dog or cat a couple of small treats while and after doing this.
- Soak ears one day, and clean them over the next day or two and then repeat. Give your dog or cat a couple of small treats while and after doing this.
- Choose which section of the pet to groom if a whole-body groom is too scary or painful. Give your dog or cat a couple of small treats while and after doing this.
- Trim coats, if warranted. Give your dog or cat a couple of small treats while and after doing this.
- A short clip can make an elderly cat or dog feel, look, and move in a more spirited manner. *The resistance to such clips is all ours; it's we who worry that the pet won't live long enough for the coat to grow again. Put the pet's needs first.*

End Notes

The suggestions discussed above are simple, and they can help repay—just a little bit—of what our best furred friends so freely and generously provide us. It's not fair that dogs and cats don't live as long as we do, but they can live well and happily even as they pass through their last years. We will become better and more humane people for ensuring that this is so.

If you wish to make note of your dog's or cat's behavioral changes as they age in a way that will help your veterinarian provide the best care possible, consider periodically completing the following questionnaire. Bring a copy of the questionnaire with you to the veterinarian's so that you can discuss noted changes and have an informed dialog about humane care for your companion.

Questionnaire to Evaluate Behaviors of Old Cats and Dogs

This questionnaire is for pets who are elderly, passing through middle age, and those who are experiencing age-related changes regardless of their chronological age. The terms "elderly" and "middle age" depend on species and breed so please make sure you understand what this means for your pet. Once you notice any alteration in any category, please re-evaluate your pet by answering all questions every 3 to 6 months so that we can monitor changes and address them as needed. We know that you cannot completely accurately assess your dog's or cat's hearing and vision, but the categories below will allow you to provide your assessment of your pet's abilities.

Behavior Screen for Age Associated Changes

1. Locomotory/ambulatory assessment (tick **only** 1)
   a. No alterations or debilities noted
   b. Modest slowness associated with change from youth to adult
   c. Moderate slowness associated with geriatric aging
   d. Moderate slowness associated with geriatric aging plus alteration or debility in gait
   e. Moderate slowness associated with geriatric aging plus some loss of function (e.g., cannot climb stairs)
   f. Severe slowness associated with extreme loss of function, particularly on slick surfaces (may need to be carried)
   g. Severe slowness, extreme loss of function, and decreased willingness or interest in locomoting (spends most of time in bed)
   h. Paralyzed or refuses to move
2. Appetite assessment (may tick **more** than 1)
   a. No alterations in appetite
   b. Change in ability to physically handle food
   c. Change in ability to retain food (vomits or regurgitates)
   d. Change in ability to find food
   e. Change in interest in food (may be olfactory)
   f. Change in rate of eating
   g. Change in completion of eating
   h. Change in timing of eating
   i. Change in preferred textures
3. Assessment of elimination function (tick **only** 1 in **each** category)
   a. Changes in frequencies and "accidents"
      1. No change in frequency and no "accidents"
      2. Increased frequency, no "accidents"
      3. Decreased frequency, no "accidents"
      4. Increased frequency with "accidents"
      5. Decreased frequency with "accidents"
      6. No change in frequency, but "accidents"
   b. Bladder control
      1. Leaks urine when asleep, only
      2. Leaks urine when awake, only
      3. Leaks urine when awake or asleep
      4. Full-stream, uncontrolled urination when asleep, only
      5. Full-stream, uncontrolled urination when awake, only
      6. Full-stream, uncontrolled urination when awake and asleep
      7. No leakage or uncontrolled urination, all urination controlled, but in inappropriate or undesirable location
      8. No change in urination control or behavior (assumes that dog was housetrained and that cat used litter appropriately)
   c. Bowel control (circle appropriate answers, if the behavior occurs)
      1. Defecates when asleep:
         a. Formed stool
         b. Diarrhea
         c. Mixed
      2. Defecates without apparent awareness:
         a. Formed stool
         b. Diarrhea
         c. Mixed
      3. Defecates when awake and aware of action, but in inappropriate or undesirable locations:
         a. Formed stool
         b. Diarrhea
         c. Mixed
      4. No changes in bowel control
4. Vision assessment (tick **only** 1)
   a. No change in vision detected by behavior—appears to see as well as ever
   b. Some change in vision **not** dependent on ambient light conditions
   c. Some change in vision dependent on ambient light conditions
   d. Extreme change in vision **not** dependent on ambient light conditions
   e. Extreme change in vision dependent on ambient light conditions
   f. Blind
5. Hearing assessment (tick **only** 1)
   a. No apparent change in hearing
   b. Some loss of/decrement in hearing
   c. Extreme loss of/decrement in hearing
   d. Deaf
6. Play interactions—if the dog/cat plays or has played with **toys** (other pets are addressed later), which situation best describes that play? (tick **only** 1)
   a. No change in play with toys
   b. Slightly decreased interest in toys, only
   c. Slightly decreased ability to play with toys, only
   d. Slightly decreased interest and ability to play with toys
   e. Extremely decreased interest in toys, only
   f. Extremely decreased ability to play with toys, only

g. Extremely decreased interest and ability to play with toys

7. Interactions with humans: Which situation best describes that interaction? (tick **only** 1)
   a. No change in interaction with people
   b. Recognizes people but slightly decreased frequency of interaction
   c. Recognizes people but greatly decreased frequency of interaction
   d. Withdrawal but recognizes people
   e. Does not recognize people

8. Interactions with other pets: Which situation best describes that interaction? (tick **only** 1)
   a. No change in interaction with other pets
   b. Recognizes other pets but slightly decreased frequency of interaction
   c. Recognizes other pets but greatly decreased frequency of interaction
   d. Withdrawal but recognizes other pets
   e. Does not recognize other pets
   f. No other pets or animal companions in house or social environment

9. Changes in sleep/wake cycle (tick **only** 1)
   a. No changes in sleep patterns
   b. Sleeps more in day, only
   c. Some change—awakens at night and sleeps more in day
   d. Much change—profoundly erratic nocturnal pattern and irregular daytime pattern
   e. Sleeps virtually all day, awake occasionally at night
   f. Sleeps almost around the clock

10. Is there anything else you think we should know?

PROTOCOL FOR PREVENTING AND TREATING ATTENTION-SEEKING BEHAVIOR

Don't All Dogs and Cats Ask for Attention?

Many dogs and cats frequently solicit attention from their people. For some of these dogs and cats, the intent is just to interact with their people. For others, the attention seeking may be more about seeking reassurance.

Unfortunately, responding to the pet's pesky behavior can contribute to worsening attention-seeking behavior and anxiety, when they are linked.

The manner in which pets seek attention can affect the manner in which the people interact with them. Pets who receive little attention from their people, those who are particularly needy for attention, and those who may never have had any guidelines set about what is acceptable behavior (and this varies among households) may resort to extremes to get attention.

Dogs may jump on their people, constantly nudge them, pull at their clothing, nip at them, or bark at them. Cats may scratch people, paw at them, pull their clothing, howl, pounce, or stroll up and down their person's body when that person is asleep. Sometimes the pets become destructive or eliminate in inappropriate places. Both cats and dogs can learn to steal objects or knock them from "forbidden surfaces" if this gets them attention. When sweet behaviors do not elicit attention, many cats will scratch furniture because they know that it will result in someone chasing them. If the cat needs this kind of a game, there are more suitable ways to meet their needs, but the human needs to be a willing partner.

When Is Asking for Attention a Sign of Distress?

It is important to remember that if an animal is severely needy for attention, for whatever reason, he will get that attention by any means possible. For an animal who craves attention—whether it's just because they want to play or because they are so anxious they need constant reassurance—even negative attention is better than none. There is a parallel with children: if the only attention a young child gets is through a kick, the child will return for that kick.

We don't want to encourage misbehavior to satisfy a need for attention. *Pets who are overly anxious are not just misbehaving, they are abnormal, and "negative" attention can make them worse.* For animals who are anxious, inadvertent "rewards" of the anxious behaviors may actually worsen the anxiety. Most often, the person giving the attention is unaware of its effect on anxiety. In fact, when people become aware of their dog's or cat's true "need" for attention, they provide reassurance for their pet without observing whether that reassurance is making their dog or cat calmer. If it is not, we need to address the problem.

Those of us who love our pets tend to automatically reach out to touch any animal who brushes against us. We are more likely to do this if we are otherwise occupied by reading a newspaper, napping, or watching TV. Particularly pushy, but normal, cats and dogs know about this and show up for attention at such times.

For anxious animals, the competing stimulus of a TV may make the dog or cat more anxious because he is not the entire focus of his human's attention. Here, the dog or cat keeps pestering the human because he *needs, not just wants,* attention, and most people are sufficiently distracted that they do not realize that their cat or dog is distressed.

Finally, please remember that *rehomed and rescued animals and those from shelters may have been abandoned because they wanted attention too much.* Unfortunately, abandonment made them more anxious and now they want attention even more. The behaviors used by these rehomed pets to seek attention often drive people away. Please don't let these dogs and cats be victimized by their own neediness and abandonment!

What Can We Do to Help Dogs and Cats Who Seek Attention Because They Are Needy and Distressed?

Treatment of attention-seeking behavior involves the same rules that succeed in preventing it. Most of these problematic behaviors can be overcome using the following instructions in combination with the **Protocol for Deference** and the **Protocol for Teaching Your Dog to Take a Deep Breath and Use Other Biofeedback Methods as Part of Relaxation.**

Although most attention-seeking behaviors are not dangerous, they are annoying, and annoying behaviors are what people complain most about. Shelters are full of animals for whom complaints about "annoying behaviors" were the only problem. *Any behavioral concern can be life-threatening, so it is critical to improve any annoying behavior.*

Specific Steps for Fixing Attention-Seeking Behavior

1. Establish a regular schedule of interaction.
   - Some degree of predictability is particularly important for anxious animals.
   - For at least 5 to 15 minutes twice daily pay attention to your cat or dog at a regular time. Scheduling this interaction will make it easier to do and will allow you both to look forward to it.
   - During this time teach your dog or cat obedience exercises (cats learn to fetch quite well for a food treat), tricks, target training (go to www.abrionline.org for some videos), relaxation exercises, walk them or otherwise encourage aerobic exercise. If you have a treadmill you may be able to teach your dog to use it.
   - If your pet's style is more sedentary, the attention can involve grooming, massage, or petting and talking.
   - Behavior modification exercises designed to teach a pet to sit, stay, and relax can help.

   These suggestions all provide an opportunity to strengthen the bond you have with your pet. Combined with an improved understanding of the pet's needs and behaviors, you'll be more patient and more receptive to your pet's needs.
2. Tailor the type of interaction to both your and your pet's needs. Very young puppies and kittens have a huge requirement for aerobic, interactive play. A walk will not fix this, but throwing a ball or Frisbee, or dragging a toy on a rope, might.

3. If your young, energetic pet eats kibble, do not "meal feed" them. Instead, use a "treat ball" or food toy (Buster Cube, Roll-A-Treat Ball, Planet Toy) filled with kibble to give your cat or dog physical exercise and mental stimulation.

4. The exuberance of youth will turn into obnoxious attention-seeking behavior if the dog's or cat's needs are not met. Structured time for play and attention provides an outlet for the pet, but also ensures that you do not feel guilty when you want some quiet, non-pet time to yourself.

All of these suggestions should decrease your pet's "need" to solicit attention through inappropriate or undesirable behaviors, while providing more calming and beneficial attention than he likely receives now.

This Makes Sense, But How Do I Discourage the Problematic Behaviors?

You will need some method to reinforce your pet's good behavior and another to discourage the undesirable behavior at times when you are not specifically focused on interaction.

If your cat or dog demands attention by using one of their problematic behaviors, ignore her. She will start to offer other behaviors as a way to ask you a question about what action of hers will gain your attention. At some point the offered behavior will involve being quiet and looking at you. As soon as your pet is quiet, ask her to sit, then tell her she is brilliant and sweet and give her a caress or treat. If you now wish to interact extensively with your cat or dog, you can, but you should be able to say "no" without being mauled or bothered.

Be aware of two relevant behavioral phenomena: extinction and resistance to extinction.

- When you do not respond to behaviors you don't like, you are using extinction (performance of behavior=no response) to encourage the dog or cat to stop the behavior.
- If you are distracted and break your "no response" rule and accidentally give the dog or cat any attention for the behavior you are trying to extinguish, your cat or dog will go right back to the old behaviors. This is resistance to extinction, and it encourages your dog or cat to continue to exhibit obnoxious behavior.

Whatever you do, do not physically push your pet down or off. If you don't want your cat or dog to struggle with you, do not struggle with her. If your dog or cat physically struggles with you, someone has encouraged such behavior, albeit often accidentally. If your pet doesn't automatically sit when you don't respond to the pesky behavior, slough her off (stand up or back up and let her slide from you) and softly say "No (or use whatever word or sound works for her as a disruptive signal), off and sit, please." As soon as the dog or cat sits, say "Good girl!" If she acts like a jack-in-the-box and comes back jumping, move further away and refuse to interact until she sits again. Then repeat the reward. If you are consistent, your cat or dog will learn that only calm behavior is rewarded with attention.

Where Are the Pitfalls?

Do not push your pet down or shove her away using your feet. Dogs, especially, will interpret this as play and will interpret this "correction" as fun and nip and grab more, not less.

Cats are very good at getting people to play with them using their feet: every time their person moves a foot, the cat plays back by grabbing it again. It is important to stand still to stop your cat from playing the foot game. If your dog or cat does not give up, walk away.

Cats will nibble on people for attention when sitting in someone's lap or when you are asleep. Gently slough these cats from your lap or move them off the bed by moving the bed covers. Ensure that the cat cannot interpret your response as play. Do not talk to the cat, just withdraw attention. Cats and dogs will use their newfound mental space to think about the situation and invariably offer another behavior. You can shape these offerings into more and more acceptable behaviors.

What If Passive Responses Fail?

If you do them correctly and consistently these passive measures will fix your problem. Occasionally they may not. If these passive measures do not stop the annoying behavior, you can try to interrupt it. Before you do this you need to consider three things:

1. you need to make sure that no one has been rewarding the pesky behavior,
2. you need to make sure that you are not angry and are not going to scare or injure your cat or dog, and
3. you need to make sure that your timing for interrupting an animal is excellent. Timing is critical here, because to stop the behavior, you need to interrupt the animal **as the behavior is starting.**

You need to use the lowest level of interruption necessary to get the pet to stop the behavior: for some dogs and cats this is a whisper, for some it's a loud "shhh." There are two rules you cannot violate:

1. you cannot scare your pet and
2. the earlier in the sequence of their attention-seeking behaviors that you interrupt your dog or cat, the better will be her response.

If you need to be reminded to pay close attention to your pet, fit them with a breakaway collar with bells (Bear Bells: www.rei.com).

As soon as your dog or cat stops the behavior that you dislike, you *must* offer her a more appropriate form of engagement (e.g., sitting for a reward, chasing a ball, a massage, et cetera).

Can Actively Disrupting the Behavior Backfire?

Yes, interrupting your pet can backfire. If your pet becomes aggressive when you try to interrupt or stop these attention-seeking behaviors you have more—and more serious—problems than you thought. *Seek help from a specialist immediately and cease any interruption or "reprimand." Continuing to attempt to interrupt such behaviors under these circumstances is inhumane and will make your pet worse.*

If your pet still persists, but is not aggressive, consider banishing her to another, neutral room. You can effectively banish pets by removing yourself to a place they cannot go. Remember that these dogs and cats are desperate for attention and the worst "punishment" that they can receive is to be deprived of the potential to get attention.

- Do not cuddle with your pet or verbally reassure her that you are not a bad person while you are leaving her behind.
- Do not leave your pet in isolation for extended periods. You wish to leave her only long enough for her to calm.
- Give your pet a chance to demonstrate that she can respond appropriately. When your cat or dog is quiet, let her out and reward a more appropriate behavior (e.g., sitting, or waiting for grooming).

Any Final Words of Wisdom? Should We Not Just Let Sleeping Dogs Lie?

The final step in this treatment of attention-seeking behavior is the *easiest and most frequently ignored step:* reward your dog or cat when she is spontaneously calm. People tend to ignore their cats and dogs when they are sleeping or being good, because they are so used to them being pesky and don't want to arouse them. This is unfortunate, because this is the perfect time to talk calmly to your cat or dog and, if she stretches out, rub her belly. Your pet is now doing exactly what you wish she would do more often—being quiet and loving—so encourage her.

Finally, especially for dogs, this type of appropriate behavior can be reinforced daily by requiring that the dog briefly defer to you by sitting and staying for anything she may want, including love, grooming, eating, going out, playing, having a leash put on, being petted, or even having a wound examined (see the **Protocol for Deference**). This is an excellent start to teaching your dog to take all the cues as to the appropriateness of her behavior from you. All dogs should learn this, and any dog older than 6 weeks of age can learn it quickly. Make sure that as soon as your dog's bottom hits the ground you tell her that she is wonderful, because she is!

Tick List

1. Regular interaction schedule, which can be playing, grooming, massaging, checking for ticks, et cetera:
   - 5 to 15 minutes in AM and
   - 5 to 15 minutes in PM.
2. Say "no" gently and slough the dog or cat off. This is the most "severe correction" you should have to use.
3. Do not push down or off.
4. If your dog or cat persists, you can try to interrupt her using a noise or action that stops the behavior but does not scare the pet. Use interruptive behaviors judiciously. Be careful: a loud noise can make a noise reactive or noise phobic animal worse. Watch your pet's behavior: If your dog or cat acts fearful, you stepped over the line. The interruption should just be enough to stop your dog or cat so she looks to you and then you *must immediately reward* with treats and praise. **You must do no harm.**
5. If still persistent, banish your pet. Release and reinforce good behavior when quiet.
6. Reward whenever quiet and calm, even when your dog is sleeping. Is this calm behavior the kind of behavior you want? If so, encourage it.
7. Reinforce, by reward, the importance of sitting and looking at you for cues about the appropriateness of your pet's behaviors at all times.

PROTOCOL FOR TREATING FEARFUL BEHAVIOR IN CATS AND DOGS

Overview of Fear

Fearful behavior can be either idiopathic (meaning that it developed spontaneously, because of something inside the animal, and that nothing external caused it) or associated with some causal event (teasing by a child, being bitten by another animal). Fear is poorly understood in both human medicine and in veterinary behavioral medicine, but it can be absolutely crippling for anyone experiencing it.

Fear and anxiety are related neurochemically and behaviorally, but they are not identical conditions or descriptions. The difference is easiest to see in the behavior. Fearful animals withdraw and signal that they do not wish to interact. If compelled to do so, they usually become more frightened and either withdraw even more (some animals freeze) or they become frantic (some animals panic). Anxious animals signal uncertainty and show many of the behavioral components we see associated with fear, but their behavior is characterized by an incomplete commitment to one behavioral outcome. They are uncertain about how they respond and may get some information about this by provoking the situation. Some anxious animals may become more reactive, while others become less reactive. Their response depends on their diagnosis and on what other individuals in the interaction do. This pattern of having a flexible response depending on the behaviors of others is also a component of normal social behavior, but when the behavior is pathological, one key aspect is changed: the provocation or solicitation for information—and the response to it—are both out of context.

Roles for Age and Development

In the first 2 months of life, both cats and dogs go through periods that have often been called "socialization periods," but might best be called "sensitive periods." During these times, kittens and puppies begin to explore the world around them. If puppies and kittens are not exposed to varying social and physical stimuli during these sensitive periods, they may be at risk for behaving inappropriately in those situations later in life.

- For example, cats who are not handled by people until 14 weeks of age may never become calm with people. In fact, to maximize the cat's potential for friendly and calm behavior they should be handled daily from 2 to 9 weeks of age.
- Dogs who don't see people until after 5 to 8 weeks of age (when they are first aware that humans exist), may become fearful of any approaches—friendly and not—by people.

In general, a very small amount of exposure to a stimulus is required during puppyhood or kittenhood to ensure that the animal does not become afraid. A good rule of thumb is that the more nontraumatic exposure that the animal can have, the better. For kittens, being exposed to people from 2 to 9 weeks of age, especially, turns out to be much more important than people anticipated. Puppies should also be exposed early, although they tend to focus more on their littermates than they do on people until they are about 4 to 6 weeks of age.

It is important to start young animals out on the right foot. The **Protocol for Basic Manners Training and Housetraining**

for New Dogs and Puppies, the **Protocol for the Introduction of a New Pet to Other Household Pets,** and the **Protocol for Preventing and Treating Attention-Seeking Behavior** can all help with this.

Helping Your Young Dog or Cat to Learn About the World

Meanwhile, please expose your cats and dogs to all the experiences you think they will routinely have.
- All cats should be comfortable walking on a harness, being bathed and brushed, having their teeth brushed, having their claws trimmed, getting into and out of a carrier, going for a car ride, going to the vet's office, and being manipulated for a veterinary exam.
- All dogs should be comfortable walking on a no-pull harness, head collar or humane collar and lead, going for a car ride, going to the vet's office, being manipulated for a veterinary exam, going to a park where there are children and other dogs, and meeting other dogs on the street. Small dogs should also be comfortable with getting into and out of carriers.

If your cat or dog is having trouble learning to be comfortable in these situations, or is already uncomfortable in these situations, please work with a veterinary professional or a certified professional dog trainer to teach your dog and cat how to enjoy these activities. The earlier you intervene, the better. Puppies and kittens who are fearful do not just grow out of it—they almost always worsen with age. Many trainers and behavioral specialists are now emphasizing how important it is to teach dogs and cats to participate in their own medical care by offering body parts for examination. Such techniques make the exam more fun and less worrisome for the dog and cat, and much less stressful for you and the veterinary staff.

When Should You Start to Worry About Your Pet's Fear?

A small amount of fear in unfamiliar situations is good and adaptive. This is what stops us from doing foolish and potentially fatal things. Fear becomes an abnormal response when it actively interferes with normal social interaction. We now know that many animals and humans who have problems with fear have an underlying abnormality with their brain chemistry. This is why so many of these animals respond so well to antianxiety medication. Some very profound fearful and panic behaviors in dogs appear to begin to be displayed at social maturity (about 18 to 24 months of age; range: 12 to 36 months of age). Humans, too, develop profound fears during social maturity. Current thought suggests that this is because the brain prunes and remodels some brain cells and shifts neurochemistry. Such modification is normal, but different aspects may go awry and contribute to fearful behavior.

Treating Fear

The keys to treating fear include:
- early recognition of your dog's or cat's fearful response (does she hide, whine, press against you, urinate, seek out another pet), so that you know when she is distressed; this

will allow you to accurately assess whether your pet improves with work and/or time,

- identification of the situations in which the cat or dog is fearful so that they can be avoided, which avoids "practicing" learning to be fearful,
- gradual desensitization and counter-conditioning of your dog or cat to the stimuli that have made her fearful, and
- rewarding your dog or cat any time she is not behaving fearfully.

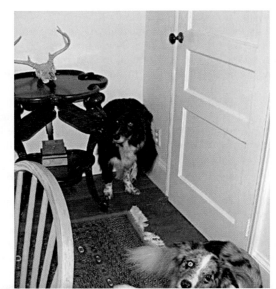

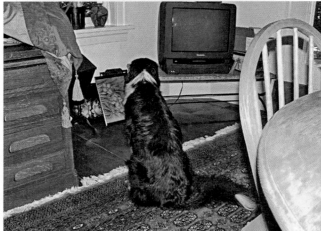

Dog who is afraid of unknown humans. Even the presence of her housemate is not enough of a "safety signal" to have her not worry. This dog either hides in corners or turns her back when faced with unfamiliar humans.

Tick List of Actions to Take to Treat Fearful Behavior

1. Practice the **Protocol for Deference,** the **Protocol for Teaching Your Dog to Take a Deep Breath and Use Other Biofeedback Methods as Part of Relaxation,** and the **Protocol for Relaxation: Behavior Modification Tier 1.** Only after you have completed these can you begin to work with the specific **Tier 2** protocols that are designed

to desensitize and counter-condition your pet to the problematic situations. And, yes, most parts of these programs are easily adapted for use in cats.

2. Until you reach the second phase of the behavior modification programs, please make sure that you **avoid** all the circumstances in which your cat or dog becomes distressed. Please make sure that you understand that you are not "giving in" to the problem. Instead, think of this as protecting the pet. Nothing renders us more helpless and distressed than to be continually put in scary situations over which we have no control and from which we cannot escape. With time and treatment, the number of situations from which your dog or cat must be protected may diminish, but this cannot happen if she is not protected from them at the outset.

3. If you must expose your cat or dog to something she finds distressing, please consider using a mild anti-anxiety agent that may have both a calming effect on the pet and a disruptive effect on learning fear. Members of the benzodiazepine class of drug have these properties when given at the appropriate dosage. See the **Generalized Guidelines for Using Alprazolam for Noise and Storm Phobias, Panic, and Severe Distress** for some guidance. Discuss with your veterinarian whether this is a good option for your pet. Often when these medications are used for particularly scary, occasional situations (e.g., going to the vet) they prevent the fearful reaction and can help start your cat or dog on the path to learning to enjoy formerly distressing situations.

4. If you have a cat who is afraid of carriers or veterinary visits, learn how to help your cat to have less stressful and more humane veterinary visits. See the following resources for additional help: Healthy Cats for Life (www.healthycatsforlife.com/clinic.html) and Catalyst Council (www.catalystcouncil.org/resources/video/?Id=88).

5. Whenever your cat or dog is calm, tell her that she is brilliant. If you can further reward your cat or dog with love, play, massage, or treats without making her more reactive, do it. The single most commonly wasted opportunity is the one that's easiest to implement: just tell your dog or cat that she is good when she is quiet and calm, even if this means talking to her when she is asleep.

6. Please do not tell your dog or cat that it is okay when it is not okay. No abnormally fearful response is truly okay for the individual experiencing it. Although your intentions are good, what you are really doing is giving your dog or cat conflicting signals. She knows it's not okay—that's why she is scared. The risk here is that you may accidentally be rewarding behaviors associated with distress by trying to reassure your pet. Unless you have taught your pet that "okay" means to take a deep breath and relax—and this can be done—avoid trying to jolly your pet from her fearful response. It won't work and will just be another failure for your pet. If your dog or cat will allow it, you can put some firm, gentle pressure on her using your hands or body. This type of closeness provides reassurance and the physical pressure, if gentle, may help your pet to relax by relaxing her muscles. If you are going to pet your dog or cat, please do so only in a slow, firm manner. Rough and fast stroking makes your dog and cat more reactive, even if you are doing it in play.

7. **Do not try to bribe any animal into not being fearful.** It will not work, and you may be doing harm. What **will** work is to teach the dog or cat to sit for a food treat and relax. Then, we can calmly and gradually introduce the fearful situation so that your cat or dog learns to associate the situation with good things. That is the principle underlying the first phases of the behavior modification programs.

8. *Please do not force any cat or dog to be in a situation where she is becoming progressively more panicked.* Many people think that if the puppy is upset, you should drag him over to the thing that's upsetting him and he will "get over it." *This is wrong.* You will make your dog or cat worse. Watch your cat's or dog's behavior: if she tries to escape in a more active manner, looks away, pants, shakes, drools, or widens her pupils, she is distressed and scared. Get her out of the situation as soon as possible. Don't try to convince anyone that it is okay, if profound fear or terror is involved. A quiet presence can be reassuring. Then, when your cat or dog is ready to take some guidance, you are there to provide it.

9. *Do not use physical punishment.* It's guaranteed to make your cat or dog worse, and possibly aggressive. Punishing someone who is fearful can only be about our own frustration.

10. Warn friends who might interact with your pet how you would like them to do so. If your dog or cat tolerates a visitor's presence, ask the visitor not to reach for or look at your pet until she solicits them. Then the visitor must be calm, quiet, and clear in all interactions. If the visitor is trustworthy, you can provide treats so that the visitor can practice having the pet sit calmly for rewards. Emphasize to your guests that it is important for them to help your pet, and that their behaviors must be in the best interests of the dog or cat needing the help. If your friends will not comply with your instructions and requests, please separate them and your cat or dog.

11. Please *do not* forcibly extract a fearful pet from an area in which she is hiding. You may be bitten, which will make the event worse for the cat or dog. Instead, speak calmly and try to coax the cat or dog. If this fails, leave a dish of food a slight distance away from the hiding hole and just sit there. When your dog or cat comes out, do not reach for her—just talk softly. She will eventually come to you. Let your dog or cat set the pace of the interaction. Be calm.

12. Some harnesses and head collars can help dogs to relax because they don't permit the dog to intensify the fearful behavior, and instead apply constant, firm but gentle pressure. Harnesses prevent cats from bolting and so may blunt some fearful behaviors. Please remember that cats recover from stressful events by hiding. After you have blunted a panicky event, let the cat recover.

13. Please remember that fearful animals may need extra protection when outside. The world is an unpredictable place, and for a fearful animal this is a nightmare.

14. Antianxiety medications can help fearful dogs and cats, and they may help you to implement the behavior modification. *Studies have shown that anti-anxiety medication increases the rate at which dogs can learn behavior modification and improve.* Some dogs or cats need anti-anxiety medication on a daily basis, some may only need it occasionally, but for profoundly affected fearful animals, humane care will involve the use of antianxiety medications plus behavior modification.

PROTOCOL FOR USING BEHAVIORAL MEDICATION SUCCESSFULLY

If your veterinarian has recommended that your dog or cat be treated with behavioral/psychotropic medication, there are a number of issues with which you should be comfortable prior to and during the treatment with this medication. These issues are discussed below by topic, and will help you to successfully use medication as part of an integrated program of behavioral modification and environmental management. This topic list is based on common client questions and on points vets always wish to ensure their clients understand.

Some of these topics are discussed in some depth and the science is explained in layman's terms. If you do not wish to understand how these drugs work, skip these parts and move on to the ones that may be more of a concern for you (e.g., the section on potential undesirable/"side" effects).

Key points with which you should be familiar are noted by: 🔺 *and you should read these.*

If you still have questions by the time you have read carefully through this protocol, please ask your veterinarian! The better you are able to monitor your dog or cat, the more helpful information you can provide to your vet, so please ask questions as soon as you have them.

Medication has made a huge difference in the quality of the lives of tens of thousands of pets and their human companions. The better your knowledge, the more successful treatment is likely to be. A good dialog with your vet and/or a specialist will help you in this treatment partnership. Good luck!

1. "Extra-label" or "Off-label" Medication vs. That with a Dog or Cat Label

All the medications prescribed for pets for behavioral problems are available for use for humans with analogous conditions. That said, most medications used for pets are used "extra-label." This means that in the United States the Food and Drug Administration (FDA) has not approved their use for the specific conditions for which they are used in treatment of pet animals. *This does not mean the medication is unsafe.* It *does* mean that the medications have not undergone the lengthy clinical trials in dogs and/or cats with targeted behavioral conditions needed to submit an application for dogs and/or cats to the FDA. Such applications take years to get approved, and unless a company thinks it can financially benefit from a veterinary label, especially if generic compounds are available "extra-label," they are unlikely to be willing to pursue this costly and lengthy exercise. This is why so many drugs used to treat cancer in pets are also prescribed "extra-label." "Extra-label" use means that the medication can legally be prescribed for the equivalent use it would have in humans. Medications tested and approved for humans almost always have toxicology data obtained from dogs on file.

Currently, medications **with a veterinary label** are available for treatment of behavioral problems in dogs. In the United States these are: Anipryl (generic = selegiline) for cognitive dysfunction (Pfizer), Reconcile (generic = fluoxetine) for separation anxiety, and Clomicalm (generic = clomipramine) for separation anxiety (Novartis). These medications have labels for other conditions and for cats in some countries outside the United States, and such uses are "extra-label" in the United States. Although there is no difference in biological effect between a brand name medication for dogs and a generic one, there may be differences in cost, size of tablet or capsule, or formulation (e.g., tablet, capsule, chewable tablet) that may be an issue for some pets. Understand these differences and, in collaboration with your veterinarian, make the best choice for you and your pet.

2. Potential Toxicity

For many of the behavioral medications, we know a lot about potential toxicity in dogs at and above routine dosage ranges because dogs are the models for human toxicology studies of these medications. Much of the toxicology and toxicity data is either published or available from the company or from poison control centers (in the United States: www.aspca.org/Pet-care/poison-control.aspx; 1-888-426-4435), should an untoward event occur. Please remember that *ingesting their human's medication* is the most common reason why pets become toxic from medication.

3. Rare Side Effects

Although we do not know the full range of side effects that could be experienced by canine or feline patients treated with these medications, we know what the potential side effects may be. Because licensing trials are small compared to the number of people ultimately treated, this same situation occurs in humans who take these medications. Because we cannot know all of the side effects that could occur, the pharmacological industry participates in ongoing reporting of side effects. Rare side effects may not be detected until tens of thousands of similar patients are treated.

This means that you should be familiar with common side effects and immediately ask questions when you are not sure if you are seeing a side effect. No dedicated veterinarian or specialist minds being asked if some behavior is a side effect of treatment, even if you think that you will sound foolish or silly. Treatment of behavioral conditions with medication requires that we stop worrying about how we sound and do what's in the best interest of our furred friends.

🔺 Rare side effects that may require stopping the medication include neurological changes that don't go away in a day (e.g., staggering, falling over, increased sensitivity to noise, crossed eyes, an inability to sleep or rest). Anything that **you** think is really weird should be reported to your vet immediately. If your vet is not available, call the emergency number ASAP, and be willing to bring your dog or cat to an emergency clinic. Although highly, highly unlikely, **in the event of a serious side effect, quick action is key,** and the more familiar you are with how to approach the situation, the less you will worry.

When your veterinarian prescribes medication, he will provide you with office and emergency phone numbers. Put these numbers somewhere accessible (e.g., taped to the telephone or entered into an automatic speed dial/address book).

- If you have a pet sitter, you should always have these numbers near the phone that the pet sitter will use or entered into her cell phone. Review all of your vet's contact information with your pet sitter.
- If you board your pet, you **must** insist that the caretakers know about the medication, are able to administer the medication, and have the numbers to call if they are the least bit concerned about any of the pet's behaviors.

- Always make sure you have the name of the medication and the amount your pet takes available. Veterinarians go on vacation and temporary veterinarians may not be able to find medication records quickly.

  ⚠ **Important point:** Emergencies, while rare, can happen. Write your vet's daytime and emergency phone numbers here:

  Daytime:

  Emergency:

  Medication (e.g., amitriptyline):

  Dose (e.g., 25 mg every 12 hours):

  In the United States, the American Society for the Prevention of Cruelty to Animals' (ASPCA) poison control center can be reached at: www.aspca.org/Pet-care/poison-control.aspx; 1-888-426-4435.

4. Relatively Common Behavioral Side Effects

The most common of the side effects for any behavioral medication include the following:
- sleepiness or sedation that wears off in a day or two,
- gastrointestinal upset that usually shows up as some mild diarrhea or some mucous in the stool,
- changes in appetite that are minor,
- licking of the lips after giving medication with increased belching or occasional vomiting,
- increased water consumption that requires you to fill the dish more frequently,
- deeper sleep,
- changes in pupil size without problems with vision,
- increased heart rate, and
- associated increased panting.

The only side effects that should cause real concern are those that last more than a few days. There are a number of actions you can take to minimize and monitor these side effects.

- Your dog or cat may always drink a little bit more because many of the medications used can cause a dry mouth. This complaint is less common in dogs and cats than it is in humans, but ensure that you start the day with full, fresh bowls of water. Watch how much your pet drinks. If you think your cat or dog is hanging over the water dish and is excessively thirsty, measure the amount he drinks (amount put in bowl at time 1 – amount left at end of day at time 2 = amount consumed if you have one pet), and talk to your vet.
- Try giving the medication in food—really good food—like cream cheese, ice cream, peanut butter, yogurt, tinned liver pate paste, et cetera. This will minimize any stomach upset, and stop most of the lip licking and vomiting. These medications are bitter, and it's the taste that causes these effects.
- Clomicalm, the tricyclic antidepressant (TCA) licensed for use as an aid in the treatment of separation anxiety in the United States, and Reconcile, the selective serotonin reuptake inhibitor (SSRI) used for the same canine condition, are made palatable by flavoring so that it can be chewed or swallowed. This is one of the biggest benefits of formulation for cats and dogs. But not all dogs can have the protein used for the flavoring. If your dog has problems with certain proteins in foods, talk to your vet about whether a chewable is the best choice.

- If your dog or cat experiences mucousy or loose stool, and it doesn't resolve in 3 to 5 days, consider using a coating agent (kaolin) before giving the medication.
- If you think your pet is sedated, chart the amount of time your pet spends asleep, noting the number of naps, and whether you think the pet is truly "awake" when he wakes up. If you do this for a few days, you will have good data that will suggest whether sedation is a problem and you can discuss your concern with your vet. Some very anxious dogs have been sleep deprived and may finally be catching up on their sleep.
- If you think that your pet is experiencing an appetite change, keep a log of how much he eats, when he eats, how long it takes him to eat, and any new behaviors associated with eating (e.g., trying to bury his food). After a week you will have enough information to discuss your concern with your vet.

  ⚠ **Important point:** Most of the medications used to help treat behavioral problems are bitter. If the pet chews through the capsule or tablet, he will salivate profusely and try to chew/lick the substance off. If this happens, you may never get your pet to take another capsule or tablet. Consider putting the medication in a terrific treat that the pet will swallow at once to minimize the bad taste and tummy upsets.

  The only potentially serious concern listed above is an increased heart rate. Have your veterinarian teach you how to take your dog's or cat's pulse or heart rate.

- If your pet is thin and likes to be handled, you can take the heart rate by putting your hand on either side of her chest under the arms. You'll feel the heart. Count the number of beats in 30 seconds and multiply by 2 for the number in 60 seconds. This is the heart rate.
- You can measure the pulse on bigger or fatter animals by taking the femoral pulse, pressing on the major vein in the back leg. If your pet is calm, you can probably run your hand over the middle of the inner thigh and find the femoral vein. Or your veterinarian can show you how to do this if your pet is calm enough to allow it, or can teach you to take the pulse on a calm dog and you can learn how to take your pet's pulse at home when she is calmer.

Normal rates can be 60 to 100 beats per minute, depending on the breed and age of dog. Cats have higher heart rates than do dogs. It's important that you know what *normal is for your pet before starting medication*. It's best to take your pet's pulse for a few days while he is sleeping or relaxing. This will give you some idea of the range of "normal" for your animal. Then, after you have started the medication, take the pulse for a few days while the pet is sleeping. *Big differences should be reported to your vet ASAP* (e.g., 70 to 140 beats per minute). Small changes generally normalize after a few days (e.g., 70 to 80 beats per minute).

If your pet seems uncomfortable and continuously pants, regardless of the change, **call your vet, please.**

⚠ **Important point:** Side effects, especially those concerned with increased heart rate, that are dramatic or that do not go away in a few days are problematic. If this happens or if you think your pet is uncomfortable in any way after starting the medication, call your vet immediately. The solution may be to change medication, decrease the drug, or tincture of time, but the key to the best outcomes is a teamwork approach based on shared information!

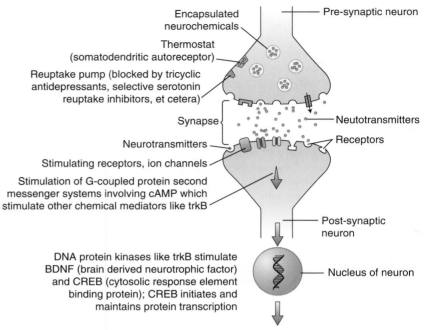

Figure 1 Schematic of how neurons work and how these medications affect neurochemicals and receptors.

5. Commonly Used Drugs/Medications

Most of the medications prescribed for the treatment of behavioral problems in pets will fall into one of a few classes:

- benzodiazepines (BZDs) and related medications like gabapentin (a GABA analog),
- tricyclic antidepressants (TCAs),
- selective serotonin reuptake inhibitors (SSRIs) and serotonin-2A antagonist/reuptake inhibitors (SARIs),
- combination TCAs/SSRIs (often called NaSSRIs for noradrenaline/selective serotonin reuptake inhibitors),
- *N*-methyl-D-aspartate (NMDA) inhibitors, like memantine,
- some alpha-adrenergic agonists, like clonidine,
- monoamine oxidase inhibitors (MAOIs), and
- some newer antipsychotic agents, which are not discussed here.

With the exception of clonidine, these compounds all act by altering levels of neurotransmitters in certain regions of the brain. They do this either by affecting activity at a neuronal receptor, or by changing the neuron's activity or metabolism by directly altering internal chemistry, or by some combination of actions. See Figure 1 for a cartoon sketch of what a neuron looks like and how it can be affected.

Benzodiazepines

BZDs work by changing the relationship between neurons that are excited/stimulated and those that are slowed/inhibited. BZDs increase the neurochemical gamma-aminobutyric acid (GABA), an inhibitory neurochemical. This means BZDs slow down or inhibit neurons that would otherwise have been stimulated. In the case of BZD, this effect is part of a balancing act: GABA is made from an excitatory amino acid that acts as an excitatory neurotransmitter, glutamate. You can think of the effects as those involved in a seesaw—as glutamate increases, the patient becomes very

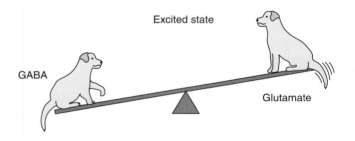

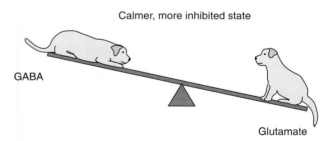

Figure 2 The relationship between glutamate, an excitatory amino acid that stimulates neurons and GABA, an inhibitory neurotransmitter that calms neurons. BZDs stimulate GABA.

excited, and then as GABA increases, the effect of inhibition becomes more apparent and the patient calms (see Figure 2).

The effects from BZDs are relatively nonspecific effects, meaning that everything calms or everything becomes excited. This is why BZDs are not commonly used as daily medications, except in cases of profound panic. BZDs also have three levels of effects depending on dosage:

- At high levels they act as true sedatives
- At intermediate levels they act as anti-anxiety medications
- At low levels they have general calming effects

When we use BZDs as part of a multi-level behavioral treatment program, we are looking for either the calming or anti-anxiety effects. Different types of BZDs have different thresholds for these different effects and affect different receptors to get the desired effect.

Please note, cats can have a very rare but *weird, paradoxical response to BZDs*: They can become extremely agitated and excited. If this happens, stop the medication and call your veterinarian, please. Dogs can also have an excitation effect, but it is rarer for them than for cats, and generally less extreme.

⚠ **Important point:** If your pet is taking a BZD and is sedated, sluggish, or really out of it for more than a day or two, call your veterinarian! This is an undesirable side effect that can usually be managed by changing the amount or type of medication your pet is given.

Do not think that one drug in this class is the same as any other drug. Each medication differs. Your pet should have *only* the dose and medication your vet prescribed: *not your medication, not one you think is the same, and not a dose that would be easier for you to give.*

If giving the medication at the suggested times in the suggested amounts is hard for you, *talk to your veterinarian*; you will be able to find a regimen that works without risking the health of your pet or the good treatment effects.

BZDs include diazepam (Valium in the United States), alprazolam (Xanax in the United States), clonazepam (Klonopin in the United States), and clorazepate (Tranxene in the United States), among other medications.

Almost all of the BZDs are abusable by humans. Dogs and cats do not have opposable thumbs and so cannot abuse these medications without human help because they cannot open the bottle at will. Accordingly, *there are households into which these medications should not be placed.* Do not be surprised if your veterinarian asks questions about *household risk.* Children, pre-teens, and teenagers also have friends, which can change the risk. If your household is one that cannot have BZD-type drugs, there are alternatives. Discuss this with your veterinarian.

For some dogs with non-specific anxieties or for those who could benefit from GABA stimulation but who may not need a BZD, gabapentin may be a good choice. Gabapentin looks like GABA and so stimulates the same pathways a GABA receptor would, but is only an analog. It's not regulated, metabolized, or otherwise converted into something that is used. As a result, it has very few side effects and can be a good choice for dogs with kidney and/or liver concerns. It may be associated with some temporary sedation and in humans has been known to very rarely cause huge behavioral shifts, so clients should be aware of a potential for profound "personality changes," although they have not yet been reported.

⚠ **Important point:** Some benzodiazepines prescribed for pets can cause or aid abuse or addiction problems in humans. Know your household and your visitors, and minimize risks.

Tricyclic Antidepressants and Related Compounds

TCAs work by inhibiting the amount of *norepinephrine*, a stimulating neurochemical, and *serotonin*, a neurochemical associated with calm, outgoing, happy behaviors that is recycled by the neuron that first releases it (the presynaptic

neuron). In other words, TCAs block the neuron's own recycling system.

The brain is a truly unique organ and not a lot of chemicals that are in the blood actually get into the brain because of something called the blood–brain barrier (BBB). The BBB's job is to maintain the overall or total brain at relatively constant conditions so only the smallest substances can go easily back and forth between the brain and the blood. This is one reason why recycling of neurochemicals is so important: This is a conservation strategy for neurochemical building blocks.

Because neurochemicals work by stimulating receptors in the next neuron (the post-synaptic neuron), the extra neurochemicals hanging around the space between the neurons (the synaptic cleft) are now available to stimulate the next receptor that becomes available. This means that you do not have to stimulate the first cell (the pre-synaptic neuron) again, to continue to stimulate the second cell. This pattern is so powerful that it overcomes the thermostatic effect experienced by the first cell. Now that you have all this neurotransmitter hanging around, the cell's thermostat (otherwise called the somatodendritic auto-receptor) tells the first cell not to move any more neurochemical to the cell's membrane because there is already more outside than is being used. Accordingly, the first cell slows down its production and movement of norepinephrine and serotonin. Because the entire point is to stimulate the receptors in the second cell so that they stimulate chemicals in the cell that affect overall activity, it's more important to have stuff available to fill the receptors than it is to have continuous supply. After a few days, a new set-point or thermostatic level is reached, and there is both high volume of neurotransmitters moved through the pre-synaptic neuron and efficient saturation of receptors on the second cell (the post-synaptic neuron).

Selective Serotonin Reuptake Inhibitors and Related Compounds

SSRIs work very much like TCAs do, but they have very, very small or virtually no effects on norepinephrine. The different SSRIs (e.g., fluoxetine [Prozac in the United States], paroxetine [Paxil in the United States], sertraline [Zoloft in the United States], et cetera) affect different types of different serotonin receptors to a greater or lesser extent, which is why sometimes a few tries are needed before choosing the best medication for your pet. Just like people, dogs and cats differ in receptor density, in receptor type distribution, in overall metabolism of the medication, and in which enzymes make them more or less sensitive to a drug. Unfortunately, the only way to learn or infer this is to try different medications if another is not working. Because of their more selective effects on receptor types, SSRIs are usually considered to have fewer side effects than many other medications, which is why they are used so often.

SSRIs and the more specific and newer of the TCAs (e.g., clomipramine/Clomicalm) do their best work by changing the metabolism of the second neuron and encouraging it to stimulate it's genetic and protein making machinery to make new and better receptors. This is also the process you go through when learning something new. *Because of this pattern, treatment with the appropriate TCA and/or SSRI can help your pets learn the behavior modification faster than they would without the medications.*

In placebo-controlled, double-blind studies, dogs treated with TCAs and SSRIs plus behavior modification compared with those treated with behavior modification, alone, improved faster and to a better level. This one of the reasons these medications are so often used in treatment programs.

⚠ **Important point:** SSRIs and some TCAs are recommended because they help dogs learn. They do this by decreasing the anxiety that interferes with learning and by using the neurochemical pathways that are already involved in learning.

Combination Selective Serotonin Reuptake Inhibitors/Tricyclic Antidepressants

Some of the newer medications (e.g., Effexor; venlafaxine) are medications that have the beneficial effects of the TCAs and SSRIs, combined, which minimizes side effects. This means that they will stimulate both the more specific and less specific neurochemical receptors, and will effect both norepinephrine and serotonin, but at different rates than would the SSRI or TCA, alone. Because of these changes, some of these medications can have fewer side effects and greater treatment effects for some patients. All of these compounds still have their patents at this writing, which can make them a little pricier than some of the other, "older" medications. The same effect may be achievable by combining the TCA and the SSRI in the animal, using two different medications, at relatively lower dosages.

Memantine and Related Compounds

Glutamate is an excitatory amino acid. It stimulates other neurons using various receptors. Increases in glutamate have been reported in a number of cognitive, epileptic, and behavioral conditions that involve explosive or impulsive behaviors. Memantine blocks the binding of glutamate with a specific receptor class and so decreases the adverse effects of glutamate.

Clonidine and Related Compounds

Clonidine is a member of the class of medications known as centrally acting, alpha-2-agonists. These medications decrease cardiac output and lower blood pressure, and so should beneficially affect the increased heart rate, tone and arousal that are reactions to stress, threats, or excitement. Medications like clonidine are thought to act by preventing the physiological effects of arousal in upsetting situations (e.g., storms, loud noises, novel situations that cause panic). Such medications should be used with care and responsibly if there is any heart disease, or if they are used with medications that increase norepinephrine (adrenalin).

Monoamine Oxidase Inhibitors

MAOIs are not widely used in veterinary behavioral medicine but one MAOI is licensed for use in the United States to treat cognitive dysfunction in dogs: selegiline (Anipryl). MAOIs work in the same way as TCAs and SSRIs, except that their focus is on the neurochemical, dopamine. Dopamine receptors are common in parts of the brain affected by aging, and increasing dopamine may help those experiencing age-related behavioral changes in cognition. Dopamine is metabolized to a version of amphetamine, so some of the desired behavioral changes we see in elderly dogs and cats treated with selegiline may be from being more active. Dopamine is a neurochemical in its own right, but it is also a precursor for norepinephrine (adrenalin), so we cannot combine TCAs or SSRIs and MAOIs because we may cause a huge pulse of adrenalin and/or serotonin.

6. Combination Treatment

BZDs can be used in combination with TCAs and SSRIs, when called for. For example, many dogs with separation anxiety are also afraid of storms. Storms may not happen every day, so we won't want to give a medication daily that the dog may not need. The dog can take a TCA like clomipramine (Clomicalm) every day, and the BZD, alprazolam, as needed. This means that for 20 days of a month the dog may get the TCA twice a day, but for 10 days she also gets the alprazolam as needed if there is a 50% chance or greater of storms. Because dogs use up alprazolam quickly and have few really sedative effects of repeat dosing if the dose chosen is correct, the dog may get alprazolam 3 or 4 times a day during those 10 days of storms.

There is currently no ideal drug to control or treat both of the chronic and sporadic types of anxieties. The best way to do this is to use the two different drugs in a rational way. This means your veterinarian needs to understand how they interact for effect and for side effects. For example, a dog whose only problem is storm phobia may need a higher dose of the alprazolam than a dog who also has separation anxiety and is already taking a TCA or SSRI. The choice has to do with the threshold that makes the dog react and how quickly the individual dog metabolizes the medications. Like humans, dogs and cats can either be slow or fast metabolizers. We know very little about this, currently.

Another kind of combination treatment is often used for the treatment of canine anxieties. As mentioned briefly above, this involves using a combination of TCAs and SSRIs (e.g., amitriptyline and fluoxetine). There are three reasons for doing this:

1. If cost is an issue, by using a less-specific medication with a more-specific one, the amount of the more-specific, and generally costlier, drug will be decreased.
2. Sometimes some amount of the less-specific drug is needed to affect receptors more-specific drugs don't. Although the problem is mainly with the receptors the more-specific drug addresses, clinical experience indicates that the behaviors differ when either medication is given, but both have desired improvements. In this case, using lower dosages of both drugs, especially if they are TCAs and SSRIs, can facilitate each other, or make each drug work better. This is especially true for drugs that share mechanisms for how they work.
3. By using lower dosages of two drugs, the side effects of each drug may be minimized.

However, caution is urged at the beginning of the combination treatment. The very, very rare animal shows an exaggerated excitation response that may be *equivalent to serotonin syndrome in humans.* These animals are quickly recognized because they don't stop moving, don't sleep, don't eat, and are generally frantic. *Medications should be stopped at once for any animal exhibiting these signs and the veterinarian should be informed immediately.* Treated appropriately, dogs and cats survive these episodes, but may never be able to take the same amounts or types of drugs again. To repeat, this is a very, very rare side effect, but in the world of side effects, knowledge is power.

⚠ **Important point:** You **cannot** give TCAs or SSRIs along with a MAOI (e.g., amitraz, Preventics, Anipryl) because both increase the amount of norepinephrine (adrenalin) available, and the combination may also increase the amount of serotonin available, increasing the risk of serotonin syndrome!

7. The Medical Aspects of Treatment with Behavioral Medications

Almost all medications used in the treatment of behavioral problems are metabolized or broken down and excreted by the liver and kidneys. Because of this, and because of the rare, but potential concerns about effects on heart function, all animals treated with any behavioral medication should have both a thorough physical examination, including at least a good listen to their heart, and a complete blood count, urinalysis, and serum biochemistry profile, just like you have when you have your annual physical, to make sure that nothing is wrong with their liver, kidney, or other organ systems, *and* that the behavioral concerns are not nonspecific signs of a physical condition.

Most behavioral signs are nonspecific and may be the result of a physiological condition. A good history will usually help clarify the diagnosis, but a good physical examination is essential. If your veterinarian has concerns, she may want to also do some radiographs and/or an electrocardiogram, but the need for such follow-up is not common.

If your pet has some liver or kidney compromise, you may still be able to give her behavioral medications but you may need to use a lower dosage or give the medications less frequently.

If your pet is treated with behavioral medications long-term—and many pets need this—you should have the physical and laboratory exams repeated at least annually, or if the pet becomes ill. As pets age, their ability to process medication may change. Again, by changing dose or frequency, these changes can usually be well managed, but you need to know the change has occurred. The only way to do this is to have a laboratory evaluation, and for some older dogs and cats this should be done 2 to 4 times a year. Remember that your pets cannot tell you when they are beginning to feel a little odd.

There are some medications that interact with the behavioral medications that your pet is taking. The common conditions that require treatment with medications that may interact with behavioral drugs include epilepsy, hypothyroidism, and, especially in cats, diabetes. Having these conditions does not mean your pet cannot be treated with behavioral drugs, but it does mean that treatment should be thoughtful. For example, treatment with a TCA can alter the level of the thyroidal hormones that are measured on routine tests. In some cases, lower doses of drugs used to treat epilepsy may be needed if the dog is calmer. However, the combination of required drugs may make some animals sluggish. Every animal is an individual and your job as your pet's best friend is to ask questions that will allow you to look out for your pet's best interests.

⚠ **Important point:** Medical conditions can affect how well your pet can utilize behavioral medications. Additionally, behavioral drugs can interfere with the metabolism of medications used for other conditions, and those medications can interfere with the ability of your pet to respond to behavioral medications. You need to discuss all of this with your veterinarian as your dog or cat ages or requires other help.

8. Length of Treatment Required

The amount of time that your animal takes behavioral medication will depend on the following four factors:

1. How long the pet was affected before beginning treatment or how early in the course of the condition the pet is treated. The longer the pet was affected, the more numerous are the neurochemical changes in the brain associated with learning the anxiety. If pets are treated early in the course of their condition, treatment is likely to be relatively short (e.g., 4 or 6 months rather than lifelong).

2. How severely the pet is affected (e.g., does your dog exhibit all of the signs of separation anxiety or a just a few of the milder ones?). The more severely affected the pet is, the more likely are pathological changes in brain neurochemistry in affected regions. Also, the more profound the fear, the more quickly it's learned and honed by practice. Severely affected pets may have a lesser probability of weaning from a medication than do mildly affected pets.

3. How well you can comply with the other aspects of the treatment. The harder people work with behavioral and environmental modification, the more likely the pet is to become well, and the less he may need medication. Because medication speeds the rate at which dogs acquire the behaviors encouraged by behavior modification, there is a synergy between effort and medication, so that people who work the best and hardest have a greater likelihood of being able to wean their pets from medication.

4. Your tolerance for giving behavioral medication to your pet. People who are frantic about potential side effects hover over their pets and make their anxieties worse. Although this isn't what they intend to do, some people are just so uncomfortable with using behavioral medication that it may not be the best, or at least the first, choice for them.

In general, the average dog or cat treated with daily medication will require treatment for 4 to 6 months before any weaning should be attempted. This not only allows for improvement to occur, but allows you and your veterinarian to gauge how reliable that improvement is as life varies. Please keep a list comparable to that kept by your veterinarian of the pet's weight, medication given, frequency given, amount given and any changes. You will also want to note dates when medication has been refilled. By keeping this list accessible (put it on the refrigerator) you will guarantee that your pet is getting the appropriate medication, as agreed with your veterinarian. A sample table (see Log for Medication) is attached.

Like humans, some dogs and cats will require lifelong medication, some will require sporadic medication, and some will require just one round of medication. Unfortunately, we do not know enough to predict in advance which dog or cat will require what. Think of these conditions like diabetes: some forms of diabetes require only lifestyle changes, some require initial treatment with insulin while implementing lifestyle changes, and some require insulin no matter what. Some dogs have neurochemical receptors that can re-regulate on their own, some will need medication forever to insure that this happens.

Regardless of how long your pet requires medication, by following the recommendations in this protocol you can assure that you are giving the medication safely and in the pet's best interests.

When stopping medication, weaning is preferred over an abrupt halt. This is because:

- abrupt halts can trigger relapses,
- by weaning you have earlier warning that the changes are going in the wrong direction,
- by weaning you can learn if your pet still needs medication, but at a lower dose, and
- clients are less worried when changes are gradual.

Some clients never wish to wean their pets from medication because they are afraid that their animals will suffer. Our incomplete ability to assess our companions' suffering is one of the real difficulties of loving dogs and cats who cannot speak. Treatment for behavioral conditions should—first and foremost—be humane and in the best interests of the pet. That said, if clients are not sure that they can tell if the animal begins to suffer or relapse, and they are worried that their pet will worsen if weaned from medication, there is nothing wrong with continuing medication as part of a treatment program involving behavior modification and environmental intervention, as long as potential physical concerns are addressed, as discussed above.

⚠ **Important point:** Discontinuation of medication abruptly is **not** recommended because of the risk of relapse and because of the potential for "discontinuation/withdrawal syndrome." That said, all of these medications can be stopped quickly if needed in an emergency, and none are addictive.

9. Other Concerns

Pets treated with behavioral medication can otherwise be treated as we do nontreated dogs and cats. Anesthesia poses special concerns, but these are easily addressed by your veterinarian by considering how the drugs your pet is taking could interact with other medications. Because of the risk of relapse and because anxiety is not helpful during anesthetic procedures, the general recommendation is to maintain the dog or cat on his or her anti-anxiety medications and alter the mix of drugs given as part of the anesthesia cocktail. If your veterinarian is not comfortable with this idea, please suggest that they speak to a specialist. The field of veterinary behavioral medicine is still relatively young, and most vets do not receive any training in behavioral medicine while they are in vet school.

10. Transdermal Patches and Gels

Clients and veterinarians, alike, would welcome a topical gel or patch for these medications. Unfortunately, the metabolism of these medications changes dramatically when absorption through the skin is compared with taking the medication by mouth. In the few studies that have been done, a much larger amount of medication is needed for the same effect, if the medication is applied to the skin. Thus far, this finding has made patches and gels impractical for behavioral treatment. Future treatments may be more flexible.

11. Last Words

Please remember that drugs are part of a treatment plan that involves changes in the environment and behavior mod: *Do not think that drugs alone will accomplish what an entire treatment plan can.* Unfortunately, like the rest of life, there are no "quick fixes."

Please do not seek to mask normal behaviors by sedating your pet. This is an inappropriate use of medication, and most of the medications discussed here will not do that anyway.

Finally, please remember safety. Any drug can be toxic if huge quantities are ingested. Dogs, puppies, and kittens often chew on pill containers. This is the most common reason for "overdose" in pets. Although the container, itself, is likely to do more damage to the animal if broken and eaten, support for these animals can require a lengthy stay in an intensive care unit. No one wants to sustain the financial or emotional costs for that. So, be a good guardian. Put medications far away from the curious hands of children and paws and mouths of puppies and kittens. Unless you have difficulty opening pill bottles, request safety lids. Safety lids are harder for dogs to open, too, but not to chew through. Common sense may not be common, but it works. In the United States, the ASPCA's poison control center can be reached at: www.aspca.org/Pet-care/poison-control.aspx; 1-888-426-4435.

⚠ **Important point:** Drugs, behavioral medications, psychotropic medications, whatever you wish to call them, **are not a quick fix.** You cannot just give a pill and expect years of anxiety to vanish. But used rationally and safely, behavioral medications actually allow you to help your pet and you to become more humane in doing so.

Summary of Commonly Asked Client Questions with Answers

Client Question	Quick Answer
What medications are used?	We use most of the same medications or classes of medication that are used for the same conditions in humans. Most commonly used medications come from the BZD, TCA, and SSRI classes of drugs.
How do these work?	All of these medications affect how brain neurons communicate with each other and the neurochemistry that appears impaired in anxiety.
What are the potential side effects?	Side effects are usually rare and transient but can include gastrointestinal distress including diarrhea and/or regurgitation/vomiting; changes in appetite, including anorexia; sedation, changes in energy level; atypical reactivity; and increased heart and respiratory rates. If any of these side effects are profound or last longer than a few days, the patient should be reevaluated. Anorexia is a rare but profound problem for some patients given SSRIs. Serotonin syndrome is a concern for any patient taking any medication that affects serotonin and who is experiencing profound increases in heart rate, body temperature, and/or agitation.
How should the client monitor for side effects?	Clients should keep a log of the worrisome behaviors, and compare them to normal. To do this, they need to know if the dog or cat occasionally has diarrhea and what their behaviors were before starting medications. Clients can learn to take patients' heart rates and report any significant increases or decreases immediately to their veterinarian. Clients can also comply with the recommendation for annual physical and laboratory evaluation for younger animals and twice annual evaluation for older animals. Evaluation should also occur if the dog or cat becomes ill.
Can these medication interact with other medications (e.g., thyroxin, anti-inflammatories, pain medications like tramadol) and, if so, how?	Yes, any medications that use the same enzyme system in the liver can have their effect exaggerated or decreased, depending on the enzyme function, and those medications can have the same effect on the behavioral drugs. This is why it is so important for clients to ensure that they tell their veterinarian every single medication and supplement that their dog or cat is being given. Clients need to understand that this list includes "homeopathic," "herbal," and "natural" products. St. John's wort, for example, is a potent cytochrome P (CYP) 34A inducer. For medications like thyroxin, there may be effects on measured blood levels of the medication or on the compounds it is intended to affect. Pain medications (e.g., tramadol), antibiotics and antiinflammatories can be given with behavioral medications if they are needed, if the dosages are appropriately adjusted, and the patient monitored, which is easy to do. Anti-inflammatories may block some effects of SSRIs, but there are no data yet for dogs and cats.
I know that I cannot use a Preventics collar (which contains amitraz) or other products containing amitraz for my dog if she is taking TCAs or SSRIs. Can I use topicals (Frontline, Advantix, pyrethrin sprays, et cetera)?	Amitraz is a MAOI that can produce a toxic response when given to a patient already taking an SSRI or a TCA. Any product containing a MAOI should be avoided if the patient is taking a TCA or an SSRI. Frontline (fipronil) and Advantix (imidacloprid, permethrin and pyriproxyfen) do not use MAOIs and instead rely on insect growth hormone inhibitors. Advantix also has a pyrethrin (permethrin), which acts as repellant and neurotoxin for insects. These medication can be used with TCAs or SSRIs. However, if the patient is a cat, you must avoid pyrethrins. They are toxic for cats.

Continued

Summary of Commonly Asked Client Questions with Answers—cont'd

Client Question	Quick Answer
What effects can be seen and when?	Dogs and cats treated with medications affecting anxiety should become calmer and less anxious. • This may mean a decrease in activity that can appear as weight gain. • Patients may actually eat more, and may finish their food treats/food toys when the clients are not with them. Contrast this with anxious patients who cannot eat when distressed and who will not eat or finish treats or food toys when alone. • Patients who are less anxious may react less quickly to a stimulus. • Less-anxiety patients may react to a certain stimulus using a lower level of reactivity than was previously possible. • Less-anxious patients may raise their threshold for reacting and so not react as readily as they had previously. Now, it takes more of a stimulus to make them react. • Patients who are improving may show a decreased amount of time between hearing the request to lie down or sit down and compliance with the request. They are less worried and so can comply more readily. • Patients who are deriving beneficial effects from their medication may pause before reacting or become more thoughtful and less concerned, in general. They may be able to attend more to cues in the environment and assess whether they need to react before reacting. • Patients may sleep longer and more soundly (more restorative sleep) as their anxiety resolves. • Patients may be more receptive to learning to change their behavior through behavior modification. • Patients may become more attentive to the helpful cues they are given, and they may solicit cues more often. • Dogs who are improving may take treats more gently rather than grabbing forcefully at them as concerned dogs often do. Here, it is important to separate poor delivery technique from patient anxiety. • Cats who are improving may become more interested in behavioral modification using food treats, and be willing to remain with the client to learn about these.
How long must the patient take the medication?	Patients affected for a long time may require or benefit from long-term treatment. Patients with relatively uncomplicated, recent concerns may require medication for only a few months. Length of treatment is determined by the patient's history, the patient's treatment response, the client's concerns, and the patient's stimulatory environment.
How do we wean or remove the patient from the medication?	If there is an emergency patients can be abruptly taken from the medication, but weaning is preferred in planned cessations. Weaning permits the avoidance of rebound syndrome and allows clients to learn if their pet would benefit from a lower dose of the medication. Be aware that some patients who are removed from a medication will not respond to it when exposed again, no matter how well they did when treated with it the first time.
What does the client do if she is scared?	The client should call her vet immediately and express the details of the concern to a member of the treatment team. If the concern is after hours and no one returns a phone call quickly, the client should take the dog or cat to an emergency service to err on the safe side and to prevent the possibility of feeling guilt.

Log for Medication

Pet's name:

Date Medication Was Provided or Refilled	Name of Medication	Dose of Medication and Schedule (for example: 1 tablet every 12 hours)	Amount Provided (for example: 60 tablets)	Weight of Pet (for example: 20 kg or 44 pounds)	Comments/Notes About Effects/ Side Effects

GENERALIZED GUIDELINES FOR USING ALPRAZOLAM FOR NOISE AND STORM PHOBIAS, PANIC, AND SEVERE DISTRESS

Dosages and Dosing

The recommended dose of alprazolam for dogs is 0.25 to 0.5 mg every 12 hours, routinely, or every 4 to 6 hours, as needed. The published dosages for dogs are extremely variable, but preferred starting range is 0.02 to 0.04 mg/kg. For most dogs this means starting with a dose of 0.25 to 0.5 mg. Alprazolam is sold in 0.25, 0.5, 1.0, and 2.0 mg tablets.

The recommended dose of alprazolam for cats is 0.0675 to 0.125 mg (¼ to ½ of the smallest tablet made) every 12 to 24 hours as needed. The published dosage for cats is 0.0125 to 0.025 mg/kg, which means that for most cats the initial dose will be ⅛ to ¼ of a 0.25-mg tablet.

All of the examples used in this handout pertain to dogs, but the pattern for use is similar for cats. *Because the medication discussed is a controlled substance and because we need to ensure that your dog or cat is healthy enough to try this medication, please use this handout in consultation with your veterinarian and make sure you understand dosing schedules and amounts.*

Three Ways to Use Alprazolam

Alprazolam is the "panicolytic" medication used in dogs and humans, and used well, it can be a godsend. There are three ways to use this:

- as a true preventative for dogs with known triggers for profound distress (e.g., storms),
- as a situational and interventional medication for distressed animals in known situations to help them not to consolidate memory about the situation and to help them in the future not to get to the level of reactivity where learning to be more fearful is a concern (e.g., your dog becomes badly scared by dogs in the park and can not enjoy the rest of her walk; the dog worries and cries when she goes to the vet), and
- in a truly panicolytic context (e.g., the storm crept up on you and now your dog is curled in a ball, drooling).
All of these can be rational uses within the same patient.

Preventative

To use alprazolam as true preventative you must be able to anticipate when there will be a provocative stimulus: a guest, the later walk in the day, a departure to go to work, a scheduled visit to the veterinarian, a known or constant pattern of storms, et cetera. With online use of Doppler radar, people can become excellent at predicting storms to which their dogs and cats might react.

The starting dose of alprazolam for most dogs is 0.25 to 0.5 mg. One choice is to give a 0.25-mg tablet 1.5 to 2 hours before anticipated event. Then repeat a full (0.25 mg in this example) or half dose (0.125 mg) 30 minutes before the event. Repeat every 4 to 6 hours as needed using either the half or full dose. Start with the half dose, as this dosing—as explained—is cumulative. If the stimulus is going to present for consecutive days (e.g., a series of storms, a house guest) you may find that giving the medication every 12 hours plus using is as needed works well. All patients are different in their responses and for clients to use this medication well they have to be willing to adjust it and watch the dog.

Situational/Interventional for Dogs with Known and Worsening Fears and Anxieties

If you find that your dog, who is already known to be fearful in certain circumstances, is reacting to some stimulus (a surprise storm, distress at discovering she is alone, meeting a scary dog or person on the street) *and she cannot return to her baseline of calm behavior within 5 minutes of you attempting to calm her* (and you should be fairly passive and just talk calmly to her), our concern is that such events will teach her to be more fearful. Every time dogs practice fear they learn to do it better and can react more quickly. So, if the dog becomes upset by the approach of a new dog in the park and is still distressed even when the dog goes away, give her a half or a whole dose at that time.

If your dog becomes distressed outside on a walk—and for dogs who also react to noise, the distress may have been triggered by a noise—you can continue or discontinue the walk, depending on her response, but you really want the dog to **not** make molecular memory of her fear and response to it, so please consider giving her the alprazolam because it interferes with consolidation or processing of memories associated with fear.

There is a fine line between whether the dog really needs the medication to stop the response or whether you can simply intervene early enough to avoid the distress that will make a molecular memory. No one is perfect at intuiting their dog's needs, so your best gauge is your dog's behaviors. If you are going to use alprazolam as an interventional, you will need to have some with you at all times or give it before you engage in the activity that may provoke the dog.

- If you know the behaviors your dog exhibits when concerned (panting, pacing, salivating, hiding, cringing, crying, et cetera) you can monitor them and medicate the dog beforehand when you think they might appear.
- If you keep a written log of your dog's behaviors and the circumstances under which they appear, this will help you to monitor the dog's behavior.

Such attention means that, in most cases, she will get the medication at the time that it will best help her.

Obviously you can do a combination of the above if you have an upsetting set of days. You could give the dog a full dose as soon as you awaken, top it off 2 hours and then again at 30 minutes before the expected event using a half dose, and continue to give a half or a full dose as needed depending on upset. *Always start as with the lowest effective dose.* If we can medicate the dog before she has any upset you will need less medication.

Panicolytic

If something happens that is truly bad and the dog has a full-blown panic attack, give the full dose immediately. If she is still distressed 30 minutes later, repeat with a half or a whole dose. Remember, the pill can be dissolved in a tiny amount of liquid or will dissolve in the dog's cheeks.

Finding the Right Dose

You may have to try different dosages to find the best dose for your dog. Alprazolam is a benzodiazepine and so can have a tremendously variable effect depending on the individual. Your first check needs to be for serious side effects. This can include serious sedation or paradoxical excitement. We do not want dogs so sleepy that they fall down the stairs or drown in their water dish, or so excited that they run through a glass door. We want to learn whether or not your dog can benefit from this medication while experiencing as few side effects as possible.

- *Checking for sedation:* When you are going to be home with the dog for at least 4 hours, give the dog at least 0.25 mg. If he is so sedated he cannot function or walk easily up and down stairs, or if he is uncoordinated (ataxic), this dose is too high for him. Halve it. If he is still sedated, we need to find another medication.

- *Checking for excitement:* When you are going to be home with the dog for at least 4 hours, give the dog at least 0.25 mg. If he starts to pant, run around, lack focus, seem wild-eyed, frantic, scared, or otherwise agitated, protect him and let the medication wear off. If you wish to try again, halve the dose. If he is still agitated, we need to find another medication.

- *The desired response when nothing is happening and you are home:* When you are going to be home with the dog, give the dog at least 0.25 mg. If there are no provocative stimuli (no scary noises or people, no upset in the household) the dog should just seem his normal self. He may sleep a bit and more deeply, but he should awaken upon request and not seem at all sedated or "drugged." In other words, you should not be able to tell he was given medication. The dog may be hungrier than on days when the medication was not given. Now we need to learn if we can find a dose that will help.
  - For a week, you can try the baseline dose.
  - If there is no effect after that, you can try doubling it.
  - After another week you can double the dose again.
  - If you are getting 2 to 4 mg into the dog and there is no effect, it's unlikely that the dog will respond to this medication. He may, however, respond to other benzodiazepines, alone or in combination with tricyclic antidepressants and selective serotonin reuptake inhibitors, or medications like gabapentin or clonidine. If you are going to try another benzodiazepine, you can work through the instructions above at a starting dose established for that particular benzodiazepine.

Tips to Remember

- Please remember that all benzodiazepines are humanly abusable and should not be placed in some households. Ensure that you keep any benzodiazepines in a secure place. In fact, if your veterinarian has any concerns about substance abuse, another medication may be suggested.

- Please do not give your dog your medication. If you think the dog would benefit from alprazolam or any other medication, you **must** talk with your veterinarian.

- If the dog has been taking any benzodiazepine for more than a few days continuously, wean the dog from the medication rather than stopping abruptly, if you have a choice. In an emergency you can stop benzodiazepines abruptly, but the concern is the development of signs of withdrawal (e.g., more anxiety).

- Regular blood work (every 3 to 6 months) can monitor how your dog is metabolizing medications.

- Note that you can give this medication twice a day, or up to every 4 hours as needed, or some combination of both of these patterns.

- If your dog or cat is going to be taking any other medication that is metabolized by the liver or is undergoing anesthesia or sedation, remind your veterinarian that the dog is taking a benzodiazepine because interactions matter.

- If you are using any benzodiazepine to treat your cat, please remember that cats metabolize these medications and their active metabolites more slowly than do dogs.

- Dogs and cats taking benzodiazepines may be hungrier than normal and if they are less anxious they may burn fewer calories.

- Finally, please remember that use of medication is not a magical solution—we are using the medication to both help modulate the anxiety, but also because it will facilitate them learning to act in new and more rational ways. These medications work best when combined with behavior modification.

INFORMED CONSENT STATEMENT—ALPRAZOLAM (XANAX)

It has been recommended that your pet be treated with a medication that is not licensed for use in domestic pet animals. This means that use of it in your pet is considered "extra label." This does not mean that the medication is dangerous to pets, just that pets were not the subjects tested for approved use. We often know a lot about potential undesirable/side effects of these medications because dogs and cats are the animals on which toxicity data have been collected by the drug company.

This medication has been chosen for your pet because it has been deemed to have the potential to be efficacious. This is not a guarantee that the medication will be efficacious in treating your pet's problem.

As with all medications, the medication that your pet will be taking may have potential undesirable/side effects. Although side effects are rare and every effort has been made to minimize them, you should know what the potential side effects are because the occasional animal may not be able to tolerate the medication. The medication prescribed for your pet, alprazolam (Xanax), is a benzodiazepine. It may cause your pet to be very slightly sedated and/or ataxic for a few days. Potential side effects may include changes in heart and respiratory rates, vomiting, diarrhea, inappetence, lethargy, and fainting. Severe depression or sedation is not to be desired or expected. If your pet becomes sedated or depressed, stop the medication and call us immediately. This medication may make some pets more assertive. Although these side effects are rare, and when experienced are usually transient, there have been reports of extremely rare cats experiencing toxic effects when given benzodiazepines. If your pet experiences any of these undesirable and worrisome effects, please call us so that we can make informed decisions about your pet's care. Please be aware that this medication is a humanly abusable substance and should not be used in some households.

After you have read this statement, please sign below indicating that you understand the statement and can comply with it. A copy will be provided for your information so that you can refer to it if needed.

Date: _____   Patient: _____

Client's name/signature: _____

Clinician's name/signature: _____

Contact number for questions/problems: _____

Emergency number: _____

INFORMED CONSENT STATEMENT—AMITRIPTYLINE (ELAVIL)

It has been recommended that your pet be treated with a medication that is not licensed for use in domestic pet animals. This means that use of it in your pet is considered "extra label." This does not mean that the medication is dangerous to pets, just that pets were not the subjects tested for approved use. We often know a lot about potential undesirable/side effects of these medications because dogs and cats are the animals on which toxicity data have been collected by the drug company.

This medication has been chosen for your pet because it has been deemed to have the potential to be efficacious. This is not a guarantee that the medication will be efficacious in treating your pet's problem.

As with all medications, the medication that your pet will be taking may have potential undesirable/side effects. Although side effects are rare and every effort has been made to minimize them, you should know what the potential side effects are because the occasional animal may not be able to tolerate the medication. The medication prescribed for your pet, amitriptyline (Elavil), is a tricyclic antidepressant (TCA). It may cause a slight increase in thirst, but it has not been associated with house-soiling accidents in pets. Potential side effects may include an increased heart rate, increased respiratory rate, vomiting, diarrhea, inappetence, lethargy, and fainting. Markedly increased heart rates may be associated with the early signs of serotonin syndrome, a potentially serious condition. Learn how to take your pet's heart rate and keep a record of it under varied conditions so that you can monitor your pet for potential marked and worrisome increases. Although these side effects are rare, and when experienced are usually transient, if your pet experiences any of them, please call us so that we can make informed decisions about your pet's care. Please do not use this medication if your pet is taking any MAO-I, including Preventics collars, and amitraz dips.

After you have read this statement, please sign below indicating that you understand the statement and can comply with it. A copy will be provided for your information so that you can refer to it if needed.

Date:_____   Patient:_____

Client's name/signature:_____

Clinician's name/signature: _____

Contact number for questions/problems: _____

Emergency number: _____

INFORMED CONSENT STATEMENT—BUSPIRONE (BUSPAR)

It has been recommended that your pet be treated with a medication that is not licensed for use in domestic pet animals. This means that use of it in your pet is considered "extra label." This does not mean that the medication is dangerous to pets, just that pets were not the subjects tested for approved use. We often know a lot about potential undesirable/side effects of these medications because dogs and cats are the animals on which toxicity data have been collected by the drug company.

This medication has been chosen for your pet because it has been deemed to have the potential to be efficacious. This is not a guarantee that the medication will be efficacious in treating your pet's problem.

As with all medications, the medication that your pet will be taking may have potential undesirable/side effects. Although side effects are rare and every effort has been made to minimize them, you should know what the potential side effects are because the occasional animal may not be able to tolerate the medication. The medication prescribed for your pet, buspirone (BuSpar), is a partial serotonin agonist and may cause a slight increase in thirst, but has not been associated with house-soiling accidents in pets. Potential side effects may include an increased heart rate, increased respiratory rate, vomiting, diarrhea, inappetence, lethargy, and fainting. Markedly increased heart rates may be associated with the early signs of serotonin syndrome, a potentially serious condition. Learn how to take your pet's heart rate and keep a record of it under varied conditions so that you can monitor your pet for potential marked and worrisome increases. This medication may make some pets more assertive. These side effects are rare, and when experienced are usually transient, but if your pet experiences any of them, please call us so that we can make informed decisions about your pet's care.

After you have read this statement, please sign below indicating that you understand the statement and can comply with it. A copy will be provided for your information so that you can refer to it if needed.

Date: _____ Patient: _____

Client's name/signature: _____

Clinician's name/signature: _____

Contact number for questions/problems: _____

Emergency number: _____

INFORMED CONSENT STATEMENT—CLONIDINE (CATAPRES)

It has been recommended that your pet be treated with a medication that is not licensed for use in domestic pet animals. This means that use of it in your pet is considered "extra label." This does not mean that the medication is dangerous to pets, just that pets were not the subjects tested for approved use. We often know a lot about potential undesirable/side effects of these medications because dogs and cats are the animals on which toxicity data have been collected by the drug company.

This medication has been chosen for your pet because it has been deemed to have the potential to be efficacious. This is not a guarantee that the medication will be efficacious in treating your pet's problem.

As with all medications, the medication that your pet will be taking may have potential undesirable/side effects. Although side effects are rare and every effort has been made to minimize them, you should know what the potential side effects are because the occasional animal may not be able to tolerate the medication. The medication prescribed for your pet, clonidine (Catapres) is a medication that acts regionally in the brain to decrease the increase in blood pressure and blood vessel tone associated with arousal. Clonidine has been potentially associated with changes in heart and respiratory rate, vomiting, diarrhea, inappetence, lethargy, sedation, and fainting. These side effects are rare, and when experienced are usually transient. If your pet experiences any of them, please call us so that we can make informed decisions about your pet's care.

After you have read this statement, please sign below indicating that you understand the statement and can comply with it. A copy will be provided for your information so that you can refer to it if needed.

Date: _____   Patient: _____

Client's name/signature: _____

Clinician's name/signature: _____

Contact number for questions/problems: _____

Emergency number: _____

INFORMED CONSENT STATEMENT—DIAZEPAM (VALIUM)

It has been recommended that your pet be treated with a medication that is not licensed for use in domestic pet animals. This means that use of it in your pet is considered "extra label." This does not mean that the medication is dangerous to pets, just that pets were not the subjects tested for approved use. We often know a lot about potential undesirable/side effects of these medications because dogs and cats are the animals on which toxicity data have been collected by the drug company.

This medication has been chosen for your pet because it has been deemed to have the potential to be efficacious. This is not a guarantee that the medication will be efficacious in treating your pet's problem.

As with all medications, the medication that your pet will be taking may have potential undesirable/side effects. Although side effects are rare and every effort has been made to minimize them, you should know what the potential side effects are because the occasional animal may not be able to tolerate the medication. The medication prescribed for your pet, diazepam (Valium), is a benzodiazepine. It may cause your pet to be slightly ataxic for a few days. Potential side effects may include changes in heart and respiratory rates, vomiting, diarrhea, inappetence, lethargy, and fainting. Severe sedation or depression is not to be desired or expected. If your pet becomes sedated or depressed, stop the medication and call us immediately. This medication may make some pets more assertive. The rare cat may suffer toxic and potentially fatal side effects. Although these side effects are usually rare, and when experienced are most often transient, there have been reports of extremely rare cats experiencing toxic effects wnen given benzodiazepines. If your pet experiences any of these side effects, please call us so that we can make informed decisions about your pet's care. Please be aware that this medication is a humanly abusable substance and should not be used in some households.

After you have read this statement, please sign below indicating that you understand the statement and can comply with it. A copy will be provided for your information so that you can refer to it if needed.

Date: _____   Patient: _____

Client's name/signature: _____

Clinician's name/signature: _____

Contact number for questions/problems: _____

Emergency number: _____

INFORMED CONSENT STATEMENT—GABAPENTIN (NEURONTIN)

It has been recommended that your pet be treated with a medication that is not licensed for use in domestic pet animals. This means that use of it in your pet is considered "extra label." This does not mean that the medication is dangerous to pets, just that pets were not the subjects tested for approved use. We often know a lot about potential undesirable/side effects of these medications because dogs and cats are the animals on which toxicity data have been collected by the drug company.

This medication has been chosen for your pet because it has been deemed to have the potential to be efficacious. This is not a guarantee that the medication will be efficacious in treating your pet's problem.

As with all medications, the medication that your pet will be taking may have potential undesirable/ side effects. Although side effects are rare and every effort has been made to minimize them, you should know what the potential side effects are because the occasional animal may not be able to tolerate the medication. The medication prescribed for your pet, gabapentin (Neurontin), is an analog of the inhibitory neurotransmitter, GABA. Gabapentin may be potentially associated with an increased heart rate, increased respiratory rate, vomiting, diarrhea, inappetence, salivation, sedation, lethargy, fainting, and atypical arousal. Although these side effects are rare, and when experienced are usually transient, you should watch your pet closely when starting this medication or changing dosages. If your pet experiences any of these worrisome effects, please call us so that we can make informed decisions about your pet's care.

After you have read this statement, please sign below indicating that you understand the statement and can comply with it. A copy will be provided for your information so that you can refer to it if needed.

Date: _____ Patient: _____

Client's name/signature: _____

Clinician's name/signature: _____

Contact number for questions/problems: _____

Emergency number: _____

INFORMED CONSENT STATEMENT—IMIPRAMINE (TOFRANIL)

It has been recommended that your pet be treated with a medication that is not licensed for use in domestic pet animals. This means that use of it in your pet is considered "extra label." This does not mean that the medication is dangerous to pets, just that pets were not the subjects tested for approved use. We often know a lot about potential undesirable/side effects of these medications because dogs and cats are the animals on which toxicity data have been collected by the drug company.

This medication has been chosen for your pet because it has been deemed to have the potential to be efficacious. This is not a guarantee that the medication will be efficacious in treating your pet's problem.

As with all medications, the medication that your pet will be taking may have potential undesirable/side effects. Although side effects are rare and every effort has been made to minimize them, you should know what the potential side effects are because the occasional animal may not be able to tolerate the medication. The medication prescribed for your pet, imipramine (Tofranil), is a tricyclic antidepressant (TCA). It may cause a slight increase in thirst, but has not been associated with house-soiling accidents in pets. Potential side effects may include an increased heart rate, increased respiratory rate, vomiting, diarrhea, inappetence, lethargy, and fainting. Markedly increased heart rates may be associated with the early signs of serotonin syndrome, a potentially serious condition. Learn how to take your pet's heart rate and keep a record of it under varied conditions so that you can monitor your pet for potential marked and worrisome increases. Although these side effects are rare, and when experienced are usually transient, if your pet experiences any of the undesirable and concerning effects, please call us so that we can make informed decisions about your pet's care. Please do not use this medication if your pet is taking any MAO-I, including Preventics collars, and amitraz dips.

After you have read this statement, please sign below indicating that you understand the statement and can comply with it. A copy will be provided for your information so that you can refer to it if needed.

Date: _____   Patient: _____

Client's name/signature: _____

Clinician's name/signature: _____

Contact number for questions/problems: _____

Emergency number: _____

INFORMED CONSENT STATEMENT—NORTRIPTYLINE (PAMELOR)

It has been recommended that your pet be treated with a medication that is not licensed for use in domestic pet animals. This means that use of it in your pet is considered "extra label." This does not mean that the medication is dangerous to pets, just that pets were not the subjects tested for approved use. We often know a lot about potential undesirable/side effects of these medications because dogs and cats are the animals on which toxicity data have been collected by the drug company.

This medication has been chosen for your pet because it has been deemed to have the potential to be efficacious. This is not a guarantee that the medication will be efficacious in treating your pet's problem.

As with all medications, the medication that your pet will be taking may have potential undesirable/side effects. Although side effects are rare and every effort has been made to minimize them, you should know what the potential side effects are because the occasional animal may not be able to tolerate the medication. The medication prescribed for your pet, nortriptyline (Pamelor), is a tricyclic antidepressant (TCA). It may cause a slight increase in thirst, but it has not been associated with house-soiling accidents in pets. Potential side effects may include an increased heart rate, increased respiratory rate, vomiting, diarrhea, inappetence, lethargy, and fainting. Markedly increased heart rates may be associated with the early signs of serotonin syndrome, a potentially serious condition. Learn how to take your pet's heart rate and keep a record of it under varied conditions so that you can monitor your pet for potential marked and worrisome increases. Although these side effects are rare, and when experienced are usually transient, if your pet experiences any of them, please call us so that we can make informed decisions about your pet's care. Please do not use this medication if your pet is taking any MAO-I, including Preventics collars, and amitraz dips.

After you have read this statement, please sign below indicating that you understand the statement and can comply with it. A copy will be provided for your information so that you can refer to it if needed.

Date: _____ Patient: _____

Client's name/signature: _____

Clinician's name/signature: _____

Contact number for questions/problems: _____

Emergency number: _____

INFORMED CONSENT STATEMENT—PAROXETINE (PAXIL)

It has been recommended that your pet be treated with a medication that is not licensed for use in domestic pet animals. This means that use of it in your pet is considered "extra label." This does not mean that the medication is dangerous to pets, just that pets were not the subjects tested for approved use. We often know a lot about potential undesirable/side effects of these medications because dogs and cats are the animals on which toxicity data have been collected by the drug company.

This medication has been chosen for your pet because it has been deemed to have the potential to be efficacious. This is not a guarantee that the medication will be efficacious in treating your pet's problem.

As with all medications, the medication that your pet will be taking may have potential undesirable/side effects. Although side effects are rare and every effort has been made to minimize them, you should know what the potential side effects are because the occasional animal may not be able to tolerate the medication. The medication prescribed for your pet, paroxetine (Paxil), is a selective serotonin reuptake inhibitor (SSRI). This medication may cause a slight increase in thirst, but has not been associated with house-soiling accidents in pets. Potential side effects may include an increased heart rate, increased respiratory rate, vomiting, diarrhea, inappetence, lethargy, and fainting. In extremely high doses, it has been associated with seizures. Markedly increased heart rates may be associated with the early signs of serotonin syndrome, a potentially serious condition. Learn how to take your pet's heart rate and keep a record of it under varied conditions so that you can monitor your pet for potential marked and worrisome increases. Although these side effects are rare, and when experienced are usually transient, if your pet experiences any of them, please call us so that we can make informed decisions about your pet's care. Please do not use this medication if your pet is taking any MAO-I, including Preventics collars, and amitraz dips.

After you have read this statement, please sign below indicating that you understand the statement and can comply with it. A copy will be provided for your information so that you can refer to it if needed.

Date: _____   Patient: _____

Client's name/signature: _____

Clinician's name/signature: _____

Contact number for questions/problems: _____

Emergency number: _____

INFORMED CONSENT STATEMENT—PROPRANOLOL (INDERAL)

It has been recommended that your pet be treated with a medication that is not licensed for use in domestic pet animals. This means that use of it in your pet is considered "extra label." This does not mean that the medication is dangerous to pets, just that pets were not the subjects tested for approved use. We often know a lot about potential undesirable/side effects of these medications because dogs and cats are the animals on which toxicity data have been collected by the drug company.

This medication has been chosen for your pet because it has been deemed to have the potential to be efficacious. This is not a guarantee that the medication will be efficacious in treating your pet's problem.

As with all medications, the medication that your pet will be taking may have potential undesirable/side effects. Although side effects are rare and every effort has been made to minimize them, you should know what the potential side effects are because the occasional animal may not be able to tolerate the medication. The medication prescribed for your pet, Propranolol (Inderal), is a non-specific, sympatholytic, beta adrenergic blocker. This medication has been potentially associated with changes in heart and respiratory rate, vomiting, diarrhea, inappetence, lethargy, and fainting. Although these side effects are rare, and when experienced are usually transient, if your pet experiences any of them, please call us so that we can make informed decisions about your pet's care.

After you have read this statement, please sign below indicating that you understand the statement and can comply with it. A copy will be provided for your information so that you can refer to it if needed.

Date: _____   Patient: _____

Client's name/signature: _____

Clinician's name/signature: _____

Contact number for questions/problems: _____

Emergency number: _____

INFORMED CONSENT STATEMENT—SERTRALINE (ZOLOFT)

It has been recommended that your pet be treated with a medication that is not licensed for use in domestic pet animals. This means that use of it in your pet is considered "extra label." This does not mean that the medication is dangerous to pets, just that pets were not the subjects tested for approved use. We often know a lot about potential undesirable/side effects of these medications because dogs and cats are the animals on which toxicity data have been collected by the drug company.

This medication has been chosen for your pet because it has been deemed to have the potential to be efficacious. This is not a guarantee that the medication will be efficacious in treating your pet's problem.

As with all medications, the medication that your pet will be taking may have potential undesirable/side effects. While side effects are rare and every effort has been made to minimize them, you should know what the potential side effects are since the occasional animal may not be able to tolerate the medication. The medication prescribed for your pet, sertraline (Zoloft), a selective serotonin reuptake inhibitor (SSRI). This medication may cause a slight increase in thirst, but has not been associated with house-soiling accidents in pets. Potential side effects may include an increased heart rate, increased respiratory rate, vomiting, diarrhea, inappetence, lethargy, and fainting. In extremely high doses it has been associated with seizures. Markedly increased heart rates may be associated with the early signs of serotonin syndrome, a potentially serious condition. Learn how to take your pet's heart rate and keep a record of it under varied conditions so that you can monitor your pet for potential marked and worrisome increases. Although these sideeffects are rare, and when experienced are usually transient, if your pet experiences any of them, please call us so that we can make informed decisions about your pet's care. Please do not use this medication if your pet is taking any MAO-I, including Preventics collars, and amitraz dips.

After you have read this statement, please sign below indicating that you understand the statement and can comply with it. A copy will be provided for your information so that you can refer to it if needed.

Date: _____ Patient: _____

Client's name/signature: _____

Clinician's name/signature: _____

Contact number for questions/problems: _____

Emergency number: _____

INFORMED CONSENT STATEMENT—TRAZODONE (DESYREL)

It has been recommended that your pet be treated with a medication that is not licensed for use in domestic pet animals. This means that use of it in your pet is considered "extra label." This does not mean that the medication is dangerous to pets, just that pets were not the subjects tested for approved use. We often know a lot about potential undesirable/side effects of these medications because dogs and cats are the animals on which toxicity data have been collected by the drug company.

This medication has been chosen for your pet because it has been deemed to have the potential to be efficacious. This is not a guarantee that the medication will be efficacious in treating your pet's problem.

As with all medications, the medication that your pet will be taking may have potential undesirable/side effects. Although side effects are rare and every effort has been made to minimize them, you should know what the potential side effects are because the occasional animal may not be able to tolerate the medication. The medication prescribed for your pet, trazodone (Desyrel), is a serotonin antagonist and reuptake inhibitor (SARI). This medication may cause a slight increase in thirst, but has not been associated with house-soiling accidents in pets. Potential side effects may include an increased heart rate, increased respiratory rate, vomiting, diarrhea, inappetence, lethargy, and fainting. In extremely high doses, it has been associated with seizures. Markedly increased heart rates may be associated with the early signs of serotonin syndrome, a potentially serious condition. Learn how to take your pet's heart rate and keep a record of it under varied conditions so that you can monitor your pet for potential marked and worrisome increases. Although these side effects are rare, and when experienced are usually transient, if your pet experiences any of them, please call us so that we can make informed decisions about your pet's care. Please do not use this medication if your pet is taking any MAO-I, including Preventics collars, and amitraz dips.

After you have read this statement, please sign below indicating that you understand the statement and can comply with it. A copy will be provided for your information so that you can refer to it if needed.

Date: _____   Patient: _____

Client's name/signature: _____

Clinician's name/signature: _____

Contact number for questions/problems: _____

Emergency number: _____

PROTOCOL FOR UNDERSTANDING AND MANAGING ODD, CURIOUS, AND ANNOYING CANINE BEHAVIORS

This handout offers advice on how to understand and manage dogs who:

- dig,
- jump, scratch, bolt, and bark at the door,
- grab you or another pet as they go through the door,
- bark and patrol outside activities,
- hump or mount you,
- roll in feces,
- eat feces, and
- never seem to stop moving.

Most of the situations discussed in this protocol pertain to management-related problems. Many people find these behaviors annoying or confusing, but they are versions of normal dog behaviors. In other words, some of these situations may be "problems" to the human, but not for the dog.

When management-related problems become an issue, some creative thinking may be required to both meet the dog's needs and keep the humans happy. Once you recognize the underlying pattern of how we can best intervene, you will be able to create your own solutions to most problems. *Remember that the keys to successful solutions always involve a humane human response that meets the pet's needs.*

The scenarios listed below—believe it or not—are all normal canine behaviors. As with all behavioral concerns, the extent to which we understand the behavior to be "normal" depends on the:

- context in which the dog exhibits the behavior,
- intensity of the behavior,
- ability of the dog to be interrupted, and
- extent to which exhibition of the behavior affects other facets of the dog's life in an undesirable way.

All of the behaviors discussed here could become so extreme that they would meet the diagnostic criteria, for obsessive-compulsive disorder (OCD). Because we do not understand the early stages of OCD and how it develops, anyone who loves their dogs should be encouraged to redirect any behaviors about which they may have concern early. That's what these instructions are intended to help you do. If these suggestions do not work, please consult your veterinarian to learn if something more serious is ongoing.

Digging

Most dogs dig, although some do so zealously. Digging can involve raking or scratching a surface a few times before sniffing, eating, defecation, urination, or turning in a few circles before sleeping.

Why Do Dogs Dig?

Dogs dig:

- to aerosolize an existing scent,
- to leave a scent mark of their own,
- because the objects they find are interesting or "play" back with them,
- to search for or find an animal that they hear or smell, and
- because they are curious and no one is paying attention to them, or because they are hot and are trying to cool down, or because they are cold and are trying to create shelter.

When dogs dig, they aerosolize scents that may have been hidden. Most of the information dogs obtain about their physical and social environments is likely done through olfactory means. This may be why dogs sometimes scratch before they eliminate: in addition to learning about who was there before them, they contribute to the olfactory environment when they eliminate and they wish to gauge how to spend their "olfactory currency."

In fact, the recent literature reports that scratching before and after elimination may convey considerable olfactory information, itself, about a dog's seasonal behaviors, estrus states, social companions, and intruders. Dogs tend to scratch more when they are not on their own property or in areas where other dogs pass frequently. Scratching is another form of marking that has both visual and olfactory components. We know little about scents that are transferred from dogs' paws, but we do know that this is one body region where dogs can "sweat," and that there are sebaceous glands between the dog's foot pads. Sebaceous glands are the source of oily secretions that may be largely invisible but heavily informative to dogs because of the sensitive canine sense of smell.

When dogs dig, hidden objects become found. It's possible that the dog buried a bone where he is digging, but while digging, dogs also discover roots of trees, rocks, old bulbs, et cetera. These are all objects that enrich the dog's intellectual and olfactory environment. In the case of roots and plants, many of these objects "play back." Remember, humans tire pretty quickly when they play a game of tug with the dog—roots of oak trees "play" for a long time.

Dogs may also dig because they hear or smell another animal. Moles, voles, groundhogs, spiders, field mice, white-footed deer mice, et cetera, all burrow to some extent. If the dog sniffs, listens, and paws a bit, and then moves on and repeats these behaviors, they are likely following cues about where another living animal has been. Some dogs may only do this in snow: Some rodents have very elaborate under-snow burrow systems and trails that interest many dogs. When people report attentive behavior, punctuated by listening, scratching, and pouncing in snow, the dog is likely trailing a rodent.

Dogs often dig just because they are curious. Attributing every behavior that annoys humans to "boredom" is simplistic and misses the point for the dogs. We have difficulty defining true boredom for people; we shouldn't just dismiss the behaviors of another species with a term that we would have even more trouble defining.

Dogs who are very social, curious, or active may just be exploring their environment whenever they dig. If their people were to play with them, these dogs might not dig. If they had a companion or went to an interactive daycare center, they might not dig. If they were provisioned with appropriate areas for digging in a manner that stimulated their mind, they'd still dig, *but* their behavior would not be distressing to the clients.

Finally, dogs can dig because it's one way they can regulate their temperature. During hot weather dogs dig because the earth is cool. Dogs can cool off by putting their belly on soil. In the winter, dogs can dig holes in the snow or dirt to create a cave-like environment where, if they curl up, they can stay warmer than they would if they were exposed.

How Can We Meet a Digger's Needs?

You can reward your digging dog in a way that stimulates his brain and gives him some exercise by burying rawhides or other treats or toys in a bucket or tub of dirt and letting him find them.

Dogs can use their digging skills with frozen toys, a particularly helpful idea in the summer. You can reuse clean, quart yogurt containers to make great digging dog toys. Fill the containers half-full with water or broth, then add a really good treat (e.g., cooked chicken liver, tiny bits of dried liver, very small pieces of cooked bacon, little pieces of apples for dogs who like fruit), then add more water and refreeze. Plunge the frozen container into hot water to release the quart-sized food toy. Now the dogs have a "food-sicle" that is mentally stimulating and helpful in the hot weather, and they can use the same skills involved in digging to focus on the toy.

For dogs who like to dig in really wet areas, fill a kiddie pool with water and add one of these frozen food toys. The frozen toy will float because ice is lighter than water and so will move and float in a way that challenges the dog to capture the food-sicle. Kongs, Planet, or other rubber and reusable food toys filled with peanut butter or cheese can also be frozen. The dogs have to really work to get to the treat, making the treat last longer. Low-calorie peanut butter may also be more palatable for the dog when frozen.

Some of the newer food toys have expanded on the idea of the original Buster Cube, providing both easier (Roll-A-Treat Ball) and harder puzzles. All of these items use the premise that when the toy is batted or moved the treats fall out. The dog is rewarded for getting the exercise of chasing the toys and for the intellectual part of figuring out how best to get the treats. These are easy ways to stimulate dogs that will help strengthen the relationship between you and your dog.

What About Dogs Who Use Digging as Temperature Control?

Some dogs dig because they are thermoregulating. Dogs can insulate themselves in snow in the winter and stay warm. This is what sled dogs do when they sleep at nights. Their tails provide the top of the "shelter" that insulates them from wind, and if snow falls on them they are even warmer because they become part of the snow cave.

Clients more commonly report (or complain) that their dogs dig in the summer. Part of the problem is that we often have breeds of dogs who were not bred for the environment in which we live. The same strategy that makes it possible for Newfoundlands to survive frigid waters off the coast of Canada to save someone, works against them closer to the equator. Understanding your pet's coat design will help you to better meet his needs. For example, some breeds of dogs have double coats, and knowing how to seasonally groom them may help your dog.

We humans can both "pant"—breathe quickly to expose a wet cavity to passing air—and sweat, and so control our body temperature by what is called *evaporative cooling*. The number of sweat glands varies with region of our body with the feet, hands, and head having the most sweat glands. Regardless, we can lose water through sweat over our entire body. **Dogs cannot.** They can only lose water for evaporative cooling from panting and from evaporation from their nose and foot pads.

Shaving the dog is *not* the answer because sunburn *can* happen in dogs, and a lack of insulation may make the dog hotter. Providing dogs with a wading pool can help. But if dogs are really hot and have no access to water, they will often dig a pit and lie with their belly and back legs fully extended and in contact with the dirt. By exposing the lightly haired area of their body to a cool surface they can transfer body heat across the gradient to the earth and cool off. Of course, they may have to move to create another cool pit if theirs heats up, which can happen in some environments.

By providing other thermoregulation choices (e.g., pools, fans, digging pits created by filling kiddie pools with wet sand and placing them under shade trees, et cetera) you can minimize the likelihood that your dog will dig in your garden to control his body temperature.

Most people are familiar with sweaters and coats for small or sparsely haired dogs to keep them warm. There are also now commercially available cooling pads and vests that functionally act as ice packs against the skin. For dogs who get too warm, these should be a serious consideration.

Are Some Breeds Likely to Be Diggers?

Indeed, many dogs dig because they are of a breed that we asked to dig. Jack Russell terriers, Glen of Imaal terriers, fox or rat terriers, et cetera, were all developed to track, chase, and kill rodents. When we decided that these breeds would be purely "pleasure pets," we did not undo the years of selection for dogs that dug well and fast. Many dogs of these breeds will even tunnel through walls in your house if you have rodents or termites! All of the above suggestions will help meet these dogs' needs, but, they may not be enough. If your dog is determined to excavate your property, and she is otherwise normal and healthy, consider getting involved in Earthdog Trials (see www.akc.org/events/**earthdog**/ for information). These are sporting events, like agility, flyball, et cetera, where the skill being directed to an appropriate venue is digging. The dogs dig to find a caged (and generally fully habituated) rodent. Timing and accuracy matter. If you are curious, just go watch one of these trials; you'll come home grateful that you have any yard left at all.

Jumping, Scratching, Bolting, and Barking at the Door

Jumping can be a normal behavior, and for some of the smaller or herding dogs we have not only encouraged that the dogs jump for work, but we have encouraged jumping in play. Sometimes we think it's cute that dogs will jump. Those small poodles who walk around on their hind legs while wearing tutus in performance situations are champion jumpers.

Jumping, barking, lunging, and bolting are all behaviors that commonly occur at doors and annoy humans. Unfortunately, humans exhibit behaviors that accidentally encourage these patterns, and teach the dogs to better perform exactly the behaviors we find most annoying.

Here are some *common situations created by humans* that turn into *problems for the dogs.*

- **Problem A:** When people open a door, they do not ask the dog to sit and be quiet before they actually open the door to whomever is on the other side. Yet the behaviors we have selected for in dogs include the barking as vocal alert that tells us someone is at the door! In fact, without breeding for and encouraging these types of attentive behaviors we would have no explosive or drug detection dogs.
- **Solution A:** Acknowledge the bark, go see what's going on, and ask the dog to sit and be quiet, then tell your dog that he is brilliant when he sits quietly. Wait until this happens. Where is it written that you *must* open the door immediately? Have the same consideration for your dog that you have for your guests. If you start a young pup off with these rules you will have no problems, but consistency is key.

  So that your guests don't think you are rude tell them you will not open the door until the dog is sitting quietly. Or, put a note on the door that says you are working to improve the dog's social and greeting skills and the door will be opened when the dog is quiet.

  For many, many dogs, quiet can be maintained by quickly offering the dog a toy and telling them they can get up when they "take it." This is like magic: They cannot bark annoyingly with their mouth full, they self-reward for being quiet, and dogs with toys are less likely to jump, and instead greet everyone by carrying a toy around and wiggling. This is so simple that, of course, few people think of it.

- **Problem B:** When dogs start to lunge at or through the doors, or jump on people who are entering, their humans tend to pull the dog back by the collar. What people do not realize is that dogs push against pressure. This means that when you grab a collar it tightens under the dog's throat and the dog lunges harder. Humans then tend to yell at the dog who, understandably, is now fairly confused.
- **Solution B:** Either teach the dog to sit quietly, as above, or, if you must use a physical cue to stop the dog, place your hand gently against the dog's chest, so that he backs up.

  If you are worried about grabbing, biting, or fleeing, you have two other choices.
  1. Isolate the dog behind a baby gate elsewhere before you expect company. The dog can then be let out to join the people when the door is closed, the greetings completed, and the people calm and sitting down.
  2. Put a head collar on your dog when you are home to supervise him and allow him to drag a light lead that slips through furniture. Then, when someone comes to the door, you can do everything recommended in this section, but also:
     - take the lead,
     - ask the dog to sit and ensure that he does so by gently pulling up on the lead, and
     - close the dog's mouth by gently pulling forward on the head collar.

  Then, the dog can have a toy. If he doesn't like toys, he can have a treat for being quiet. The dog must have a reward once calm and quiet, and praise is not enough.

  If you truly think that the dog might snap at or bite the person at the door, unless you are specifically working on some prescribed behavior modification, *you should not have the dog at the door.* The dog should be behind a baby gate, in a crate out of the way, or locked behind another door. And your guests should know that the dog might snap or bite and not be able to interact with them.

- **Problem C:** People tell dogs what **not** to do, but never tell them what **to do.** The situation at the door is a perfect example of this pattern in the extreme. The dog wants to ensure that his people pay appropriate attention, while the people are telling the dog "no." The dog is saying "yes, yes, yes…there is someone here," while the human is saying "no, Roscoe, down." The result is some profound cross-communication which results in the humans raising their voices.

  There is no need to yell at the dog—the problem is not deafness, it is inadequate signaling. There is an additional liability associated with yelling at the dog: the human becomes upset. This bodes poorly for the dog.

- **Solution C:** This problem is *so* easy to address.
  - The dog barks.
  - You verbally acknowledge the bark ("Good boy, Flash!").
  - You go see what the dog sees or hears ("You're right, Flash, FedEx is here.").
  - You thank the dog ("Thanks for letting me know, Flash.")
  - You ask the dog to sit and be quiet ("Can you sit and give me a smooch, boy?").

  The second the dog sits you tell the dog that he is brilliant and you reward him with praise, with a treat, or with a toy ("Oh, you are so wonderful, take your toy!"). You repeat as necessary.

- **Problem D:** Dogs bolt through doors because they take advantage of opportunity. If the dog is always ready to bolt, what canine needs might not be being met?
- **Solution D:** Make sure that the only exercise, outdoor stimulation, or interaction the dog gets is **not** restricted to what he can steal. Dogs who get adequate access to the outdoors are pretty happy to stand quietly by a door when appropriate. To make this work, you need to know how much and what type of exercise your dog needs. On weekends, learn what schedule of outdoor time and what type of exercise will stop the dog from bolting. Use that schedule to meet the dog's needs. Some dogs always bolt because this behavior ensures that they have the opportunity to go out and eliminate. You can avoid bolting by taking the dog out often. Dogs should get all of the following:
  1. off-lead exercise, if safe and possible,
  2. on-lead walks of a good length and of sufficient social and intellectual interest, and
  3. quick pit stops for bladder and bowel comfort. Canine metabolisms are a lot like yours, so if you are home, you may wish to give the dog a quick pit stop every time you take one yourself.
- **Problem E:** Dogs who are without behavioral pathology scratch at the door because:
  - there is someone on the other side of it,
  - they have to go out, and
  - they get some attention for doing so anyway.
- **Solution E:** Consider putting a Plexiglas shield on the door if damage is a concern. These shields are now commercially available from pet product catalogs. Once you stop worrying about damage you'll have more mental space left to meet the dog's needs.

If the dog is trained to "knock" to go out, or if she trains you that this is what scratching means, you must let her out. You can creatively take advantage of the scratching at the door by putting sandpaper over the part of the door where the scratching occurs. This will keep the dog's nails smooth while also stopping him from damaging the door.

Even if you are not going to let the dog out, unless you wish the behavior to become worse and more intense, you *must* go to the door immediately to see if anyone is there. Dogs will intensify their behavior until you finally get up. By that time you are annoyed and you have taught your dog to be persistent. Tell the dog "thank you," take a good look, and then if there are no further interactions to occur at the door, tell the dog that "that will do." You can hasten the dog's understanding of his role in starting or stopping this type of "door alert" by using a reward for being quiet. A treat or a toy could be a reward here. It's a good idea to keep a treat jar or toy basket by the door for these purposes.

Make sure that the dog is not training you, unless you wish to be trained. Dogs will learn quickly about the treats and alert all the time. If you only reward the dog when the "door alert" is real, the dog will work with you.

If you want your dog to have a different signal at the door for "I have to go out to wee" from "there is someone at the door," hang bells from the door. Take the dog's paw, tap the bell, say "good dog," open the door (with the dog on a lead, if needed for safety or to get the dog back), and take the dog out. Because going outside is so rewarding it will take very few replications of this behavior for your dog to "get it." And, yes, if you are not otherwise meeting their exercise needs, some dogs will tap the bell often, but this should tell you how to meet your dog's needs. The dog will learn that when no one is home the bell is not answered.

Grabbing You or Another Dog or Cat When You Go Through the Door

Many dogs who grab humans, and who are normal, are just excited. Some dogs who grab humans are not normal and may need to control humans in order to have some sense of security. *We are not discussing the latter group of dogs here.* They are discussed in the **Protocol for Understanding, Managing and Treating Dogs with Impulse Control Aggression.**

The dogs who are excited are similar to humans who are excited, but without opposable thumbs. Opposable thumbs are what allow you to grab people, pick up a coffee cup, and hold someone's hand. Dogs use their mouth for behaviors where humans use thumbs.

Many dogs who grab humans or other dogs as they go through doors are dogs from herding breeds. This makes sense: Grabbing someone as they move through the environment is the very definition of herding behavior. Not everyone understands that the dog is "just herding you," and many other pets become frightened or injured.

The rule for these dogs is simple: You have a toy basket inside every door, you have a toy basket outside every door, and the dog must take a toy and sit quietly before any door is opened (see photo). Continue to request that the dog stay as you open the door, then quickly release her and get out of the way.

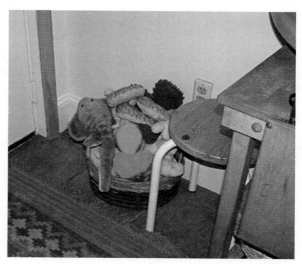

Toys in a basket placed by the door so that dogs can be handed the toys before going through the door. This prevents the dogs from grabbing humans in their excitement to go outside.

Barking and Patrolling Activities That Occur on the Street

Dogs will watch what's happening in their world by looking through windows or doors. If your dog has nothing else to stimulate him, like the caricatured nosey, old lady down the street, he will spend more time watching activities outside the house. If you are not home, these behaviors will become reinforced because they are self-reinforcing: your dog sees someone, he barks, he becomes stimulated by his own barking, and then whoever was in the street moves on and the situation changes. If the dog is inclined to be protective, the situation is even more self-rewarding: he alerted, he protected, and the person who threatened his home left! He succeeded!

If it is important for you that your dog *not* exhibit these behaviors when you are *not* home, you will have to make it impossible for your dog to patrol and alert.

Please do not even consider using a shock collar to stop this behavior. This is like saying you'll chop off a dog's leg to stop him from jumping.

Instead, use blinds, curtains, barriers, gates, large and spacious crates, et cetera, to provide an environment that protects your dog from the stimulus, and then make sure that the dog has other kinds of stimulation. This is where the food puzzles discussed in the section on digging can be useful.

If you are home, treat this behavior in the same way you do rowdy behavior at the door, which is discussed above. Additionally, figure out ways to keep your dogs stimulated and/or closer—but not glued—to you. You can practice asking the dog to sit at the door, and then calling him away. If you give him a treat every time he leaves the door, calling him from the door will become much easier. By doing this and providing stimulation that does not rely on those who pass by, you will make it easier to interrupt your dog's alerting behavior and to redirect him to a preferred behavior (e.g., carrying a rope toy).

Mounting and "Humping"

Mounting and humping are behaviors that trigger more mythical and pseudoscientific explanations than any other behaviors. The most common incorrect explanation is that the dog is being "dominant" to the human, dog, cat, stuffed animal, et cetera, that he is mounting. Think about that for a minute and you'll realize that it makes no sense.

The second explanation that is usually offered is that this is about sex. This statement is almost always followed with "but he is neutered" if you live in the United States.

Here's what we know:
- Both intact and neutered/desexed dogs can mount.
- Both males and females can mount.
- Unless this behavior is part of a sequence in a dog fight or antagonistic interaction, in which case the actual behaviors are very different, such behaviors are stiff, directed toward the shoulders and neck, and the dog is very focused and quiet. Most mounting is about affiliation or wanting to be with others and/or is used as an attempt to get the others to pay attention to you.
- Dogs will hump people when they are happy and want the people to interact with them.
- Humping is involved as a part of the sequence involved in sex or masturbation. The form is very different from the affiliative form: sex and masturbation involve fast, repetitive motions, leaning with the face and neck on the object of desire, and facial signal changes. Both males and females, neutered and intact dogs can masturbate.
- It's a normal behavior.

Now that you know what's normal, also understand that dogs will work for information and a salary. If you do not wish to be humped or mounted, ask the dog to stop, to sit, and reward that behavior instantly. If the dog goes back to mounting you, get up and walk away. When the dog pays attention to you, ask him to stop, to sit, and, again, reward sitting instantly. If the mounting behavior continues, the dog is either not being rewarded quickly enough, or the reward is not good enough when compared to humping your leg. Learning is also involved in this behavior: many dogs have learned that humping feels good and that at some point you liked it because you laughed. Think about this.

Rolling in Feces

Many dogs roll in feces. The feces chosen is usually that of other dogs or of other species, and not the dog's own feces. We must remember that our sense of smell is very "impaired" compared to that of dogs so that we cannot fairly understand this behavior. Hypotheses about why dogs do this include:
- rolling to disperse, and so lessen, the effect of the original scent,
- covering the original scent with the dog's own,
- making a visual statement about the other animal's mark,
- covering themselves in another animal's scent for camouflage,
- using the scent as an insect repellant,
- obtaining chemicals from the feces that help nervous system development and immune health, and
- gaining information from the scent about who the animal was, when he last passed through, and what he had recently eaten.

For now, it's probably safe to say that any or all of these could be true in different contexts, and that there are likely other reasons that we do not understand.

If you find rolling in feces obnoxious, please remember:
- dogs are washable,
- if unsupervised, dogs who like to do this will do it more,
- dogs share this information with other dogs and can introduce another dog to the joys of rolling, and
- if you wish the dog to stop doing this you must interrupt them as early in the sequence as possible. In other words, if you have a dog who does this and you see her beginning to focus her sniffing in a specific area, you know that she will take a dive. The time to call her to you and reward her for coming without rolling is when she begins to focus her sniffing.

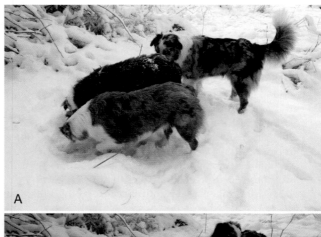

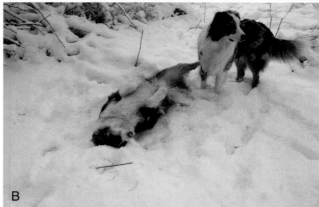

Dogs who roll in feces can find feces, even under snow, as shown in **A**. One dog, shown in **B**, rolls in the feces, dispersing it, and leaves a large visual snow signal that the feces were found by a dog who dispersed them.

Eating Feces of Other Species

Ingestion of other's feces can either be a normal behavior or one of desperation.

Starved animals will eat the feces of others. Puppies kept in pet stores and those bred in puppy mills/farms may not be fed enough if the pet store or puppy dealer wishes to keep them small, and so may be both hungry enough to eat their own feces, and under-stimulated enough to use feces as toys. This is one very good reason why dogs and cats should never be purchased from pet stores. Please remember that virtually all pet store puppies and dogs come from puppy mills/farms and likely received inadequate food, care, exercise, et cetera.

Dogs who are inappropriately punished for elimination may become ultra-fastidious as a way to avoid the pain and anxiety that they have come to associate with elimination. Some of these dogs will ingest their urine or feces immediately after elimination or as they are eliminating.

Finally, some dogs ingest feces (coprophagia) as a manifestation of OCD. These dogs all need more than just management-related help, and would benefit from a visit to a specialist in veterinary behavioral medicine.

That said, many dogs enjoy snacking on the feces of other individuals. They may enjoy cat feces because they are actually high in protein and animal muscle that is not fully digested. Dogs often love the feces of herbivores (e.g., deer, rabbits, cows, horses), and it has been suggested that this is because these species all use bacteria in their digestion and the bacteria form a source of protein. Additionally, this can be a good way to get partially digested herbs and grains, like oats.

Ingestion of feces is not a behavior that is easily amenable to change because it is *normal*.

The keys to **controlling** eating of feces are simple and difficult to continuously implement:
- don't let the dog ingest the feces to begin with and
- keep a sharp eye so that you see the feces before the dog does and can call him away.

In a worst case scenario, this activity will improve both your and the dog's reflexes as you continually race each other to the feces. It may be easier to brush the dog's teeth every day, which has other benefits.

If you know your dog ingests feces, please be aware that they can contract parasites this way and that they should be screened by your veterinarian for these at least every 6 months. Please also know that some of these parasites may be transmissible to humans if the dog gives lots of kisses and saliva is exchanged. This is more common and worrisome with small children, and dogs in urban areas, but you should know that this is one way dogs can pass disease to humans.

If the dog ingests only canine feces, the solution is easy: clean up all dog feces found, including those deposited by other dogs. It is harder to know where the feces of squirrels, rabbits, deer, foxes, raccoons, cats, et cetera, are, and so more difficult—and in some cases, impossible—to remove them.

Some people use muzzles to help control the ingestion of feces. You should know that some dogs can eat feces through muzzles. Muzzles may send other messages to the neighbors about your dog; consider whether this is what you wish. Some dogs become incredibly unhappy in a muzzle and the quality of their life declines. Muzzles should be reserved for situations where they are mandated by pressing health concerns.

Mouthing and Biting

Mouthing and biting are common complaints of people who have, inadvertently, played too roughly with their dog or cats. No puppy should be encouraged to mouth. Puppies will "mouth" naturally because they use their mouths much as we use our hands. It is a simple matter to abort this behavior when it is first starting, but mouthing can be tremendously difficult to stop it if it has been ongoing for a long time.

- Think about the behaviors that you see in your pup and ask if you wish to see the same behaviors when that puppy is an 85-pound (~45-kg) adult dog.
- Ask yourself if the behaviors you see in the pup would be desirable if you are rushing around like crazy during the holiday season and the house is full of people.

If the answer to either of those questions is "no," you can and should take preventative action to avoid or abort potentially undesirable behaviors by learning about age-related normal behavior and how you can best shape appropriate and desirable behaviors, given the breed and adult size of the dog you have.

People are more tolerant of troublesome behaviors with dogs who will still be small as adults than they are with dogs who will be larger, but for the complaints of mouthing and biting, tolerance can produce an obnoxious and difficult to handle little dog. No dog, regardless of size, should feel that he has to mouth or bite someone to get anything that he needs, including attention.

- The first thing clients can do to stop this annoying and potentially dangerous behavior is to stop interacting with the puppy and freeze as soon as you are mouthed or grabbed. If you pull your hand away from the puppy or kitten, even if you are doing so to avoid a prick, you are encouraging him to pursue the "game."
- You can use a *gentle* verbal cue to signal that the interaction is finished (say "no," "stop," "uh-uh," "all done"), and *gently* extricate or remove your body part while *gently* holding the body of the animal. These are babies. They make mistakes. They can be injured easily. They may have hurt you, but you don't have to hurt them.
- Then, quickly offer the puppy something on which she can chew (e.g., a stuffed toy, a ball, a chew toy) and tell her that she is good.
- When puppies play with toys that you hold, they may mouth you again. Be prepared to redirect the mouthing back to the toy and repeat this as often as necessary.
- If your puppy persists, you can make a sharp noise (e.g., a whistle) as a distraction. Remember that the only reason you wish to distract him is so that the behavior stops. *You do not have to scare the dog to stop him from mouthing. If you scared your dog, then the behavior you used to interrupt him was inappropriate or the timing was wrong.*
- As soon as the undesirable behavior stops, you need to encourage an appropriate behavior. In the absence of this information, puppies will again offer mouthing, if it worked in the past, or more intense behaviors like biting. By offering these behaviors, puppies learn if these are the behaviors that will get you to interact with them. *Puppies and kittens are asking for information; you provide information when you respond to their behaviors and by the way you respond.*
- Stopping the behavior is important. **It is equally important to REWARD the cessation of the undesirable behavior with a behavior that is fun, but more appropriate (i.e., chewing on a toy).**
- Remember, puppies are hugely energetic and will tire the average human almost instantly. You have to be vigilant. If you are not willing to be vigilant, consider placing the puppy in a safe area (his own room, a crate, a pen) with a safe chew or food toy until you feel that you have the energy again to face the onslaught of play.
- If you don't feel like you can honestly face this type of activity day after day, please consider whether a pet sitter

or dog walker can help. Perhaps there is a responsible child in your neighborhood who is not allowed to have a pet but who might be happy to learn to play appropriately with your puppy. Children can be excellent at teaching pets tricks and teaching pets manners, if they are given some guidance.

- The bottom line is that puppies and kittens need lots of exercise and mental stimulation. Both of these activities can be geared to teaching them safe, socially acceptable behaviors.

If you have done all of the above, and the puppy or dog is still grabbing, mouthing, or biting people or other animals and you are sure no one has encouraged this behavior, consider seeing your veterinarian or a specialist in veterinary behavior for an evaluation. Dogs who are worried or anxious will take treats more roughly than they would have otherwise and may grab people or dogs to stop them. Dogs use their mouths as hands. If the dog needs to control everything, this is a problem. The earlier you seek help the better. With newer, humane head collars and harnesses it has never been easier to redirect mouthing, grabbing behavior, but you have to see them clearly for what they are—points of concern—first.

Some breeds or lines of dogs, like herding dogs, may grab more readily than others because they have been selected to do so. This does not mean that you must tolerate being grabbed if your dog is a breed selected for herding and guarding. Instead, you need to know that this can be a normal behavior for them and that they can learn to exhibit it only in appropriate contexts. Inappropriate herding behavior is a common complaint, and almost always starts early in the dog's life. Redirection is possible. Inhibition is possible. For the best outcome, early recognition and intervention is essential because behaviors that have been selected for are easily and naturally rewarded.

There are more ideas for how to manage rough play, including mouthing and biting, in the handout **Protocol for Teaching Kids—and Adults—to Play with Dogs and Cats.**

Energy, Energy, Energy

Most dogs that people think are hyperactive are not; they are high-energy dogs whose needs are unmet. Both you and you dog likely get less exercise than you need. Almost all dogs can benefit from increased **aerobic** exercise. Tired dogs are happy dogs and they have ecstatic people!

Think of the needs of your dog in terms of breed, age, and individual temperament or personality. Young border collies from working lines are not good candidates for couch potato status. Meet the needs you identify in your dog.

Suggestions for increasing aerobic exercise include leash walks, running with your dog, and playing with toys indoors and out. Many frisbees and balls are now made from fleece, which can cause minimal damage if the toys are thrown indoors. That said, if you have priceless and fragile art objects, find another place to play indoors with the dog. Regardless, this type of exercise, alone, is unlikely to fatigue a dog.

If you want a calm dog you need to know what is necessary to encourage the dog to stop on his own. Learn what causes the dog to fatigue. It may be 30 minutes of running, it may be 3 hours of running. It may be that you never learn the limit because you collapse before the dog does, but all of these data are clues.

Still, there is hope.

If you want your dog to be exhausted there is no replacement for play with another dog. Indoor and outdoor play with other dogs is intellectually challenging, aerobic, and usually contextually appropriate. Take advantage of this. If you do not have another dog, see if one of your neighbors has a dog who plays well and also needs exercise. Join, or start, a doggie play group.

Intellectual stimulation, clear and kind rules, and opportunities for dogs to know that they can succeed and will be rewarded for succeeding are important. As dogs begin to improve, become more attentive, and are calmer, consider adding clicker training for tricks, or sports like agility and herding. Just do not push your dog faster than she can or wishes to go, and realize that she may not like all sports. If you decide to engage in these activities, please insure that you have had your vet check your dog to ensure she is healthy enough for such work, and that you have discussed your dog's problems and needs with the organizer or instructor. Your dog may not be suitable for the class you had in mind, or it may not be suitable for her. Many dog clubs run smaller or quieter classes for needier dogs. Please be realistic; to not do so may be injurious to your dog, and your dog's well-being has to be your first concern.

Finally, there are sports where you—the human—can do almost nothing, but the dog runs like crazy: with flyball you get to sit while the dog does all the work. If your dog likes this activity, there are also automated ball baskets that you can program to send a tennis ball into the air on a regular basis. If you are a couch potato with an energetic young dog, swallow your embarrassment and do what's necessary to help him out.

Final Words

Remember that *the simplest way to encourage a desired behavior is to reward it,* even if it happens without your instructions. So when your dog is sleeping, tell her she is incredibly beautiful and brilliant! Repeat early and often.

PROTOCOL FOR UNDERSTANDING ODD, CURIOUS, AND ANNOYING FELINE BEHAVIORS

Evolutionary Overview of Cats, Diets, and Social Interactions

We actually have little knowledge of what constitutes normal feline behavior, and there are many myths about cats. For starters, cats are not small dogs and it's important to understand this. The story of dogs is the long history of cooperative work with humans. The story of human–cat relationships is the story of disease control and passive tolerance of cats because of the important feline characteristic of feeding on rodents. The domestic cat was attracted to human settlements because a rodent is a meal for one cat. Had cats had to co-operatively hunt, as did ancestral dogs, as do wolves, and as do some of the larger wild cats, their integration into human society would likely have been slower because, unlike dogs, their social system is not like ours, and they are considered obligate carnivores, meaning that they must eat meat. Some small wild cats like Margay cats eat a lot of fruits, as do many pet cats, but cats are still viewed as mainly meat eaters.

When cats live in our households we need to realize that, if the decision was theirs, cats would *not* choose to live in such a solitary state. It's interesting that humans have no trouble comparing dogs to wolves, and repeatedly refer back to wolf behavior to explain dog behavior, *often with error,* yet we seldom think about ancestral cats and their social systems. To treat our cats most humanely and to best meet their needs, we need to remember that the domestic cats who live with us have, in history, lived very, very differently.

Cats live in matrilineal (mother run and focused) family groups and most of the females in a group are likely to be related to each other. Females may nurse the young of other females, and there is shared care of young among females. Males may help care for the young until they become socially mature (~2 to 4 years of age), and then most males leave their family group and either enter another or become "bachelor" males.

Knowing about the range of normal behaviors that cats exhibit that are different from ours and dogs will help prevent the development of serious behavioral problems and will allow redress of any management-related issues. A discussion of a few of the common problems that can occur with cats follows, and shows how the unique history of the domestic cat affects these concerns.

Eating Plants

Although we tend to think of cats as "obligate carnivores," animals who must eat meat and eat only meat, they will chew on and eat other substances. Most cats will eat plants if they have access. Cats appear to enjoy fresh grass. Whether this is because of a taste preference or because the cats want or need the roughage is unknown. We know that roughage can be important and may help cats who are routinely constipated, and there are some studies that show that adding fiber to a diet can help regulate some feline diabetics who are poorly regulated. For cats with these medical conditions, discuss the addition of measured amounts of fibrous bulking agents (e.g., psyllium) with your veterinarian.

The needs of cats who like and seek out plants to ingest can and need to be met safely. There are now commercially available "grass gardens" that can be grown indoors for cats. Certain herbs and mints will also grow indoors and are favored by many cats. Some aromatic plants may also act as anti-parasite agents, so their choice may be a healthy one.

Concerns about eating plants focus primarily on toxic issues. **Many houseplants are far more toxic to cats than they are to dogs.** For example, any plant in the lily family can kill a cat. Stargazer lilies, Easter lilies, and amaryllis are commonly grown indoors and are common ingredients in commercial bouquets. Ingestion of these plants is serious and potentially life-threatening for cats, and you should contact your veterinarian immediately if you think that the cat has eaten any of them. Go to www.aspca.org/Pet-care/poison-control/plant-list-cats.aspx for more information. Pesticides, chemicals used in lawn treatments, and fertilizers can also threaten the health of your cat. For this reason, if you have a cat who likes to eat plants, grass, vegetables, or fruit, PLEASE either grow these specifically for the cat, or know the source of your herbage, et cetera, and wash them before allowing the cat to snack on them.

You may want to grow catnip for your cat, thinking that this will make the cat happy. Catnip contains compounds that may act as mood elevators in cats, but the behaviors exhibited by cats are extremely variable. If your cats enjoy catnip, this can be used as a special treat for the cats who react strongly and recover slowly. You should know that the ability to respond to catnip is genetic: the cat either responds or doesn't. For example, cats in Australia don't respond; the "catnip gene" apparently never arrived. So if your cat does not respond to catnip, please do not assume that something is wrong. Not responding to catnip is a variant of normal. Some cats can become quite forceful after eating catnip. This is not a desirable response for some households, but it can be a variant of a normal response to catnip.

Vomiting may follow ingestion of plants. This can be a normal behavior. If your cat is vomiting excessively or seeking out plants and eating until she vomits, seek your veterinarian's advice immediately.

Spraying and Other Pungent Marking Behaviors

The bad news for humans is that spraying is a normal behavior. The good news is that it is facilitated by hormones and some social conditions, and that we can manipulate both of these.

Spraying urine communicates a huge range of information through both postures and olfactory signals. Information communicated likely includes individual identity, sex, reproductive status, recent meal contents, stress level, et cetera. Humans have a terribly impaired sense of smell compared with cats, so we need to accept that we are not going to appreciate the scent of cat urine in the same way a cat does. Spraying occurs more often if new cats enter the environment, if a female is in heat, if another intact male courts a female, and in stressful situations. To fully understand these patterns you should know that when cats spray they are not only putting information into the environment, but they are provoking the environment, hoping to get information back.

Cats spray over other cats' urine marks; this pattern communicates important information.

Removing the testicles or uterus and ovaries decreases the amount of spraying significantly. The type of spraying that neutering/desexing decreases is that associated with sex or sexually related behaviors. Neutered cats can still spray for the other social reasons listed above. It is in this context that it is important to remember that under "normal" conditions, domestic cats would live in family groups headed by related females.

By working to manage "unnatural" social groupings—those that we construct by adding unrelated cats who are of ages and social composition that would not occur were the cats grouping themselves—we can decrease the spraying. This is best done by gradually introducing a new cat (see the **Protocol for Introducing New Pets**), providing attention and some private time for each cat, providing more litterboxes than there are cats, and using a good odor eliminator. The best odor eliminators contain enzymes that break down the compounds in urine and other substances that make the particles with the scent too heavy to be sniffed up and aerosolized. These two mechanisms alter the information in the urine and should decrease spraying. Recommended odor eliminators include Nature's Miracle (available at pet supply stores), FON (available at pet supply stores), PON (available at pet supply stores), Urine-Off (available online and elsewhere), Get Serious! (www.getseriousproducts.com), Elimin-Odor (available from veterinarians), The Equalizer (available from veterinary supply companies), Anti-Icky Poo/AIP (www.antiickypoo.com), and KOE/AOE (broadly commercially available). The last four have a reputation for being particularly effective. Febreeze was first marketed for its potent odor-elimination properties , especially with respect to urine, feces, and other bodily fluids and products. If an odor eliminator is good, the cat pays less attention than he otherwise would to the soiled area. All odor eliminators should first be tested on a small patch of the target fabric to ensure that they will not damage it.

If the spraying is about the change in social groups, it may be transient. If the spraying continues, it may be a nonspecific sign of anxiety, and you should consult your veterinarian. *Most anxiety in cats shows up as behaviors that you may not see as "aggressive" but which for cats represent profound aggression.* This is another scenario where knowing what "normal" is makes a huge difference. If you think you are having an ongoing or worsening problem see the **Protocol for Understanding and Treating Cats with Elimination Disorders and Elimination Behaviors That May Be of Concern.**

Cats also mark their turf using feces and urine that is **not** sprayed. If cats are doing this, they will often continue to mark in a litterbox if one is provided in the area the cats have been using. If moving a litterbox does not help, see your vet.

Scratching Behavior

Cats scratch objects for two main reasons: (a) to remove the layered sheaths that comprise their claws and (b) to leave visual and olfactory marks. Like spraying, the act of scratching is also a behavior that is very obvious and can be seen by any watching cats. *Were cats given their choice, they would never have their claws and the end segment of their toes surgically removed*—they would scratch in materials like tree

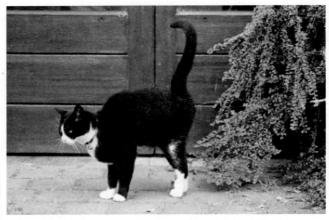

A cat spraying against a shrub outside his house. (Photo courtesy of Anne Marie Dossche.)

trunks, lawns, fabric-like surfaces of peeled bark, et cetera. In fact, the scratches left by the behavior then act as a mark to inform other cats who was there and when the tree was last scratched! Cats have glands between their toes that leave a scent that other cats can smell. Removing the claws and a section of their toes doesn't change this, so declawed cats can still "scratch" and leave the scent and, in some cases, a visual residue.

Scratching on furniture can be done for either of the reasons cats commonly scratch, but it occurs because the fabric resembles the natural surfaces that the cat would otherwise seek out. If you provide all cats with appropriate scratching surfaces when they enter the household and encourage the cats to use them, rewarding them when they do so, scratching that is inappropriate will not occur unless there are other behavioral concerns in the household.

- You can buy commercial scratching posts that are covered in carpet or hemp, and some kitty condos have a scratching post built into them.
- You can make one of these yourself with wood and fabric scraps and rope.
- You can add a scratching panel that is made of sandpaper so the cat can file his own nails.
- You can bring in logs.

You may still need to clip the ends of cat's nails, but if you start to do this when the cat is a kitten, the cat will not fear you and will learn that nail trimming is also a time to get treats, massages, et cetera. Have your vet demonstrate how to cut your cat's nails, and buy good clippers and keep them sharp. The extent to which you can meet the cat's needs for scratching is limited only by your imagination.

The conventional wisdom regarding declawing (onychectomy) is changing. In Canada, Australia, and most European nations, declawing is not considered a valid or legal veterinary procedure unless injury is involved (i.e., the procedure is done only when medically warranted). Most declawings in the United States are elective, meaning that there is not a medical reason for the procedure. Attitudes are changing in the United States and more veterinarians, welfare groups, and veterinary groups now feel that declawing should be a last resort, not a first choice.

When cats are declawed—and the method used may include anything from scalpels to lasers—the end bone in the

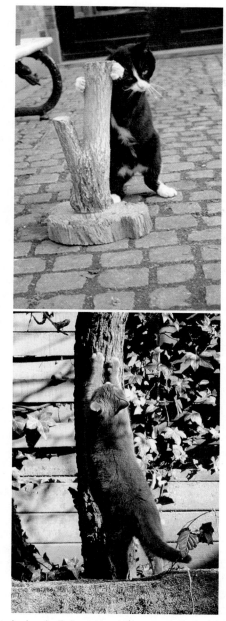

Scratching behavior is important for removal of old sheaths on claws and because it leaves visual and olfactory marks. The cat in the *top photo* is using a "homemade" scratching post crafted from tree branches. The cat in the *bottom photo* is using a real tree in the yard. (Photos courtesy of Anne Marie Dossche.)

finger/toe is removed. If this bone is not removed, the nails continue to grow. In order to scratch, cats have to extend their claws. As part of the basic posture of cat toes, nails are retracted. This is why you can always tell whether a cat or a dog walked across the snow in your yard: if there are only pad marks and no nail indentations in front of them, the animal passing through was a cat; if there are nail marks in front of the pads, the animal was a dog.

Because this ability to retract claws uses tendons, newer methods for controlling destructive scratching include tenectomy, which is the severing of the tendon. In this case, claws continue to grow and must be routinely trimmed, but the cat cannot extend the claws to scratch on furniture or other living things.

Pain can be involved with both of these procedures, but according to published reports, tenectomy appears to have faster recovery and fewer long-term side effects. Long-term pain and discomfort is, in general, the exception, but no good **behavioral** studies have been done that compared cats' personal behaviors, activity, and interactions before and after declawing. Done correctly, these studies are likely to be extremely informative.

Finally, when considering declawing ask yourself if you are subjecting your cat to a procedure where blood loss and pain can be considerable just because you find it more convenient than trimming nails. We are moving into a new age of improved animal welfare and humane care. When we give more serious and generous thought to meeting the needs of those animals dependent on us, we benefit, too.

Hunting and Caching

Indoor–outdoor cats or outdoor cats may hunt. Cats have to learn to hunt and they are generally taught to do so by their mother. If you want your cat to have fewer hunting skills, obtain a kitten from a mother who has never hunted. That said, starved cats can learn to hunt. Even well-fed cats will hunt if they are "hunters." They may or may not eat their prey, even if they are well-fed.

Hunting is an intellectual endeavor. Consequently, the more we stimulate our cats and provide them with lives rich with opportunities to problem solve, the less likely they are to hunt. Teach your cats all the tasks, tricks, and signals that are taught to dogs! Cats can learn to jump through hoops and over fences that are used in agility! Watch the videos on YouTube. Imagine—intellectual stimulation and exercise all rolled into one feline activity!

Cats eat one small meal multiple times per day, so rodents are the feline version of a boxed or "takeout" meal. The mental stimulation involved in this activity is not trivial. When we "meal feed" cats, they not only don't get to hunt, they get all their calories in one setting. After they empty their dish, they have 23 hours and 55 minutes of their day to fill.

Cats fed dry food can be encouraged to mimic hunting behaviors by having all their food placed in treat balls: as the cats bat these, one or two pieces of kibble come out. Filling these with a tiny amount of food 3 to 5 times a day can mimic the native hunting behavior.

If you feed wet food you can create food puzzles: Small amounts of food can be put into holes in peg boards or small Kongs and other food toys; a cafeteria tray can be outfitted with small flower pots covering food, or rocks and large pebbles that hide food. Again, only your imagination limits how your cat's needs are met.

You may be distressed and confused if your cat brings you not-quite-dead-yet prey or prey that has been decapitated. In a free-ranging situation, cats will return injured prey to the group to share with the more dependent cats and to teach hunting, and they will cache dead prey. Start seeing yourself through your cat's eyes; your cat is only trying to help and provide for his extended family.

One last concern about hunting needs to be discussed: the issue of wildlife. In many parts of the world, cats have been responsible for the extinction of native species. Many island species are particularly victimized and large extermination programs are necessary to control the cat population if we are to have any wildlife left in these areas. As sad as it is to discuss this topic, we need to realize that feline overpopulation is the result of irresponsible human behavior, unnatural provisioning, and, on islands, a result of humans abandoning cats. More countries, provinces, states, and townships are legislating the extent to which cats are allowed to roam. Sharing the world is a lesson with which we humans seem to struggle.

Rubbing

Cats rub people, cats, other animals, walls, and inanimate objects. Rubbing is a normal behavior that has tactile, social, and olfactory components. Cats rub when they are exhibiting "affiliative" behavior—these are behaviors associated with being close, with being in relaxed and friendly social circumstances.

Because cats have large numbers of glands that secrete a waxy and—to cats—odoriferous substance, they actually leave deposits wherever they rub. We think that these compounds differ depending on the region of the body, which may explain why certain patterns of rubbing seem to occur more frequently in some environments than others.

When cats rub against humans they may rub with only their tail and their hind end, or they may "bunt." Bunting is the behavior where the cat pushes his head up into someone and rubs the area just in front of the ears across the individual being rubbed.

Cats will also rub the sides of their cheeks, the area in front of the ears, and their chin on corners of walls or furniture. You can learn if your cat has been doing this by looking at hallways, entrances, et cetera, at cat height—you'll see the slightly waxy deposit. This behavior has created a market for "corner combs," devices that can be attached to edges of walls and where cats can rub and groom their facial hair at the same time.

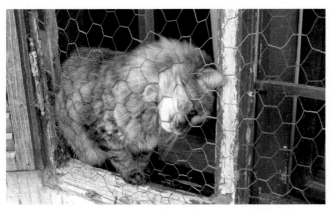

A cat rubbing her cheeks and whiskers across a metal screen, which leaves behind some waxy secretions and odor.

Cats will also move back and forth along edges while pressing the base of their tail and their rump against them. These are normal behaviors. When patterns of these marking behaviors begin to change, the change may indicate difficulties in the feline social environment. *Again, you cannot*

recognize when something changes without knowing what normal is. Please watch your cats to learn what they do so that when something changes, you'll notice it.

Nocturnal Activity

Cats are solitary predators of animals who are awake at night (e.g., mice, voles, et cetera). Hence, cats are much more nocturnal than we or dogs are. Cats do not have to swing from chandeliers at 2 AM, but if they are young, are left alone all the time, get little attention, and have learned that you will give them attention if they bother you enough, they can learn to swing from chandeliers. *Meet your cat's needs.*

If you have an only cat who is running around like crazy at night, try playing games with the cat before you go to bed. If this doesn't work, consider another cat with the same playful temperament. A dog can also help exercise a cat if you don't want two cats.

If you wish for your cats to match your sleeping pattern, you need to be reasonable. This is another reason why leash walks can be so good for cats—they can actually accompany you much of the time and will be on a more similar schedule.

Remember that cats generally sleep for a few hours after they eat. Feed them so that this 3- to 4-hour hiatus starts at a time that helps encourage a realistic sleeping schedule for both of you.

For any change to occur, you **must** be meeting your cat's intellectual and exercise needs. Unless you wish the cat to get you up to play or eat, do not encourage these behaviors as a way of shutting the cat up. All you have done is shown the cat what will get him attention or food. Instead, get earplugs, ignore the commotion (unless it's a danger to the cat) and wake up the next morning prepared to meet the cat's needs and change the way you have been interacting.

If your older cat begins to show a change in her nocturnal behavior, such as a change in sleep cycle or nocturnal vocalization, please have your veterinarian assess the cat immediately. Nocturnal vocalization and changes in activity are two of the most common signs of age-related cognitive decline/dysfunction in cats. Medications, diet, and exercise can help.

Ingestion of Non-food Items That Are NOT Plants

Ingestion of non-food items like fabric or rocks is called pica. Many cats try to lick or eat non-food objects, but do not do so religiously. If cats begin to seek out and focus on chewing, sucking, or ingesting non-food items, they have a true behavioral disorder and you need to seek help.

In addition to the concern about a potential intestinal obstruction please understand that this form of ingestion is a variant of obsessive-compulsive disorder (OCD) and will worsen without treatment. OCD runs in both family and breed lines. Sucking, licking, and ingesting non-food items are all separate forms of OCD. Any item can be involved, but many cats suck or chew wool. In fact, when Siamese and other Oriental breed cats have behavioral conditions, they often have an OCD involving chewing and ingestion of wool. Some cats generalize to other fabrics, and some cats are only attracted by one type of fabric.

If your cat occasionally licks clean plastic (it would make sense to lick plastic containers that previously had food in them), sucks on a pillow or a toy, or chews on a pen, it's not a big deal. Make sure that the cat cannot injure herself, especially if the cat's preference for an afternoon snack involves electrical cords, by sequestering appealing objects or sequestering the cat when unsupervised. Ensure that the objects sucked and chewed are not toxic. If you notice you cannot distract the cat when "caught in the act," have your cat evaluated. Tasting and sampling can be normal, obsession is not.

Roaming and Cat Enclosures

Roaming cats who defecate in neighbors' gardens are nuisances. The aesthetic aspect is one problem, the public health one is more severe. Illness is a concern in areas where humans garden in soil in which cats have defecated, or where children play in sand boxes also used by cats. The soil or sand may harbor fecal parasites that can make humans ill. In young children, one of the most common cat-caused illnesses is caused by the larval stage of a fecal worm and the child can become blind. This is **not** a trivial concern in many, many urban regions, and as such, it is a public health issue that requires people who have feline partners to take responsibility for the actions of their cats (www.petsandparasites.org./cat-owners; www.cdc.gov/parasites/toxoplasmosis/gen_info/pregnant.html).

- Neutering cats renders them more likely to stay close to home and less likely to roam.
- Having an entertaining and stimulating environment at home will keep cats closer to home.
- Providing cats with physical exercise and mental stimulation will keep the cats closer to home.
- Finally, keeping cats indoors can keep them safe and they will live longer than do outdoor cats.

However, if you want your cats to have some outdoor exercise but are concerned about these other issues, there is a way to simultaneously meet all needs: cat enclosures. Custom-made enclosures are more commonly seen in Europe than in the United States, and they can be wonderful. These enclosures are made from various kinds of fencing and mesh, can be built into a window or a cat door, and can even be designed to include most of a tree so that the cats can see the birds, but not snack on them (www.catsondeck.com; http://habitathaven.com; http://catnet.stanford.edu).

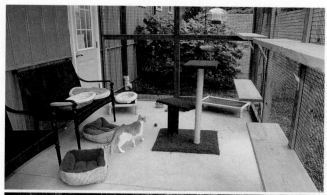
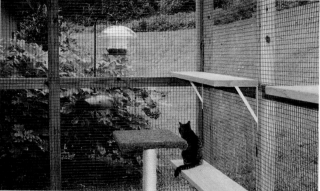

Cat pens made from enclosing a concrete slab porch. This is a safe way for cats to be outdoors and experience mental stimulation.

There are also some fencing additions that can restrict your cats to their own backyard safely and humanly (www.kittyfence.com; www.catfence.com; www.purrfect fence.com).

These are two ways to bring the rich stimulation of the outside world to the stay at home cat, and make everyone happy while meeting the cat's needs.

PROTOCOL FOR CHOOSING COLLARS, HEAD COLLARS, HARNESSES, AND LEADS

Identification

One of the main objectives that collars accomplish is identification. All cats and dogs should be "labeled." There are three main ways to do this and they are not exclusive: (1) collars with tags or embroidered information, (2) tattoos in ears or on thighs, or (3) microchipping.

Tags on a collar can provide information about the client (name, address, and phone number), veterinarian (primarily the phone number), and vaccination status (current rabies vaccine). Embroidered collars usually have the pet's name and a phone number.

Tattoos are usually made up of the client's social security number in the United States or of some code. They require at least sedation to execute. The dog or cat then usually wears another tag on its collar indicating the telephone number to call should the animal be separated from its people and need to find its home.

Microchipping is becoming more broadly available, but in Europe and the United Kingdom, the systems are more universal than they are in the United States. Microchips are easy to install, but require the widespread availability of microchip readers. Long-term effects of an implanted, digitally coded device have not been fully evaluated, but—compared to the benefits—the risks appear small in preliminary tests. The general principle behind microchips is that, when scanned, a number is displayed for which ownership data can be obtained by calling a central depot. The animal generally, but not always, wears a tag that indicates that it has been implanted with a chip. The chips are radiopaque, meaning that they will be displayed on a radiograph or X-ray. Microchips may migrate and no long-term studies are available that have investigated or substantiated any common adverse health effects.

Whatever method the client chooses, two factors should be certain: (a) the tags are up-to-date, and (b) they are on a collar that fits safely and comfortably. The latter means that the collar either is a breakaway collar through which one or two fingers can slip comfortably, or that the collar is fitted to be sufficiently loose so that it remains on the animal when the dog or cat puts her head down, but if the collar become entangled, the animal can pull her head out of the collar. If clients are not cautious about the fit of collars, animals can strangle or collars can become imbedded in their skin, resulting in morbidity or mortality. Breakaway collars are particularly important for cats, who are very good at forcing their bodies into small places where a collar could become entangled.

If animals are lost or stolen, labeling may be their only hope of getting home again. And if the township in which the pet lives requires a tag license, the animal's "label" could be the only thing that saves the animal from impoundment, quarantine, or death.

Control

Collars, harnesses, et cetera are generally used in dogs for control, but a few words about harnesses and leads for cats will be helpful.

Cats need to be "restrained" when they go to the veterinarian and, if they are indoor cats, when they are out-of-doors.

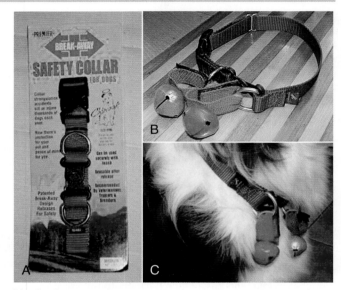

Photo 1 A, A breakaway safety collar that is adjusted to the dog's neck, but with an additional clasp *(center)* that will release if the collar catches on anything or is grabbed. This collar can be turned into a regular collar simply by clasping the lead to both rings over the clasp.
B, The breakaway safety collar with two Bear Bells added by the client so the client can hear the dog, Picasso, as he moves away.
C, The collar in **B** on Picasso, the dog who had a tendency to escape the property. Here the bells help alert the clients to the dog's movements, while the collar protects the dog from hanging from any bush or tree in the woods behind the clients' property.

They should also be "restrained" when in a car so that they do not become a projectile. Placing them in a crate can accomplish this, but more freedom and exercise can be an excellent idea. All kittens should be fitted with a harness so that they can be encouraged to explore the world. A harness is preferable to a collar because, if fitted correctly, it will not injure the cat, and the cat cannot slip out of it. The younger the cat is when the client fits the cat with a harness, the easier it will be to accustom the cat to it. Once on the harness the cat should be taken for trips in cars, on walks, and for visits to the vet. These activities should occur frequently—they will pay off later when the cat needs care and needs to be tractable. Also, if the cat can safely be taken outside, the cat's life and the interaction between the cat and client will be enriched. Finally, if cats can safely and comfortably wear harnesses, they can wear seat belts and gain all the stimulation of car rides that was previously the domain of dogs and humans.

Choker Collars

Dogs are often routinely fitted with something like a choker collar as part of a training program. Choker collars are usually either made from chain, leather, or a rolled, braided nylon. When used correctly, choker collars are actually one of the best examples of true "negative reinforcement": when the dog pulls, the collar tightens and either the sound or smallest amounts of pressure indicate that dog has engaged in an undesirable behavior; when the dog stops, that pressure is released (and in the case of a chain the sound of slippage occurs) *and* the dog is unimpeded. It is the release from the negative stimulus (the tightening of the collar) that is the reward.

Unfortunately, virtually no one uses choke collars in the described manner. Instead, most dogs placed on chokers "choke." When they are allowed to pull on the collar and permitted to sustain the pull, these dogs learn to override the choker. In doing so, they are also at risk for laryngeal damage, esophageal damage, and ocular damage (change in the blood vessels in the eye). The dog who pulls harder has no choice: dogs will always push against pressure, which means they will pull harder.

Traditional choke collars are an idea whose time has passed. When clients can get past their own misconceptions about how they look or what they mean, they will, with ever-increasing frequency, choose a head collar or a no-pull harness for their dog. Used correctly, these are safer, easier to use, and help teach the dog better behaviors. They are a winning solution that could, and perhaps should, eclipse the choker.

For people whose dogs don't bite but who dislike the idea of harnesses and head collars, a modified neck collar with a baffle is now available. The Scruffy Guider has two neck straps that can be adjusted for a snug fit. The collar tightens when the dog pulls in a manner similar to a fabric choke collar, but there is a baffle that prevents the collar from tightening beyond the point where it is just flush to the neck. This is not the solution for an out-of-control dog, but it is another tool that may work for some dogs.

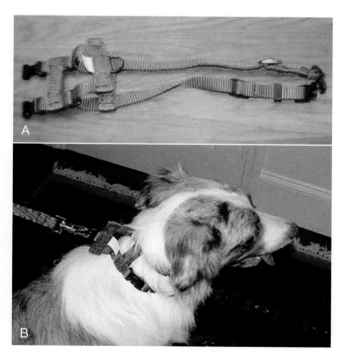

Photo 2 **A**, An unattached Scruffy Guider. **B**, Linus is modeling a fitted Scruffy Guider.

Head Collars

Head collars are very much like horse halters: they act as a basket that holds the dog's cheeks and jaws and stay on the dog by fastening high on the back of the neck. There is generally at least one strap that fits over the bridge of the dog's nose, and one that fits over the back of the neck. The lead is attached in the middle of the halter, to the nose strap, but under the chin. This is just like how a lead is attached to a horse halter, but is a major change for many people accustomed to attaching a lead directly to something around a dog's neck. The two major versions of the head collar are the Halti (Photo 3) and the Gentle Leader Canine Head Collar, although there are a growing number of choices, including the Canny Collar (Photo 4). The Halti (Photo 3) is intended to be fitted with a second collar because it fits loosely. It also cannot be as easily tightened by pulling forward, but it fits some very jowly breeds well and snugly. The Gentle Leader and the Blackdog Training Halter give most dogs a better, more secure fit, require no second collar, and can be used with a lead to redirect a dog from inappropriate behaviors and prohibit biting. Most head collars have undergone many improvements in their first decades, including narrower nose straps and ergonomic buckles that resist breakage.

Blackdog makes two styles of wonderfully flexible head collars: the Infi8 (see Photo 5), which is simple to fit and uses a nose piece that softly wraps around the muzzle, allowing easy movement of the dog, and the Training Halter, which allows snug but humane closure of the dog's mouth (see Photo 6). At this writing, these collars must be ordered from Australia (www.blackdog.net.au).

Because the manufacturer of the Gentle Leader, Premier Pet Products, sold their company in 2010 to Radio Systems Corporation/RSC, the largest manufacturer of electronic and shock collars, a number of trainers, vets, behaviorists, and clients have been looking for other sources of head collars and harnesses from companies that do not use, endorse, or sell products that involve electric shock. A number of alternative products from the growing range of those available are listed here. There are also many head collars and harnesses that are humane and helpful, but only available locally.

At this writing, unless the dog is fat-faced, *two collars best close an aggressive dog's mouth when used appropriately:* the Gentle Leader (an RSC product) (Photo 7) and the Blackdog Training Halter (www.blackdog.net.au) (Photo 6, *D*).

Head collars are wonderful for most dogs and people. They spare the dog's larynx and esophagus, and so are one of the ideal choices—along with harnesses—for dog's with laryngeal damage, tracheal collapse, or cervical (neck) damage involving disks, bones, nerves, or muscles. Head collars also ride high on the back of the dog's neck so that when the lead is pulled forward or the dog pulls in the direction opposite to that of the lead, this part of the collar tightens a bit and puts a small amount of steady pressure on this area of the upper neck near the head. Not only is this generally very safe, but this pressure is the exact kind of signal that dogs communicate to other dogs when they wish to control them or stop. So, when the dog is signaled using constant, gentle pressure on the lead, the head collar communicates a "doggy" signal to the dog to stop. No translation is necessary, and the response is quick. For clients who are already working with a behavior modification program, this type of helpful, kind device can be a godsend. If the dog has a mouthing or biting problem, some head collars can be gently pulled forward to firmly, safely, securely, and humanely close the dog's mouth. When used correctly the collar cannot injure the dog and will allow the client to control most of the dog's behaviors and stop the dog's biting.

The best thing about head collars is that anyone—truly anyone, no matter how inexperienced or inept they are with dogs—can safely and humanely walk a dog using a head collar and have it be a mutually enjoyable experience. The leverage that a head collar provides allows children and people with arthritis to walk even unruly dogs—*and* to enjoy it. If dogs get more exercise, they are calmer, and if people enjoy being with their pets more, they will be more motivated to work with them.

Head collars are a win-win situation, and are increasingly becoming the first collar of choice for a puppy. They are certainly appropriate for **all** life stages and have another advantage over chokers: **they encourage humane behavior from people.** We can use all the kindness and humanity we can learn.

Used incorrectly, as is true for any device, injury can occur. The most common complaint about head collars involves loose-lipped dogs who chew on their lips because the nose piece of the collar fits too tightly. Hair on the nose can also be damaged if this occurs. A good fit is important, and some practice might be needed before the best adjustment of the neck strap and the nose strap is found. Dogs fitted with head collars should be able to comfortably eat, drink, pant, and even bark and bite, if not corrected. There are excellent instructional videos for fitting most head collars. These are **not** muzzles, they are **not** rubber bands around the dog's nose, and they are **not** cruel or inhumane. They are great. Now that these head collars come in designer colors, people should accept them more readily.

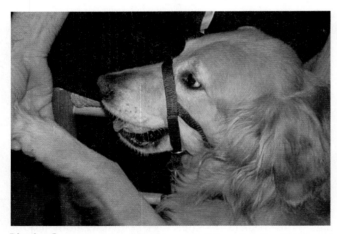

Photo 3 Austin demonstrating a Halti head collar. This head collar has a jaw strap that many dogs find more comfortable, and it fits many fat-faced dogs, like mastiff breeds, more comfortably than do one-nose-strap head collars. Unless it fits snugly, it may come off (and there is now a martingale adaptation to prevent this risk), and you will not be able to tightly close the dog's mouth, if desired. The lead attaches under the throat with the Halti collar.

The Blackdog's Training Halter does an excellent job of closing a dog's mouth and maintaining it closed (see Photo 6). This head halter is actually among the easiest to fit, is well tolerated by dogs, and communicates well with the dogs. The webbing is cotton, which means that it doesn't slip once sized. Photo 8 shows a leather version of a quickly adjustable head collar and lead designed for dogs who only sometimes pull, or who may also need to switch between collars quickly. This

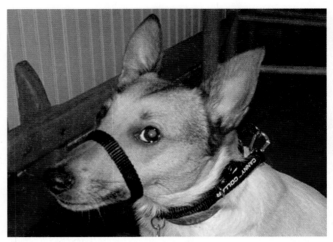

Photo 4 Snap demonstrating a Canny Collar, a type of convertible collar where the nose loop can be incorporated into the collar so that the dog can quickly be wearing a type of flat buckle collar without having to disconnect or remove the head collar. This is a boon to people who have enthusiastic dogs who also may wish to go to a dog park. The lead attaches at the back of the neck with this head collar.

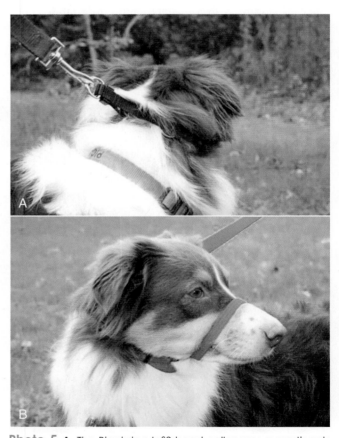

Photo 5 **A**, The Blackdog Infi8 head collar uses a martingale type of attachment for the lead at the back of the neck. **B**, The nose loop of the Infi8 head collar wraps around the nose then clips to the side of the collar allowing the collar to easily adjust to the dog's movement and head shape. These head collars are made of cotton webbing and so are unlikely to slip.

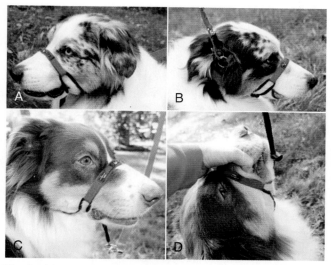

Photo 6 **A,** The Blackdog's Training Halter has a nose loop that is padded and held in place by easily adjustable mouth and neck pieces (control cords) that are secured under the neck. The lead attaches under the neck so that the dog's mouth can be gently closed, if needed.
B, The Blackdog Training Halter fits snuggly behind the neck and the lead attaches under the throat to the adjustable control cords, which lock after adjustment to the dog's size and head shape.
C, The Blackdog Training Halter used on a dog at rest.
D, The Blackdog Training Halter used to hold the mouth shut. The toggle that adjusts to securely fit the nose loop is shown.

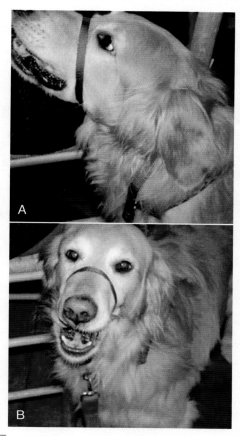

Photo 7 Austin demonstrating two views of a Gentle Leader head collar.
A, Austin showing the snug fit at the top and back of his neck, and the correct placement of the nose loop so that it sits **behind** the corners of the mouth. In this case, the lead attaches under the throat.
B, A front-on view of Austin showing an appropriate fit. The dog can open his mouth, yawn, lick his lips, eat and drink, and even bite someone when no pressure is put on the lead. This snug fit allows the person with the lead to close the dog's mouth and stop or prevent a bite. Premier Pet Products is now wholly owned by Radio Systems Corporation, the largest manufacturer of electronic and shock collars, so many will not wish to purchase their products. For those wishing to buy products from companies that do not use, endorse, or sell products that involve electric shock, see **Photo 6** for an alternative head collar made by Blackdog that can close the dog's mouth.

collar does not permit the mouth to be closed but is well tolerated by dogs who pull, likely because of the ease and flexibility of fit. Leather must be oiled and maintained to withstand strain.

No-Pull Harnesses

No-pull harnesses fit under the dog's front legs and loop over the dog's shoulders so that when the dog pulls, its front legs are pulled back and it slows its pace. A number of these harnesses exist: the Lupi, the Sporn/No Pull Harness, the DreamWalker Harness (Photo 9), the Easy Walk Harness (Photo 10), the SENSEation harness (the original no-pull harness; Photo 11), the Blackdog Balance Training Pack (Photo 13), and the Freedom No-Pull Harness from Wiggles, Wags and Whiskers (Photo 12).

The No Pull Harness has a special collar that is sewn with two different-size metal tabs. The loose, leadlike part of the harness fits through one of the loops, and then goes under and around the legs, and is attached to the other loops, under the neck, using a clasp. The lead is then attached to the loose part of the harness over the dog's back. The back part of the harness can be tightened for a better, more responsive fit. The Lupi doesn't have any clasps or tabs, instead relying on a system of concentric loops that are fitted around the dog's front legs and over the back. The lead is then again affixed to the back portion, which slips to tighten if the dog pulls. The Lupi is a little easier to fit to very hairy dogs and for people whose hands are very arthritic. Both of these fitting patterns sound complex and like topological puzzles. They are not. Once clients have the devices in their hands, the fit becomes self-explanatory. Care must be taken with both of these harnesses to ensure that hair is not caught or broken and skin is not abraded.

The SENSEation Harness, the New Freedom Harness, the Balance Training Pack, and the DreamWalker Harness are all "power-steering for dogs." The Blackdog Flyball Racing Harness provides a different type of control and leverage for some dogs and provides a handle, which for some rambunctious dogs is a safety measure. Some of these harnesses are more complex than others to fit. The DreamWalker Harness can challenge anyone's spatial skills, but the instructions are so good and logical that, with a small amount of practice, fitting it makes complete sense. The handle is a little bulky and people accustomed to traditional leads may take a while to get used to it, but for anyone who needs instantaneous control over a dog's movement, this is a great solution. This product is still around but hard to find, as it is being

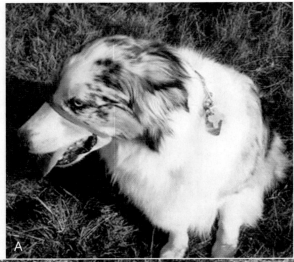

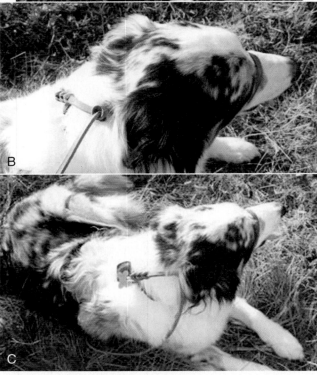

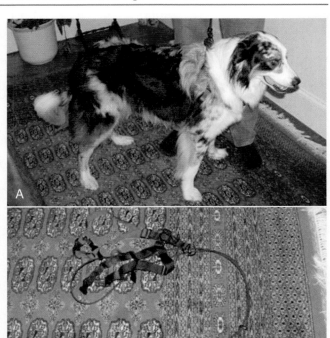

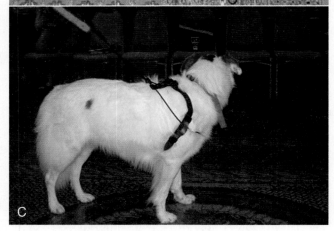

Photo 8 **A** to **C,** An easy-to-use and fit version of a leather figure 8 head collar, The Infinity Lead, is being made as a prototype by Service Dog Designs, which makes custom equipment for service/assistant dogs and their partners. This simple head collar is designed so that the lead attaches at the top of the neck, behind the head. A lanyard attaches it to the dog's neck collar for additional security. Leather requires special care, and anyone using leather leads, harnesses, collars, or head collars should know and meet these care needs. This prototype has huge potential, given its simple on–off assembly, its ease of fitting, how readily dogs take to it, and how well it manages pulling. **A,** The nose loop is snuggly fitted over Toby's nose by adjusting a leather connector under Toby's chin. **B,** The back part of the figure 8, the neck loop, is slipped over the head behind the ears and gently snugged at the bottom of the skull/top of the neck using the leather ratchet. The lanyard attachment that can hook to a regular neck collar is seen in **A** and **B. C,** the entire lead and head collar as it would be used is seen, complete with lanyard attached to a regular neck collar.

Photo 9 **A,** Toby demonstrating the DreamWalker Harness. The instructions make this fit easy to understand, and if the harness is stored correctly, putting it on the dog each time is not a challenge.
B, Toby's already fitted/sized DreamWalker Harness as it comes off the dog. You can see why reading the instructions and practice are so important for getting this on the dog correctly and quickly.
C, A DreamWalker Harness that is well fitted to a border collie showing the set of cords that help with steering.

"orphaned." The concepts are so good that one should expect to see a reinvention of it soon.

No-pull harnesses are wonderful for dogs who pull or lunge. These are **not** appropriate devices to fit to a dog whose biggest problem is biting, nipping, or grabbing as they do nothing to control the dog's mouth or head. Furthermore, reaching around the dog's head and neck to fit these harnesses could be dangerous if the dog is aggressive to people.

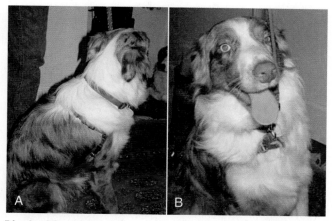

Photo 10 **A** and **B**, Linus models the Gentle Leader Easy Walk Harness. **A** shows the adjustable straps that go across the back and under the chest. **B** shows the adjustable strap that fits across the front of the chest and that can tighten to put mild pressure on the dog's shoulders, telling him he should slow. Note in **B** that Linus's lead is attached to a ring in the center of the chest strap. Sizing can be tricky with these harnesses and the amount of hardware in the front can cause the harness to sag on some dogs. For these dogs, the SENSEation harness or custom-fitted ones from Wiggles, Wags, and Whiskers may be preferable. Because the manufacturer of the Gentle Leader, Premier Pet Products, sold their company to Radio Systems Corporation/ RSC, the largest manufacturer of electronic and shock collars, a number of trainers, vets, behaviorists, and clients have been looking for other sources of head collars and harnesses from companies that do not use, endorse, or sell products that involve electric shock. A number of alternative products from the growing range of those available are listed here.

When fitted correctly, these harnesses will easily allow children and people with arthritis to pleasurably and calmly walk their dogs **if** the dogs are not huge and strong. Huge, strong dogs, especially those who are poorly or unmannered can override these and end up dragging their person down the street while inflicting self-induced rope burns. These "no-pull" harnesses, like head collars, spare the dog's neck so that dogs with laryngeal, tracheal, esophageal, or spine problems can be more safely exercised.

Caution is urged against fitting no-pull harnesses too tightly: too tight a fit could impede circulation in the dog's front legs. Fortunately, this is difficult to accomplish.

Regular Harnesses

Regular harnesses fit around the dog's chest, and avoid any pressure on the neck when the lead is pulled. They are purely devices to attach the dog to the lead, and offer no chance for correction of undesirable behaviors. Many dogs do not pull or lunge when walked, and just need to be protected from the world and to comply with lead laws. For these dogs regular harnesses are fine. They can also work well for small dogs who perform undesirable lead behaviors, but who are too small to really cause what the client would consider to be a problem. In fact, some of the harnesses for smaller dogs have built-in "handles" so that the dog can be picked up by the client should they need to be removed from a situation or placed in a car.

Regular harnesses are **not** good choices for large dogs who are not absolutely perfectly behaved because they provide the

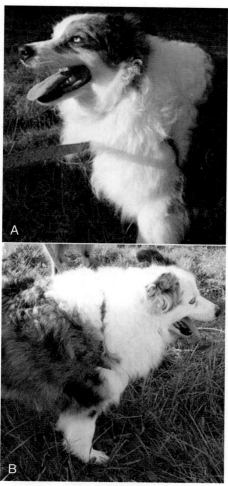

Photo 11 **A**, Bunny is wearing a SENSEation Harness. The front attachment is clear. The hardware in this no-pull harness is not bulky and fits smoothly against the chest. Bunny is older, arthritic, and small, so this is helpful. **B**, You can see that the SENSEation Harness is fitted so that the angles on the shoulders are as recommended in the instructions, which are excellent. This fit allows fully unimpeded shoulder and forelimb girdle motion.

client with little control. In fact, big, highly motivated dogs will actually be able to use the harness to push into the situation from which their people are trying to drag them because their shoulders are unrestrained. This is only beneficial if a sled is involved in the exercise you give your dogs. Clients often choose harnesses because they want to protect the dog's neck. This is a good idea, but head collars and no-pull harnesses are a better solution for dogs who feel the call of the wild and absolutely "must" pull.

Prong or Pinch Collars

Prong collars are subject to all of the same criticisms as chokers. Furthermore, they can do incredible damage to the dog's neck because they can become imbedded in the skin if the dog learns to override them. Most dogs learn to override these collars and people who use them often voluntarily comment that they need to use some degree of pain to control their animals under some circumstances. These collars, if sharpened, as is often the case, are intended to employ pain to encourage the dog to attend to the person. If left

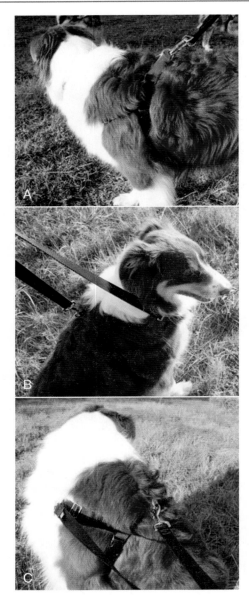

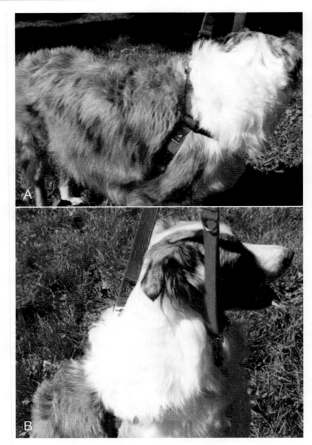

Photo 13 A, Linus is wearing the Blackdog version of a no-pull harness that fits across the chest below the neck and behind the front legs. **B,** The double-ended lead can attach only in one location or both on the dorsum and under the neck.

Photo 12 A, The back lead attachment of the Wiggles, Wags, and Whiskers Freedom No-Pull Harness with both leads attached to it is shown. A single lead could also attach here. Note that the buckle is well away from the shoulder and front arm motion. **B** and **C** show Picasso with one of the leads attached to the back lead attachment and one to the front lead attachment for more control.

unsharpened, these collars are intended to provide more uniform pressure than a choke collar. Oddly, prong collars were intended to be a safer improvement over choke collars. That's not how it has worked. For aggressive dogs, this uniform pressure response—especially if accompanied by pain—can worsen their aggression, and for dominantly aggressive dogs, this response can not only worsen their aggression, but can endanger the client. Were people to understand more about how dogs communicate and how these collars work, they would appreciate that responses other than pain and pressure are more desirable for changing an animal's behavior. These collars are no substitute for early intervention and the treatment of problem behaviors. For every situation involving reactivity and/or aggression for which clients claim control is provided by a prong collar, a head collar is the better, safer, and more humane choice, although it requires some investment of time to use correctly.

Some dogs are fitted with prong or spike collars because they make the dog look "tough." The problem, here, does not lie with the dog.

Shock Collars

Shock should not be used to "train" dogs or as a treatment for behavioral concerns. The use of shock collars for this purpose is now illegal in numerous locations worldwide (e.g., Wales and the state of New South Wales, Australia).

Based on the peer-reviewed, scientific literature consisting of multiple, data-based studies of both laboratory and owned dogs, study authors and specialists have recommended that *no dog should wear a shock collar to correct an inappropriate behavior except on the qualified recommendation of a specialist in behavioral medicine.* This conclusion is based on situations where the shock was well controlled and tested in a controlled setting—circumstances considerably more conservative than the "real world." This means that such recommendations apply even more strongly to the "real-world" situation, and that a recommendation by a qualified specialist will be rare, indeed. This is equivalent to saying that **no dog should wear**

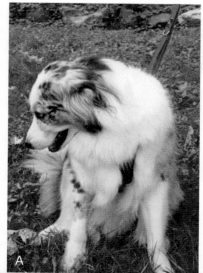

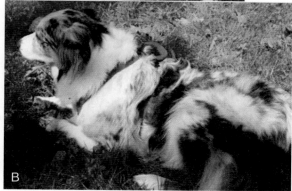

Photo 14 **A,** By providing a solid Y-front against Toby's chest, the Blackdog Flyball Racing Harness provides additional guidance for the dog and encourages the dog to pull less. **B,** This harness provides the safety of a handle so that the dog can be stopped, if needed.

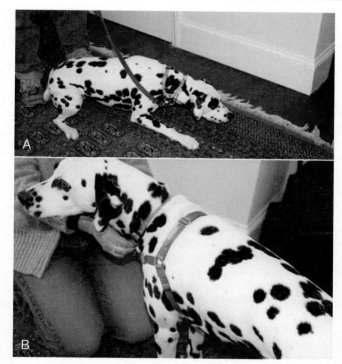

Photo 15 **A,** The dog is wearing a prong collar and acts more uncertainly when on it. **B,** The same dog when fitted with a no-pull harness. These profound behavioral changes are common.

a shock collar. *Certainly, no client should self-prescribe a shock collar for their dog to control an unruly or aggressive behavior.* In at least one clinical specialty practice of veterinary behavioral medicine, dogs who were "treated" with shock prior to assessment all were euthanized for worsening behavior that could be linked to the shock administered.

Given the correct reward and timing circumstances, and the appropriate level of shock, all animals can learn avoidance behaviors from the application of a painful shock. There is an entire literature in the psychology of learning that is based in shock. However, the application of shock (and shock collars are intended to be painful) is an absolutely inappropriate treatment for aggression and fear because it hurts and is scary and because it teaches the recipient only to avoid or cease an associated behavior without teaching them what behavior is appropriate and desirable. The use of shock collars will invariably make problematic behaviors worse, render the dog less predictable, and potentially endanger the client.

There is no role for shock in basic training and manners training of dogs and cats.

Even police and attack dogs are now seldom trained using shock. In these most valuable of dogs positive reinforcement, including clicker training, has largely replaced compulsion training. Data show that all dogs who are shocked experience adverse alterations in the neurochemicals involving stress and distress, leading researchers to conclude that it is painful for the dogs receiving shocks, and that the shocks affect how dogs respond to people long-term. Such findings were noted even in the most flawless of police dogs. Simply, every time a dog is shocked that dog and its neurochemistry are damaged.

Most people who use shock collars either want a quick fix or need to absolutely control their dog. The former will not work for dogs with problem behaviors. The latter is problematic for other reasons.

There *may* be some ***rare theoretical exceptions*** where shock collars *may* be used rationally to change or shape a dog's behavior *if and only if that behavior is dangerous to the **dog** and if the behavior is recently acquired.* Under these extremely restrictive and rare conditions, the scientific literature shows that very few (1 to 3) shocks would be sufficient to cause an avoidance or cessation response. An easier, cheaper alternative to shocking the dog is to simply protect the dog from the behavior that is injurious. By the time most people learn that shock is not helpful, they have done profound harm.

Anyone considering using a shock collar for their dog needs to seek professional help from a specialist in behavioral medicine immediately. No specialist recommends shock collars, but if the client's concern is sufficiently severe that they are considering shock, the specialist can provide competent assessment and alternative humane and effective solutions.

Neither shock collars nor prong collars should be the training collar of first resort—to do so is inhumane and negligent. Dogs who are troubled respond especially poorly to shock and so these collars should not be the choice of last resort, either. People who wish to use these collars require the help of a specialist and should get that help as soon as possible before injury or death occurs. Clients need to remember that good behavior is not based on compulsion, brutality, fear, or domination; it is based on a willingness to acquiesce to another's desires. Where pets are concerned, that's a two-way interaction.

Leads

Finally, a few words on lead choice will be useful.

- Avoid metal/chain leads. They will absolutely injure your hands. They are heavy. They can become weapons when yanked free. If the dog chews on the lead and you are there, you can ask him to stop and redirect him to an appropriate chewing vehicle. If the dog chews and you are not present, the dog should not be leaded or tied. In some areas of the United States, tying a dog is illegal. The American Veterinary Medical Association (AVMA) has finally taken a stand, saying that tying is not an appropriate form of restraint for dogs. Tied dogs can choke, become more aggressive, injure themselves, and generally just have a miserable life. Why would you tie a companion you chose for its sociability?
- Leather leads are soft—if kept cleaned and oiled with leather products—and have a good weight, but may be too thin for children or anyone with arthritis. Also, the stitching in leather leads can let go as the leather ages and cracks: one hard tug from the dog and the lead is broken and the dog is gone. If you like leather leads, maintain them and check for strength and damage often.
- Nylon fabric (webbing/mesh) leads have truly come of age. They come in a variety of widths, colors, and designs and are washable and durable. One drawback to nylon fabric is that it can slip with time and pressure. Equipment should be checked frequently. The Blackdog products are made of cotton webbing so that they do not slip. If cotton becomes wet, it is difficult to adjust, so the situation in which the tool is to be used should be considered. Both nylon and cotton webbing are harder to chew through than is a leather lead. That said, any head collar or harness can fail. Occasional defects occur even in well-maintained tools (see Photo 16). Responsible manufacturers will repair or replace equipment that does not perform as promised, as was the case for the pictured head collar.
- Retractable leads have become very popular. They are fine **only if** your dog is either (a) tiny enough to be picked up in one arm **and** (b) sufficiently well-behaved to come when you ask him to do so. If your dog meets these conditions, you don't need a retractable lead and will do better with one of light webbing. Otherwise, **retractable leads are weapons.** The mechanism by which the lead is held is heavy and not appropriate for people with arthritis or any strength-sapping condition or for small children. If the lead is pulled from your hand, it can wedge into something, resulting in a harsh, abrupt, and potentially injurious stop for the dog. The mechanism can also hit another dog or human and do damage. If the dog is poorly behaved

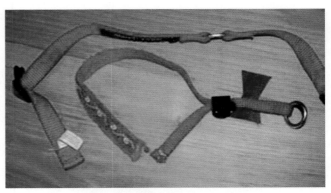

Photo 16 As with all equipment, check your leads, harnesses, collars, and head collars routinely for damage and replace anything that is questionable. Nothing lasts forever, defects occur, and wear is normal. This head collar suddenly tore across a stitched area, but no one was injured. Most companies will replace products that fail like this one did.

or just clueless, the ever-extending lead can result in a literal tie-up of people and dogs. These situations are just ripe for dog fights. Finally, just because the dog can run out further, does not mean that they will return. Unless the dog has good recall skills these leads are not useful unless they come equipped with a winch. None do. In a poorly behaved dog, these leads are an invitation to behave even more poorly. Addressing such behaviors is more fully covered in the ***Protocol for Teaching "Sit," "Stay," and "Come."***

Final Suggestions

Whatever style of lead you get, please think about the following.

- Have more than one lead, especially if you have children. When you most need it you will not be able to find the lead. A dog without a lead is just waiting to get hit by a car, and if you can't take the time to look for the lead, you are likely pretty agitated and rushed. No lead, no time, no patience—it's a guaranteed recipe for disaster. Keep a spare lead in a reliable place, whether it's a hook by the door, a drawer, a glove bin, the car, et cetera. In fact, with kids, encourage them to have their own color leads and head collars for walking the dog so that they always know where the lead is.
- If you are using a head collar, hang the lead and the collar up as a unit when not in use. In an emergency you can find it quickly. Again, a spare complete set is reasonable and one can be kept in every car.
- Put an extra lead, along with a dish, a blanket, and a bottle of water in each of your cars. Someday someone will just put the dog in the car, the car will break down, it will be hot, and you will have no control of the dog on a busy highway without this "emergency backup." Why risk the tragedy?
- Never, ever leave a dog tied, restrained, or with the potential to be ensnared with a lead/collar. Even if you are just crating a dog for 30 minutes, take the collar off unless it

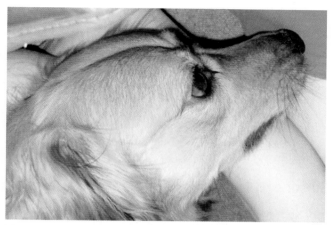

Photo 17 Hemorrhage in the sclera of eyes of a dog whose ID collar became entangled with her housemate's collar during a play bout. A human was present and quickly disentangled the dogs, but this damage was already done. Had the dogs been unattended, one or both of them could have died. These dogs will no longer wear collars when indoors. (Photo courtesy of Dr. Soraya Juarbe-Diaz.)

slips over the dog's head or is a breakaway. Do not allow anyone to place your dog in a run with a lead, which will catch on something, or with a collar that cannot release or come off. Do not leave your dog in the car unless the collar can release or come off, and do not leave the lead attached to the collar while the dog is alone in the car. Do not allow your dog to play with other dogs unless his collar can somehow release. By now, you can see the pattern of concern: every year dogs strangle, hang, die painfully, or become severely injured by collars or other animals with whom they become ensnarled. Such tragedies can be minimized by forethought.

- Your standard walking lead will be 4- to 6-feet long. Please remember that this is shorter than the average inter-personal approach distances for any but toy dogs. The average inter-personal approach distance or "personal space" for most dogs is 1 to 1.5 body lengths. If your dog is worried about other dogs or people, the short lead will not allow them to find a space where she can get away. If you aren't walking the dog in a congested urban area, consider a longer lead; leads come in increments up to 50 feet. This way, if the dog is on a head collar or a no-pull harness, the lead can be slack enough that they can have enough space to safely withdraw from the individual who distresses them, while you still have control because of the head collar.

- If you need to teach your dog to come back to you, use a long lead and roll up the slack in big loops in one hand. People make the mistake of letting their dog off-lead and expect the dog to magically return. Why? The dog can always come back—he cannot always run free. A very long lead allows the dog to run variable distances and to receive a slight physical signal (the tug on the head collar), coupled to a verbal signal, to return. Briefly, if the dog is leaded

and on a head collar, you can throw a toy 5 feet and tell Muffy to "get it." When she stops to pick it up, tell her she's great, slap your thigh or whistle or click, et cetera, and ask her to "come." If she doesn't return immediately, tug gently on the lead so that she is looking at you and repeat your request in an encouragingly exciting manner. If Muffy hasn't already been taught by you to ignore you, she'll likely come. When she's back, tell her she's brilliant, reward her with a treat or a pat, and throw the toy. When she is perfect for 5 feet, let her have a little more lead. If you increase the recall distance she'll likely not need to be reeled in, but if she does need to be reeled in, you can gently gather the lead hand-over-hand while encouraging her to "come."

- Only when she is always perfect should you consider letting her off-lead. Even then—think carefully. Assess the risks of cars, ill-mannered or dangerous dogs, enticing stimuli (e.g., cats, squirrels, deer, the neighbors' kids), bratty children, horses, et cetera. In urban areas, there has been a movement to create fenced dog runs where nice dogs can run together. When done correctly this is a brilliant and humane idea.

Product Sources

SENSEation harness
  www.softouchconcepts.com/products/harness-over
  view.php
Locatis
  http://locatis.typepad.com/home/2005/11/front_clip_
  harn.html
The Freedom No-Pull Harness from Wiggles, Wags, and
  Whiskers
  www.wiggleswagswhiskers.com/newsite/freedom-no-
  pull-harness.htm
Blackdog Gear:
  Balance Harness and Balance Training Pack (with 2 leads):
    www.blackdog.net.au
  Infi8 Halter and Training Halter (go to the website and
    watch the videos to choose):
    www.blackdog.net.au
Canny Collar
  www.cannyco.co.uk
Scuffy Guider
  www.mistypinesdogpark.com
Halti head collar
  www.companyofanimals.us/products/halti/halti-har
  ness
*Custom products, including prototype leather head collars, service
  dog harnesses, and many other humane products that require
  custom approaches*
  www.servicedogdesigns.com; www.boldleaddesigns.com
Gentle Leader
  www.premier.com (parent company: Radio Systems Cor-
  poration/RSC www.petsafe.net)
Easy Walk Harness
  www.premier.com (parent company: Radio Systems Cor-
  poration/RSC www.petsafe.net)

PROTOCOL FOR HANDLING "SPECIAL-NEEDS PETS" DURING HOLIDAYS AND OTHER SPECIAL OCCASIONS

Your pet has been diagnosed with a behavioral condition, so it's helpful to think of the pet as a "special-needs" animal. Dogs and cats with special needs almost always improve, largely because we have helped you to provide them with a stable, kind, humane, non-abusive rule structure that relieves their anxieties by anticipating problems. As part of this rule structure, pet dogs and cats are asked to sit, relax, breathe calmly and deeply, and look to you for information that tells them that you will guide and reward them (see the **Protocol for Deference** and the **Protocol for Teaching Your Dog to Take a Deep Breath and Use Other Biofeedback Methods as Part of Relaxation**). Most patients and clients do so wonderfully well that the clients often forget that the dog or cat was ever abnormal.

Unfortunately, novel, exciting, or busy social circumstances can often be provocative for the special-needs pet. Clients are often very hurt and upset when their pet experiences a breakthrough event under such circumstances. In the rare circumstance, the situation results in the death of the pet. More commonly, though, an otherwise happy circumstance becomes a sad, awkward, or stressful one. There is no need for this to occur. A relatively small amount of anticipation and thinking the potential problems through in advance can relieve your anxieties, and provide a more compassionate, less stressful experience for your pet.

Situations Involving Food

* If you know that your pet is aggressive or otherwise reactive around food, remember that holidays are big food events. Either do not have buffet-style meals, or baby gate or lock the pet in another room with an interactive toy or another pet to keep her occupied and to signal that she is not being punished. During the party visit the pet, and bring a small treat if this is something you can safely and routinely do. Make sure that the room can be locked and is locked from the outside. A very high hook-and-eye latch or a small sliding bolt can accomplish this. For adults, this will act as a signal not to open the door and allow the pet to escape; for children, it will prevent them from doing so. You can also post a note at adult eye level that explains why the door is locked and why you want your dog or cat to stay in the room so that you do not have to remember to remind everyone not to let her out. When people ignore or disbelieve the note, the lock at the top of the door will emphasize why they should comply.

Fearful Pets

* If you have a cat or dog that is fearful of new people, crowds, or noise, again, sequester her. This is not inhumane, exclusive, or unfair—**it's the better choice for the pet.** We understand that everyone wants to include pets in family events without worry. This is simply not realistic in most human families, so we should not expect our pets—especially those with special needs—to be able to accomplish this. Think of this as protecting or guarding your pets from circumstances that could be behaviorally injurious to them. And remember that every time your pet has an

adverse or negative experience involving fear or aggression, she learns from this and reinforces her inappropriate behavior. If one of the first steps of our treatment paradigm is to avoid all circumstances that provoke the pet, it makes sense that a logical step in the continued treatment and improvement of your pet should be to avoid placing her in a situation in which she may not be able—or should not be expected—to cope.

Situations Involving Visitors and Guests

* If your house is going to be full of visitors, please consider boarding the pet. If you are going to do this, you will need to plan ahead. First, boarding facilities book and fill early at holidays. Second, you want to make sure that the facility you choose will not make your pet worse—that the facility will be kind and humane and that it can meet the needs of your special pet. Third, you may want to see how your pet does when boarded under "no stress" circumstances, rather than introducing her to the situation during a busy holiday that is very stressful. If your pet doesn't tolerate boarding—and **many special-needs pets do not board well**—and she won't eat, loses weight, becomes withdrawn and unkempt, or becomes more fearful or aggressive, see if someone else in your family with whom your pet already has a good relationship can "pet sit." Alternatively, you can establish a good relationship with a professional pet sitter. Check for members of the national organization in your area. If this is not an option, consider having all seasonal celebrations elsewhere—you could still host them—so that your pets can be happy and healthy in their own home while you party with your friends and relatives.

A Note About Pet Sitters

* Please consider only using pet sitters who are bonded and/or about whom you can get recommendations and with whom you have some innate comfort level. A good source for pet sitters for special-needs pets is your veterinarian, a certified professional dog trainer, or a client with another special-needs pet. Regardless, when looking for a pet sitter you want him to have two character traits for your special-needs dog or cat: he must be **responsible and reliable.**
  * The pet sitter *must* understand that loving the animal is not enough and that you have created a strategy for helping the dog or cat function as well and happily as she can, and that this strategy keeps everyone sane, safe and healthy.
  * If the pet sitter has a question, the sitter must call you, regardless of where you are in the world or the time of day.
  * If the problem behaviors begin to appear, the sitter must call you.
  * If something seems a little off, the sitter must call you.

When you can get this degree of responsibility and reliability from someone, hire them. Special-needs pets are not well served by being cared for by some random, well-meaning neighbor, especially if that neighbor is not an adult.

Special-needs pets are also not well served by being cared for by people who do not appreciate the behavioral needs in the way that you do.

Noise: Fears, Phobias, and Reactivity

- If your pets are afraid of noise—holidays like New Year's, Mardi Gras, Guy Fawkes Day in the United Kingdom, and, in the United States, the 4th of July, are hellish, nightmarish situations for these animals. The best prevention and treatment involves repeated medication with a short-acting anti-anxiety medication before and during the expected raucous explosion. This may not be possible with some aggressive pets. You will benefit from the information in the handout on **Protocol for Understanding and Treating Dogs with Noise and Storm Phobias.** Please make sure you get, read, and implement this handout if your dog or cat reacts to noises. Meanwhile, if you can decrease the dog's or cat's sensory perception in a way that is safe and helps them, this is worth considering. There are now eye goggles that fit many pets and that come with tinted lenses for those that react to visual displays (www.doggles.com); some dogs and cats will tolerate eye masks primarily intended for beauty treatments or air travel; and ear muffs exist that will help cancel out noise (www.muttmuffs.com). Such tools may have a place in your toolbox.

Situations Involving Children

- If your pets have never seen children and families with multiple kids plan to visit, *caution is urged.* Cats should either be elsewhere and safe or on harnesses, if they are accustomed to them, and dogs should be on head collars at the first introduction to the children. The children should be of an age and temperament that they will follow your instructions and not deliberately or inadvertently provoke the pet. If the children cannot or will not do this—or if their parents are not willing or able to supervise them **or** think that you are overly and unreasonably concerned—sequester the pet as above. Don't worry about what anyone thinks of you and don't let anyone bully or embarrass you: You know you are being humane to and protective of the pet, and you are the only one responsible for that pet's continued well-being and improvement. Please also remember that children who have been well-behaved and non-threatening one-on-one may not behave the same way in a group. Here, the way the pet responds to them will be more than the sum of the parts. Caution is urged. If you have children, even if they have a good relationship with your pet, please remember that your children will not behave the same way when the house is full of people during a holiday as they would during a regular day. This means that their relationship with the pet may change and, or their behavior may change in a way that scares the pet. Again, err on the side of minimizing the cost of error to the pet.

Protective and Territorial Pets

- Please remember that many pets who are excessively or inappropriately protective or territorial will be made more anxious and worsened by the frequent coming and going of delivery people and guests. Accordingly, they will be more reactive. The busier you are, the more likely you are to be unable to accurately assess the pet's concern. Again, sequestering the pet—even if just behind a baby gate—will allow you to proceed at a more realistic and safer pace.

The Role of Exercise

- Please make sure—particularly if you have a special-needs dog—that your pet is well exercised before the big event. The more aerobic exercise your pet gets, the calmer she will be. Exercise her early in the day before a party and again just before it. Use the pet's standard for real aerobic exercise and tiredness, not yours. You will tire first. Using the pet's standard will take more time, but tired pets are less anxious and more calmly behaved.

Food, Diet, and Schedules

- Try to stick to as regular a schedule as possible for your pet and try to stick to the pet's regular diet. The more disruptions, the more unstable the pet will be. Also, if she has an upset stomach, vomiting, or diarrhea because of too many rich foods, she will be more unstable, more reactive, more anxious, and more unpredictable. Neither you nor your pet need this.

Problems with Yards and Kennels

- Please remember that putting an aggressive or fearful dog in the backyard is not a solution.
  - First, the dog is not protected from others—dogs or humans—who can enter the yard or look over the fence.
  - Second, if people are milling around—particularly children—they can and will open the door to the yard. This could be tragic and it can absolutely be avoided.

Under no circumstances should dogs of any kind be left chained or "tied out." These dogs are trapped and will be more reactive. In fact, dogs maintained under these conditions are overrepresented on some sets of dog bite statistics. This is beyond dangerous—it is inhumane for the dog.

Can a Crate Help?

- Please remember that unless your pet is already comfortable in a crate, enjoys it, and cannot be disturbed by others when in it, the use of a crate will actually make the situation more stressful for you and your pet. Also, remember that some dogs with separation anxiety cannot bear to be locked up and panic when trapped. The crate is an entrapment for these dogs. Finally, many animals in crates or behind fences or grates are more—not less—aggressive than when they are loose. That barrier gives them a physical boundary which they may feel they have to defend, but which also prevents them from choosing the option of withdrawal. People have the foolish tendency to reach through gates or over gates. Never, ever let anyone do this, stare at an animal that is crated, or get close enough to stick anything through the crate. If you decide to crate your pet and your pet has a known history of enjoying the crate, make sure that the crate is in a quiet area that prohibits deliberate or inadvertent tormenting of what is now a trapped animal.

Inviting the Pet to the Party

- If you think your pet is sufficiently improved that she can be "invited" to the party, pick your parties. Smaller groups of controllable adults who know of the problem, like pets, and are willing to comply with your instructions on how to interact with the pet are your best bet. You can introduce dogs on leashes and head collars and cats on leashes and harnesses, if they are accustomed to them. The first time your dog or cat acts distressed or a human responds in a way that worries you, put the pet in a safe place. Whatever you do, please remember that people who are afraid of pets or uncertain about them or who have never had them, people who are physically or behaviorally impaired (alcohol ingestion comes to mind), and children pose the worst risks for distressed, special-needs pets. Please remember that many abandoned and rehomed pets have experienced abuse when near someone who is chemically impaired and so may react with anxiety or fear to the smell of substances like marijuana or alcohol.

Stress, Stress, and More Stress

- Please remember the law of multiple stressors: The more often you and your pet are subjected to stressful or unexpected situations, the more likely the pet will react inappropriately to the situation. Watch your pet—if your social life during the holidays is too much for your pet, please consider some of the other options recommended in this handout. A small amount of attending to your pet's signals and anticipation of their needs and concerns can avoid tragic disasters.

Guilt, Love, and Guardianship

- Finally, do not feel that by sequestering your pet away you have let your dog or cat down, or that she is paying dearly for your social life. You would be letting her down only if you placed her in an upsetting situation where she became more fearful or aggressive. These recommendations are compromises that allow you to work with difficult situations with as little worry as possible. If you give yourself the time to sit down and list the circumstances in which you think your pet might become distressed during these very social times, you will be able to anticipate how to avoid them. Timing is critical here: do not wait until the last minute when you are forced to react rather than to plan or prevent. If you err on the side of caution, you will find that you and your pet will have a far more enjoyable holiday, and one that is relatively risk-free.

PROTOCOL FOR BASIC MANNERS TRAINING AND HOUSETRAINING FOR NEW DOGS AND PUPPIES

The steps below are designed to help you begin to train and housetrain any dog. They are divided into two sections: puppies and older dogs.

Puppies

Sensitive Periods for Social Exposure

Puppies become adept at interacting with to other dogs between the ages of 4 and 8+ weeks and with people between the ages of 5 and 10+ weeks. They are especially able to learn to explore complex new surroundings between 5 and 16 weeks, and if they are not exposed to such stimuli by about 10 weeks of age, they can become *neophobic* (fearful of the unfamiliar). Because of these "sensitive periods"—periods where puppies learn quickly about new social and physical experiences—the recommended time for bringing a new puppy home starts at about 8.5 weeks. Before this, dogs are really honing their dog–dog skills and need the stimulation and solace of their parents and littermates. Dogs with a good social background have more tools for understanding increasingly complex worlds.

If a breeder is willing to expose the dog to all new environments and new people, and housetrain the pup, the pup can stay at the breeders through 12 weeks of age without detrimental effects. The real advantages of having the dog stay with the breeder all have to do with social experiences with other dogs. As long as the puppy is engaged in an active vaccination and preventative healthcare program, there are other ways for this interaction to be achieved, including puppy play parties, play dates, puppy daycare, and puppy kindergarten. If there is an adult dog in the home already, the pup will learn best and fastest from that dog, so anyone who already has a dog and is bringing home a puppy needs to make sure their adult dogs are well behaved before adding a pup.

Dogs who miss these sensitive periods for interaction and development do not *necessarily* develop problems associated with lack of experience, but may be more *at risk* for developing such problems. Dogs may not get adequate exposure because they are kept in isolation at the breeder's or because they are sent to their new home too early. The more we learn about effects of the early learning environment, the more justification we have for trying to *minimize risk* for young puppies in terms of the social and environmental exposure. Doing everything right does not guarantee you a perfect dog, but *not* doing what we know helps puts your dog at risk for behavioral problems.

Exposing the Dog to Try to Minimize the Development of Fear

So, in the first 2 months that you have your puppy you should make sure that the pup interacts with other dogs and people of all ages and sexes, experiences cars and traffic, meets other animals the puppy lives with, such as farm animals, and gets accustomed to most of the situations in which the adult dog will be expected, by you, to function. The key to producing a behaviorally healthy and happy puppy is to understand and recognize fear.

- It **is** okay if the dog is a little startled by the new experiences, as long as the puppy recovers quickly. This means

that the pup is willing to continue exploring and maintains his curiosity and willingness to interact, even if he is a little uncertain.

- It's **not** okay if the experience upsets the puppy so much that he cries, urinates, defecates, and wants to hide.
- It's **not** okay if the puppy does not recover quickly—within a few minutes—when startled by a normal, but unfamiliar event or object.
- It's **not** okay to deliberately scare a puppy to make him "tougher." You will just behaviorally damage the pup.
- It's **essential** to seek veterinary help as soon as possible if you begin to see a pattern of when the puppy reacts fearfully to new things, people, and events and does not recover quickly in a way that allows the puppy to enjoy his life.

If you intend to show the dog in conformation, agility, or obedience, take the pup to shows early, even before he is old enough to be entered. This is possible with outdoor shows. This way you ensure that the pup has experience with vans, crates, pens, runs, rings, food smells, many dogs, the chaos of shows, and—maybe most importantly—with the various options used for allowing a dog to eliminate within the confines of dog show rules and events. Please remember that *if the pup shows any signs of fear or anxiety* (crying, whining, withdrawal, salivation, avoidance, shaking/trembling, nonstop panting, salivation, scanning, vigilance, inappetence, vomiting, diarrhea, uncontrolled urination/defecation, et cetera) that do not quickly stop, *you must remove the dog from the situation to one where he is calmer.* Please do not think that by continually exposing the dog to something worrisome that the dog "will get over it." In fact, the opposite is true: you will render your pup truly fearful and do long-term harm.

Teaching Puppies to Eliminate Outside

The best time to start teaching a dog to eliminate in a desired location is when the puppy is between 7.5 and 8.5 weeks of age. At about 8.5 weeks the puppy is best able to start to choose a preferred substrate (grass, dirt, cement) *and* to act upon that choice. This is the first age at which the pup can cognitively make the connection between the scent and feel of the place they are eliminating and the act of elimination, *and* that they are able to control the act of eliminating. Before about 8 weeks of age most puppies just do not have the neurological control to inhibit elimination. Housetraining a pup has two parts:

1. getting the pup to use the "right" place and
2. encouraging the pup to *wait to eliminate* until he gets to the "right" place.

This means that puppies need both the neuromuscular control and the cognitive component for housetraining to succeed. Working well with an 8.5-week-old puppy does not guarantee that the puppy will not have accidents after that time: they will, but the foundations for easier housetraining are best laid at that age.

Some puppies are not as developmentally advanced as others at the same age and may do well forming a preference for an area for urination and defecation, but they may not have the physical muscle and nervous control necessary to endure extended periods without accidents. There is a lot of variation in the rates at which puppies develop, just as is the case for human children. This control will come with age if the puppy is appropriately reinforced and if there is no physical problem. This is important to know because for puppies, as for human children, the first incident of abuse often comes with house- and toilet-training.

If you have truly done everything "right" and the 6- to 9-month old puppy is still not completely housetrained, it is important to look for an underlying medical problem, like an infection, that may be contributing to or causing the problem. Sometimes, a slight amount of dribbling, particularly if the dog is excited, can be normal. For example, although not true for every dog, it is not uncommon for female puppies to dribble urine because of some of the hormonal and anatomical differences that distinguish them from male dogs. The dribbling usually resolves or improves with age, but in some cases when it doesn't, the puppy may respond to the hormones that become abundant during an estrous or heat cycle. Heat cycles usually start at about 9 months of age and will recur about every 6 months if the puppy is not spayed/ neutered (ovariohysterectomized).

Housetraining a puppy is time-consuming, because it requires attention to the puppy's signals and consistent action. Housetraining a puppy when young is a lot easier than trying to correct inappropriate elimination behaviors that could have been avoided by the right approach at the start. If you do not have the knowledge or energy to housetrain a puppy kindly and humanely, please consider adopting an adult dog who is known to be housetrained.

Should You Neuter/Desex Your Puppy?

A word on spaying and castration is in order. Spayed and castrated (neutered/desexed) pets are often considered healthier pets for several reasons:

- They are less likely to roam. This is especially true for intact or non-castrated males. Roaming exposes dogs to other dogs with whom they may fight, traffic, and, possibly, to areas of infectious disease.
- Castrated male dogs have decreased risk of prostatic and testicular cancer and infection.
- Spayed females are not at risk from dying of uterine infections or unintended pregnancies.
- Spayed females have a greatly decreased risk of mammary cancer if spayed by no later than 1.5 years of age.

In the United States, most dogs and cats are neutered to prevent the births of unwanted pets. There is some developing evidence that suggests neutering of some animals *may* be associated with increased risk of illnesses not directly linked to the reproductive tract. The data are few, but it should be understood that we may make different decisions for dogs coming from shelters, and those people can and will supervise. Early neutering (5 to 8 weeks vs. the traditional 6 months of age) is now common for shelter and rescue dogs. Studies show that long bone growth is greater in early neutered animals so they will be taller.

If the decision is made to allow the female puppy to have a heat cycle, the owner is absolutely responsible for always keeping the puppy on a leash, in sight, and away from male dogs for the extended period of time before, during, and after the actual discharge phase of the cycle. Otherwise, the puppy will become pregnant.

Although the numbers have decreased in the past decade, at least 10 million unwanted pets are killed annually in humane shelters in the United States. No one needs unwanted and unplanned puppies, and it is not a kindness to allow a puppy to bear puppies. Even if the dog is a superior quality breeding dog, no responsible breeder would encourage or allow a **puppy** to be bred and have babies while she is still a baby.

Castrated dogs are thought to fight less with other dogs, urine mark less frequently, and roam and wander less. It is important to remember that every behavior has a learned component and hormones may just act to facilitate some behaviors. Taking away the hormone source doesn't take away the memory that certain behaviors were interesting or fun.

If your dog is not an absolutely top-quality breeding animal (i.e., all of your dog's parents and "grandparents are free of any genetic disease or problem" *and* your dog's "temperament" and that of your dog's parents and grandparents is flawless, *and* you are willing to take back and humanely home animals who do not work out in others' homes), **do not breed the animal:** either neuter your dog or ensure that the dog will not breed. This is a kindness; most of the dogs turned in to humane shelters are purebred dogs, and 60% of all breedings result in the death of either the mother or one or more of the puppies.

Managing Puppy Chewing and Other Developmental Issues

Decide whether you are going to crate-train the puppy. Using a crate (a cage or kennel) can be an excellent idea for most puppies and can be an essential step in the housetraining process. Small, enclosed areas encourage the pup to develop conscious muscle control to inhibit elimination at inconvenient times.

Crates are available from pet stores and online, and some kennel clubs may rent them. If you are planning to travel by air with the pet, buy an airline-approved crate. Airlines require crates (although please think carefully about whether you need to fly your pets and research the best ways to do so safely) and you can even check in to some of the finest, fussiest hotels if you are willing to crate the dog when you're not in the room.

Some pups immediately feel more secure when left alone in a crate with blankets, toys, food, water, and, **if** large enough, an area for paper for urination and defecation. Get a bigger crate if the pup is to spend all day crated, but please consider having a pet sitter exercise the dog if you have to spend this much time away from your pet. Young (8-week-old) puppies need to eliminate **at least** every hour (more if eating, playing, or just awakening) and will need an area they can start to use for this. If the crate is small, an older puppy will be unlikely to soil it; however, no puppy can be expected to last 8 to 10 hours without urinating or defecating.

Please note: Even better than a crate for pups that must be left for long periods (>4 hours) is a dog sitter, doggie daycare, or taking the dog with you to work, if possible.

Crates should always be placed in family areas, not in the damp basement or the garage. You want the puppy to learn to love going into the crate. Feed the puppy in the crate with the door open: ask the puppy to sit and wait (see **Protocol for Deference** and **Protocol for Relaxation: Behavior**

Modification Tier 1), put the food inside, and release the puppy. Teach the puppy to wait to go in by using biscuits to reward the puppy for having some restraint and not charging the crate.

Correctly **reward** with treats or toys—**do not bribe.** Remember, a bribe is an action taken to lure the dog away from an undesirable behavior that rewards the animal before the animal offers the undesired behavior; a reward is an action taken after the dog has willingly complied with a request. A reward is a salary; a bribe is blackmail.

Each day, give the puppy a toy, a blanket, and something to chew (a biscuit, a big sterilized bone that has been stuffed with peanut butter, a stuffed Kong, Planet Toy, or a Nylabone) and put the puppy into the crate for some quiet time. This is quiet time for all of you and will provide you with the ability to give the dog a safe place to relax and calm down ("time out") any time the puppy is driving you nuts and you do not have the patience to work with the pup.

Puppies are babies and need their own quiet time, too. During these short (2 to 5 minutes to start) sessions, stay quietly in the room with the pup, but don't respond to attempts to get your attention. The puppy is capable of amusing himself. As the pup becomes more accustomed to the crate, extend the period of time that he is in it and go to other areas of the house.

Before you release the pup from the crate, ask the pup to sit and praise her when she sits. When the puppy is let out of the crate, don't fuss over the pup for a few minutes—she could learn to associate release from the crate with lots of attention. You can give the pup all the love and attention you wish a few minutes after releasing her from the crate. Some of the attention you give the pup should consist of practicing a few really helpful "good manners" behaviors like "sit, please" and "down, please" and "take a deep breath, please" (see the **Protocol for Teaching "Sit," "Stay," and "Come"** and the **Protocol for Teaching Your Dog to Take a Deep Breath and Use Other Biofeedback Methods as Part of Relaxation**).

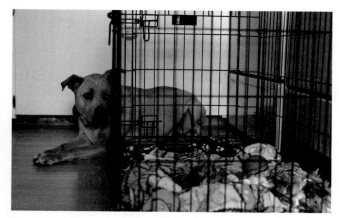

This puppy is next to and outside of her crate. The crate is in the kitchen and has toys and bedding. This pup would spend more time in the crate than is good for her. (Photo courtesy Kristen Penkrot.)

Keeping Crates and Puppies Safe and Clean

The crate should be kept clean. If soiled, use hot water and non-irritating soap or baking soda and vinegar and **rinse well** and dry. Use an odor neutralizer (Elimin-odor, PON, FON, The Equalizer, AIP), let sit for a bit, rinse well, and dry again. Crates should be placed in well-lit areas, but not in those that will get the heat of the afternoon sun—the puppy could easily overheat and die. Timers can be placed on lights so that the pup isn't left alone in the dark. Radios and TVs can be left on for auditory company and to mask scary street sounds.

Never, ever leave **anything** around the pup's neck, like a loose buckle or choker collar, that can tangle and hang on any part of the cage or anything in it. The puppy could strangle and die a painful death.

The crate has three main purposes:

1. to encourage the dog to start inhibiting the urge to eliminate,
2. to keep the puppy safe from all the disasters from electric cords to toxic substances that lurk in the average home, and
3. to keep you sane when the puppy is too rambunctious.

Puppies **are** rambunctious. They need an **aerobic** outlet for all that energy. The crate is **not** meant to keep them incarcerated or to substitute for that need for aerobic exercise. **Do not** think that you can keep the puppy in the crate 8 to 10 hours per day and then not have to play energetic games at night. **If you need an animal you can keep caged for most of the animal's young life, please consider a gerbil.**

Alternatives to Crates

If you are not going to crate your puppy, confine him to one area (kitchen, den, heated or air-conditioned sun porch) at first. This may give the dog a greater sense of security when you're not home, and minimize damage. Leave a radio and a light on for the pup. Expand the areas to which the pup has access gradually, only when the puppy has not eliminated or destroyed anything in the area to which he was previously confined. Baby gates can help with this. If you are going to be gone for more than 2 to 3 hours, the puppy will have to urinate or defecate, so you'll have to provide the pup with an area to do this (litterbox or newspaper; see below). Make sure that the room is puppy-proof: no cupboards with chemicals or toxic substances into which the dog can get—no strings, ropes, slippers, magazines, or mail the dog can shred and/or ingest, possibly causing an intestinal obstruction. Just as for a crate, the dog should have a blanket, water, toys, and a biscuit or two.

Caution is urged in confining puppies to bathrooms, where they have been known to drown in toilets, or in kitchens, if they can reach and turn on the stove accidentally.

Elimination Paradigm

Puppies develop substrate preferences for urination and defecation. "Substrates" are the surfaces on which dogs wee and poo. This means that if you teach a dog to urinate on newspaper, the pup will learn to seek out **that** substrate. Although it is tougher to teach a puppy to go outside to urinate and defecate after he has learned to use newspaper, it is not impossible. It **is** preferable to teach the dog to go outside at the outset, but this may not fit into your schedule.

Directly Training the Puppy to Urinate (Wee) and Defecate (Poo) Outside

1. Every 1 to 2 hours take the puppy outside. Puppies have *high* metabolisms—meaning that they make a lot of urine

quickly—and *small* bladders—meaning that they cannot store all that urine for long. The basic Labrador retriever puppy has a bladder the size of a lemon when full; the basic Yorkie pup's bladder is the size of a small apricot when full.

2. When you take the pup out, let him sniff a bit. Don't just pull him away from what he is sniffing and keep walking. Sniffing is an important part of the elimination sequence in dogs.

3. If the dog is just rampantly plowing ahead sniffing, consider stopping and walking a bit quickly back and forth. This movement simulates normal dog elimination precursor behavior. The pup will eventually squat—pay attention and praise him. When the dog is finished, tell him that he is brilliant.

4. Use a fixed-length, short lead so that you can quickly encourage your puppy and respond to her cues. You can give the pup a little piece of biscuit or another small treat as she squats on a substrate you both like (grass). A reward may help encourage the association between squatting on that substrate and good experiences. Urinating or defecating is physiologically self-rewarding—you are rewarding the behavior exhibited in the location chosen.

5. Regardless of the frequency of your other walks, take the pup out 15 to 45 minutes after *each time he eats.* This is the time range for eating to stimulate intestines to move feces. "Food" means all meals, including biscuits and rawhides, both of which will stimulate elimination.

6. Watch for behaviors that tell you the dog may be ready to eliminate—pacing, whining, circling, a sudden stopping of another behavior—and intercept the pup. If you pick the pup up and she starts to leak, or the act of picking up the pup starts the leak, get a cloth and clamp it to the pup's genitals. This will help to stimulate the pup to associate inhibition of elimination with those muscle groups. It also keeps the floor cleaner. Again, praise the pup as he is squatting and **immediately** after he has finished. *Do not punish any leaks.*

7. Take the puppy out immediately after any play **and** naps or if he awakens at night.

8. Prepare for the first walk of the day by having your clothes ready to put on before you approach any crated puppy. Puppies who have waited through the night cannot wait long once you are awake!

9. Watch the puppy between walks—pups often get caught short, especially if they encounter and play with a water dish or they become superfocused or distracted. Any puppy who is moving around and suddenly stops, needs to eliminate. You can make monitoring easier by putting a bell on the dog's collar: any time the puppy's bell stops, get the pup and take her outside immediately. If you are going to do this, you need to use a breakaway/quick-release collar that will come undone if the dog catches it on anything.

10. If you have an older dog that is housetrained, take this dog with you when you take the pup out. Dogs learn extremely well by observing, and this may speed the process.

11. Dogs are generally faster to housetrain for defecation than urination. This may be, in part, because puppies urinate more frequently than they defecate. For some very clueless dogs it can help to take either a urine-soaked sponge or a piece of feces to the area you would prefer

the pup use. This may help the pup to learn to associate her scent pattern with the area, but it cannot be used in the absence of the other steps above.

Paper or Litterbox Training the Puppy Inside

1. If you must train the pup to paper or a litterbox, put the box or paper in one place, preferably close to a door. Take the puppy to the paper frequently and praise him when he squats.

2. You may want to put heavy-gauge plastic under the newspaper to protect flooring and rugs in case the pup misses or the urine soaks through the paper.

3. Getting the puppy outdoors **still** requires you to be home for a while. Although the dog is being trained to paper, you still have to take him out at least 3 to 4 times a day (after meals, awakening, play). Praise the puppy immediately during and after the squat.

4. To wean the puppy from the paper, gradually start to move the paper 1 to 2 inches per day closer to the door. Spy on the puppy during weekends and as he begins to squat on the paper, rush him outside and **wait** for him to urinate or defecate. This also helps stop him from being fearful outside. Enthusiastically praise the pup when he pees or poos outside.

5. Know that paper training may slow the process of getting the puppy to develop an outdoor substrate preference. It may be, however, your only option.

6. Some people with small dogs elect to have the dog permanently trained to paper or a litterbox. Litterboxes are now commercially available that are suitable for large dogs. Litterboxes are easier to handle for small dogs, but if you do not want the dog to rely on these, you must go through the amount of work described here.

7. **Caution: Litterboxes are not intended as devices to relieve you of "having" to take your dog out and about.** *Please* **do not use these as an excuse to not exercise your dog, to let him or her explore the world, or to prevent free play with other dogs.**

8. If you have an older dog who is housetrained, take this dog with you when you take the pup out. Dogs learn extremely well by observing, and this may speed up the process.

9. Dogs are generally faster to housetrain for defecation than urination. This may be, in part, because puppies urinate more frequently than they defecate. For some very clueless dogs it can help to take either a urine-soaked sponge or a piece of feces to the area you would prefer the pup use. This may help the pup to learn to associate his scent pattern with the area, but it cannot be used in the absence of the other steps above.

A Word About Cleaning

You must clean any indoor area where the dog has urinated or defecated.

1. If the dog soiled a rug, be aware that you may ultimately need to clean the rug pad and subfloors. Start with soaking up urine and removing feces.

2. Then soak with club soda, let sit a minute or so, and blot.

3. You can repeat this as often as needed until there is no scent and clear liquid is being blotted.

4. Then use one of the odor eliminators suggested above, or Febreze or a similar product. Always test the floor or rug

to make sure that whatever you put on it is not going to discolor it. Use just enough odor eliminator to cover the area—remember you are trying to stop the odors from being smelled by the dog by changing them. This is a chemical process. Washing odors away or diluting them is a physical process. You need to do both.

5. If the dog revisits used spots or sniffs at them, there is still odor that the dog can detect. Start over with the club soda.

What About the Older Puppy Who Does Not Seem to Understand That There Are Preferred Places for Elimination?

For puppies who are older (7 to 9 months) and who still seem to have no awareness of appropriate elimination behavior, diapers can help. This is **not** a substitute for the steps above, but an addition to them. Dog diapers or britches are available at pet-care outlets and are sold primarily for females in season/heat. The uncomfortable sensation of a damp diaper next to the skin may help to teach some dogs to control themselves. You have to be willing to bathe and powder any dog who might soil himself to prevent urine burns or fecal contamination. A thin layer of Vaseline can help to provide a protective coating.

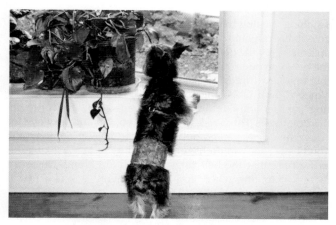

A young, male dog who is not completely housetrained and who also engages in some marking wearing a "belly band," a type of diaper for male dogs. The wrap is fabric and washable, and it holds an absorbent pad over the dog's prepuce.

What About Just Letting the Dog Roam and Housetrain Himself?

In addition to all the steps above it is important to note that even if you have 120 acres and the dog will have free range, **you** need to be standing there, next to the dog, rewarding him for eliminating on an appropriate substrate or the association will not be made. It is not acceptable to wave at the dog through a window or to praise the pup when he returns. This is **not** a reward structure. Remember that free-range dogs learn to eliminate anywhere. This is not what you want.

Essential Role for Play in Training a Puppy

Reward the puppy with a longer walk and play outside **after** *he eliminates.* Do not play with the puppy or allow him to play with other dogs before he eliminates. In essence, you want to reward eliminating outside with carefree play. If the only time that the pup has to watch the air, chase leaves, and hear birds

is when he is out to eliminate, you may be making your housetraining problems worse. If the pup is yanked back inside right after eliminating, he can learn to avoid or postpone elimination outside and to save walks for exploration. After all, the pup can always eliminate indoors.

Can We Use a Word to Tell the Dog to Wee or Poo?

Finally, if you want your dog to start to learn to eliminate "on command," request that the dog eliminate as she does so. Say "empty," "potty," or "go wee," and make sure the last repetition of your cue coincides with a squatting event. Then tell the dog that she is brilliant. Use this with play after elimination and your pup will be more than willing to do your bidding.

Punishment

You will notice that no mention of punishment for housetraining has been made. That is because **punishment has no role in housetraining any dog.** Animals and people make associations between acts and consequences; this is how we learn. Coming downstairs to find a puddle of urine on the rug and the dog cringing **does not** mean that the dog **knows** he erred. What he is probably telling you is that this has happened before: you have come home, grabbed the dog, dragged the dog to the urine, and whacked him. The dog **has** made an association: you come home and the dog gets whacked, but it's the wrong association (or at least one you did not intend for the dog to learn). In fact, if you have punished the pup, the pup probably cringes when you come home even if he hasn't urinated on the rug, but you don't notice.

You **must** couple any "correction" exactly with the action that needs "correcting." If you see the puppy start to squat or find her in the act of urinating or defecating on the rug et cetera, interrupt the dog if you think you can do so successfully. She should just stop the behavior but not be terrified. Saying "uh, uh," inhaling sharply, or softly clapping your hands will interrupt most pups. Use the lowest level of stimulus necessary to achieve the interruption. If you don't think you can interrupt the pup as she starts to piddle so that she stops and is able to go outside to eliminate, forget it. After you clean up make a mental note to take the dog out in 30 minutes and frequently thereafter, each time rewarding the dog for eliminating in the more desirable (from your viewpoint) place. For some very meek pups **any** "correction" can make them more timid, so caution is urged. If you are able to successfully interrupt the pup, take her outside and praise her as soon she urinates or defecates on an appropriate substrate. Psychologists have shown that we learn best and most quickly if we are interrupted in an unexpected context, so disrupting undesirable elimination can help you to dissuade the pup from eliminating in the wrong place *if and only if you do not scare the dog.*

Reminder: No matter how distressed you are about the dog's accidents, there is **never any** excuse to hit or beat a dog. *Never.* Please remember that dog abuse and child abuse are associated and both often begin when training the individual to eliminate in a preferred location, on a preferred schedule.

What If You Have Done Everything "Right" and the Puppy Is Still Having "Accidents"?

If you have done all of the above and are still having problems, keep a log for a week to tell you how frequently the dog is out, for how long the dog is out, what happens when the dog eats, plays, sleeps, snacks, et cetera. Review the log for any patterns associated with elimination in the house. Chances are something will jump out at you.

However, if you review your log and see no patterns, bring the dog and the log to your veterinarian so that they can review the history and double-check the dog for medical or developmental concerns. Something will make sense.

Early Training for Manners

No puppy is too young to learn to earn what he wants by sitting and staying. All pups should be taught to sit and stay for walks, food dishes, water, play attention—anything. The fastest way to teach this is with food treats—tiny pieces of really good biscuits, treats, jerky, or cheese. This technique allows you to only use voice signals so that your moving hands do not distract the pup. Later—when the dog is flawless for your verbal requests, you can add hand signals and other cues, if you wish.

Teaching sit is like teaching any other behavior: take advantage of normal, freely offered behaviors to reward the pup. Then you can teach the pup to offer the behavior in response to a cue. The puppy will accidentally sit the first time you attempt this: hold the treat in one hand in front of the dog's nose; gradually move him close to the ground and repeat "sit" when his bottom touches the ground. **Instantly open your hand for the treat and say "good pup."** As the puppy matures you can begin to expect him to distinguish between "sit" and "down" by using those words to only mean what they say; at first, the pup only has to get his bottom on the ground, however it's done (see **Protocol for Relaxation: Behavior Modification Tier 1**). At first use the words "sit" and "down" to mean exactly that, but reward the pup if he does either; reinforce them to distinguish between the commands by being particularly enthusiastic if they do. You will gradually shape their behavior. Later, as the pup is more mature, you only reward him for "down" when he lies down and "sit" when he sits instead of lying down. The earlier you start to teach a dog to look to you for cues and to defer to you for anything he desires, the better off you'll be. *All* dogs should be taught manners and to respond to their owners' requests. This is particularly true for large-breed dogs who can be unpleasant, at best, and dangerous, at worst, when out of control. *No* dog needs to be hit to do this.

Older Dogs

The same basic training and housetraining rules apply to older dogs that apply to puppies, but older dogs can be more difficult to housetrain because they may have to unlearn some less-favorable behaviors. Older puppies or dogs who have been kenneled for extensive periods may have developed a preference for the substrate on which they were kept. You may be able to use this (e.g., there might be cement in your neighborhood) or you may be able to shift the preference to a broader range of substrates.

- For older dogs—even as you repeat all of the steps involved in housetraining a pup—you will have to be very vigilant any time that the dog is around substrates she had used in the past.
- Expect to have to do a lot of monitoring and redirecting.
- Spying on the dog can be made easier by putting a bell on the dog's collar.

- Incarcerate the dog any time you cannot monitor her.
- **BE PATIENT.** If you have ever tried to lose 5 pounds you know how hard it is to change behavior.
- As soon as you see the dog squat in an inappropriate area, calmly shuffle the dog outside and reward any act of elimination.
- If the dog startles and will not eliminate, take the dog on a long-leash walk and reward sniffing and acts of elimination.
- If the dog will not eliminate on a lead, take her to a fenced outdoor area with the scents of other dogs and wait. Bring coffee. Reward any elimination behaviors.
- Finally, consider borrowing a dog who is good at eliminating in the outside, desired places as a demonstration model. Dogs do observational learning quite well and are interested in the scent of the urine and feces of other dogs. Praise and reward the other dog every time he eliminates. Your dog will catch on with exposure.
- On the positive side, these older dogs are usually so grateful that they were rescued and can now be loved, they will work wonderfully for praise and interaction. Use this.

Tips the Pros Use: Teaching a Dog to "Knock"

Teaching the dog that he has some control over the ability to go outside can help. Put a cow bell, sleigh bells, or jingle bells on a string by the door and teach your dog that when he baps the bell, you open the door and let him out. Demonstrate this the first few times by taking the dog's paw and saying "knock," and whacking the bells. Then tell the dog "good dog" and let him out (on a lead, if needed for safety or to get the dog back). This process will give you an auditory cue for when the dog has to go out, so you can further reinforce the good behavior. You **do** have to be willing to take the dog out every time that the bell rings and you are home. Dogs can learn not to ring when you are not there. This is a useful technique for older puppies, too.

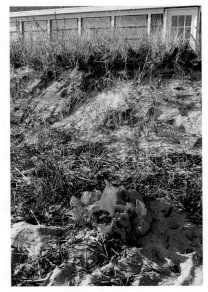

One week at the beach with 4 dogs produced 42 bags of poo. All dogs should have their feces cleaned up and disposed of properly.

Checklist for Housetraining a Puppy

1. Bell the puppy so you know where she is at all times; this way you can interrupt elimination and take her to the desired spot
2. Crate
3. Times to take to desired area
   - Immediately upon awakening
   - Immediately after playing (especially if the puppy voluntarily slows play)
   - Fifteen to 30 minutes after any food
   - Minimum of 6 to 8 times per day
   - Every 1 to 2 hours is optimal
4. Restrict access
5. Regular feeding times; no free access; take up food after 20 minutes
6. Leash walk!!!!!
7. No play until he has eliminated
8. Fifteen- to 20-minute walks
9. Permit sniffing
10. Concentrate in one area—small steps
11. Allow play/exploration after
12. Reward
13. Appropriate interrupts—do not make the dog afraid or wary of you
14. Reinforce scent (older dog, feces in correct area)
15. Variety of substrates (show or traveling dogs)
16. Verbal signal/cue (empty, potty, go wee, et cetera)
17. Patience
18. Odor eliminators and appropriate cleaning
19. Non–elimination-associated aerobic play—LOTS

Checklist for Housetraining the Older Dog

1. See puppy checklist
2. Identify preferred substrate
3. Gradually switch preferred substrate
4. Concentrate on rewarding appropriate behavior
5. Interrupt when the dog starts to eliminate in an undesirable spot, then take the dog to a place more acceptable to you
6. Crate—use natural inhibition
7. Short lead for leash corrections
8. Walk and reinforce frequently; teach "knock"

PROTOCOL FOR ASSESSING PAIN AND STRESS IN DOGS

The tables contained in this handout were developed by veterinarians to assess pain and stress in dogs. These conditions may not be independent. Some behavioral complaints are the result of stress and/or pain, *or* may cause more stress and/or pain.

By using these scales, which are used in hospital and shelter settings, clients can evaluate their dogs when they first have a concern and seek help, and then repeatedly evaluate the dogs using the same scales during treatment. Treating behavioral problems is a process, so it is very useful to have a series of objective measures that can be evaluated repeatedly on a regular basis over time.

For clients whose dogs are not yet having problems, these scales can and should be used to evaluate all household dogs once or twice a year, and when anyone in the household dies or there are any additions to the household. Any changes or concerns should be discussed with your veterinarian.

There are four scales relevant to all dogs, and three additional scales that pertain only to certain situations (blood drawing, imaging, nail trimming). Clients may benefit from assessing their dogs during veterinary procedures. The clients' observations may help their vet to address fear as it appears, and may help protect the dog from becoming worse when repeatedly undergoing a set of procedures. Use of such scales is in keeping with meeting the dog's cognitive and behavioral needs while delivering the most humane care possible.

By recording the dog's responses at each visit, veterinarians and clients can detect changes in the dog's behavior, which will be relevant to ensure that the dog receives the best care.

The total score possible for scales one to four is 51. Dogs with a zero score are happy to go to the vet. Dogs with high scores likely need help.

Clinic Dog Stress Scale 1: Entry to the Clinic

Dog's behavior upon entering the veterinary practice and in the waiting room (this section can be completed by a member of the reception staff). A total of 5 points are possible. Dogs with a score of 5 are distressed and need help. Dogs with zero scores are calm.

Stress Level	Dog's Behavior/Demeanor
0	Extremely friendly, outgoing, solicitous of attention
1	Calm, relaxed, seemingly unmoved
2	Alert, but calm and cooperative
3	Tense, but cooperative, panting slowly, not very relaxed but can still be easily led on lead
4	Very tense, anxious, may be shaking or whining, will not sit or lie down if exposed (may do so behind owners' legs), panting, difficult to maneuver on lead
5	Extremely stressed, barking/howling, tries to hide, needs to be lifted up or forced to move

Clinic Dog Stress Scale 2: Weighing the Dog

Dog's behavior upon being weighed (this section can be completed by the veterinary nurse or technician who weighs the dog). A total of 5 points are possible. Dogs with a score of 5 are distressed and need help. Dogs with zero scores are calm.

Stress Level	Dog's Behavior/Demeanor
0	Extremely friendly, outgoing, solicitous of attention, eagerly gets onto scale
1	Calm, relaxed, seemingly unmoved, and walks easily onto scale and sits
2	Alert, but calm and cooperative, can get onto scale but not sit on it
3	Tense, but cooperative, panting slowly, not very relaxed but can still be easily led on lead, gets onto scale only with encouragement
4	Very tense, anxious, may be shaking or whining, will not sit or lie down if exposed (may do so behind owners' legs), panting, difficult to maneuver on lead, must be helped/encouraged to get on or stay on scale for 10 seconds to get reading
5	Extremely stressed, barking/howling, tries to hide, needs to be lifted up or forced to get onto or stay on scale for 10 seconds to get reading

Clinic Dog Stress Scale 3: Entering the Exam Room

Dog's behavior upon being brought into the exam room (this can be completed by whomever guides the client and dog to the room). A total of 5 points are possible. Dogs with a score of 5 are distressed and need help. Dogs with zero scores are calm.

Stress Level	Dog's Behavior/Demeanor
0	Extremely friendly, outgoing, solicitous of attention
1	Calm, relaxed, seemingly unmoved
2	Alert, but calm and cooperative
3	Tense, but cooperative, panting slowly, not very relaxed but can still be easily led on lead
4	Very tense, anxious, may be shaking or whining, will not sit or lie down if exposed (may do so behind owners' legs), panting, difficult to maneuver on lead, avoids room
5	Extremely stressed, barking/howling, tries to hide, needs to be lifted up or forced to move into room

Clinic Dog Stress Scale 4: Examining the Dog

Dog's behavior upon examination (this chart can be completed by the veterinary nurse or technician, and if needed, in consultation with the veterinarian). This chart evaluates body regions that are involved in the stress response. Having as much information as possible enables the veterinary staff to suggest interventions and to use the behaviors noted to assess improvement or debility. Rather than trying to remember if the dog is "worse" or "better" than at previous visits, this tick sheet allows the veterinary team to collect actual data and to use it to improve the quality of the dog's and client's experience. A total of 36 points are possible. Dogs with high scores are showing signs of stress and may be distressed. Dogs with low scores may be less distressed. Dogs with zero scores are calm.

Stress Level	Body Posture	Tail Posture	Ear Posture	Gaze	Pupils	Respirations	Lips	Activity*	Vocalization
0	Relaxed and moves on own	At rest for that breed or high	High and softly forward	Will look steadily at vet	Normal response to light	Normal—jaw relaxed	Relaxed	Flexible	None
1	Tense—can manipulate	Lower than at rest but not down	Moving back a bit	Looks only intermittently at vet	Normal to slight dilated	Normal—jaw tense	Firm	Inactive	Whine, cry
2	Rigid—hard to manipulate and a bit lower	Completely down	Fully back	Will not look at vet but scans room	Dilated, large amount of iris	Panting—dry	Licking lips	Paws flexed, may tremble	Whimper
3	Hunched—hard to see or examine belly and low posture	Tucked between legs	Ears back and down	Not scanning, looking steadily at distance or owner	Dilated, small amount of iris	Panting—dripping	Yawning and licking	Periodic trembling	Snarl, snap
4	Curled—completely withdrawn and belly maximally tucked	Clamped hard up to belly	As low and back as is possible	Staring fixedly and steadily at immediate fore-distance	Completely dilated—no iris	Profound panting, salivating, gasping		Uncontrollable trembling	Bite

Note if urinates, defecates, or releases anal sacs at any point.

Clinic Dog Stress Scale 5: Taking Blood from the Dog

This scale will only be used if blood is taken. The circumstance under which blood is taken should be noted below.

1. Laboratory evaluation: routine or because dog is ill? (circle one)
2. Tourniquet used? Y/N (circle one)
3. Vein from which blood was taken: _____
4. Restraint level: (circle one)
   a. None—dog sat still and butterfly catheter with digital pressure used
   b. Mild—vein held off manually
   c. Moderate—dog gently and minimally restrained physically while vein held off
   d. Severe—dog held down and restraint great

Stress Level	Body Posture	Respirations	Lips	Body Activity*	Forearm	Vocalization
0	Relaxed and moves on own	Normal—jaw relaxed	Relaxed	Flexible	Allows vet to pick up feet and forearm; forearm not stiff	None
1	Tense—can manipulate	Normal—jaw tense	Firm	Inactive	Allows vet to pick up feet and forearm; forearm stiff	Whine, cry
2	Rigid—hard to manipulate and a bit lower	Panting—dry	Licking lips	Paws flexed, may tremble	Allows touch but tries to withdraw forearm or body	Whimper
3	Hunched—hard to see or examine belly and low posture	Panting—dripping	Yawning and licking	Periodic trembling	Avoids all touch and needs leg held still	Snarl, snap
4	Curled—completely withdrawn and belly maximally tucked	Profound panting, salivating, gasping		Uncontrollable trembling	Avoids all touch and needs leg and body held still	Bite

Note if urinates, defecates, or releases anal sacs at any point.

Clinic Dog Stress Scale 6: Radiographing or Ultrasounding the Dog

Stress Level	Body Posture	Respirations	Lips	Body Activity*	Body	Vocalization
0	Relaxed and moves on own	Normal—jaw relaxed	Relaxed	Flexible	Allows vet to place as needed and remains loose and pliant	None
1	Tense—can manipulate	Normal—jaw tense	Firm	Inactive	Allows vet to place as needed but is stiff	Whine, cry
2	Rigid—hard to manipulate and a bit lower	Panting—dry	Licking lips	Paws flexed, may tremble	Allows vet to place by stretching out or manipulating areas and is rigid	Whimper
3	Hunched—hard to see or examine belly and low posture	Panting—dripping	Yawning and licking	Periodic trembling	Avoids manipulations by moving and stiffening, needs some restraint	Snarl, snap
4	Curled—completely withdrawn and belly maximally tucked	Profound panting, salivating, gasping		Uncontrollable trembling	Not possible to do without stretching and controlling head and legs	Bite

Note if urinates, defecates, or releases anal sacs at any point.

Clinic Dog Stress Scale 7: Trimming the Dog's Nails

Stress Level	Body Posture	Respirations	Lips	Body Activity*	Feet/legs	Vocalization
0	Relaxed and moves on own	Normal—jaw relaxed	Relaxed	Flexible	Allows vet to pick up feet and manipulate without resistance	None
1	Tense—can manipulate	Normal—jaw tense	Firm	Inactive	Allows vet to pick up feet, but stiff	Whine, cry
2	Rigid—hard to manipulate and a bit lower	Panting—dry	Licking lips	Paws flexed, may tremble	Allows touch to feet, but tries to withdraw them	Whimper
3	Hunched—hard to see or examine belly and low posture	Panting—dripping	Yawning and licking	Periodic trembling	Avoids all touch and needs foot/leg held	Snarl, snap
4	Curled—completely withdrawn and belly maximally tucked	Profound panting, salivating, gasping		Uncontrollable trembling	Avoids all touch and will not permit any access to feet without extreme restraint of body and feet	Bite

*Note if urinates, defecates, or releases anal sacs at any point.

The tables and scales used in this handout and the text were inspired by and/or adapted from: Döring D, Roscher A, Scheipl F, Kuchenhoff H, Erhard MH. Fear-related behavior of dogs in veterinary practice. Vet J 2009;182:38-43; Hellyer P, Rodan I, Brunt J, Downing R, Hagedorn JE, Robertson SA. AAHA/AAFP pain management guidelines for dogs and cats. J Am Anim Hosp Assoc 2007;43:235-248; and Hernander L. Factors influencing dogs' stress level in the waiting room at a veterinary clinic. SLU Student report 190, 2008; 29 pp; ISSN 1652-280X.

PROTOCOL FOR ASSESSING PAIN AND STRESS IN CATS

The two tables in this handout were developed by veterinarians to assess pain and stress in cats. Unfortunately, these conditions may not be independent in cats. Furthermore, when cats are exhibiting behavioral concerns, those concerns may be the result of stress and/or pain, *or* may cause more stress and/or pain.

By using these scales, which are used in hospital and shelter settings, clients can evaluate all the cats in their house when they first have a concern and seek help, and then repeatedly evaluate the cats using the same scales during treatment. Treating behavioral problems is a process, so it is very useful to have a series of objective measures that can be evaluated repeatedly on a regular basis over time.

For clients whose cats are not yet having problems, these scales can and should be used to evaluate all household cats once or twice a year, and when anyone in the household dies or there are any additions to the household. Any changes or concerns should be discussed with your veterinarian.

REFERENCES

Hellyer P, Rodan I, Brunt J, Downing R, Hagedorn JE, Robertson SA. AAHA/AAFP pain management guidelines for dogs and cats. JAAHA 2007;43:235–248.

Hellyer PW, Uhrig SR, Robinson NG: Canine Acute Pain Scale and Feline Acute Pain Scale, Fort Collins, 2006, Colorado State University Veterinary Medical Center. www.cvmbs.colostate.edu/ivapm/professionals/members/drug_protocols/painscale-caninenobandagesPAH.pdf.

Kessler MR, Turner DC. Stress and adaptation of cats (*Felis sylvetris catus*) housed singly, in pairs and in groups in boarding catteries. Anim Welf 1997;6:243–254.

McCune S: Temperament and welfare of caged cats. Doctoral dissertation, Cambridge, UK, 1992, University of Cambridge.

TABLE 1

Cat Pain Assessment Scale

Pain Score	Behavioral Patterns	Response to Palpation	Body Tension
0	Content and quiet when unattended. Comfortable when resting. Interested in or curious about surroundings.	Not bothered about palpation anywhere.	Minimal
1	Signs are often subtle and not easily detected in a hospital setting but are more likely to be detected at home by clients *(if the clients are asked to monitor the cat and schooled in how to do so)*. Earliest signs at home may be withdrawal from surroundings or change in the cat's normal routine. In the hospital, the cat may be content or slightly unsettled. The cat is less interested in the surroundings but will look around to see what is ongoing.	May or may not react to palpation of wound or surgery site.	Mild
2	Decreased responsiveness, seeks solitude. Quiet, loss of brightness in eyes. Lies in a curled up posture or sits tucked up with all 4 feet under body, shoulders hunched, head held slightly lower than shoulders, tail curled tightly around body. Eyes partially or mostly closed for either posture. Hair coat appears rough or fluffed up. May intensively groom an area that is painful, sensitive or irritating. Decreased appetite, not interested in food.	Responds aggressively or tries to escape if painful area is palpated or if that area is approached. Tolerates attention, may even perk up with petting if painful area is avoided.	Mild to moderate: reassess analgesic plan

TABLE 1

Cat Pain Assessment Scale—cont'd

Pain Score	Behavioral Patterns	Response to Palpation	Body Tension
3	Constantly yowling, growling, or hissing when unattended. May bite or chew at wound, but unlikely to move if left alone.	Growls or hisses at nonpainful palpation. The concern here is that the cat may be experiencing allodynia,* "wind-up,"† or fear that the pain could be made worse.	Moderate: reassess analgesic plan
4	Prostrate. Potentially unresponsive to or unaware of surroundings. Difficult to distract from pain. Receptive to care—even pretty awful cats and wild and feral cats will be more tolerant of contact.	May not respond to palpation. May be rigid to avoid pain induced by movement.	Moderate to severe: reassess analgesic plan

Modified from Hellyer et al., 2006.
*Allodynia—pain caused by a stimulus that does not normally result in pain (Hellyer et al., 2007).
†Wind-up pain—heightened sensitivity that results in altered pain thresholds both peripherally and centrally (consider using antianxiety agents) (Hellyer et al., 2007).

TABLE 2
The Seven-level Cat Stress Score*

Score	Body	Belly	Legs	Tail	Head	Eyes	Pupils	Ears	Whiskers	Vocalization	Activity
1 Fully relaxed	I: laid out on side or on back A: NA	Exposed, slow ventilation	I: fully extended A: NA	I: extended or loosely wrapped A: NA	Laid on the surface with chin upwards or on the surface	Closed or half open, may be slowly blinking	Normal (consider ambient light)	Normal (half back)	Normal (lateral)	None or soft purr	Sleeping or resting
2 Weakly relaxed	I: laid ventrally or half on side or sitting A: standing or moving, back horizontal	Exposed or not exposed, slow or normal ventilation	I: bent, hind legs may be laid out A: when standing extended	I: extended or loosely wrapped A: tail up or loosely downward	Laid on the surfaces or over the body, some movement	Closed, half opened or fully/ normally opened	Normal (consider ambient light)	Normal (half back) or erect and moved to front	Normal (lateral or forward)	None	Sleeping, resting, alert or active, may be playing
3 Weakly tense	I: laid ventrally or sitting A: standing or moving, back horizontal	Not exposed, normal ventilation	I: bent A: while standing extended	I: on the body or curved backward, may be twitching A: up or tense downward, may be twitching	Over the body, some movement	Normally opened	Normal (consider ambient light)	Normal (half back) or erect and moved to front or back and forward on head	Normal (lateral) or forward with small amount tension	Meow or quiet	Resting, awake or actively exploring
4 Very tense	I: laid ventral, rolled or sitting A: standing or moving, body behind lower than in front	Not exposed, normal ventilation	I: bent A: when standing hind legs bent, in front extended	I: close to the body A: tense downward or curled forward, may be twitching	Over the body or pressed to the body, little to no movement	Widely opened or pressed together	Normal or partially dilated	Erected to front or back, or back and forward on head	Normal (lateral) or forward with tension	Meow, plaintive meow or quiet	Cramped sleeping, resting or alert, may be actively exploring, trying to escape
5 Fearful, stiff	I: laid ventrally or sitting A: standing or moving, body behind, lower than in front	Not exposed, normal or fast ventilation	I: bent A: bent near the surface	I: close to the body A: curled forward, close to the body	On the plane of the body, less or no movement	Widely opened	Dilated	Partially flattened	Lateral (normal) or forward and back	Plaintive meow, yowling, growling, or quiet	Alert, may be actively trying to escape
6 Very fearful	I: laid ventrally or crouched directly on top of all paws, may be shaking A: whole body near to ground, crawling, may be shaking	Not exposed, fast ventilation	I: bent A: bent near the surface	I: close to the body A: curled forward close to the body	Near to surface, motionless	Fully opened	Fully dilated	Fully flattened	Back	Plaintive meow, yowling, growling, or quiet	Motionless alert or actively prowling
7 Terrorized	I: Crouched directly on top of all fours, shaking A: NA	Not exposed, fast ventilation	I: bent A: NA	I: close to the body A: NA	Lower than the body, motionless	Fully opened	Fully dilated	Fully flattened back on head	Back	Plaintive meow, yowling, growling, hissing or quiet	Motionless alert

*A further development of the Cat-Assessment-Score by McCune, 1992; from Kessler and Turner, 1997.
A, Active; I, inactive; NA, not applicable.

PROTOCOL FOR INTRODUCING A NEW BABY AND A PET

The addition of a new baby to a household can upset the social environment of that household and can upset the pets in the household. Steps can be taken to greatly reduce the probability of distress, and the potential risk that may go with distressed dogs and cats. The stepwise instructions below are primarily designed for two-parent families. However, it is possible to implement most of the instructions if only one parent is available, and notations for single parents have been made throughout the instructions.

Please remember that no animal should be left alone unsupervised with an infant for any reason. This is not because most animals are innately aggressive toward infants—they are not. But no infant would be capable of pushing an animal away if that animal cuddles up to them either for love or for heat. Until the child is old enough to behave absolutely appropriately with the pet (and that could be as old as 10 to 12 years), do not let children interact alone with the pets until you know how they will respond in a wide range of circumstances. This cautious behavior protects both the child and the pet.

Step 1

Before the baby comes, get your pet used to a regular schedule that you believe is realistic and that will be manageable when the baby is initially present. Start using the feeding, grooming, and walking schedules that your pet will experience once the baby is home. These schedules will probably be radically different than your current schedules, and it is best that your pets do not experience all baby-related changes at once when the baby arrives. Planning and practicing before the baby is born will make all the difference to your stress level and to how well you and your pet learn to adapt to the presence of a new child.

Include in your schedule a 5- to 10-minute period daily when you will attend only to your pet's needs. This period will provide your pet with quality time and can occur either in one bout or in two. During this time, pet your dog or cat, groom and scratch him, play with toys, use quiet and calm massage, talk to your pet—do all of the things your cat or dog likes but in a short, condensed session. This plan will allow you to rotate through various enjoyable activities by scheduling time to do so. Try to maintain this schedule no matter what (emergencies excepted), and make it one that can be implemented in the presence of the infant.

To accomplish this plan you may need to set your alarm 5 minutes earlier. You may have to have someone else watch the baby just in case the baby cries. You may also be able to watch over the baby while still giving your pet attention without terminating your session with your dog or cat unless the baby is distressed. How you choose to handle a crying baby will vary, but if you think about how this could affect your cuddle session with your pet, you will be able to make a sane and workable plan. Please remember that some pets are truly distressed by a child's cries. In this case, you will have the complex task of diminishing the pet's distress while attending to the baby's needs. The easiest way to do this may be to put your dog or cat on the other side of a door or gate.

Think of this time with your pet as time that you can set aside for you to relax also—the grooming, massage, and conversation with your pet can also be a respite for you. Be realistic and do not feel guilty. Five or 10 minutes of concentrated attention is probably more time than you give your dog or cat as a block now. Although everybody will have to adjust to an infant's schedule, providing your pet with scheduled time for attention is one way that you can tell your dog or cat that he is still important to you. Realize that if you have multiple pets, each will need at least 5 minutes of undivided attention each day. If you have pets who get along particularly well with each other, you can certainly team them up to play with or to talk to them, but remember that the more animals you have, the more difficult it will be to give them all of the things that they need. This is one reason why no one recommends adopting a pet (especially a kitten or puppy) just before or after a new child is added to the household.

Step 2

Make your schedule realistic and implement it before the arrival of the child. It would be preferable if the schedule changes could be made as early as possible before the arrival of the child. This is a good time to consider changing the mechanism you use to walk your dog. If you are using a choke collar or a regular buckle collar and your dog is not flawlessly responsive without ever pulling you, please consider teaching the dog to walk on a head halter or a no-pull harness (see the **Protocol for Choosing Collars, Head Collars, Harnesses, and Leads** for photos and specific examples). *The time to ensure that your dog can pose no risk to you or the baby even if the dog is startled, or there is traffic, or the walk is icy, or when another dog approaches, is before the baby arrives.* Ideally, you will want to be able to take your dog with you everywhere you go with the baby where dogs are welcome, and you want the dog to behave well. In addition, you do not want to struggle with a baby in a backpack or in a stroller and a dog who is pulling. Pulling dogs may create a potentially dangerous scenario for all three of you. You may want the protection of the dog, the company of the dog, and the necessary exercise for the dog when you are with the baby. A well-behaved dog will give you this. And, if you are unable to take the dog everywhere you take the baby, the dog may feel that he has been displaced by the baby, which could cause the dog to withdraw or otherwise alter his behavior. Although it is inappropriate to use terms such as jealousy when discussing the manner in which the pet treats the baby, any dog or cat recognizes changes in attention. Pets will also realize that attention has been transferred to another individual, possibly promoting attention-seeking behaviors that will detract from both the time budget you have created and the enjoyable relationship you'd hoped for. The more often you can exercise the dog or cat—physically and cognitively—with the child, the better everybody's relationship will be. As soon as you learn that an infant will be arriving, obtain and learn to use one of the more modern head collars or harnesses.

Step 3

Before the baby arrives, allow your pet to explore the baby's sleeping and diaper-changing area. For the same reasons discussed previously, you do not wish to wholly exclude any dog or cat from every place the baby will be. These areas will provide smells that are interesting to the dog or cat, so allow the pets to become familiar with them. By acclimating your dog or cat to the baby's room and items before the baby's arrival, you will avoid worrying about or yelling at your pet to get off the baby's items when the dog or cat is simply exploring a very interesting circumstance and environment. You will be using baby powder, lotions, diapers, and baby objects before you have the baby. Allow your cat or dog to become accustomed to these objects by sniffing, pawing, or nosing at them.

If the dog or cat tries to drag away any baby items, gently tell him that this is not okay, and ask the dog or cat to relinquish the object. If you are unable to get your pet to relinquish the object, now is the time to start teaching more appropriate manners, such as "sit," "stay," "drop," "down," "take it," and "drop it." Both cats and dogs can learn these cues, but we tend to worry more about dogs because of their size and the manner in which they interact. *If your dog cannot demonstrate success with these simple requests before the arrival of the baby, consider that you are likely to have serious management problems.* Now is the time, when you have some time, to address your pet's manners. It is insufficient to say that your dog has been to an obedience class if the dog still does not quickly and accurately respond to your request.

All dogs should have an emergency "stop" signal where they disengage from any activity and just stand still. Such a signal can save the dog's life in traffic, around wildlife and in an emergency situation. And it can also ease everyone's concern for accidents that could happen with a baby. If you do not know how to teach this request, and it requires only a special, protected word and the instructions provided in the **Protocol for Teaching Cats and Dogs to "Sit," "Stay," and "Come,"** please consider getting help from an excellent and humane trainer, such as those who are members of the Pet Professional Guild (www.petprofessionalguild.com). Mechanisms for teaching dogs these types of behaviors are also discussed in the **Protocol for Deference** and the **Protocol for Relaxation: Behavior Modification Tier 1.**

Do not let your dog or cat make a habit of sleeping in or on any of the baby's furniture simply because it will only seem like a further estrangement when you do not allow the pet to do so once the baby arrives. Dogs and cats can become familiar with the area and explore it, but they cannot camp out there as if it was a newly designed perch spot just for them.

If your pet has toys that are stuffed, these may look just like infant or baby toys, so expect that your pet may think that he can play with the baby's toys. If you are willing to wash the baby and dog/cat toys, there is nothing wrong from a health standpoint. The big problem is that the pet—usually the dog—may round up and take all of the infant's toys. As the baby ages, the dog may drag the toys from the baby's hand. Babies can be unintentionally, but tragically, injured under such circumstances. It may be preferable to shift the dog to toys that do not closely resemble the toys the baby may have. Such toys can have different scents or different sounds associated with them. Alternatively, you can establish some rules for using and storing toys (e.g., toys on floor are the dog's and cat's, toys not on the floor are the baby's). If your dog can "sit" and "stay" and take an object and "drop it" at your request now, you can use that behavior to teach both the baby and the dog how to interact appropriately with each other later in life.

Step 4

When the baby is born, have whomever has been caring for your pet at the time take home some articles of clothing that the baby has used. Having access to the baby's clothes/blankets/towels will teach your pet not only that these new clothing smells are part of the new repertoire, but also that there is an infant involved. Dogs and cats can easily identify individuals and families by scent, so help them to use this skill to learn that there is a new human who is part of their family. Allow the pet to smell any relevant items. Distribute them around the house to incorporate the baby's odor into the entire household. In this way, you will facilitate what will be a natural canine and feline behavior.

It is also best to make arrangements for your pet to be cared for in your home in advance of the arrival of the infant. Advance notice is good because dogs and cats are rushed around in a surprising manner, left with strangers and shifted quickly from one place to another, only to return home to discover the infant. For special-needs dogs and cats, such upheaval can be truly mentally traumatic. It is preferable to have your pets cared for in your home because familiarity will decrease their overall stress level. Any pet, especially if he does not like being in a kennel or has never been kenneled, may become more anxious and fearful when removed to the kennel. Your pet could then learn to associate the advent of this fear and anxiety with the advent of a new arrival. You can wholly avoid this concern with advance planning.

Step 5

When the baby comes home, you will need help. Someone should hold the baby while you go in to greet the dogs and cats. You have been missing from the household while either having or going to meet the baby, and the pets will have missed you. You should be able to greet and pay attention to all pets without having to tell them to go away and without having to risk them inadvertently knocking you over or scratching the baby. If you have a dog who jumps, that dog should be put in another room until everything is calm and you can get inside and have the time to greet him in a way that is meaningful and helpful. You may want to introduce any jumping dogs, dogs who are difficult to control, or those exuberant to the rest of the family, on a lead, if the lead provides more control, but first you should greet your dog or cat as exuberantly as you are greeted. Remember that you have been gone and that is potentially scary for pets. After the greeting process, the baby should be held by someone else and kept out of the way. When you are ready to start introducing the pets to the new baby, harnesses and leashes can be very helpful. Introductions should only be begun once all pets are already quiet and calm and everything is back to a more normal situation. This could take 15 to 30 minutes. During this time, the pets might be curious about the baby, but they must first calm down from the earlier rambunctious mode.

Step 6

Once the initial pandemonium has ceased, you are ready to start formally introducing the pets to the new baby. Your partner, spouse, or a friend who is helping you, should sit comfortably on the couch with the baby. You can then be responsible for controlling and monitoring your pet. The pet should be able to smell the baby and explore. Pets should be leashed or otherwise restrained in case they make any sudden movements toward the baby. If your pet is fearful of the baby, talk to him gently; use calm strokes while encouraging your dog or cat to quiet and to smell the baby. *Do not hold or dangle the child in front of the pet.* Such behavior could cause your pet to lunge simply to see the baby and is potentially dangerous. Dogs and cats and the baby will get used to each other on their own terms, but any infant that is dangling over a pet is in an abnormal social circumstance. If you are alone, you can put a harness on the pet and tie the harness to solid, stationary pieces of furniture with a leash. If you do this, you can then sit down at a distance where your pet can sniff the infant but not lunge. You can still verbally reward your cat or dog while enforcing this safe distance.

Remember to be calm at all times. Although one lick might be acceptable, you should be able to tell any dog or cat to cease licking and he should comply. If your dog or cat is unable to respond to a verbal request, licking is not acceptable simply because the risk that enthusiastic licking could injure an infant is high.

If your pet hisses or growls at the baby, you must be able to verbally stop those behaviors. If you cannot encourage your dog or cat to stop and come quietly to you, put him in another room until everyone is calm. As soon as everyone is calm, you can try this again in the same circumstances. Do not reassure your pets that it is "okay" and that "mommy" and "daddy" still love the pet—a truly unprovoked, aggressive behavior toward an infant is not okay. Most pets who are just worried readily learn that if they would like to be part of this expanded social circle and receive favorable attention, they must behave in a favorable manner toward the newest addition to the family.

If you have trouble getting your dog or cat to calm, in an emergency you can toss a towel or blanket over the cat or dog or toss some water on your pet simply as a disruptive stimulus. Then, you can remove your dog or cat to a quiet room and gradually work up to having her become accustomed to the baby. If your dog or cat does not respond to a verbal request to cease the threatening behavior as it starts, interrupt and remove the cat or dog, or interrupt the interaction and remove the child. You want to use the most humane interrupter possible that will allow you to safely protect and rearrange everyone. Most dogs and cats stop what they are doing if a blanket or towel is thrown over them, and this also allows feistier cats and dogs to be safely escorted from the room.

The next time this cat or dog approaches or is introduced to the baby, watch carefully to ensure a risky pattern is not developing. Remember that the point of any "correction" is to interrupt the dog or cat so that she aborts the worrisome behavior. You can then reinforce a more appropriate behavior, by rewarding—verbally, with a toy or with a treat—any other behavior that you find acceptable. The point of such interventions is not to terrify your pet. In fact, terrifying your dog or cat or brutally punishing her will grossly misfire and will teach your dog or cat that any time the infant is present horrible things happen. "Corrections" are best done immediately, or within the first 30 seconds *of the beginning* of the behavioral sequence, and that behavioral sequence usually starts with a look. For example, cats' eyes usually become huge, their ears move back, their hair is up, and she might arch the back, duck the neck, and retract the lips or sound nasty. Please do not wait for a pounce or a swat to interrupt, redirect, and remove any animal who is telling you that she is uncertain and worried. Tincture of time and gradual exposures are better than immersing any dog or cat in non-stop interaction with infants.

Step 7

When there is only one adult human at home with the infant during the first few weeks, pets should be restrained or confined in the presence of the infant. It is impossible for you to be sitting on the couch, ministering to a baby, and prevent an accident or attack involving the dog or cat, if the situation arises. The key for safe interactions is to avoid any aggression or any circumstances in which the dog or cat is uncertain and distressed. Both dogs and cats can be fitted with comfortable harnesses that can help keep them out of the range where they could even accidentally injure a baby.

Baby gates also work well for some dogs and cats. If the dog is prone to run through baby gates, a new baby is a potent stimulus. If you are tethering a dog or cat using a harness or using a gate, make sure that the full extent of the dog's or cat's reach, including the extent of the neck and head, is at least one dog/cat length away from the baby. Remember that you will invariably be nursing the baby, using your laptop, talking by phone, and the doorbell will ring at the same time. Any dog or cat who is problematic may wait for a moment when your guard is lowered to lunge at the baby. Most of the time these dogs and cats are just trying to get information helpful to them about household changes, but they could still injure an infant. Dogs and cats do not object to being banished from a room for short periods of time if their needs are otherwise met.

Step 8

If, after 3 weeks or so, your pet accepts the baby with no untoward behavior, try unleashing the dog or cat in the presence of another person who can help if anyone becomes startled. Regardless, you will still need to closely supervise and observe. It is best if one partner/spouse tends to the pet while the other tends to the baby. It is important that if two people are to share caretaking duties and the responsibility for reinforcing appropriate behavior, that one person does not always reinforce the dog or cat. Sharing and trading off the attention for the dog and the baby is critical for both people so that the dog or cat learns to associate the warm, loving environment with everybody. For dogs or cats who do not respond well to voice requests and for whom the baby is a strong stimulus, consider never leaving him alone with the child, even in passing, until the child can fend for herself. In some cases, dogs or cats should not be alone with the child if only one adult is available until the dog or cat can be taught to react more appropriately to the child.

Please do not believe that a muzzle will protect an infant or a young child from damage by a dog. Muzzles may prevent bites, but they do not dissuade the dog from lunging and pushing on the child. Infants and young children are particularly susceptible to crush injuries and, in many cases, skulls have been fractured by a dog that lands on a child in play, and without the intention to do damage. True accidents can still be tragic.

Step 9

If your pets do not pose a hazard (e.g., tripping, falling, jumping, grabbing) and they are truly just being social, there is no reason, once they are accustomed to the new baby, that they cannot accompany the parent around the house and be with the baby while she is being changed, bathed, and so on. In fact, this helps facilitate the future interaction between the child and the pet, and may help the child become a kinder, more humane individual by learning age-appropriate pet behavior. Regardless, any dog or cat so treated should be very responsive to voice requests so that no struggle should ever ensue in getting the dog to comply with a desired behavior.

Step 10

Under no circumstances should any pet be allowed to sleep in a room with an unattended infant or young child. Use a baby monitor, an intercom, or a room monitor, and close the door. Predatory tendencies are far less of a concern than is the fact that a dog or cat could inadvertently smother a child. The amount of guilt associated with a tragedy would be unbearable for both the new parent and the pet.

Step 11

If your pet is aggressive or frightened around the child, you should start exposing the pet to children very gradually. Go back to Steps 5 and 6. Such pets must be supervised in all interactions with children. Remember that even muzzled animals can harm infants. Predatory aggression is the most common form of aggression shown by dogs to very young infants, whereas aggression caused by pain or fear is frequently associated with older children (18 to 36 months of age). These children are often uncoordinated and may inadvertently hurt a pet by their play or their ambulatory capabilities. Older pets who may be arthritic or that have painful hips or shoulders are particularly at risk, as are those with chronic ear conditions. These are body regions that children frequently grab. Young children should be taught to treat pets gently: no pulling, no tugging, and no pounding on them. Again, this is especially important if the pet is old, ill, or arthritic because any dog that is in pain may use a bite as its only defense against a rambunctious child. For more information see the **Protocol for Teaching Kids—and Adults—to Play with Dogs and Cats** and the **Protocol for Handling and Surviving Aggressive Events** for a list of age-specific behaviors that children may exhibit with pets.

Finally, there has been a well-documented link between animal abuse and child abuse. Children who abuse animals will progress to abuse of other individuals and will abuse their own children in the future. In turn, many children who are abused will abuse pets. If your child has a problem complying with age-specific, appropriate, humane, and gentle handling conditions of pets, it could be that the child has a problem or has observed this behavior from friends. If so, this potential problem should be explored. On the very positive side, appropriate pet-child behavior can be a wonderful experience and can help make the children more humane and socially well-adjusted.

PROTOCOL FOR THE INTRODUCTION OF A NEW PET TO OTHER HOUSEHOLD PETS

This handout has a tick sheet at the end that summarizes the main points. If you are an experienced pet person, you may not need to read the entire handout in detail if the tick sheet makes sense to you. If you have questions, the answers are likely in the handout.

Adjustment and Transition

When you first bring home a new pet, expect a period of transition and adjustment for the other pets in the household. You may find that some of your pets hide from the new addition, while others might try to push him around. Sometimes, the original pets will start to do behaviors designed to get your attention, including barking, pawing, stealing items, or pushing the new addition out of the way and jumping all over you. Cats may mark with urine, feces, or their claws. All of these behaviors can be normal and are not worrisome if they change within a week or two. If you have a younger animal, or one who is going through social maturity, you may find that he "regresses" a bit and reverts to younger behaviors for a short while. He will recover and catch up quickly.

If the animals in the household do not revert to normal within a short time, or if they become aggressive, you have a problem that will not go away on its own. Short, temporary changes in appetite may be normal; not eating or only eating at odd hours or in certain circumstances is not normal. The sooner you seek help from your veterinarian and/or a qualified specialist, the better off you will be.

Before Introducing the New Pet

Before introducing **any** new pet, make sure she is healthy and up-to-date on **all** relevant vaccinations, make sure that tests for fecal parasites are negative, and that the pet is flea-free. It is particularly important that all new cats are checked for their viral titer (feline immunodeficiency virus [FIV], feline leukemia virus [FeLV]) status. The conventional wisdom is that positive cats should not be brought into negative households.

Gradual Introductions

You can make the transition easier for new pets by using gradual introductions. This means that, unless it is "love at first sight," the new pet should be kept separate from the other pets whenever they are not closely supervised. This advice may be a bit extreme, but it is designed to ensure both that no injuries occur and that the social system of the original pets isn't suddenly fragmented. The original pet or pets should have access to the same areas of the house as previously. If the original dog was crated, the crate can still be used. If access was restricted to the first floor, this pattern should continue to be followed.

The new pet should be placed in a neutral area (e.g., a den, finished basement, or brightly lit bathroom) with toys, a blanket, water, a litterbox if the new pet is a cat, and anything else that she might need. It is important that the new pet **not** be placed *only* in an area that is considered highly desirable by the other pets. Areas of high value usually include places where the people spend a lot of time with the pets (bedrooms)

or where the pets choose to stay when alone (around food dishes, window sills that are good perch sites). If you restrict the new pet to a highly valued and preferred area and exclude the other pets from it, you may be provoking anxieties that accompany rehoming on all sides.

Introduce the new pet gradually. First, spend some time alone with the new pet. Then bring the new pet out on a leash or harness and let the other pets explore her. If you anticipate problems, the other animals can be on leashes or harnesses, too. If you have too many animals to adequately monitor under these circumstances, the new pet can be placed in a crate or cage in the center of a room and the other pets can *sequentially* explore the caged pet. *Please note that you can only place a dog or cat in a cage or crate if he is comfortable in it. If you see any signs of panic or freezing behavior, do not use the enclosure. By doing so, you will cause behavioral harm.* Ensure that if the resident pet is hostile, the new pet cannot feel "trapped" by removing any hostile animal and placing the crate in an area where the crated animal cannot be victimized. Animals newly introduced to other animal households need to have some quiet, secure time.

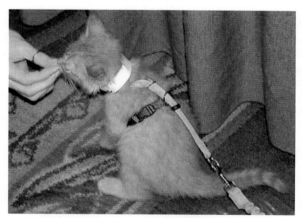

A commercially available harness and lead for cats that could help facilitate introductions.

Crates

If you have a dog that is always crated, you can accustom her quickly to a new dog by crating the new dog at a distance where she can be seen by the original dog, but where they cannot directly interact through the crates. As the dogs become more accustomed to each other, their crates can be moved gradually closer together until they are side-by-side.

"Pet-Proofing" Your Home

Beware that the area in which you are confining the new pet should be "pet proof." This means that toilet seats should be down, electric cords should be up and put away, sockets should be protected with child-guards, and any valuable or fragile items should be moved. New pets will explore and that exploration should not put them in danger. If the new pet is a very young puppy or kitten you may wish to crate her for her own protection (see handout on **Protocol for Basic Manners Training and Housetraining for New Dogs and Puppies**). Crates do not afford total protection from willful and determined claws and teeth of an un-crated animal, but they do greatly minimize the risk of damage.

What About "Recycled" Pets?

Many newly adopted pets are "recycled" pets who are being rehomed. You may have some knowledge of their reasons for rehoming, but it is unlikely that you know all the triggers that will cause such dogs or cats distress. If you try to separate the new pet by placing him in a crate or a separate room and he becomes more distressed, please consider using leads, harnesses, and baby gates, rather than true separations, to control interactions. One of the common problems with recycled pets is panic that is associated with confinements. If the distress is as described, you will not overcome it by repeating the isolation; instead, you will make the animal more anxious. If you note a problem associated with extreme distress or panic, please consult your veterinarian and/or a specialist in veterinary behavioral medicine sooner rather than later.

Where Might There Be Problems?

Whenever any animal is isolated for any reason, it is critically important that the dog or cat still receives a lot of social attention. "Separate" does not have to mean "deprived." This is especially true for new pets. When you come home, greet the original pets (ask them to sit and look at you first) and let them out, if this is your normal routine. Do not rush—when people are stressed and rushed they may either facilitate undesirable interactions between the pets or fail to attend to the dog's or cat's cues about impending problems.

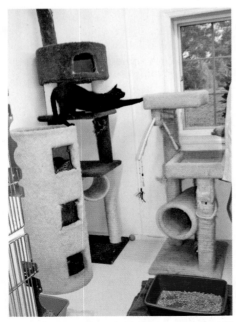

This set of cat condos built for a rescue group provides for both "separate" and "shared" space use during introductions. Similar solutions may help in homes.

Please remember that the dogs in your household do not live in a true "pack," nor do the cats live in a true "pride." In a true pack, new additions are neither abrupt nor adult: puppies are born into groups of known animals and grow knowing them. For the vast majority of humans, this is not a pattern reflected in their canine or feline household, and to expect the resident animals not to react is just not realistic. When we add a new pet, we are disrupting the social structure. Think about it: We bring in an unannounced, unrelated stranger—maybe even an alien species—and expect everyone to be instantly happy. How would most of us react under the same circumstances?

The best times to perform gradual introductions are when the animals are calm. Start by petting the original pets and telling them that it is "okay" **only** if it is truly okay—do not reward hissing, growling, or biting. When you tell a pet it is "okay" when he is upset, you are not calming him down— you are rewarding his inappropriate behavior. If the animals in the household are calm, and either ignore each other or act friendly despite the new addition, you can feed them within sight of the new pet. This distance should be close enough that they can easily see and watch each other, but not so close that they exhibit any signs of distress (e.g., not eating, eating at a faster rate, hissing, growling, snarling, et cetera). Once you find this distance you can move their food dishes closer together by an inch a day until they are side-by-side. If you ever have an aggressive encounter, back off from that distance and return to the last distance where neither pet reacted. Leave the dishes there for a few days and then gradually start to move them again. Feeding and petting the animals in each other's presence can teach them that good things happen when they are together and calm. This will not happen if either participant reacts violently.

Problems That Start Between the Old and New Pets Now That a New One Is in the Household

If one animal responds to a gradual introduction with frank and forceful aggression, remove the aggressor to a neutral zone **immediately** and try again when she is calm. It can take anywhere from seconds to hours for the aggressor to calm. When you go to reintroduce the animals again, if the same animal again behaves aggressively in the same manner, separate the animals for the rest of the day or evening, and try later in the day or during the next morning. The separation must ensure that the animals cannot physically interact, and this includes preventing them from staring at each other.

Much posturing involving behaviors associated with aggression—hissing, growling, showing teeth, circling, piloerection (hair lifting on scruff, neck, or back)—is part of a normal way for animals to provoke social systems with other animals to obtain information. You may not like these behaviors, but they can be normal. If this is the only antagonistic type of behavior you witness, just keep calling the animals to you, and when they come, reward them for doing so and again for sitting and being quiet. Chances are animals who behave like this will work it out.

If there is actually physical grabbing and wrestling, call the animals to separate them. If a verbal signal succeeds in separating them, *and* after the antagonistic event the animals do not seem worried about or fearful of each other, *and* no physical damage was done, don't interfere the next time they interact. Some aggressive and undesirable interactions are not violent, but are still not conducive to the development of a good relationship between the pets.

If, on the other hand, when you try to separate the animals the behaviors intensify, one animal is clearly afraid, or if there is any damage, you have at least one animal exhibiting excessive aggressive behavior. This is the animal with whom you will have to work to gradually accustom the animals to each other.

You can learn to watch for subtle behaviors that can signal potential problems. In dogs, these behaviors include piloerection (hair lifting on scruff, neck, or back), staring, snarling, stalking, side-by-side posturing with growling or lip lifting, and pinning the other animal by grabbing his neck. Watch the recipient of such agonistic encounters. If the recipient is unable to respond to the agonistic individual in a way that decreases the exhibition of potentially threatening behaviors, you may wish to go slowly. You do not want one dog to feel helpless in the presence of another, and some dogs may not read or handle antagonistic signals as well as other dogs.

Cats are masters of subtle threats and their biggest nonvocal threats include a direct stare and an elevation of the rump and base of the tail with or without piloerection. Hissing, snarling, and pouncing are also threats, but are less intimidating to many animals than a direct stare accompanied by an elevated or humped rump. Again, watch for the response of the recipient of the stare. If the recipient of the stare can behave in a way that causes the staring cat to behave in a less-threatening manner, terrific. If you feel that the new cat is losing the contest, is terrified, or is becoming so aggressive she might injure the original pet, separate the animals.

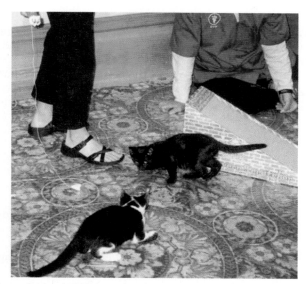

Normal wary behaviors of two rescue kittens who do not know each other while being introduced on "neutral" turf. Note that each cat stares at the other.

When separating animals, please **do not** put your hands or other body parts between the animals! This is the single most common way people are injured by pets. Use cardboard, brooms, blankets thrown over them, loud noises, or, if you are desperate, water (from a hose, bowl, bucket, open a shaken bottle of seltzer) to separate the animals. If you can

identify the aggressor, banish **that** animal to neutral turf. If you cannot identify one aggressor, banish everyone to different pieces of neutral turf.

If the new pet is sitting in close proximity to the other pets and everything seems to be going well, tell all the animals that they are good and give them all small food treats and petting; they like to be petted. This works best if you have two people so one person can hold the new pet while the other deals with the other animals. If you are working with two people, switch roles so that the new pet doesn't just associate her rewards with one person. If you are only one person, this can still be accomplished by using leashes and harnesses and crates. Leashes can be tied to furniture or door knobs that are at a distance that will allow the pets to sniff each other and react, but not permit them to lunge at and injure one another. **Never** leave a tied pet unsupervised even for a minute: an unsupervised, tied dog or cat can strangle and die.

For the entire time that you are doing the above—and it could take hours or weeks—make sure that each pet has 5 to 10 minutes alone with you each day, when all you do is pay attention to that pet. This attention could be grooming, playing with a toy, petting and massage, or just sitting in the grass next to you. Make sure that the pet is happy and relaxed at these times. If you know in advance that you are getting a new pet, you may want to set these periods of individual attention up in advance of the new arrival. If these periods follow a regular schedule the pets will learn to anticipate them. Because they can rely on these set periods, it may decrease their anxiety about the new addition.

Once you are able to get the pets to react to each other in a positive manner, or not to react at all when restrained, take away the restraints. Be vigilant, and be ready to interrupt any dangerous situations. A raised voice, a whistle, or clapped hands will stop most minor skirmishes, but if you need a more forceful stimulus you also need more help.

If the pets are all being good, remember to reward them with praise and treats.

Once you have done the above, you are ready to let the animals out of your sight. Bell the new animal by attaching a bell to her collar so that you and the other animals always know where they are (see Bear Bells at www.rei.com). Consider using a breakaway collar that will release if snagged on furniture or grabbed by another animal. Use of a collar and a bell will allow you to spy on any potentially problematic interactions and to interrupt them before they get out of hand. During this period when you are beginning to provide the pets with free access, remember to provide additional water dishes, litterboxes, beds, toys, et cetera, so that you minimize competition and the potential aggressive interaction.

The keys to making this all work are patience and observation. It is critical that the animals are not inadvertently encouraged to become hostile or nervous in each other's presence by well-meant but misplaced reassurance for inappropriate behaviors. Expect that the social system may shift. For example, the dog that *you* always thought of as the "boss dog" may not only be relegated to what *you* perceive as a lower position, but may prefer not having to be the dog who always makes all the decisions. Let your pets set their own pace and forge their own relationships. In many cases the pets never become close companions, but are reasonably content leading separate lives under the same roof. This is far preferable to frank aggression. Do not push the animals too hard, or push for relationships they clearly do not want; this could backfire and you could undo most of the good you had previously done.

Problems That Start Between or with the Old Pets Now That a New One Is in the Household

If you have pets who have lived in the same household, but have begun to have some problems with interaction, the above protocol can also help them (for more detailed information for dogs, see **Protocol for Understanding and Treating Dogs with Interdog Aggression** or the **Protocol for Understanding and Treating Feline Aggressions with an Emphasis on Intercat Aggression**). **Regardless, the general rule in managing these situations is to reward the pet who is behaving the most appropriately, given the context.** The pet who is the victim of the aggressive behavior should be fed, walked, and given attention before the aggressor. This will help to reinforce his right to be able to live unmolested.

If confinement of one pet becomes necessary, confine the aggressor in a neutral or lower-quality room. Do not confine the aggressor in the place where she would rather spend her time—this will only convince her that their contest is meritorious.

When you start to reintroduce the pets, do it gradually, as described above. Move from introductions under controlled circumstances to ones where they are being monitored from a distance. Let the animals' behaviors tell you when you are ready to progress. This time, put a bell on the collar of the aggressor. At the first sign of any aggressive behavior, and definitely within 30 to 60 seconds of the *onset of the behavioral progression,* use whatever minimum level of startle or disruption necessary to get the animals' attentions and to abort the interaction. For some animals this will be clearing your throat or calling their name; for others you'll need something more intense (e.g., clapping your hands). This means that you do not wait to interrupt the cat until he has pounced on the kitten, but that you interrupt him as soon as he stares at her. Timing is everything. The disrupted stimulus must be sufficient that the behavior is aborted. At that time reassure the victim, and after everyone has calmed down, engage them both in behaviors that are incompatible with aggression (i.e., feeding and petting). If the aggression persists, banish the aggressor until he is calm, and then try again. If the aggression continues, banish the aggressor until later in the day or the next morning.

The Concept of Flooding

If the aggression, either between new pets or pets already in the household, continues, someone will likely have recommended a behavioral modification technique called "flooding." You need to think clearly about whether this is something that can be done safely in your household. **In the vast majority of cases, flooding is a terrible, traumatic, and damaging idea.** Because flooding is almost never a good idea, anyone considering it should consult a behavioral specialist to see if

it is even wise to consider using this technique. Flooding **can** be a last resort in truly exceptional circumstances, but you really must ensure that you are reading the animals' signals correctly or you will do irreparable harm. Remember that flooding is almost always done incorrectly, that it works best in mild, very specific situations, and that it can permanently damage animals. The technique is discussed here only because it's such a commonly—**and wrongly**—recommended panacea.

In flooding, one animal is kept confined or otherwise restrained, while he is reacting inappropriately in the presence of the other animal. He is kept in that restrained or confined situation until the level of the inappropriate reaction diminishes by at least 50%. You must measure the changes in behavioral and physiological reactions before and during the process. Obviously, you could not keep an animal on leash for days on end without respite, but an aggressive animal can be crated for an extended period with food, water, toys, litterbox, if necessary, and a blanket, while the other animal is either locked in a room with him or placed in a similar cage facing him. If one animal is loose, you should know that she could injure the caged animal, or be injured by him, by sticking her paws through the crate. **If the animals become more aggressive and upset, flooding is failing, is counterproductive, doing harm, and should be stopped.**

Honest assessments should render the consideration and use of flooding as the exceptional case. **Do not attempt any flooding methodologies without qualified advice from a specialist.** Other strategies are likely to be much more helpful and successful.

Medication?

Finally, pharmacological intervention may succeed in helping create a harmonious household where other interventions have failed. There are many newer anxiolytics available, which, when used correctly and prescribed by qualified individuals, may be useful adjuvants to behavioral and environmental modification. In very extreme cases of inter-animal aggression, in which all other therapies, including pharmacological, have failed, the best, kindest, and safest solution may be to place one of the animals in a new home.

Tick List

☐ 1. Separate the pets when they are unsupervised.
☐ 2. Crate one or more of the pets.
☐ 3. Pet proof the home.
☐ 4. Gradually introduce the pets using food and rewards.
☐ 5. Introduce the pets during quiet times using leashes and harnesses.
☐ 6. Use whistles, water, blankets, et cetera, to interrupt any ongoing and potentially injurious aggression.
☐ 7. Be familiar with physical signs of impending aggression, and know how to safely interrupt such behavior.
☐ 8. Bell the new animal when you are ready to introduce her to the household unsupervised.
☐ 9. **Reward, reward, reward any calm or happy behavior.**
☐ 10. New home? This will be an exceptional outcome to adding a new animal if the above are done well.

PROTOCOL FOR TEACHING CATS AND DOGS TO "SIT," "STAY," AND "COME"

There are three signals/requests that, if your dog or cat knows them, will make your life a pleasure. In fact, in certain cases *these signals will save your pet's life.* These signals are "sit," "stay," and "come," and they are all easy to teach. If you teach your pet to respond to these signals early in your relationship, they can become the foundation for anything else you wish the pet to do and for further "collaboration and cooperation."

Notice that here these signals are not called "commands." Calling them commands puts us in an adversarial relationship with our pets. We don't want this type of relationship. An adversarial relationship, coupled with the anger it often carries, is one reason why dogs and cats who know these signals choose to ignore them.

Humans act in a unique kind of social guardianship relationship with their pets, and so we should realize that our pets are totally dependent on us. We need to be patient and clear in our signals to our pets. It's likely that our pets speak "human" better than we speak "dog" or "cat." If we teach our dogs and cats these three basic signals as soon as they come to live with us, there will be no chance for them to learn undesirable behaviors.

Older, rescued, or rehomed animals can learn these requests, too, but it may take a little more patience. For animals with a prior history, positive reinforcement, praise, and rewarding what you want the cat or dog to do—not punishing what you don't want them to do—are the keys to success.

Notice that this protocol can be used for both cats and dogs. Cats can be taught to "sit," "stay," "come," "lie down" (or "down"), "roll over," "salute," give "high fives," et cetera, just as dogs can, and they, too, will benefit from the mental stimulation. You may have to choose different treats for your cats than you do for your dogs, but many cats and dogs like the same things: cheese, liver, shrimp, sardines, and chicken. Tiny slivers of these are easy to prepare, cheap, and can be frozen in plastic bags to be available as "single servings." Many cats love yeast spreads—Marmite and Vegemite—making tiny amounts easy to use as rewards.

Teaching "Sit"

The easiest way to teach a cat or dog to "sit," "stay," and "come" is to use food treats. Please consider using a food reward or salary, particularly if the dog or cat has been rehomed and needs to reshape behaviors. Many humans have a tremendous resistance to using food rewards for dogs. The charitable explanation for this is that they do not understand that a food reward is **not** a bribe, but rather a salary. It is important to understand the difference and to avoid bribes.

- A *bribe comes before* the desired behavior, as a lure to distract the dog or cat from a behavior we don't like.
- A *reward/salary comes after* a behavior is perfectly executed. Rewards show that when the dog or cat attends to our requests, we recognize his good behavior and provide him with an *earned* reward.

A reward structure sets the standard for compassionate, but disciplined guidance as part of guardianship or partnership relationship.

Food rewards may not be necessary to teach and enforce behaviors for dogs that already know how to sit—happy, calm petting and praise may be sufficient. Food rewards can be extremely useful in teaching puppies who do not know how to sit how to do so. Puppies are babies and have short attention spans. Food will help focus them.

Few people teach cats to sit so even if you adopt a rehomed cat, no one has likely ruined the sit request for you.

If the food treat is held in one of your hands between two fingers, and if that hand is first placed in front of the pup's (cat's, kitten's, adult dog's) nose and then raised up and back, the pup's head will begin to move to follow it. Gradually the pup will sit because it is easier and more comfortable to do so. If you say "sit (2- to 3-second pause), sit (2- to 3-second pause)," et cetera, while doing this, and as soon as the puppy accidentally sits, say, "Good **sit**!" and **instantly** give the treat, the pup will be reinforced in the appropriate time period.

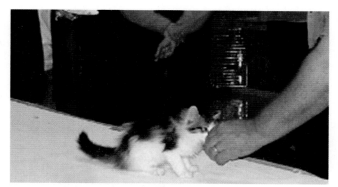

Kitten being taught to sit using a table (for ease of reaching the kitten by the human) and a food treat.

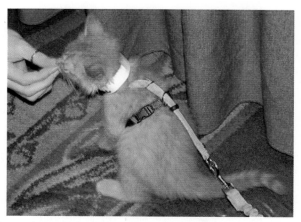

Using a harness to keep a rescue kitten from roaming while teaching him to sit for a treat. As soon as the kitten's bottom touched the floor, the treat was put into his mouth.

This pattern of behavioral requests, responses and rewards must be repeated until the puppy does it flawlessly and without hesitation. This will generally take less than 5 minutes for a pup or kitten that has not yet developed bad or inattentive behaviors. If you practice by asking the puppy or kitten to sit once or twice every 15 or 30 minutes the puppy or kitten will not forget what's learned. Now, if you ask the puppy or kitten to sit for everything (e.g., to be petted, groomed, fed, to have a leash put on, et cetera) you will have encouraged a very calming behavior and created a nicely mannered pet!

Is it necessary to push on the puppy's or kitten's bottom to "make the puppy sit"? **No,** and given how big we are and how small the puppies and kittens can be, it might be unwise to force them to sit. We could injure their hips or spines, and some breeds of cats and dogs who are predisposed for hip problem may have a special risk.

There are **at least three other choices** for teaching "sit," **none of which involve force.** Here are three suggestions.

1. You can gently put a hand behind the kitten's bottom. As the kitten backs up, their bottom hits the hand. Now you can gently shape the kitten to sit for a reward by following the instructions, above, by having the kitten follow a treat. When the head is tipped up, the kitten moves down and back. If it is not possible to move back because of the hand, the kitten will sit.
2. You can have another person stand behind the pup with their feet near the pup's haunches; as the pup backs up the person's feet and legs will shape the puppy's body in the sit position. This technique also works for cats.
3. A head collar can help you to teach puppies to sit and may help with big, fast, or overly exuberant pups. More information on these pups is found in the handout **Protocol for Choosing Collars, Head Collars, Harnesses and Leads.** This technique is the only one that is difficult to implement for cats because there are no great kitty head collars, but a good harness can at least prevent a rambunctious kitten from running and help her to focus.

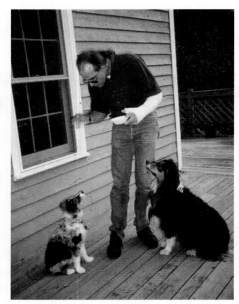

Using an older dog as a model to teach "sit" to a 9.5-week-old puppy.

Teaching "Stay"

While cats tend to stay and observe more than dogs do, "stay" can still be more difficult to teach than "sit" because we humans forget that puppies and kittens have a different attention span than we do. We want our pets to learn more quickly than they are sometimes able.

There is a lot of variation in dogs' abilities to relax and stay, and we often, without realizing it, give inconsistent signals with our body language. For example, most humans talk to dogs over their shoulders as we walk away and then wonder why the dog did not "stay." Dogs who do not know "stay" won't learn it if you are walking away when you are talking to them. They will, instead, follow you. If we become angry, the dog becomes scared and we did harm, all because we didn't understand how dogs read body language! When working with animals, children, your friends, and yourself, try to remember that the first and most important rule is **do no harm.**

Starting to Teach "Stay"

First, your dog or cat needs to know how to sit.

If your dog is physically more comfortable lying down, that's fine. If you decide to show the dog in obedience, you will soon enough teach him that "sit" and "stay" differ. We want the dog in a posture of "deferential" behavior, where he is calm and can pay attention to you.

Sitting is a less reactive posture than is standing, lying down is less reactive than is sitting. Some dogs are calmer or more comfortable when lying down, so this is the preferred posture for them. Please keep the age, physical condition, and attention span of your dog or cat in mind when asking him to assume any posture. Cats can have hip pain and dysplasia as do dogs, so the position requested may affect compliance.

Next, ask your dog or cat to "sit," verbally praise him, say "stay," and take a tiny step—a few centimeters—backward. Almost instantly repeat "stay," go back to the dog or cat, repeat "stay," and reward. A sample sequence looks like this.

"Bonnie—sit—good girl! (treat)—stay—good girl—stay (take a 2-cm step backward while saying "stay"—then stop almost instantaneously)—stay Bonnie—good girl—stay (return quickly while saying "stay"—then stop)—stay Bonnie—good girl (treat)—okay (is the release and she can get up)!"

Note the Following

1. Please use your dog's or cat's name—this will get her to attend to you. You can use your pet's name frequently, unlike in obedience, **as long as she is paying attention to you.** Pets who have not been taught to ignore their names will look at you when you use their names. If your pet doesn't look at you immediately when you say her name, put the treat near your eye. You need her to focus. Ask her to "look" when the treat is near your eye. If you do this regularly, your dog or cat will begin to look to your face whenever you say the word "look." Watch the video, *Humane Behavioral Care for Dogs: Problem Prevention and Treatment,* for a demonstration of how to do this. If your dog or cat has learned or been taught by yelling to ignore you, you may need another sound to get your pet's attention. Try clicking with your tongue, whistling, et cetera. Failing this, clickers are commercially available that are not so loud that they startle anyone as a whistle might.
2. Repeat the requests/signals as the dog or cat requires and when she is paying attention to you. With improvement, you will repeat the signals less frequently and at greater intervals. This is a process known as "shaping" behavior.
3. Reward your dog or cat appropriately: use small, high-quality treats **every single time** he exhibits the desired

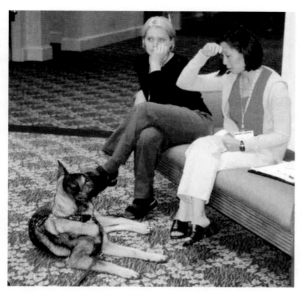

Here, the person is teaching the dog to look at her and be calm while lying down. Some dogs, like this one, are calmer when lying down than they would be when sitting.

behavior. Eventually, the food treats will appear less predictably, but we learn best when we are rewarded every time we do something right.

4. Remember to use one or two words consistently as a releaser (e.g., "okay," "all done"). Then remember that if you use those words while talking to your dog, he will get up. If he gets up before being released, ask him to "sit" and "stay" again, and wait 3 to 5 seconds—without a treat—then repeat "stay" and treat. Now you can either continue with the practice session or release the dog or cat. By repeating the "stay" signal and having a very short interval where the pet is not rewarded until the second "stay," you will prevent jack-in-the-box behavior that will otherwise accidentally be taught by rewarding the dog or cat every time she sits, regardless of staying.

As your pet becomes more experienced and masters staying at a short distance, **gradually** increase the distance between you and your dog or cat. **Do not** go from having your pet stay within 1 meter of you to walking across a 20 meter room. This is too great a distance and too quick a transition for a cat or dog who may not be sure what you want. The temptation will be great for you to do this, but remember that **this isn't about you: it's about teaching the dog or cat to be less anxious.** If you move too quickly, you have just signaled unclearly and provoked anxiety.

You can also practice these signals on lead, using a head collar or a harness (but see **Protocol for Choosing Collars, Head Collars, Harnesses, and Leads**). Using a head collar or harness permits you to reinforce sitting long-distance and to more quickly "correct" the dog or cat if he gets up. A note about "correction" is essential.

• The "correction" we are talking about here is not brutal; it's a gentle "un-uh" or any soft sound that will allow your pet to stop and look to you for cues about what he should be doing. A harness and a lead allow you to slowly and gently keep your pet's attention so that he can again focus on the task. Think of what you need as an interruption

that encourages the animal to look to you for further information.

Remember that the younger the dog or cat, or the longer you have been working in the session, the shorter your pet's attention span becomes. If you find that your pet is making more mistakes as the session progresses, you are better off practicing for a few minutes 6 times a day rather than once a day for 30 minutes.

Teaching "Come"

"Come" is the easiest of the requests to teach because it uses your dog's or cat's natural curiosity and willingness to follow you. If your pet is older, you may be able to accomplish this as simply as starting with the animal sitting and paying attention to you, and then your walking away while patting your thigh and saying "come!" in a happy voice. You can make the transition more clear by sitting with your cat or dog, using a treat to encourage him to "look," and then getting up and moving away as discussed while holding the treat at his eye level.

Young puppies and kittens can be taught "come" almost instantly. All you do is have them "sit," stand right in front of them, take one step back and say "come," and as soon as the puppy or kitten stands they will have "come." Reward and praise them! You can then walk slowly around patting your thigh and doling out treats while repeating "come." If your dog or cat is doing this well, you may want to add the signal "wait": All you have to do is stop, say "wait," and put your hand out, palm facing the pet. After your dog or cat has paused, tell him he is brilliant, and resume the "come" sequence with the rewards.

You can use a leash to make sure the puppy or kitten cannot run off, but if your puppy or kitten walks away and doesn't respond to "come," just ignore him. **Do not** tug on a leash or collar or drag the dog or cat: dogs and cats push against pressure so if you drag them there is pressure on the back of their neck. This pressure will make them stop and stay away from you, not come to you.

If you continue to use a technique that is not working you will confuse or scare the pet. If after starting over a couple of times you still cannot get the pet to pay attention to you, leave it for later. Puppies and kittens have short attention spans. You will gain more from working with your pet in many small bursts than in one long one.

A Cautionary Word on Food Treats

Remember that the treats are to be used as a salary or reward—*not as a bribe.* If you bribe a dog or cat, you are sunk before you start. *Bribes* come *before* the dog or cat executes the desired behavior to lure him away from an undesirable behavior; *rewards* come *in exchange* for a desirable behavior. It is often difficult to work with a problem dog or cat who has learned to manipulate bribes, but there are creative ways around this.

First, find a food that your pet likes, and that he does not usually experience. Suggestions include boiled, slivered chicken or tiny pieces of cheese. Boiled, shredded chicken can be frozen in small portions and defrosted as needed. Individually wrapped slices of cheese can be divided into tiny pieces (0.5 × 0.5 cm) suitable for behavior modification through the plastic, minimizing waste and mess. Whatever you choose, the following eight guidelines apply:

1. Foods that are high in protein may help induce changes in brain chemistry in some animals that may help with relaxation.
2. Dogs and cats should not have chocolate because it can be toxic.
3. Some dogs and cats do not do well with treats that contain artificial colors or preservatives.
4. Dogs or cats with food allergies or those taking medications that are monoamine oxidase inhibitors (MAOIs) may have food restrictions (cheese, for dogs taking or using MAOIs such as Anipryl and Preventics collars).
5. Dog biscuits and dog and cat kibble generally are not sufficiently interesting for learning new behaviors but some foods are so desirable that the dog or cat is too stimulated by them to relax; you want something between these two extremes.
6. Treats should be tiny (less than one-half of a thumbnail) so that the dog or cat does not get full, fat, or bored with them.
7. If the dog or cat stops responding for one kind of treat, try another.
8. Do not let treats make up the bulk of the dog's or cat's diet; they need their normal, well-balanced ration.

The Reward Process

There is an art to rewarding dogs and cats with food treats. Learning to do so correctly will help the dog or cat to focus on the exercises and will keep everyone safe. If you keep the already-prepared treats in a small cup or bag behind your back, or in a treat bag at your waist, you always have easily available treats. By keeping only one or a few treats in your hand at a time, you will be able to prevent dogs and cats from lunging for treats. The hand that you will use to reward your pet can then be kept behind your back so that the dog or cat doesn't stare at the food, or you can move your hand to your

eye so that you can teach the pet to look at you. The food treat must be small: the focus of the pet's attention must be you, not the food. Bring your hand, with lightly closed fingers, to the dog or cat, just under his mouth and open your hand flat. You want to move quickly enough to ensure that your pet gets the reward a second or two after successfully completing the task, but not so fast or forcefully that you scare or threaten your pet. Animals who have been hit or beaten may need to have the food treats gently dropped in front of them at first. Otherwise, they may shy from the hand with the treat.

Avoiding Problems

Please do not push or pull on your dog or cat or tug on her collar to get the dog to sit. These types of behaviors can be viewed as challenges by some dogs and may make them potentially dangerous. Use the methods discussed above.

Please do not wave your hands or the treat around in front of the dog. This will just act as a distraction and confuse the dog or cat. Part of the point of this program is to help your pet become calmer and less confused. Excitable behavior or unclear signals can make your pet more anxious. This will not help. If it is important to you to use hand signals, these can be added later. *Please do not try to do everything at once.*

Please be calm. Your dogs and cats will make mistakes. This doesn't have to reflect on you. Problem pets and new puppies or kittens require a lot of patience. The people who have the most success are the people who work the hardest and the most consistently.

Finally, **please remember** that we and our pets all learn best when we are rewarded every single time we perform the new behavior. We remember the new behavior if we practice it often, and get the rewards. We retain that memory best when the rewards are intermittent. Rewards should **only** become intermittent or sporadic after a long period where the behaviors were perfectly performed. Be generous and clear. You will benefit from a closer, kinder, and less-stressful relationship with your pet.

PROTOCOL FOR TEACHING KIDS—AND ADULTS—TO PLAY WITH DOGS AND CATS

One reason why we have pets is so that we can cuddle and play with them. Such interactions should be the source of much joy, but they often lead to injury to the pet or the person. Rough play can also worsen a behavioral problem that is developing. Some basic guidelines on how to appropriately play with cats and dogs can minimize these problems while leading people to more fully appreciate the intricacies of canine and feline communication.

Puppies and kittens, like young children, are energetic, can quickly progress to out-of-control and exhausted play, and make mistakes in both the objects and the intensity of their play behaviors. Unlike human children, puppies and kittens do not have hands with opposable thumbs (a purely primate trait). Instead, they have a jaw and tooth structure that allows them to carry and manipulate a variety of objects. Hence, much play between young cats and dogs involves the use of the mouth. Kittens and puppies will box and rear and pounce on each other as part of play. They will transfer these behaviors to people unchanged.

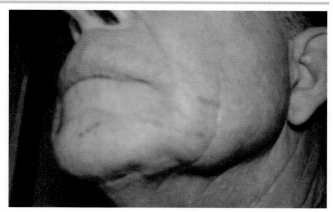

Scratches due to an exuberant greeting of an 11-month-old rescue dog who uses his paws to grab at people and who was relinquished because he was "too much dog for a family with kids."

Boxing, Mounting, Rearing, and Pouncing

Boxing, mounting, rearing, and pouncing are normal kitten and puppy behaviors. These behaviors function to allow closeness and energetic play between animals, and may help to shape adult social behaviors and communication skills.

By their second month of life, both puppies and kittens will begin to pay a lot of attention to humans and will use the same behaviors that they use to communicate with other animals to communicate with humans. All social mammals play and so we are able to recognize signals from puppies and kittens that they wish to play and to act on these impulses.

Human children do not exhibit exactly the same form of play that puppies and kittens do, in part, because humans can manipulate objects and each other with their hands. The tendency is for puppies and kittens to play with humans exactly as they would play with other puppies and kittens, and for humans to mimic the puppy and kitten behaviors using their hands.

When dogs and cats are little and do not weigh much these wrestling and boxing behaviors tend to be non-injurious to people. As the animal grows, the pouncing and boxing can injure a child, or, in the case of a large-breed dog, an adult human. Very exuberant, large-breed dogs can knock a human toddler to the ground and fracture the toddler's skull. Tragic deaths and injuries are no less tragic because the animal "didn't mean to do it." In fact, accidental injury to a child caused by an animal who is wonderful will cause more guilt for the humans involved than will injury by a dangerous animal. Appropriate play behavior minimizes the risk of injury.

Puppies and kittens remain youngsters until they are socially mature beginning at around 2 years of age. Accordingly, they cannot be expected to show the judgment and restraint that an older dog or cat might. It is impossible to know whether a dog or cat understands how fragile infants, young children, or aged, frail humans can be. It is absolutely unfair to make the puppy or kitten solely responsible for the decisions about the directions that play will take. Guidance needs to be provided by you, the responsible human.

Tackling, pawing, mounting, et cetera by young animals **can be** acceptable if and only if you can (a) always stop the behavior by saying "no" or by withdrawing, (b) redirect the behavior to another focus, like a toy, and (c) gently change the behavior so that it decreases in the future, should the behavior be too rough.

If the animal's response to a gentle "correction" of standing up or withdrawal of your leg is to attack more forcefully, **a serious problem already exists and you need to talk to your veterinarian.** Either the animal is already displacing some undesirable tendencies related to aggression and control, or the cat or dog has been taught or encouraged to play too roughly. Appropriate correction for forceful tackles or pouncing includes stopping, saying "no," redirecting the animal's attention to a toy, and asking the cat or dog to exhibit a more appropriate behavior. Preferred behaviors include sitting and waiting for a toy, or being redirected to pounce on a preferred object (e.g., a feather on a string for the cat who lurks around corners and chases feet, shoes, or shoe laces).

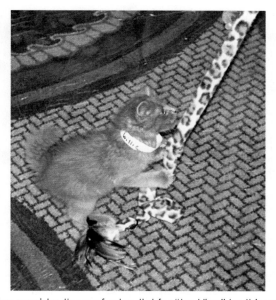

This toy provides the perfect outlet for "tackling" by this rescue kitten.

You should not "correct" animals by swatting them in the face or thumping them on the rump. This will only encourage them to play more roughly or to be frightened. This is **not** the message you need to send.

You also should refrain from exhibiting what too many humans think of as human versions of feline or canine "correctional" behaviors. These include hanging a kitten by its scruff; rolling a dog over forcefully and lying on it while growling in its face; shaking a dog by the jowls, scruff, or neck; swatting a dog across the ears; slapping a dog under the chin, et cetera.

- First, these behaviors are not exact mimics of behaviors that adult dogs and cats use to control play that is too rough in puppies and kittens.
- Second, even to the extent that these behaviors overlap with how a normal dog or cat may respond, there is a real danger in over-doing them and causing the pet injury. This is particularly true for cats. Cats are tiny, and although adult cats frequently bite at or carry young cats by the nape of the neck, cats also have pressure sensors under their teeth and can use just the right amount of control. People don't have this ability and could injure or scare the cat.
- Finally, these forceful kinds of correctional behaviors exhibited by humans towards their pets may encourage physical solutions for problems which are better solved using intellectual solutions. We shouldn't have to manhandle a cat or dog to convince them to alter their behavior; we should be smart enough to change their behavior in ways that can be mutually satisfying. The best emotional relationships with our pets are founded on a basis that is devoid of fear and injury. We need to protect both our children and our pets so that they can have those relationships.

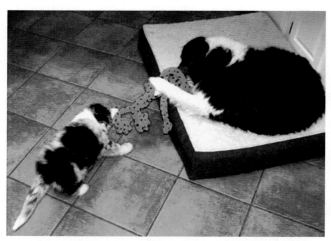

Normal play between an adult dog and a young puppy, using a toy. Note that the puppy determines how hard the play will be and that the toy chosen by the adult dog is very large compared to the puppy's mouth. Together, these strategies— which humans can mimic—keep both the puppy and the adult safe and happy.

One final comment on physical discipline and pets is warranted. Not only will physical discipline cause the animal to respond by increasing their potentially aggressive responses, but it will send the message to any other individuals watching (i.e., your children, friends, or spouse) that the way you

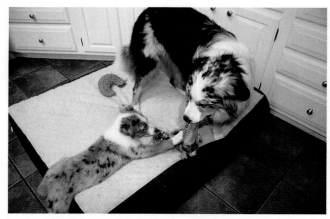

The puppy in the previous photo is shown as an adult, using the same techniques that were used for him on a new puppy in the household. All of the Australian shepherds pictured in this handout are happy rescue dogs.

solve conflicts is through physical intervention and violence. Ask yourself if this is the message that you wish to send. The American Humane Association (AHA), the Humane Society of the United States (HSUS), and the Latham Foundation have all demonstrated that **child abuse and pet abuse are linked.** People who are abused as children will hone their abuse skills on their pets before then continuing the cycle by abusing their own children. In turn, pets who are abused may act as a flag for child abuse. The concepts of abuse and discipline are changing as we learn more about ourselves and our pets. Harsh punishment of our pets may act as guides to other problems that we have not previously understood.

That said, recent research shows that people who are best able to play and signal as dogs and cats would have the best relationship with their pets and report few behavioral complaints. By allowing our pets to teach us how to better play and communicate with them we engender better relationships.

Claws and Scratching

Kittens are not able to reliably retract their claws prior to 4 weeks of age, but can learn to do so after that. If they are allowed to snag at humans using their claws, they will continue to do so as adults. Cat scratch disease (CSD) is a serious problem for people who have been scratched by cats. Most of the cats who communicate this bacterial disease are young kittens infested with fleas, but any cat can potentially transmit CSD. Cat bites are a serious problem in human health because cats' teeth are curved, small, and sharp. A cat bite provides the ideal environment for infection.

Kittens who are hand- or bottle-reared will play more roughly with both their claws and teeth than will those who have been naturally weaned by and kept with their mothers. This is because their mothers and other siblings will not tolerate overly rough play. Early correction as the kitten begins to get bigger is invaluable and involves not just the tendency to modulate or control rough behaviors, but also the ability to use signals that communicate when the play is getting too rough. That "early correction" is best coming from another cat. This is why we recommend that kittens stay with their mothers as long as possible. If they can be kept with their mothers until 9 to 14 weeks of age, she will monitor all the play and the kittens won't learn to play roughly. Part of the problem with bottle-fed or orphaned kittens is that they may not learn to inhibit their aggression using either their claws or teeth because there is no adult present who can read the early signals that the play is rougher than needed. Fortunately, the adult cat who raises the kitten needn't be the mother. If you have an early orphaned kitten please try to find a caring, normal older cat—male or female—who is good with kittens and is nurturing and can help the kittens play more gently. These cats are not rare, and even a few hours of exposure a day may make a difference.

A second part of the problem has to do with social development and the evolution of cat behavior: cats who are weaned early exhibit predatory behavior earlier than do cats who are allowed to spend extended amounts of time with their mothers and siblings. Clients who take on these orphaned kitties need to be realistic and to learn to read their kitten's signals well: no rough play should be tolerated, toys should always be substituted for swatting at people, "corrections" should include distractions (like a whistle) followed by a substitute focus (e.g., a toy), and if the cat persists in her aggressive behavior, that cat should be abandoned unceremoniously or dumped from the client's lap (just stand up and let the cat fall off; do not dangle any body parts in front of the cat) and ignored until she has calmed down. Be aware that some cats arouse easily and may require 24 to 48 hours to calm. Once the cat has become calm, play can be reintroduced using a toy.

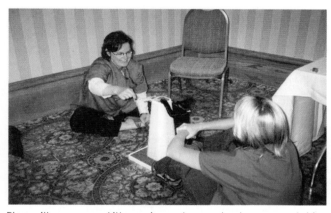

Play with a rescue kitten using a toy and a hemp scratching post. Notice that this cat is very physical in the use of his paws and claws and that this mode of play keeps everyone safe, while encouraging the kitten to use his claws on the scratching post.

Claw use is less of an issue for clients with dogs, but this can still be problematic for dogs that bat and swat with their feet. These dogs do well with Kong toys, Buster Cubes, Boomer Balls, Planet Toys, et cetera, that redirect their foreleg movements to something that will not be injured. Caution is urged: Dogs in hot pursuit of a toy can knock over another animal, a child, or small human adult without realizing that they have done so or that they caused injury. Appropriate supervision is always necessary.

Finally, keeping any dog's or cat's nails trimmed should be mandatory. Nail trims become easier for both pet and

human with practice. Clients should start to trim nails as soon as they get their pet. Even if the nails do not need trimming clients should routinely handle the feet of all dogs, cats, puppies, and kittens. Nail care will get easier with time, render the pet easier to handle, and make it safer and more comfortable for the pet to run, and for the person to interact with the pet. Furthermore, if puppies and kittens learn to tolerate such care early and then begin to resist, clients have an early warning sign that there is a problem and they can seek help before a huge behavioral crisis arises. If you dislike trimming your cat's or dog's claws, please consult a good dog trainer who uses only positive and humane techniques to teach you how to condition your dog or cat to "file" his own nails on sandpaper boards.

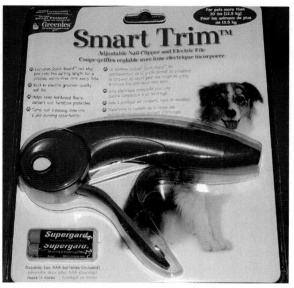

One of a series of new nail clipper designs that makes it easier and safer to trim your cat's and dog's nails frequently. Kittens and puppies who have their nails painlessly trimmed frequently become very easy to handle.

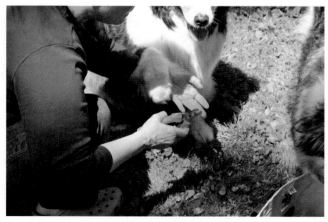

This adult dog has been taught to offer his paw for nail trims. If puppies and kittens are taught to offer their feet for care, they are very easy to work with as adults.

Mouthing and Biting

Mouthing and biting are common complaints of people who have, inadvertently, played too roughly with their dog

or cats. **No puppy or kitten should be encouraged to mouth.** Puppies and kittens will "mouth" naturally because they use their mouths much as we use hands. It is a simple matter to abort this behavior when it is first starting, but mouthing can be tremendously difficult to stop it if it has been ongoing for a long time.

- The first thing you need to do when your puppy or kitten mouths you is to gently say "no" and freeze. If you pull your hand away from the puppy or kitten, even if you are doing so to avoid a prick, you are encouraging him to pursue the "game."
- Softly say "no" to signal that the interaction is stopping, stop, and then gently extricate or remove your body part while gently holding the puppy's or kitten's body.
- Then quickly offer something on which your pet can safely chew or chase (e.g., a stuffed toy, a ball, a feather on a string) and tell your dog or cat that she is good. When puppies or kittens play with toys that you hold they may mouth you again. Be prepared to redirect the mouthing back to the toy and repeat this as often as necessary.
- If your kitten or puppy persists, you can make a sharp noise (e.g., a whistle) as a distraction. Remember that the only reason that you wish to distract him is so that the behavior stops. *You do not have to scare the dog or cat to get them to stop mouthing. If you scared your pet, then the behavior you used to interrupt her was inappropriate or the timing was wrong.*
- As soon as the undesirable behavior stops you need to encourage an appropriate behavior. In the absence of this information, the puppy or kitten will again offer mouthing or more intense behaviors like biting to learn if these are the behaviors that will get you to interact with them. *Puppies and kittens are asking for information: you provide information when you respond to their behaviors.*
- Stopping the behavior is important. **It is equally important to REWARD the cessation of the undesirable behavior with a behavior that is fun, but more appropriate (i.e., chewing on a toy).**
- Remember that puppies and kittens are hugely energetic and will tire the average human almost instantly. You have to be vigilant. If you are not willing to be vigilant, consider placing the puppy or kitten in a safe area (his own room, a crate, a pen) with a safe chew or food toy until you feel that you have the energy again to face the onslaught of play.
- If you don't feel like you can honestly face this type of activity day after day, please consider whether a pet sitter or dog walker can help. Perhaps a responsible child in your neighborhood is not allowed to have a pet but might be happy to learn to play appropriately with your puppy or kitten and wear them out. Children can be excellent at teaching pets tricks.
- The bottom line is that puppies and kittens need lots of exercise and mental stimulation. Both of these activities can be geared to teaching them safe, socially acceptable behaviors.

Puppies and kittens need energetic, positive attention. If they are not able to get attention through positive means, they will get it through ones you will consider negative. You are responsible for shaping your pet's behavior. Young puppies and kittens are just like young children: If the only interaction they get is negative, they will still learn to crave negative attention, and will learn to intensify the negative behaviors to get ever increasing amounts of response.

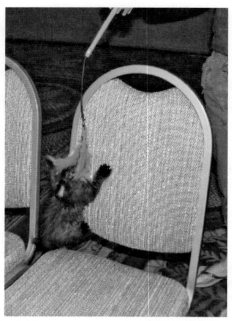

A rescue kitten playing appropriately with a human and toy, and demonstrating one of the skills characteristic of kittens—climbing!

People often feel that they do not have to manage puppy nipping and mouthing because it is not injurious and does not hurt. **This is absolutely incorrect.** These dogs are going to get bigger: the bigger the dog, the more powerful the jaws, and the more damage that the dog will do if he bites. The time to help your dog learn to not mouth and nip humans is when the dog is young. If your dog is allowed to "mouth," he will learn that this is an acceptable way to interact with people. It is much harder to unlearn a behavior than to teach an appropriate one at the beginning.

People (often adult human males) often feel that they can teach their dogs to be protective by wrestling with them. This is anthropomorphic, wrong, and dangerous. If a dog is going to protect you or your family when a threat is present, he will do so regardless of whether or not he plays roughly. The only thing that this kind of "training" will accomplish is to teach your dog to treat you roughly. This is not what you want. If you want to help your dog to avoid mistakes in grabbing people during play, use dog toys 4 times larger than the dog's mouth and 2 times larger than the dog's head. Even if the dog has lousy aim, this size difference makes it tough for dogs to mistake human body parts for toys.

Some puppies who are raised with other energetic dogs can play very roughly. Dogs of all ages can learn to distinguish between rough play between dogs and more gentle play with people. One of their first clues is that you do not use your mouth to grab the ruff of their neck. Do not tolerate rough play from your puppy or kitten just because you assume that this is the way the puppy or kitten plays with your other pets. As long as none of the animals in the house is becoming injured in their energetic play, they can play as roughly as they want with each other, but must be encouraged through the use of interruptions, toy substitution, and ignoring them that this same quality of play will not be tolerated by you or other humans.

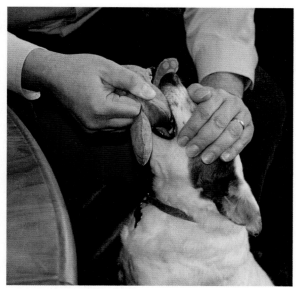

The importance of toy size is show here where this Jack Russell both ingests and protects toys. The toy needs to be large enough to safely retrieve.

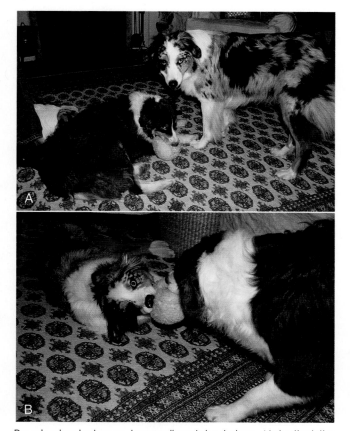

Rough play between two well-matched dogs. Note that the toy, while at the lower end of the recommended size range, is big enough that the 11-month-old puppy (the red dog) can play tug safely with the older dog (the blue merle). The older dog is allowing the younger dog to decide how the game will be played.

If you have pets that vary widely in size, energy level, or judgment about how to play with younger or smaller pets, **you are responsible for supervising them.** Bigger pets can and do kill smaller ones by accident. Some older animals have problems with smaller ones and may exhibit predatory behavior toward them (see the **Protocol for Introducing a New Baby and a Pet**). It is not necessary that your pet be "problematic" for her to injure a younger or smaller puppy or kitten in play. Only when you are certain that the animals play well and safely together should they be left alone, and then only for short periods of time. If you think that your new puppy or kitten plays too roughly with you after playing with another pet, consider limiting her time together to short, supervised periods and working with her on leash or harness immediately after playing with the other pet.

Teaching Tug

Clients often want to play energetic tug with their pets. Many training manuals will tell you not to do so because doing so will make the pet aggressive. **This is not true.** If the goal is to play appropriately, energetically, and interactively, you can play tug with your pet **if you observe the following seven rules:**

1. The dog must sit and wait until you are ready to start the game and until you offer the toy. This way you are clear about the rules for starting a game and the signal that the activity is a game.
2. You must say "take it" and the dog will wait to take the toy until you give the request.
3. You and the dog both pull on the toy, you are gentle and don't swing the dog around the room (which could injure its neck) and the dog is gentle and does not grab any of your body parts.
4. If the dog so much as grazes any of your body parts you act as if if you are mortally wounded, stop the game, ask the dog to sit, or preferably lie down, be calm, and the dog complies.
5. You again offer the toy as in step 1, above.
6. You decide when the game is over by announcing that the game is "over" or "done." The dog then sits and drops the toy into your waiting hand. This step provides a clear rule

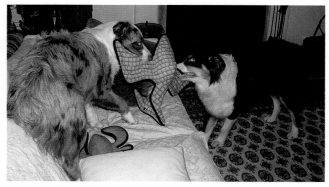

A game of tug involving only dogs. The size of the toy they chose suggests that these young dogs (6 and 11 months) understand that tug requires objects both participants can easily manipulate.

for stopping. Remember, humane rules provide practical guidance and decrease anxiety and uncertainty.

7. You release the dog and he goes off to do something else without charging you.

If you cannot honestly execute all of the steps above flawlessly, you do not get to play tug. You and your pet will be safer for this.

Remember that dogs and cats—like humans—make mistakes. You cannot afford to lose your temper with an animal, particularly one that is a baby. Not only could you seriously injure a young pet by behaving irresponsibly, but you will set the tone for future interactions and could teach that dog or cat to be fearful, aggressive, or simply just too rough. Also, you damage trust, and recovery of trust in never easy.

PROTOCOL FOR CHOOSING TOYS FOR YOUR PET

Young cats and dogs are social and energetic—they need to play. The current scientific literature indicates that play is not really all about learning to hunt. Pet dogs and cats don't have to hunt to eat and if they did, practicing on a toy that does not itself "behave" will not help.

Instead, play seems to be about two important lessons: (1) learning to make mistakes, and (2) learning to recover from those mistakes. The most common mistakes are those involving communication, and good play skills can lead to good communication—an essential feature in social dogs and cats. Growing up for cats and dogs, as for people, is not about **not** making mistakes—it's about learning how to make mistakes **successfully.** The ability to learn creatively and to rebound from mistakes is the quality that allows social dogs and cats to deal appropriately with changing and complex social and physical situations. Cats, dogs, and humans who have difficulty with this quality often seem to have behavioral conditions, most commonly anxiety disorders.

Many of the principles of play are discussed in a companion handout, **Protocol for Teaching Kids (and Adults) to Play with Dogs and Cats.** The focus of this handout is on teaching about specific toys.

If we can teach puppies and kittens to play appropriately with toys, we will have minimized the chance of injury to humans that is often the unfortunate outcome of overly boisterous or rambunctious play. People with large, exuberant dogs—or with puppies who will become large, exuberant dogs—need to realize that these dogs are capable of inadvertently causing extreme injury or death. It doesn't matter if the dog "did not mean to do it" and that the dog was just "playing" or "saying hello." If the puppy or dog knocks down an older person, a person with a disability, or a young child, and that person is seriously injured or dies (and death can be the result of falling and hitting one's head), it will not matter to the dog that the injury is accidental. The dog will be blamed for the injury and his people will be held accountable. Teaching dogs appropriate outlets for their energy and play can minimize the chance of a tragedy, while simultaneously making the dogs a lot more fun to be around and making them happier.

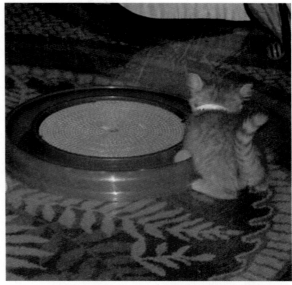

A chase toy that allows a very young kitten to play safely, whether or not people are involved in the play.

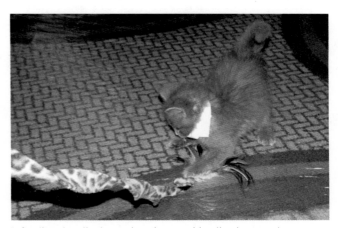

A feather toy that can be dragged by the human to encourage normal, safe, aerobic play for a very young kitten.

Puppies and Kittens—The Role of Teething

Young puppies and kittens are learning about coordination and modulation or moderation of their behaviors, and *are teething.* They should have toys that will meet these needs. Most people understand that this is true for dogs, but many people do not believe the same thing is true for cats. **Both puppies and kittens can benefit from the same chew toys.**

- Food toys made from animal parts can be excellent outlets for chewing behaviors. These toys include rawhides, pig's ears, pizzle sticks, cow hooves, et cetera. Rawhides can provide good exercise for the teeth and massage for the gums. Rawhides can also be soaked and softened for small puppies or kittens. Potential problems exist, though, for pets who rip off huge hunks and swallow them without chewing them. For these cats and dogs, choking or

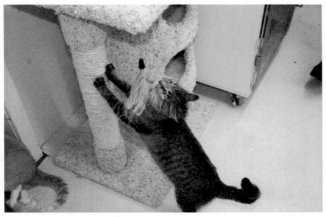

A stationary version of a toy that plays back for a young cat.

intestinal obstructions may be problems. You can avoid these risks by watching your pets when they chew and intervening if you are concerned. Some dogs and cats can have rawhides only until the rawhides become a certain size and then they have to be replaced with a fresh one to stop the pet from swallowing the remaining piece whole.

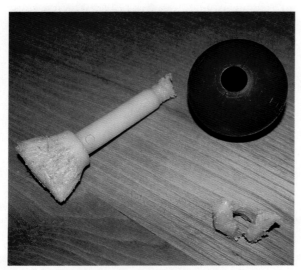

The importance of maintaining and checking toys. This Bouncy Bone is a synthetic bone inside a ball. Once worn, it can come apart and the pieces of synthetic bone can pose a choking hazard. By checking such toys regularly dogs can enjoy many hours of stimulating chewing with minimal risk.

- Some dogs and cats are allergic to the meats from which these food "toys" are made. Some dogs react to the flavorings or coatings with which some rawhides are processed. Dogs and cats who may be experiencing allergic responses to their food toys may vomit, have gas and/or diarrhea, or become very itchy and scratch a lot. Cats in particular scratch their face and lose hair. Also, please remember that in recent years there have been some serious concerns about health effects of some additives to some "treats" and dried food products. Know what you are buying and what the original source is. This will help you to avoid potentially toxic additives (e.g., melamine) and help you to avoid potential pathogens (e.g., *Escherichia coli*). The *Whole Dog Journal* (www.wholedogjournal.com) routinely reviews foods and treats.
- Finally, some dogs and cats become very aggressive around any food treats. Please remember that rawhides, pig's ears, pizzle sticks, cow hooves, et cetera are *not* true toys for pets that are omnivorous or carnivorous: *they are food* and if the pet cares so much about them that the pet becomes aggressive, the situation is worsened by allowing the pet access to these toys. A companion handout, **Protocol for Understanding and Managing Dogs with Aggression Involving Food, Rawhide, Biscuits, and Bones,** addresses these concerns and makes specific suggestions for how to avoid associated problems.

- Kong, Planet, and numerous other manufacturers make rubber toys that have holes into which food can be placed. The rubber comes in two hardnesses, generally red for dogs that chew with fairly normal vigor, and black/blue for the heavy-duty chewers. These toys all come in a variety of sizes, some suitable for *cats*. The rule for any toy should be that it is 2 times bigger than the dog's or cat's mouth. If you follow this general rule of thumb, you will avoid toys on which dogs and cats can choke. Of course, dogs and cats can still chew off pieces of these toys and choke on the pieces or have them get stuck in their intestines. If you are observant and check the toys frequently, you will minimize these risks. Blue Kongs also contain a substance that will show up on radiographs (X-rays) if eaten. All of the members of this class of toys bounce in unpredictable directions when the dog or cat (yes, these come in small sizes and kittens love them) tries to get the food or when they bat at the toy. This action helps keep the pet stimulated, gives him more exercise, and makes it harder to obtain the food. In essence, these toys, whether used with food or not, "play back." Almost any kind of food can be used to stuff the toys. Kibble can be mixed with wet food or damped and then stuffed into the toy. Special biscuits that are big and get stuck in the toy can keep the dog or cat busy for hours. For really rambunctious dogs, the toys can be stuffed with wet or tinned food, peanut butter (consider using all-natural, extra chunky—it sticks their mouths together better, or low-calorie peanut butter for chunky pets), or cream cheese, and then frozen. The dogs and cats will then chew the toy for hours. If soft food is used with these toys, they must be cleaned regularly. Bamboo skewers work well to poke food from crevices. In addition, the toys can go into the dishwasher, although this will shorten the life of the rubber. Toys should be frequently checked for loose or missing rubber pieces and should be replaced when damaged to lessen the chance of choking or obstructing.

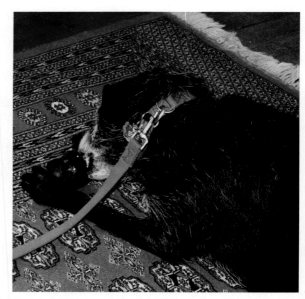

A dog enjoying a peanut butter–stuffed Kong during her appointment.

- Raw bones from sheep, cows, et cetera are seldom recommended for dogs in our modern times (unless one subscribes to a "raw diet" and there are cautions about *Salmonella* and *E. coli* transmission and shedding that should be discussed with respect to raw diets), but they can be given to dogs and cats if the decision to do so is well considered. Although chickens sent to slaughter are young, their bones splinter and unless the cat or dog was a street animal who learned early how to deal with these, chicken bones are to be avoided. Bones from sheep, goats, cows, and pigs may be given if they are the long, thick leg bones. Other bones splinter and should be avoided. Many people prefer to give their dogs raw bones with meat, tendons, and sinews attached. If you decide to do this you need to know your butcher very well. There are public health concerns for humans and pets involved with raw meat; some strains of *Salmonella* and *E. coli* can cause a fatal illness, and even if the dog is asymptomatic he can shed the bacteria, infecting humans. Immunocompromised humans are especially at risk. Unless you butcher your own meat and subscribe to and test for the highest hygienic standards, you may wish to consider avoiding raw bones. Bones can be cooked, but should be examined well after the pet has removed the meat and marrow. Many bones are brittle and can splinter. The tendency to splinter worsens with cooking. The dog or cat will be getting off lightly if all that occurs is a little diarrhea and vomiting. Slabs and splinters of bones can break teeth, pierce intestines, and become lodged somewhere in the stomach or intestines, all of which will require surgery.
  - Large, hard, sterilized leg or shank bones are now sold as pet toys. These are much harder than bones you would cook yourself. Like the rubber toys, they can be stuffed according to the directions listed above. These bones also freeze well, and if you are using a soft food to stuff them, their length makes it a challenge for the pet to get all the food. Again, busy kittens and puppies have happy people, so any toy that the pet will work on for hours is a great idea. However, these bones can also splinter with time, and they can cause pets' teeth to crack if the animal chews hard. They are not for everyone. There is no substitute for watching your pets and learning how they chew. This allows responsible decisions to be made. If you notice the bone splintering or chipping, replace the bone.
  - Finally, please remember that some dogs and cats are very aggressive about food toys, especially "real" bones. The aggression may be directed toward humans or other dogs and cats in the household. A companion handout, **Protocol for Understanding and Managing Dogs with Aggression Involving Food, Rawhide, Biscuits, and Bones,** addresses these concerns and makes specific suggestions for how to avoid associated problems.
- Nylabones, Gummi-bones, and Booda-bones are other options for teething dogs and cats. Nylabones are synthetic hard plastic polymers that come in a variety of shapes from those resembling bones to those resembling funky shapes with nipples. They don't splinter, and hunks are less often able to cause gastrointestinal problems. They can be great gum massagers; however, they are very hard and can cause some pets dental, gum, and mouth injury.

Like all toys, they are not for everyone. Gummi-bones are a softer, more pliant version of these. Their softness means that the dog can chew off and swallow hunks, and many larger pups can destroy one of these in an hour. Smaller puppies, though, benefit from the softer massage to their gums, and the more manageable texture. Booda-bones are pressed bones that often involve flavoring and a potato starch. They are relatively risk-free as far as injury goes, but **they are food** to the dog or cat. Accordingly, if the pet has any allergies or problem aggression involving food, these may not be the teething toys of choice.

- There are a variety of dental bones and rope toys available that have been developed to massage gums. The twisted rope toys are strong enough to use for pulling matching between pups and for using in appropriate games of "tug" with humans (see the **Protocol for Teaching Kids (and Adults) to Play with Dogs and Cats**) and have been made in a way that minimizes raveling of the toy. This is important, because long, loose threads can become lodged in an animal's intestines and cut through them. When such damage occurs you have a true medical emergency that requires *immediate* attention. Any client whose pet is "splinting" with a hunched back as if their belly hurts, vomiting—especially if nothing comes up—or frequently straining to defecate, should check their pets' toys and bring the toys and the pet to the vet immediately. Knowing what the object could be is a great help to a vet trying to treat an obstruction.

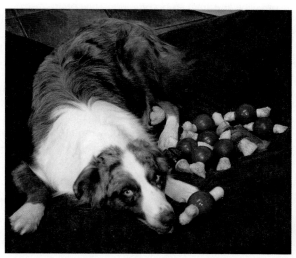

This dog enjoys chew toys, including ones that are dental toys and softer Gummi-bones. Toys for chewers like this dog should be checked daily to ensure that they do not pose a risk to the dog.

All Dogs and Cats

All of the suggestions discussed for teething puppies and kittens can also be used for older dogs and cats. In addition, there are other toys that are better suited to non-teething dogs and cats that should be discussed.

- Food balls and puzzles can be great ways to feed puppies or kittens and adult cats or dogs who are left alone a lot and who eat dry food. The Roll-a-Treat Ball (Play and Treat Ball for cats) and the Buster Cube are just two examples of these types of toys. Dry kibble is placed in them and the pet has to move the toy around for the kibble to drop out. Both of these toys have adjustments so that the food can be made to come out more easily or with more difficulty. This is a great way to feed a pet who eats dry food while giving them some exercise. These toys also prolong mealtimes, which has health and behavioral benefits. You can also make very clever homemade food puzzles for pets who gulp their food and then ask for more. These puzzles can be particularly beneficial for overweight, under-stimulated pets. All you need is a large tray, some large stones, and some fairly sturdy, non-breakable containers that the pet can move with some effort. Then, you need to hide the food in a number of spots in the puzzle. If the cat or dog has to take his or her paw and move things around or tip them over, eating will be a long-lasting, more aerobic activity. Also, these puzzles are intellectually stimulating. Most of us are wasting our dogs' and cats' brains and intellect, so anything that helps to stimulate problem-solving skills is good.

- Squeaky and fuzzy toys now come in thousands of sizes and combinations and most dogs and cats love them. As long as the toy is a pet toy—and not a human child's toy—the immediate risk from parts that can injure dogs or cats is minimized. However, many dogs and cats will dismember these toys to get to the squeakers and these squeakers can cause obstructions. **Check the toys frequently!**
  - If the soft latex toys are ripped—throw them out. The ripped latex can cause the animal to choke or obstruct.
  - If the plush toys are ripped—repair them or throw them out. The stuffing can become the focus of an obstruction.
- The dog or cat doesn't care about the cosmetic aspect of the plush toys—that's for you, the consumer—they care about the soft texture and the fact that they can grab and squish or throw around the toy. Again, get plush and squeaky toys that are 2 to 4 times bigger than the pet's head: if you are going to play with the toy with your pet, this size allows you to have your hands on the toy without the dog or cat having his or her teeth on you. Wash plush toys frequently—they can become fetid sources of bacteria. Check for and trim loose strings. Cats and dogs can swallow these, causing obstruction and cutting of the intestine.

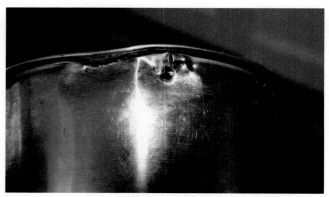

An inappropriate choice for a toy: a metal water dish. Dogs who chew on metal can damage their teeth and gums.

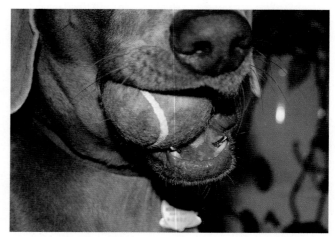

Tennis balls, when enjoyed too much by some dogs, can be abrasive for their teeth. The young Weimaraner in the photo has already has two of his canine teeth capped because of damage to them from the ball.

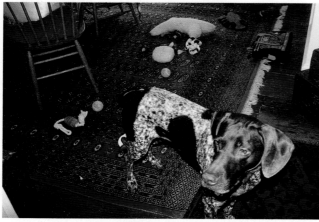

A sample of toys chosen by this German short-haired pointer during her appointment. She has chosen tennis balls, Bouncy Bones, large and small squeak toys, soft and Tuff toys, soft toys that make animal sounds (duck and cow) and a chew toy on a rope.

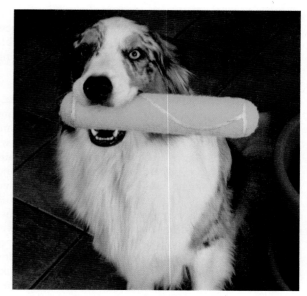

A tennis ball toy that can allow two dogs to play safely or a dog and human to play without risking anyone's fingers.

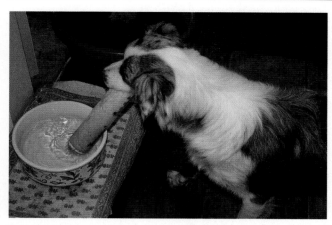

Remember, dogs will not always play with toys the way you think that they should. This dog is using the same toy shown above to play with the water. Puppies often play with water. Most of them outgrow this, but some puppies benefit from being redirected to a toy from the water.

Toys for the Children vs. Toys for the Dogs

People often worry about how they can get the dogs to play with their own toys and not those belonging to the kids. This is simple: make a rule that can be enforced in your house about where each set of toys is kept.

- If, after play, the kids' toys go in a chest or on a shelf and the dogs' toys go in a basket, the rule is clear.
- The rule could also be that, any stuffed toy on the floor is fair game for the dog or cat, but if it's on a chair it is not. This rule can protect stuffed dogs and cats about which the humans care.
- Children must learn never to play tug with their own toys with the pets.
- All of these rules have two things in common:
  - They require the supervision of an adult human who is watching to avoid and prevent a mishap; and
  - They assume that it is much easier to prevent a bad or undesirable behavior from developing than to reteach the dog or cat to "unlearn" it. Prevention is easiest and best, but requires time upfront.
- If you are willing to invest this time, you will have very few, if any, toy tragedies. If you are not willing to invest this time, you should realize that you may not be meeting your pets' needs.
- Finally, big balls and flying discs now come in plush versions. These toys can be played with indoors with little risk to the human, pet, or furniture, although you may want to move anything fragile. Certainly, these toys are way more appropriate for indoor play than are tennis balls.
- Interactive toys like those on strings and ropes and those involving feathers can be terrific for housebound dogs and cats or those whose people are very busy. Kittens and puppies will chase toys that are dragged around on bungee cords and move when the people move. Many of these can be tied to your waist so that when you move so do the toys. Some exotic scratching posts for

cats involve spring and feather setups that keep the cat moving. These can also be rigged to provide the occasional treat if the cat really plays. The same principle of interactive play is involved in the plastic toys that have balls within them that cats or dogs can move and chase on a built-in track. These are all relatively safe toys as long as none of the parts are chewed off and swallowed. These types of toys are played with best if people get involved.

Specialty Toys

Many people want their pets to play flyball, chase and catch Frisbees, retrieve sticks, hunt, herd, or to participate in some competitive event. To do any of these well requires work and maturity on the part of both the animal and the human. Advanced play requires further skills than those used in basic play. Before any animal becomes engaged in flyball, Frisbee, et cetera, it is important to make sure that these activities are not doing the dog harm. Dogs with bad hips or knees should not be jumping up in the air to catch a Frisbee, no matter how elegant it looks when the person next door does it. These activities should not be performed on hard surfaces like asphalt, should not occur in slick weather like extreme wet or ice, should not occur on sloped or uneven terrain, and should not be required of any dog with arthritis, disk disease, degenerative conditions, or those involving chronic luxations. Remember, dogs should work up to the most challenging posture by learning how to do the early ones leading to it first. People are often more ambitious for their dogs than they are for themselves. This may not be a great idea.

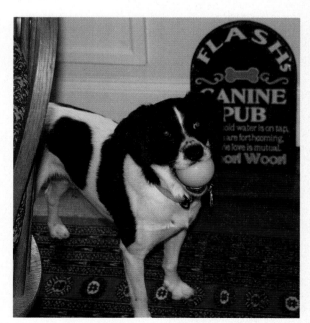

This dog's preferred game is to catch balls. Notice the size of this ball. It was specifically chosen because even when she grabs it while running, she cannot swallow it. Size of toy matters.

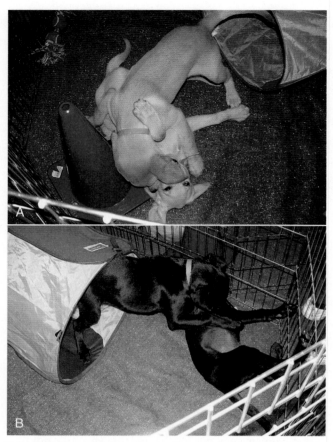

In both of these photos above, the puppies have lots of toys. None of these toys entertain them as much as does another dog. Puppies need play with other dogs, and humans will benefit from the aerobic effect of this play.

Other Kinds of "Toys"

Finally, people often forget that **the best toys are those that play back**—*and the ones that play back best are other dogs and cats.* If your pet is social, look for or create play groups that match your pet's temperament, physical size, and age needs. Dogs and cats that can play aerobically with other dogs and cats are tired dogs and cats. Tired dogs and cats are happy dogs and cats and they have ecstatic human guardians.

Cool Toys

Make notes about cool toys you have discovered here.

PROTOCOL FOR ACTIVITIES FOR CLIENTS TO PRACTICE WITH PUPPIES AND KITTENS

The chart below outlines recommended handling for puppies and kittens beginning at 8 weeks of age. You can start this earlier, if needed or wanted, but you should know that you may have difficulty engaging in many of these activities with kittens older than 12 weeks. Kittens should be handled extensively between 2 and 9 weeks of age if they are to be as calm as possible with handling. If you have an older kitten who is resistant to these manipulations, *please talk to your veterinarian about ways to teach your kitten that handling is a good thing.* Puppies are fairly flexible, but the earlier you gently handle them, the better. Please note that all of these activities are done very slowly and gently. *If at any point your puppy or kitten becomes distressed, resists any touch, or you begin to worry, please make an appointment to see your veterinarian.*

Activity	How Frequently to Do It	When to Call the Vet
Firmly but gently stroke the kitten or puppy starting at the top of the head to the tail, and continue more gently to the tip of the tail. 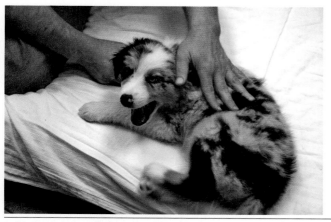	Multiple times daily	Become familiar with how your pet feels and report any lumps, bumps, scabs, changes in coat texture or behavior.
With the puppy or kitten supported in your lap or gently supported on the floor, pick up their tail and look at their rectal area. Put the tail down and gently touch around this area. (Wash your hands afterward!)	Once a day as a kitten or puppy, at least weekly as an adult	If you see any swelling, or the dog or cat suddenly doesn't want you to touch around her tail base, or the tail is being held oddly, or there is feces caked to the pet's bottom.
Run your hands gently over the pet's face, and gently pick up each ear and look in it. 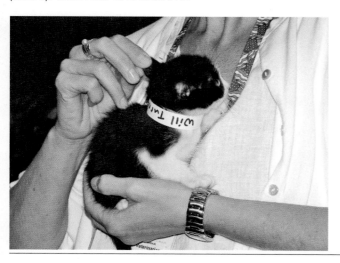	Once a day as a kitten or puppy, and once a week as an adult	If the pet shies away before you get to the ear, yelps, cries, hisses, et cetera, or if there is swelling, discharge or an odor. Normal ears are clean and pink and without odor.

Continued

Activity	How Frequently to Do It	When to Call the Vet
Run your hands gently over the pet's face, and gently wipe the corners of the pet's eyes while looking at the eyes.	Once a day as a kitten or puppy, and once a week as an adult	If the pet doesn't let you touch his face, moves away from you as you clean the corners of his eyes, vocalizes, or there is a bad smell, something oozing from the eye, or the eye is swollen or red.
Stroke the pet slowly from head to tail until the dog or cat lies down ("settles"), then slowly stroke his sides, until he is relaxed, and finally, move his legs gently and stroke his belly, gently rolling him onto his back ("puppy/kitty belly"). Gently run your hands over all of the nipples.	Once a day as a kitten or puppy, and once a week as an adult	If the cat or dog cries when any pressure is exerted, if you feel lumps, bumps, changes in texture, see wounds, see a rash, feel a swelling or hard area under a nipple, or smell anything foul.

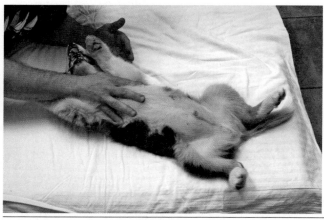

When the kitten or puppy is relaxed in your lap ("settled"), gently move your hands from his side or belly and down each leg. Gently spread and flex all toes and claws.	Once a day as a kitten or puppy, and once a week as an adult	If the cat or dog won't let you touch the leg or paw, the pads are swollen or cut, nails are broken, there is any discharge, the pads are cracked, or there is any odor or blood.

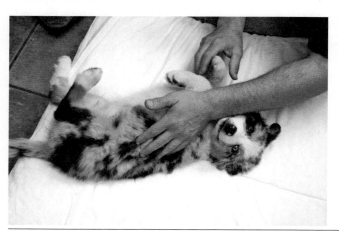

Activity	How Frequently to Do It	When to Call the Vet
Learn to file or trim the nails with the appropriate nail clipper and do this frequently, taking off the tiniest amount of nail when the pet is young so that the pet learns nail trimming isn't scary; putting treats on the towel your pet is sitting on can help.	Multiple times a week as a kitten or puppy and once a week as an adult.	If you could previously trim the dog's or cat's nails and now you cannot; this change could be due to a behavioral or physical problem.

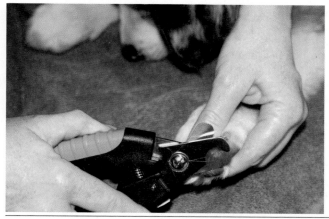

Activity	How Frequently to Do It	When to Call the Vet
Using pet toothpaste and a soft, pet toothbrush, finger brush, or cloth, rub all the teeth and the nearby gums.	At least weekly, but daily is better	If the gums bleed; if the cat or dog will not let you touch or open her mouth; if the dog or cat bites, growls, or hisses; if there is any fouls smell or discharge.
Give the puppy or kitten a "pill." Accustoming the pet to taking medication is essential for minimally stressful care. Normal, healthy animals can be given a "blank" daily. This "blank" can be a small amount of cream cheese, peanut butter, sausage, hot dog, sardine, Marmite/Vegemite, cheese, or a pill pocket that is soft enough to be molded around a pill.	Daily	By encouraging the dog or cat to take a "pill"/"blank" made of something the pet really loves as a treat daily, when the pet needs real medication, you will have a way to get the pet to swallow it without being overly suspicious. The ideal "blanks" are wolfed down without chewing.

RESOURCES FOR INFORMATION, TOOLS, BOOKS, PRODUCTS, AND OTHER HELP

Further Training

Board certification (Diplomate) in the United States and Canada is through the American College of Veterinary Behaviorists (ACVB: www.dacvb.org). Certification requires the publication of original research, participation in an approved or conforming program, successful completion of case reports, and passing an exam. Details about the process and about conforming and nonconforming training programs can be found on the website.

In Europe, the European Society of Veterinary Clinical Ethology (ESCVE) (www.escve.org/about.htm) determines the standards for certification as a specialist in companion animal behavior (EVCBM-CA).

In Australia, the Australian College of Veterinary Scientists in Animal Behaviour oversees a Fellowship process and exam. Fellows are equivalent to board certified specialists. This group also is in charge of the Membership exam, the first step in the Fellowship process. Membership represents a level of certification not available in the United States, Canada, and Europe, allowing practitioners to attain a credential indicating a greater level of training and expertise above that of standard continuing education and veterinary school (http://acvsc.org.au/info). The University of Sydney also offers a distance education course in behavioral medicine through the Centre for Veterinary Education (www.cve.edu.au/debehaviouralmedicine).

Dog trainers can become certified by the Certification Council for Professional Dog Trainers as Certified Professional Dog Trainers (CPDT) (www.ccpdt.org) in a series of exams that require demonstration of theoretical and practical knowledge.

Other certifications for trainers and other professionals exist. The International Association of Animal Behavior Consultants (www.iaabc.org) is an organization of veterinary and non-veterinary professions. The Peaceable Paws Academies offer different types of certification for trainers (www.peaceablepaws.com). The Animal Behavior Society (ABS: www.animalbehaviorsociety.org) has a certification procedure for those who are veterinarians and/or have master's or doctoral degree. They provide a list of Associate and Certified Applied Animal Behaviorists who will help with pet behavioral issues.

Organizations

The American Veterinary Society of Animal Behavior (AVSAB) has a member website, which is restricted to professionals, and a public website, which contains lots of helpful information. This public website lists the position statements agreed upon by AVSAB (such as the ***AVSAB Position Statement on Puppy Socialization***: www.avsabonline.org/avsabonline/images/stories/Position_Statements/puppy%20socialization.pdf and the ***AVSAB Dominance Position Statement***: www.avsabonline.org/avsabonline/images/stories/Position_Statements/dominance%20statement.pdf), some handouts, and a list of Internet help and books (www.avsabonline.org). A similar group, the Companion Animal Behaviour Therapy Study Group (CABTSG: www.cabtsg.org), is affiliated with the British Small Animal Veterinary Association (BSAVA).

The ACVB is the group of board-certified veterinary specialists in the field of veterinary behavior in the United States and Canada. Its website contains position statements and a listing of specialists with their contact information (www.dacvb.org). The equivalent European organization, the ESCVE (www.escve.org/about.htm) provides resources for veterinarians and the public.

Veterinary technicians with a focus on veterinary behavioral medicine and veterinary behavior in the United States can become members of the Society of Veterinary Behavior Technicians (SVBT: www.svbt.org). SVBT sponsors educational seminars and has a members forum for ongoing information exchange. SVBT worked towards and has attained the option of pursuing specialty status in behavior for technicians.

In the United States, the Association of Pet Dog Trainers (APDT) sponsors conferences and continuing education for dog trainers. They also provide some online resources (www.apdt.com) and links to dog trainers certified by the Certification Council for Professional Dog Trainers as Certified Professional Dog Trainers (CPDT) (www.ccpdt.org).

Because CPDTs are not required to avoid forceful training, the Pet Professional Guild (PPG) (www.petprofessionalguild.com) was established to guarantee that clients can find help from well-schooled professionals who are committed to force-free behavioral education for pets and their people. Furthermore, this organization seeks to act as a bridge between veterinarians, trainers and all others engaged in the team effort of providing humane education for pets and for the people who partner with them.

In Europe, the Pet Dog Trainers of Europe (PDTE) (www.pdte.org) provides online resources and educational seminars. The PDTE specifically notes that it ***does not*** *support training methods that use prong, choke, spike, spray or electronic collars, physical corrections, and coercive methods including pinching, pushing and holding down, or fear and aversive techniques, including discs, cans of stones, throwing water.*

The Blue Dog Trust (www.thebluedog.org) is responsible for the interactive Blue Dog video and booklet for preventing dog bites to young children. Their video and booklet program are licensed to a number of organizations, including the American Veterinary Medical Association (AVMA: www.avma.org) and information is available at their site (www.avma.org/bluedog). Other, extremely helpful information to educate children about humane care of and kind interactions with dogs can be found at the Blue Dog website.

Websites

- Good Internet sources to obtain current and appropriate information for *cats* include:
  - For information on creating the best indoor environment http://indoorpet.osu.edu/cats/basicneeds/informedowners/index.cfm; http://fabcats.org/behaviour/cat_friendly_home/info.html
  - Creative use of vertical habitats www.moderncat.net/2010/07/26/singapore-flat-has-cats-living-in-style

- For information on enrichment for cats
  http://indoorpet.osu.edu
  www.catvets.com/healthtopics/wellness/?Id=213
  www.fabcats.org/behaviour/cat_friendly_home/
    Environmental_enrichment_JFMS%20article%20
    for%20website.pdf
  www.fabcats.org/behaviour/cat_friendly_home/
    info.html
  www.tufts.edu/vet/behavior/feline.shtml
  http://vet.osu.edu/assets/pdf/hospital/behavior/
    evironmentalEnrichmentForIndoorCats.pdf
- For information on one toy, the Pipilino, that encourages normal **active** feline feeding behavior
  www.pipolino.ca/eng/faq.html;
    www.pipolinoUSA.com; www.pipolino.net
- For ideas wheels that may provide exercise for some cats (not all cats will be suitable for this intervention, but the site may encourage clients to think creatively)
  www.moderncat.net/2012/01/15/
    city-the-kitty-loves-the-cat-wheel
- For information on "feline personalities"
  http://fabcats.org/behaviour/understanding/
    personalities.html
- For continually updated information on humane care of cats and studies supporting it
  http://fabcats.org and http://catalystcouncil.org/
    resources/health_welfare/categorical_care
- For information on helping cats to have less stressful and more humane veterinary visits
  Healthy Cats For Life: www.healthycatsforlife.com/
    clinic.html
- For videos to help with vet visits
  Catalyst Council: www.catalystcouncil.org/resources/
    video/?Id=88; www.catalystcouncil.org/resources/
    video/?Id=89; www.catalystcouncil.org/resources/
    video/?Id=102.
- For information on creating perching locations for cats
  Hide-Perch Go box: www.spca.bc.ca/welfare/
    professional-resources/catsense/CatSense-Hide-
    Perch-Go-Box.html
  Catswall Design Co., Ltd: www.catswall.com
  This company produces modular cat walls, creative nesting/sleeping areas, innovative design spaces that are physically and intellectually stimulating for cats and a novel cat scratching board.
- For information on various types of cat fences and enclosures
  www.purrfectfence.com, www.catfencein.com,
    www.catterydesign.com
- Good example of an internet source for food toys for *dogs* and *cats*:
  www.aikiou.com
- Good Internet sources to obtain current and appropriate information for *dogs* include:
  - For books and training videos
    www.dogwise.com
  - For training information and courses, including the different types of certification
    www.peaceablepaws.com
    www.patriciamcconnell.com
    www.clickertraining.com
    www.apdt.com

- www.iaabc.org/suchen
  www.puppyworks.com
  www.raisingcanine.com/Professionals/Pro_main.htm
  www.dogstardaily.com
- For dog bite prevention
  www.thebluedog.org
  www.livingwithkidsanddogs.com
  www.preparingfido.com/http://www.avma.org/
    animal_health/brochures/dog_bite/dog_bite_
    brochure.asp
- For information on environmental enrichment for dogs
  http://indoorpet.osu.edu/dogs/environmental_
    enrichment_dogs/index.cfm
- For humane care for dogs and myth-busting, the Dog Welfare Campaign
  www.dogwelfarecampaign.org
    (www.dogwelfarecampaign.org/why-not-
    dominance.php)
- For downloadable videos, expert commentary and a range of behavioral help options for dogs *and* cats
  The Animal Behavior Resource Institute (ABRI):
    www.abrionline.org
- Product sources for head collars, leads and harnesses for dogs (some of which will also work for cats), and other materials:
  SENSEation harness: www.softouchconcepts.com/
    products/harness-overview.php
  Locatis harness: http://locatis.typepad.com/
    home/2005/11/front_clip_harn.html
  The Freedom No-Pull Harness from Wiggles, Wags, and Whiskers: www.wiggleswagswhiskers.com/
    newsite/freedom-no-pull-harness.htm
  Blackdog Gear: www.blackdog.net.au
  Balance Harness and Balance Training Pack (with 2 leads), Infi8 Halter, and the Training Halter (go to the website and watch the videos to choose which tool best meets the dog's needs; all gear in heavy durable cotton webbing that does not stretch or slip)
  Gentle Leader Canine Head Collar and Easy Walk Harness: www.premier.com (note that the parent company develops, manufactures and distributes aversive devices that deliver electric shock: Radio Systems Corporation; www.petsafe.net)
  Canny Collar: www.cannyco.co.uk
  Scuffy Guider: www.mistypinesdogpark.com
  Halti head collar: www.companyofanimals.us/
    products/halti
  Halti harness: www.companyofanimals.us/products/
    halti/halti-harness
- Custom products, including prototype leather head collars (Infinity Lead): If you do not see what you need, contact this company. They provide truly custom products for service and pet dogs, alike
  www.servicedogdesigns.com;
    www.boldleaddesigns.com
- For dogs who are deaf, vibrational collars may help. Various sources are discussed at:
  www.deafdogs.org/resources/vibramakers.php.
    Many electronic collars have a vibrational feature that does not require that the shock application be activated.

Scuffy Guider (a baffle-protected double neck collar that humanely distributes any pressure and may be ideal as a second secure device for people who worry a head collar or harness could break): www.mistypinesdogpark.com

Calming caps: www.trishking.net; www.thundershirt.com/calmingcap

Thundershirts: www.thundershirt.com

Anxiety wraps: www.anxietywrap.com

Ear/hearing protection: Mutt Muffs, www.muttmuffs.com

- Product source for a nonrestrictive walking harness for cats:
www.kittyholster. com/?gclid=CKn_rfmXnLACFQaxnQodezxmYQ

Index

Page numbers followed by "f" indicate figures, "t" indicate tables, and "b" indicate boxes.

A

Abnormal behaviors. *See* Canine behaviors, abnormal; Feline behavior, abnormal
Acepromazine, 35-36, 282, 474
Acetate, 459t
Active defense, signaling behavior involved in, 150
Adaptive fear, 9
Additive genetic variance, 174-175
Adenyl cyclase, 485
Adjacent marking by dogs, 159
Affective defense behavior, 391
Aggression. *See also specific type of aggression*
  anxiety and, 657, 673
  canine. *See* Canine aggression
  damage caused by, 189t-190t
  definition of, 172, 605
  feline. *See* Feline aggression
  phenomenologically diagnosis for, 45
  phenotypic diagnosis for, 45
  Protocol for Handling and Surviving Aggressive Events, 605-611
Aging, 8
Agonistic behavior
  aggressive components of, 148
  vocal sounds associated with, 156
Aktivait, 270-271, 438, 464-465
Allelomimetic behavior, 130, 131b
Allogrooming, 331t-343t
Allorubbing, 355
"Alpha", 673
Alpha agonists, 186, 471
Alpha-2 agonists
  description of, 190
  fear treated with, 234
  pain-related aggression in cats treated with, 406
Alpha-adrenergic agonists, 485-486

Alpha-casozepine, 440, 466
Alpha-enolase, 463
Alpha-lipoic acid, 459t
Alprazolam, 185-186, 263, 281, 413, 477b, 478t-480t, 498, 507t-510t, 714-716
Alzheimer's disease, 462
American College of Veterinary Behaviorists, 39
American Society for the Prevention of the Cruelty to Animals, 2
American Veterinary Society of Animal Behavior, 38
Amino acids, 460, 460t, 466-467
Amitriptyline, 413, 482t, 483, 507t-510t, 717
Amygdala
  in aggression, 390
  anatomy of, 68-69, 71
  extracellular environment of, 71
  facial social cues and, 487-488
  fear and, 69
β-Amyloid plaques, 432
Anal sac secretions, 158
Anesthesia, 498-499
Animal Behavior Resource Institute, 38
Anticipatory anxiety, 239
Anticipatory guidance, 57, 288
Anxiety. *See also* Generalized anxiety disorder
  aggression and, 657, 673
  anticipatory, 239
  appeasement, 61-62
  arousal's role in, 49
  behavioral signs of, 60
  definition of, 60
  fear and, 60-61, 231
  learning affected by, 53
  neurophysiological signs of, 60
  non-specific signs of, 46, 47b, 576b, 580b

Anxiety *(Continued)*
  pre-anesthetic medications for, 36
  reinforcing of, 221-222
  selective serotonin reuptake inhibitors for, 488-490
  signs of, 46, 47b, 60
  situational, 60
  tricyclic antidepressants for, 488-490
  triggers for, 612
  weighing of patient as cause of, 16
Anxiety Wrap, 98-99, 98f-99f
Apolipoprotein E, 464
Appeasement, 61-62, 148-150, 186-187
Appointments
  frequency of, 2, 3t
  information discussed in, 6
  length of, 2-7
  older pets, 8
  quality information provided at, 7-8
Arachidonic acid, 459t, 462
Arched back posture, in cats, 331t-343t, 345
Arginine vasopressin antagonists, 220-221
Arousal levels, 60-62
  in anxiety, 49
  description of, 9
  effects of, 60
  fear and, 9
  physical environment effects on, 62
  reduction of, 9, 11
Aspartate, 475
Association of Pet Dog Trainers, 38
Associative learning, 68
Astrocytes, 463
Attention-seeking behavior
  in cats, 396, 698-700
  in dogs, 236, 306-308, 698-700
Auditory barriers, 104-105
Autonomic nervous system, 74
Autoshaping, 78-79
Autosits, 78
Aversive conditioning, 75

Aversive stimuli
   differential effects of, 71
   molecular level of, 71-72
Averted gaze by dogs, 132t-140t
Avoidance, 75

B

Back-chaining, 79
Barbiturates, 476
Bark collars, 88-90, 105
Barking
   context/circumstance for, 132t-140t,
      156
   problematic, management of,
      164-166
Barriers
   auditory, 104-105
   indications for, 104
   visual, 104-105, 104f
Bartonella henselae, 361
Bathrooms, 25
Bear Bells, 424
Behavior
   canine. *See* Canine behavior
   clients' views of, 2, 3f
   endogenous hormones effect on,
      467-469
   feline. *See* Feline behavior
   modeling of, 114-116, 115f-116f
   reasons for caring about, 2
   rewarding of, 59
Behavior modification, 66-67
   attention-seeking behavior treated
      with, 307
   canine post-traumatic stress
      disorder treated with, 262-263
   characteristics of, 66
   cognitive dysfunction/cognitive
      dysfunction syndrome treated
      with
      in cats, 437
      in dogs, 269-271
   depression treated with
      in cats, 440
      in dogs, 274
   elimination complaints in cats
      treated with
      location preference, 378
      non-spraying marking, 389
      spray urination, 386
      substrate preference, 374
      substrate/location aversions, 381
   examples of, 66-67
   excessive urination treated with,
      306
   fear aggression treated with
      in cats, 400
      in dogs, 185

Behavior modification (*Continued*)
   fear treated with
      in cats, 428
      in dogs, 234
   feline aggression treated with,
      395
   feline hyperesthesia treated with,
      448-449
   food-related aggression treated
      with, 206
   generalized anxiety disorder treated
      with, 236-237
   hyperactivity treated with, 291
   hyper-reactivity treated with, 294
   impulse-control aggression treated
      with
      in cats, 419
      in dogs, 220
   incomplete housetraining treated
      with, 298-299
   inter-cat aggression treated with,
      424-425
   inter-dog aggression treated with,
      199, 201
   marking behaviors involving urine
      or feces treated with, 301
   maternal aggression in cats treated
      with, 410
   neophobia treated with, 255
   noise phobia treated with, 259,
      651-652
   obsessive-compulsive disorder
      treated with
      in cats, 445
      in dogs, 281
   overactivity treated with, 287
   pain-related aggression treated
      with
      in cats, 403-405
      in dogs, 188
   panic disorder treated with, 284
   phobia treated with, 253
   play aggression treated with
      in cats, 397-398
      in dogs, 182
   possessive aggression treated with,
      208-209
   predatory aggression treated with
      in cats, 415
      in dogs, 213
   re-directed aggression treated with
      in cats, 412
      in dogs, 204
   REM sleep/sleep behavior disorder
      treated with, 309
   separation anxiety treated with
      in cats, 430
      in dogs, 246-248
   steps in, 82-84

Behavior modification (*Continued*)
   storm phobia treated with, 259,
      651-652
   submissive urination treated with,
      304
   territorial aggression treated with
      in cats, 408-409
      in dogs, 193-194
Behavior patterns, 48b
Behavioral adjustment training, 79-80
Behavioral concerns
   Protocol for Generalized Discharge
      Instructions for Dogs with
      Behavioral Concerns, 599-604
   treatment for. *See* Treatment
Behavioral development
   in dogs, 123-124, 124t-127t
   sensitive periods in, 124t-127t
Behavioral domestication, 312
Behavioral environments
   arousal levels affected by, 62
   manipulation of, 64-65
Behavioral interventions, 59-66
Behavioral medicine
   benefits of, 2-3
   diagnostic terminology, 45-46
Behavioral ontogeny
   in cats. *See* Feline ontogeny
   in dogs, 123-130, 124t-127t
   play, 124-128
Behavioral problems. *See also specific
      behavioral problem*
   no-fail steps for, 58-59, 59b
   pets abandoned because of, 2, 45
Behavioral tools, 6f
Behavior-centered practices
   description of, 2-7
   questionnaires for, 39, 40f-42f
   tips for ensuring, 39-42
Belly bands, 301, 301f
Belly presented position, 132t-140t
Benzodiazepines
   atypical responses, 492-493
   barbiturates versus, 476
   canine post-traumatic stress
      disorder treated with, 263
   characteristics of, 476-478, 479t-480t
   classification of, 476
   cognitive dysfunction/cognitive
      dysfunction syndrome treated
      with, 271
   cross-tolerance, 477
   depression treated with
      in cats, 440-441
      in dogs, 275
   description of, 25
   disinhibition, 493-494
   elimination complaints in cats
      treated with

Benzodiazepines *(Continued)*
  location preference, 378
    spray urination, 387
    substrate/location aversions, 382
  extreme responses to, 493-494
  fear aggression in dogs managed
      with, 185-186
  fear treated with
    in cats, 428
    in dogs, 234
  feline hyperesthesia treated with,
      449
  food-related aggression treated
      with, 206
  generalized anxiety disorder treated
      with, 237
  half-life of, 478, 478t
  hyper-reactivity treated with, 295
  impulse-control aggression treated
      with, 419
  indications for, 472
  inter-cat aggression treated with,
      425
  intermediate metabolites, 492-493
  liophilicity of, 493
  metabolic pathways of, 481f
  noise phobia treated with, 259-260,
      714-715
  obsessive-compulsive disorder
      treated with, 281
  panic disorder treated with, 285
  pharmacokinetics of, 478t
  physiological tolerance, 477
  protocols for, 706-707
  rebound syndrome, 477-478
  sedative use of, 472
  separation anxiety treated with, 248
  side effects of, 476-478, 491
  storm phobia treated with, 259-260,
      714-715
  submissive urination treated with,
      304
Beta-adrenergic receptor antagonists,
    485
Bethanechol, 486
Binocular vision, 26, 131
Biofeedback, 82-83
Biting
  by cats, 331t-343t, 354
  by dogs. *See* Dog bites
  inhibition of, 169-170
Black Dogs Training Halter, 87,
    87f-88f, 743f
"Blank", 30t-32t
Bleach, 27
Blood pressure, 485-486
Blood samples, behavior-centered
    approach to collection of, 22-25,
    24f

Blood-brain barrier, 460
Boarding, 37, 37f
Body wraps, 98-99
Bolting, 164-165
Border collies, 257f, 258
Bounding, 150
Brain
  development of, in puppies,
      123-124, 129-130
  in learning, 68-69
Brain-derived neurotrophic factor, 9,
    70-71, 263, 436, 463
Breakaway collars, 424
Bridging stimuli, 78
Bunting, 352-353
Buspirone, 382, 387, 389, 425, 483-484,
    507t-510t, 718
Butterfly catheter, 24-25, 25f

C

Cages
  for cats, 37, 37f
  flooring in, 15
CALM Diet, 430-431, 466
Calming Caps, 35-36, 36f, 104,
    105f
cAMP response element binding
    protein, 70-71
Canine aggression. *See also* Dog bites
  assessment of, 172
  castration effects on, 176
  client monitoring of, 228-230
  diagnosis issues, 222-228
  dominance, 214-215
  fear-related, 183-187, 223t-224t,
      663-665
  food-related, 204-207, 223t-224t,
      666-669
  human selection's role in, 174-179,
      175f-176f
  idiopathic, 222, 223t-224t
  impulse-control, 214-222, 223t-224t,
      625-627, 657-662
  intensity of, 173b
  inter-dog, 194-203, 196f-197f, 196t,
      223t-224t, 670-676
  maternal, 179-180, 223t-224t
  neutering effects on, 176
  non-specific signs of, 223t-224t
  objective monitoring of, 228-230
  overview of, 172-173
  pain-related, 187-191, 197,
      223t-224t
  play-related, 181-183, 223t-224t
  possessive, 207-209, 223t-224t
  predatory, 181, 209-214, 211f-212f
  protective, 191-194, 223t-224t,
      677-680

Canine aggression *(Continued)*
  Protocol for Handling and
      Surviving Aggressive Events,
      605-611
  provocation of, 172, 227
  reacting to, 608-609
  reasons for, 172
  re-directed, 203-204, 223t-224t,
      686-687
  screening of, 225t, 229f
  signals associated with, 173b
  territorial, 191-195, 210, 223t-224t,
      677-680
  water-related, 207, 209
Canine Behavioral Assessment and
    Research Questionnaire, 227
Canine behaviors
  abnormal
    attention-seeking behavior,
        306-308, 698-700
    canine post-traumatic stress
        disorder, 261-264, 265f-266f,
        309, 648
    cognitive dysfunction/cognitive
        dysfunction syndrome. *See*
        Cognitive dysfunction/
        cognitive dysfunction
        syndrome
    depression, 273-275
    excessive urination, 305-306
    fear, 231-235
    feces, marking behaviors
        involving, 299-301, 302f
    generalized anxiety disorder,
        235-238, 655-656
    human selection's role in,
        174-179, 175f-176f
    hyperactivity, 170-171, 238,
        289-291
    hyperkinesis, 170-171, 289-291
    hyper-reactivity, 238, 292-295
    incomplete housetraining,
        295-299
    marking behaviors involving
        urine or feces, 299-301,
        302f
    maternal aggression, 179-180,
        223t-224t
    neophobia, 253-256
    noise phobia, 256-261, 650-654,
        714-715
    obsessive-compulsive disorder.
        See Obsessive-compulsive
        disorder
    overactivity, 285-289
    panic disorder, 283-285, 647-649
    phobia, 251-253
    REM sleep/sleep behavior
        disorder, 308-309

Canine behaviors (Continued)
    separation anxiety. See Separation anxiety
    storm phobia, 256-261, 256f-257f, 650-654, 714-715
    submissive urination, 301-305
    urine, marking behaviors involving, 299-301, 302f
aggression. See Canine aggression
early, 130
overview of, 122-130
problematic
    barking, 164-166
    biting, 168-170. See also Dog bites
    bolting, 164-165
    classification of, 162
    digging, 162-164
    eating of feces, 167-168
    grabbing, 168-170
    grabbing people and/or other pets as they go through the door, 165
    "humping", 166
    hyperactivity, 170-171
    jumping, 164-165
    mounting, 166, 467-468
    mouthing, 168-170
    overview of, 162
    patrolling activities, 165-166
    rolling in feces, 166-167, 167f-168f
    scratching, 164-165
psychopharmacological agents for, 509t-510t
questionnaire for monitoring changes in, 42, 42f-44f, 544
Canine chew toy consultant, 4t-5t
Canine collar, harness, head collar, and lead consultant, 4t-5t
Canine eye shade/ear muff consultant, 4t-5t
Canine food puzzle consultant, 4t-5t
Canine housetraining consultant, 4t-5t
Canine post-traumatic stress disorder, 261-264, 265f-266f, 309
Canine vision, 26, 131
Canine vocal communication, 154-157
Canine wrap consultant, 4t-5t
Canny Collar, 85, 86f, 742f
Capes, 99-100
Carbamazepine, 483, 492t, 509t-510t
Cardiomyopathy, 426
Carotenoids, 459t
Case-control studies, 46-49
Castration. See also Neutering
    canine aggression reduced through, 176, 219, 670
    chemical, 469
    urine marking by dogs reduced after, 300-301

Cat-Assessment-Score, 345, 346t-347t
Catechol O-methyltransferase, 474
Cats, domesticated. See also Feline behavior; Kittens
    aggression in. See Feline aggression
    agonistic behaviors, 355
    arthritis in, 403
    behavioral domestication in, 312
    behavioral ontogeny in. See Feline ontogeny
    biting by, 331t-343t, 354
    color discrimination by, 327
    communication by
        auditory, 327, 347-351
        body positions, 345
        call, 347
        chirr, 347, 351t
        head rubbing, 352
        hiss, 66-67, 349, 351t
        meow, 347-351, 351t-352t
        methods of, 327-351
        murmur, 351t
        olfactory signals, 327, 352-354
        posture, 313t, 329-345
        purr, 347, 351t
        shriek, 351t
        spit, 351t
        tactile signals, 327, 354
        tail position for, 313t, 329-344, 330f, 331t-343t
        vibrissae position for, 345
        visual, 327-347
        vocal, 347-351, 351t
        yowl, 351t
    containment fences for, 109
    direct stare at, 329
    distress in, 429
    domestication of, 312-313, 360
    dominance in, 355-356
    early neurobehavioral development in, 315-318, 316t-317t
    enclosures for, 453
    estrus cycle of, 314-315
    evolutionary history of, 312-313
    examination of, 19
    fearful behavior in, 426-429, 701-703
    feeding behaviors in, 318, 322
    food toys for, 106-107, 107f
    foraging mode of, 326
    gestation in, 314
    habitats for, 109
    harnesses for, 90-91, 90f
    hiding place for, 37, 37f
    history questionnaire about, 547
    home range for, 358-359
    housing for, 37, 37f-38f
    hunting by, 321, 451-452
    light detection by, 26

Cats, domesticated (Continued)
    linear dominance hierarchies in, 356-358
    litters in, 315, 318
    males, 314
    meal patterns of, 106-107
    nipples of, 314
    ontogeny. See Feline ontogeny
    ovulation in, 315
    pain assessments, 764
    pain scale for, 349t, 402t
    perching by, 407, 408f
    "personality types", 326-327
    play behavior in
        description of, 319-322, 320t
        inappropriate, 454-455, 454f
    playing with, 779-784
    posture of
        arched back, 331t-343t, 345
        belly-up, 344-345
        communication uses of, 313t, 329-345
        description of, 67
        head-up, straight-back, 328f, 344
        spraying, 384, 384f
        sternal crouch, 331t-343t, 344
        straight legs, 344
        submissive, 399
    predatory behavior in, 319-322, 320t, 328f
    proestrus behavior of, 314
    puberty in, 314
    pupils in, 329
    queens, 314-315, 319
    reactivity in, 54-55
    relatedness in, 315
    reproductive biology in, 313-315, 313t
    scent marking by, 353
    scratching behavior by, 331t-343t, 355, 450-451, 450f-451f, 780-781
    sebaceous glands in, 352
    as "sit-and-wait" predators, 360
    social cohesion in, 355
    social grouping of, 313-315, 407f
    social maturity of, 423
    social play in, 320-321
    spatial structure, 358-359
    spray urination by, 331t-343t, 353, 369, 371f
    stress assessments, 764
    stress score for, 346t-347t, 348b, 404t-405t, 766t
    urine marking by, 353
    vibrissae of, 345, 354
    vision of, 327-345
    weaning in, 315, 320t

Cats, non-domesticated
    allogrooming by, 331t-343t
    arched back posture in, 331t-343t
    bites by, 331t-343t
    crouch position in, 331t-343t
    cuff behavior by, 331t-343t
    defecation by, 331t-343t
    ears in, 331t-343t
    flehman response in, 331t-343t, 352,
        629f
    gape behavior in, 331t-343t
    hiss behavior in, 331t-343t, 351t
    licking by, 331t-343t
    lordosis in, 331t-343t
    mouth threat behavior in, 331t-343t
    napebite behavior in, 331t-343t
    nuzzling by, 331t-343t
    object rubbing by, 331t-343t, 352
    pounce behavior by, 331t-343t
    pupils in, 331t-343t
    raking behavior by, 331t-343t
    scratching behavior by, 331t-343t
    snapbite behavior in, 331t-343t
    sniffing by, 331t-343t
    social grooming by, 331t-343t
    social grouping of, 407f
    social play in, 331t-343t
    social roll by, 331t-343t
    social rubbing by, 331t-343t
    spray urination by, 331t-343t, 353,
        369, 371f, 628f
    squat urination by, 331t-343t
    stalk behavior by, 331t-343t
    swat behavior by, 331t-343t
    tactile behaviors in, 331t-343t
    touching noses by, 331t-343t
    visual behaviors in, 331t-343t
    yawn behavior in, 331t-343t
Cat-scratch disease, 361-362
Central alpha agonists
    generalized anxiety disorder treated
        with, 237
    panic disorder treated with, 285
    separation anxiety treated with, 248
Central nervous system, 123
Centrally acting alpha agonists, 471
Certification Council for Professional
    Dog Trainers, 38
Certified Pet Dog Trainer, 248
Chaining, 79
Chains, 109
Cheeks, 132t-140t
Chemical castration, 469
Children
    developmental stages of, 177t-178t
    dog bites in, 174, 177t-178t, 608
    fearful aggression and, 663
    warning signs of dog distress with,
        178t

Chirr, 347, 351t
Chlordiazepoxide, 509t-510t
Chlorpheniramine, 507t-508t
Choker collars
    description of, 84-85, 740-741
    as negative reinforcement, 77
Cholecystokinin B receptors, 447
Chondroitin sulfate, 71, 459t
Citalopram, 509t-510t
Citronella collars, 88-90
Classes
    packets/bags for, 7-8
    quality information provided at, 7-8
Classic conditioning, 76, 77b
Clicker training, 409
Clients
    compliance by, 58
    frequency of visits, 2
    generalized instructions for,
        58-59
    listening to, 7
    outcomes affected by, 58b-59b
    packets/bags given to, 7-8
    questions to ask, 7
Clomipramine, 248, 281, 425, 445,
    482t, 483-484, 507t-510t
Clonazepam, 281, 478t-480t, 492t,
    507t-510t
Clonidine, 25, 260, 281-282, 309,
    485-486, 509t-510t, 653, 708, 719
Clorazepate, 479t-480t, 492t, 507t-510t
Closed-ended questions, 7
Cod liver oil, 459t
Cognitive dysfunction/cognitive
    dysfunction syndrome
    in cats, 432-439, 434f-435f
    in dogs, 235
        behavior screen for, 267f-268f
        client questions commonly asked
            about, 269
        diagnostic criteria for, 264
        epidemiology of, 268-269
        etiology of, 268-269
        myths associated with, 269
        risk groups, 268-269
        rule outs, 266-268
        signs of, 264-266
        treatment of, 269-273, 272f
Cognitive function, 464
Cognitive therapy, 116-117
Collars
    bark, 88-90, 105
    breakaway, 424
    choker, 84-85, 85f
    head, 85-88, 86f-89f
    prong, 84-85, 85f
    purpose of, 84-90
    selecting of, 740-749
    shock, 113f

Color vision, 131
"Come", 775-778
Communication
    canine, 130-161
        auditory signals, 156-157
        basic signals, 141-154
        non-vocal signals, 130, 132-141,
            132t-140t
        tactile signaling, 160f, 161
        visual, 131
        vocal signals, 132t-140t, 154-156
    feline
        auditory, 327, 347-351
        body positions, 345
        call, 347
        chirr, 347, 351t
        head rubbing, 352
        hiss, 66-67, 349, 351t
        meow, 347-351, 351t-352t
        methods of, 327-351
        murmur, 351t
        olfactory signals, 327, 352-354
        posture, 313t, 329-345
        purr, 347, 351t
        shriek, 351t
        spit, 351t
        tactile signals, 327, 354
        tail position for, 313t, 329-344,
            330f, 331t-343t
        vibrissae position for,
            345
        visual, 327-347
        vocal, 347-351, 351t
        yowl, 351t
Compulsive disorder, 276
Conditioned stimulus, 75
Conditioning
    aversive, 75
    classic, 76, 77b
    counter-conditioning, 66
    definition of, 77
    description of, 76-80
    instrumental, 77-78
    operant, 78t, 81, 106
    Pavlovian, 76, 77b
Constructional aggression treatment,
    79-80
Containment fences, 109
Continuing education, 38
Continuous reinforcement schedule,
    81
Coprophagia, 167
Copulation, 357
Cortical development, 124
Cortisol, 9, 71
Counter-conditioning
    attention-seeking behavior treated
        with, 307
    description of, 66

Counter-conditioning (*Continued*)
  Protocol for Desensitizing and
    Counter-Conditioning a Dog or
    Cat From Approaches From
    Unfamiliar Animals, Including
    Humans, 614-617
  submissive urination treated with,
    304
Countermarking, 159
Courses, fees for, 6
Crate(s)
  description of, 100, 751
  housetraining use of, 100-101
  responses to, 102-103, 102f-103f
  size of, 101
Crate training
  considerations for, 100
  for separation anxiety, 246
Crying, 132t-140t
Cuff behavior, 331t-343t
Cyproheptadine, 497, 507t-510t
Cytochrome P-450, 479t, 494-496,
    495t

D

Daycare, 37
Death, 37-38
De-barking, 110
Deep breathing, protocol for, 82-83,
    580-584, 581f-584f
Defecation, 239, 240t, 331t-343t
Defensive aggression
  in cats, 390
  description of, 60
  in dogs, 196
Deferential behaviors, 575-576
"Demo" dog, 28, 28f
"Departure cues", 247
Depression
  in cats, 439-441
  in dogs, 273-275
Desensitization, 73
  attention-seeking behavior treated
    with, 307
  description of, 66
  Protocol for Desensitizing
    and Counter-Conditioning
    a Dog or Cat From Approaches
    From Unfamiliar Animals,
    Including Humans,
    614-617
  submissive urination treated with,
    304
Desipramine, 482t
Deslorelin, 469
Destruction, 239, 240t
Dexmedetomidine, 498
Dextroamphetamine, 509t-510t

Diagnosis
  accurate, role for, 470-471
  phenotypic, 45-46, 47t, 48b, 60
Diagnostic terminology, 45-46
Diazepam, 425, 478t-480t, 492-493,
    492t, 507t-510t, 720
Diet
  behavior affected by, 466-467
  description of, 458, 504
Dietary compounds, 458, 459t
Digging, 162-164
Digital scale, 16
Diphenhydramine, 509t-510t
Direct gaze by dogs, 132t-140t
Dishabituation, 73
Displacement activity, re-directed
    aggression versus, 203
Distress
  description of, 27
  in dogs, 178t, 238
Docosahexanoic acid, 409, 459t, 462,
    467
Dog(s). *See also* Puppies
  aggression in. *See* Canine
    aggression
  behaviors in. *See* Canine behaviors
  cognitive function in, 464
  communication by, 130-161
    auditory signals, 156-157
    basic signals, 141-154
    non-vocal signals, 130, 132-141,
      132t-140t
    tactile signaling, 160f, 161
    visual, 131
    vocal signals, 132t-140t, 154-156
  countermarking by, 159
  distress in, 178t, 238, 681
  dominance in, 130
  examination of, 19-21, 20f
  fearful behavior in, 231-235, 701-703
  harnesses for, 91, 91f-93f
  hearing by, 154-156
  history questionnaire about, 558
  light detection by, 26
  nail trimming training in, 33,
    33f-34f
  no-pull harnesses for, 91, 91f-93f
  object relinquishment by, 622-624
  olfactory signaling by, 157-159
  play in, 151-154, 151f-155f
  playing with, 779-784
  posture of, 67
  reactivity in, 49-54, 50f-52f, 173, 230,
    249b-251b
  relinquishing objects by, 622-624
  scent marking by, 158
  social systems in, 574-575
  staring at, 579
  stress in, 11, 11t, 760-763

Dog(s) (*Continued*)
  tactile signaling by, 160f, 161
  vocalizations by, 156-157, 157f
  waiting area/room for, 17-18, 17f
  weight bearing by, 15-16
Dog bites
  children as victims of, 174,
    177t-178t
  damage caused by, 189t-190t
  epidemiology of, 173-174
  fatalities caused by, 173
  inter-dog aggression as cause of,
    200f
  management of, 168-170
  prevention of, 177
  studies of, 174
Dog parks, 110-111
Dolichocephalic dogs, 131
Domestication
  canine, 122, 174
  feline, 312-313, 360
Dominance
  in cats, 355-356
  definition of, 355-356
  displays of, 218
  in dogs, 130, 198-199, 218-219, 673
Dominance aggression, 214-215, 468
Door entryway, of veterinary practice,
    10-11, 10f-11f
Dopamine, 474-475
Doxepin, 281, 445, 449, 507t-510t
DreamWalker harness, 91, 744f
Drug Enforcement Administration,
    501t
Dying, 37-38

E

Early-phase long-term potentiation,
    70
Ears, communication uses of, 132t-
    140t, 327-329, 331t-343t
Eating plants, by cats, 450
Eicosahexanoic acid, 409, 462
Eicosapentaenoic acid, 459t, 467
Elimination, 295-299
  in cats
    description of, 318-319, 363-369
    feline aggression and, 637-641
    location preference, 376-379
    Protocol For Understanding and
      Treating Cats With
      Elimination Disorders and
      Elimination Behaviors That
      Concern Clients, 628-631
    spray urination, 369, 371f,
      383-387
    substrate preference, 370-376,
      371b, 371t

Elimination (Continued)
  substrate/location aversions, 379-383
  complaints about, 296b
  incomplete housetraining, 295-299
  by puppies, 100-101
Elizabethan collars, 282, 446
Enclosures
  for cats, 453
  indoor, 101f
  outdoor, 101f, 200f
Endocrinopathies, 231-232
Endogenous hormones, 467-469
Environmental manipulations
  advantages of, 64
  behavioral environment, 64-65
  effects of, 65-66
  neurochemical environment, 65
  pharmacological environment, 65
  physical environment, 59-60, 62-65
  social environment, 64-65
Epileptic seizures, 486
Epileptiform seizures, 278
Epimeletic behavior, 130, 131b
Essential fatty acids, 459t
Estrogens, 486
Et-epimeletic behavior, 130, 131b
Euthanasia, 113-114
Exam rooms
  flooring in, 21
  layout of, 21
  lighting of, 21
  noise in, 21
  space in, 19, 19f
  toys in, 6
Exam tables, 19-21, 19f-20f
Examination
  of cats, 19, 20f
  of dogs, 19-21, 20f
  stress caused by, 12b-14b
Excessive urination, 305-306
Excitability, 306
Excitatory amino acids, 221, 475
Exercise
  for geriatric pets, 690
  for hyperactive dogs, 170-171
  suggestions for, 8
Extended outpatient work-ups, 34-35, 35f
Extinction, 73, 307
Eye masks, 35f, 36, 104, 104f
Eye radius, 131

F

Facial expressions, 145, 146f
Faraday cage, 99
Fast mapping, 116-117

Fear
  adaptive nature of, 68
  amygdala's role in, 68-69
  anxiety and, 60-61, 231
  appeasement, 61-62
  arousal levels and, 9
  in cats, 426-429
  criteria for, 61
  definition of, 60-61
  diagnostic criteria for, 231
  in dogs, 231-235
  early, 9
  learning of, 9, 25, 69
  non-adaptive arousal as, 60
  physiological signs of, 183
  in puppies, 128-129
  signs of, 231
  visits and, 8-9
Fear aggression
  behaviors associated with, 61
  in cats, 399-401, 638
  criteria for, 61
  in dogs, 144-145, 144f, 183-187, 223t-224t, 663-665
Fearful behavior, 61
  in cats, 426-429, 701-703
  in dogs, 231-235, 701-703
Feces
  covering of, 363-369
  eating of, 167-168
  marking behavior involving
    in cats, 369, 384
    in dogs, 299-301, 302f
  rolling in, 166-167, 167f-168f
Feeding, 7
Feeding puzzles, 106-108
Fees
  bundling of, 6
  course-specific, 6
  disclosure of, 6
Felbamate, 492t
Feline aggression
  affective defense behavior, 391
  concerns involving, 390-426
  covert, 390
  defensive, 390
  description of, 356-357
  diagnoses involving, 391
  fear-related, 399-401
  impulse-control, 416-420, 639-640, 644-646
  inter-cat, 420-426, 421b, 422f-423f, 637-643
  lack of socialization as cause of, 391-395, 637
  maternal, 410-413, 638
  medications for, 643t
  offensive, 390
  overt, 390

Feline aggression (Continued)
  pain-related, 401-406
  phenotypic patterns of, 421b, 422f, 641t
  play-related, 395-401, 635-638
  predatory, 413-416, 639
  protocols for, 635-643
  re-directed, 411-413, 639, 686-687
  screening for, 392f-393f
  territorial, 406-409, 637-638
Feline behavior
  abnormal, problematic, and undesirable types of aggression. See Feline aggression
  cognitive dysfunction/cognitive dysfunction syndrome, 432-439, 434f-435f
  depression, 439-441
  elimination-related. See Feline behavior, elimination-related
  fear/fearful behavior, 426-429
  hyperesthesia. See Feline hyperesthesia
  inappropriate play behavior, 454-455, 454f
  marking behaviors, 369, 371f
  obsessive-compulsive disorder, 361, 441-446, 442f-444f, 688-689
  separation anxiety, 429-432, 431t
  spray urination, 369, 371f
  aggression, 356-357
  caching, 451-452
  eating plants, 450
  elimination-related
    confinement as treatment for, 382-383
    description of, 363-369, 364f-369f
    feline aggression and, 637-641
    location preference, 376-379
    non-spraying marking, 387-390
    Protocol For Understanding and Treating Cats With Elimination Disorders and Elimination Behaviors That Concern Clients, 628-631
    spray urination, 369, 371f, 383-387, 628f
    substrate preference, 370-376, 371b, 371t
    substrate/location aversions, 379-383
  evolutionary history of, 312-313
  geriatric-onset, 433-436
  hunting, 321, 451-452
  litterbox, 363-369, 367f-369f, 370t
  nocturnal activity, 453
  in non-domesticated cats, 331t-343t
  overactivity, 455f, 456

Feline behavior (Continued)
   overview of, 312-313, 360-361
   "personality type" in, 326-327
   predatory, 312
   psychopharmacological agents for,
      507t-508t
   questionnaires about, 39, 40f-42f,
      364f-366f, 540
   roaming, 453
   rubbing, 331t-343t, 352, 452-453,
      452f
   scratching, 331t-343t, 355, 450-451,
      450f-451f, 780-781
   social behavior, 354-359
   social distance, 358
   spatial structure, 358-359
   submissive, 356-358
   tactile, 331t-343t
   veterinarians and, 363
   visual, 331t-343t
   zoonotic diseases that affect
      cat-scratch disease, 361-362
      overview of, 361-363
      toxocariasis, 362-363
      toxoplasmosis, 362
Feline catus, 312-313
Feline harness and carrier consultant,
   4t-5t
Feline hyperesthesia, 441-449
Feline kitten toy consultant, 4t-5t
Feline litter environment and hygiene
   consultant, 4t-5t
Feline lower urinary tract disease,
   372, 376, 389
Feline ontogeny
   deprivation effects on, 318
   early neurobehavioral
      development, 315-318,
      316t-317t
   elimination behaviors, 318-319
   feeding behaviors, 318, 322
   litter size effects on, 318
   play behavior, 319-322
   predatory behavior, 319-322
   reproductive biology, 313t
   social behavior, 319-322
   social grouping, 313-315
Feline scratching consultant, 4t-5t
Fences
   containment, 109
   as feline boundaries, 407, 407f
   invisible, 108-109
   live wire, 108
   safety uses of, 108
   standard, 108
   static shock, 108-109
Figure 8 head collar, 89f, 744f
Flehman response, 331t-343t, 352, 629f
Flight distance, 358

Flooding
   description of, 74-75, 110, 774
   fear aggression in dogs treated
      with, 185
Flooring
   in cages, 15
   in exam rooms, 21
   in runs, 15
   in veterinary practice, 11-16, 15f
Flumazenil, 478, 493, 507t-510t
Fluorescein, 385
Fluoxetine, 248, 445, 484, 507t-510t
Flurazepam, 507t-510t
Fluvoxamine, 507t-510t
Flyball harness, 94
Follow-up examinations, 4-6
Food
   for cats, 322
   questions about, 7
Food toys, 106-108, 106f-107f, 164,
   437f, 438, 439f, 452f
Food treats, 579, 586, 600-601
Food-related aggression, 204-207,
   223t-224t, 666-669
Forepaw raising, 132t-140t
Freedom No-Pull harness, 93f
Front fit no-pull harness, 96f
Front-control harness, 22f
Furniture scratching, 451

G

G protein-coupled receptor, 158, 485
GABA receptors, 475, 475f
Gabapentin, 190
   canine behavioral diagnoses treated
      with, 509t-510t
   feline behavioral diagnoses treated
      with, 507t-508t
   feline hyperesthesia treated with,
      449
   GABA effects, 478
   generalized anxiety disorder treated
      with, 237
   impulse-control aggression treated
      with, 419
   informed consent for, 721
   mechanism of action, 492t
   neurogenic pain treated with, 406
   obsessive-compulsive disorder
      treated with, 281, 445
   panic disorder treated with, 285
   re-directed aggression treated with,
      413
   separation anxiety treated with, 248
   side effects of, 480
Gamma-aminobutyric acid, 475,
   478-480
Gape behavior, 331t-343t

Gates, 103-104, 104f
Gene by environment effects, 45,
   325-326
Generalized anxiety disorder
   description of, 60
   in dogs, 235-238, 655-656
Genetic diagnoses, 48b
Gentle Leader Easy Walk harness, 92f,
   745f
Gentle Leader head collar, 87, 87f, 89f,
   743f
Ginkgo biloba, 459t
Glasgow pain scale, 188, 189t-190t
Glial cell-derived neurotrophic factor,
   494
Glucose, 464
Glutamate, 217, 417, 459t, 463, 475
Glycogen, 464
Glycolysis, 464
GPS, 96-98, 97f-98f
Grabbing behaviors, 168-170
Gradual departures, Protocol for
   Desensitizing and Counter-
   Conditioning Using, 618-619
Greeting of patients, 28
Grimace, 148, 149f
Grin, 132t-140t, 148, 149f
Group classes, 6
Growling
   by cats, 349, 351t
   by dogs, 132t-140t, 156
Guanfacine, 485-486

H

Habituation, 72-73
Halti head collar, 85, 86f, 742f
Hand signals, 601
Handouts, 8
Harmonease, 466
Harnesses, 90-94
   cat, 90-91, 90f
   no-pull, 91, 91f-93f, 744, 746f
   selecting of, 740-749
Head collars, 22, 22f, 85-88, 86f-89f,
   190, 740-749
Hearing, 154-156
Herding behavior, 192
Herding dogs, 279
Hippocampus, 53
Hiss, 331t-343t, 349, 351t
History questionnaires, 56, 547
Holidays, 750-752
Homeopathy, 504
Hormonal response element, 71
Hospitalization, 35
Housetraining
   incomplete, 295-299
   protocol for, 753-759

Howling, 132t-140t, 156, 351t
"Humping" behavior, 166
Hunting, by cats, 321, 451-452
Hydrocodone, 507t-510t
5-Hydroxyindoleacetic acid, 218, 474
5-Hydroxy-L-tryptophan, 465
Hyperactivity, in dogs, 170-171, 238, 289-291
Hyperkinesis, 170-171, 289-291, 486-487
Hyper-reactivity, in dogs, 238, 292-295
Hypersensitivity to touch, 293
Hyperthyroidism, in cats, 396
Hypothalamic-pituitary-adrenocortical axis
    anxiety and, 60
    stress and, 26, 53
Hypothyroidism, 217, 232

I

Idiopathic aggression, 222, 223t-224t
Imipramine, 482t, 507t-510t, 722
Immersion, 110-111
Imprinting, 68, 322-323
Impulse-control aggression
    in cats, 416-420, 639-640, 644-646
    in dogs, 214-222, 223t-224t, 625-627, 657-662
Incomplete housetraining, 295-299
Indoleamine 2,3-dioxygenase, 461
Indoor enclosures, 101f
Inflammatory bowel disease, 235
Informed consent
    for alprazolam, 716
    for amitriptyline, 717
    for buspirone, 718
    for clonidine, 719
    for diazepam, 720
    for gabapentin, 721
    for imipramine, 722
    for nortriptyline, 723
    for propranolol, 724-725
    for trazodone, 726
In-house animals, 27-28
In-house work-ups, 35
Initial examinations, 4
Instrumental conditioning, 77-78
Insulin-like growth factor-1, 459t
Intellectual curiosity, 163
Inter-cat aggression, 420-426, 421b, 422f-423f, 637-643
Inter-dog aggression, 194-203, 196f-197f, 196t, 223t-224t, 670-676
Intermediate medial hyperstriatum ventrale, 68
Intermittent reinforcement, 73, 81
Introducing New Baby and a Pet, 767-770

Invisible fences, 108-109
Irritable bowel syndrome, 235

J

Jumping, by dogs, 164-165

K

Kennels, 100-104
    noise levels in, 27
    requirements for, 100
Kittens. *See also* Cats
    activities to practice with, 30t-32t
    clicker training of, 409
    early handling of, 323-325, 325t
    early neurobehavioral development in, 315-318, 316t-317t
    elimination behaviors in, 318-319
    exploratory behavior in, 322-326
    eye opening in, 317
    feeding behaviors in, 318, 322
    friendliness of, 322-326
    hand-reared, 394
    imprinting in, 322-323
    massaging of, 32f
    medication administration practice with, 30t-32t
    play behavior in, 319-322, 320t
    play postures in, 321
    preventive care consultant for, 4t-5t
    preventive veterinary care for, 29
    Protocol for Activities to Practice with, 791
    reactivity in, 55
    social development of, 322-326
    socialization of, 323-326
    tactile sensitivity in, 319
    teething in, 785-787
    vaccinations for, 22-23, 23f
    vocalizations by, 350
    weaning in, 315, 319, 320t, 322
Kneading, 331t-343t

L

Lactate, 464
Late-phase long-term potentiation, 70
L-carnitine, 459t
Leads, 94-95, 740-749, 748f
Learned helplessness, 74-75
Learned pain, 25
Learning
    anxiety effects on, 53
    aspects of, 68
    associative, 68
    basics of, 68
    brain structures involved in, 68-69
    cellular aspects of, 69-70

Learning (*Continued*)
    definition of, 68
    molecular aspects of, 69-70
    task, 71
Learning theory, 72-76
    aversive conditioning, 75
    avoidance, 75
    counter-conditioning, 74
    desensitization, 73
    extinction, 73
    flooding, 74-75
    habituation, 72-73
Leash walking, 690
Levetiracetam, 492t
Licking
    description of, 331t-343t
    of lips, 132t-140t, 148, 149f
Lighting
    of exam room, 21
    stress response caused by, 35
    of veterinary hospital, 26
Limb removal, 109
Linear dominance hierarchies, 356-358
Lips
    communication uses of, 132t-140t
    licking, 132t-140t, 148, 149f
Listening to clients, 7
Lithium, 509t-510t
Litterbox, 363-369, 367f-369f, 370t, 373-374, 379-380
Live wire fences, 108
Local enhancement, 79
Location devices, 96-98, 97f
Long-term potentiation, 69-71, 488-489
Look at that, 80
Lorazepam, 479t-480t, 507t-510t
Lordosis, 331t-343t
L-theanine, 459t, 466
Lupi, 91
Lure, 76-77

M

Marking behaviors
    feces, 299-301, 302f, 369
    non-spraying, 369, 387-390
    urine, 299-301, 302f, 369
Maternal aggression
    in cats, 410-413, 638
    in dogs, 179-180, 223t-224t
Maternal stress, 53-54
Mechanistic diagnoses, 46-49, 46f
"Mediator dogs", 116, 199, 199f
Medications
    accidental overdose of, 498
    administration of, 499-501
    adverse effects of, 472
    ancillary concerns for, 472-473

Medications (*Continued*)
  attention-seeking behavior treated
    with, 307-308
  behavioral conditions treated with,
    471-472
  benzodiazepines. *See*
    Benzodiazepines
  canine post-traumatic stress
    disorder treated with, 263
  client questions about, 506t-507t,
    711t-712t
  client selection considerations,
    499
  cognitive dysfunction/cognitive
    dysfunction syndrome treated
    with
    in cats, 437-438
    in dogs, 271
  depression treated with
    in cats, 440-441
    in dogs, 274-275
  dosing of, 499
  Drug Enforcement Administration
    schedule information, 501t
  efficacy of, 471
  elimination complaints in cats
    treated with
    location preference, 378
    non-spraying marking, 389
    spray urination, 386-387
    substrate preference, 374-375
    substrate/location aversions,
      381-382
  estrogens, 486
  excessive urination treated with,
    306
  extra-label use of, 471
  fear aggression treated with
    in cats, 400-401
    in dogs, 185
  fear treated with
    in cats, 428
    in dogs, 234
  feline aggression treated with, 395
  feline hyperesthesia treated with,
    449
  first-pass effects, 492
  food effects on, 491
  food-related aggression treated
    with, 206
  frequently used types of, 471-472
  generalized anxiety disorder treated
    with, 237
  half-lives of, 488t
  hyperactivity treated with, 291
  hyper-reactivity treated with,
    294-295
  impulse-control aggression treated
    with

Medications (*Continued*)
  in cats, 419
  in dogs, 220-221
  inter-cat aggression treated with,
    425
  inter-dog aggression treated with,
    202
  log for, 511f, 713t
  marking behaviors involving urine
    or feces treated with, 301
  maternal aggression in cats treated
    with, 411
  neophobia treated with, 255
  noise phobia treated with, 259-260,
    714-715
  obsessive-compulsive disorder
    treated with
    in cats, 445-446
    in dogs, 281-282
  overactivity treated with, 287
  overview of, 469-470
  pain-related aggression treated
    with
    in cats, 405-406
    in dogs, 188-190
  panic disorder treated with, 284-285
  patient monitoring of, 490-491
  phobia treated with, 253
  play aggression in cats treated with,
    398
  possessive aggression treated with,
    209
  predatory aggression treated with
    in cats, 415
    in dogs, 213
  progestins, 486
  protocol for, 704-710
  re-directed aggression treated with
    in cats, 412-413
    in dogs, 204
  REM sleep/sleep behavior disorder
    treated with, 309
  seizure activity and, 492, 492t
  separation anxiety treated with
    in cats, 430-432
    in dogs, 248
  serotoninergic, 473
  side effects of, 704-705
  storm phobia treated with, 259-260,
    714-715
  submissive urination treated with,
    304
  summary of, 504-505
  territorial aggression treated with,
    194
  tranquilizers, 476
  weaning of, 491b
Medium-chain triglycerides, 464
Melatonin, 465

Memantine, 281, 445, 449, 475, 486,
    509t-510t, 708
Meow, 347-351, 351t-352t
Methylphenidate, 291
Methysergide, 497
Microchipping, 84
Midazolam, 285, 406, 479t-480t,
    507t-508t
Moans
  by cats, 351t
  by dogs, 132t-140t
Mobius strip model, 294f
Molecular diagnoses, 48b
Monoamine oxidase inhibitors
  characteristics of, 480-481
  depression treated with, 275
  elimination complaints in cats
    treated with, 378
  polypharmacy concerns, 494
  protocols for, 708
  selective serotonin reuptake
    inhibitor contraindications,
      484
Motivation, 69
Mounting behavior
  by cats, 331t-343t
  by dogs, 166, 467-468
Mouth threat behavior, 331t-343t
Mouthing behaviors, 168-170
Mutt Muffs, 36f, 104, 105f
Muzzles
  description of, 95-96
  eating feces through, 168
Myelination, 124t-127t

N

Nail trimming
  in cats, 781
  in dogs, 33, 33f-34f
Naloxone, 391, 486, 509t-510t
Naltrexone, 507t-508t
Napebite behavior, 331t-343t
Narcotic agonists/antagonists, 486
Neck, 132t-140t
Negative punishment
  definition of, 75
  "time outs" as, 100
Negative reinforcement, 75-76
  description of, 68
  neurochemical systems involved in,
    69t, 70
Negative stimuli, 72
Negotiated settlements
  benefits of, for clients, 56
  considerations for, 57b
  creation of, 56
  description of, 56
  keys to, 57-59

Negotiated settlements (Continued)
  outcome of, 56
  rules for, 57
Neophobia, 253-256
Neuroanatomical diagnoses, 48b
Neurochemical diagnoses, 48b
Neurochemical environment, 65
Neurochemical systems
  in negative reinforcement, 69t,
    70
  in positive reinforcement, 69, 69t
  in punishment, 69t, 70
  in rewards, 70t
Neurochemicals, 458-462
  tryptophan, 458-461, 459t
Neurodevelopment, in dogs, 124t-127t
Neurofibrillary tangles, 264
Neuronal membranes, 462
Neuropathic pain, 190
Neurophysiological diagnoses, 48b
Neuroprotective agents, 462-463
Neutering. See also Castration
  canine aggression reduced through,
    176, 202, 468
  early, 468
  health effects of, 468
  overactivity and, 287
  spray urination reduction through,
    383
New pets
  Protocol for Introducing New Pet
    to Other Household Pets,
    771-774
  questions to ask owners of, 7
Nicergoline, 271, 438, 507t-510t
Nitric oxide, 475
NMDA receptor antagonists, 406, 419,
  486
Nocturnal activity, 453
Noise
  in exam room, 21
  in veterinary hospitals, 26-27
Noise desensitization, 258, 620-621
Noise phobia, 256-261, 650-654,
  714-715
Non-spraying marking behaviors,
  387-390
Nonsteroidal anti-inflammatory
  drugs, 494
Nonthyroidal illness syndrome,
  491-492
No-pull harnesses, 77, 91, 91f-93f, 744,
  746f
Noradrenaline, 474
Noradrenergic receptors, 237
Nordic breed dogs, 212
Norepinephrine, 474
Norepinephrine receptors, 237
Normal behaviors, 8-9

Nortriptyline, 413, 425, 482t, 507t-
  510t, 723
NOVIFIT, 271, 438, 465
Nuclear magnetic resonance
  spectroscopy, 464
"Nuisance" barking, 88-89
Nutraceuticals, 194, 234, 248, 465-466,
  467t, 474, 504

O

Object rubbing, 331t-343t, 352
Obsessive-compulsive disorder
  in cats, 441-446, 442f-444f, 688-689
  in dogs
    behaviors associated with,
      277-278, 277f
    client questions commonly asked
      about, 280
    co-morbidities, 279, 282-283
    diagnostic criteria for, 276
    epidemiology of, 278-279
    etiology of, 278-279
    handouts for, 282
    myths associated with, 279-280
    non-specific signs of, 277-278
    protocol for, 688-689
    risk groups for, 278-279
    rule outs for, 278
    schematic diagram of, 276f
    self-mutilation, 282
    signs of, 277-278, 277f
    treatment of, 280-282, 689
Obsessive-compulsive disorder
  spectrum disorders, 279
O-desmethyltramadol, 494
Offensive aggression, 60, 390
Older pets
  appointments for, 8
  behavior screening for, 696-697
  car trips with, 692
  diet for, 693
  elimination behaviors in, 693-694
  food-related aggression in, 668-669
  grooming of, 695
  interactions with other animals, 694
  inter-dog aggression by, 197
  leash walking of, 690-697
  massage for, 695
  physical manipulation for, 695
  protocols for, 690-697
  questionnaire for, 696-697
  sleeping by, 694
  supplements for, 693
Olfaction
  description of, 36
  digging and, 163
Olfactory epithelium, 501-502
Olfactory neurons, 27

Olfactory receptors, 158
Olfactory signaling
  canine, 157-159
  feline, 327, 352-354
Olfactory system
  in cats, 352-354
  development of, 123
Omega-3 fatty acids, 419, 492
Omission training, 77
Onychectomy, 450
Operant conditioning, 78t, 81, 106
Outcomes
  client-driven factors that affect,
    58b-59b
  measuring of, 83-84
  patient-driven factors that affect,
    59b
Outdoor enclosures, 101f, 200f
Ovariohysterectomy, 176, 468
Overactivity
  in cats, 455f, 456
  in dogs, 285-289
Overlearning, 78
Overmarking, by dogs, 159
Overshadowing, 78
Oxazepam, 413, 478t-480t, 507t-510t
Oxidative stress, 463-464
Oxytocin, intranasal, 263, 487

P

p11, 494
Pain
  fear aggression secondary to,
    184
  protocol for assessing, 760-763
  signs of, 187
Pain scales, 187, 349t, 402t, 764t-765t
Pain-related aggression
  in cats, 401-406
  in dogs, 187-191, 197, 223t-224t
Panic disorder, 283-285, 647-649
Paroxetine, 507t-510t
Partial serotonin agonists, 483
Passive aggression, 421
Passive defensive behavior, 150
Patient monitoring, 490-491
Pavlovian conditioning, 76, 77b
Paws, communication uses of,
  132t-140t
Pentazocine, 509t-510t
Peripheral nervous system, 123
Permission to evaluate and treat, 539
Pet Dog Trainers of Europe, 38
Pet sitters, 750-751
Petting, 584
Pharmacological environment, 65. See
  also Medications
Phenobarbital, 278, 492t, 507t-508t

Phenomenologically diagnosis, 45-46, 48b
Phenothiazines, 474-476
Phenotypic diagnosis, 45-46, 47t, 48b, 60
Phenylalanine, 460t
Phenylpropanolamine, 509t-510t
Phenytoin, 492t
Pheromonal analogue collars, 129
Pheromones, 501-502
Phobia
    in dogs, 251-253
    neophobia, 253-256
    panic disorder versus, 647
Phosphatidylserine, 459t
Physical environments
    arousal level affected by, 62
    definition of, 62
    elements of, 62
    manipulation of, 59-60, 62-65
    perception of, 62, 64
Piloerection, 132t-140t, 152
Pindolol, 485, 509t-510t
Plants, eating, 450
Play
    in cats, 319-322
    digging as form of, 163
    in dogs, 151-154, 151f-155f
    for geriatric pets, 690
    open-mouth response to, 153, 153f
    role of, 124-128, 153-154
Play aggression
    in cats, 395-401, 635-636, 635f
    in dogs, 181-183, 223t-224t
Play posture, 151, 151f
Polydipsia, 305
Polypharmacy, 494-501
    accidental overdose caused by, 498
    anesthesia concerns, 498-499
    sedation concerns, 498-499
    serotonin syndrome, 494, 496-498
Polyunsaturated fatty acids, 234, 270, 395, 437-438, 459t, 462
    depression treated with, 274
Positive punishment, 75
Positive reinforcement
    description of, 68, 77
    neurochemical systems involved in, 69, 69t
Possessive aggression, 207-209, 223t-224t
Post-surgical environments, 35-37
Post-traumatic stress disorder
    canine, 261-264, 265f-266f, 309
    description of, 129-130
Posture
    in cats
        arched back posture, 331t-343t, 345

Posture (Continued)
    belly-up posture, 344-345
    communication uses of, 313t, 329-345
    head-up, straight-back posture, 328f, 344
    sternal crouch posture, 331t-343t, 344
    straight legs posture, 344
    in dogs
        communication uses of, 132t-140t, 142f-143f
        fear aggression, 183-184
        play, 151, 151f
        T-threat, 148, 149f
Pounce behavior, 331t-343t
Predatory aggression
    in cats, 396, 413-416, 639
    in dams, 181
    in dogs, 209-214, 211f-212f, 223t-224t
Predatory behavior
    in cats, 319-322, 320t, 328f
    predatory aggression versus, 414
Pregabalin, 492t
Pre-surgical environments, 35-37
Progestins, 387, 486
Prognosis
    client-driven factors that affect, 58b-59b
    patient-driven factors that affect, 59b
Prong collars, 84-85, 85f, 747f
Propentofylline, 271, 438, 507t-510t
Propofol, 499
Propranolol, 485, 497, 509t-510t, 724-725
Prostatic disease, 468
Protected spaces, 102-103, 103f
Protective aggression, 191-194, 223t-224t, 677-680
Protocols
    for Activities to Practice with Puppies and Kittens, 791
    for Attention-Seeking Behavior, 698-700
    for Canine Panic Disorder, 647-649
    for Collars, 740-749
    for Deference, 82, 574-579
    for Desensitizing and Counter-Conditioning a Dog or Cat From Approaches From Unfamiliar Animals, Including Humans, 614-617
    Impulse-Control Aggression, 625-627
    To Noises and Activities That Occur By the Door, 620-621
    To Relinquish Objects, 622-624

Protocols (Continued)
    Using Gradual Departures, 618-619
    for Elimination Disorders in Cats, 628-631
    for Fear/Fearful Aggression in Dogs, 663-665, 701-703
    for Feline Aggressions, 635-643
    for Food-Related Aggression in Dogs, 666-669
    for Generalized Anxiety Disorder, 655-656
    for Generalized Discharge Instructions for Dogs with Behavioral Concerns, 599-604
    for Geriatric Animals, 690-697
    for Handling and Surviving Aggressive Events, 605-611
    for Harnesses, 740-749
    for Housetraining, 753-759
    for Impulse-Control Aggression, 625-627, 644-646, 657-662
    for Inter-Cat Aggression, 637-643
    for Inter-Dog Aggression, 670-676
    for Introducing New Baby and a Pet, 767-770
    for Introducing New Pet to Other Household Pets, 771-774
    for Leads, 740-749
    for Manners Training, 753-759
    for Medications, 704-710
    for Noise Phobia, 650-654, 714-715
    for Obsessive-Compulsive Disorder, 688-689
    for Pain Assessments
        in Cats, 764
        in Dogs, 760-763
    for Play Aggression in Cats, 635-636
    for Protective Aggression, 677-680
    for Redirected Aggression, 686-687
    for Relaxation, 83-84
        Behavior Modification Tier 1, 175f-176f, 585-598
    for Separation Anxiety, 681-685
    for Special-Needs Pets, 750-752
    for Status-Related Aggression, 644-646
    for Storm Phobia, 650-654, 714-715
    for Stress Assessments
        in Cats, 764
        in Dogs, 760-763
    for Teaching Kids and Adults to Play with Dogs and Cats, 779-784
    for Teaching "Sit", "Stay", and "Come" to Dogs and Cats, 775-778

Protocols (*Continued*)
  for Teaching Your Dog to Take a
    Deep Breath and Use Other
    Biofeedback Methods as Part
    of Relaxation, 82-83, 580-584,
    581f-584f
  for Teaching Your Dog to Uncouple
    Cues About Your Departures
    From the Departure, 612-613
  for Territorial Aggression, 677-680
  for Toy Selection for Pets, 785-790
  For Understanding and Treating
    Cats With Elimination
    Disorders and Elimination
    Behaviors That Concern
    Clients, 628-631
  For Understanding and Treating
    Feline Aggressions With An
    Emphasis on Intercat
    Aggression, 637-643
  For Understanding and Treating
    Play Aggression in Cats,
    635-636
Protriptyline, 507t-508t
Pseudocyesis, 179-180
Psychopharmacological agents,
    507t-508t
Punishment
  critical factors in, 75
  fear aggression and, 184
  negative, 75
  neurochemical systems involved in,
    69t, 70
  nonphysical, 75
  physical, 575
  positive, 75
Puppies. *See also* Dog(s)
  activities to practice with, 30t-32t
  behavioral development in,
    123-124, 124t-127t
  brain development in, 123-124,
    129-130
  cortical development in, 124
  early adoption of, 127b-128b
  elimination by, 100-101
  examination of, 20f
  fear in, 128-129
  food guarding, 666-668
  housetraining of, 753-759
  maternal aggression toward,
    179-180, 223t-224t
  medication administration practice
    with, 30t-32t
  mouthing by, 168-169
  predatory aggression against, 181
  preventive care consultant for, 4t-5t
  preventive veterinary care for, 29
  Protocol for Activities to Practice
    with, 791

Puppies (*Continued*)
  Protocol for Desensitizing and
    Counter-Conditioning Dogs To
    Relinquish Objects, 622-624
  social maturity of, 129-130
  socialization period for, 123-124,
    150
  teething in, 785-787
  vaccination programs for, 128-129
  vaccinations for, 22-23
"Puppy belly", 33f
Puppy classes, 128-129
Purr, 347, 351t
Pyroxidine, 459t

Q

Questionnaires
  behavioral changes in cats
    monitored using, 39, 40f-42f,
    540
  behavioral changes in dogs
    monitored using, 42, 42f-44f,
    544
  description of, 4-6
  feline behavior, 39, 40f-42f, 540, 547
  history, 56, 547, 558
  note taking use of, 7
  staff review of, 7

R

Rage, 222
Raking behavior, 331t-343t
Reactive oxygen species, 458
Reactivity
  in cats, 54-55
  in dogs, 49-54, 50f-52f, 173, 230,
    249b-251b, 650-651
Reception desk, 18f
Recognition memory, 69
Re-directed aggression
  in cats, 411-413, 639
  in dogs, 203-204, 223t-224t, 686-687
Rehabituation, 73
Reinforcement
  definition of, 77
  negative, 68, 75-77
  neurochemical systems involved in,
    69t
  positive, 68-69
Reinforcement schedules, 81-82, 81f
Relaxation protocol, 82-84, 580-584,
    581f-584f
REM sleep/sleep behavior disorder,
    308-309
Remote devices, 105-108
  food toys, 106-108, 106f-107f
  operant conditioning, 106

Remote devices (*Continued*)
  positive reward use of, 106-108
  punishment use of, 105
Resistance to extinction, 73, 307
Resource guarding, 666
Resources, 794-796
Response generalization, 78
Response surfaces, 46, 46f, 48f, 65-66,
    65f
Resveratrol, 459t
Retinal ganglion cells, 131
Rewards, 67-68
  behavior modification uses of, 600
  components of, 69-70
  description of, 59, 67-68, 579,
    586-587
  differential effects of, 71
  habituation affected by, 72
  molecular processes affected by,
    70-71
  neurochemicals involved in, 70t
  remote devices used to deliver,
    106-108
  timing and, 81-82
  types of, 67b
  value of, 81
Rhodopsin, 131
Ribonucleic acid, 123
Rigid stance, 132t-140t
Rolling in feces, 166-167, 167f-168f
Routine care, 29-34, 30t-32t
Rubber mats, 15-16
Rubbing, 331t-343t, 352, 452-453,
    452f
Rule structures, 575
Runs
  construction of, 15
  flooring in, 15

S

Salmon oil, 459t
Scale
  digital, 16
  walk-through, 16, 16f
Scat Mats, 111-113, 415
Scent marking
  in cats, 353
  in dogs, 158, 163
Scratching
  by cats, 331t-343t, 355, 450-451,
    450f-451f
  by dogs, 164-165
  scent marking through, 163
Scruffing, 76
Scruffy Guider, 85, 86f
Second-order reinforcers, 81
Sedation, 498-499
Seizures, 492, 492t

Selective serotonin reuptake inhibitors
  anxiety disorders treated with,
    488-490
  attention-seeking behavior treated
    with, 307
  buspirone with, 484
  characteristics of, 483-484
  depression treated with, 274-275
  elimination complaints in cats
    treated with
    location preference, 378
    spray urination, 386-387
    substrate preference, 375
    substrate/location aversions,
      382
  fear aggression treated with, 401
  fear treated with
    in cats, 428
    in dogs, 234
  food-related aggression treated
    with, 206
  generalized anxiety disorder treated
    with, 237
  hyper-reactivity treated with, 294
  impulse-control aggression treated
    with, 419
  indications for, 484t
  inter-cat aggression treated with,
    425
  monoamine oxidase inhibitor
    contraindications, 484
  neuropathic pain treated with, 406
  obsessive-compulsive disorder
    treated with
    in cats, 445
    in dogs, 281-282
  pain treated with, 190
  panic disorder treated with, 284
  patient monitoring of, 490
  phases of, 489
  protocols for, 707-708
  re-directed aggression treated with,
    412-413
  REM sleep/sleep behavior disorder
    treated with, 309
  renal and hepatic measures affected
    by, 500t
  separation anxiety treated with, 248
  side effects of, 472
  submissive urination treated with,
    304
Selegiline
  canine behavioral diagnoses treated
    with, 509t-510t
  cognitive dysfunction/cognitive
    dysfunction syndrome treated
    with, 271, 438
  depression treated with, 275, 440
  dopamine specificity of, 480-481

Selegiline (Continued)
  feline behavioral diagnoses treated
    with, 507t-508t
Selenium, 459t
Senelife, 270, 438
SENSE-action harness, 91, 93f
Sensory integration dysfunction/
    sensory processing disorder, 293
Separation anxiety
  behavior modification for, 246-248
  in cats, 429-432, 431t
  client questions about, 244
  co-morbid conditions, 240-242
  daily/weekly schedule for, 245t
  description of, 62, 114-115, 238-249
  diagnostic criteria, 238
  epidemiology of, 240-242
  etiology of, 240-242
  handouts for, 249, 249b-251b
  myths associated with, 242-244
  protocol for, 681-685
  quantifying changes in behavior for
    dogs treated with, 249b-251b,
    250t
  risk groups for, 240-242
  rule outs for, 239-240
  signs of, 238-239, 239b, 240t, 242b
  treatment of, 245-249, 245t, 246f,
    483, 653, 684
  triggers for, 242b
Serotonin
  description of, 473-474
  impulse-control aggression treated
    with, 220-221, 417
Serotonin-2 antagonist reuptake
    inhibitors
  characteristics of, 485
  fear treated with
    in cats, 428
    in dogs, 234
  generalized anxiety disorder treated
    with, 237
  hyper-reactivity treated with, 294
  impulse-control aggression treated
    with, 419
  panic disorder treated with, 284
  separation anxiety treated with,
    248
Serotonin norepinephrine reuptake
    inhibitors, 484-485
Serotonin receptors, 473, 473t
Serotonin syndrome, 494, 496-498
Sertraline, 507t-510t
"Settle", 33f
Sexual dimorphism, 159, 467-468
Shaping, 78-79
Shock, 111-113
Shock collar, 113f, 746-748
Sibling rivalry, 202-203

Sick euthyroid syndrome, 482-483,
    491-492
Single nucleotide polymorphisms,
    46-49
"Sit", 775-778
Situational anxiety, 60
Skylights, 26
Slow-adapting epidermal units,
    354
"Smart-pet", 82-83
Smells, in veterinary hospitals, 27
Snapbite behavior, 331t-343t
Snarling
  by cats, 349, 351t
  by dogs, 132t-140t
Social development, 123
Social distance, 358
Social environment, 64-65
Social grooming, 331t-343t
Social maturity, of puppies, 129-130,
    197
Social roll, 331t-343t
Social rubbing, 331t-343t
Social systems
  in cats, 644
  in dogs, 574-575
Socialization
  for kittens, 323-326
  lack of, feline aggression caused by,
    391-395, 637
  for puppies, 123-124, 150
Society of Veterinary Behavior
    Technicians, 38
Somatosensory cortex, 123
Spaying
  hemangiosarcoma risks, 468
  maternal aggression and, 180
"Special-needs pets", 750-752
Spontaneous recovery, 73
Sporn No Pull Harness, 91, 91f
Spray urination
  in cats, 369, 371f, 383-387, 628f
  in dogs, 331t-343t, 353
Squat urination, 331t-343t
Staff
  behavior of, 28-29
  educational resources for, 38-39
Stalk behavior, 331t-343t
Static electricity, 99
Static shock fences, 108-109
Status epilepticus, 278
"Stay", 775-778
Stimulants, 295, 486-487
Stimuli
  bridging, 78
  negative, 72
Stimulus generalization, 73, 78
Storm phobia, 256-261, 256f-257f,
    650-654, 714-715

Stress
in cats, 346t-347t, 348b, 404t-405t, 766t
cortisol levels, 71, 72f
in dogs, 11, 11t, 760-763
hypothalamic-pituitary-adrenocortical axis signs of, 26, 53
laboratory evaluations affected by, 25
maternal, prenatal exposure to, 53-54
protocol for assessing, 760-763
rating system for, 11t
scales for evaluating, 12b-14b, 404t-405t
waiting room as source of, 10-11
Submissive behaviors
in cats, 356-358, 399
in dogs, 296
Submissive urination, 301-305
Supplements
Aktivait, 464-465
behavior affected by, 466-467
description of, 504
NOVIFIT, 271, 438, 465
recommended amounts of, 467t
roles for, 458
Swat behavior, 331t-343t
Sympathomimetics, 486-487

T

Tactile signaling
in cats, 331t-343t, 354
in dogs, 160f, 161
Tail
in cats, 313t, 329-344, 330f, 331t-343t
in dogs, 132t-140t, 141
removal of, 109
Tail-wagging
aggression and, 173
context/circumstance for, 132t-140t
in puppies, 123
Target, 76-77
Task learning, 71
Technicians, as consultants, 4t-5t
Teething, 785-787
Temazepam, 285
Tenectomy, 450-451
Territorial aggression
in cats, 406-409, 637-638
in dogs, 191-195, 210, 223t-224t, 677-680
Testosterone, 219
Thermoregulation, digging for, 164
Thundershirt, 98-99, 99f
Thyroidal illness, 491-492
Thyrotoxicosis, 217

Thyrotropin-releasing hormone, 491-492
Thyroxine, 217, 232
Tie-outs, 109
Tongue, communication uses of, 132t-140t
Tooth removal, 109
Topiramate, 492t
Touching noses, 331t-343t
Toxocariasis, 362-363
Toxoplasma gondii, 362
Toxoplasmosis, 362
Toys
in exam rooms, 6
Protocol for Selecting, 785-790
Tramadol, 375, 494, 497
Tranquilizers, 476
Trazodone, 281, 413, 445, 449, 485, 509t-510t, 726
Treading, 331t-343t
Treatment
goals of, 56
negotiated settlement approach to. See Negotiated settlements
thought process for, 118b-119b
Treats, food, 579
Triazolam, 478t-480t, 507t-510t
Tricyclic antidepressants, 54f, 482-483
algorithm for, 484b
anxiety disorders treated with, 488-490
attention-seeking behavior treated with, 307
contraindications, 482
derivatives of, 483
effects of, 482
elimination complaints in cats treated with
location preference, 378
spray urination, 386
substrate preference, 374-375
substrate/location aversions, 381-382
fear aggression treated with, 401
fear treated with
in cats, 428
in dogs, 234
feline hyperesthesia treated with, 449
generalized anxiety disorder treated with, 237
hyper-reactivity treated with, 294
impulse-control aggression treated with, 419
indications for, 484t
inter-cat aggression treated with, 425
neuropathic pain treated with, 406
norepinephrine affected by, 482

Tricyclic antidepressants (Continued)
obsessive-compulsive disorder treated with
in cats, 445
in dogs, 281-282
pain treated with, 190
panic disorder treated with, 284
phases of, 489
protocols for, 707
re-directed aggression treated with, 413
REM sleep/sleep behavior disorder treated with, 309
renal and hepatic measures affected by, 500t
selective serotonin reuptake inhibitors as derivatives of. See Selective serotonin reuptake inhibitors
separation anxiety treated with, 248
sick euthyroid syndrome caused by, 482-483, 491-492
side effects of, 472, 482
submissive urination treated with, 304
Tryptophan, 458-461, 459t-460t
Tryptophan 2,3-dioxygenase, 461
T-threat, 148, 149f
Tug, 783-784
Tyrosine, 460t

U

Unconditioned response, 76
Unconditioned stimulus, 75
Unfamiliar animals, Protocol for Desensitizing and Counter-Conditioning a Dog or Cat From Approaches From, 614-617
Urination, 240t
excessive, 305-306
spray. See Spray urination
squat, 331t-343t
submissive, 301-305
Urine, covering of, 363-369
Urine marking
by cats, 353, 369
by dogs, 159, 299-301, 302f

V

Vaccinations
behavior-centered approach to collection of, 22-25
of kittens, 22-23, 23f
of puppies, 22-23
Value, 81

Venipuncture
   restraint for, 23-24
   in unrestrained dog, 24f
Venn diagrams, 426
Venous stasis, 25
Ventromedial hypothalamus, 390
Vests, 94, 94f
Veterinarians, 363
Veterinary care, patient behaviors
      affected by, 9
Veterinary hospitals
   lighting in, 26
   noise in, 26-27
   other animals in, 27-28
   smells in, 27
   staff behavior in, 28-29
Veterinary practice
   door entryway of, 10-11,
      10f-11f
   flooring of, 11-16, 15f
   waiting room of, 10-11, 11f
Viciousness, 173
Vision
   in cats, 327-345
   in dogs, 26, 131
Visit frequency, 2, 3t

Visual barriers, 104-105, 104f
Vitamin C, 459t
Vocal communication
   by cats, 347-351, 351t
   by dogs, 154-157
Vomeronasal organ, 501-502

W

Waiting, 25-26
Waiting area/room
   description of, 17-19
   design of, 18
   illustration of, 11f
   images of, 17f-18f
   stress caused by, 10-11
Walk-through scale, 16, 16f
Water, canine aggression toward, 207,
      209
Water bowl, guarding of, 209
Weaning, 315, 319, 320t, 322
Web Master Harness, 98-99, 99f, 185
Websites, 794-796
Weighing
   anxiety associated with, 16
   stress caused by, 12b-14b

Wellness appointments
   frequency of, 2, 3t
   length of, 3-4
Whimpering, 132t-140t
Whining, 132t-140t, 156
Wolves, 147, 147f
Work-ups
   extended outpatient, 34-35,
      35f
   in-house, 35
Wraps, body, 98-99

Y

Yawn behavior, 331t-343t
Yoga mats, 15-16

Z

Zonisamide, 492t
Zoonotic diseases
   cat-scratch disease,
      361-362
   overview of, 361-363
   toxocariasis, 362-363
   toxoplasmosis, 362